AF182432

Gardner and Sutherland's

Chromosome Abnormalities and Genetic Counseling

OXFORD MONOGRAPHS ON MEDICAL GENETICS

General Editors:
JUDITH G. HALL PETER S. HARPER LOUANNE HUDGKINS EVAN EICHLER CHARLES J. EPSTEIN (DECEASED 2011)
ARNO G. MOTULSKY (RESIGNED 2011)

1. R. B. McConnell: *The genetics of gastrointestinal disorders*
2. A. C. Kopéc: *The distribution of the blood groups in the United Kingdom*
3. E. Slater and V. A. Cowie: *The genetics of mental disorders*
4. C. O. Carter and T. J. Fairbank: *The genetics of locomotor disorders*
5. A. E. Mourant, A. C. Kopéc, and K. Domaniewska-Sobezak: *The distribution of the human blood groups and other polymorphisms*
6. A. E. Mourant, A. C. Kopéc, and K. Domaniewska-Sobezak: *Blood groups and diseases*
7. A. G. Steinbert and C. E. Cook: *The distribution of the human immunoglobulin allotypes*
8. D. Tills, A. C. Kopéc, and R. E. Tills: *The distribution of the human blood groups and other polymorphisms: Supplement I*
10. D. Z. Loesch: *Quantitative dermatoglyphics: Classification, genetics, and pathology*
11. D. J. Bond and A. C. Chandley: *Aneuploidy*
12. P. F. Benson and A. H. Fensom: *Genetic biochemical disorders*
13. G. R. Sutherland and F. Hecht: *Fragile sites on human chromosomes*
14. M. d'A. Crawfurd: *The genetics of renal tract disorders*
16. C. R. Scriver and B. Child: *Garrod's inborn factors in disease*
18. M. Baraitser: *The genetics of neurological disorders*
19. R. J. Gorlin, M. M. Cohen, Jr., and L. S. Levin: *Syndromes of the head and neck*, third edition
21. D. Warburton, J. Byrne, and N. Canki: *Chromosome anomalies and prenatal development: An atlas*
22. J. J. Nora, K. Berg, and A. H. Nora: *Cardiovascular disease: Genetics, epidemiology, and prevention*
24. A. E. H. Emery: *Duchenne muscular dystrophy*, second edition
25. E. G. D. Tuddenham and D. N. Cooper: *The molecular genetics of haemostasis and its inherited disorders*
26. A. Boué: *Fetal medicine*
27. R. E. Stevenson, J. G. Hall, and R. M. Goodman: *Human malformations*
28. R. J. Gorlin, H. V. Toriello, and M. M. Cohen, Jr.: *Hereditary hearing loss and its syndromes*
29. R. J. M. Gardner and G. R. Sutherland: *Chromosome abnormalities and genetic counseling*, second edition
30. A. S. Teebi and T. I. Farag: *Genetic disorders among Arab populations*
31. M. M. Cohen, Jr.: *The child with multiple birth defects*
32. W. W. Weber: *Pharmacogenetics*
33. V. P. Sybert: *Genetic skin disorders*
34. M. Baraitser: *Genetics of neurological disorders*, third edition
35. H. Ostrer: *Non-Mendelian genetics in humans*
36. E. Traboulsi: *Genetic factors in human disease*
37. G. L. Semenza: *Transcription factors and human disease*
38. L. Pinsky, R. P. Erickson, and R. N. Schimke: *Genetic disorders of human sexual development*
39. R. E. Stevenson, C. E. Schwartz, and R. J. Schroer: *X-linked mental retardation*
40. M. J. Khoury, W. Burke, and E. Thomson: *Genetics and public health in the 21st century*
41. J. Weil: *Psychosocial genetic counseling*
42. R. J. Gorlin, M. M. Cohen, Jr., and R. C. M. Hennekam: *Syndromes of the head and neck*, fourth edition
43. M. M. Cohen, Jr., G. Neri, and R. Weksberg: *Overgrowth syndromes*
44. R. A. King, J. I. Rotter, and A. G. Motulsky: *Genetic basis of common diseases*, second edition
45. G. P. Bates, P. S. Harper, and L. Jones: *Huntington's disease*, third edition
46. R. J. M. Gardner and G. R. Sutherland: *Chromosome abnormalities and genetic counseling*, third edition
47. I. J. Holt: *Genetics of mitochondrial disease*
48. F. Flinter, E. Maher, and A. Saggar-Malik: *Genetics of renal disease*
49. C. J. Epstein, R. P. Erickson, and A. Wynshaw-Boris: *Inborn errors of development: The molecular basis of clinical disorders of morphogenesis*
50. H. V. Toriello, W. Reardon, and R. J. Gorlin: *Hereditary hearing loss and its syndromes*, second edition
51. P. S. Harper: *Landmarks in medical genetics*
52. R. E. Stevenson and J. G. Hall: *Human malformations and related anomalies*, second edition
53. D. Kumar and S. D. Weatherall: *Genomics and clinical medicine*
54. C. J. Epstein, R. P. Erickson, and A. Wynshaw-Boris: *Inborn errors of development: The molecular basis of clinical disorders of morphogenesis*, second edition
55. W. Weber: *Pharmacogenetics*, second edition
56. P. L. Beales, I. S. Farooqi, and S. O'Rahilly: *The genetics of obesity syndromes*
57. P. S. Harper: *A short history of medical genetics*
58. R. C. M. Hennekam, I. D. Krantz, and J. E. Allanson: *Gorlin's syndromes of the head and neck*, fifth edition
59. D. Kumar and P. Elliot: *Principles and practices of cardiovascular genetics*
60. V. P. Sybert: *Genetic skin disorders*, second edition
61. R. J. M. Gardner, G. R. Sutherland, and L. C. Shaffer: *Chromosome abnormalities and genetic counseling*, fourth edition
62. D. Kumar: *Genomics and health in the developing world*
63. G. Bates, S. Tabrizi, and L. Jones: *Huntington's disease*, fourth edition
64. B. Lee and F. Scaglia: *Inborn errors of metabolism: From neonatal screening to metabolic pathways*
65. D. Kumar and C. Eng: *Genomic medicine*, second edition
66. R. Stevenson, J. Hall, D. Everman, and B. Solomon: *Human malformations and related anomalies*, third edition
67. R. Erickson and A. Wynshaw-Boris: *Epstein's inborn errors of development: The molecular basis of clinical disorders of morphogenesis*, third edition
68. C. Hollak and R. Lachmann: *Inherited metabolic disease in adults: A clinical guide*
69. V. P. Sybert: *Genetic skin disorders*, third edition
70. R. J. M. Gardner and D. J. Amor: *Gardner and Sutherland's chromosome abnormalities and genetic counseling*, fifth edition
71. G. Neri, L. Boccuto, and R. E. Stevenson: *Overgrowth syndromes: A clinical guide*
72. E. I. Traboulsi, V. M. Utz, and A. O. Khan: *Genetic diseases of the eye*, third edition
73. D. J. Amor and R. J. M. Gardner: *Gardner and Sutherland's chromosome abnormalities and genetic counseling*, sixth edition

Gardner and Sutherland's Chromosome Abnormalities and Genetic Counseling

Sixth Edition

David J. Amor
Lorenzo And Pamela Galli Chair
University of Melbourne
Victorian Clinical Genetics Services
Murdoch Children's Research Institute
Royal Children's Hospital, Melbourne, Australia

R. J. McKinlay Gardner
Adjunct Professor
The Laboratory for Genomic Medicine
University of Otago, Dunedin, New Zealand

OXFORD
UNIVERSITY PRESS

OXFORD
UNIVERSITY PRESS

Oxford University Press is a department of the University of Oxford.
It furthers the University's objective of excellence in research, scholarship,
and education by publishing worldwide. Oxford is a registered trade mark of
Oxford University Press in the UK and in certain other countries.

Published in the United States of America by Oxford University Press
198 Madison Avenue, New York, NY 10016, United States of America.

© Oxford University Press 2026

All rights reserved. No part of this publication may be reproduced, stored in a retrieval system, transmitted, used for text and data mining, or used for training artificial intelligence, in any form or by any means, without the prior permission in writing of Oxford University Press, or as expressly permitted by law, by license or under terms agreed with the appropriate reprographics rights organization. Inquiries concerning reproduction outside the scope of the above should be sent to the Rights Department, Oxford University Press, at the address above.

You must not circulate this work in any other form
and you must impose this same condition on any acquirer.

CIP data is on file at the Library of Congress

This material is not intended to be, and should not be considered, a substitute for medical or other professional advice. Treatment for the conditions described in this material is highly dependent on the individual circumstances. And, while this material is designed to offer accurate information with respect to the subject matter covered and to be current as of the time it was written, research and knowledge about medical and health issues is constantly evolving and dose schedules for medications are being revised continually, with new side effects recognized and accounted for regularly. Readers must therefore always check the product information and clinical procedures with the most up-to-date published product information and data sheets provided by the manufacturers and the most recent codes of conduct and safety regulation. The publisher and the authors make no representations or warranties to readers, express or implied, as to the accuracy or completeness of this material. Without limiting the foregoing, the publisher and the authors make no representations or warranties as to the accuracy or efficacy of the drug dosages mentioned in the material. The authors and the publisher do not accept, and expressly disclaim, any responsibility for any liability, loss or risk that may be claimed or incurred as a consequence of the use and/or application of any of the contents of this material.

ISBN 978–0–19–774772–8

DOI: 10.1093/med/9780197747728.001.0001

Printed by Integrated Books International, United States of America

The manufacturer's authorized representative in the EU for product safety is
Oxford University Press España S.A., Parque Empresarial San Fernando de Henares,
Avenida de Castilla, 2 – 28830 Madrid (www.oup.es/en or product.safety@oup.com).
OUP España S.A. also acts as importer into Spain of products made by the manufacturer.

MIX
Paper
FSC FSC® C183721

This book is dedicated to Jocelyn, Geoffrey, and Craig, their parents, and all other families who seek our "chromosomal advice."

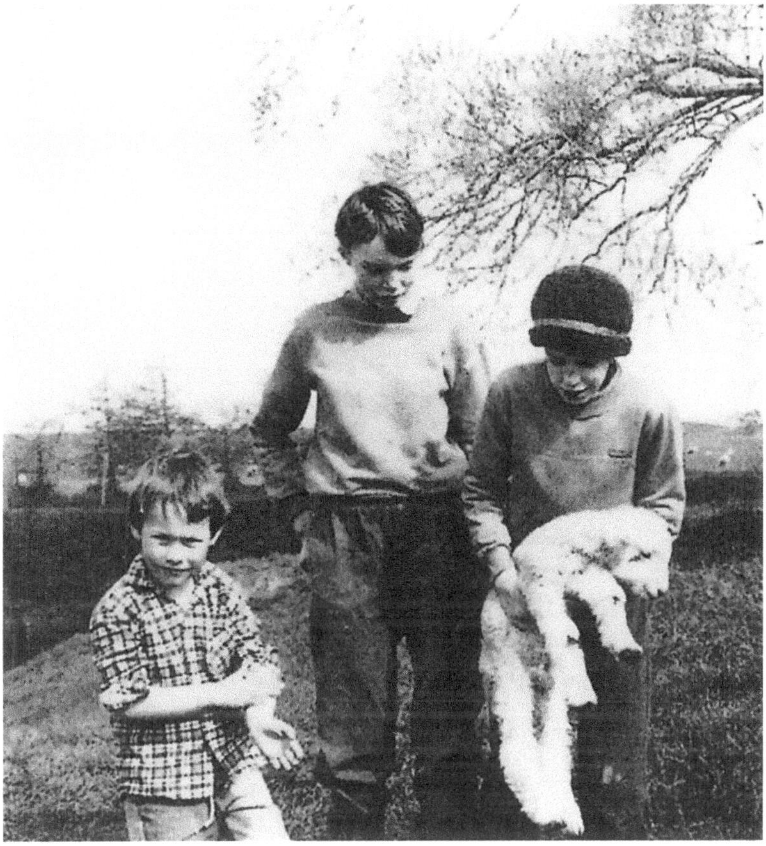

Jocelyn and Geoffrey (with lamb) have a partial trisomy for chromosome 4 long arm, and Craig, the youngest, had a 46,XY result on amniocentesis. Their father is a translocation carrier (see Figure 5–1, lower). Craig, since married, came to the genetic clinic for confirmatory advice about his low genetic risk.

Heredity

Inescapably, this is me—the diagnosis
is cause for anger at those
who brightly say we choose our destinies.
There is no store
of courage, wit or will
can save me from myself and I must face
my children, feeling like
that wicked fairy, uninvited
at the christening, bestowing on my own,
amidst murmurs of apprehension, a most
unwanted gift—that
of a blighted mind. No one
could tell me of this curse when I
was young and dreamt of children
and the graces they would bear. Later,
it seemed that a chill morning
revealed deeper layers
of truth. For my romancing
there is a price to pay—
perhaps my children's children
will pass this tollgate after me.
My grandmothers gaze down from their frames
on my wall, sadly wondering.

—Meg Campbell

Dear DNA

In real life you're just
a tangle of white filaments
captured in a test-tube,
and your first photo is not flattering:
grey smudges like tractor tracks,
or a rusty screw. Yet
many say you are beautiful.
Online for a night
with a hundred fantastic portraits
and I'm head over heels
In love with you, DNA,
bewitched by your billions
coiled in my cells, transcribing,
replicating, mutating.
I see your never-ending dance.
A length of twisted ladder
briefly unwinds,
both strands duplicate,
each copy drifts away
on its secret mission
to make a thought, feel sunshine,
or digest this morning's porridge.
Two winding parallel threads,
a tiny tangle of gossamer
designing my life.
DNA, you are astonishing
and I am yours truly.

—Winifred Kavalieris

Genes pass on our kind
But our selves are transmitted
In words left behind.

—J. Patrick Gookin

Curiosity is a virtue, perhaps an
unsung and undervalued virtue,
which should be the energizing fuel
to the thinking geneticist.

—Willie Reardon

Where is the wisdom we have lost in knowledge?
Where is the knowledge we have lost in
information?

—T. S. Eliot

PREFACE TO THE SIXTH EDITION

A book growing into its sixth edition might be seen as having achieved a certain maturity. Certainly, the discipline upon which it is based has matured enormously, and indeed the centenary of "clinical chromosomology" in 2058 does not now sound so far away that it cannot, on a distant horizon, be glimpsed. The lifetime thus far of this book (1980s to 2020s) has followed much of this evolution, witnessing the increasing clinical scope for which chromosome testing can be applied, the precision with which chromosome abnormalities can be recognized, the extraordinary methodologies applied to the analysis of chromosomes, and the growing sophistication that the counselor must bring to her/his understanding of the issues facing those who seek our advice.

Maturity, yes, but equally we have been aware of a need to avoid an age-related ossification, and we have kept in mind Sir Peter Harper's admonition that a genetic document should grow by attrition, not accretion. Nevertheless, some growth is—to our very considerable satisfaction—entirely warranted, given the remarkable advances made even since the previous edition of 2018. The reader must decide how well we may have balanced Sir Peter's criteria.

Melbourne D.J.A.
Dunedin R.J.M.G.
October 2025

ACKNOWLEDGMENTS

We thank Gabby Atlas, Naja Becher, Amber Burgess, David Francis, Wayne Gillett, Jessie Jacobsen, Ida Charlotte Bay Lund, Sharyn Stock-Meyer, Mark Pertile, Stephen Robertson, and Ida Vogel; the book is the better for their advice. Grant Sutherland has reviewed, and advised upon, most of the chapters. Several of the new Figures have been drawn by Kelley Gardner. The index was compiled by Max McMaster, and Cushla McKinney and Frances Dawson helped with proof-reading. We thank many colleagues worldwide, and their publishers, who have kindly allowed us to use illustrations from their work (the reader will note very frequent use of the expression "Courtesy of" in Figure legends). Some authors we were unable to contact, and we hope that they may allow the liberty we have taken, nevertheless, of using their work. The chromosomal imaging from the Genome Browser of the University of California, Santa Cruz, has been invaluable in drawing many of the diagrams. We owe a remarkable debt to the National Center for Biotechnology Information: their hosting of PubMed has enabled ready access to the world literature that would otherwise have been a Herculean task.

CONTENTS

PART FOUR DISORDERS ASSOCIATED WITH ABERRANT GENOMIC IMPRINTING

PART FIVE REPRODUCTIVE CYTOGENETICS

PART SIX DISORDERS OF SEX DEVELOPMENT

PART SEVEN PHENOTYPES

PART EIGHT NOXIOUS AGENTS

PART NINE ETHICS

APPENDIXES

Several commonly used abbreviations appear throughout this book. As well as the cytogenetic abbreviations listed in Appendix B, these include also:

ABT	Apparently balanced translocation
ADHD	Attention deficit hyperactivity disorder
cfDNA	Cell-free DNA
cFTS	combined first-trimester screening
CNV	Copy number variant
CPM	Confined placental mosaicism
CVS	Chorionic villus sampling
dn	De novo
DNA	DNA
DS	Down syndrome
FDIU	Fetal death in utero
GRCh	Genome Reference Consortium human [followed by build number]
gw-NIPS	Genome-wide cell-free DNA-based non-invasive prenatal screening
hg	human genome [followed by build number]
ICE	Interchromosomal effect
ICM	Inner cell mass (also called embryoblast)
ICSI	Intracytoplasmic sperm injection
IUFD	In utero fetal demise
IUI	Intrauterine insemination
IVF	In vitro fertilization
kb	kilobase of DNA
LRS	Long read sequencing
Mb	Megabase of DNA
NAHR	Non-allelic homologous recombination
NHEJ	Nonhomologous end-joining
NICS	Noninvasive chromosome screening
NGS	Next-generation sequencing
PGT	Preimplantation genetic testing
PGT-A	PGT for aneuploidy
PND	Prenatal diagnosis
POC	Products of conception
POF	Premature ovarian failure
POI	Premature ovarian insufficiency
RAT	Rare autosomal trisomy
RIF	Recurrent implantation failure
RPL	Recurrent pregnancy loss
SNP	Single nucleotide polymorphism
SRS	Short read sequencing
TAD	Topologically associating domain
TFM	True fetal mosaicism
UPD, upd	Uniparental disomy
wcp	whole chromosome painting
WGA	Whole genome analysis

PART ONE

BASIC CONCEPTS

1
ELEMENTS OF MEDICAL CYTOGENETICS

CHROMOSOMES WERE FIRST SEEN and named in the late 19th century. *Chromosome* is a combination of Greek words meaning colored (*chrom*) body (*soma*); the word was coined by the illustrious German anatomist Heinrich Wilhelm Gottfried von Waldeyer-Hartz. It was eventually appreciated that these brightly staining objects appearing in the cell nucleus must be the "stuff of heredity," the very vessels of our genetic inheritance, and Thomas Hunt Morgan received the Nobel Prize in 1933 for having proved the "chromosome theory of inheritance."

Most observers had concluded, in the earlier part of the 20th century, that the human chromosome count was 48. It was not until the 1950s, due to technical advances—and in particular the use of a hypotonic solution to swell the cells, giving an uncluttered view of the chromosomes—that Joe Hin Tjio and Albert Levan could recognize that 46 was the correct number. This discovery spurred research into conditions in which a chromosomal cause had hitherto been suspected, and in 1959 ("the wonderful year of human cytogenetics") came the first demonstrations of a medical application of the new knowledge, with practically simultaneous discoveries of the chromosomal basis of Down syndrome, Klinefelter syndrome, and Turner syndrome (Lejeune et al. 1959[1]; Jacobs and Strong 1959; Ford et al. 1959); these were followed soon thereafter by the recognition of the other major aneuploidy syndromes. Harper (2006) records the history, and the personalities behind the history, in his book *First Years of Human Chromosomes*—a book that should be read by every student of medical cytogenetics with an interest in how their discipline came to be. Harper points out that the practice of genetic counseling came into its own essentially upon the basis of these chromosomal discoveries. So to speak, geneticists now had "their organ." The value in this chromosomal knowledge lies in diagnosis and management—of the index case, and of the family.

"Colored bodies" became an especially apt derivation with the development of various different staining techniques in the 1980s and 1990s, showing different parts of chromosomes in many different colors, whether true or computer-generated false colors. The images produced by this kaleidoscopic karyotyping could be rather beautiful (Figure 1–1). Black-and-white photographs were less splendid but often sufficed (Figure 1–2). Although molecular methodologies have substantially taken over from classical cytogenetics, providing a different view of the genetic material (Miga and Eichler 2023), the word *chromosome* will surely last forever.

[1] Among the "al." was Marthe Gautier, who recounted, half a century following this report, her own less than fully acknowledged role in the endeavor; and Sir Peter Harper, in a commentary and in his role as historian to the genetics community, takes an interpretative perspective on this pioneering discovery (Gautier and Harper 2009).

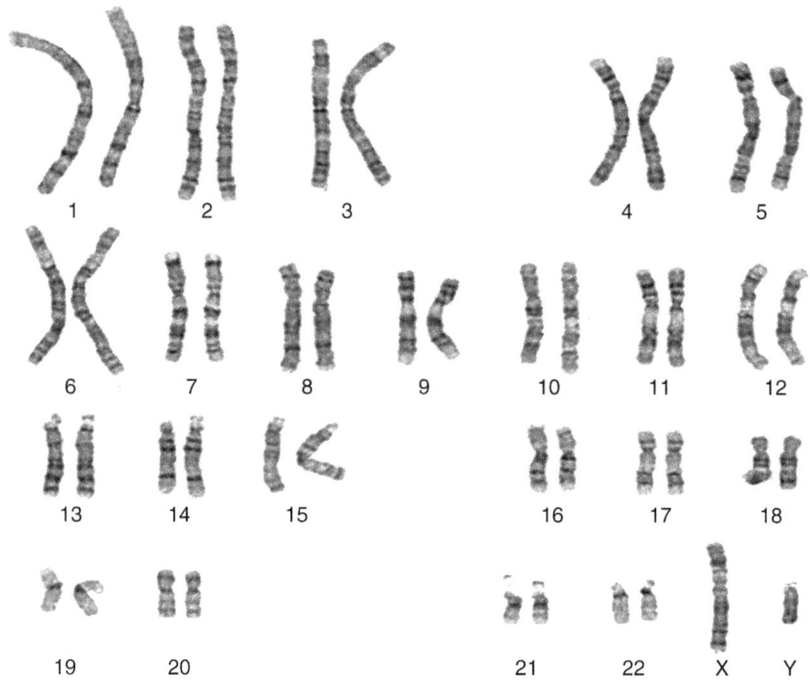

Figure 1–3. Chromosomes arranged as a formal karyotype, from a classical cytogenetic study based upon a mitotic cell.

example, chromosomes 10 and 11 are shorter than chromosome 12, and chromosome 21 is smaller than 22).

The classical format of a chromosome display, the *karyotype*, has the chromosomes lined up with p arms upward, in their matching pairs (Figure 1–3). Those coming from a DNA-based view may see the chromosome lying on its side, and microarray reports usually show a horizontal depiction of the chromosome arms, with the graph indicating duplications and deletions by a rise or a fall compared to baseline, respectively (although no one is proposing that short and long arms be renamed as left and right!). Karyotypes are described according to a shorthand notation, the International System of Human Cytogenetic Nomenclature (ISCN 2024); an outline is given in Appendix B.

In this age of "molecular karyotyping," chromosomes are more readily being thought of as lengths of DNA, rather than as segments of stainable chromatin. A laboratory report may be couched in terms of the actual DNA content of an imbalance (Chapter 2). It is almost as though we can "see" the genes, rather than just knowing intellectually that this is—of course—what a chromosome consists of. Table 1–1 and Figure 1–4 set out the amounts of DNA and the number of genes carried by each chromosome.

CHROMOSOMAL STRUCTURE

Chromatin exists in differently condensed forms: the less condensed *euchromatin* and the more condensed *heterochromatin*. Euchromatin contains the coding DNA—the genes—while heterochromatin comprises non-coding DNA. Chromosomes are capped

Table 1-1. The Lengths of the Chromosomes in Megabases, the Number of Genes per Chromosome, and the Density of Genes per Chromosome

CHROMOSOME	LENGTH IN Mb	GENES	GENES PER Mb
1	249.3	1959	7.86
2	243.2	1184	4.87
3	198.0	1029	5.20
4	191.2	721	3.77
5	180.9	835	4.62
6	171.1	1002	5.86
7	159.1	855	5.37
8	146.4	638	4.36
9	141.2	748	5.30
10	135.5	714	5.27
11	135.0	1236	9.16
12	133.9	987	7.37
13	115.2	305	2.65
14	107.3	577	5.37
15	102.5	547	5.33
16	90.4	783	8.67
17	81.2	1111	13.68
18	78.1	257	3.29
19	59.1	1332	22.53
20	63.0	518	8.22
21	48.1	213	4.43
22	51.3	418	8.15
X	155.3	806	5.19
Y	59.4	65	1.09

Notes: The relative sparsity of genes on the three classic "trisomic" chromosomes, 13, 18, and 21 (and as also evident in Figure 1-4) is to be noted. In contrast, chromosome 19, although one of the smallest, carries an extraordinary load of genes. This, presumably, is the basis of the extreme lethality of trisomy 19 (see Figure 20-22). The lengths here (from hg19,[a] of the time) differ slightly from those listed in Table A-1, based upon hg38.

[a]"hg"—human genome—refers to the UCSC (University of California Santa Cruz) Genome Browser assembly number. The similar GRCh (Genome Reference Consortium, human) database now uses the same numbering system, both currently 38; previously they had had different numbers, and hg37 matched CGRh19. These two databases are "reference genomes" that are periodically updated.

Source: After S Scherer, *Guide to the Human Genome*, Cold Spring Harbor Laboratory Press, Woodbury, New York, 2010.

at the terminal extremities of their long and short arms by *telomeres*, specialized DNA sequences comprising many repeats of the sequence TTAGGG, that can be thought of as "sealing" the chromatin and preventing its fusion with the chromatin of other chromosomes. The *centromere*[3] is a specialized region of DNA that, at cell division, provides the

[3] When considering the physical structure of rearranged chromosomes, it is useful to keep in mind the absolute requirement for a centromere to be present on every chromosome. There is also the need for each chromosome to have two telomeres, the single exception being when the rearranged chromosome forms a ring.

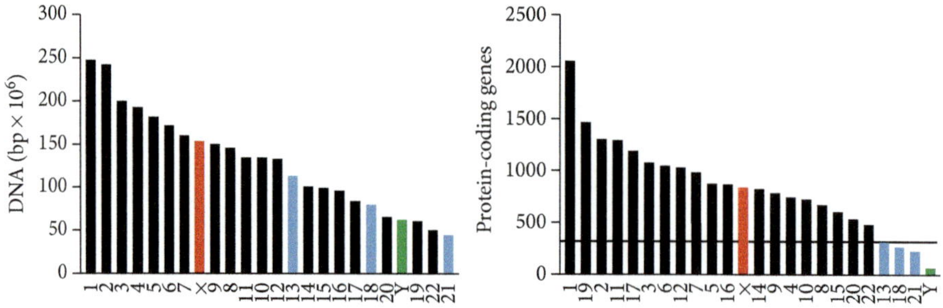

Figure 1–4. A Display of the DNA Content, and the Gene Load, of Each Chromosome.

Notes: Chromosomes are ordered by size (*left*) and gene content (*right*). The "viable" autosomes, 13, 18, and 21, are shown in blue, and the sex chromosomes in red and green. The low gene content of the viable autosomes is evident; the bar (*right*) is set at 327 genes.

Source: From EM Torres, Consequences of gaining an extra chromosome, *Chromosome Res* 31:24, 2023. Courtesy EM Torres, and with the permission of Springer Nature.

site at which the spindle apparatus can be anchored and draw each separated chromatid[4] to opposite poles of the dividing cell. Centromeric heterochromatin contains "satellite DNA," so called because these DNA species have different buoyant densities and produce distinct humps on a density gradient distribution. (These are not to be confused with the satellites on acrocentric chromosomes.) A separate issue, of considerable academic interest (but which we shall take no further here), is the "packaging question": how the centimeters of DNA are compacted into micron-length chromosomes, and which parts of the nucleus each chromosome occupies (Figure 1–5) (Sehgal et al. 2016; Sedat et al. 2022; Labade et al. 2024). Neither do we delve into the molecular anatomy of the chromosome, while it did not escape our notice[5] that the DNA sequences within, now so well documented (Nurk et al. 2022), are, of course, their *sine qua non*.

CHROMOSOME ABNORMALITY

Chromosomes are distributed to each daughter cell during cell division in a very precise process—precise, but prone to error. From our perspective, the two cell divisions of *meiosis*, during which the gametes are formed, are of central importance. Much of the discipline of medical cytogenetics focuses on the consequences of disordered meiosis having produced a chromosomally abnormal gamete, causing a chromosomal abnormality in the *conceptus*. A chromosome abnormality that is present from conception and involves the entire body is a *constitutional* abnormality. If an additional cell line with a different chromosomal complement arises before the basis of the body structure is formed (that is, in embryonic or pre-embryonic life) and becomes an integral part of the organism, *constitutional mosaicism* results. In this book, we concern ourselves practically solely with constitutional abnormalities. Acquired chromosomal abnormality of course exists, and indeed it is a major initiating and sustaining cause in most cancers, a fact first proposed by Boveri in 1914 and voluminously attested in the work

[4] Chromatids separate at mitosis and at meiosis II, and at "predivision" in meiosis I.

[5] A nod to Watson and Crick.

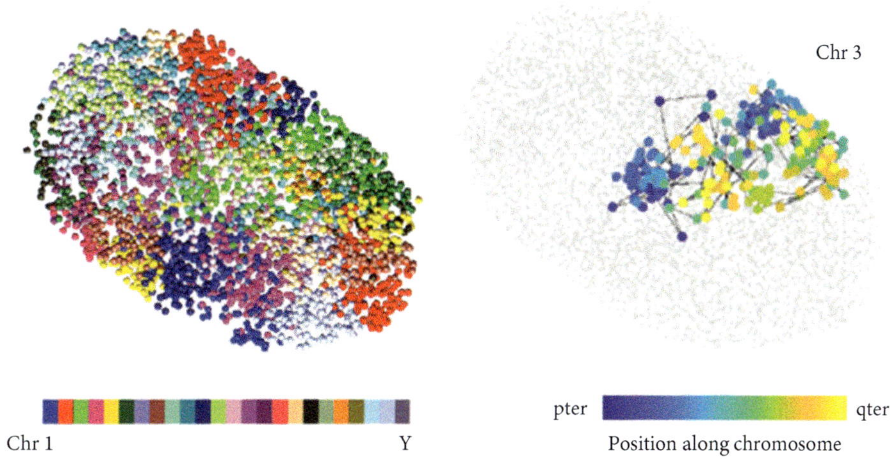

Figure 1–5. The Spatial Arrangement of Chromosomes within the Nucleus.

Notes: The color coding indicates which part of the nucleus each chromosome occupies, in a human fibroblast. The figure at *left* is a composite from the analysis of all 23 chromosomes. At *right*, chromosome 3's territory is outlined, which can be discerned in the green coloring in the composite image. This study is based on expansion in situ genome sequencing (ExIGS).

Source: From AS Labade et al., Expansion in situ genome sequencing links nuclear abnormalities to hotspots of aberrant euchromatin repression, bioRχiv 2024.09.24.614614, 2024. Courtesy of JD Buenrostro and Colleagues, and with their permission.

of Mitelman et al. (2024); but this is more the field of study of the molecular pathologist than the genetic counselor.

An incorrect amount of genetic material carried by the conceptus disturbs and distorts its normal growth pattern (from zygote → blastocyst → embryo → fetus). In *trisomy*, there is three of a particular chromosome, instead of the normal two. In *monosomy*, only one member of the pair is present. Two of each is the only combination that works properly! It is scarcely surprising that a process as exquisitely complex as the development of the human form should be vulnerable to a confused outflow of genetic instruction from a nucleus with a redundant or incomplete database.

Trisomy and monosomy for a whole chromosome were the first cytogenetic mechanisms leading to an abnormal phenotype to be identified. More fully, we can list the following pathogenetic mechanisms that arise from chromosomal abnormalities:

1. A dosage effect, with a lack (deletion) or excess (duplication) of chromosomal material, whether for a whole chromosome or a part of a chromosome. This is by far the predominant category.
2. A direct damaging effect, with disruption of a gene at the breakpoint of a rearrangement.
3. A position effect, whereby a gene in a new chromosomal environment functions inappropriately.
4. An effect due to the incongruent parental origin of a chromosome or chromosomal segment (genomic imprinting).
5. Combinations of the above.

We discuss these mechanisms in more detail in following chapters.

AUTOSOMAL IMBALANCE

As noted earlier, imbalance may involve the gain or loss of a whole chromosome—*full aneuploidy*—or of part of a chromosome—*partial aneuploidy*. Full aneuploidies are trisomies and monosomies; partial aneuploidies are duplications (*dup*) and deletions (*del*). The abnormality may occur in the non-mosaic or mosaic state. Loss (that is, monosomy/deletion) of chromosomal material typically has a more devastating effect on growth of the conceptus than does an excess of material (that is, trisomy/duplication). Smaller dups and dels are referred to as copy number variants (CNVs), and Collins et al. (2022) document, at the level of individual dosage-sensitive genes within the CNV segments, which loci are critical to the generation of phenotypic abnormality; they speak of haploinsufficient (deletion intolerance) and triplosensitive (duplication intolerance) imbalance.

Certain imbalances lead to certain abnormal phenotypes. The spectrum is listed in outline in Box 1–1. Most full autosomal trisomies and virtually all full autosomal monosomies set development of the conceptus so awry that, sooner or later, abortion occurs—the embryo "self-destructs" and is expelled from the uterus. This issue is further explored in Chapter 20. A few full trisomies are not necessarily lethal in utero, and many partial chromosomal aneuploidies are associated with survival through to the birth of an infant.

Characteristically, "survivable imbalances" produce a phenotype of widespread dysmorphogenesis, and there may be malformation of internal organs and limbs. It is often in the facial appearance (*facies*) that the most recognizable physical abnormality is seen, with Down syndrome the classic example, although the physical phenotype in

Box 1–1. The Spectrum of Effects, in Broad Outline, Resulting from Constitutional Chromosomal Abnormality

1. Devastation of blastogenesis, with transient implantation or non-implantation of the conceptus.
2. Devastation of embryogenesis, with spontaneous abortion, usually in the first trimester.
3. Major disruption of normal intrauterine morphogenesis, with second or third trimester abortion/fetal death in utero, stillbirth, or early neonatal death.
4. Major disruption of normal intrauterine morphogenesis, but with some extrauterine survival.
5. Moderate distortion of normal intrauterine development, with substantial extrauterine survival and severe intellectual disability.
6. Mild distortion of normal intrauterine development, with substantial extrauterine survival and considerable intellectual compromise.
7. Minimal physical phenotypic effect, varying degrees of intellectual compromise; possible compromise of fertility.
8. No discernible physical phenotypic effect; cognitive function within the normal range, but less than expected from the family background.

some cases of subtler deletion or duplication may be rather "bland." The most complex organ of all, the brain, is the most vulnerable to a less-than-optimal genetic constitution, and some compromise of mental and intellectual functioning, usually to the extent of an obvious deficit, is nearly invariable, at least in imbalances of classical size. With several of the (much smaller) imbalances due to copy number variants, flawed neurodevelopmental progress or intellectual disability,[6] with an outwardly normal physical phenotype, is well recognized as a chromosomal presentation. Thus, the central concern of most people seeking genetic counseling for a chromosomal condition is that of having a child who might have a physical, intellectual, or severe social handicap.

Historically, the chromosomal basis of many syndromes was identified following analysis of groups of patients with similar phenotypes. This "phenotype-first" approach led to the identification of many of the well-known microdeletion syndromes (and of course such classic conditions as Down syndrome). With the advent of molecular karyotyping, new syndromes came to be identified based on their DNA aberration, a "genotype-first" approach. Representative examples of these newer syndromes are reviewed in Chapter 14.

SEX CHROMOSOMAL ABNORMALITY

Sex chromosome (gonosome) imbalance has a much less deleterious effect on the phenotype than does autosomal aneuploidy. The X chromosome is one of the larger and is gene-dense; the Y is small, comprising mostly heterochromatin, and carries very few genes (the key one being *SRY*, which determines maleness). In both male and female, one, and only one, completely functioning X chromosome is needed. X chromosomes in excess of one are inactivated, as the normal 46,XX female exemplifies; her second X does, however, maintain some segments genetically active.

With X chromosome excess or deficiency, a partially successful buffering mechanism exists whereby the imbalance is counteracted, in an attempt to achieve the same effect as having a single active X. In such states as, for example, XXX, XXY, XXXX, XXYY, and XXXXX, excess X chromosomes are inactivated. In the 45,X state, the single X remaining is not subject to inactivation. If an abnormal X chromosome (e.g., an isochromosome, or a deleted X) is present, then, as a rule, cells containing this abnormal chromosome as the active X are selected against, perhaps due to preferential growth of those cells in which it is the normal X that is the active one. In X imbalance, the reproductive tract and brain are the organs predominantly affected. The effect may be minimal. As for Y chromosome excess, such as XYY, there is a limited phenotypic consequence—but again, the brain may be a vulnerable organ.

[6] Words can be powerful, and choice of language can help, or hinder, a counseling consultation: Facts are to be conveyed clearly but also sensitively. The term "mental retardation," once widespread in the genetics literature, has acquired a pejorative and somewhat harsh sense over the years, and we now prefer such expressions as "intellectual disability" or "cognitive impairment." "Developmental delay" is a widely used term, and it can be perfectly appropriate in early childhood setting, but less so in dealing with a school-age child or adult; this distinction acknowledges that prediction of intellectual capacity is more precise in older children. As we write elsewhere, counselors will need to know to whom they speak, and what language is best to use.

Functional Imbalance

A correct amount of chromatin does not necessarily mean the phenotype will be normal. Inappropriate inactivation, or activation, of a segment of the genome can compromise the genetic message. Some segments of the genome require only monosomic expression, and the homologous segment on the other chromosome is inactivated. If this control fails, both segments can become activated or both inactivated, and the over- or under-expression of the contained loci can cause phenotypic abnormality. The classic example of this is genomic imprinting according to parent of origin, and we discuss this concept in Chapter 19. A rather specialized example arises with the X-autosome translocation. A segment of X chromosome can fail to be inactivated or, conversely, X-inactivation can spread into an autosomal segment, and in each case to deleterious effect (Chapter 6).

THE FREQUENCY AND IMPACT OF CYTOGENETIC PATHOLOGY

According to the window of observation (Figure 1–6), chromosomal disorders make a greater or lesser contribution to human mortality and morbidity. Looking at prenatal existence, the earliest window has been provided by the in vitro fertilization (IVF) clinic, from the procedure of preimplantation genetic testing (Chapter 23), at which cells taken from 5-day-old embryos are subjected to genetic analysis, and an extraordinary fraction are chromosomally abnormal. After implantation (about day 6), and through the first trimester of pregnancy (to week 13), chromosomal mortality is very high, and aneuploidy is the major single cause of spontaneous abortion (Chapter 20). Perinatal and early infant death have a significant chromosomal component, of which trisomies 18 and 21 (although the latter less so in more recent times) are major elements.

In Table 1–2 we set out the birth incidences of the various categories of (classical) chromosomal abnormality; these data are from a Danish study, one of a number that have examined this question in the later decades of the 20th century with largely similar findings in each. Overall, around one in 135 liveborn babies have a classical chromosomal abnormality, and about 40% of these are phenotypically abnormal due to the chromosome defect.

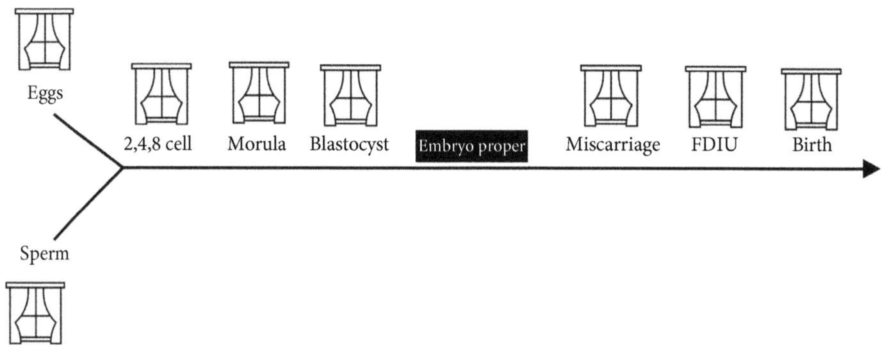

Figure 1–6. The windows of observation open to chromosomal study.
Note: Obviously, time on the *x* axis is depicted asymmetrically. FDIU, fetal death in utero.

Table 1-2. Classical Chromosomal Rearrangements and Imbalances, Recorded in 34,910 Live Newborns in Århus, Denmark, Over a Total 13-Year Period, 1969–1974 and 1980–1988

	NO. OF CASES	PER 1,000[a]	BIRTH FREQUENCY PER GROUP
Sex Chromosomes			
Klinefelter Syndrome and Variants			
47,XXY	20	1.12[b]	
47,XXY/46,XY	7	0.39	
46,XX ♂	2	0.11	
			1 in 616 ♂
XYY			
47,XYY	18	1.01	
47,XYY/46,XY	2	0.11	
			1 in 894 ♂
XXX			
47,XXX	17	1.00	
			1 in 1,002 ♀
Turner Syndrome and Variants			
45,X	1	0.06	
45,X/46,XX and 45,X/47,XXX	3	0.18	
45,X/46,X,r(X)	1	0.06	
45,X/46,X,i(Xq)/47,X,i(Xq),i(Xq)	1	0.06	
Other Turner Variant	2	0.12	
			1 in 2,130 ♀
Other			
45,X/46,XY	1	0.06	
46,XX/47,XX,del(Yq)	1	0.06	
46,XX/46,XY	1	0.06	
Total	77	2.21	1 in 453
Autosomes			
Unbalanced Forms			
Trisomy 13	2	0.06	
Trisomy 18	7	0.20	
Trisomy 21	51	1.46	
Trisomy 8	1	0.03	
Supernumerary marker, ring	25	0.72	
Deletions, duplications	6	0.17	
			1 in 379
Balanced Forms			
Robertsonian 13/14 translocation	34	0.97	
Other Robertsonian	9	0.26	
Reciprocal translocations	50	1.43	
Inversions (other than of chromosome 2)	4	0.11	
			1 in 360

(continued)

Table 1-2. Continued

	NO. OF CASES	PER 1,000[a]	BIRTH FREQUENCY PER GROUP
Combined sex plus autosomal totals	266	7.62	1 in 131
Combined totals, excluding balanced autosomal forms	169	4.84	1 in 207

Notes: Not included in the 34,910 live newborns listing are four cases of induced abortion due to sex chromosome prenatal diagnosis, involving the karyotypes 47,XXY, 47,XYY, 47,XXX, and 45,X/46,X,del(Xq), and 15 cases of autosomal-diagnosis induced abortions, involving the karyotypes +21, +13, +18, and three different derivative chromosomes. Had these pregnancies proceeded to term, the frequencies in the relevant group category would have been marginally increased.

These figures might continue to be broadly valid into this century, except that the category of deletions and duplications will substantially increase due to the more powerful detection now offered by molecular technology (Table 1-3).

[a]Per 1,000 male, per 1,000 female, or per 1,000 both, as appropriate. The gender-specific denominators in this study were 17,872 males and 17,038 females.

[b]An increasing incidence of XXY in recent years has been suggested, and an Australian study, including data up to 2006, arrived at a figure of 1.91 per 1,000 (Herlihy and Halliday 2008; Morris et al. 2008; Herlihy et al. 2010).

Source: From Nielsen and Wohlert (1991)

The finer the cytogenetic focus, the greater the incidence, and it is now a task for the cytogenetic (or molecular genomic) epidemiologist of this century, in the microarray/molecular era, to derive new estimates of cytogenetic abnormalities in the different populations (Rosenfeld et al. 2013). While the incidence of classical data remains stable, the subtler del/dups have been increasingly observed in more recent years (Figure 1-7). A useful start has been made by Smajlagić et al. (2021) in their analysis of a population of newborns and their parents, in whom they tested for the presence of 13 of the recurrent deletions and duplications that have become well recognized as causative of known phenotypes/syndromes and are associated, in particular, with a neurodevelopmental component. They were able to make a distinction between those del/dups inherited from a parent, and those arising de novo (Table 1-3). In this population, the notable figure of one in 200 children were born with a recurrent deletion or duplication; in other words, these abnormalities are not uncommon. And if we combine the overall estimates of Tables 1-2 (1 in 207) and 1-3 (1 in 200), and if we may extrapolate these Scandinavian data more generally, we approach a broad figure that about one in 100 individuals, at least in a newborn population, are chromosomally imbalanced and with an associated abnormal phenotype, whether of severe, moderate, mild, or barely discernible degree.

Adolescence is a period during which many sex chromosome defects come to light, when pubertal change fails to occur, and in young adulthood when chromosomal causes of infertility are recognized. If the target population is fertile adults (ascertained incidentally), a much lower frequency of sex chromosome aneuploidy is observed (Samango-Sprouse et al. 2016). If we were to study a population of 70-year-olds, we could expect to see very few individuals with an unbalanced autosomal karyotype (but loss of the Y chromosome is a common observation in older men; p. 472).

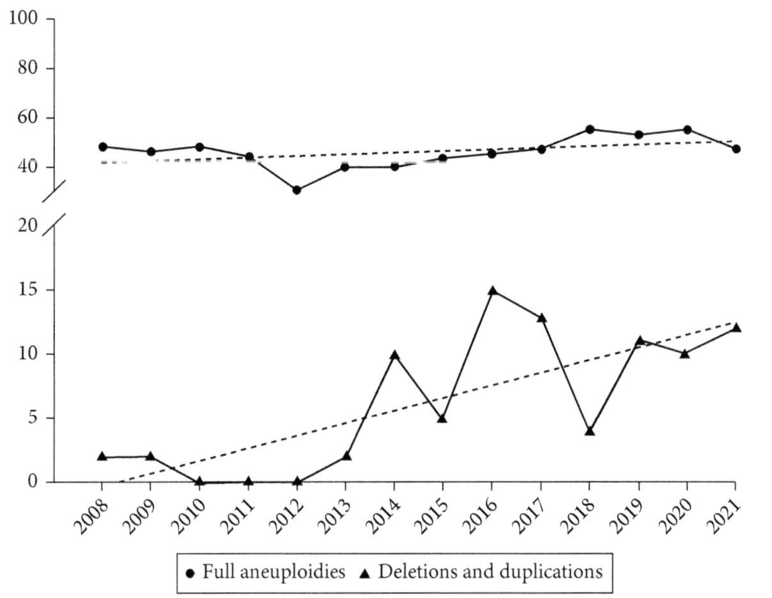

Figure 1–7. The Increasing Detection of Deletions and Duplications.

Notes: Shown are the numbers (*y*-axis) of terminations in central Denmark over the period 2008–2021 (*x*-axis), for the indications of an aneuploidy (*upper line*), and for a deletion or duplication (*lower line*). The baseline birth rate in this population is c. 14,000 per annum. Termination on the grounds of a fetal abnormality was available from 12 to 22 weeks gestation, but required approval from a local Regional Abortion Council.

Source: From L Raaby et al., Has the introduction of increased genetic prenatal testing affected rates of termination of pregnancy due to fetal abnormality? *Prenat Diagn* 44:280–288, 2024. Courtesy L Raaby, and with the permission of John Wiley & Sons.

While few classic cytogenetic defects come to attention later in adult life, many children with an aneuploidy can survive well into adulthood and some into old age, and some require lifelong care from their families or from the state. This latter group imposes a considerable emotional and financial burden. While some parents and caregivers declare the emotional return they experience from looking after these individuals, for others this responsibility is a source of continuing, unresolved, if attenuated, grief.

As for morbidity, the brain, as mentioned above, is the most vulnerable organ, and chromosomal defects are the basis of a substantial fraction of all intellectual deficit. Many of these affected individuals will also have structural malformations that cause functional physical disability. Among an intellectually disabled population, Down syndrome is the predominant contributor in the fraction who have a classic chromosome abnormality (Phelan et al. 1996). Development of the heart is particularly susceptible to chromosomal imbalance, and in a population study from the US National Center on Birth Defects, 1 in 8 infants with a congenital heart defect had a chromosomal abnormality with, again. trisomy 21 the most common of these (53%), followed by trisomy 18 (13%), 22q11.2 deletion (12%), and trisomy 13 (6%) (Hartman et al. 2011).

Table 1–3. The Population Prevalences of Some of the More Notable Deletions and Duplications, Derived from the Norwegian Mother, Father, and Child Cohort Study, 1999–2008

RECURRENT CNVs		DE NOVO CNVs		ALL CNVs	
Position (hg38)	**Del/Dup**	**N**	**Parental**	**N**	**Prevalence**
1:147,107,276-147,924,476	del1q21.1 distal	2	pat ×2	6	4.9
1:147,107,276-147,924,476	dup1q21.1 distal	0		4	3.26
3:196,033,055-197,619,681	del3q29	1	pat	1	0.82
3:196,033,055-197,619,681	dup3q29	0		0	0
7:73,331,825-74,731,095	del7q11.23 (Williams-Beuren)	0		0	0
7:73,331,825-74,731,095	dup7q11.23	0		0	0
15:23,123,715-28,325,372	del15q11.2-13.1 (Prader-Willi/Angelman)	0		0	0
15:23,123,715-28,325,372	del15q11.2-13.1	2	mat ×2	3	2.450
15:30,783,588-32,154,652	del15q13.3	1	pat	5	4.08
15:30,783,588-32,154,652	dup15q13.3	1	pat	6	4.9
16:28,811,768-29,035,413	del16p11.2 distal	1	mat	3	2.45
16:28,811,768-29,035,413	dup16p11.2 distal	2	mat	8	6.53
16:29,639,423-30,183,727	del16p11.2 proximal	4	mat ×3, pat	6	4.9
16:29,639,423-30,183,727	dup16p11.2 proximal	0		5	4.08
17:1,344,540-2,685,615	del17p13.3 (Miller-Dieker)	0		0	0
17:1,344,540-2,685,615	dup17p13.3	0		0	0
17:16,908,429-20,313,519	del17p11.2 (Smith-Magenis)	0		0	0
17:16,908,429-20,313,519	dup17p11.2 (Potocki-Lupski)	0		0	0
17:36,460,758-37,856,053	del17q12	3	mat, pat ×2	3	2.45
17:36,460,758-37,856,053	dup17q12	0		2	1.63
17:45,628,753-46,087,790	del17q21.31 (Koolen-deVries)	0	0		0
17:45,628,753-46,087,790	dup17q21.31	0	0		0
22:19,037,347-21,114,846	del22q11.2 (DiGeorge)	1	mat	1	0.82
22:19,037,347-21,114,846	dup22q11.2	2	mat, pat	6	4.9
22:21,566,197-23,310,015	del22q11.2 distal	0		0	0
22:21,566,197-23,310,015	dup22q11.2 distal	0		0	0
Total		20	16/10,000	59	48/10,000

Notes: The extents of the del/dups are shown in molecular detail, at the level of the nucleotide. “hg38” refers to Human Genome build, version 38, also referred to as GRCh38 (Genome Reference Consortium human build 38). Prevalences are per 10,000. The study was based upon a material of 12,252 newborns and their parents.

Eur J Hum Genet 29:205–215 2021.

The Research Application of Cytogenetic Pathology

The phenotypes that result from chromosome abnormalities can point the way to discovery of the causative genes. An early example of deletion mapping is the recognition that the gene for retinoblastoma was on chromosome 13, given the association of this cancer with the 13q− syndrome. Another cancer gene to be similarly mapped was *APC* (adenomatous polyposis coli), following the observation of polyposis of the colon in an individual with intellectual disability and del(5)(q22q23) (Hockey et al. 1989). The triple dose of chromosome 21 in Down syndrome (DS), and knowing that Alzheimer disease almost invariably affects DS persons aged 40 and older (Hithersay et al. 2019), was a signpost on the way to finding the β-amyloid precursor protein (*APP*) gene as one of the major Alzheimer loci; and the DS adult population may prove a valuable resource in the assessment of new dementia treatments (Rafii and Fortea 2023).

A translocation with one breakpoint at 7q11.23 was found to disrupt the elastin gene in a family segregating supravalvular aortic stenosis. Further investigation of this locus in Williams syndrome proved this to be the site of deletion in this condition (Nickerson et al. 1995). The gene for CHARGE[7] syndrome, *CHD7*, was discovered due to two patients with an 8q12 microdeletion (Vissers et al. 2004). David et al. (2023) studied two men presenting with infertility, of otherwise normal phenotype, in whom a balanced chromosome rearrangement had been identified: t(5;9)(q32;p21.1) and t(4;21)(p15.1;q22.3), respectively, leading them to propose *YIPF5* near the 5q32 breakpoint, and *SPATC1L* within 21q23 as candidates contributory to the control of spermatogenesis. We have conducted reviews of chromosomal conditions in which epilepsy and kidney disease are features, with the aim of providing leads to epilepsy genes and renal genes (Singh et al. 2002a; Amor et al. 2003).

> The precision of microarray analysis, coupled with access to genome databases, now allows a much finer focus in the pursuit of causative genes. Ou et al. (2008) proposed, and Ballesta-Martínez et al. (2013) supported, that one of the genes *SIX1, SIX6*, or *OTX2* might be the basis of one form of branchio-oto-renal syndrome, from their study of a child with a duplication of 14q22.3q23.3; *SIX1* was eventually revealed as the culprit gene. We have shown *WDR35* to be the gene for a short rib–polydactyly syndrome, having found a microdeletion on chromosome 2p24 by single nucleotide polymorphism (SNP) and copy number variant (CNV) analysis (Mill et al. 2011); and *RAB39B* was found to be the basis of a syndrome of early-onset Parkinson disease and intellectual disability, a 45 kb deletion at Xq28 leading us to this discovery (Wilson et al. 2014).

It is a general principle that many important scientific discoveries are made serendipitously—or, as Louis Pasteur put it, "chance favors the prepared mind" (*le hasard ne favorise que les esprits préparés*). Voullaire et al. (1993) identified a small supernumerary marker chromosome (sSMC) in a child with a nonspecific picture of physical abnormality and intellectual deficit, which had no C-band positive centromere

[7] CHARGE = coloboma, heart, choanal atresia, retardation, genital, ear.

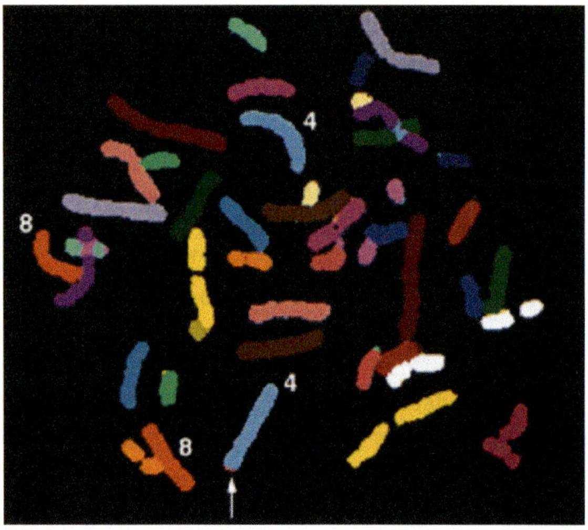

Figure 2–2. Spectral karyotyping.

Notes: Every chromosome is of a different color. Chromosome 4 stains light blue, and chromosome 8 is orange. In this example, a child with Wolf-Hirschhorn syndrome (p. 392) manifests a distal 4p deletion with a very small segment from chromosome 8, the orange tip only just discernible (arrowed), in its place, from the karyotype 46,XY,der(4)t(4,8).

Source: From T Ried et al., Chromosome painting: a useful art, *Hum Mol Genet* 7:1619–1626, 1998, with the permission of Oxford University Press.

known by computer analysis. Some commercial microarrays combine CGH and SNP detection on the same array.

> Not that classical cytogenetics is likely to fade altogether from view: There are two crucial reasons for its continuing use in the laboratory. First, not all array results can give a definitive construction, and FISH is sometimes necessary to elucidate the cytogenetics. Second, the array cannot detect balanced rearrangements,[1] and recognition of the carrier state will continue to need an old-fashioned chromosome test. And third, a rather subjective "reason" is that, by continuing to work with chromosomes, the molecular cytogeneticist/cytogenomicist will not lose the intuitive understanding of what chromosomes are really like, rather than seeing them merely as theoretical constructs or computer-screen displays. As mentioned above, the reporting of microarray results is a sophisticated exercise, and counselors need to be sophisticated readers of these reports. Many laboratories now use depictions from one of the genome browsers—with a classic chromosome ideogram laying on its side at the top—to illustrate the precise extent of the imbalance, and noting the genes contained within this segment.

Comparative Genomic Hybridization

The fundamental principle is essentially the same as in chromosomal CGH, noted above, but using the array, rather than the metaphase spread, as substrate. Patient and

[1] Albeit that whole genome sequencing is being used to address this shortcoming (Ordulu et al. 2016; Redin et al. 2017).

control DNA are labeled in two different fluorophores, usually one that appears red and one that appears green. These labeled DNAs are applied to the microarray, and hybridization takes place. Typically, if the number of copies between the control and the patient are the same, the spot looks yellow (produced from an overlapping of equal amounts of red and green). The fluorescent intensities of each dye are measured. If the patient has an excess at a locus (due to duplication or aneuploidy), the hybridization will more reflect the dye of the patient's DNA. If the patient has a deficiency at a locus (loss due to deletion or unbalanced translocation), the hybridization will more reflect the dye of the control DNA (see the cover art of this book).

Single Nucleotide Polymorphism (SNP) Array

SNP arrays detect the number of alleles in a specimen (Figure 2–3) and provide two types of information. First, the intensity of the signal arising from each SNP can be measured to produce a $\log_2$ ratio: A relative increase in signal intensity corresponds to copy number gain, and a decrease in signal intensity corresponds to deletion. Second, SNP arrays produce genotyping information: Heterozygosity, with two distinct alleles, can be distinguished from homozygosity, and from the presence of three alleles. Apparent homozygosity may indicate a loss of DNA, such as a deletion, while three alleles may indicate a gain of DNA copy number, such as a duplication or trisomy. SNP-based microarrays have the added advantage of detecting uniparental disomy when the

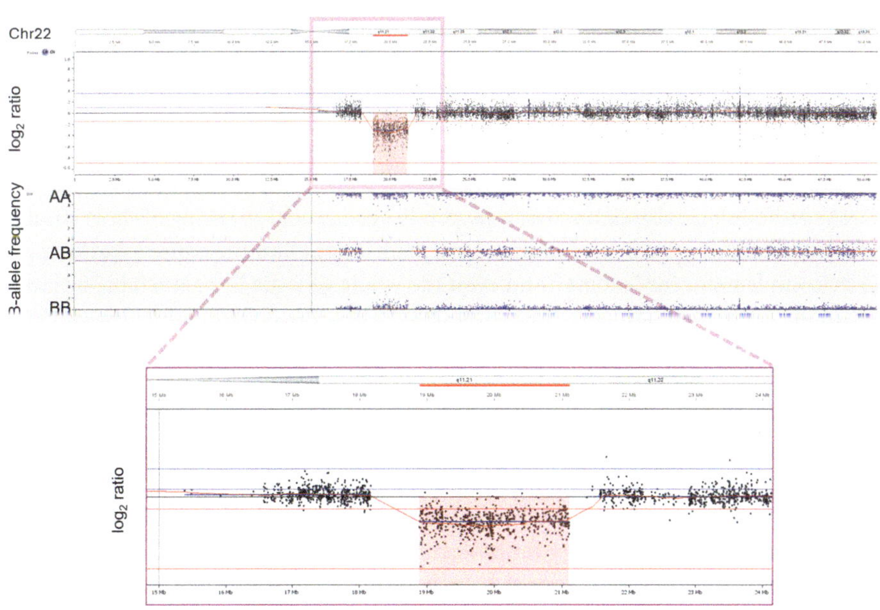

Figure 2–3. SNP-based Microarray.

Notes: Plot of chromosome 22 in a patient with a 22q11 deletion, using a SNP-based microarray that combines copy number ($\log_2$ ratio) and genotyping (B-allele frequency, blue dots) data. The copy number is reduced to a single copy in the region of the deletion, shown by the deviation of the $\log_2$ ratio (black dots) towards minus 1. The genotyping plot (blue dots) demonstrates an absence of A/B heterozygous probes in the deleted region, showing only hemizygosity for the A or B alleles, thus also allowing inference of a deletion (indicated by pink shaded region). Courtesy DI Francis.

versus causative genomic changes. A pedantic but important point is that the genome "build" be noted.

GENETIC COUNSELING CONSIDERATIONS

Mostly, the abnormalities found by molecular technologies have clear clinical relevance for the patient and the family. However, higher resolution strategies may uncover DNA changes of unclear clinical significance (as we discuss at length in Chapter 18). Such findings may lead to testing of additional family members, parents, grandparents, and sometimes siblings, to understand the relationship, if any, between the DNA alteration and the clinical phenotype or medical condition of the patient. The possibility of findings of unclear clinical significance should be discussed when ordering the test, especially in the prenatal setting. Because these molecular-based tests have the ability to interrogate the entire genome, the pretest genetic counseling should include information about uncovering unwanted information, such as loci that could predispose to cancer, or to adult-onset disorders. The use of SNP arrays may uncover substantial stretches of homozygosity due to consanguineous or even incestuous relationships (Schaaf et al. 2011). These counseling caveats notwithstanding, the higher resolution potential of these new technologies will increase the detection rate of chromosome abnormalities, and will much improve our ability to make diagnoses, and to provide the answers that families seek. The counselor need not be expert in the nature of the technologies outlined above, but should have a broad understanding of the different applications and of what each can, or cannot, offer in the clinical setting.

3

THE ORIGINS AND CONSEQUENCES OF CHROMOSOME PATHOLOGY

"WHAT WENT WRONG? And might it happen again?" These are the common questions from "chromosomal families" that bring people to the genetic clinic. We can recast these questions: "Did I, or one of us, produce an abnormal gamete? If so, why? What gamete might be produced next time? Or, if the chromosomes were normal at conception, what went wrong thereafter?" To deal intelligently with these questions, the counselor needs a broad knowledge of how gametes form, how chromosomes behave, and how the early conceptus grows.

The *classic chromosome disorders* are the full aneuploidies and the partial aneuploidies. These partial aneuploidies are of sufficient size (albeit some have been called "microdeletions" and "microduplications"[1]) that they are detectable on 20th-century microscope cytogenetics; the phenotypes are practically always abnormal. In 21st-century molecular karyotyping, the challenge arises of dealing with very small imbalances (*microdeletions, microduplications, copy number variants*), which may not always lead to overt clinical abnormality. *Mosaicism* has been recognized since the earliest days of clinical chromosomology; more recently, the concepts of *incomplete penetrance* and polygenic (or at least oligogenic) inheritance have become of practical relevance. Finally, *errors of imprinting* contribute a small fraction to the whole.

The broadening scope of medical cytogenetics—some now say medical cytogenomics—following advances in molecular methodologies has led to the distinction between chromosomal and other genetic causes of disease, formerly so clear-cut, now being somewhat blurred at the margins. One practical definition of a chromosomal disorder might have been based on the methodology used for diagnosis—that is, any condition typically diagnosed by classical cytogenetics or by microarray. But with next generation sequencing (NGS) that distinction would fail: NGS can be widely applied, diagnostically, to the generality of genetic disease. "Genomic imbalance" may be a more suitable, and a more fundamental, definition: too much, or too little, chromosome material. Even so, the line cannot be drawn with absolute clarity between chromosomal and Mendelian disease. A Mendelian condition may be due to a duplication (e.g., Charcot-Marie-Tooth neuropathy,

[1] For the most part, we confine our use of the expressions "microdeletion" and "microduplication" to those pathogenic imbalances detectable only on molecular karyotyping, and to which the expression "pathogenic copy number variant" is also often applied. The word *microdeletion* had been applied to some conditions of the classical cytogenetic era, such as Prader-Willi syndrome and Smith-Magenis syndrome; these certainly were, by the standards of the day (the 1980s), very small deletions, and only just visible to very experienced microscopists. However, by molecular criteria they would now be seen as rather large, of megabase size, whereas several of the pathogenic microdeletions and microduplications of molecular karyotyping are measured in kilobases.

Chapter 14) or to a deletion of a gene (e.g., Pitt-Hopkins syndrome, Chapter 14), and thus diagnosable on cytogenomic technology. The analysis of copy number variants (CNVs)—short segments of genomic material in excess or deficiency—is generally regarded as a chromosomal exercise. We will largely confine ourselves (Chapter 18) to those CNVs which are known to be pathogenic; but there is also blurring, here, in terms of CNVs, whose harmlessness (or not) is uncertain.

We focus first upon the classic chromosomal disorders. Most of these arise at meiosis. A gamete from a 46,N person may acquire an extra (but normal) chromosome, and this would lead to a *full aneuploidy* in a conceptus of theirs: a trisomy. Or, *partial aneuploidy* may be due to meiotic malsegregation having taken place in gametogenesis of a 46,rea (rea = rearrangement) parent carrying a balanced rearrangement. De novo ("of new"; that is, with normal parental karyotypes) partial aneuploidies may have been generated at a meiotic division, or at a premeiotic germ cell mitosis; where there is normal/aneuploid mosaicism, a postmeiotic event in the embryo is implicated. While it may not be possible to presume with reasonable confidence where the original error lay, a theoretical consideration of the point at which a chromosomal defect arose—before, during, or after meiosis—can underpin a useful understanding. It thus behooves us to appreciate the broad processes of meiotic and mitotic cell divisions.

MEIOSIS

Meiosis in Chromosomally Normal Persons

The purpose of meiosis is to achieve the reduction from the diploid state of the primary gametocyte ($2n = 46$) to the haploid complement of the normal gamete ($n = 23$); and to ensure genetic variation in the gametes. The latter requirement is met by enabling the independent assortment of homologs (the physical basis of Mendel's second law)[2] and by providing a setting for recombination between homologs. While we do not dwell on recombination per se, this is, to the classical geneticist, a raison d'être of the chromosome: "From the long perspective of evolution, a chromosome is a bird of passage, a temporary association of particular alleles" (Lewin 1994).

The mature gamete is produced after the two meiotic cell divisions: meiosis I and meiosis II, the cells going through stages of oögonium/spermatogonium → primary gametocyte → secondary gametocyte → mature gamete (or polar body).

As per the *classical description* (Figure 3–1), the chromosomes of the (diploid) primary gametocyte entering *meiosis I* do not divide at the centromere, and they remain, following cell division into secondary gametocytes, as double-chromatid chromosomes. With only one of each homolog, the cell is in the haploid state. In *meiosis II*, the chromosomes of the secondary gametocytes separate into their component single chromatids, and this cell division gives rise to the (haploid) gametes. In the male, the cells produced from one primary gametocyte are the four spermatids, which mature into spermatozoa. In the female, the cells are the mature ovum and its polar bodies. (In fact,

[2] The law of independent assortment: During gamete formation, the segregation of the alleles of one allelic pair is independent of the segregation of the alleles of another allelic pair. The exception: If two loci are close together—"linked"—on the same chromosome.

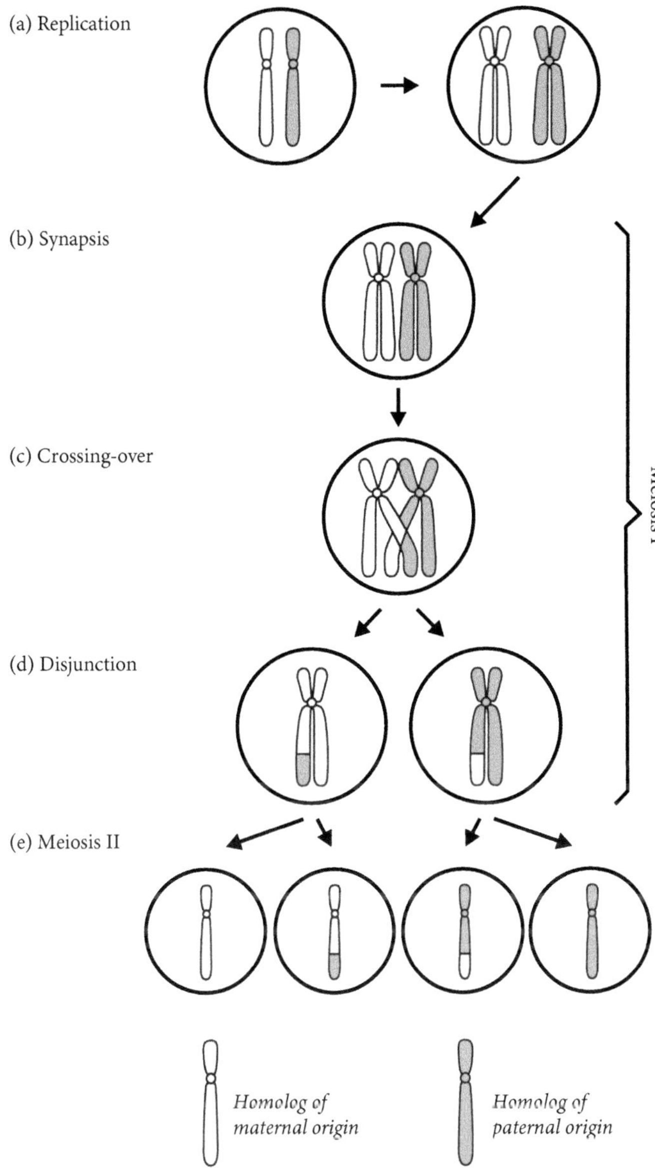

Figure 3–1. Meiosis I.
Chromosomal behavior during meiosis I, according to the classical model. Circles represent germ cells: at (*a*) oögonia and spermatogonia (gonocytes); at (*b–d*) primary oöcytes and spermatocytes (gametocytes); and at (*e*) secondary oöcytes and spermatocytes. One crossover has occurred between the long arms of one chromatid of each homolog. Following meiosis I, the chromosome number has halved (reduction division). In oögenesis, one of the two cells at (*d*) would be the first polar body, and would typically not enter meiosis II.

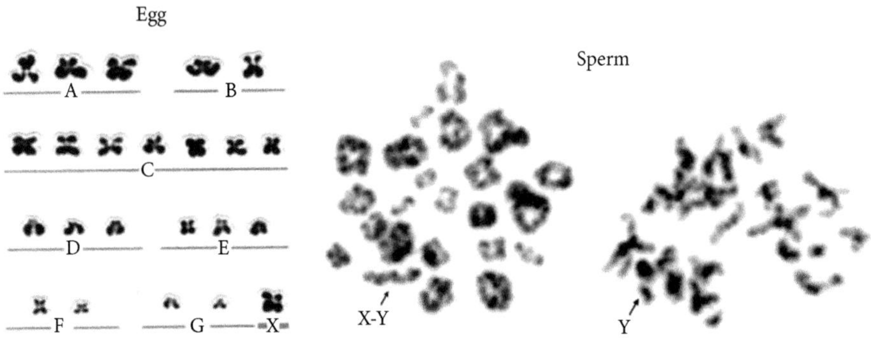

Figure 3–2. The Chromosomes in Human Gametes.

Notes: The karyotype from a 23,X egg (*left*), showing the haploid set of double-chromatid chromosomes following the completion of the reduction division of meiosis I (cf. Figure 3–1d). The chromosome spread (*center*) from a 46.XY spermatocyte, the homologs having come together as bivalents in mid-meiosis I (cf. Figure 3–1b,c). The autosomal bivalents have their homologous segments aligned, whereas the X-Y bivalent aligns only at the tips of Xp and Yp. The single-chromatid chromosomes of a 23,Y sperm (*right*) at meiosis II (cf. Figure 3–1e).

Sources: From O Samura et al., Sperm and oocyte chromosomal abnormalities, *Biomolecules* 13:1010, 2023; and L Uroz and C Templado, Meiotic non-disjunction mechanisms in human fertile males, *Hum Reprod* 27:1518–1524, 2012. Courtesy O Samura, and with the permission of MDPI; and courtesy L Uroz and C Templado, and with the permission of the European Society of Human Reproduction and Embryology and Oxford University Press.

it is not until sperm penetration that meiosis II in the ovum is completed.) Figure 3-2 shows the appearances of the chromosomes at these different stages of meiosis.

Each gamete thus contains a haploid set of chromosomes. The diploid complement is restored at conception, with the union of two haploid gametes. The moment of conception, as the embryologist sees it, is not at sperm penetration but only when the two pronuclei have fused to form a single nucleus ("syngamy").

Note that spermatogenesis divides the cytoplasm evenly, so that after meiosis II there are four gametes of equal size. The sperm head that penetrates the ovum comprises almost entirely nuclear material; the tail is cast off. In oöcytes, cytoplasmic division is markedly uneven, producing a secondary oöcyte and first polar body after meiosis I, and the mature ovum and second polar body at meiosis II.[3] The ovum and the polar bodies each have a haploid chromosome set, but the ovum retains almost all of the cytoplasm.[4]

Another major sex difference concerns the timing of gamete maturation. In the female, meiosis is partway through, in the late prophase of meiosis I, by the eighth month of intrauterine life (the actual process of recombination taking place during weeks 16–19 of fetal life). At birth, a female baby has around a third of a million oöcytes (Figure 20–30). Most of this pool is gradually lost, but those eggs destined to mature stay in a "frame-freeze" until they enter ovulation some one to five decades thereafter,[5] and meiosis recommences. Testicular stem cells (spermatogonia), on the other hand,

[3] The first polar body does not normally undergo (a biologically pointless) meiosis II.

[4] Cytoplasm contains the mitochondria, and transmission of mitochondrial DNA is maternal. The mitochondrial genome has been described, somewhat whimsically, as chromosome 25, or the M chromosome. In not otherwise referring to this "chromosome" we are not seeking to deny its importance or interest!

[5] As Eichenlaub-Ritter (2012) points out, oöcytes are one of the longest-lived cells in the body.

do not begin to enter meiosis until the onset of puberty. Thereafter, millions of mature sperm are continuously produced.

Meiosis in Detail. We now examine more closely the details of meiosis, according to the classical model. During the final mitotic division in the primary gametocyte, the homologous pairs of chromosomes have (as with any mitosis) replicated their DNA to change from the single-chromatid to the double-chromatid stage. They now enter into the meiotic cell cycle (Figure 3–1a). As meiosis I proceeds to prophase, chromosomes conduct a "homology search" and come together and pair, with matching loci alongside each other (Figure 3–1b). This process—*synapsis*—continues with a more intimate pairing of the homologs, starting at the tips of the chromosomes and proceeding centrally, and the synaptonemal complex is formed (Barlow and Hultén, 1996). The paired chromosomes themselves are called *bivalents*.[6] Synapsis sets the stage for an exchange of matching chromosome segments; this is the process of *recombination*, or *crossing-over* (Figure 3–1c). Next, desynapsis occurs (the diplotene stage), with dissociation of the synaptonemal complex and the formation of chiasmata.

Now, the two homologous chromosomes *disjoin* and go to opposite poles of the cell. This is the anaphase stage; the orderly movement of chromosomes during this sequence is facilitated if synapsis, recombination, and chiasmata formation have proceeded normally. Finally, the cell divides into the two daughter cells (Figure 3–1d). How the chromosomes are distributed—which chromosome goes to which pole—is called *segregation*. Normally, each daughter cell gets one of each of the pair of chromosomes, and this is referred to as one-to-one (1:1) segregation. Uniquely in the meiosis I cell division daughter cells are produced with double-chromatid chromosomes.

These gametocytes then enter meiosis II (with the exception of the first polar body). In this cycle, the chromosomes do not replicate because they are already in the double-chromatid state. The chromosomes separate at the centromere, and the resulting single-chromatid chromosomes disjoin, one going to each pole, resembling a mitotic division (Figure 3–1e).

The foregoing, classical construction held sway since practically the beginning of human cytogenetics, and it remains very useful conceptually; but its primacy has since been challenged. One alternative description puts the events of meiosis I and II in the reverse order: That is, the chromosomes separate into chromatids at meiosis I and then segregate into daughter cells at meiosis II (Figure 3–3). This has been called *reverse segregation* (Ottolini et al. 2015; Webster and Schuh 2017).

The other, very important, retelling of the events of meiosis is *premature separation of sister chromatids* (PSSC). This is, in fact, the predominant mechanism in the female, and is important in the male (Ottolini et al. 2015; Sakakibara et al. 2015). It refers to the "precocious" separation of chromatids during meiosis I, as initially proposed by Angell (1997), and involves three sequential events (Figure 3–4). First, the (double-chromatid) homologs fail to pair during meiosis I; or, if they do pair, they separate again before meiosis I is complete. In other words, instead of the two (double-chromatid) chromosomes existing as a conjoined bivalent, they exist as two separate univalents. Second, these univalents are prone to "predivide"—that is, the separation of the two chromatids that should (on the classical plan) happen

6 Since, at the level of the chromatid, the bivalent pair contains four elements, the word *tetrad* can also be used in this setting; in this sense, the cell at this stage of the cycle has $23 \times 4 = 92$ chromatids.

Malsegregation and Nondisjunction in Meiosis

Malsegregation (or missegregation) is remarkably frequent at meiosis, and in consequence many human conceptions are trisomic or monosomic. Malsegregation is a "catch-all" term; in principle, nondisjunction specifically refers to the failure of homologous chromosomes to segregate symmetrically at cell division, although in practice it is often considered (and we sometimes do) as "the inclusion of both daughter chromosomes in the same nucleus, by whatever mechanism" (Miller and Therman 2001).

The process of malsegregation is described according to two models: the classical description of nondisjunction (Figure 3–5), and a modern description based upon the PSSC model as described above. While the classical model has long been seen as the typical process, in fact, as Gabriel et al. (2011) write, "it appears to be a relatively minor player" and "the received wisdom that non-disjunction [sensu stricto] is the primary mechanism leading to human aneuploidy should be reconsidered." Nevertheless, and taking a conservative viewpoint,[7] we first set out in detail the model that has appeared in textbooks for generations, but then pay due attention to the more recent knowledge.

The *classical description* of the mechanism of meiotic nondisjunction is as follows: In a chromosomally normal person, if the pair of homologs comprising a bivalent at meiosis I fail to separate (fail to disjoin[8]), one daughter cell will have two of the chromosomes, and the other will have none. This is 2:0 segregation (Figures 3–5 and 3–6, upper). In other words, one gametocyte is disomic for that homolog, and the other is nullisomic. Or, nondisjunction may occur in meiosis II, meiosis I having proceeded normally. In meiosis II, it is the chromatids that fail to separate (Figure 3–5b). Following these nondisjunctional errors, the conceptus, at fertilization, ends up trisomic or monosomic, assuming the other gamete to be normal (Figure 3–7a, b). Trisomy or monosomy in the offspring of normal parents is called primary trisomy or primary monosomy.

Concerning meiotic malsegregation following the alternative *premature separation of sister chromatids* scenario Figure 3–4 sets out the picture. As the oögonium and spermatogonium enter meiosis, one double-chromatid homolog "pre-divides" and now consists of a pair of single-chromatid chromosomes. If these chromosomes were then to segregate symmetrically, at meiosis I, the primary gametocytes resulting would have a balanced constitution; but if it is asymmetric—as in the example in Figure 3–4—one gametocyte has an extra chromatid, while the other has only one. As meiosis II proceeds, giving rise to the secondary gametocytes, it transpires that two are normal haploid, one is diploid, and one "nulliploid." The oöcyte in Figure 3–6 (lower) may be an example of asymmetric segregation due to this process, having received a double-chromatid and a single-chromatid chromosome 21.[9] Polar body and embryo studies in the IVF laboratory suggest that, at least at an older maternal age, half of all aneuploidy in the oöcyte results from meiosis I,[10] about a third from meiosis II and a small fraction from meiosis I nondisjunction (Verdyck et al. 2023).

[7] "Be not the first by whom the new are tried, Nor yet the last to lay the old aside." Alexander Pope, *An Essay on Criticism*, 1711.

[8] Note that disjunction is a normal process, and nondisjunction is not; there is no such word as *dysjunction*.

[9] Certain terminologies and nomenclature may be mentioned here. A gamete with an extra chromosome is *hyperhaploid*, with a karyotype written as, for example, 24,X,+21. A gamete missing a chromosome is *hypohaploid* (e.g., 22,Y,–21). If, at meiosis I, the extra chromosome is present only as a single chromatid (e.g., the asterisked oöcyte in Figure 3–4), the abbreviation cht (for chromatid) is used: thus, 24,X,+21cht. The ISCN (2024) provides nomenclature for meiotic cells, and an extra 21 at meiosis I, present as a univalent, would be denoted as MI,24,+I(21).

[10] This category may also have included examples of reverse segregation.

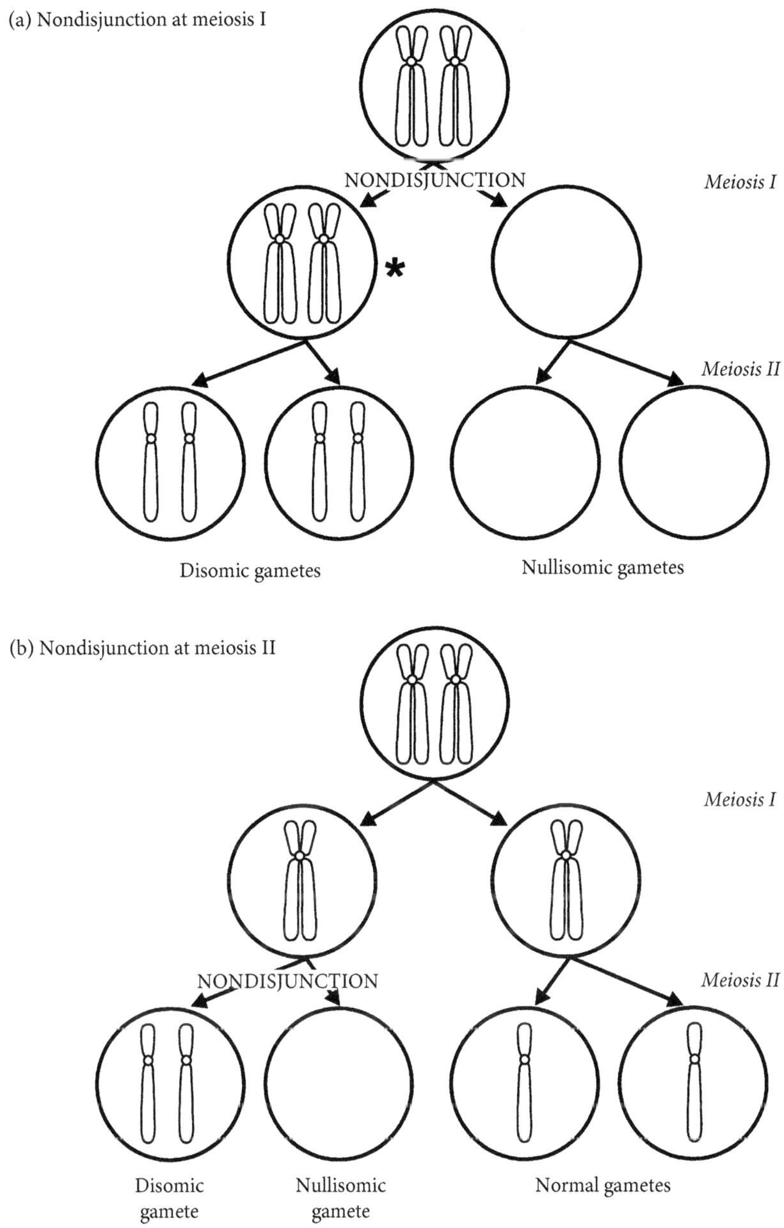

Figure 3–5. The classical view of the mechanics of nondisjunction. The asterisked gamete reflects the complement of the oöcyte in Fig. 3–6 (*upper*), with respect to one of the G-group chromosomes. In oögenesis, one of the two cells following meiosis I would be the first polar body, which typically does not proceed to meiosis II.

A process somewhat intermediate between these two major mechanisms is *achiasmate nondisjunction*, in which the homologs had never joined and then segregate together to the same daughter cell. The end result is the same as if classical nondisjunction had occurred, but without any recombination (Uroz and Templado 2012).

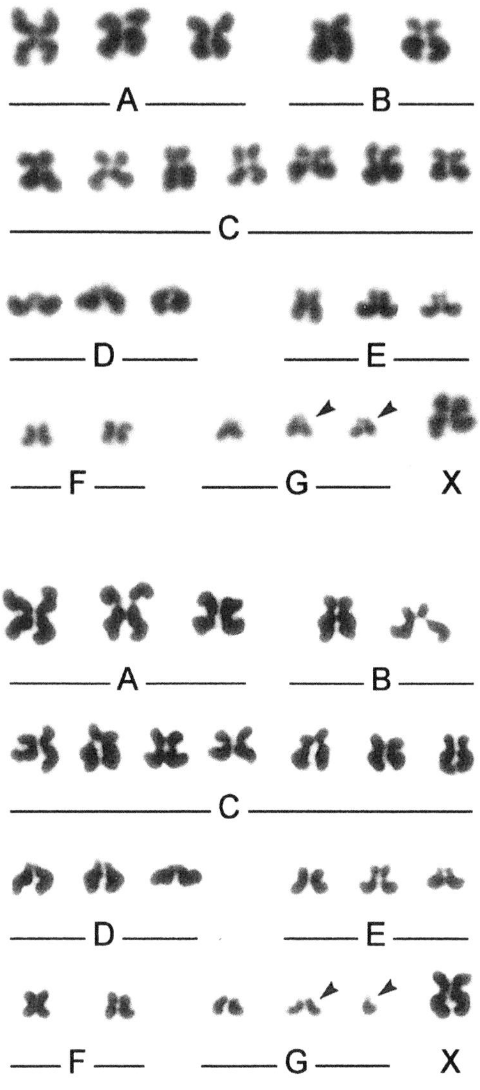

Figure 3–6. Oöcyte chromosomes at metaphase of meiosis II, showing nondisjunction of a G-group chromosome having occurred at the preceding first meiotic division. *Upper*, oöcyte with classical nondisjunctional disomy, showing an additional G-group double-chromatid chromosome. Possibly the arrowed pair are chromosome 21s, and the karyotype 24,X,+21. *Lower*, oöcyte with "predivisional" disomy, showing an additional G-group single chromatid. The arrowed pair may be chromosome 21s, and the karyotype 24,X,+21cht.
Source: From Kamiguchi et al. Chromosomal analysis of unfertilized human oocytes prepared by a gradual fixation-air drying method, *Hum Genet* 90:533–541, 1993. Courtesy Y Kamiguchi.

Figure 3–8 summarizes these several scenarios, with particular reference to the more vulnerable gamete, which is to say, the egg.

Frequencies of Meiotic Malsegregation

The very considerable majority of human aneuploidy due to meiotic malsegregation, takes place during *oögenesis.* Remarkably high fractions of mature oöcytes are

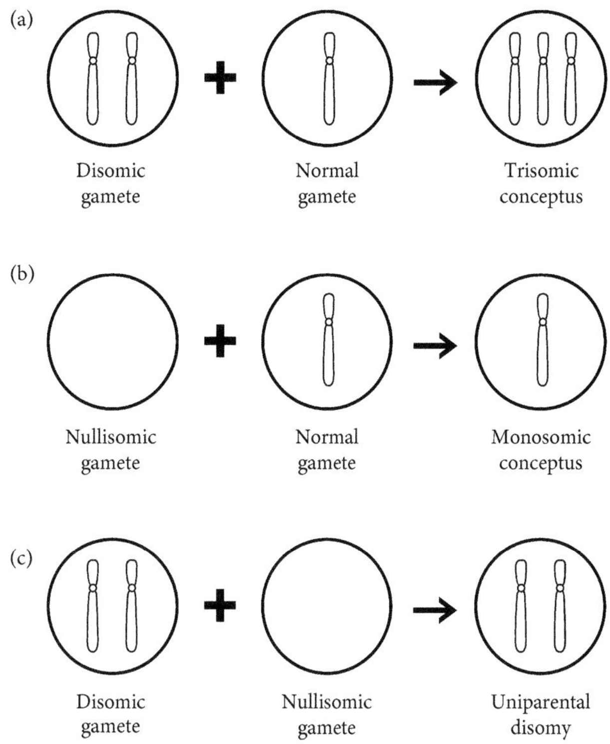

Figure 3–7. Aneuploid gametes producing an aneuploid conceptus (*a* and *b*), and aneuploid gametes producing uniparental disomy (*c*).

aneuploid, at least as measured in a population of women presenting to an in vitro fertilization (IVF) clinic (Figure 3–9). In women aged 28–37 years, nearly half of eggs are disomic or nullisomic, whereas in 38- to 47-year-olds the figure rises to three-quarters (Fragouli et al. 2013). In a different population—women from teenage to mid-30s presenting for cryopreservation of eggs due to a diagnosis of cancer, and otherwise perhaps more representative, of the general population—Nikiforov et al. (2020) determined a rather smaller fraction, one-third of oöcytes at the second meiotic division being aneuploid.

If we look at the immediate downstream consequence of these abnormalities, which is to say, the picture in preimplantation embryos at day 3 to 4, again we see a very striking maternal age effect, aneuploidy rates ranging from about 10% to 70% from ages 20s through early 40s (Figure 3–10). By day 5—that is, at the appearance of the blastocyst—aneuploidy figures have reduced somewhat, likely reflecting lethality due to the most severe aneuploidies, and range from about a quarter (maternal age under 35) to a half (over age 35) from IVF data (Kubicek et al. 2019). The maternal basis of aneuploidy is again very apparent, with only minor contributions from paternal meiotic error or postmeiotic mitotic error (Figure 3–11).

Certain aneuploidies show predilections for one or other meiotic stage. For example, essentially all trisomy 16 may be due to a maternal meiosis I error, whereas most trisomy 18 reflects meiotic II malsegregation. In those aneuploidies which are capable of carrying on through to birth, it is the classic trisomies of chromosomes 21, 18, 13, and of the sex chromosomes, which have a strong advanced maternal age association, but not triploidy and monosomy X (Elmerdahl Frederiksen et al. 2023).

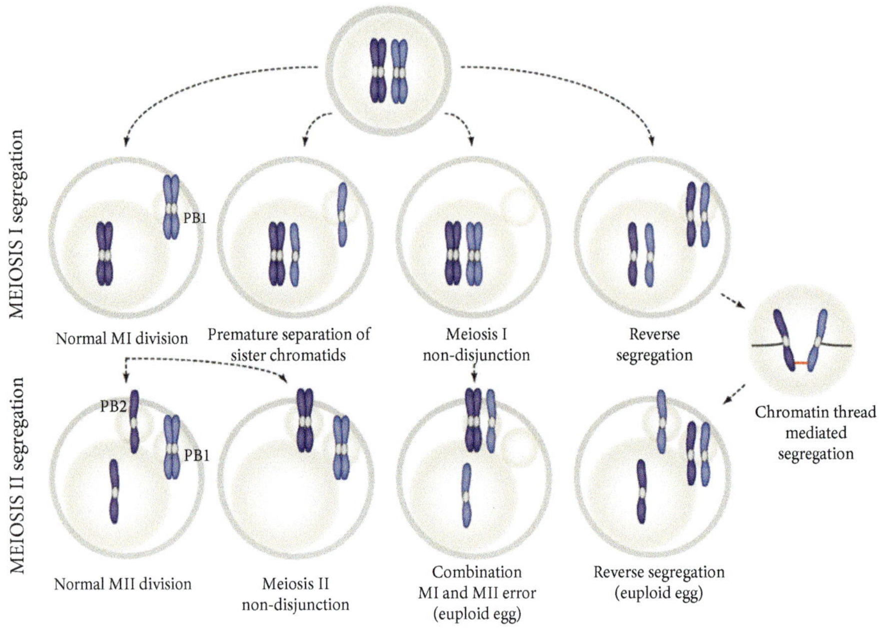

Figure 3–8. Different Ways in which Meiotic Error may Happen in the Egg.

Notes: Some errors at meiosis I can be corrected at meiosis II, resulting in the egg being euploid. In the case of reverse segregation, this correction may be mediated by chromatin threads.

Source: From L Wartosch et al., Origins and mechanisms leading to aneuploidy in human eggs, *Prenat Diagn* 41:620–630, 2021. Courtesy ER Hoffmann, and with the permission of John Wiley and Sons.

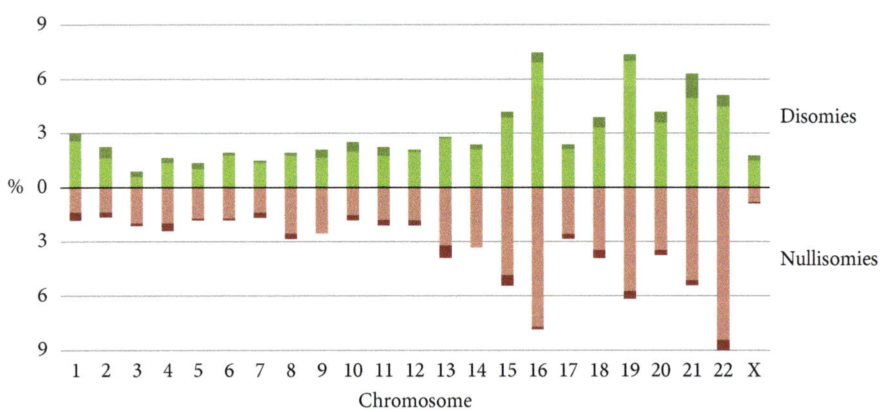

Figure 3–9. Aneuploidies in Oöcytes of Women of Ages 36–40.

Note: Disomies per chromosome are shown above the 0% baseline, nullisomies below These findings are based on inferences from the analysis of the first and second polar bodies in 676 oöcytes, from women undergoing PGT-A. The mirror-like appearance, above and below the line, reflects the agency of meiotic error, with essentially equal likelihoods of the missegregating chromosome going to the egg (for disomy), or to the polar body (for nullisomy); the similar observation of equal numbers of disomies and nullisomies in seen in Oberle et al. (2024). Light green = chromatid gain, darker green = 2-chromatid chromosome gain; Light red = chromatid loss, darker red = 2-chromatid chromosome loss.

Source: Adapted from P Verdyck et al., Aneuploidy in oocytes from women of advanced maternal age: analysis of the causal meiotic errors and impact on embryo development, *Hum Reprod* 38:2526–2535, 2023. Courtesy P Verdyck, and with the permission of Oxford University Press.

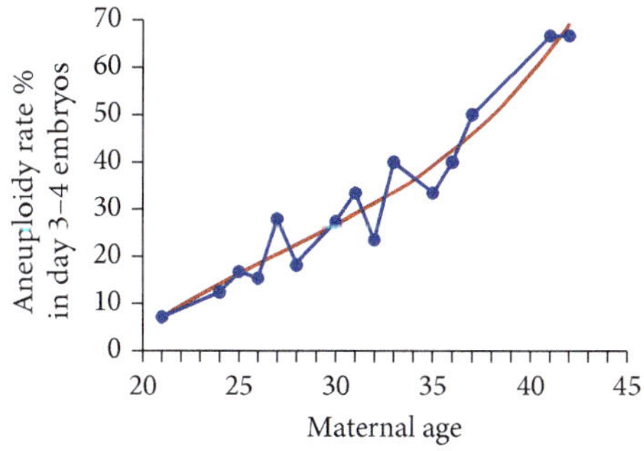

Figure 3–10. Aneuploidy Rates in Day 3 to 4 Embryos.

Note: These data were derived from material at day 3 to 4 (the morula stage), through different maternal ages, in patients from an IVF clinic. Observe the near straight-line upward slope of the smoothed data (in red) of the graph, attesting to the strong correlation of aneuploidy of the embryo cf. maternal age.

Source: From J Li et al., Chromosome aneuploidy analysis in embryos derived from in vivo and in vitro matured human oocytes, *J Transl Med* 19:416, 2021. Courtesy Y Xu, and with the permission of Springer Nature.

Spermatogenesis makes very little contribution to meiosis-based aneuploidy (Dviri et al. 2021; Ivanova and Semenova 2023); a reason may be the existence of a postmeiotic checkpoint excluding most aneuploid spermatozoa from full maturation (Uroz and Templado 2012). Figure 3–12 sets out the range of abnormality in a very large sample; the comparison with oöcytes (Figure 3–9), in terms of overall fractions, comparing the scales of the *y* axes, is notable.

Given the frequency with which nondisjunction happens, it is not at all surprising that instances of *multiple aneuploidy* are known, the observed numbers during stages of pregnancy reducing as nonviability takes its toll. In spontaneous abortions toward the end of the first trimester, double autosomal combinations, from simultaneous nondisjunctions, may be seen in the analysis of products of conception

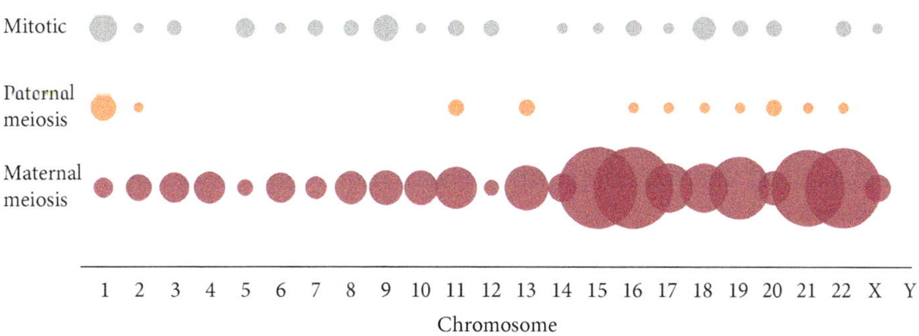

Figure 3–11. Aneuploidies in Day 5 to 6 Blastocysts.

Note: This is a display of the relative frequencies of the different origins, in day 5-6 blastocysts, of uniform (non-mosaic) aneuploidies of the different chromosomes. Maternal meiotic error is very much the predominant, with only very small contributions due to paternal meiotic error, or from mitotic error in the conceptus. These maternal meiotic data closely resemble the similar data in Figure 20–12. The data are from an analysis of SNP genotyping from 2,277 trophectoderm biopsies, of which 29% were aneuploid, from women of a wide maternal age range.

Source: From B Rana et al., Identifying parental and cell-division origins of aneuploidy in the human blastocyst, *Am J Hum Genet* 110:565–574, 2023. Courtesy NR Treff, and with the permission of Cell Press.

(a)

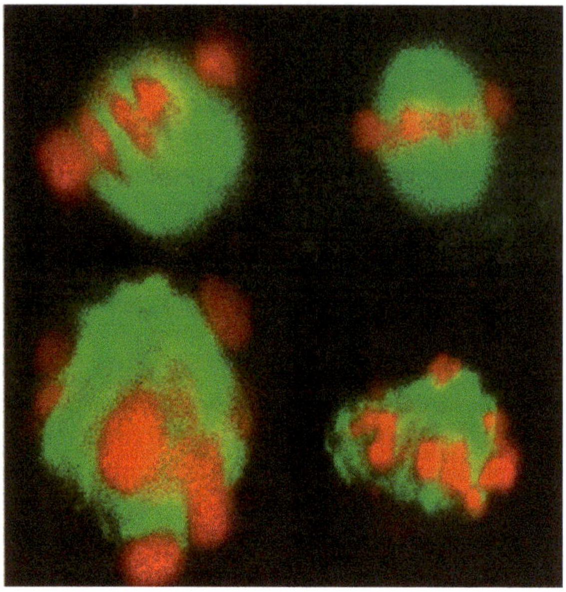

(b)

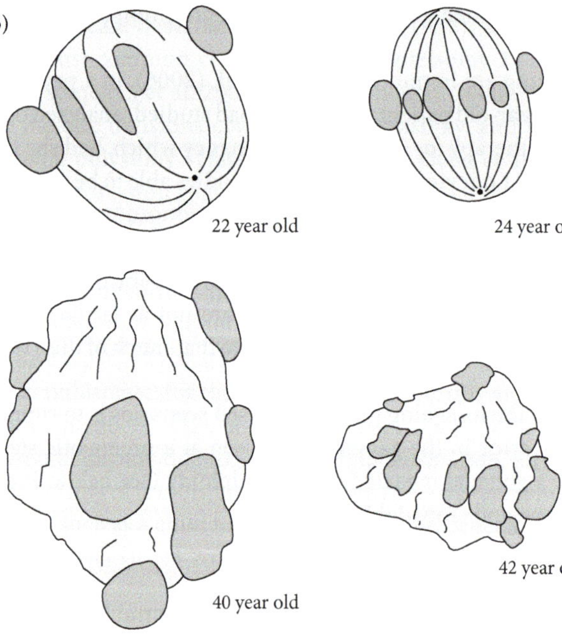

Figure 3–13. Oöcytes in Younger and Older Women.

Notes: The disposition of the chromosomes at meiosis II in the oöcytes from younger and older women is shown, illustrating what may be the physical basis of the maternal age effect. Meiosis II oöcytes (*a*) from younger and older women, illustrating what may be the physical basis of the maternal age effect. The microtubules of the spindle stain green, and the chromosomes stain orange. The tracing (*b*) identifies these components, and the smooth or wavy lines suggest, respectively, an intact or a degenerating spindle apparatus (the ages of the women indicated). The chromosomes are well organized at the metaphase plate at the equator of the cells in the younger women (the 22-year-old's oöcyte, on the upper left, is viewed on a tilt). In contrast, the 40-year-old's oöcyte shows the chromosomes in disarray. The 42-year-old woman's oöcyte has one chromosome, at the top, dislocated from the metaphase plate, and the disposition of the other chromosomes at the equator is not as regular as in the younger women.

Source: From Battaglia et al., Influence of maternal age on meiotic spindle assembly in oöcytes from naturally cycling women, *Hum Reprod* 11: 2217–2222, 1996. Courtesy DE Battaglia, and with the permission of the European Society of Human Reproduction and Embryology and Oxford University Press.

will deal in detail with each situation in separate chapters, but we consider the broad principles here.

BALANCED CARRIERS OF CLASSIC STRUCTURAL REARRANGEMENTS

In heterozygotes for some balanced rearrangements involving only small segments, the chromosomes may "ignore" the nonhomologous material they contain, and pair (this is *heterosynapsis*) and segregate, much as would happen at a normal meiosis. In other balanced rearrangements, the inherent tendency to pairing dictates that homologous segments of rearranged chromosomes will align, as well as they are able, in order to achieve full pairing (*homosynapsis*). This may require the chromosome to be something of a contortionist, forming complex configurations such as multivalents and reversed loops. According to either scenario, the stage is set for the possibility of unbalanced segregation.

The gametes produced—and therefore the conceptuses that arise—are frequently imbalanced. In this context, a segmental aneuploidy is usually involved—that is, a part of a chromosome is present in the trisomic or monosomic state; or, quite frequently, a combination of trisomy for one segment and monosomy for another. Partial trisomy and partial monosomy are also referred to as *duplication* and *deletion*, respectively.

In some rearrangements, recombination presents a further hazard. Inversions and insertions may produce a new recombinant (*rec*) chromosome that has a different genetic composition from that of the original rearrangement. A conceptus forming from a gamete containing it would inevitably be genetically unbalanced.

CARRIERS OF COPY NUMBER VARIANTS

These imbalances, typically detectable only on molecular karyotyping, are small relative to chromosome length, mostly of kilobase size. CNVs are not known to interfere with normal cell division; thus, meiosis is typically symmetric, 1:1—an even probability of transmitting the abnormal chromosome (although the resultant phenotype is far less predictable). These microdeletions and microduplications are to be distinguished, in practice, from the partial aneuploidies (deletions and duplications) of classical cytogenetics noted above.

FULL AND PARTIALLY ANEUPLOID INDIVIDUALS

In the individual who him- or herself has a full aneuploidy and in whom gametogenesis is able to proceed, in theory a trivalent may form, or a bivalent and an "independent" univalent. Either could lead, effectively, to a 2:1 segregation. This appears actually to be the case in trisomy 21, whereas in sex chromosomal states (XXX, XXY, and XYY) the "third" chromosome is, as it were, disposed of, and most gametes are normal. In the person with a classic partial aneuploidy due to an unbalanced rearranged chromosome, whether 46,(abn) or 47,+(abn), the abnormal chromosome may have an even (or near-even) chance to be transmitted in the gamete.

Nondisjunction in Mitosis and the Generation of Mosaicism

The purpose of a mitotic cell division is faithfully to pass on an intact and complete and balanced copy of the parental cellular genome to the progeny cells. An error in this process can lead to an aneuploid cell. If the error occurs in a mitosis during gametogenesis, mosaicism of the gonad is the consequence, and this is a *premeiotic mitotic error.* An error in early embryogenesis, perhaps as early as the very first mitosis after conception, can lead to a constitutional mosaicism of the embryo, typically comprising a mix of normal and aneuploid cells. This is a *postmeiotic mitotic error.* An early error typically leads to a widespread mosaicism, affecting many and possibly all tissues of the embryo. An error in later embryogenesis typically affects a lesser fraction of the soma, and may be restricted to certain tissues, and the expression "low-grade mosaicism" is used. If the mosaicism affects a cell line destined to give rise to both some somatic tissue and gonadal tissue, this is somatic-gonadal mosaicism.

> The mitotic cycle consists of the following sequence: gap-1 period (G1) → synthesis period (S) → gap-2 period (G2) → mitosis (cell division). The G1 → S → G2 components together comprise the interphase period of the cell cycle. During the S period, the chromosomes replicate their DNA, thus converting from the single-chromatid to the double-chromatid state. Genetically active segments of chromosomes replicate earlier during the S period, while inactive segments, which include almost the entire inactivated X chromosome in the female, are late-replicating. The cell division period is further subdivided into prometaphase → metaphase → anaphase → telophase. The chromosomes condense to enter prometaphase, and condensation continues into metaphase. Metaphase chromosomes align on the equatorial plate (Figure 3–14), and the spindle apparatus becomes attached to the centromere of each chromosome, consisting of its two kinetochores. Pulled at the kinetochores (centromeres), the chromatids of each chromosome then separate (disjoin) and are drawn in opposite directions (anaphase) and arrive at the opposite poles of the cell (telophase). Then the chromosomes decondense, the nuclear membrane reconstitutes, the cytoplasm constricts and divides, and two daughter cells now exist.

PreMeiotic Mitotic Error in the Gamete, and Gonadal Mosaicism

A mitotic error occurring in a primary gametocyte, oögonium or spermatogonium, prior to its entering into meiosis, can produce an aneuploid cell, which could then lead to a lineage containing this abnormality and comprising a "wedge" or an "island" within the gonad—in other words, *gonadal mosaicism* with a mix of normal and aneuploid gametocytes. As the abnormal gametocytes enter meiosis, the mature gametes then resulting from them would[11] be aneuploid. Note that the conceptus resulting from such an aneuploid gamete would be uniformly (that is, non-mosaic) aneuploid.

We now consider the case in more detail. Cells destined to give rise to gametocytes originate from the yolk sac in early embryogenesis and migrate to the gonadal ridge on the dorsal wall of the abdominal cavity, where, along with the supporting cells, they come to comprise the tissue of the gonad (De Felici 2013). In doing so, gametocytes

[11] Barring a "correction" during meiosis (Maiato and Silva 2023).

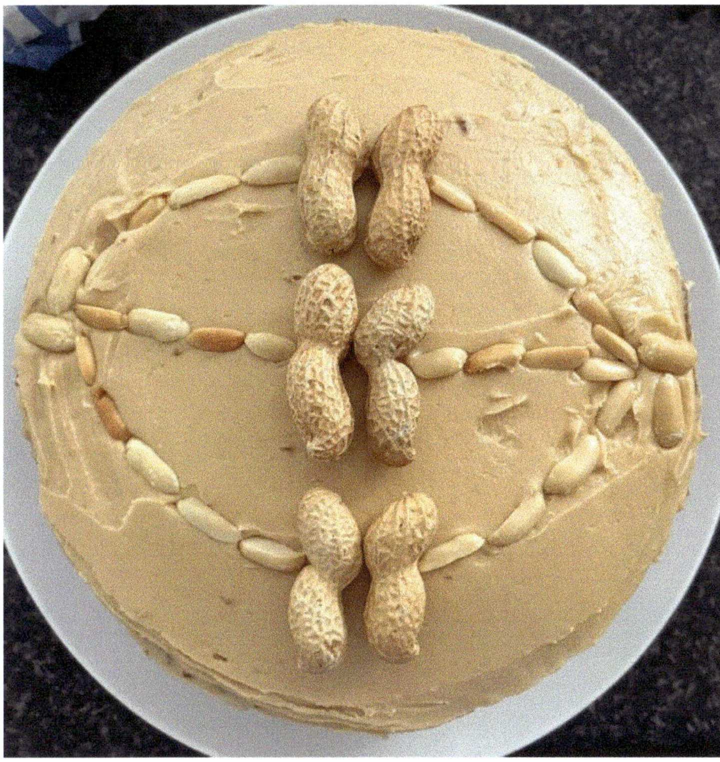

Figure 3–14. Mitosis.
A culinary whimsy. The cake is a cell about to undergo a mitotic division. The peanut pairs are three double-chromatid chromosomes, submetacentric and metacentric; the reader will need to imagine the other twenty. The other nuts are the spindle mechanism and kinetochores. Courtesy Dr Nooshin Sheidaei.

must replicate over and over. Looking at the male case, going through about 30 cycles of division produces 2^{30} (about 1,000,000,000) progeny spermatogonia, and the potential for error exists at each cell division contributing to this population. These errors could be nondisjunctions, or the production of structural rearrangements.

Consider this startling statistic: The total length of the seminiferous tubule in a man is about half a kilometer, a third of a mile (Johnson et al. 1998). If a mutation were to occur in a spermatogonium in, for example, the 20th cycle of division, its progeny would then go through 10 more cycles and comprise 2^{10} (about 1,000) cells. This would be only a millionth (1,000/1,000,000,000) of the ½ km of tubule—a mere ½ mm. So a man mosaic in such a way would have a risk of only one in a million to father a conception with this particular abnormality, given the improbability of the fertilizing sperm coming from this imperfect ½ mm. From similar reasoning, a defect arising at the tenth cycle could affect half a meter of tubule and carry a risk of 1 in 1,000. Oögonia need go through a lesser number of mitotic cycles (about 22), but the same principles broadly apply.

If the error took place in embryonic existence before gonadal precursors had formed, and may thus have involved a cell giving rise to both gonadal and somatic tissue, this is *somatic-gonadal mosaicism*. If a significant fraction of the soma carries the aneuploid cell line, an abnormal phenotype may result; but if not, the fact of a somatic component may not become known until a gonadal event—that is to say, a child born with the (non-mosaic) aneuploidy—has come to notice (e.g., Figure 3–23).

Given the huge number of premeiotic mitoses, and, as noted above, opportunity thus for mitotic error, gonadal mosaicism might, in theory, be expected to be common. This indeed seems to be so, and direct analysis of gametes gives similar results for male and female, with premeiotic aneuploidy[12] (disomy or nullisomy) rates around 10% (Ghevaria et al. 2022; Zhu et al. 2022b).[13] Findings from family searches for gonadal mosaicism have had mixed results. Nimmakayalu et al. (2013) report a case from molecular karyotyping: two siblings with macrocephaly and intellectual disability with a 399 kb 19p13.13 microdeletion, this the only case of gonadal mosaicism being recognized in a cohort of 1,800 patients studied. Campbell et al. (2014) undertook a systematic analysis of parents from a prospectively collected cohort of 100 children with a microdeletion, and they showed four parents to be mosaic for their child's deletion (the mosaicism level, on blood, was from <1% to 9%). Four out of 100 is a quite surprising number, but perhaps more widely indicative. (These latter cases represent somatic-gonadal mosaicism, and thus could equally have had mention in the following section.)

PostMeiotic Mitotic Error and Constitutional Mosaicism

A mitotic error can cause phenotypic abnormality by generating, in an initially normal conceptus, an abnormal cell line at some point during early embryogenesis. If we focus on the end result, the feature distinguishing post-conception mitotic from meiotic (or premeiotic mitotic) errors is that the post-conception error typically produces a mosaic conceptus, whereas meiotic/premeiotic errors lead to non-mosaic abnormality.

We define *constitutional chromosomal mosaicism* as the coexistence, within the one conceptus, of two (or, rarely, more) distinct cell lines which are otherwise genetically identical except for the chromosomal difference between them, these cell lines having been established by the time that embryonic development is complete (the point at which the embryo becomes a fetus, around eight weeks post-fertilization). Thus, the different cell lines are fixed in the individual and are a part of his or her chromosomal constitution. The earlier in embryogenesis that a mitotic error occurs, the greater the likelihood for a substantial fraction of the soma to be aneuploid, leading to increasing departure from normality of the phenotype. But it is probable that many mitotically arising abnormalities lead to cell death, leaving no trace, as we go on to discuss.

Mosaicism may involve any type of chromosomal abnormality. In a large study in Pham et al. (2014), these authors identified 57 cases of somatic mosaicism among just over 10,000 patients, who had presented with a wide range of phenotypic abnormality (and so, naturally, a selected population). The abnormalities included classic

[12] Note that detection of premeiotic aneuploidy requires analysis of immature oöcytes, or alternatively, the analysis of both the metaphase II oöcyte and its corresponding first polar body.

[13] Hultén et al. (2013) controversially suggest mitotic errors during ovariogenesis are inevitable and that "most women may be trisomy 21 ovarian mosaics."

autosomal and sex chromosomal aneuploidy, isochromosomes, ring chromosomes, marker chromosomes, single del/dups, multiple del/dups, and unbalanced translocations. The level of mosaicism in these cases ranged from low (5%) to high (80%).

Mosaicism may affect a cell destined to give rise to both soma and gonad: this is *somatic-gonadal mosaicism* (quite likely the case in some of the patients in Pham et al. above). If the proportion of abnormal cells in the mosaic parent is higher or differently distributed, that parent may manifest some signs of the partial aneuploid state. The father reported in Kennedy et al. (2001) had a dup(8)(p23.1p23.1) in mosaic state, in the ratio normal:duplication of 17:8 on blood sampling, and he himself had a heart defect, as did his non-mosaic dup(8) daughter. Her defect was, however, rather more severe than his. Notably, the daughter was described as "achieving top grades in school," a very unusual phenotypic commentary in a child with a non-mosaic classical chromosome duplication. A mother and daughter in Freitas et al. (2012) carried a 6.2 Mb deletion at 2q36.1q36.3, mosaic (~15% on blood) in the mother, non-mosaic in the daughter. The intellectually disabled daughter presented an obvious facial dysmorphism, but in the mentally normal mother this was very mild, and only appreciated in retrospect.

While "clinical chromosomology" is widely seen as a discipline of application particularly to a pediatric or obstetric population, older age groups are beginning to get a look-in.[14] The quite common finding of acquired loss of an X or a Y chromosome in an occasional cell in an older female or male population (and more notably in centenarians) may reflect "normal" age-related anaphase lag (Russell et al. 2007). Mosaicism involving an X or an autosome is linked to advanced maternal age, and inferentially to an increased risk for infertility (Kouvidi et al. 2021). The potential significance of the observation of mosaic loss of a Y chromosome (mLOY) as a marker of biological aging, and an associated risk for a number of common diseases of aging (Sano et al. 2023; Kuznetsova et al. 2023), is discussed in Chapter 15 (p. 472). The suggestion that Alzheimer disease might have a basis in mosaic trisomy 21 or X aneuploidy of some brain tissue is intriguing, but leaves open the question of the time in life at which the putative aneuploid cell line may have become incorporated (Graham et al. 2019; García-González et al. 2023). The bowel, an organ constantly replenishing its epithelium, accumulates microdeletions and microduplications with age, which are not necessarily harmful (Hsieh et al. 2013). Finally, we make mention, but no more than that, of the role of shortening of the telomeres (the chromosomal "caps") in aging, and potentially in the diseases of aging (Chakravarti et al. 2021); but this is not what we usually think of as being a part of the repository of classic chromosomal abnormality.

Vulnerability to Error in the First Few Mitoses in a Euploid Zygote or Early Embryo

The first few mitotic divisions from the normal (46,N) one-cell zygote, the fertilized egg, are particularly vulnerable to error, and especially the very first, the number-one

[14] Actually, the classic example of disease due to acquired somatic chromosomal mosaicism is, of course, cancer, usually an age-related condition; and a textbook of much larger size than this one would be needed to review the role of tissue-confined aneuploidy apropos (Oromendia and Amon 2014); we make no further mention here.

46,XX cell line: Most are 45,X/46,X,i(Xq). This is what would be expected if the error happened at the very first mitosis of the initially 46,XX zygote. If it happened at the next two or three divisions, a 46,XX cell line would also have been present, and thus three cell lines, 45,X/46,XX/46,X,i(Xq). The presence of three cell lines in Stefanou et al. (2006), who describe an abnormal infant with diploid/aneuploid trisomy 20 mosaicism on blood, but with a monosomic 20 cell line identified in urinary epithelial cells, similarly allows the inference of an initiating error at, or a little later than, the second mitosis.

Actually, about 5% of standard apparently non-mosaic 47,+21 is due to a postmeiotic mitotic defect from a 46,N zygote (Antonarakis et al. 1993), with the "third" chromosome 21 equally likely to be maternal or paternal. In 3% of apparently non-mosaic 47,XXY and 9% of 47,XXX, the error was post-zygotic, presumably prior to the formation of the inner cell mass[18] (MacDonald et al. 1994). As noted above, the nature of the mosaicism can indicate the likely time of its generation. More than one mitotic error can happen, separate in time and place; for example, DeBrasi et al. (1995) identified concomitant 45,X, 46,X,+8, and 47,XX,+8 in a woman with clinical features of both trisomy 8 and Turner syndrome, in whom the molecular study supported the hypothesis of an originally 46,XX conception.

Mosaicism Arising from Error at Later Mitoses in a Euploid Embryo

The categories of mosaicism described above are associated with phenotypes of varying degrees of severity, and with the mitotic event having caused the mosaicism of early occurrence during embryogenesis. But if the aberrant mitosis takes place later in embryogenesis, perhaps some thousands or millions of cell divisions along the way to the establishment of the fetal, and thus, eventually, post-natal anatomy, the effect upon the phenotype may be minimal, indiscernible, or without any effect at all.[19] Perhaps, as we now go on to discuss, every apparently 46,XX or 46,XY person is, somewhere in their anatomy, a mosaic.

Consider the following. A classic chromosome test on any normal person—a routine analysis from a sample of peripheral blood, or from a "spit" sample—would probably get a normal result (46,N). We would conclude from an analysis of a dozen or so cells from one particular tissue that the rest of the soma is also 46,N. In most of the person's tissue, this will be truly the case. But the body comprises a vast number of cells—ten trillion (10^{13}) or so—which required a vast number of mitoses for their generation. The dozen cells checked in the laboratory are only a ten-billionth of a percent of all the person's cells, and we routinely (and, for practical purposes, not unreasonably) regard this minute fraction as a valid representative of the remaining 99.9999999999%. Notwithstanding, we can surely suppose that one or more errors will have happened during one or some of the many mitoses, and these will have produced a chromosomally abnormal cell line, and the person is really a chromosomal mosaic. It seems plausible to

[18] The "inner cell mass" is seen as a clump of cells on part of the inner wall of the blastocyst, and these cells are destined to form the embryo (Figure 23–6). The remaining cells, comprising the shell of the blastocyst, are trophoblasts, and will form the placenta.

[19] But not overlooking, as noted above, that some chromosomal mosaicisms of restricted extent, or of late acquisition, can lead to certain adult-onset diseases.

imagine that unrecognized islets of mosaicism, involving a tiny number of cells—only a few thousand, perhaps—could well be a frequent state. Almost certainly, somewhere in their soma, everyone may be such a mosaic; but this fascinating academic matter is not a question of much practical relevance in the genetic counseling clinic.

Classical cytogenetics can (if the tested tissue is representative) show mosaicism unequivocally, with the recognition of two different karyotypes, but this is dependent on there being enough cells in the less frequent line for the observation to be made. In molecular karyotyping, detection is a subtler exercise, and it is based on an appreciation of a quantitative shift in the log_2 graph, or, if single nucleotide polymorphism array is the methodology, the genotyping pattern may be revealing; but in principle, mosaicism that might otherwise have slipped through on classical analysis can be picked up (Repnikova et al. 2012). The practicalities of this question are discussed below, Tissue Sampling in the Detection of Mosaicism.

Mosaicism Arising from Error in an Aneuploid Zygote or Embryo

Nondisjunction can occur in a post-zygotic mitosis in a conceptus that is initially trisomic for an autosome (for example, 47,+21). Thus, one copy of the homolog in question is lost. The same result may be due to the mechanism of anaphase lag.[20] This converts the trisomy in this cell to 46,N and is sometimes referred to as "correction" or "rescue." Its descendant cells are 46,N, and the karyotype of the conceptus is, for example, 47,+21/46,N (Figure 3–15c). Most mosaic trisomy/disomy 13, 18, 21, and X, arises in this way: for example, 47,XXY → 46,XY/47,XXY (Robinson et al. 1995).

A conceptus with what might be called *interchange tertiary trisomy*—that is, a 47-chromosome count, with the two translocation chromosomes and an additional copy of one of the derivative chromosomes—might generate a cell line with the balanced state, if one of the derivatives is lost post-zygotically. Thus, a zygote with, for example, a 47,t(1;2),+der(1) karyotype might acquire a cell line with 46,t(1;2). If this cell line included blood-forming tissue, but if much of the soma otherwise consisted of cells with the unbalanced state, a phenotypically abnormal child could have, on blood sampling, a balanced translocation karyotype. Such a case is presented in Dufke et al. (2001) concerning an abnormal child who, on blood, had a familial balanced karyotype 46,t(17;22), but who on skin biopsy karyotyped 47,der(22)t(17;22), and was thus shown to be duplicated for segments of 17 and 22. These authors speculate that this scenario might be a rare contributor to the apparent slight excess of abnormal children among the balanced carrier offspring of translocation carrier parents (p. 123).

Gonadal mosaicism can arise due to this mechanism, and again the classic example comes from mosaic trisomy 21, in which a 47,+21 embryo at a very early post-zygotic

[20] In this latter case, the chromosome fails to connect to the spindle apparatus, or is tardily drawn to its pole, and fails to be included in the reforming nuclear membrane. On its own in the cytoplasm, it will form a micronucleus and soon be lost.

stage discards the extra chromosome in one cell, thus giving a 46,N lineage. This 46,N line then contributes to most tissues, and an apparently normal physical phenotype results; but the gonad is not so fortunate, as it were, and may receive a larger fraction of 47,+21 cells (Kovaleva 2010). A clinical observation supporting this conclusion is that the low-level mosaic mothers (who had presented due to their having had a non-mosaic Down syndrome child) are of a typical maternal age range, whereas *their* mothers—the *grand*mothers of the Down syndrome children—were of older maternal age at the time their daughters had been born. This is consistent with their daughters having been conceived as (maternal-age-influenced) trisomy 21, but subsequently, at least in their soma, "corrected."

Post-zygotic "Correction" of Aneuploidy and Uniparental Disomy. If the conversion of trisomy to disomy occurs prior to the formation of the inner cell mass, and if the 46,N line then gives rise to the inner cell mass, the embryo will be non-mosaic 46,N. According to which one of the three chromosomes was lost, normal biparental disomy in the embryo could be restored, or uniparental disomy (UPD) could result (Figure 3–16). This is much the usual mechanism of formation of UPD. It is at prenatal diagnosis, typically, that the fact of this rescue mechanism comes to be discovered, with trisomy seen at chorionic villus sampling (CVS) and disomy at a subsequent amniocentesis (Sirchia et al. 1998). Chromosome 15 is of particular concern, and Purvis-Smith et al. (1992) and Cassidy et al. (1992) provide historic illustrations in pregnancies showing 47,+15 at CVS, with conversion to 46,N at amniocentesis—but the infants had UPD(15)mat, and so they were born with Prader-Willi syndrome. A contemporary example is the diagnosis of UPD(15)mat following the detection of trisomy 15 at noninvasive prenatal testing (NIPT) (Hong et al. 2023).

An inference of "rescue" may be made in the case of UPD discovered because of isozygosity for a recessive gene, and an example of this is deafness due to the connexin-26 gene. Yan et al. (2007) report a child presenting with deafness due to homozygosity for the common 35delG mutation, for which his father, but not his mother, was a carrier. As it transpired, the child had UPD(13)pat, with isodisomic and heterodisomic segments of chromosome 13. The segment in 13q12.1, which contains the connexin-26 locus, was one of the regions of isodisomy. Quite possibly, this had been a trisomic 13 conception but rescued due to discarding one of the chromosomes, which happened to be the maternal chromosome 13. Had it not been for the coincidence of the father's heterozygosity for the 35delG mutation, the rescue would have been entirely successful.

Post-zygotic correction can also happen in the other direction, as it were: to convert a monosomic zygote into a disomic one. It is very rarely recognized (Schinzel et al. 1993). Quan et al. (1997) report a girl, 46,XX, with Duchenne muscular dystrophy due to a homozygous deletion of exon 50 of the dystrophin gene. She had homozygosity of the X chromosome for all of the tested marker loci, apparently a complete maternal uniparental isodisomy X. Even a meiosis II nondisjunction would likely have had some heterozygosity, due to recombination at meiosis I; and so Quan and colleagues propose a mitotic mechanism. A 45,X0 conception, from a "22,0" sperm + 23,X egg at syngamy, underwent duplication, or possibly nondisjunction, of the single X chromosome. Unfortunately, this X chromosome carried a de novo Duchenne mutation.

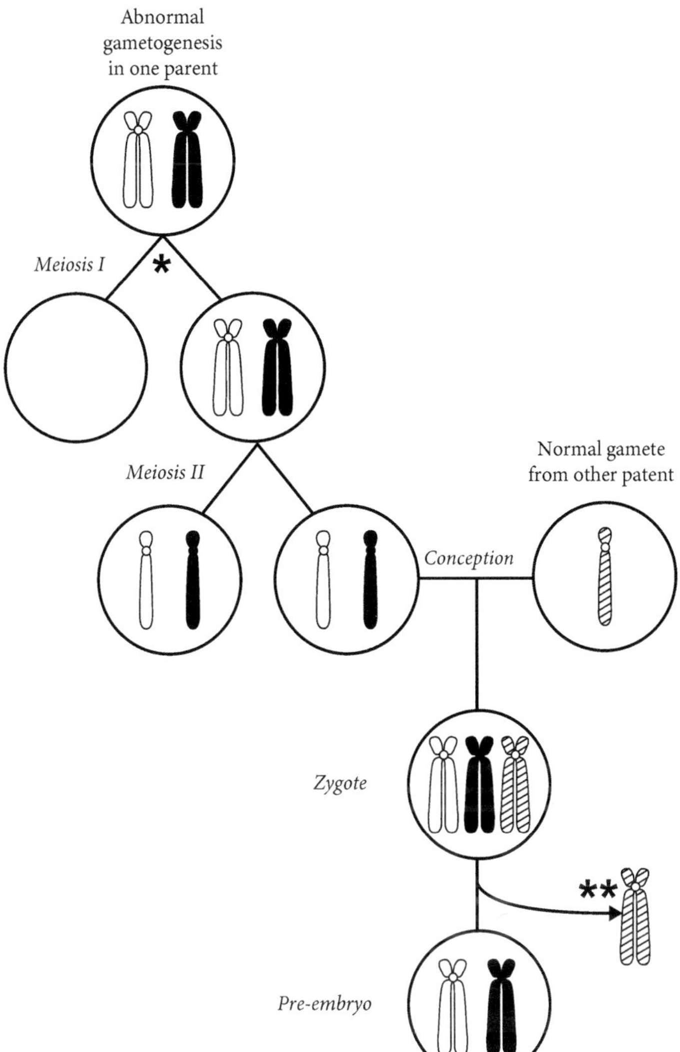

Figure 3–16. Uniparental disomy from "correction" of a trisomic conceptus by loss of a homolog. Nondisjunction* at meiosis I, followed by postzygotic loss** of one homolog, causes uniparental heterodisomy. (If, for example, this were chromosome 15, and the meiotic nondisjunction occurred in the mother, the child would have Prader-Willi syndrome.) Nondisjunction at meiosis II would cause uniparental isodisomy.

Mosaicism Due to Somatic Recombination in Homologs

Genetic exchange can take place as a normal event during a mitotic cycle, involving either the pair of homologous chromosomes or the sister chromatids of one chromosome. The cytogenetic demonstration of sister chromatid exchange (SCE) is rather dramatic (Figure 16–3). Should the SCE be unequal, tandem duplication and deletion lines may be generated. If the deletion line is lost, a normal/duplication mosaicism results (Rauen et al. 2001). According to the somatic extent of the abnormal cell line, the phenotype may or may not be affected.

CHIMERISM

Chimerism, which is to be distinguished from mosaicism, is the coexistence of more than one cell line in an individual due to the union of two originally separate ("sibling") conceptions (Chen et al. 2013f; Madan 2020).[21] It could be imagined that dizygotic twin blastocysts happen to make contact and then fuse, and this may be the more typical scenario. Since four gametes will have contributed to the person, we may hear the expression "tetragametic" chimerism. Alternatively, but rarely, there might have been two sperm fertilizing an ovum and a polar body. A 46,XX//46,XX or 46,XY//46,XY chimera would most probably present as a normal female or male, whereas 46,XX//46,XY could manifest an abnormality of sexual differentiation (Wimmer et al. 2022).

> The discovery of chimerism can cast a most remarkable light in certain cases in which parenthood is being tested. A mother apparently "could not have been" the mother of two of her three sons, when she and the family underwent HLA (immune histocompatibility) testing ahead of a planned kidney transplant. But it transpired that she was a tetragametic 46,XX//46,XX chimera. Her ovaries presumably comprised tissue from both fused conceptuses, but blood-forming tissue came from only one. Thus, she could have children who had neither of her blood-test HLA haplotypes (Yu et al. 2002). Similarly, a father who "failed" a paternity test from a son conceived at IVF—could this have been a laboratory mix-up?—turned out himself to be a tetragametic 46,XY//46,XY chimera. The child came from sperm due to tissue deriving from the father's absorbed fraternal co-twin, and his genetic profile was that of a nephew of his father (Baird et al. 2015).

The more usual form is "confined" chimerism, in which only one tissue—that is, blood—possesses the two cell lines. This is due to twin-to-twin (or feto-fetal) transfusion, when dizygous twins have intimately opposed placentae, allowing vascular connections ("anastomoses") to form between them, with marrow colonization by the other twin's hematogenous cells. Sudik et al. (2001), for example, describe a woman typing XY in almost all (99%) of peripheral lymphocytes, but she was 46,XX on three other tissues, including ovarian; she had had a twin brother who had died as a neonate. Somewhat stretching the analogy, Bianchi (2000) makes the intriguing suggestion that, due to the retention and persistence of fetal blood cells following delivery, every mother is, in a sense, a hematologic (micro)chimera.

TWINNING

Dizygous twinning is more frequent in mothers in their late 30s, and so it is not remarkable that occasionally twins are born, one with normal chromosomes and the other with a maternal-age-related aneuploidy. Monozygous twinning could happen in an abnormal conception just as in a normal one, and the occasional instance of twins concordant for an abnormal karyotype is to be expected (Schlessel et al. 1990). Rather more remarkable is the case of monozygous (MZ) twins discordant for karyotype—clearly,

[21] For the record, the chimera of classical mythology was "in the forepart a lion, in the hinder a serpent, and in the midst a goat." Note the // descriptive format.

the adjective "identical" is inappropriate here! Rogers et al. (1982) studied monochorionic twin brothers, one 46,XY and the other 47,XY,+21 with Down syndrome, in whom genetic analysis supported a diagnosis of monozygosity; similarly, Chanes et al. (2021) describe MZ twins, one normal, the other with ring(13) mosaicism. In this type of twinning, the assumption is that either a mitotic nondisjunction or a mitotic rearrangement occurred in one of the two monozygous embryos from an initially normal conception; or, vice versa, an initially 47,XY,+21 conceptus underwent splitting, with loss of a chromosome 21 then occurring in one of the newly created embryos. A number of similar cases are on record,[22] including monozygous twins of opposite gender (Lewi et al. 2006; Stemkens et al. 2007; Zech et al. 2008).

> Perhaps the most extraordinary circumstance of chromosomal discordance in monozygous twins concerns the acardiac (that is, lacking a heart) fetus. Trisomy 2 is one of the aneuploidies observed (Mihci et al. 2009). An initially normal conceptus might generate a trisomy 2 cell line that then separates and produces the co-twin, or an initially trisomic conceptus gives rise to a "corrected" lineage. It is only the presence of the normal twin that allows the acardiac co-twin to survive, at least temporarily, with placental vascular connections providing blood circulation (twin reverse arterial perfusion, TRAP) from normal to abnormal twin. We have seen such a case due to trisomy 3, with the affected acephalic, acardiac fetus surviving through to the second trimester, of barely recognizable human form (and see Figure 20–24).

STRUCTURAL REARRANGEMENT

The following classical structural rearrangements may be listed: translocations, insertions, inversions, isochromosomes, duplications, deletions, rings, and complex rearrangements. These may be very obvious on classical karyotyping or, for smaller deletions or duplications (3–5 Mb), may have required high-resolution banding for identification. With molecular karyotyping, imbalances of submicroscopic size, typically measured in kilobases, are detectable: these are referred to as "microdeletion" and "microduplication," or alternatively, as "copy number variants" (CNVs). In general parlance, the terms microdeletions and microduplications are often used in a setting of assumed pathogenicity, whereas CNV may need a qualifying adjective of benign, pathogenic, or of uncertain status.

All arose de novo at one point—whether with the index case in whom the abnormality was discovered, or in a parent or more distant ancestor, with a balanced or unbalanced form transmitted thereafter in the family. Jacobs (1981) derived the following mutation rates for the generation of de novo classical rearrangements: 1.6×10^{-4} per gamete for the balanced reciprocal translocation, and 2.9×10^{-4} per gamete for unbalanced rearrangements.[23] Concerning CNVs, the mutation rate for larger (>500 kb) microdeletions/duplications is 6.5×10^{-3} per gamete (Itsara et al. 2010). In other words, out of 100,000 gametes, on average 16 will have a balanced and 29 an unbalanced de novo classical rearrangement, while 650 will have a de novo larger CNV.

[22] It is plausible that in some instances, the presence of different cell lineages contributes to the monozygotic twinning process.

[23] These conclusions were derived from data of several studies of pregnancies that were able to "survive long enough to give rise to a recognized pregnancy": in other words, from clinical miscarriage and newborn data. Jacobs acknowledges that these figures will surely be underestimates.

still there; they are still perfectly capable of being read. If a sequence of pages is inserted upside down (an inversion), one need only turn the book around to read them.

If a phenotypically abnormal person has a rearrangement that is balanced on classical laboratory study, one can only speak, at the cytogenetic level, of the rearrangement being "apparently balanced." In the case of an associated cognitive impairment, one can suggest (and more so in a de novo case), but not necessarily state with certainty, that the observed phenotype may be due to the identified karyotype. Modern methodologies can clarify such cases as being either indeed truly balanced, or with very subtle imbalances. A rearrangement that is balanced at the genomic level may yet lead to a phenotypic consequence, due to gene disruption or due to "position effect."

As an example of *gene disruption*, consider the well-known *PMP22* gene at 17p11.2, the basis of Charcot-Marie-Tooth and pressure-sensitive neuropathy (Chapter 14). Nadal et al. (2000) studied a mother and son, both of whom presented with pressure-sensitive neuropathy. The classical cytogenetic study showed them to be heterozygotes for the apparently balanced translocation t(16;17)(q12;p11.2). Applying the technology of the day, the chromosome 17 breakpoint was shown to have been sited actually within the *PMP22* gene. This disruption would have led to a functional haploinsufficiency, which is known to be the basis of pressure-sensitive neuropathy. Another such example is described in Dupont et al. (2013), who identified a *COL2A1* disruption in a family with Stickler syndrome, the affected persons having inherited a rcp(12;15)(q13;q22.2); *COL21A* is located at 12q13.11. Redin et al. (2017) and Lowther et al. (2022), applying molecular methodology, address the question in the study of large cohorts of translocation carriers. Comparing those with a normal (n = 304) and those with an abnormal (a developmental disorder) phenotype (n = 406) in Lowther et al., those with an abnormal phenotype had a sevenfold increased likelihood, compared to the normal group, to have the breakpoint disrupt a known developmental gene. As one such example, the *TCF4* gene (Chapter 14; Pitt-Hopkins syndrome) at 18q21 was disrupted in some of the phenotypically abnormal cases but none of the normals.

Concerning *position effect*, one of the earliest examples is of the *SOX9* gene at 17q25.1: Chromosomal rearrangement in the vicinity can result in loss of long-range regulation and hence non-expression of the (intact) gene, with sex reversal, campomelic dysplasia, and Pierre Robin syndrome possible phenotypic consequences (Gordon et al. 2014) (Figure 3–18). Sophisticated methodologies can reveal in closer detail the

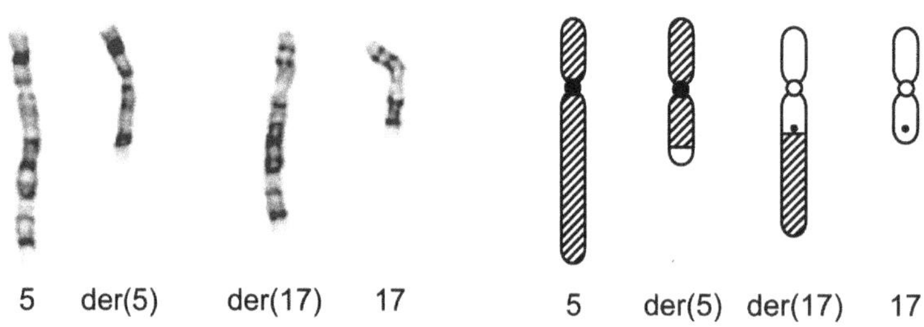

Figure 3–18. Position Effect in an Apparently Balanced Translocation.

Notes: An apparently balanced translocation causing the syndrome of campomelic dysplasia (which includes skeletal, genital, and brain defects). One breakpoint is at 17q25.1, on or close to the *SOX9* locus (shown as dot on the cartoon karyotype), where the basis of the syndrome lies. One possibility is that the gene is disrupted. Or, an influence of adjacent chromosome 5 chromatin ("position effect") leads to inactivation of the *SOX9* gene on the der(17), the functional *SOX9* haploinsufficiency then being responsible for the phenotype.

Source: From R Savarirayan and A Bankier, Acampomelic campomelic dysplasia with de novo 5q;17q reciprocal translocation and severe phenotype, *J Med Genet,* 35:597–599, 1998.

pathogenetic mechanism in some such cases, in which a region of influence—a "topologically associated domain" (TAD)—is implicated. Wallis et al. (2021) studied a family with a history of lymphedema and distichiasis (LDS), segregating a rcp(16;22)(q24;q13.1), and showed that the (normal) LDS locus at 16q24.1, *FOXC2*, this locus lying within 16q24, had been separated from its normal control due to the translocation breakpoint being close by, 120 kb upstream. This compromise of genetic control led to the appearance of the syndrome. There may be no loss or gain of DNA in such cases; in other words, the rearrangement is genomically balanced, but functionally unbalanced.

MICRODELETIONS, MICRODUPLICATIONS, AND COPY NUMBER VARIANTS OF INCOMPLETE PENETRANCE AND VARIABLE EXPRESSIVITY

While the classic chromosome disorders are characterized by complete penetrance,[24] the picture with the molecular-defined microdeletions/duplications is different. Some carriers may display no clinical abnormality, and yet a child of theirs may have presented with obvious symptomatology. If the "normal" parent is studied more closely, microsigns of the phenotype associated with that imbalance may be discerned; but they remain within the range of what is considered normal in the general population, and they can function as independent, productive adults. These "normal" parents are considered to be nonpenetrant with respect to the imbalance in question. It is more particularly with autism (Chapter 25) and non-dysmorphic cognitive impairment that these matters apply.

The basis of this variation may lie in the coexistence of different CNVs or SNP variants, most likely on another chromosome, and inherited quite coincidentally. Each imbalance might not suffice to cause a phenotype on its own, but the two together may add up to abnormality. This is the "two-hit" hypothesis (Girirajan et al. 2010; Atli et al. 2022). Most often, one hit (the first hit) will be the more important, and the second hit could be due to any one of a number of different "lesser" imbalances, which typically would warrant being called no more than a "VUS" (variant of uncertain significance).[25]

It might be more accurate to speak of two or more hits multiplying together, rather than adding up, to produce a phenotype of combined effect. Multiple hits contribute to a "liability threshold" beyond which a phenotype emerges (Pizzo et al. 2019; Jensen et al. 2021; Smolen et al. 2023). This concept is illustrated in study of the well-known 16p12.1 deletion (Figure 3–19). These further hits comprise CNVs, rare sequence variants of variable impact, or the combined effect of multiple common variants (in other words, polygenic inheritance).

Rosenfeld et al. (2013) reviewed a number of the more common microdeletions/duplications ("first-hit" imbalances), establishing penetrance estimates ranging from 10% to 62% (the 62% referring to the 16p11.2 microdeletion just mentioned). Their

[24] *Penetrance* is a quantitative descriptor and refers to the percentage fraction of a particular genetic cohort who show phenotypic abnormality. In such a population, in which the fraction is less than 100%, we may speak of *incomplete* penetrance; in a single individual showing no abnormality, this is *nonpenetrance*. *Expressivity* is qualitative, and reflects the range of clinical manifestation in those in whom a condition has been penetrant. It may sometimes become a matter of semantics whether a subtly abnormal person is considered to represent nonpenetrance, or penetrance with very mild expressivity.

[25] A rare and different form of two-hit mechanism concerns the "unmasking" of a recessive allele on a normal homolog, due to a deletion of that segment on the other chromosome (Poot 2012; Paciorkowski et al. 2013).

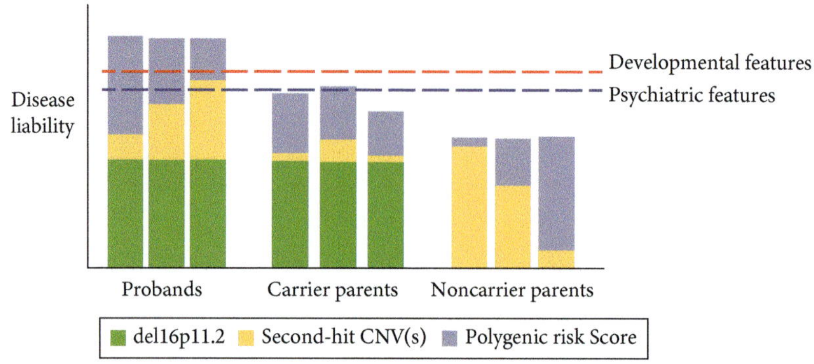

Figure 3–19. The 16p12.1 Deletion in a Proband, and in the Carrier and Non-Carrier Parent.
Notes: The thresholds are shown for developmental and psychiatric manifestation, according to an individual's genetic load: the presence of the 16p deletion; the carriage of second-hit variants; and the load otherwise of variants relating to an autism polygenic risk score. The deletion is carried by the proband and the carrier parent. Some carrier parents may manifest a relatively mild psychiatric phenotype. The non-carrier parent may have a number of different rare variants (blue), which of themselves, in this setting, are harmless, along with a variable polygenic load. But the combination, then, in the child, of the 16p deletion, along with a number of rare second-hit variants (yellow), combined with a polygenic load (polygenic risk score, blue), combine to cross a threshold sufficient to convey a developmental phenotype.

work was since followed up by others (Coe et al. 2014; Kendall et al. 2019; Redaelli et al. 2019), and culminating in the review of Goh et al. (2025) as listed in Appendix C.

EPIGENETICS AND GENOMIC IMPRINTING

A formal definition of an epigenetic effect includes these points: The DNA sequence of a particular gene remains unaltered, but the capacity of this gene to be expressed is altered. The expression "genomic imprinting" is applied in the setting of epigenetic effects that are imposed during germline transmission. Some parts of some chromosomes are subject to genomic imprinting as a normal occurrence, and this imprinting is parent-specific; that is, genes in the chromosomal segment are expressed, or not expressed, according to whether the chromosome had been transmitted in the sperm or in the ovum ("parent-of-origin effect"). An imprinted segment takes up an "epigenetic mark," and the gene or genes in this segment are not expressed, leaving it to the corresponding locus or loci on the homologous chromosome from the other parent to be the only source of expression. When the phenomenon was first appreciated in humans, it was naturally suspected that many forms of congenital abnormality might be due to aberrant imprinting. As it has transpired, however, the practical application of genomic imprinting appears to be confined to a rather small number of cytogenetic conditions (Chapter 19). Nevertheless, the theoretical interest is considerable.

Most of the autosomal genome is not subject to imprinting, and it is functionally disomic. That is, with each locus having a pair of alleles, each of the pair is functionally active, contributing more or less equally to the genetic output from that locus.[26] This is *biallelic gene expression*. A minority of the genome is subject to imprinting and requires only one of the pair of alleles to be active, while the other one becomes inactivated

[26] But exceptions exist, and approximately 5% of autosomal genes are randomly expressed from only one or other parental allele (Gimelbrant et al. 2007).

("silent"); in other words, the locus is functionally monosomic, with a genetic output from only one allele. This is *monoallelic expression.*

If the allele of maternal origin is inactivated, only the allele of paternal origin is functionally active, and vice versa. Following conception, the imprint remains through cycles of post-conceptional somatic mitoses: The chromosome "remembers" the sex of the parent who contributed it (put differently, it retains its epigenetic mark). The imprinting pattern may be specific to a certain tissue or to a certain developmental stage (Ideraabdullah et al. 2008). Thus, in some tissues a gene may express monoallelically, whereas in other tissues biallelic expression is retained; or a gene may express monoallelically in a specific tissue at one stage in embryogenesis, and biallelically thereafter. X chromosome inactivation is a special case.

Parent-of-origin imprinting is a normal mechanism of gene regulation. It is mediated through a process taking place during gametogenesis, of which the physical basis includes methylation of cytosine bases within the gene(s) or in controlling sequences upstream of it. This process is reversible, and in the "life" of an autosomal allele or chromosomal segment, as it passes from individual to individual down the generations and across the centuries, imprinting—the epigenetic mark—will be acquired, maintained, lost ("erased"), reacquired ("reset"), and lost again, according to the sexes of the individuals through whom it is transmitted. Throughout, it retains the same DNA sequence.

Mechanisms Whereby Functional Genetic Abnormality Can Arise

In the context of imprinting, we may consider three categories of functional genetic defect. These are as follows: uniparental disomy with overexpression or non-expression of genes in certain chromosomal segments; deletion with non-expression; and relaxation of imprinting with overexpression. *Uniparental disomy* will lead to either biallelic expression, or to no expression, at the locus or loci within the imprintable segment. If a *deletion* removes a chromosomal segment that would otherwise have been "silenced," all that is lost is a nonfunctioning genetic segment, and there is no untoward consequence. On the other hand, if the deletion removes the segment on the active chromosome, the corresponding part of the other homolog is inactive, and so neither chromosome will be genetically functioning in this segment; in a sense, the silent allele is unmasked. *Relaxation of imprinting* allows a segment that should be non-expressed to lose its imprint. The locus or loci contained therein will be operating biallelically, which will be, theoretically, at double normal capacity. These mechanisms are dealt with in detail in Chapter 19.

CONSEQUENCES OF GENETIC ABNORMALITY

Structural Imbalance

Our physical anatomy is due to our chromosomes (Gardner 2016; Anastasiadou et al. 2024). Chromosome imbalances are harmful because of the fundamental reason that many genes are dosage-sensitive. And if megabase amounts of chromatin are involved, it is highly likely dosage-sensitive genes will be included in the imbalanced segment(s). In duplications, there is 150% of the normal amount of this chromosomal segment, and in the deletion there is 50% of the normal amount. The imbalance involves a whole chromosome (full aneuploidy) or a part of a chromosome. From classical cytogenetics, the latter state is described as partial or segmental aneuploidy, a deletion or a duplication. In molecular karyotyping, in which the focus is on much smaller segments, the terms used are *microdeletion* and *microduplication*, or CNV deletion or duplication.

An incorrect amount of dosage-sensitive genetic material in every cell of the conceptus distorts its development to a greater or lesser extent. As discussed above, large losses or gains almost invariably set early anatomical development so awry that natural abortion occurs. Lesser imbalances may be compatible with continued intrauterine survival, but with the eventual production of a phenotypically abnormal child. Very minor partial aneuploidies may cause defects that are not readily detectable in early infancy; and some chromosomal "defects" may be without phenotypic effect. However, as a first principle, anything but 100% of the normal amount of genetic material (in classical, megabase cytogenetic terms) produces a less than 100% normal phenotype. Cognitive impairment is the almost universal consequence of classical autosomal imbalance, while much intellectual disability is due to a chromosome abnormality.

On the other hand, imbalances detectable only by molecular karyotyping (CNV del/dups) may be so small that no dosage-sensitive material is affected, and the phenotype is unaffected; or, the imbalance may only lead to phenotypic abnormality when it exists in the company of another micro-imbalance elsewhere in the genome ("second-hit" effect, as discussed above). The distinction between very small classical and larger molecular imbalances is not as clear-cut as the foregoing might suggest, and indeed some cases could carry either description; but it is useful nevertheless to consider these as two categories.

It is generally too simplistic to think of deletions and duplications leading to opposite qualities of phenotype (Neri and Romana Di Raimo 2010). But in some instances the concept of "type and countertype," originally proposed by Lejeune (1966), may be invoked. Deletion of 7p15 may cause the cranial bones to fuse prematurely (craniosynostosis) due to abnormal behavior of osteoblasts at their periphery, whereas duplication leads to underdevelopment of the skull, with a large and confluent fontanelle (Stankiewicz et al. 2001) (Figure 14–31). Deletion of 15q26.1qter (which removes the growth factor locus *IGFR1*) is associated with intrauterine growth retardation, whereas dup(15)(q26.1qter) may cause a syndrome of post-natal overgrowth (Faivre et al. 2002; Nagai et al. 2002). Similarly, carriers of reciprocal CNVs at 16p11.2 exhibit mirror phenotypes of obesity/macrocephaly (deletion) and underweight/microcephaly (duplication) (Loviglio et al. 2017).

Assessment of Imbalance

With respect to classical degrees of cytogenetic imbalance, the blunt quantitative tool of haploid autosomal length (HAL; see Appendix A) measurement can be applied, although this may now be of somewhat historic interest in the molecular era. The largest chromosome, no. 1, comprises 8.66% of the HAL, whereas chromosome 21, the smallest, is 1.77% (Table A–1). As a very general rule, if the imbalance consists of less than 1% of HAL (corresponding to ~30 Mb), the conceptus is often viable in utero, and live birth frequently results. If the excess is greater than 2%, in utero lethality, with spontaneous abortion, is likely. Imbalance involving autosomal deficiency (partial monosomy) is generally much less survivable than is duplication (partial trisomy).

A qualitative assessment is more to the point: chromosomal segments vary considerably in respect of their genetic content. Insight is gained on the empiric observations of phenotypes. Some large segments (e.g., 9p, all of 21) appear to have a substantial pre- and post-natal survivability in the trisomic state, whereas a lesser number of segments (e.g., distal 4p) are often viable when monosomic. Chromosome 13 provides the most impressive examples of viability for a large autosomal imbalance. Trisomy for the whole of chromosome 13—fully 3.7% of the HAL—frequently goes through to live birth, and in the 13q− deletion syndrome, monosomy occurs for up to 2.5% of HAL. This reflects the low gene density on this chromosome, only 6.5 genes per Mb (Table 1–1). The same principle applies to chromosomes 18 and 21.[27] On the other hand, chromosome 19, although small, carries a high concentration of genes, indeed the highest per length (Figure 1–4), and segmental imbalances are thus rarely viable.

Occasionally, imbalance detectable classically is so "small" that the effect on the child's physical phenotype is only very minor, and intellectual function can remain within the normal range, albeit toward the lower end of that range. Indeed, there are some segments of Mb size which, when duplicated or deleted, appear to cause no abnormality at all (Stumm et al. 2002; Barber 2005; Atli et al. 2022). The concept of heritable "euchromatic deletions and duplications without phenotypic effect" is discussed in Chapter 17.

Molecular karyotyping has enabled a finer view of the genome, and microdeletions and microduplications of kilobase size are routinely detectable. These imbalances may impose a phenotype in which cognitive and behavioral abnormality is the predominant observation. Dysmorphism may be evident, but can be of quite minor degree. This may reflect that these small imbalances affect only a few or even a single gene, or regulatory factor. Since the organ commanding the largest component of a person's genome is the brain, it is plausible to suppose that "brain genes" will be the most likely type of gene to reside within the microdeletions/duplications concerned.

Differing lengths of deleted or duplicated segments enable a dissection of the specific segmental contributions to components of an abnormal phenotype. A broad-brush "malformation map" can be produced from documenting the association of certain congenital defects or known syndromes with particular segmental aneusomies (Brewer et al. 1998, 1999; Carey and Viskochil 2007) (Figure 3–20). Specific malformations can be interrogated: van Karnebeek and Hennekam (1999) document imbalances associated with congenital heart disease, as do Thorsson et al. (2015); Tyshchenko et al. (2009) have assembled a (very preliminary) brain list; Marcelis et al. (2011) record chromosomal segments associated with anorectal malformations; and we have undertaken phenotype mapping studies with respect to epilepsy (Singh et al. 2002a) and to kidney defects (Amor et al. 2003). Catelani et al. (2009) have searched for molecular imbalances in children with syndromic deafness.

The chromosome regions thus illuminated may serve as candidate regions for the discovery of culprit genes. Note that a one-to-one connection between a deleted/duplicated segment and a specific trait cannot necessarily be drawn; and, for example, we have proposed that the particular nervous system malformation of periventricular

[27] Chromosome 21 has a similar density, at 6.7 genes/Mb, whereas chromosome 18 is the least dense, at 4.3 genes/Mb (Nusbaum et al. 2005).

The distribution of the abnormal cells in hypomelanosis of Ito, and thus of dyspigmentation, follows the lines of Blaschko, and Magenis et al. (1999) use the expression "Blaschkolinear malformation complex." Asymmetry is a further clinical pointer (Woods et al. 1994).

An interesting category of mosaicism for a structural rearrangement is that in which two lines of opposite imbalance coexist, with or without a normal cell line as well. Here, the error must have happened at a very early stage, and quite possibly, in those cases lacking a normal cell line, at the very first mitosis of the zygote. Such a case is described in Morales et al. (2007a), who analyzed a boy with the karyotype at birth of 46,XY,del(7q)/46,XY,dup(7q), although by age 12–14 months, the deletion cell line had disappeared, at least from blood and exfoliated urinary epithelial cells. Presumably, the karyotype at conception was 46,XY, but then the two chromosome 7 homologs underwent an unequal exchange of q21.1q31.3 material, generating, in the two daughter cells from the first mitosis, the deletion and duplication lineages. If, for example, the error had occurred one division later, at one of the two second mitotic divisions, a normal cell line might have been retained and have contributed to the inner cell mass.

Tissue Sampling in the Detection of Mosaicism

Clearly, detecting—or failing to detect—a mosaic state will depend upon which tissue is studied and how many cells are counted/analyzed. Blood, buccal cells, amniocytes, chorionic villi, trophectoderm, skin fibroblasts, and urinary sediment cells have been the usually tested tissues. A normal blood result in a child with an indicative phenotype, or following an abnormal prenatal test, might then warrant testing other tissues. Blood is a specialized tissue, and an abnormal cell line, otherwise widespread through the soma, can potentially be excluded from blood marrow following untold numbers of mitoses and if normal cells exert a superior survivability. Presumably this was the case, for example, in the child described in De Ravel et al. 2001 above, in whom skin fibroblasts, but not blood, retained the aneuploidy. Skin fibroblast analysis has been a mainstay of mosaicism detection since the earliest days of cytogenetics (and actually predated the use of blood).

Another tissue of historic provenance is the buccal mucosa, the inner lining of the cheek obtained from a "cheek swab," and this was the basis of a simple analysis of X chromosome aneuploidy via the demonstration of a compacted inactivated X (the Barr body)—a methodology little used these days. But this tissue has come to the forefront in the current century with the development of technologies to extract DNA from buccal mucosal cells that are contained in saliva, the "spit sample." The buccal mucosal cells present in a saliva sample are representative of ectodermal tissue: the tissue from which, among others, the nervous system derives. There is an obvious practical attraction in the ability to avoid even the (for most people) minor pain of a venipuncture, especially with children; no more is involved than simply spitting into a tube. The DNA can then be subjected to a methodology such as single nucleotide polymorphism (SNP) chromosome microarray (CMA).

The suitability of this approach was demonstrated in a landmark study in Francis et al. (2023), who compared the diagnostic utility of saliva-based against blood-based

CMA. In the analysis of 370 patients in a pediatric setting, including 224 presenting with syndromic or non-syndromic intellectual disability, in whom both types of testing were applied, the saliva-based test picked up 20 cases of mosaicism, a CNV or a trisomy, which were missed on the blood sampling. Notably, these mosaic cases were confined to the group of patients presenting with a syndromic intellectual disability. (For non-mosaic results, the blood and saliva samples were completely concordant.) These observations lead to the conclusion that saliva-based chromosome analysis should be a first-tier test, at least in the case of syndromic intellectual disability: that is to say, intellectual disability in the context of such other observations as organ malformation, facial and other dysmorphism, or growth disturbance.

Gonadal (and Somatic-Gonadal) Mosaicism

Gonadal mosaicism is suspected upon the observation of a chromosomally normal couple (at least on blood testing) having had two or more children with the same abnormal karyotype. Molecular analysis can allow an inference of who is the carrier parent, such as Tosca et al. (2010) show in the family study of two children with a dup(4)(q22.2q32.3), in which the microsatellite pattern indicated a maternal origin. In Kuroda et al. (2014), even though chromosome studies on the mother were normal, a maternal origin could be assumed in two siblings with Angelman syndrome due to a chromosome 15 inversion, which had deleted (among other genes) the *UBE3A* gene (Chapter 19).

Direct proof is provided by analysis of gametes. For example, in a case that had come to notice through an IVF clinic, Somprasit et al. (2004) report a couple having had a 21q duplication in two embryos subjected to PGT, and then showed the same duplication in 6.6% of 1,002 of the father's sperm. The abnormality was not present in his blood. Similarly, Alkaya et al. (2020) describe a father of three children with cri du chat syndrome (Chapter 14) due to an unbalanced translocation t(5;19)(p13.3;q13.4); the translocation was present in his sperm, but in neither blood nor skin biopsy.

Somatic-gonadal mosaicism can be inferred on the observation of one parent of an aneuploid child carrying, in mosaic state, the same aneuploidy. Sachs et al. (1990) studied a mother who had had one Down syndrome child and three other trisomic 21 pregnancies, and her blood karyotype was 47,+21[3%]/46,N[97%]. Ovarian biopsies showed almost half the cells in each ovary to be 47,XX,+21. We have seen a similar case, a woman who presented having had two trisomic 21 pregnancies. On blood with a 60-cell count, she and her partner were non-mosaic 46,N. She recounted a story that her own mother had had an amniocentesis when pregnant with her, which had shown a single + 21 cell. Given this information, "spit sample" microarray was done, and she proved to have ~5% of cells trisomic, inferentially revealing her state of somatic-gonadal mosaicism.

Figure 3–23 shows an example of somatic-gonadal mosaicism for a structural rearrangement, del(1). The index case was identified with a small intrachromosomal del(1) at routine prenatal diagnosis. The father was mosaic for this deletion in 20% of lymphocytes. Of his two other children, one had normal chromosomes, and the other had the same deletion. The father is phenotypically normal, and the older child with the deletion has an IQ in the low normal range. A similar circumstance is recorded in Fan et al. (2001): A university-educated man working as a financial planner, having the blood karyotype 46,XY,dup(8)(p21.3p23.1)[6]/46,XY[24], fathered two daughters risk estimate has a greater or lesser degree of precision depending on how much data has been accumulated upon which the estimate is based.

2. *Mendelian risks.* If a clear model of inheritance is known, risk figures derived by reference to that theory may be used. In practice, only Mendel's law of segregation is applied in this context. When a pair of homologous chromosomes segregates at meiosis, which chromosome enters the gamete that will produce the conceptus is typically a random matter. Each has an equal chance: a probability of 0.5. Thus, a parent who carries a microdeletion 16p11.2 has a 50/50 likelihood to transmit this chromosome to a child, a 1:1 segregation. This is assumed to be a *true* risk, not an estimate: It is 0.5 exactly.

Consider, for example, the common situation of a young couple having had a child with Down syndrome. Nothing is known about nondisjunction that could provide a theoretical model on which to base a recurrence risk figure. We therefore use empiric data—that is, information obtained from surveying large numbers of other such families. It may be observed, for example, that in these families about one pregnancy in 100, subsequent to the index case of Down syndrome, produced another child with Down syndrome. Formally expressed, this is a segregation analysis. From this rate of 1/100 we can derive a risk figure of 1%, which we then have as the basis for advising patients. (Actually, it is not quite as straightforward as this in Down syndrome; see Chapter 13.)

If a theoretical construct can be applied, this may allow a more precise calibration of the empiric figure. The del 17q21.31 of Koolen-de Vries syndrome (Chapter 14), which has a population frequency of 1/16,000, offers an example. This particular deletion may have, as a necessary but not sufficient basis for its generation, a 17q inversion encompassing the length of the deleted segment (chr17:45.6-46.1 Mb). The risk is related to the inversion status of the parents, the dimorphism referred to as H1 (normal 17q21.31 sequence, *N*) and H2 (inverted 17q21.31 sequence, *V*). Koolen et al. (2012) apply some fundamental genetic concepts in order to tailor the risk figure according to the possible parental inversion genotypes, NN, NV, and VV, and thus the six possible mating combinations: NN × NN, NN × NV, NV × NV, NN × VV, NV × VV, and VV × VV. The adjusted risk figures of 0.03% (for VV × VV parents) and 0.008% (NN × NV parents), versus the population figure of 0.006%, barely dent the >99.9% chance of non-recurrence, but the principle behind the exercise is to be acknowledged.

A somewhat similar approach may apply to the inverted duplication of 8p (inv dup 8p), as discussed on Chapter 14. An inversion polymorphism at chr8:7.6-12.3 Mb, which has a high (26%) frequency in the general population, predisposes to a misalignment during meiosis (Giglio et al. 2001). Indeed, generation of the rearrangement may only be possible in the setting of this parental inversion. However, the absolute risk among this quarter of the (at least European) population must remain extremely low, given the rarity with which the inv dup 8p is seen, and the absence of any report of recurrence. The risk to the non-carrier may be a true 0.0%.

Likewise, for the circumstance of the parent heterozygous for a chromosomal rearrangement, the counselor can consult data that have been accumulated by workers in the field, foremost among whom, in respect of reciprocal translocations, are Stengel-Rutkowski et al. (1988), Cohen et al. (1992, 1994), and Midro et al. (2000). Since almost all reciprocal translocations are unique to one family, it is not necessarily simple to estimate a figure for a family with a "new" translocation, but an attempt can be made (see Chapter 5). On the other hand, for the Robertsonian translocations, each type of which can generally be regarded as the same between families, extrapolation of risk figures from historical data to a current family is usually valid.

Risk may apply more generally in the sense of a successful or unsuccessful outcome. Consider the case of couples having had a previous aneuploid pregnancy and now seeking blastocyst testing to be sure of avoiding a recurrence: What are their odds of having a euploid blastocyst, suitable for transfer? In an observational study, L Zhang et al. (2023b) saw a 30% rate of an aneuploid blastocyst in this group, substantially above the 21% rate of those presenting with no previous aneuploidy history. These authors caution that these rates were derived from a population of women who were able to produce at least four blastocysts, and who had good ovarian reserve; hence they should be applied as risk estimates only to those in this same category.

Hook and Cross (1982) note the importance of distinguishing between the *rate* (which may be thought of as "past tense") and the *risk* (which is "future tense"). They emphasize that although geneticists routinely extrapolate from rates in one population at one point in time, and may use these figures as risk estimates in another population and certainly at a later point in time, they should be on their guard for any evidence that a condition varies with time, geography,[2] or ethnicity. But actually, there is little indication that any important variation exists. Chromosomal biology appears to be rather consistent throughout the human race and across the centuries.

Doing a Segregation Analysis

Segregation analysis is essentially a simple exercise. A farmer who surveys a flock of newborn lambs and notes that 3 are black and 97 are white has done a segregation analysis. In human cytogenetic segregation analysis, the exercise involves looking at a (preferably large) number of offspring of a particular category of parent: parents who carry some particular chromosome rearrangement, or those who have had a child with a chromosomal abnormality while they themselves are karyotypically normal. The proportion of these parents' children who are abnormal is noted (say, 3 out of 100), and this datum serves as the point estimate of the recurrence risk (thus, 3%).

Although segregation analysis is simple in principle, there are potential pitfalls in its application, the most important of which is *ascertainment bias*. We will deal with this problem only briefly. It is important that the counselor know of ascertainment bias, and recognize whether it has been accounted for in the published works consulted. But it is not necessary to understand the complex and sophisticated mechanics of segregation analysis in detail. The reader wishing fuller instruction is referred to Murphy and Chase (1975), Emery (1986), and Stene and Stengel-Rutkowski (1988). The classic example of ascertainment bias is that of the analysis of the sex ratio in sibships of military recruits in World War I. Adding up the numbers of brothers and sisters, there was a marked excess of males. But of course (in 1914–1918) the recruit himself *had* to be male. Once he was excluded from the total in each sibship, the overall sex ratio was normal, namely

[2] A curious difference in the types of chromosome abnormality from prenatal testing in different regions of China (J Zhang et al. 2023a) remains unexplained.

1.0. Likewise, in a cytogenetic segregation analysis, the individual whose abnormality brought the family to attention—the proband—is excluded from the calculation. That person *had* to be abnormal. Furthermore, for very many classical chromosomal scenarios, that individual's carrier parent, grandparent, and so on in a direct vertical line, had to be phenotypically normal to have been a parent. These individuals must also be excluded from an analysis of their own sibship, if that generation is available for study. Other sibships may be included in full.

These manipulations—dropping the proband and the heterozygous direct-line antecedents—are the major steps to be taken to avoid the distorting effects of ascertainment bias. Another potential methodological confounder for the aficionado is *ascertainment probability*. For example, families with more affected members may be more likely to come to medical attention, which would unduly weight the data. There are means to overcome this problem.

Family/population studies on the microdeletions, microduplications, and copy number variants (CNVs) of 21st-century chromosomology present a more difficult problem. Non-penetrance and variable expressivity, and phenotypes confined to intellectual/behavioral traits and in some of mild degree, complicate the picture. Where is the threshold to be taken as affected/unaffected? The pioneers in this field are Vassos et al. (2010) and Rosenfeld et al. (2013), who compared prevalences of CNVs in affected cohorts versus a presumed normal population. The work of Vassos et al. was focused specifically on schizophrenia. Goh et al. (2025) undertook a formal review of several published studies, calculating penetrance values for many CNVs, and these data are listed in Appendix C. We discuss these conditions in Chapter 14 and Chapter 18.

Essential to a good analysis is good data, or at least as good as possible. Some retrospective information may be uncertain. In a family translocation study, did a phenotypically abnormal great uncle who died as a child in 1930 have the "family aneuploidy"? (Old photos may be very helpful in this respect.) Some family skeletons may remain in cupboards unopened to the interviewer. Particularly in the follow-up of prenatal diagnosis results, it is important to know the endpoint of data collection of the child and how the data were collected: at birth or until school age, by formal examination or by anecdotal report. The investigative zeal, clinical judgment, and personal qualities of the researcher are crucial in getting the right information, and getting it all.

THE DERIVATION OF A "PRIVATE" RECURRENCE RISK FIGURE

We will demonstrate some of the previously noted principles in estimating a private recurrence risk figure for the hypothetical family depicted in Figure 4–1. Six sibships are available for analysis: one in generation II, two in generation III, and three in generation IV. We determine the segregation ratio in each. It is conventional to form a table with a row for each sibship, noting the numbers of phenotypically normal (carrier, non-carrier, unkaryotyped) and phenotypically abnormal offspring (Table 4–1). The figures in parentheses give raw totals in these sibships, but then the proband (IV:4) and his heterozygous antecedents (II:1 and III:1) are excluded from their sibships.

Note that I:1's heterozygosity must be inferred from his wife's and children's karyotypes. (It is a subtle question whether his offspring should properly be included in the analysis, which we will not pursue here.) We see that the offspring of heterozygous parents total 14, the proband and the heterozygous antecedents having been excluded. The proportion of abnormal children is 3/14 (0.21). This, then, is a point estimate of the risk for recurrence in a future pregnancy of a heterozygote. The reader should know intuitively

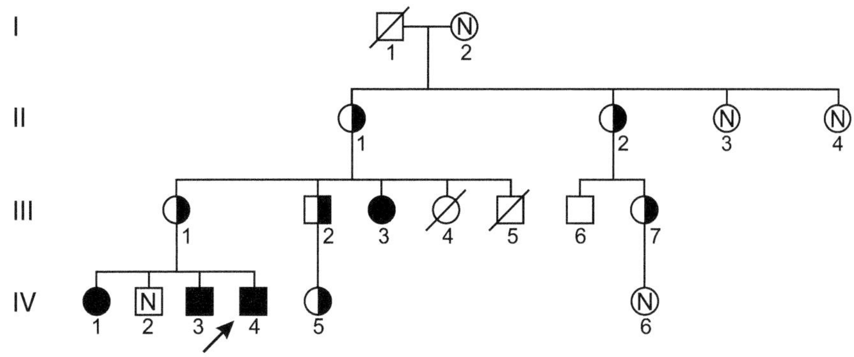

Figure 4–1. A Family Study.

Notes: Hypothetical pedigree in which a chromosomal rearrangement is segregating. Filled symbol, abnormal individual with unbalanced karyotype; half-filled symbol, balanced carrier; N in symbol = 46,N. The proband is, as is conventional, indicated by an arrow.

that an estimate based on just 14 children is not going to be very precise (but not to be discarded). And what of children who had died before the family cytogenetic study was done? Let us suppose this was the case with III:4 and 5. If there was good historic evidence for their having been chromosomally abnormal, a better estimate would be 5/14 (0.36).

> VanDerwerken (2015) takes the sophistication of a "private" risk assessment to a further level, in applying the principles of Bayesian analysis. He proposes that a prior probability due to relevant literature data is usefully to be taken into account, and that this can fine-tune the accuracy of advice given. The mathematically sophisticated reader is referred to his paper.

Genetic Heterogeneity and the Use of Empiric Risk Data

It is not necessarily valid to extrapolate from one family's experience to a prediction for another. Different factors may cause an abnormality in different families. As an obvious example, it would be misleading to "lump" all Down syndrome families to determine

Table 4–1. Calculating a Recurrence Risk Due to a Familial Translocation

PARENT OF SIBSHIP	SIBSHIPS				
	AFFECTED	CARRIER	NON-CARRIER	UNKARYOTYPED	TOTAL
I:1	0	1 (2)	2	0	3
II:1	1	1 (2)	0	2	4
II:2	0	1	0	1	2
III:1	2 (3)	0	1	0	3
III:2	0	1	0	0	1
III:7	0	0	1	0	1
Total	3	4	4	3	14

Notes: These data come from the family shown in Figure 4–1. The numbers in brackets refer to the raw totals, before the removal of the proband and the heterozygous antecedents.

a recurrence risk figure. We need to "split" into the different karyotypic classes of standard trisomy, familial translocations, and de novo translocations. The standard trisomic category requires further splitting in terms of maternal age. In a unique case, a woman had three trisomy 21 conceptions and displayed a tendency to produce multiple cells with differing ("variegated") aneuploidies in at least skin, blood, and gonad (Fitzgerald et al. 1986). She required unique advice. And in reciprocal translocation families, uniqueness is the rule!

It is generally reasonable (and often all that is feasible or possible) to apply a risk figure derived from the study of families with a similar, albeit not exactly identical, chromosomal arrangement. But occasionally a family is large enough for a "private" estimate of the recurrence risk to be made from the family itself. This estimate, if it is precise enough (see the later discussion of confidence limits and standard error), is the most valid to offer that family.

Pregnancy Outcomes to which the Risk Figures Refer

With particular reference to the situation of a parent heterozygous for a chromosomal rearrangement, risk figures are generally presented in terms of "the risk that a liveborn child would have a chromosome imbalance related to the parental translocation." The numerator is the number of aneuploid babies, and the denominator is the number of all babies. Thus, considering the example of the common t(11;22)(q23;q11) translocation (Chapter 5), Stengel-Rutkowski et al. (1988) accumulated data on a total of 318 births (the denominator) to carrier parents, of whom, after ascertainment correction, nine (the numerator) had the 47,+der(22) aneuploidy, and 9/318 gives the risk expressed as a percentage, 2.8%. Separating out mothers and fathers, the respective risk figures are 3.7% (9/241) and <0.7% (0/77).

For those choosing prenatal diagnosis, the risk figure of interest relates to the timing of the procedure, generally chorionic villus sampling (usually done at 10–12 weeks) and amniocentesis (15–17 weeks). In other words, they want to know how likely it is they will have to face the actuality of a decision about termination. The risk here is likely to be higher (7% in the case of the 11;22 translocation), given that some of the abnormal pregnancies would have spontaneously aborted some time after that period of gestation. Table 4–2 sets out these and other possible ways of considering risk.

Table 4–2. Different Ways of Looking at the Quantum of Reproductive Risk Due to a Parent Being a Carrier of a Chromosomal Rearrangement

NUMERATOR	DENOMINATOR
Abnormal liveborn baby	All liveborns
Abnormal liveborn baby	All recognized pregnancies
Abnormal amniocentesis result (early second trimester)	All pregnancies at ~16 weeks
8–14 week miscarriage	All recognized pregnancies
Abnormal embryo on biopsy	All embryos from one in vitro fertilization procedure

Association: Coincidental or Causal?

The counselor not infrequently encounters the problem of a chromosomal "abnormality" discovered in a phenotypically abnormal individual but in whose family, others—who are quite normal—are then shown to have, apparently, exactly the same rearrangement. Does a genetic risk apply, then, to children of the carrier, to whom the same rearranged chromosome may be transmitted? From classical cytogenetics, the familial paracentric inversion is a good example. In a review of 69 probands, Price et al. (1987) list the phenotypic abnormalities that led to these individuals coming to a chromosome study. There was a collection of various clinical indications, with no consistent pattern (other than that intellectual disability was frequent), and several ascertained quite by chance at prenatal diagnosis. By definition, one parent carries the same inversion; and if the net is widened, often other relatives do so as well (Groupe de Cytogénéticiens Français 1986a). In this context, and provided of course that the carrier relatives are phenotypically normal, one would reach the conclusion that the chromosome rearrangement was balanced, with no functional compromise of the genome, and that it was coincidence that led to its discovery (Romain et al. 1983).

But when some very unusual clinical picture is associated with a paracentric inversion that is rare or previously undescribed (as many inversions are), some writers are skeptical of coincidence and propose a causal link (Fryns et al. 1994; Urioste et al. 1994). Similarly, Wenger et al. (1995), noting the coincidence of children with an apparently balanced familial translocation and being phenotypically abnormal, wrote that "the chance that two rare events in the same individual are unrelated seems unlikely to us." Here, there is a risk of deception due to "Kouska's fallacy"—Kouska was a fictional 19th-century philosopher who concluded that the combination of unlikely events that led to his parents meeting was too implausible to believe, and that therefore he himself could not exist (Lubinsky 1986). As does Lubinsky, we must insist on the point: The proband *had* to be phenotypically abnormal, and the coexistence of a subsequently discovered different abnormal event (the karyotype) need not be seen as necessarily remarkable. (Having made that point, we cannot, nevertheless, discount the alternative interpretation that these authors may indeed have concluded correctly.)

A similar question arises when two rare karyotypes are seen in the same family, or when one individual has more than one aneuploidy. A double aneuploidy such as Klinefelter plus Down syndrome, 48,XXY,+21, could be interpreted as two separately arising nondisjunctions but with each occurring on the basis of the same underlying predisposing factor (such as maternal age). The two conditions occur together more often than the product of the frequency of each singly, which would be consistent with that interpretation. Alternatively, if the XXY component could be shown to reflect a paternal meiotic error, while the trisomy 21 was of maternal origin, then the association could be seen as coincidental.

Two different types of abnormality, such as Klinefelter plus Prader-Willi syndrome (a handful of cases of which have been published; see Nowaczyk et al. 2004), might also be judged to reflect two unrelated abnormal events, at least for the deletional form of Prader-Willi syndrome, given that the mechanisms leading to nondisjunction and to deletion are quite different. The prior probability of two abnormal karyotypes coinciding might be a very small figure (1/2000 × 1/15,000 = 1/30,000,000 in the foregoing example); but recalling that the range of abnormal karyotypes is very wide, it should not necessarily be seen as reflecting some extraordinary predisposition when two abnormalities are diagnosed in the one individual or family. Coincidences do happen, and interesting coincidences are publishable (Schneider et al. 2004).

In the molecular era, the matter of CNVs brings the question of causality into a sharp focus, although some of the answers may be less than sharp. A small molecular duplication, for example, which might at first sight appear to be a plausible candidate as explanation for a child's abnormal phenotype, may be judged less likely as culpable if the same observation is made on the DNA sample from a parent. And yet, in the complexity that CNVs present, there may yet remain a possibility that such a duplication could contribute to abnormality when existing on a different genetic background. In other words, and as discussed above, a particular CNV may be nonpenetrant in a parent but penetrant in the child—a concept that hitherto has had little relevance in clinical cytogenetics. We can expect that CNV associations and their causing, or not, of abnormality will continue to be an active area of study (and see Chapter 18, Chapter 25, and Appendix C).

PRESENTATION OF A RISK FIGURE

A risk figure is a probability statement, and it should be presented as such to the counselee in everyday language—for example, "There is a 50/50 chance for such and such an event," and "The risk for such and such to happen is around one chance in 10." The raw probability figure may not of itself be sufficient, and it is a test of the counselor's skill to interpret figures so as to provide empathic guidance rather than presumptuous direction. Loaded interpretative comments such as "The risk is quite high that . . ." or "There is only a small chance that . . ." should be used with great care. The perception of a risk figure as high or low may vary greatly according to an individual's personality and life experiences, and the way he or she uses the language of numbers; the very act of discussing the risk may help the client see it in a less threatening light (Kessler and Levine 1987). Some counselors use diagrams with cartoons showing a crowd of 100 people, with the risk fraction shown in a different color.

Dealing with risk advice in a pregnancy, in particular, can be anxiety-inducing. Nagle et al. (2009) examined the views of 294 Australian mothers in the postpartum period and recorded preferences for how these women felt, in retrospect, that a risk of having a child with Down syndrome might best have been conveyed. The choices were as follows, with the fractions of the women choosing each category shown:

1. As a number in percentage, such as "1%" or "0.05%"	13%
2. In words such as "no increased risk" or "increased risk"	13%
3. As numbers such as "1 in 10" or "1 in 1000"	37%
4. In words such as "high risk" or "low risk"	19%
5. Other (please specify)	0%
A combination of the above	18%

None of these stood out as an obvious best to help the counselor decide on the most appropriate approach. People are different!

And people can see the same risk from different positions. For example, older women having an increased age-related risk (say, 1 in 100) for a child with Down syndrome may decide against an amniocentesis if a screening test gives a risk (say, 1 in 200) that is above the cut-off for access to amniocentesis (1 in 250) but lower than their "starting figure"; whereas a younger woman with an age-related risk of, for example, 1 in 500 is likely to opt for amniocentesis if she were to have the same 1 in 200 result from the screening test (Beekhuis et al. 1994).

Responses to risk figures might not always be what we, as scientifically trained professionals, would necessarily consider objective. This is in the nature of the human condition! Urquhart (2016), a folklorist, gives her own perspective on the counseling she received during the course of prenatal diagnosis (in this case not for a chromosome condition, but rather for a Mendelian disorder, albinism). She had

> "always had an insatiable urge to know the future. Coupled with a keen interest in the supernatural—as a folklore scholar and as a layperson—this has led me to forms of soothsaying like tarot cards and runes but also to the people who trade in clairvoyance."

When she was about to hear the results of her amniocentesis test, she writes, "First, she [the counselor] tells me the odds. But the numbers never meant anything to me. I put as much faith in those predictions as I might in a palm reading. This child will either have albinism, or he will not." In the event—to her initial consternation, but then fierce acceptance—he did not.

PRECISION OF THE RISK FIGURE

As noted above, theoretical risk figures are true, and empiric risk figures are estimates; the former are exact, and the latter are not. For an empiric figure we have a point estimate (e.g., 10%) and a likely range (e.g., 5%–15%) of where the risk actually is. The more data that have been gathered, the more accurate the estimate and the narrower the likely range—and the more confidently, therefore, can the counselor present the figure. The likely range can be measured in different ways. The standard error, which formally measures the precision of the estimate, can be used to give a sense of the region within which the true risk can realistically be considered to lie. The 95% confidence limits define the broad range that very probably ($p = 0.95$) encompasses the true risk.

PART TWO

PARENT OR CHILD WITH A CHROMOSOMAL ABNORMALITY

5
AUTOSOMAL RECIPROCAL TRANSLOCATIONS

RECIPROCAL TRANSLOCATIONS ARE common, and about one or two people per 1,000 are carriers. Every counselor can expect to see translocation families. The usual form is the simple, or two-way, reciprocal translocation: Only two chromosomes, usually autosomes, are involved, with one breakpoint in each. It is this category we consider in this chapter. The special cases of translocations involving sex chromosomes, and of complex translocations, are dealt with in separate chapters.

The translocation heterozygote (carrier) may have a risk to have a child who would be intellectually and physically abnormal due to a "segmental aneusomy": that is, segments that are not euploid. Typically, the imbalance is due to a segment of one of the participating chromosomes being duplicated and a segment of the other chromosome being deleted. This confers a partial trisomy and a concomitant partial monosomy. A few translocations are associated with a high risk, as much as 20% or, very rarely, up to 50% or more, to have an abnormal child. Many translocations imply an intermediate level of risk in the region of 5%–10%. Some carriers have a low risk, 1% or less; but the woman who is a carrier, or the partner of a male carrier, may have a high miscarriage rate. Others imply, apparently, no risk to have an abnormal child, but the likelihood of miscarriage is high. Yet others, discovered fortuitously, seem to be of no reproductive significance, with carriers having no difficulties in conceiving or carrying pregnancies and having normal children. The counselor needs to distinguish these different functional categories of translocation, in order to provide each family with tailor-made advice.

BIOLOGY

Simple reciprocal translocations (*rcp*) arise when a two-way exchange of material takes place between two chromosomes. This event might, for example, occur in one gamete of a 46,N parent, who then has a child who carries this de novo translocation. Or, the translocation could have been familial, transmitted through generations, and sometimes of centuries-long duration. For example, Koskinen et al. (1993) trace a t(12;21) in western Finland back to a couple born in 1752.

The process of formation follows the physical apposition of a segment of each chromosome, which may have been promoted by the presence in each segment of a similar DNA sequence. A break occurs in one arm of each chromosome, and the portions of chromosome material distal to the breakpoints switch positions. The distal portions exchanged are the *translocated segments*; the rest of the chromosome (which includes the centromere) is the *centric segment*. The rearranged chromosome is called a *derivative* (der) chromosome. It is identified according to which centromere it possesses, as in the der(5) and der(10) depicted in Figure 5–1. When no loss or perturbation of genetic

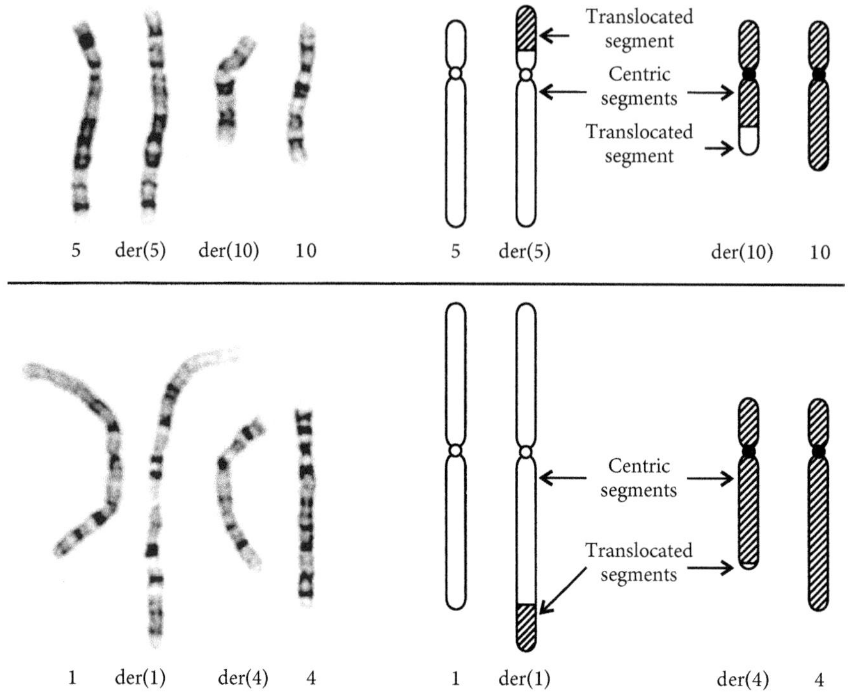

Figure 5–1. The Reciprocal Translocation.
Reciprocal translocations demonstrating (*above*) double-segment and (*below*) single-segment exchange. The translocations are t(5;10)(p13;q23.3) and t(1;4)(q44;q31.3). (Cases of MA Leversha and NA Adams.)

material occurs—in other words, the translocation is balanced—the phenotype of the heterozygote is normal, other things being equal.

When one of the translocated segments is very small and comprises only the telomeric cap of a chromosome arm—and thus we suppose contains no genes—this is regarded as being, effectively, a *single-segment* exchange. The t(1;4) translocation shown in Figure 5–1, involving a substantial piece of chromosome 4 long arm exchanging positions with the terminal tip of a chromosome 1 long arm, exemplifies single-segment exchange. On the other hand, when both translocated segments are of substantial size, we refer to this as a *double-segment*[1] exchange. The translocation shown in Figure 5–1 between a chromosome 5 and a chromosome 10, with breakpoints in about the mid-short arm of chromosome 5 and a little below the middle of the chromosome 10 long arm, is an example of a double-segment exchange. The translocation involving breakpoints right at, or actually within, the centromere, with

[1] There is scope for confusion in the use of these terms: Of course, all reciprocal exchanges, by definition, involve two segments. A true single-segment exchange—that is, a one-way translocation—is generally considered not to exist, in that a segment of chromosome cannot attach to an intact telomere, although there are rare exceptions to this rule. The distinction begins to break down when a translocated segment is very small (subtelomeric) but could still contain genes. Be this as it may, the terms double- and single-segment exchange, used knowledgeably, serve a practical purpose.

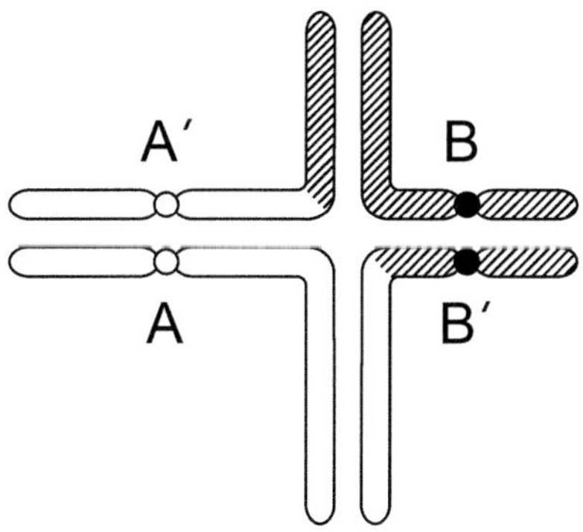

Figure 5–2. Meiotic Behavior of the Reciprocal Translocation.
Pachytene configuration, simplified outline. The two normal (A, B) and the two translocation (A′, B′) homologs align corresponding segments of chromatin during meiosis I.

an exchange of entire arms, is a particular and rare type of double-segment exchange known as a *whole-arm* translocation.

Details of Meiotic Behavior

At meiosis I in the primary gametocyte, the oöcyte or spermatocyte, the four chromosomes with segments in common come together as a foursome: a *quadrivalent.* In order to match homologous segments, the four chromosomes must form a cross-shaped configuration. This is most clearly seen when the chromosomes are at the pachytene stage (Figure 5–2). As meiosis progresses, the four components of the quadrivalent release their points of attachment except at the tips of the chromosome arms, and they form a ring. If attachment fails, or if one of the terminal pairings releases, a chain forms instead of a ring (Oliver-Bonet et al. 2004). With breakdown of the nuclear envelope, spindles forming at each pole of the cell can track to the equator and seek attachment to the centromeres. A cellular motor comes into play, and each chromosome travels to one or other pole.

According to which spindle attaches to which centromere—and this may in part be influenced by the configuration of the ring or chain—the distribution of the four chromosomes to the two daughter gametocytes is determined. Which chromosomes go to which pole is referred to as *segregation.* The expression *2:2 segregation* describes two chromosomes going to one daughter cell, and two to the other. In *3:1 segregation*, three chromosomes go to one daughter cell, and one to the other. In *4:0 segregation*, all four chromosomes go to one daughter cell, and none to the other.

Modes of Segregation

Within these three broad categories we can list the particular modes of segregation, according to which chromosomes actually go where. Referring to the four chromosomes of the quadrivalent as A, B, A′, and B′ (Figure 5–2), the modes of segregation are summarized as follows (Table 5–1):

Table 5–1. Modes of Segregation of Reciprocal Translocations

ONE DAUGHTER GAMETOCYTE WITH:	OTHER DAUGHTER GAMETOCYTE WITH:	SEGREGATION MODE
2:2 Segregations		
A and B	A′ and B′	Alternate segregation
A and B′	B and A′	Adjacent-1 segregation
A and A′	B and B′	Adjacent-2 segregation
3:1 Segregations		
A B and A′	B′	3:1 segregation with tertiary trisomy or monosomy
A B and B′	A′	
A′ B′ and A	B	3:1 segregation with interchange trisomy or monosomy
A′ B′ and B	A	
4:0 Segregation		
A B A′ B′	None	4:0 segregation with double trisomy or monosomy

Figure 5–3 depicts five of the possible pairs of daughter gametocytes. Other things being equal, the chromosomal combination is conserved through meiosis II, and the mature gamete forms. From one primary gametocyte, one ovum and its polar bodies, or four spermatozoa, are thus produced. Gametes from alternate segregation are normal or balanced, and the conceptions from them likewise normal or balanced, other things being equal. Conceptions from adjacent-1 gametes have a partial trisomy (duplication) of one translocated segment and partial monosomy (deletion) of the other. Adjacent-2 conceptions have a duplication of one centric segment and deletion of the other. Tertiary aneuploidies have duplication, or deletion, with respect to the combined chromosomal content of one of the derivative chromosomes. Interchange aneuploidies have a full autosomal trisomy or a full monosomy. In 4:0 segregation, there is a double trisomy or a double monosomy. Some of the gametes with these unbalanced combinations may be "viable" in the sense of being "capable of giving rise to a conceptus, which would proceed through to the birth of a child." Mostly, in fact, they are not.

Recombination at meiosis I, and asymmetric segregation at meiosis II, can complicate the story, although not often does this have a practical implication. If recombination occurs in the interstitial segment (between the centromere and the breakpoint), further unbalanced combinations are generated, most of which would not be remotely viable. This phenomenon may possibly have some relevance in preimplantation genetic testing, because testing is done at a stage where there has been little opportunity for selective pressure to have had an effect. Scriven et al. (1998) list various of these recombination possibilities, and Van Hummelen et al. (1997) diagram the process with respect to a particular translocation on which they had undertaken sperm studies (and also illustrate the interesting point that a normal/balanced gamete can be restored following recombination in adjacent-1 segregation). The most telling evidence that recombination can happen comes from the observation of a meiosis I chromosome having one normal and one derivative chromatid, and polar body analysis has enabled such an observation to be made (Munné et al. 1998a). At meiosis II, asymmetric segregation may lead to two copies of a derivative chromosome being transmitted, as noted below in the section "Meiosis II Nondisjunction."

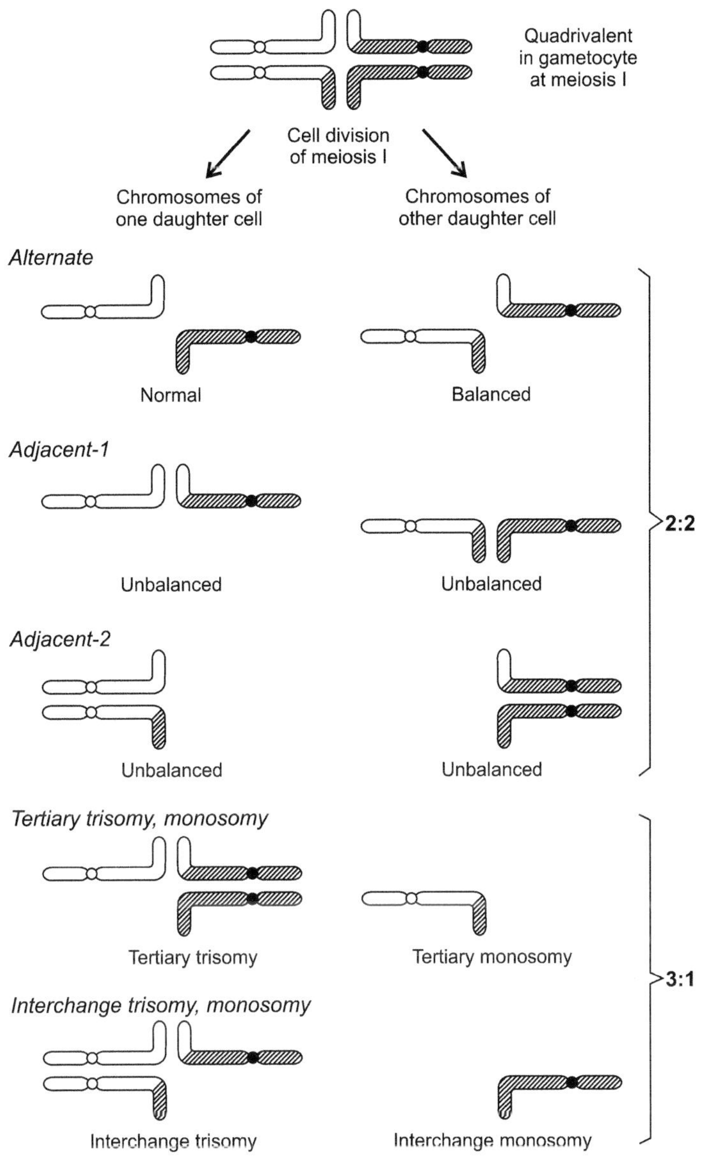

Figure 5–3. Segregation at Meiosis.
The categories of 2:2 and 3:1 segregation that may occur in gametogenesis in the translocation heterozygote. In the four 3:1 categories, only one of the two possible combinations in each category is depicted (both of each are shown in Fig. 5–4).

ALTERNATE SEGREGATION

In 2:2 alternate segregation, looking at each centromere in turn around the quadrivalent, one centromere goes to one pole, and the next centromere goes to the other pole. In other words, each centromere goes "alternately"[2] to one or the other pole. Thus, the two daughter cells come to contain, respectively, the two normal homologs in one, and the

[2] Not "alternatively," as some publications erroneously use.

two derivative chromosomes in the other. Note that alternate segregation is essentially the only mode that leads to gametes with a complete genetic complement—one with a normal karyotype, the other with the reciprocal translocation in the balanced state. All other modes can be classified as *malsegregation.*

ADJACENT SEGREGATION

In 2:2 adjacent segregation, adjacent centromeres travel together ("adjacent" in the sense of centromeres being next to each other in their positions around the quadrivalent). There are two categories. In *adjacent-1* segregation, adjacent chromosomes with unalike (nonhomologous) centromeres travel to the same daughter cell (an aide-mémoire: in adjacent-*1*, the daughter cells get *one* of each centromere). Overall, adjacent-1 is the most frequently seen mode of malsegregation in the children of translocation heterozygotes. In *adjacent-2* segregation, which is rather uncommonly seen, adjacent chromosomes with like (homologous) centromeres go to the same daughter cell (another aide-mémoire: in adjacent-*2*, the *two* homologous centromeres go *to*gether).

3:1 SEGREGATION

This is also referred to as 3:1 nondisjunction. Gametes with 24 chromosomes and 22 chromosomes are formed, and the conceptuses therefore have 47 or 45 chromosomes. Almost always in autosomal translocations, the 47-chromosome conceptus is the only viable one. Two categories exist: Either the two normal chromosomes of the quadrivalent plus one of the translocation chromosomes go together to one daughter cell (*tertiary trisomy*) or, rarely, the two translocation chromosomes and one of the normal chromosomes segregate together (*interchange trisomy*). Tertiary monosomy, with a 45-chromosome conceptus, is very rare. Interchange monosomy is never seen, except at preimplantation genetic testing.

4:0 SEGREGATION

In autosomal translocations, 4:0 segregation has been regarded as being of academic interest only. But it may have some practical relevance in preimplantation genetic testing.

Segregant Outcomes

In theory, 16 possible chromosomal combinations could be produced in the gametes of the autosomal translocation heterozygote. In terms of a consideration of the risk for a liveborn child, four of these we can, for the most part, ignore (3:1 interchange monosomies and 4:0 segregants) because they are never viable. The two balanced gametes (2:2 alternate segregants) are always viable, other things being equal. Of the remaining 10 possibilities, it is common for none to be viable, with non-implantation or spontaneous abortion the inevitable outcome.

If, however, a translocation heterozygote does have the potential for viable imbalance in an offspring, it is most likely that there will be only one such combination (this was the case in 99% and 100% of translocations, respectively, in the considerable experience of two groups; see Scriven et al. 1998). Usually, this sole survivable imbalance will be one that endows a partial trisomy. Infrequently two, and very rarely more than two, of the imbalances may be viable. Figure 5–4 depicts the various combinations that may be considered (using the previously discussed t(1;4) translocation as an example). In a review

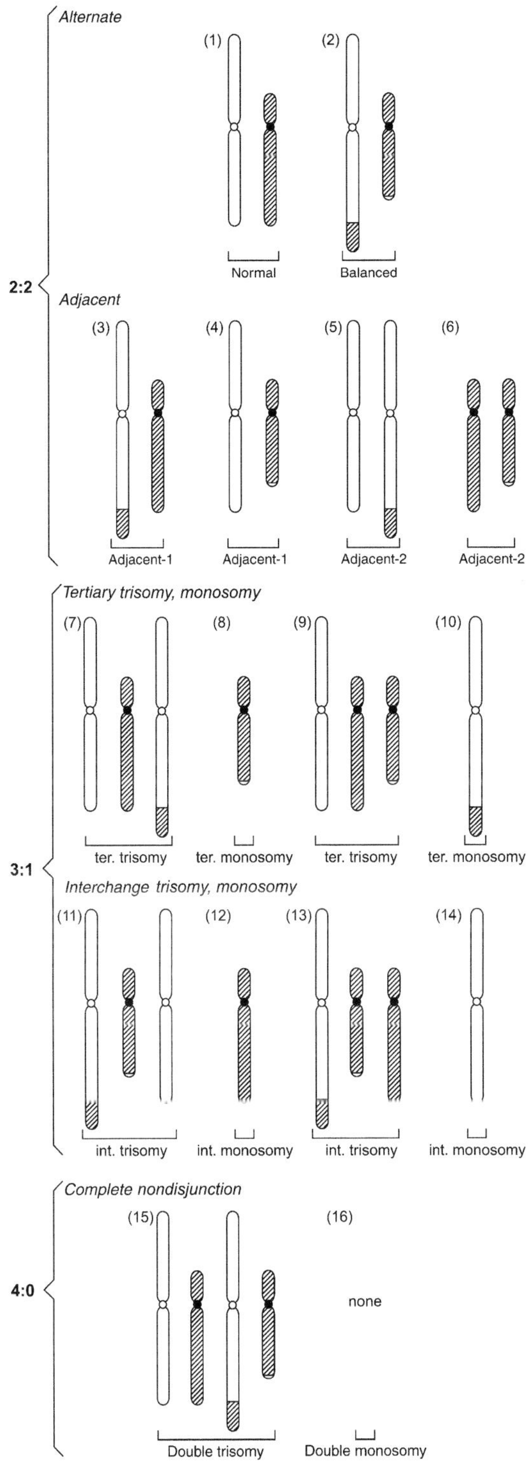

Figure 5–4. The Range of Segregant Gametes.
The full range of segregant gametes that may be produced by the translocation heterozygote, using the t(1;4) depicted in Figure 5–1 as an example. Chromosome 1 chromatin is shown open; chromosome 4 chromatin is cross-hatched.

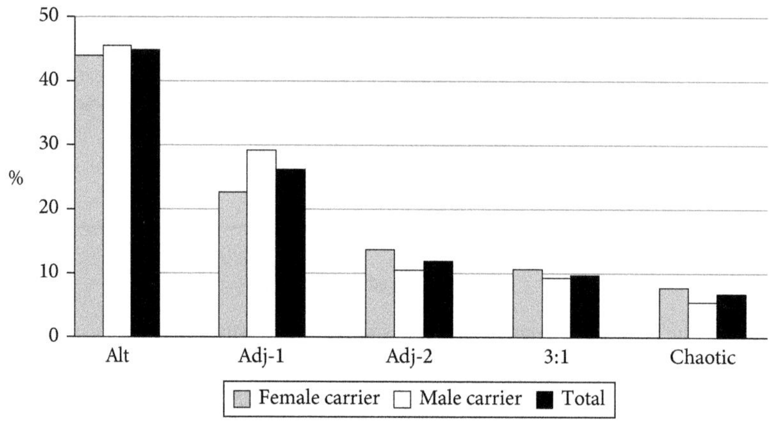

Figure 5–8. Chromosomal Segregations in Day-3 Embryos of Translocation Carriers, According to the Parental Gender.

Source: From J Wang et al., Analysis of meiotic segregation modes in biopsied blastocysts from preimplantation genetic testing cycles of reciprocal translocations, *Mol Cytogenet* 12:11, 2019, with the permission of Springer Nature.

increase is seen in the average normal fraction for embryos (45%) versus gametes (30%), although the oöcyte numbers upon which the 30% figure is based are very small, and this difference should not be unduly weighted. For male translocation heterozygotes, for whom the numbers of gamete observations are substantial, the average normal fraction of embryos (41%) is very similar to that of gametes (44%). Thus, we might infer that balanced and unbalanced gametes have very similar fertilizing/fertilizable capacities and that little selective pressure applies, at least in the first three days of development of the partially aneuploid embryo.[4] There appears to be little difference according to the gender of the translocation parent (Figure 5–8). However, a selective pressure apparently does apply in the short period from the day-3 embryo to the day-5 blastocyst, in particular with respect to 3:1 malsegregants and, in consequence, the relative fractions of alternate and adjacent segregants increase from day 3 to day 5 (Figure 5–9).

Acrocentric Chromosomes. Acrocentric chromosomes participating in a reciprocal translocation might be expected to hinder normal segregation, due to the very small lengths of their short arms and thus a marked asymmetry of the quadrivalent, and more so in the direction of 3:1 malsegregation; and indeed, this is what is observed. In Verdoni et al. (2021), among 196 autosomal translocation couples, one-third involved an acrocentric, but fully half of the instances of 3:1 malsegregation were seen in these cases. Figure 5–10 shows data from Xie et al. (2022), who analyzed over 10,000 blastocysts from 2,253 translocation couples, teasing out the influence of gender and whether or not the translocation included an acrocentric chromosome. The tendency to 3:1 malsegregation in the female carrier, and more particularly so with an acrocentric-related translocation, is well illustrated. The early (day 3 to day 5) lethality of many 3:1 conceptions is noted in Figure 5–9.

[4] And yet, not all studies support such a conclusion. In a study based upon 10 male rcp heterozygotes, Haapaniemi Kouru et al. (2017) made the curious observation that the proportions of unbalanced forms seen at the day-3 embryo stage (52%) were very substantially greater than the fractions at sperm analysis (21%) might have suggested. The authors conclude that sperm FISH is not a reliable indicator of PGT outcome.

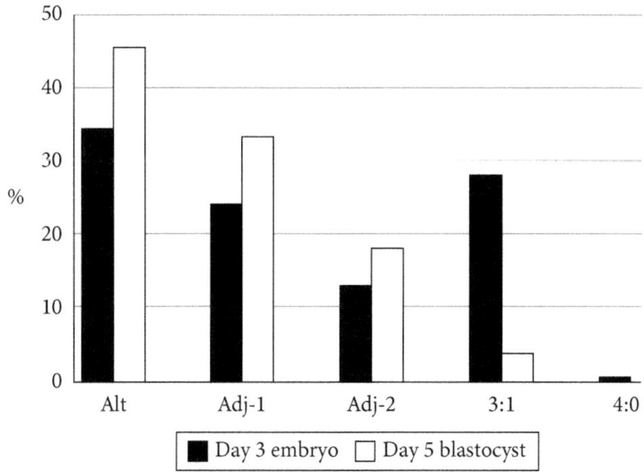

Figure 5–9. Comparing Chromosomal Segregations in Day-3 and Day 5 Embryos of Translocation Carriers.

Notes: Segregant categories from rcp carriers, comparing observations at day 3 embryos cf. day 5 blastocysts. The substantial fall-off of 3:1 from day 3 to day 5 leads to higher relative fractions of alternate and adjacent conceptions remaining. The difference in the Day 3 fractions cf. Figure 5-8 lies in the proportions, in the two studies, of 3:1 cases.

Source: From ZN Tonyan et al., Assessment of quadrivalent characteristics influencing chromosome segregation by analyzing human preimplantation embryos from reciprocal translocation carriers, *Comp Cytogenet* 18:1–13, 2024. Courtesy ZN Tonyan, and with the permission of Pensoft.

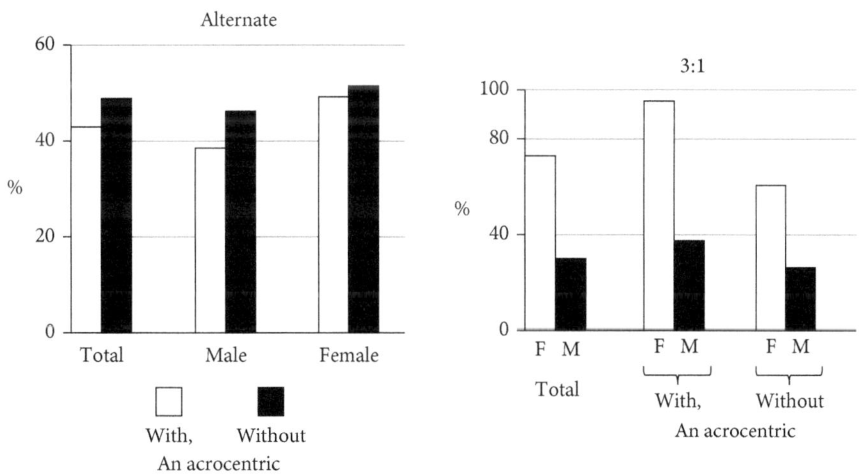

Figure 5–10. The Influence of Parental Gender on Translocation Segregation, as Observed at the Blastocyst Stage.

Notes: The fractions of segregation types are shown according to the gender of the translocation carrier parent, and according to the participation, or not, of an acrocentric chromosome in the rearrangement. Note that alternate segregation is slightly favored in the absence of an acrocentric, while 3:1 is markedly favored when an acrocentric is present. F = female, M = male, y axis is % of all embryos in this series. Compare the data in Figure 5–7, based upon day-3 embryos, at which earlier stage the parental gender has apparently had little influence upon 3:1 malsegregation.

Source: Adapted from P Xie et al., Risk factors affecting alternate segregation in blastocysts from preimplantation genetic testing cycles of autosomal reciprocal translocations, *Front Genet* 13:880208, 2022. Courtesy G Lin, and with the permission of Frontiers in Genetics.

Viability In Utero. Further along in pregnancy, most unbalanced combinations would produce such enormous genetic imbalance that the conceptus would be lost very early in pregnancy (occult abortion), or even fail to implant. Moderate imbalances could, following implantation, proceed to the stage of recognizable miscarriage or to later fetal death in utero. Only those conceptuses with lesser imbalances might eventually result in the birth of an abnormal child.

Viability is much more likely in the case of effective single-segment imbalance, with only one segment of substantial size, as discussed above. This is of particular relevance in adjacent-1 segregation. Consider, for example, gamete (3) in Figure 5–4. The material missing from the telomeric tip of chromosome 1 long arm—the telomeric cap—is so small that its loss is, as far as we can tell, of nil or insignificant phenotypic effect. For practical purposes, we can ignore this partial monosomy. Thus, the significant imbalance reduces to a partial 4q trisomy (dup 4q31.3qter). This, as it happens, is well recognized as being a viable complement (and it is the imbalance in the children whose photograph appears in the frontispiece). On the other hand, in the double-segment exchange, the imbalance contributed by each segment must be taken into account. Thus, adjacent-1 gametes have both a partial trisomy and a partial monosomy to a significant degree and would produce a "phenotypic hybrid." Very frequently, such a combination is nonviable.

Predicting Segregant Outcomes

How can we determine, for the individual translocation carrier, which segregant outcomes, if any, might lead to the birth of an abnormal child? What might be the relative roles of an inherent tendency for a particular type of segregation to occur, and of in utero selection against unbalanced forms? A useful approach is to imagine how the chromosomes come to be distributed during meiosis. Following Jalbert et al. (1980, 1988) we may draw, roughly to scale, a diagram of the presumed pachytene configuration of the quadrivalent, and then deduce which modes of segregation are likely to lead to the formation of gametes, which could then produce a viable conceptus. The following, and with reference to Figure 5–11, are the ground rules:

1. We assume that alternate segregation is (a) frequent and (b) associated with phenotypic normality.
2. The least imbalanced, least monosomic of the imbalanced gametes is the one most likely to produce a viable conceptus.
3. If the translocated segments are small in genetic content, adjacent-1 is the most likely type of malsegregation to be capable of giving rise to viable abnormal offspring (Figure 5–11a).
4. If the centric segments are small in content, adjacent-2 is the most likely segregation to give a viable abnormal outcome (Figure 5–11b).
5. If one of the whole chromosomes of the quadrivalent is small in content, typically a small derivative chromosome, 3:1 disjunction is the most likely (Figure 5–11c).
6. If the quadrivalent has characteristics of both Rules 3 and 5, or of Rules 4 and 5, then both adjacent and 3:1 segregations may give rise to viable offspring.
7. If the translocated and centric segments both have large content, no mode of segregation could produce an unbalanced gamete that would lead to a viable offspring (Figure 5–11d).

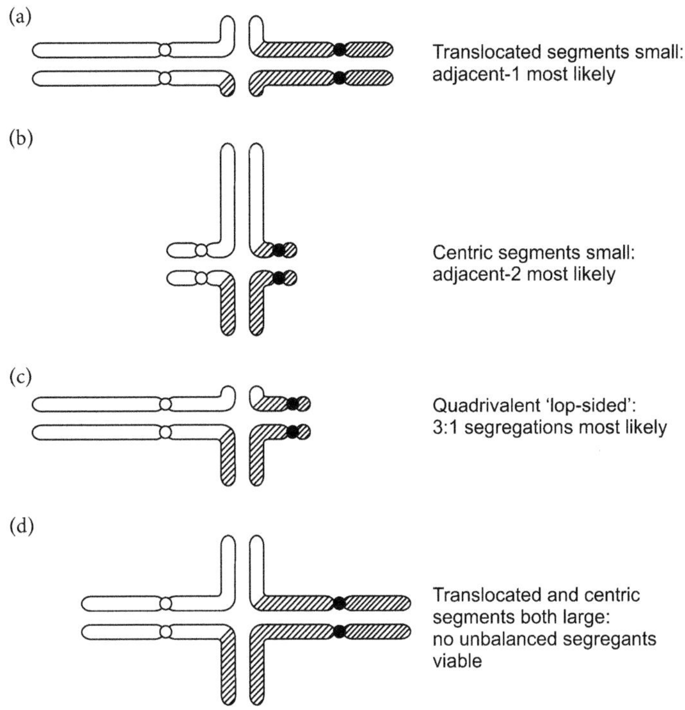

Figure 5–11. Predicting Segregant Outcomes.
Prediction of likely viable segregant outcomes by pachytene diagram drawing and assessment of the configuration of the quadrivalent.

8. If the translocated segments are both very small (subtelomeric), the chromosomes may not necessarily form a quadrivalent, and the pairs of homologs might simply join up as bivalents as if they were normal, each pair then segregating independently.

Some examples to illustrate these points follow.[5]

ADJACENT-1 SEGREGATION, SINGLE-SEGMENT EXCHANGE

Many translocations involve an effectively single-segment exchange, with the "single" translocated segment comprising a fairly small amount of chromatin (1%–2% of the haploid autosomal length, or HAL). This is the classical scenario for adjacent-1 segregation to occur, and to produce a phenotype capable of post-natal survival. The family with the t(1;4) in Figure 5–1, whose children with partial 4q trisomy are shown in the frontispiece and as discussed above, provides an example.

Consider now the family whose pedigree is depicted in Figure 5–12a, in which the individuals shown as heterozygotes have the balanced translocation t(3;11)(p26;q21). A segment of chromatin consisting of almost half of the long arm of chromosome 11, and comprising 1.4% of the HAL, is translocated to the tip of chromosome 3 short arm

[5] The reader wishing to study further worked examples is referred to Midro et al. (1992), who analyze in some detail a series of translocations of differing risk potentials.

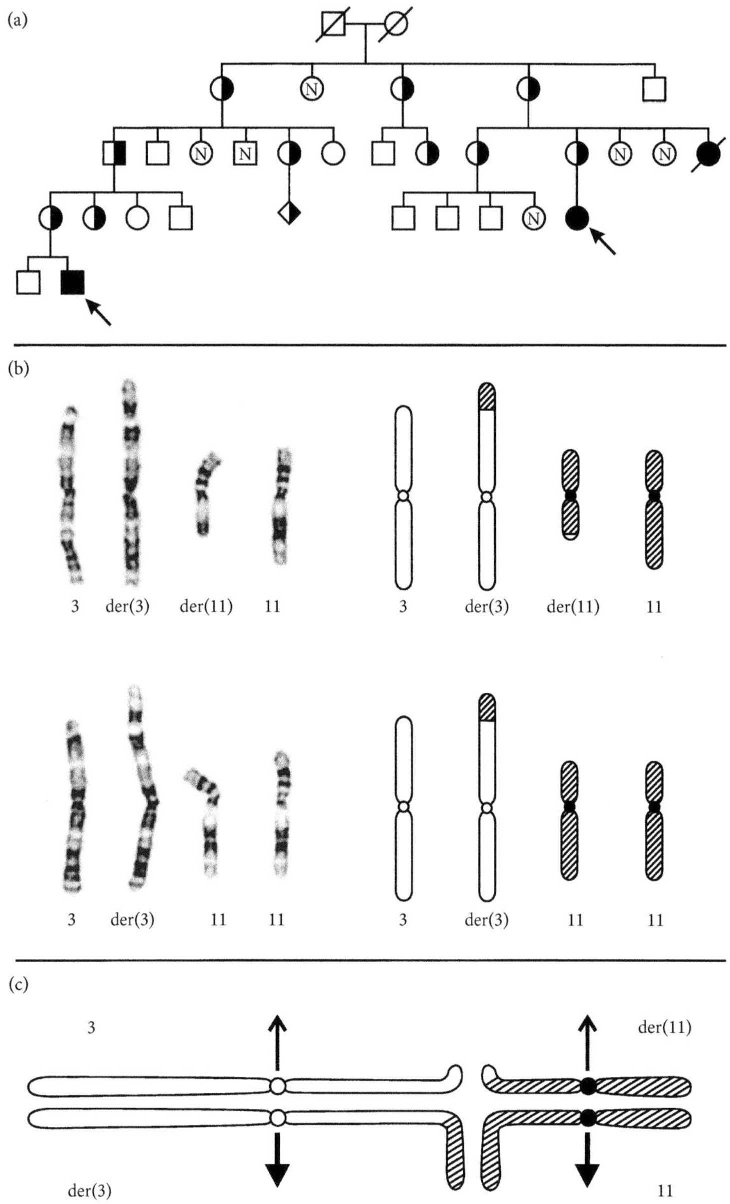

Figure 5–12. Adjacent-1 segregation.
(*a*) Pedigree of a family in which there segregates a t(3;11)(p26;q21) having the characteristics associated with adjacent-1 malsegregation. Two independently ascertained probands have a partial 11q trisomy, and a deceased relative, who died at age 18 years in an institution for the retarded, had a similar appearance from photographs, and so very probably had the same karyotype. Filled symbol, unbalanced karyotype; half-filled symbol, balanced carrier; N in symbol = 46,N; small diamond, prenatal diagnosis; arrow, proband. (*b*) Partial karyotype of a translocation heterozygote (*above*), showing the 3;11 translocation, and a child with the unbalanced complement (*below*). (Case of AJ Watt.) (*c*) The presumed pachytene configuration during gametogenesis in the heterozygote (chromosome 3 chromatin, open; chromosome 11 chromatin, cross-hatched). Arrows indicate movements of chromosomes to daughter cells in adjacent-1 segregation; heavy arrows show the combination observed in this family.

(Figure 5–12b). The telomeric tip of chromosome 3 short arm, which we imagine to comprise little or no phenotypically important genetic material, has moved reciprocally across to chromosome 11.

The presumed pachytene configuration during gametogenesis in the heterozygote would be as drawn in Figure 5–12c. The adjacent-1 segregant gamete with der(3) plus normal 11 (heavy arrows) produces a conceptus that has a partial 11q trisomy, since the der(3) carries the segment 11q21qter. The loss of the 3p telomeric tip in this der(3) we suppose to have no effect. Two, probably three children in the family had been born with this karyotype. No individuals are known having the other adjacent-1 combination (Figure 5–12c, light arrows), that is, the 46,+der(11) karyotype, which would endow a partial 11q monosomy. Consulting Schinzel (2001), viability for the segment 11q21qter in monosomic state is recorded in only two cases. We assume, therefore, that it has a very high lethality in utero.

The scenario of a single survivable imbalanced form due to a partial trisomy from adjacent-1 segregation in a "single-segment" translocation, as in this t(3;11) example, is, as mentioned above, much the most commonly encountered circumstance in translocation families at risk for having an abnormal child.

Infrequently, both the partial trisomic and the partial monosomic forms are observed in families segregating a single-segment rcp. A good example of this is given by distal 4p translocations: Both deletion and duplication for this segment are well recognized as capable of going through to live birth. Consider the translocation t(4;12)(p14;p13) described in a family study in Mortimer et al. (1980). The breakpoints of the translocation are in distal 4p and at the very tip of 12p (12pter). A number of family members over three or more generations were balanced carriers, and abnormal children had been born with typical Wolf-Hirschhorn syndrome (all dying in infancy), while others presented the syndrome of partial 4p trisomy (all surviving at least well into childhood).

The presumed pachytene configuration would be as drawn in Figure 5–11a (imagining the chromosome 4 chromatin open and chromosome 12 chromatin cross-hatched). With such short translocated segments (and very long centric segments), adjacent-1 segregation is the only possibility for viable imbalance. If we ignore the tiny contribution of a duplication or deletion for telomeric 12p—in other words, if we interpret this as an effective single-segment imbalance—the situation reduces to the two possible adjacent-1 outcomes being a partial 4p trisomy and a partial 4p monosomy. Both of these are recognized entities, as noted above, and apparently both have substantial viability in utero. The abnormal karyotypes would be written 46,der(12)t(4;12)(p14;p13) and 46,der(4) t(4;12)(p14;p13).

If the "other segment" can actually be proven not to contain any coding genes, the case for considering the translocation as a single-segment entity is particularly valid, with the resulting imbalances being demonstrably "pure." Martínez-Juárez et al. (2014) allowed such a conclusion to be drawn in the case of two children born from a translocation carrier mother, 46,XX,t(2;12)(p24.2;q24.31). The 12q breakpoint was at chr12:132,960,869, and the 12q translocated segment, which comprised only 300 kb, was beyond the distalmost gene on that chromosome.[6] Thus, the children's abnormal phenotype was due purely to trisomy for the large segment chr2:1-32,745,624

[6] The final nucleotide on chromosome 12, at 12qter, is number 133,275,309.

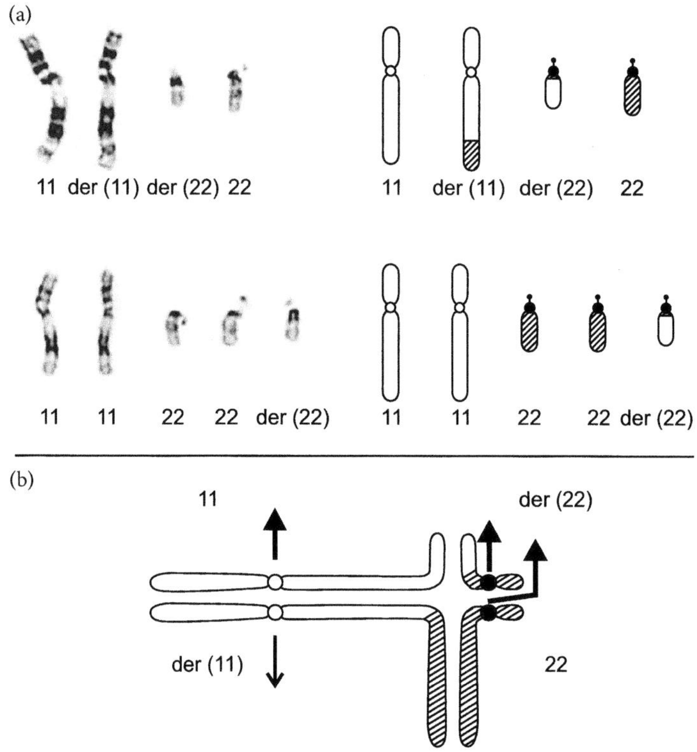

Figure 5–16. Tertiary Trisomy and Emanuel Syndrome.
(*a*) The common t(11;22)(q23;q11) in the heterozygous state (*above*) and in the typical unbalanced state, associated with Emanuel syndrome (*below*). (*b*) The presumed pachytene configuration during gametogenesis in the heterozygote (chromosome 11 chromatin, open; chromosome 22 chromatin, cross-hatched). Arrows indicate movements of chromosomes to daughter cells in a 3:1 tertiary segregation; heavy arrows show the viable trisomic combination.

the requirement for the derivative to have a small short arm, acrocentric chromosome 22 easily qualifies), and its major genetic composition is accounted for by the distal 11q segment. The presence of this 47th chromosome does not necessarily impose a lethal distortion upon intrauterine development, and a pregnancy could continue through to the birth of a child with a 47,+der(22) karyotype, with trisomy for the segment 11q23qter (and for the very small segment 22pter-q11).

The male t(11;22) heterozygote produces other types of unbalanced gamete as shown on sperm chromosome study, but none of these is ever viable.[8] On embryo study, in fact the most frequent category of malsegregation is adjacent-1, with as high as 68% from the male heterozygote and 50% from the female, but none of these will survive; the survivable 3:1 combination accounts for only 5% of embryos (Zenagui et al. 2019).

[8] Except in the extraordinary setting of post-zygotic rescue. Kulharya et al. (2002) report a t(11;22) carrier mother having had a child from presumed adjacent-1 segregation with 46,XY,der(22) at conception, and then mitotic loss of the der(22) in one cell and duplication of the normal 22, leading to 46,XY,der(22)/46,XY mosaicism.

This t(11;22) is the spectacular exception to the rule that, in different families, translocations arise at different sites. The great majority of families have a "private translocation," and many may represent the first and only case in the whole of human evolution. Apparently, few predispositions for specific rearrangement exist. Equally apparently, 11q23 and 22q11 show a remarkable predisposition, which may reflect a physical proximity between the two chromosomes during meiosis (Ashley et al. 2006). Kurahashi and Emanuel (2001) studied normal volunteers and, being able to test very large numbers of sperm, they could show that de novo t(11;22)(q23;q11) translocations must be being generated from time to time; and Ohye et al. (2010), studying eight de novo cases, showed the translocation in each to have been of paternal origin.

Supernumerary Marker Chromosomes. The point is to be noted that probands in whom a supernumerary marker chromosome (SMC) is discovered are often found, on parental study, to have a derivative chromosome reflecting a tertiary trisomy (Stamberg and Thomas 1986). Braddock et al. (2000) describe a family in which an SMC due to 3:1 malsegregation had initially escaped recognition as such. In the family, a child with "atypical Down syndrome" had been karyotyped as trisomy 21. On attending a Down syndrome clinic at age 9 years, the clinical picture raised doubt, and his chromosomes were restudied. He turned out to have a tertiary trisomy for a der(21), which comprised much of chromosome 21 and a small part of distal 5p. His mother and several other relatives carried a t(5;21)(p15.1;q22.1), and a similarly abnormal aunt had the same tertiary trisomy, 47,+der(21). A rather similar account comes from Valetto et al. (2013). A young woman with a mild intellectual disability and what looked like 47,XX,+21 on classical karyotyping proved actually to have 47,XX,+der(21) due a maternal t(8;21)(q24.21;q21.1), and the imbalance precisely defined as dup chr8:128,493,142-145,054,634, dup chr21:13,045,202-22,115,024. In the family in Oubោukss et al. (2024), a child presenting with dysmorphism and psychomotor delay karyotyped initially as having a small SMC due to dup(14). Family studies revealed his mother and brother to carry a t(8;14)(p22.3;q21), and thus the SMC in the child could be seen as a dup14q/dup8p chromosome, from a tertiary trisomy of maternal origin. These stories have lessons both for cytogeneticists and for genetic counselors, although modern methodology will usually allow a "SMC" to be properly identified.

3:1 SEGREGATION WITH TERTIARY MONOSOMY

If one derivative is very small, and the amount of material that is missing is "monosomically small," the countertype 3:1 22-chromosome gamete may lead to a viable conceptus. Consider the 12;13 translocation t(12;13)(p13.32;q12.11) shown in Figure 5–17a. The large derivative chromosome is not far from being a composite of the two complete chromosomes. It is missing only subterminal 12p and pericentromeric chromosome 13. This is a "small" loss, and thus the 45,der(12) conceptus is viable (Figure 5–17b).

Any initially 45-count karyotype obliges consideration that there may, in fact, be a tertiary monosomy. For example, Courtens et al. (1994) describe an infant who died at birth with, at first sight cytogenetically, monosomy 21 (45,–21). But on further study, a 45,+der(1) from a maternal 1;21 translocation was discovered. In Nur et al. (2015), a baby with multiple abnormalities who died at age 5 months had a 45-chromosome count, with a der(18;22) comprising most of chromosomes 18 and 22. Her mother proved to carry a t(18;22)(p11.2;q11.2), enabling a diagnosis in her child of tertiary monosomy for

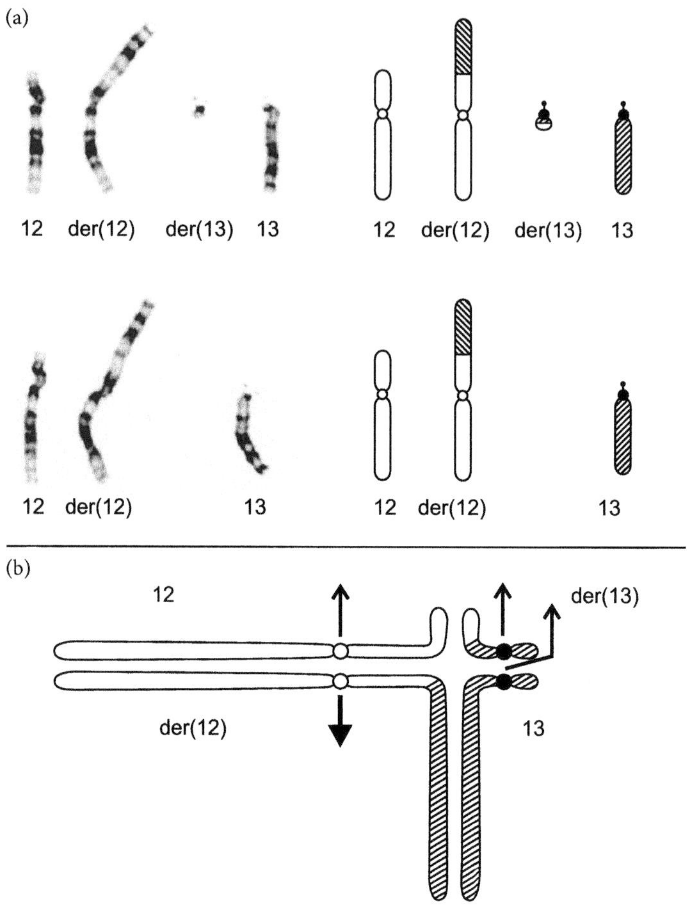

Figure 5–17. Tertiary Monosomy.
(*a*) Mother (*above*) has a reciprocal translocation between nos. 12 and 13, 46,t(12;13)(p13.32;q12.11). Two children (*below*) inherited the derivative 12, but no normal chromosome 12 or 13 from the mother, and have the karyotype 45,der(12). They are thus monosomic for the tip of 12p and pericentromeric 13 (and show only a mildly abnormal phenotype). Chorionic villus sampling in a subsequent pregnancy gave a 46,XX result; an elder sister was a balanced carrier. (Case of MD Pertile) (*b*) The presumed pachytene configuration during gametogenesis in the heterozygote (chromosome 12 chromatin, open; chromosome 13 chromatin, cross-hatched). Arrows indicate movements of chromosomes to daughter cells in a 3:1 tertiary segregation; heavy arrow shows the monosomic complement. Alternatively, the three large chromosomes might form a trivalent, and the tiny der(13), being unattached, might segregate at random.

most of 18p and the DiGeorge critical region of 22q. Prenatal diagnosis at a subsequent pregnancy gave a normal result.

Sometimes the two phenotypes of the two contributing monosomies can be separately discerned. Thus, Reddy et al. (1996) describe children with a combined DiGeorge (DGS) and Wolf-Hirschhorn (WHS) phenotype, having the karyotype 45,der(4)t(4;22)(p16.3;q11.2)mat. The large derivative chromosome comprised almost all of 4 and almost all of 22q, but it lacked the WHS and DGS critical segments. Cases in which one of the deleted segments includes the Angelman region at 15q13 are reported in Wenger et al. (1997) and Torisu et al. (2004), and in which this syndrome is seen in 3:1 malsegregant children of the carrier mother. An interesting historical example, in that it provided a key observation toward the discovery of the *TSC2* locus, is that of a child with 45,der(16), who had monosomy for the segment 16p13pter, and who had both tuberous sclerosis complex and polycystic kidney disease due to loss and disruption, respectively, of the adjacent *TSC2* and *PKD1* loci. The heterozygous 46,t(16;22) family members had polycystic kidney disease, due to the disruption of *PKD1* (European Polycystic Kidney Disease Consortium 1994).

Almost all conceptions with a tertiary monosomy are expected to be lethal preimplantation or in early embryogenesis. A direct demonstration of this circumstance is illustrated in the case of a 3:1 malsegregation of a maternal t(11;22) in a spontaneous abortus at seven weeks gestation with 45,der(11), which resulted in monosomy for distal 11q and monosomy for proximal 22q (Jobanputra et al. 2005).

3:1 SEGREGATION WITH INTERCHANGE TRISOMY

This mode of segregation can only produce a liveborn child when a "trisomically viable chromosome" (i.e., 13, 18, or 21) participates in the translocation (Figure 5–18a). This chromosome accompanies the two translocation (interchange) elements of the quadrivalent to one daughter cell (Figure 5–18b). Interchange trisomy 21 is rare, interchange trisomies 13 and 18 are extremely rare, and interchange trisomy 9 is barely recorded (Table 5–2). Concerning other (nonviable) autosomes, interchange trisomy can be seen at PGT (Lim et al. 2008) or upon analysis of abortus material, such as the trisomy 2 in a pregnancy from a t(2;17)(q32.1;q24.3) carrier discussed in Lorda-Sánchez et al. (2005).

Theoretically, uniparental disomy can be a consequence of interchange trisomy, if one of the "trisomic" chromosomes is subsequently lost post-zygotically and if this chromosome had come from the non-carrier parent. If this chromosome is one that is subject to imprinting according to parent of origin, phenotypic abnormality will be the consequence notwithstanding the apparently balanced karyotype, the same as the parent's. Thus, for example, a 46,t(8;15) father could have a 46,t(8;15) child with Angelman syndrome, or a mother could have a child with Prader-Willi syndrome. Actual examples of this type of mechanism are extremely rare (Table 19–6).

3:1 SEGREGATION WITH INTERCHANGE MONOSOMY

Autosomal monosomy is typically associated with very early arrested development of the embryo. Only with PGT does a practical relevance of interchange monosomy emerge, since there may not yet have been the chance for selection pressure to have operated. In the PGT case reported in Conn et al. (1999) noted earlier, the woman being a t(6;21) heterozygote, a transferred embryo that implanted only transiently may have had an interchange monosomy 6. Sperm capable of giving rise to interchange monosomy can certainly be produced in numbers, as Midro et al. (2006) show in a man heterozygous for a t(7;13)(q34;q13), from whom 2.8% of sperm showed interchange nullisomy 7 and 8.0%

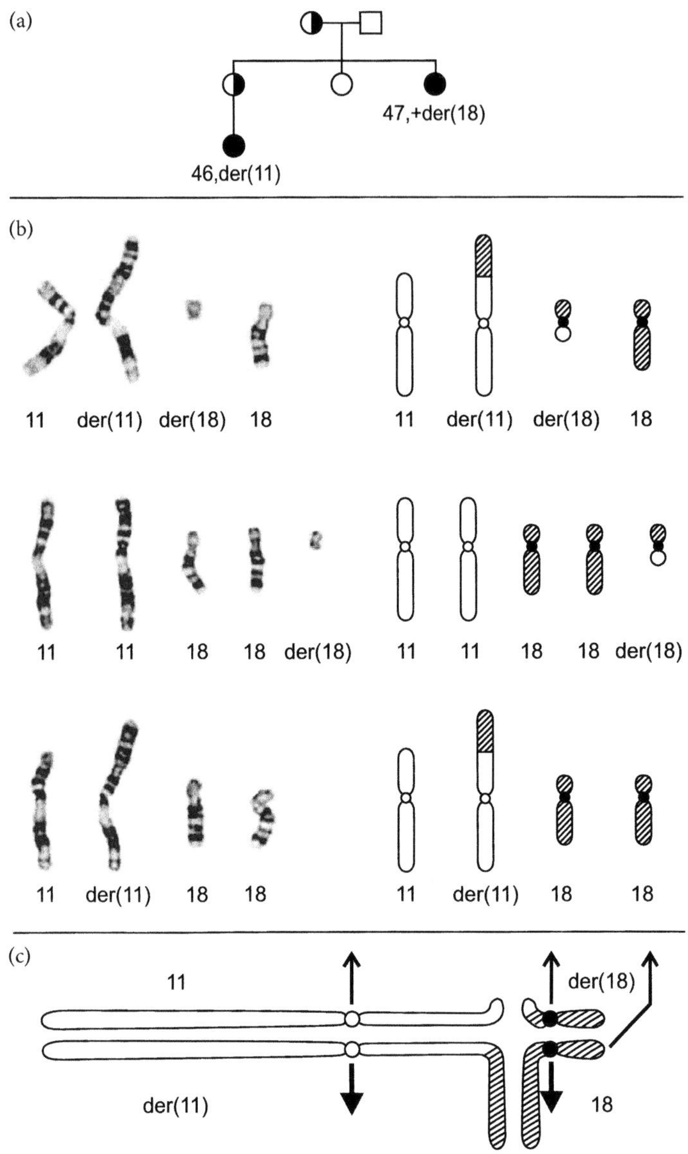

Figure 5–19. More than One Viable Malsegregant Form.
(*a*) Pedigree. Filled symbols, unbalanced karyotype, as shown; half-filled symbols, heterozygote. (*b*) Mother and one daughter have a reciprocal translocation of chromosomes 11 and 18, t(11;18)(p15;q11) (*upper*). Each had one unbalanced offspring, one having 47,+ der(18) due to 3:1 tertiary trisomy (*middle*), and the other 46,+der(11) from adjacent-1 segregation (*lower*). The former had a complete trisomy 18p and the latter a partial 18q trisomy. (Case of C Ho and I Teshima.) (*c*) The presumed pachytene configuration during gametogenesis in the heterozygote (chromosome 11 chromatin, open; chromosome 18 chromatin, cross-hatched). Heavy arrows indicate one adjacent-1 segregant movement of chromosomes, and light arrows indicate movements of chromosomes to daughter cells in a 3:1 tertiary trisomy segregation, each of which occurred in this family.

Source: From RJM Gardner et al., Autosomal imbalance with a near-normal phenotype: The small effect of trisomy for the short arm of chromosome 18, *Birth Defects Orig Artic Ser* 14: 359–363, 1978.

First, the translocated segments are small: 18q is known to be viable in the trisomic state, and the tip of 11p contributes a minimal/nil imbalance (thus, this is regarded as a single-segment imbalance). Accordingly, one of the adjacent-1 segregants is presumed to be viable. Second, two component chromosomes of the pachytene configuration, the der(18) and chromosome 18, are of small overall genetic content. Thus, 3:1 segregation with either tertiary trisomy or interchange trisomy is possible. In the event, the two unbalanced karyotypes in this family reflected adjacent-1 and 3:1 tertiary trisomy segregation.

Rather more spectacular is the translocation illustrated in Figure 5–20. A mother had the karyotype 46,XX,t(18;21)(q22.1;q11.2): these breakpoints are toward the end of 18q and immediately below the centromere in 21q. She had a stillborn child with tertiary monosomy, a miscarriage with adjacent-1 malsegregation (and two other unkaryotyped miscarriages), and a surviving child with tertiary trisomy. These three karyotyped

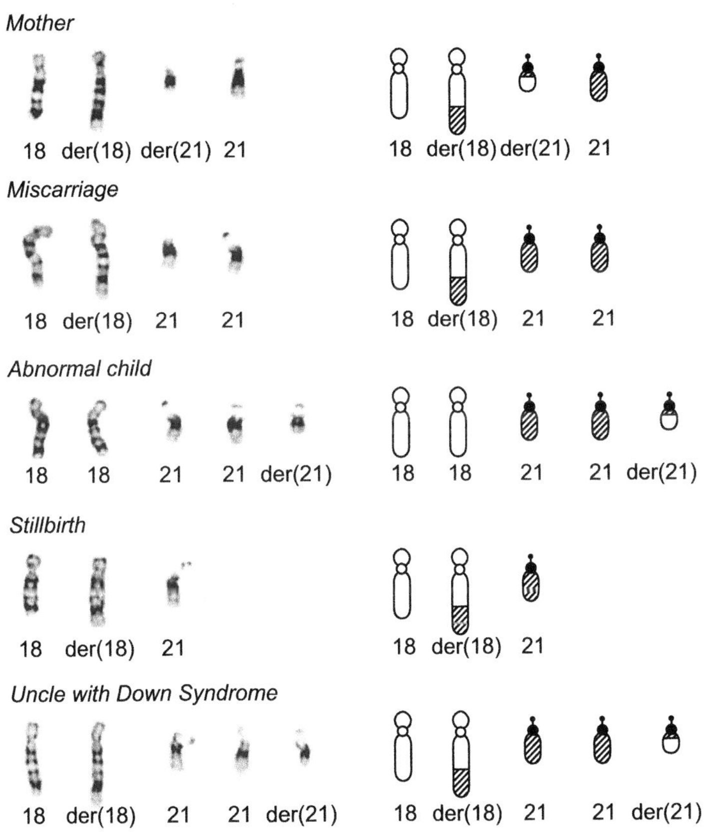

Figure 5–20. Several Viable Unbalanced Forms.
The karyotype is illustrated (*top*) of a mother carrying the translocation t(18;21)(q22.1;q11.2). She had a miscarriage due to adjacent-1 segregation, an abnormal child with a tertiary trisomy, and a stillborn child with a tertiary monosomy, as depicted in the cartoon karyotypes. An uncle with Down syndrome may have had the same adjacent-1 karyotype as in the second row, or possibly interchange trisomy 21, as depicted in the bottom row. (Case of MD Pertile.)

pregnancy outcomes were, respectively, 45,der(18), 46,der(18), and 47,+der(18). An uncle said to have had Down syndrome may have had the 46,der(18) karyotype (the der(18) includes the segment of 21 that contributes substantially to the Down syndrome phenotype), or possibly interchange trisomy with 47,+21,t(18;21). Some of the other possible imbalanced segregants could theoretically be viable, and the reader may wish to determine which ones these would be. This is due to the fact that many of these combinations have a genetically "small" imbalance. All partial trisomies and some partial monosomies for segments of chromosomes 18 and 21 can be viable as a single imbalance; and when two different imbalances occur in combination, for example, partial trisomy 21 plus partial monosomy 18, a pregnancy may still be capable of proceeding substantially along its course.

Failure to Form Quadrivalent

Where very small segments are involved, the imperative may lack for the coming together of the four chromosomes with segments in common, and they might simply synapse as bivalent pairs along their matching lengths and then segregate independently. In that case, a segregation ratio of 1:1:1:1 would presumably operate for normal, balanced, and the two imbalanced outcomes—clearly a high-risk circumstance. This likely applies to the general case of the subtelomeric translocation, such as the t(3;4)(p26.3;p16.1) in Iype et al. (2015) referred to above, in which the derivative chromosomes comprise almost a complete copy of the normal. The opposite, in which the der consists almost entirely of chromatin of the *other* chromosome, is exemplified in the t(14;15)(q12;q12) in Burke et al. (1996), in which the derivative chromosomes each comprise near to an entire chromosome 14 and chromosome 15, respectively (Figure 5–21).

Different grounds for the non-formation of a quadrivalent may exist if one chromosome is a very small one. While the three other chromosomes could have come together as a trivalent, the fourth very small one might fail to be captured by the meiotic mechanism. That being so, it could then segregate at random (a variation on the theme of 3:1 segregation; see "Acrocentric Chromosomes" above).

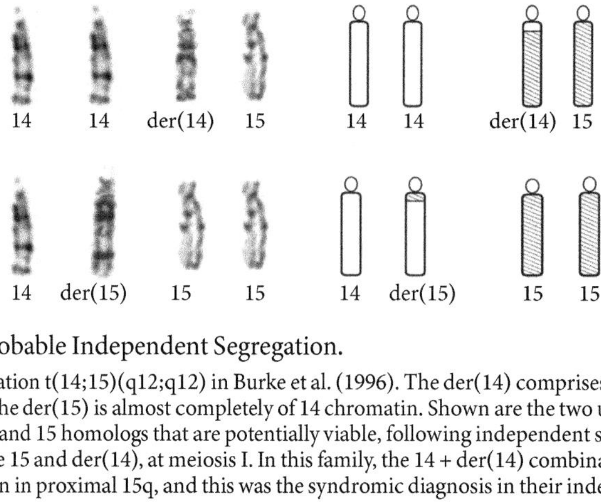

Figure 5–21. Probable Independent Segregation.

Notes: The translocation t(14;15)(q12;q12) in Burke et al. (1996). The der(14) comprises almost completely 15 chromatin, and the der(15) is almost completely of 14 chromatin. Shown are the two unbalanced gametic combinations of 14 and 15 homologs that are potentially viable, following independent segregation of the 14 and der(15), and the 15 and der(14), at meiosis I. In this family, the 14 + der(14) combination (upper) lacked the Angelman region in proximal 15q, and this was the syndromic diagnosis in their index case.

No Unbalanced Mode Viable

Finally, for the translocation in which the quadrivalent is characterized by long translocated and long centric segments, no mode of segregation could produce a viable unbalanced outcome. We emphasize the point that many reciprocal translocations (including whole-arm translocations, see below) are in this category.

Consider the family depicted in Figure 5–22, in which a 4;6 translocation t(4;6)(q25;p23) was discovered by chance at amniocentesis. The quadrivalent would have the form depicted in Figure 5–11d. It possesses none of the criteria that would allow a viable imbalance to result, by whatever mode of segregation. The translocated segments are both large (leading to double-segment imbalance); the centric segments are very large; and the content of all four chromosomes is large. Miscarriage is as far as any unbalanced conceptus could ever get, and in some such instances pregnancy loss will be the presenting complaint. The large kindred of Madan and Kleinhout (1987) graphically illustrates this circumstance: 11 carriers of a t(1;20)(p36;p11) had had two or more miscarriages and numerous normal children, but none had had an abnormal child. In some such translocations identified fortuitously—for example, at amniocentesis for maternal age—there may be little or no history of apparent reproductive difficulty.

Meiotic Drive. The nature of the quadrivalent may, of itself, influence segregation. The propensity for a particular segregation outcome may reflect a particular geometry of the quadrivalent and what sort of ring or chain it forms. Quadrivalents that have translocation chromosomes with short translocated segments more usually form a ring, and have the quality of being more likely to generate adjacent-1 gametes, while those with short centric segments, more often existing as a chain, may have a predisposition to the

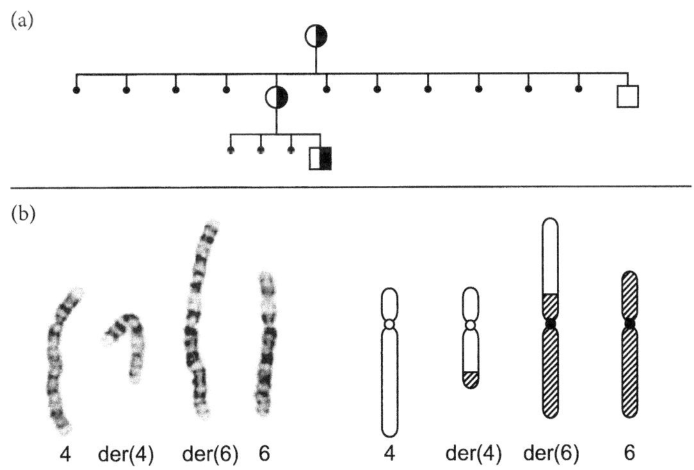

Figure 5–22. No Unbalanced Product Viable.
(*a*) Pedigree of a kindred in which mother and daughter have had multiple miscarriages, each having (*b*) the karyotype 46,XX,t(4;6)(q25;p23). (Case of AJ Watt.) The presumed pachytene configuration during gametogenesis in the heterozygote would be as in Figure 5–11d (chromosome 4 chromatin, open; chromosome 6 chromatin, cross-hatched) and, with large centric and translocated segments, the translocation has none of the features that enable viability of any unbalanced segregant combination.

sibship, five miscarriages, alongside three abnormal individuals with proven or probable dup17p13.3 syndrome, very likely reflected the opposite del17p imbalance.

Oögenesis is not, however, immune to the translocation obstacle, and indeed in the rcp series of Verdoni et al. (2021), women outnumbered men as the carrier in those couples whose presentation had been through recurrent pregnancy loss. Chen et al. (2005d) studied a number of "translocation couples" and compared ovarian responses between those where the male or the female partner was the heterozygote. The 28 female rcp carriers did worse than the women whose male partner was the heterozygote, as measured by estradiol levels following human chorionic gonadotrophin (HCG)[9] stimulation: 23% were "very low responders" compared with 7% where the female was not the carrier. It remains true, however, that oögenesis in most female carriers is apparently unscathed.

The sex difference in susceptibility is striking in the family of Paoloni-Giacobino et al. (2000b). A mother was a t(6;21)(p21.1;p13) heterozygote, and she had eight children—four sons and four daughters—and two miscarriages. The four sons, each 46,XY,t(6;21), were all married, (one three times), and none had any children. Each had severe oligospermia or oligoasthenoteratospermia, and the two having testicular biopsies manifested spermatogenic arrest at meiosis I prophase, with extensive asynapsis of several chromosomes. Two sisters were 46,XX,t(6;21), and the one who was married had had two children (and two miscarriages).

The Practical Problem of the Apparently Balanced Translocation

The ABT is not uncommon in the general population, about 2 to 5 per 1,000 persons. When an ABT has been discovered in the course of investigation of a child with a nonspecific picture of cognitive compromise and sometimes also some dysmorphic signs, and particularly when de novo, this raises the question: Is the translocation causative, or simply coincidental? If an ABT co-segregates faithfully with a consistent abnormal phenotype in a good number of individuals in a family, a conclusion can reasonably be drawn that the ABT is indeed the cause, and that the translocation is, in fact—at least functionally—unbalanced. A de novo case, however, cannot so readily be interpreted. The abnormal phenotype could be coincidental, unrelated to the ABT.

Families such as those reported in Hussain et al. (2000) offer useful illustration: in this example, an ABT that was co-segregating with a phenotype of "varying degrees of behavioral and learning difficulties." Presumably this translocation, a t(1;17)(p36.3;p11.2), had been de novo at some prior point, possibly with the 65-year-old grandmother of their index case. In this family, there were children and grandchildren (seven of them) to bear witness to the apparent harmful role of the translocation, notwithstanding an inability, given the methodology of the day, to show (as these authors suspected) an imbalance.

With the improving technology of this century, it is usually possible to make the distinction between an actually balanced versus a truly unbalanced ABT. In a paper attesting to the international collegiality of the profession, from over 100 institutions, Redin et al. (2017) accumulated data on 248 subjects in whom a spectrum of congenital anomalies and neurobehavioral disability had been presented, and each with an apparently

[9] HCG is very similar functionally to luteinizing hormone (LH). FSH and LH promote egg production and estrogen output.

balanced rearrangement. Most were de novo. Whole genome sequencing led to a revision of the interpretation in terms of the cytogenetic band(s) involved, in as many as 93% of karyotypes.

In what way might an ABT lead to phenotypic abnormality? (1) A very small, submicroscopic deletion, but containing an important gene or genes, is one obvious candidate. (2) A more complicated submicroscopic rearrangement may happen, with losses and gains. (3) Numerous cases have been shown due to the breakpoint occurring actually within a gene, disrupting it and making it nonfunctional, thus leading to an effectively haplo insufficient state. (4) Otherwise, the genomic landscape may put an intact gene within a region of inappropriate influence: "position effect." (5) Mosaicism with a concealed unbalanced cell line is a theoretical, and very occasionally proven, possibility. Finally (6), uniparental disomy with a functional imbalance is a rarely seen basis for abnormality in a structurally balanced rearrangement (Chapter 19).

An example of *gene disruption* is provided in Kurahashi et al. (1998). A child with lissencephaly (a severe structural brain abnormality; Figure 14–68) had a de novo t(8;17)(p11.2;p13.3). The p13.3 breakpoint on the chromosome 17 was sited within intron 1 of the *LIS* gene, with the gene being split between the two derivative chromosomes, its 5′ part on the der(8) and the remainder on the der(17). The gene could not, in consequence, function, and this functional haplo insufficiency at the *LIS* locus affected brain development. An example of one case from the series of Redin et al. (2017) is shown in Figure 5–25.

A *position effect*—a "disrupted long-range regulatory interaction"—may be the consequence of an inappropriate apposition of "topologically associating domains"[10] (TADs) in this part of the chromosome. A well-known example of position effect is campomelic dysplasia with sex reversal due to a chromosome 17q25.1 translocation, whose breakpoint is up to a megabase away from the (intact) *SOX9* locus; but the activity of this gene, within this new landscape, is nevertheless compromised (Figure 3–18) (Fonseca et al. 2013).

A similar phenotype may result via either of the above two mechanisms: In the study of Redin et al. mentioned above, a number of patients with a phenotype consistent with the 5q14.3 deletion syndrome (Chapter 14) had a breakpoint within (disruption) or close to (position effect) the *MEF2C* locus. Loci that were definitely or plausibly the basis of phenotypic abnormality, by whichever mechanism, in the 242 cases in Redin et al. (2017) are depicted in Figure 5–26. Likewise, in the international breakpoint mapping consortium presented in Tommerup et al. (2017) and comparing NGS findings in phe notypically normal and abnormal carriers of ABTs, breakpoints in the abnormal cases are more likely to occur within known autosomal dominant genes, genes that are susceptible to loss of function, or within TADs.

The case reported by Dufke et al. (2001) illustrates the possible scenario of *mosaicism*. An abnormal child with the same balanced t(17;22)(q24.2;q11.23) as his mother on peripheral blood analysis showed, on skin fibroblast culture, a 47,t(17;22),+der(22) karyotype. This mosaic picture may reflect there having been an interchange tertiary trisomy complement in the conceptus, with post-zygotic loss of one of the two der(22)s

[10] A topologically associating domain is a segment of chromatin, the DNA of kb to Mb size, within which physical interactions can take place. A spatial folding brings enhancers into closer proximity to their client genes (which might otherwise be quite apart in linear genomic distance), thus enabling a long-range regulatory control. A 3-D genome browser enables interrogation apropos: http://promoter.bx.psu.edu/hi-c/ (Wang et al. 2018).

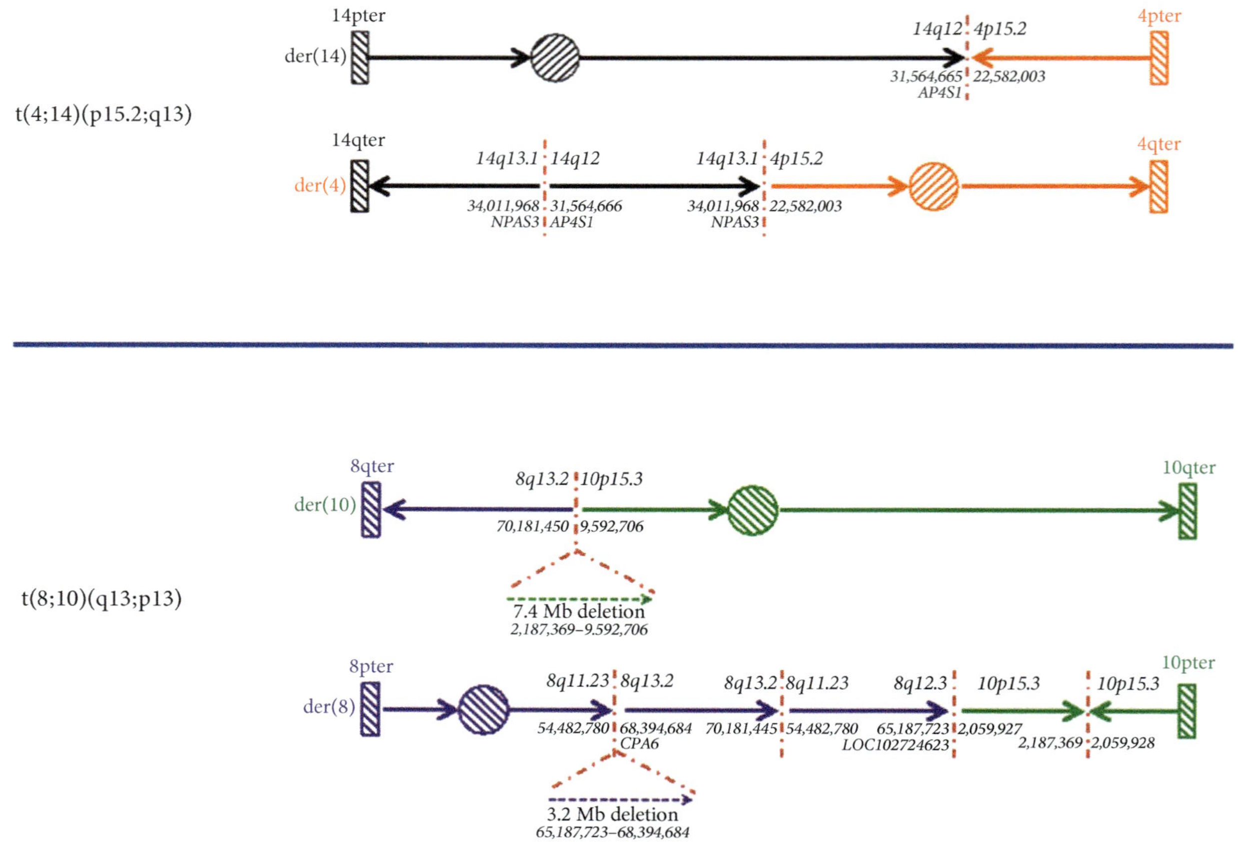

Figure 5–25. Two Apparently Balanced Translocations that were Not.

Notes: The translocation *above* was initially reported as t(4;14)(p15.2;q13)dn. Black = chromosome 14, orange = chromosome 4, circles = centromeres, rectangles = telomeres. Red dot-and-dash lines = breakpoints. Array-CGH was normal, and chromosome 4 and 14 DNA is present in the correct amount. In the der(4), a short ~2.5 Mb segment of chr 14 is inserted in an opposite direction, and genes *NPAS3* and *AP4S1* at the two breakpoints are disrupted, and in consequence, a functional imbalance.

The translocation *below* was initially reported as t(8;10)(q13;p13)dn. Purple = chromosome 8, green = chromosome 10. Red dot-and-dash lines = breakpoints. Two submicroscopic deleted segments, of 10p and 8q, are shown as green and purple dashed lines respectively. Following the nucleotide numbering will enable the reader to piece together the several breakages and rejoinings.

Source: From C Redin et al., The genomic landscape of balanced cytogenetic abnormalities associated with human congenital anomalies, *Nat Genet* 49: 36–45, 2017. Courtesy ME Talkowski, and with the permission of Springer Nature.

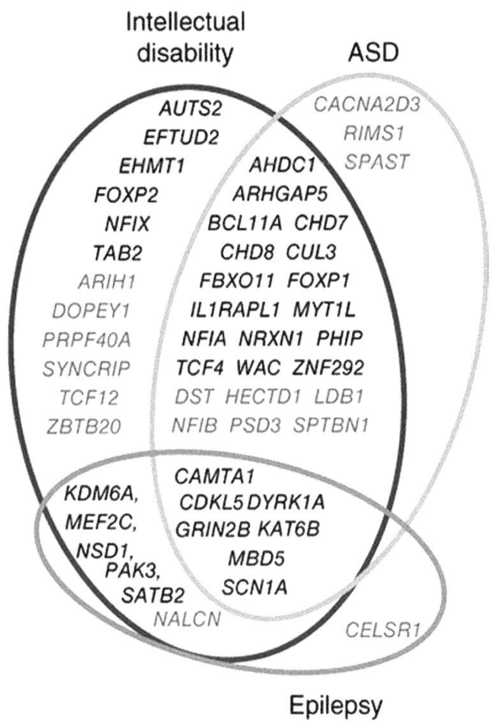

Figure 5–26. Loci Affected in Apparently Balanced Translocations.
Apparently balanced rearrangements subjected to analysis by whole genome sequencing, from a study of 248 cases. At the molecular level, the loci depicted were compromised, due to their residence at or near a chromosomal breakpoint. Those loci in bold are presumed to have been, by virtue of their structural/functional haploinsufficient state, definitely pathogenic; those in gray are likely pathogenic. The Venn diagram shows phenotypes associated with these several loci. ASD, autism spectrum disorder.
Source: From C Redin et al., The genomic landscape of balanced cytogenetic abnormalities associated with human congenital anomalies, *Nat Genet* 49: 36–45, 2017. Courtesy ME Talkowski, and with the permission of Springer Nature.

in blood-forming tissue. A similar scenario is documented in Prontera et al. (2006): A mother carrying a t(1;15)(q10;p11) had an abnormal child, in whom the same apparently balanced karyotype had been shown at prenatal diagnosis. In view of the abnormal phenotype, a stringent post-natal analysis was done, which revealed a small fraction of cells, 4% (on blood), with trisomy 15; the conclusion is thus drawn that the initial conception had been from a 3:1 malsegregation with interchange trisomy, and a mitotic "correction" thereafter resulted in loss of the additional chromosome 15 in a substantial fraction of cells, but obviously not all.

In the extraordinary coincidence of a recessive mutation being on the intact homolog, a translocation breakpoint that disrupted a gene would lead to the appearance of the recessive syndrome, as Kuechler et al. (2010) exemplify in a teenage girl with gonadal failure, who received an apparently balanced t(2;8)(p21;p23.1) from her mother that removed two exons from the *FSHR* gene (FSH receptor gene, which is located at 2p21) and a point mutation in that same gene on her paternal chromosome 2.

The possibility of a coincidental genetic abnormality is to be borne in mind. Aristidou et al. (2022) reanalyzed four kindreds in which an ABT co-segregated with phenotypic abnormality. They made the case, applying whole exome sequencing, that particular Mendelian mutations, actually on another chromosome, were likely candidates to have produced the observed pathological states. Coincidences can happen. Indeed, in some of the cases studied in De Gregori et al. (2007), coincidental de novo deletions were identified at chromosomal sites other than on the translocation chromosomes.

The discovery of a de novo ABT at prenatal diagnosis is a particular case, which we review in Chapter 22.

Rare Complexities

Double Translocation Carrier. The double two-way rcp translocation comprises, essentially, two coincidental simple rcps (Phelan et al. 1990; Yardin et al. 1997). Presumably, two separate and independently operating quadrivalents can form. Burns et al. (1986) record sperm karyotypes in a man with a double two-way rcp(5;11)(p13;q23.2),rcp(7;14)(q11.23;q24.1), whose wife had had four miscarriages, a child with cri du chat syndrome, and a normal son carrying the rcp(7;14). Only four of 23 sperm analyzed had an overall balanced complement, and the majority (13) had adjacent-1 segregants for one or the other translocation. Another five showed 3:1, and one sperm showed 4:0 segregation.

Bowser-Riley et al. (1988) proposed that the risk of having an abnormal child would be approximately the sum of the figures derived separately for each rcp. They acknowledge that might be an overestimate due to nonviability of doubly imbalanced combinations, notwithstanding that each on its own might be viable. We have seen a couple, the husband having a double two-way translocation t(2;20)(p25.1;p11.23),t(4;8)(q27;p21.1), who presented following four first-trimester miscarriages, although their first pregnancy had produced a normal (but unkaryotyped) son. Of 320 theoretically possible karyotypes, only four (1.25%) would be balanced (thus raising a glimmer of hope that their first fortunate pregnancy might reflect a tendency toward a balanced combination). Following the collection of 25 eggs, of which 23 were subjected to intracytoplasmic sperm injection (ICSI) and with 18 embryos then resulting, biopsy was achieved in 15 embryos, but none had a balanced constitution.

A triple two-way balanced translocation carrier is extremely rare. In one such case, Gupta et al. (2019) describe 46,XX,t(1;3)(q44;p11),t(2;14)(q11.2;q13),t(9;11)(p22;p15) in a woman presenting with infertility, herself physically and mentally normal.

Carrier Couple. Since reciprocal translocation heterozygotes are not uncommon in the population, on rare occasions both members of a couple will, by chance, carry a translocation (Neu et al. 1988b). We have seen, for example, a couple who had had several miscarriages, from 5 weeks to 9 weeks gestation. The husband's karyotype was 46,XY,t(7;11)(q22;q23) and the wife's 46,XX,t(7;22)(p13;q11.2). Presumably, their history of miscarriage reflected at least one parent transmitting an unbalanced gamete with each pregnancy— as the reader can determine, rather many unbalanced karyotypes are possible! A normal child is possible if each contributes a normal or a balanced gamete to the same conceptus. It should, in theory, be reasonably likely in a given conception for the two contemporaneous gametes to have arisen from alternate segregation—as an educated guess, the chance might be about 20%—although at the time of our seeing this family, only miscarriage had occurred. A child of theirs having each parental translocation would qualify as having a "double two-way translocation."

If a translocation is in a family and a couple are related, the possibility is open that they might both be carriers. Such a scenario is illustrated in Kupchik et al. (2005), who report a consanguineous husband and wife with the same t(16;18)(p13.3;p11.2). Their child received two copies of the der(18) and one of the der(16), due to alternate segregation in one parent and adjacent-1 in the other. As the reader may determine, the end result was a duplication of distal 16p and a deletion of 18p. In Martinet et al. (2006), a first-cousin couple each carried a t(17;20)(q21.1;p11.21), and their severely malformed fetus was homozygous for the translocation. The phenotype may have been due to a recessive gene. Similar histories with respect to a Robertsonian translocation, and to an inversion, are noted in Chapter 7 and Chapter 9, respectively.

Mosaicism. Almost all balanced reciprocal translocations are seen in the non-mosaic state. This reflects either that the translocation had been inherited from a carrier parent, or that the rearrangement had arisen preconceptually in one or other parental gamete. Rarely (or at least rarely recognized), a balanced translocation can be generated as a post-zygotic event, and the person is a 46,rcp/46,N mosaic (Garzo et al. 2020). Most often, the clinical presentation is due to multiple miscarriage or infertility, or in the pursuit of a family study following the discovery of a non-mosaic (balanced or unbalanced) case. In these cases, the mosaicism is necessarily, at least inferentially, somatic-gonadal. An incidentally discovered case could be somatic-gonadal, or purely somatic.

The infrequency with which a mosaic rcp is recognized is attested in the analysis of Park et al. (2022), who reviewed chromosomal findings in 399 female and male rcp carriers presenting with recurrent pregnancy loss. In only one—0.25% of the whole group—was mosaicism for a rcp seen: mos 46,XX,t(11;22)(q23;q11.2)/46,XX(50%). We have seen this same mosaic translocation in 40% of cells of a man whose partner had presented with a miscarriage due to trisomy 22. (Mosaicism for an *un*balanced translocation is well recorded [e.g., Choi et al. 2015], but our concern here is with the balanced state.)

Unstable Familial Translocation. Tomkins (1981) documents a family in which a mother with 46,XX,t(11;22)(p11;p12) had one daughter with the same translocation and another daughter with 46,XX,t(11;15)(p11;p12), and a very few other similar cases are on record. Typically, the translocation breakpoints are at telomeres, centromeres, or in nucleolar organizing regions. There is some sequence similarity in these regions between different chromosomes, and this may set the stage for these very rare "second translocation" events (and see "Jumping Translocation," Chapter 12).

Homologous Translocation. A reciprocal translocation between each of a pair of homologs is extremely rare, and only three such cases are reported in Almeida et al. (2012), all phenotypically normal persons presenting with infertility/repeated pregnancy loss. The karyotype description has the notable observation that the homologs in the first set of brackets are the same: for example, 46,XY,t(2;2)(p23;q21.2). All heterozygotes would necessarily have been of de novo generation. Such translocations would be expected inevitably to lead to an unbalanced state in the conceptus—a 100% genetic risk—and only the possibility of gonadal mosaicism (which actually was so in the t(2;2) man in Almeida et al.) would offer the prospect of a successful pregnancy.

Whole-Arm Translocation. When entire arms of chromosomes are translocated (whole-arm translocation), it is almost always so that the unbalanced segregants would be unviable, and infertility is the usual presentation (Vázquez-Cárdenas et al. 2007; Yunchun et al. 2023). Rare exceptions exist. Czakó et al. (2002) report a t(18;20)(p11.1;p11.1), in which the abnormal child of a carrier father was effectively trisomic for all of 20p and monosomic for all of 18p.

GENETIC COUNSELING

The counselor may have to deal with these questions:

1. Is there a risk of having an abnormal child?
2. If so, what is the magnitude of the risk?
3. What would be the abnormality, and would the child survive?
4. Could there be miscarriage?
5. What testing in pregnancy is open to us?
6. Could we avoid the risk by testing an embryo in the IVF laboratory?
7. What if the same translocation that I have is found at prenatal or preimplantation testing?
8. Anything else I should know?

Does a Risk Exist of Having an Abnormal Child?

If a family is ascertained through a liveborn aneuploid child, that very fact demonstrates viability for that particular aneuploid combination. It could happen again.

If, on the other hand, the family was ascertained by miscarriage or infertility, or fortuitously, and there is no known family history of an abnormal child, the picture is less clear. Most likely, no aneuploid combination is viable. Alternatively, a viable imbalance may be possible, but it has not yet happened; or an imbalance could occasionally be viable, but usually it is not, and (so far) has led only to abortion. The approach here is to determine the potentially unbalanced segregant outcomes, according to the favored mode of segregation—adjacent-1, adjacent-2, or 3:1—and to check to see whether any of these is on record in a pregnancy that produced an abnormal child. Valuable sources of information include Schinzel's (2001) catalog and sites such as Decipher, ClinGen, and the CNV morbidity map.

Where a single-segment imbalance from adjacent segregation is a potential outcome in a conceptus, and if the potential imbalance comprises an aneuploidy equal to or less than one of these segments on record, viability must be assumed to be possible. If the potential imbalance comprised an aneuploidy greater than any on record, viability would be unlikely, especially if the aneuploidy is much greater. The great majority of double-segment imbalances from adjacent segregation due to a translocation, ascertained other than by a liveborn aneuploid child, would be expected to lead to lethality in utero. Nearly always, a "new" double-segment exchange presenting at the clinic will truly be new, and there will be no literature record of exactly the same thing to which the counselor may appeal. In many instances one has to make an educated guess, erring on the side of caution, whether the combination of imbalances from a derivative chromosome might, in sum, be viable.

The Magnitude of Risk

The lowest risk for a surviving abnormal child, namely zero, applies in the case of imbalances of large genetic content, in which in utero lethality would be seen as inevitable. This essentially no-risk circumstance may apply to a considerable fraction, perhaps the great majority of "translocation couples."

If, in a family, it is judged that there does exist a risk to have an abnormal child, a broad estimate of the level of risk may be derived from a consideration of these factors: the assessed imbalance of potentially viable gametes; the predicted type of segregation leading to potentially viable gametes; the mode of ascertainment of the family; and in 3:1, the sex of the transmitting parent. Most risk figures fall in a range from 0% to 30%; higher risks are rare. These percentages are expressed in terms of abnormal live births as a proportion of all live births, although there are other ways of looking at the risk: the risk for an unbalanced embryo at preimplantation diagnosis; risk at prenatal diagnosis; the risk for miscarriage. Overall, the livebirth risk is higher in cases ascertained through an abnormal child, versus those identified through other routes; in the review of Youings et al. (2004), the respective pooled figures were 19% and 3%.

A precise risk estimate needs to be based on the actual cytogenetic, or molecular cytogenetic, imbalance.[11] Different chromosomal segments contain, of course, different genomic information. Some segments, in the imbalanced state, impose a lesser degree of compromise on the process of embryonic development, and the pregnancy may proceed through to live birth. Other segments, although they may be shorter but carrying more "important" genes, are lethal during early pregnancy and lead to miscarriage. Different segments associated with different translocations are associated with differing outcomes (Figure 5–27). It is scarcely possible to come up with a unifying format, given that chromatin is not uniform; as Cohen et al. commented in 1994, "it would be hazardous to suggest a simple mathematical relationship between unbalance length and viability" (Cohen et al. 1994).

Nonetheless, attempts have been to calculate a correlation of quantitative chromatin imbalance with risk to have a liveborn affected child. Daniel et al. (1989), Cans et al. (1993), and Cohen et al. (1994) have compared the HAL with viability in translocation families. Most (96%) viable imbalances comprise up to 2% monosomy and up to 4% trisomy, with combinations of monosomy/trisomy viable only when the additive (or multiplicative) effect of *x*% monosomy plus *y*% trisomy falls within a triangular area defined by joining the 2% and 4% points on the *x* and *y* axes of a graph (Figure 5–28). A few (4%) fall outside of this area, and these cases define the boundaries of a "surface of viable unbalances," reflecting the effects of qualitative differences in different segments of chromatin.

For routine practice in the genetic clinic, and if the counselee wishes to have a good idea of the level of risk, we suggest starting off with the unvarnished empiric data for individual chromosome segments collected by Stengel-Rutkowski and colleagues, as set out in their invaluable monograph (Stengel-Rutkowski et al. 1988), and discussed in a review and further illustrated in practice (Stene and Stengel-Rutkowski 1988; Midro et al. 1992), and to which we have already referred several times above. The figures set out in Tables 5–4, 5–8, and 5–9 for the three major categories of malsegregation are

[11] Translocation breakpoints mapped using only G-banded karyotype can also be surprisingly inaccurate when compared to molecular data, differing by as much as 50Mb (Ordulu et al. 2016) and adding another layer of imprecision to risk estimation.

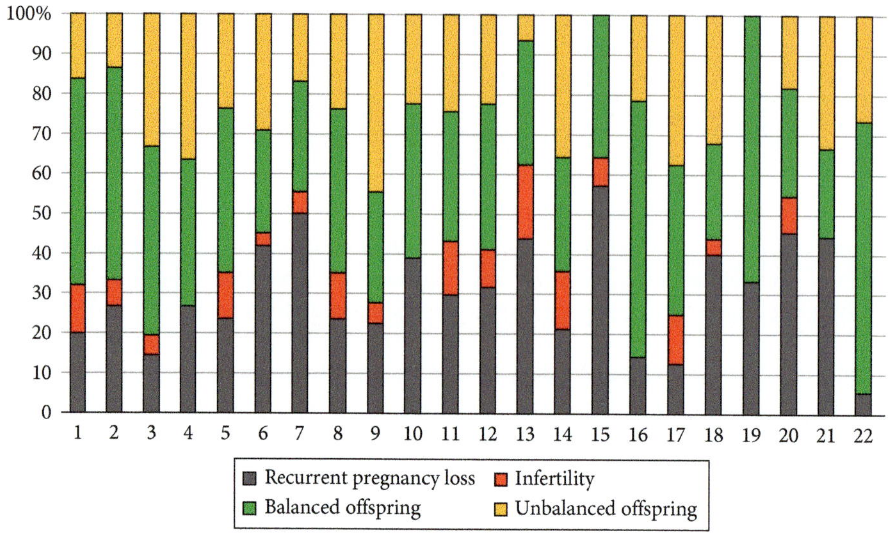

Figure 5-27. Differing Outcomes from Different Translocations.

Notes: Different translocated chromosomes have different associations with reproductive outcomes, presumably reflecting, in part at least, the number and nature of the genes within translocated segments. The gene-sparse nature of parts of chromosomes 4, 9, 18, and 21 may be a factor behind their quite substantial fractions in the survivable "unbalanced offspring" category (albeit that the very small fraction due to gene-sparse chromosome 13 might seem inconsistent; but this may simply be a matter of the numbers in this study). Colored segments indicate proportions (*y* axis) associated with particular reproductive outcomes, for each chromosome (*x* axis).

Source: From A Verdoni et al., Reproductive outcomes in individuals with chromosomal reciprocal translocations, *Genet Med* 23:1753–1760, 2021. Courtesy SA Yatsenko, and with the permission of Elsevier and the American College of Medical Genetics and Genomics.

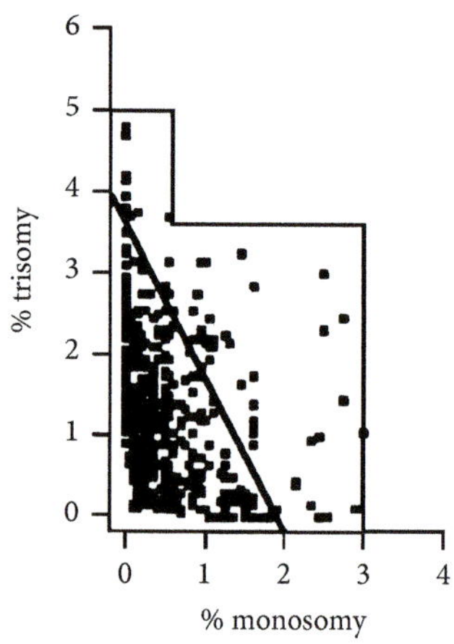

Figure 5-28. Assessing Viability of Unbalanced Forms.

Viability of combined duplication/deletion states, according to amount of imbalance, measured as % HAL. Most (96%) fall within the triangular area whose hypotenuse lies between 4% duplication/0% deletion and 2% deletion/0% duplication, and a few outliers define an envelope of viable imbalances.

Source: From O Cohen et al. 1994, Viability thresholds for partial trisomies and monosomies. A study of 1,159 viable unbalanced reciprocal translocations, *Hum Genet* 93: 188–194. Courtesy O Cohen, and with the permission of Springer-Verlag.

Table 5–4. Risks in the Case of Adjacent-1 Segregation, with Single-Segment Imbalance

Specific Risk Figures, Based upon Empiric Data, for Having a Liveborn Aneuploid Child or a Child Stillborn or Dying as a Neonate[a] Because of Single-Segment Imbalance from 2:2 Adjacent-1 Segregation[b]

TRANSLOCATED SEGMENT THAT WOULD BE IMBALANCED[c]		RISK		
		% LIVEBORN	S.D.	+ % STILLBORN, NEONATAL DEATH[e]
1.	1pter→1p11–p34	0		
	1p35	?		
	1qter→q11–q22	0		
	q23–q32	<1.3		+ 5.1
	q42	13.6	5.2	
2.	2pter→p11–p12	0		
	p13–p16	<2.5		+ 15.0
	p21–p23	5.7	3.9	+ 14.3
	2qter→q11–q23	0		
	q31–q32	<1.7		+ 6.7
	q33	20.0	8.9	
	q34–q35	22.9	7.1	+ 11.4
3.	3pter→p13–p14	0		
	p21	<2.3		+ 13.6
	p22–p25	28.6	17.1	
	3qter→q12–q13.2	0		
	q21–q27	<1.1		
4.	4pter→p11	7.7	5.2	+ 38.5
	p14	15.4	4.5	+ 7.7
	p15	28.6	12	+ 7.1
	4qter→q11–q13	?0		
	q21–34	0.8	0.8	+ 14.1
5.	5pter→p11–p12	3.3	2.3	+ 13.1
	p13	7.0[d]	2.6	+ 4.0
	p14	29.4	11.1	
	5qter→q13–q21	?		
	q22–q33	7.7	7.4	+ 7.7
	q34	25.0	7.2	
6.	6pter→p11–p12	?		
	p21.2–24	1.3	1.3	+ 11.8
	6qter→q11–q16	?0		
	q21–q24	20.0	17.9	
	q25–q26	33.3	15.7	+ 33.3
7.	7pter→p11–p13	4.4	3.0	+ 4.4
	p15–p21	19.1	8.6	+ 4.8
	7qter→q11–q21	?0		
	q22–q35	<0.8		+ 7.9

(*continued*)

Table 5-4. Continued

TRANSLOCATED SEGMENT THAT WOULD BE IMBALANCED[c]		RISK		
		% LIVEBORN	S.D.	+ % STILLBORN, NEONATAL DEATH[e]
8.	8pter→p11–p23	9.1	3.5	
	p23.1	40[e]	12.6	+20
	8qter→q11–q13	2.0	2.0	
	q21.2–q24.2	11.1	6.1	
9.	9pter→p11.2	11.8	3.7	+9.2
	p13	25	8.8	+4.2
	p22	21.2	4.4	+2.4
	9qter→q11–q13	0		
	q21–33	<0.8		+ 8.3
10.	10pter→p11.1	4.7	2.6	+ 4.7
	p12–p14	18.8	9.7	+ 18.8
	10qter→q11–q21	?0		
	q22–q23	<1.4		+ 5.7
	q24	5.9	2.6	+ 9.4
	q25–q26	14.0	4.9	+ 12.0
11.	11pter→p11–p13	?0		
	p14	<3.1		+ 6.3
	11qter→q13–q22	<2.6		
	q23	7.0	3.9	+ 18.6
12.	12pter→p11.1	9.4	5.2	+ 3.1
	p12	9.1	8.7	+ 18.2
	12qter→q11–q15	0		
	q21–q24.3	<1.5		+ 3.8
13.	13qter→q11–q33	1.6	1.1	
14.	14qter→q11.1–q31	1.0	1.0	
15.	15qter→q11–q15	0		
	q21–25	2.7	2.7	
16.	16pter→p11.11	8.3	3.6	
	16qter→q11–q13	6.2	6	+ <3.1
	q21–q23	<5.4		+ <5.4
17.	17pter→p13.3	18.9	3.5	+ 7.1
	p11.1	<2.7		
	17qter→q11–12	?0		
	q21–23	10.0	6.7	
18.	18pter→p11.1–p11.2	? (probably high)		
	18qter→q11.1–q12	2.5	2.5	
	q21	2.9	2.8	+ 6.7
	q22	15.0	7.8	+ 15.0
19.	19pter→p11–p13.2	?0		
	19qter→q11–q12	?0		
	q13.2–q13.3	11.1	6.1	

Table 5–4. Continued

TRANSLOCATED SEGMENT THAT WOULD BE IMBALANCED[c]		RISK		
		% LIVEBORN	S.D.	+ % STILLBORN, NEONATAL DEATH[e]
20.	20pter→p11.1–p11.2	20.0	8.0	
	20qter→q11.1	?0		
21.	21qter→q11.1–q22	13.8	6.4	
22.	22qter→q11.1–q13	<2.6		

[a]Figures are expressed as a percentage of all karyotyped liveborn infants, typically considered as a baby of >28 weeks gestation, with survival at least beyond the neonatal period. Where there are data relating to unkaryotyped stillbirths or neonatal deaths, the figures for these are indicated with a + sign in the third column under "Risk," as a probable additional component of the overall risk, on the assumption that many, at least, of these cases would have been karyotypically abnormal. The maximum estimate of risk will thus be given by the sum of the two percentage figures. This combined figure may be an overestimate but if so, likely of small degree, and this may be the more useful figure to consider.

[b]One specific translocated segment is of substantial genetic content (the one shown here), and the other is judged to be of minimal content. For adjacent-1 segregation, the risk does not differ between male and female heterozygotes. For segments not listed here, no specific data are recorded in Stengel-Rutkowski et al. (1988).

[c]Some segments are noted precisely (e.g., 1pter→1p35). Most are given as a pair of breakpoints encompassing a range (e.g., 1pter→1p11–34), extending from a maximum length of terminal-to-proximal breakpoint to a minimum length of terminal-to-distal breakpoint. Thus, 1pter→1p11–p34 refers to an imbalanced segment comprising anywhere from a maximum of 1pter→1p11 (the whole of the short arm) to a minimum of 1pter→1p34 (about one-third of the short arm).

[d]In one reported large family with several cases of "pure" deletion or duplication of this segment (the other segment being derived from acrocentric short arm), the risk was very high: 54% (De Carvalho et al. 2008; and see text).

[e]When the combined live birth + neonatal death figure approximates 50%, this may suggest that the single-segment imbalance is fully viable in utero in either the duplicated or deleted state, with approximately equal numbers of offspring due to alternate and to adjacent-1 segregation.

S.D., standard deviation; ?, Rare cases have occurred, but data too few to derive a figure; ?0, Probably no risk; <, No additional aneuploid child has been born apart from the proband, figure is estimate of upper limit of risk interval.

Sources: From Stengel-Rutkowski et al. 1988, with further entries/amendments from Pollin et al. 1999 (17p13.3), Stasiewicz-Jarocka et al. 2000 and 2004 (1q42, 2q33, 16q), and Panasiuk et al. 2007 and 2009 (4p, 9p), and personal communications A Midro (8p23.1) and M Ozaki (5p14). We are unaware of any more recent such studies; perhaps there is an opportunity for updating from services with large databases, and now in the more subtle molecular age.

summarized from their monograph and from additional subsequent data. It would give a false sense of precision to use decimal points; a rounded figure will suffice. The paucity of information for some chromosomes has necessitated lumping of data for considerable lengths of a chromosome arm; the risk figures derived in this way are, naturally, composites, and indicative rather than definitive. We assume that, in different families with the same translocation (Table 5–5), the genetic risks will likely be the same, regardless of what may have been the mode of ascertainment. And of course, the principle always applies: If the counselee's family is large enough, do a segregation analysis to derive a "private" recurrence risk, as well exemplified in Šumanović-Glamuzina et al. (2017).

The figure given for a segment, say, q31/q34qter—in other words, a lumped figure applying to a segment extending anywhere from q31qter to q34qter—might be given as, say, <0.8%: in other words, a very small risk. (The "less than" sign in the risk data tables is used for estimates in those translocations where no additional aneuploid child

Table 5-5. Recurrent Translocations

TRANSLOCATION	TYPICAL PHENOTYPE OF UNBALANCED STATE	REFERENCES
t(11;22)(q23;q11)	Emanuel syndrome	Carter et al. 2009
t(4;8)(p16;p23)	Wolf-Hirschhorn syndrome and *	Giglio et al. 2002
t(4;11)(p16.2;p15.4)	*	Ou et al. 2011
t(8;22)(q24.13;q11.21)	*	Sheridan et al. 2010
t(5;11)(p15;p15)	Beckwith-Wiedemann syndrome	Slavotinek et al. 1997
t(6;20)(p21;p13)	*	Berner et al. 2012
t(1;12)(q43;q21.1)	Vascular	Luukkonen et al. 2018

Notes: The phenotypes in the unbalanced state due to the asterisked translocations are relatively nonspecific, with intellectual compromise in all. In the case of the t(1;12)(q43;q21.1), the phenotype is due to locus disruption, in the apparently balanced state.

has been born apart from probands.) But this figure might have been based mostly on data from families having a q31 breakpoint. A breakpoint at q34 might happen to exclude a dosage-sensitive region of major effect within q33, and thus imbalance for the slightly smaller segment q34qter might be of considerably greater viability. The risk figure needs to be interpreted intelligently in the light of what is otherwise known from the literature and Web resources about the segments in question, and naturally from observation within the same family.

The reader consulting and using these figures, imperfect though they may be, will gain a good sense of the practical principles of estimating risk. Additional data may come to hand. For example, Stasiewicz-Jarocka et al. (2004) assembled data from 65 new pedigrees involving 16q, to add to the original 35 pedigrees from Stengel-Rutkowski and colleagues, and their combined risk calculations are included in the Tables. As expected, the new data continue to be consistent with the notion that the risk for viable unbalanced offspring increases with decreasing length of the segments. In another study, the methods of Stengel-Rutkowski et al. were applied to a large pedigree segregating a double-segment t(7;13)(q34;q13). Midro and colleagues (2006) were able to predict the chance of a miscarriage or stillbirth from carriers in this family to be 13% and 30%, respectively. The high rate of selection against abnormal karyotypes, applying in particular in the latter part of pregnancy with this particular translocation, resulted in a very low presumed risk (0.3%) of the abnormal outcome of a surviving liveborn.

A determination of precise genetic risk in couples in whom the translocation implies a negligible risk of having a liveborn unbalanced child, may be, for some, less important now that genome-wide NIPT can be used to detect unbalanced segregants of translocations that have at least one large segment (Flowers et al. 2020). This approach allows couples to avoid the risks of invasive testing and to receive reassurance at 10 to 12 weeks' gestation that the pregnancy is balanced. However, invasive testing remains a high priority for translocations in which both segments are very small, as these have the highest risk of leading to a liveborn unbalanced child, and the reliability of NIPT in this setting remains under assessment (Srebniak et al. 2021). For these couples, a precise risk assessment remains useful.

RISK AT THE TIME OF PREIMPLANTATION GENETIC TESTING

PGT for a reciprocal translocation has been available for much of this century. Initially, it was the day-3 cleavage-stage embryo at IVF that was analyzed, but latterly it has been the day-5 blastocyst that is chosen (Chapter 23). In terms of the relative detection rates at these two timeframes, there is a small but definite increase in the normal/balanced detection rate, from 25% to 28% (Tian et al. 2022); this likely reflects a lethality of embryos with a substantial monosomic load during the day 4 to day 5–6 period. PGT requires a very different viewpoint, since in utero (in other words, post-implantation) lethality has not had the chance to operate; hence a wide range of imbalances may be seen, the great majority of which could never survive to term, and indeed, many would fail even before implantation.

The numerator/denominator of the risk figure becomes the fractions of euploid and aneuploid embryos out of all created embryos. The overall figure of about one-quarter to one-third, for the fraction of day-5 embryos that are euploid, is consistently seen across a number of studies in which large numbers (thousands) of blastocysts have been analyzed (Xie et al. 2022; Oğur et al. 2023; Zhou et al.2024). A typical range of findings is shown (Table 5–6) in the smaller study of Shetty et al. (2022). In the series of Xie et al., in which over 2,000 rcp carrier couples were studied—all of whom had presented with histories of infertility, recurrent spontaneous abortion, or having had a pregnancy with a chromosomal abnormality—the segregation ratios were as follows: alternate, 46%; adjacent-1, 31%; adjacent-2, 12%; and 3:1, 30%. A proportion of these embryos may have other aneuploidies unrelated to the translocation, and more so in the case of an older mother. In the series of Zhou et al. (2024), one-fifth of blastocysts had an abnormality unrelated to the translocation.

The subtleties of the range of potential imbalances here may be, to some counselees, a little beside the point: the aim is, naturally, to select a normal/balanced embryo, and whatever the abnormal ones are, they can be disregarded. What really matters, of course, is the take-home baby rate (Lledó et al. 2010). Overall, the proportion of successful pregnancies per embryo transfer, after PGT, is around one-half. In the series of Oğur et al. (2023), that figure was 43% for mothers under age 35, and 58% for those over that age; interestingly, the respective miscarriage rates, at 12% and 5%, were actually less than the general population risk.[12] Xie et al. (2022) reported an overall delivery rate, per embryo transfer, of 50%. A similar livebirth figure (56%) comes from Zhou et al. (2024) in couples who had a single embryo transfer. If the chances of an embryo at PGT being normal is one-third, and the odds for a successful transfer one-half, only one in six fertilized ova will, on average, result in a baby. Tong et al. (2022b) propose that four or more embryos would need to be created in order to improve the odds of having at least one euploid embryo. The absence of any effect on the outcome due to parental gender is confirmed in Tan et al. (2025).

Of the euploid embryos, essentially one-half are non-carriers of the translocation (Zhou et al. 2024). It is possible to distinguish between a carrier and a normal embryo via haplotype analysis, using genotype data generated from SNP arrays (Treff et al. 2016; Xu et al. 2017), whole genome sequencing (Zhai et al. 2022), or long-read nanopore sequencing (Madjunkova et al. 2020). While this may be an attractive option to parents who will be only too aware of the complicated reproductive implications of

[12] The numbers in each age group were not large, 52 cf. 22, and so the apparently better outcomes for older mothers should not be over-interpreted.

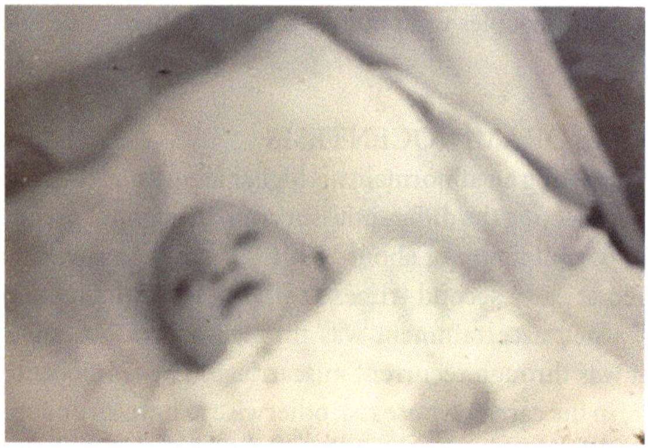

Figure 5–29. Photograph of a Baby who had Died in Infancy Years Before, from a t(4p;12p) Family.

Note: A retrospective diagnosis of Wolf-Hirschhorn syndrome is reasonably proposed.

Source: From JG Mortimer et al., A further report on a kindred with cases of 4p trisomy and monosomy, *Hum Hered* 30:58–61, 1980.

with a figure of 25%, which is sufficiently close to 23.1% to provide reassurance as to its accuracy.

The risk at preimplantation testing is naturally seen through a different lens. Here, the full range of malsegregation may be observed. As noted above, around one-quarter to one-third of blastocysts will be euploid, while the remainder majority are imbalanced due to malsegregation of the translocation or to an unrelated aneuploidy.

ADJACENT-1 SEGREGATION, DOUBLE SEGMENT

Every double-segment translocation is likely to be a unique case (or at least no other described family is known), and risk assessment is less precise. One known recurrent double-segment translocation, the t(4;8)(p16;p23), has been seen in sufficient numbers for a useful risk estimate to be derived (Table 5–5), and some other examples are listed. Of course, if the family is large enough, a private segregation analysis will provide the best estimate. If no literature data is available, and in the absence of a family study, Stengel-Rutkowski et al. (1988) otherwise recommend considering each segment separately. They propose the rule of thumb that the risk will be half that of the smaller of the two risk figures. Even this may be an overestimate. Consider the t(4;9)(p15.2;p13) family listed in Table 5–7. The smaller of the risks is that applying to 9p13, as a single-segment, and which is given at 25% (from Table 5–4); this halves to 12.5%. But from an actual family study, the empiric figure was only 3.2% (Midro et al. 2000). And in many cases, the duplication/deficiency from a double-segment imbalance will be invariably lethal in utero—a risk of 0%—notwithstanding that each segment separately is on record with viability in the single-segment state.

When the translocated segments are of small content, one or possibly both of the dup/del and del/dup combinations could be viable. Segregation may be due to the adjacent-1 format, or possibly simply an independent 1:1 segregation of each normal homolog and its derivative chromosome, as discussed above. The family history may well be informative, as illustrated in Midro et al. (2014). Two large kindreds were segregating apparently the same t(1;11)(p36.22;q12.2); and although no familial link was known between the kindreds, who both came from the same region in Poland, it would not be surprising were

Table 5-7. Risks in the Case of Adjacent-1 Segregation, with Double-Segment Imbalance

TRANSLOCATION	RISK[c]		
	% LIVEBORN	S.D.	+ % STILLBORN, NEONATAL DEATH
t(1;2)(q42;q33)	6.8		
t(1:3)(q42.3;p25)	63.6	14.5	
t(1;11)(p36.22;q12.2)	6.2	3.5	<1.1
t(2;13)(p25.1;q32.3)	14.5	7.6	+ 4.8
t(3;10)(p26; p12)	24.0	8.5	
t(3;15)(q21.3;q26.1)	?0		+ 17
t(4;5)(p15.1;p12)	1.6		
t(4;8)(p16.1;p23.1)	18.8	9.7	
t(4;8)(p16.3;p23.1)	41.2	11.9	
t(4;9)(p15.2;p13)	3.2	3.2	+ 6.5
t(4;19)(p15.32;p13.3)	3.7	3.6	+ 7.4
t(7;9)(q36.2;p21.2)	30	14.5	+ 10
t(7;13)(q34;q13)	0.3*		+ 29.0
t(12;14)(q15;q13)	?0		+?0
t(16;19)(q13;q13.3)	1.2		
t(16;20)(q11.1;q12)	1.1		

Notes: Empiric risk figures for having a liveborn aneuploid child, or a child stillborn or dying as a neonate,[a] because of double-segment imbalance from 2:2 adjacent-1 segregation, in 14 specific translocations[b]

*Plus another 0.2% to account for a theoretical risk for interchange trisomy 13. The considerable gap to the next risk figure, 29%, reflects the several instances in this family of unkaryotyped stillbirths and early neonatal deaths.

[a]Figures are expressed as a percentage of all karyotyped liveborn infants, as described in the legend in Table 5-4.

?0 indicates probably no risk, albeit that the 17% risk figure above for stillbirth/neonatal death in the t(3;15)(q21.3;q26.1) indicates viability of the unbalanced state through to the end of pregnancy.

[b]Families published in Kozma et al. (2004), Midro et al. (2000, 2006, 2014, 2016), Nucaro et al. (2008), Stasiewicz-Jarocka et al. (2000, 2004), Tranebjaerg et al. (1984), Wiland et al. (2007), and Šumanović-Glamuzina et al. (2017), and personal communication, AT Midro.

[c]Some figures come from direct segregation analysis, and in others from applying this rule: Halving the risk for the lesser of the two risks, which would otherwise have applied to each translocated segment when viewed as a single-segment imbalance (and see text).

this indeed the case. The only viable imbalanced outcome was taken to be the adjacent-1 combination, with monosomy 1p36.22→pter, and trisomy 11q12.2→qter (Figure 5-30). The no. 11 segment was not small in terms of length, but is apparently small in content, such that trisomy for most of 11q is a viable imbalance. The risk for this outcome was calculated at 6%, which is rather more than might have been drawn from Stengel-Rutkoski et al. (1988). As with the t(4;12) family above, retrospective assumptions had to be made, since all the presumed affected babies had died, with similar neural tube malformations. Carriers had an increased risk for miscarriage, 35%. Sperm studies in one heterozygote showed gametes of alternate, adjacent-1, adjacent-2, and 3:1 malsegregation, of relative fractions 40%, 38%, 5%, and 11% respectively.

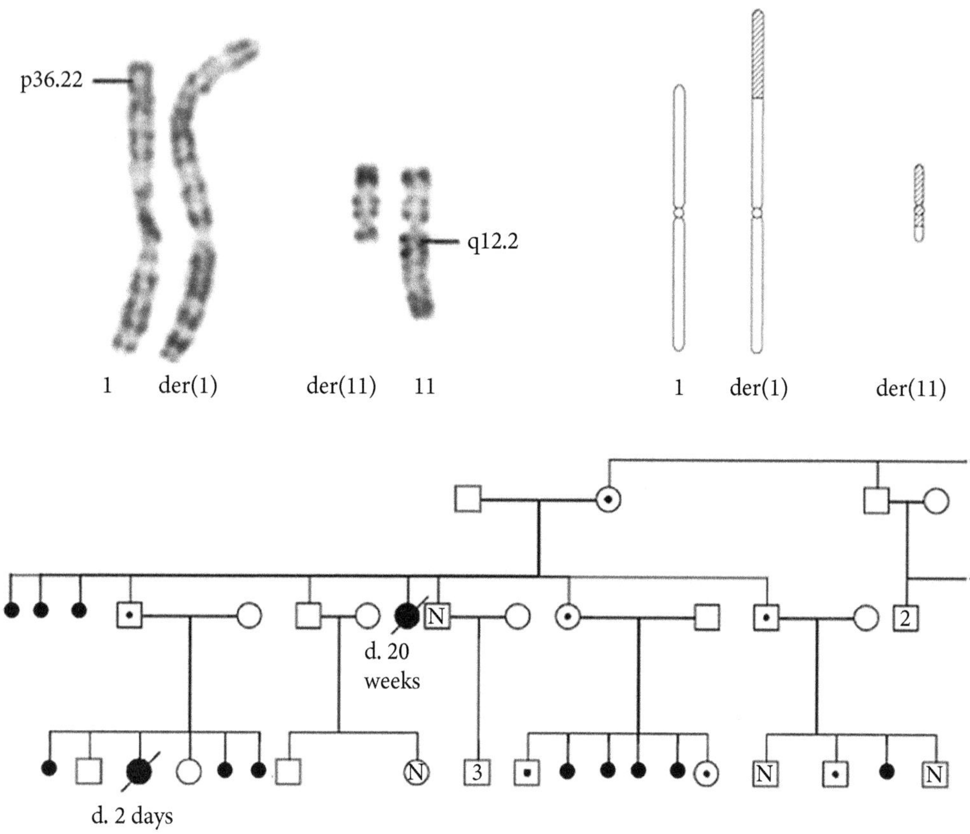

Figure 5–30. A Double-Segment Translocation Seen in Two Extensive Kindreds.

Notes: This double-segment translocation, t(1;11)(p36.22;q12.2), was studied in two extensive four-generation pedigrees, the two quite possibly connected. The larger of the two is depicted here; the balanced translocation carriers are shown with bulls-eye symbol. The large numbers enable the derivation of a quite precise risk estimate (see text). The only viable imbalanced combination from this translocation was the adjacent-1 malsegregant leading to monosomy for distal 1p and trisomy for much of 11q. As the reader may determine, such a karyotype would be 46,der(1)t(1;11): that is, the der(1) in the company of two no. 11 chromosomes. The malformative phenotype was lethal in early infancy, as shown with the filled symbols. The many miscarriages (the small black circles) presumably reflect unviable malsegregant outcomes.

Source; From AT Midro et al., Recurrence risks for different pregnancy outcomes and meiotic segregation analysis of spermatozoa in carriers of t(1;11)(p36.22;q12.2), *J Hum Genet* 59:667–674, 2014. Courtesy M Gajęcka, and with the permission of Springer.

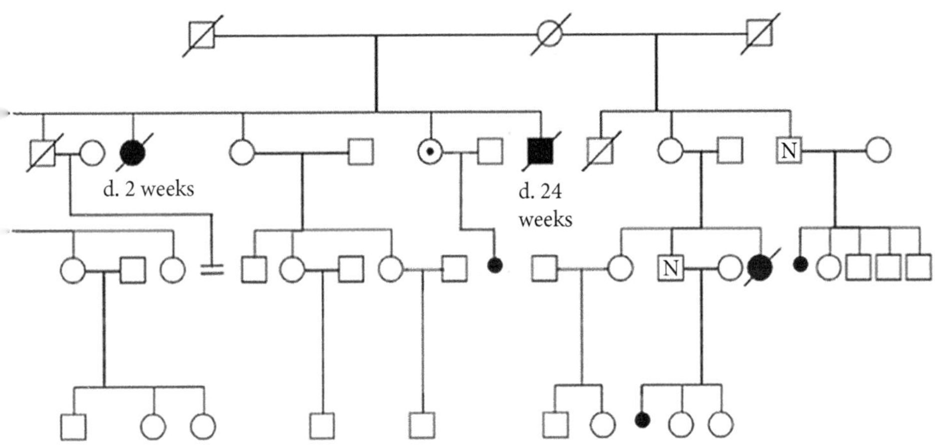
d. 2 weeks
d. 24 weeks
N
N

The different scenario implied by preimplantation analysis is seen, by way of example, in the double-segment translocation t(3;11)(q27.3;q24.3) carried by a brother and sister (Coonen et al. 2000). At least 15 out of 18 embryos of the brother were karyotypically unbalanced, and only one was normal or balanced. This one embryo was transferred, amniocentesis showed 46,XX,t(3;11), and a healthy carrier daughter was in due course born. His sister, a carrier of the same translocation, underwent two treatment cycles, with two out of six embryos apparently normal, but neither transferred successfully. In another PGT case, relating to a couple one of whom carried a t(2;17)(qter;qter), 13 of 18 embryos showed 2:2 segregation for the translocation (six alternate, seven adjacent-1) consistent with either two independent 1:1 events or 2:2 disjunction from a quadrivalent (McKenzie et al. 2003). The remaining five malsegregants displayed 3:1 segregation.

ADJACENT-2 SEGREGATION

Very few translocations are capable of producing viable adjacent-2 segregant products, and the data on specific risk levels are limited (Table 5–8). Where the potential imbalance has considerable viability (for example, trisomy 9p and trisomy 21q) the risk is likely to be substantial and may be in the range of 20%–30%. The t(9;21) carrier mother in Figure 5–14, for example, would have, from Table 5–8, an 18% risk for the recurrence of trisomy 9p.

3:1 SEGREGATION, TERTIARY ANEUPLOIDY

In contrast to 2:2 segregation, the probabilities for unbalanced 3:1 outcomes differ between the sexes, with the female (and especially if of older maternal age) having the

Table 5–8. Risks in the Case of Adjacent-2 Segregation
Specific Risk Figures for Liveborn Aneuploid Child due to Imbalance from 2:2 Adjacent-2 Segregation

CENTRIC SEGMENT THAT WOULD BE IMBALANCED	RISK	
	%	S.D.
4pter→q11–q13	?0	
8pter→q12–q13	?	
9pter→q11–q13	18.4	4.5
10pter→q11–q21	?	
12pter→q11–q13	?	
13pter→q14–q21	?	
14pter→q21–q22	?	
15pter→q13–q24	11.8	7.8
20pter→q11.1	27.3	13.4
21pter→q11.1–q22	?	

Note: Figures are expressed as a percentage of all live births. No obvious difference exists according to sex of parent. For the very many segments not listed, no specific data are recorded in Stengel-Rutkowski et al. (1988).
?, Rare cases have occurred, but data are too few to derive a figure; ?0, Probably no risk.

Source: From Stengel-Rutkowski et al. (1988).

greater risk (Figure 5–10). For translocations other than the common t(11;22)(q23;q11), the risk is generally small and less than 2%. Nevertheless, each translocation is entitled to its individuality, and atypically higher risks are possible, as may be exemplified in the t(12;13) noted earlier and shown in Figure 5–17, in which two out of four children had a tertiary monosomy. In this case, it could be that the tiny derivative segregated independently, at random.

The Common t(11;22). Practically the only segregation mode to produce a viable abnormal baby in the common t(11;22)(q23;q11) is 3:1 with tertiary trisomy (Emanuel syndrome) (Figure 5–16). Different figures have been proposed for the level of risk. From the data of Stengel-Rutkowski et al. (1988) as listed in Table 5–9, the risk is 3.7% and <0.7%, respectively, for the female and the male carrier. In a very large collaboration, with data from 110 families seen in 15 countries (there being some overlap with the material in Stengel-Rutkowski et al.), Iselius et al. (1983) arrived at risk figures for the female and male heterozygote, respectively, of 2.1% and 1.8%. Notably, in most of these families the index case was the only one known definitely to have the unbalanced karyotype. However, it could be supposed that reported malformed stillborn infants in these families were rather likely also to have had the unbalanced karyotype, and if this assumption is accepted, the risk figures for a live- or stillborn affected infant would increase to 5.7% and 5%, respectively. A rather higher risk figure for the female carrier, namely ~10%, is due to Zackai and Emanuel (1980). These authors also observed that the chance of transmitting the translocation in balanced state is significantly greater than the theoretical 50%, with a probability of >70% in the families studied (a form of meiotic drive). An earlier concern about a breast cancer risk to the heterozygote has since been dismissed (Carter et al. 2010).

3:1 SEGREGATION, INTERCHANGE ANEUPLOIDY

The risk to have a child with Patau, Edwards, or Down syndrome from an interchange trisomy is remarkably small. It may be in the vicinity of 0.5% in the female, and less than this in the male (Stengel-Rutkowski et al. 1988). Upper limits of the estimated risks are given in Table 5–9. The figures for PGT can be much higher: 5.4% in the survey of Xie et al. (2022), and as illustrated by the case of Conn et al. (1999) noted above, in which a woman with the karyotype 46,XX,t(6;21)(q13;q22.3) had 9/9 embryos with chromosome imbalance, including two with interchange trisomy 21 and one with probable interchange monosomy 6.

MORE THAN ONE UNBALANCED SEGREGANT TYPE

It is prudent to assume that where more than one mode of segregation can lead to a viable outcome, the overall risk will be cumulative and will be given by the sum of the individual risks. Thus, the carrier mother of the t(11;18)(p15;q11) shown in Figure 5–19 would have a risk comprising three components: duplication 18q11qter due to adjacent-1; tertiary trisomy 18pter-q11 due to 3:1; and trisomy 18 due to 3:1 interchange. From Tables 5–4 and 5–9, and choosing the closest listed segments, these risks are 2.5%, <1.3%, and <0.2% respectively, for a total of up to 4.0%.

IMPRINTABLE CHROMOSOMES AND UNIPARENTAL DISOMY

Any translocation of which a participating chromosome has an imprintable segment is to be considered from this specific perspective. Here, the gender of the transmitting parent becomes relevant. But in practice, this is a very rarely observed circumstance

Table 5–9. Risks in the Case of 3:1 Segregation, with Double-Segment Imbalance
Specific Risk Figures for Liveborn Aneuploid Child due to Imbalance from 3:1 Single-Segment Segregation

A. TERTIARY TRISOMY OR MONOSOMY		
Segment That Would Be Imbalanced	**RISK**	
	%	**S.D.**
4pter→q12–q13	?	
8pter→q12–q13	?	
9pter→q11–q32	1.7 (mat) ?0 (pat)	1.7
10pter→q11.1–q21	?	
11qter→q23*	3.7% (mat) <0.7% (pat)	
12pter→q11–q13	?	
13pter→q12–q33	2.6 (mat) 0 (pat)	1.8
14pter→q11.1–q24	2.6 (mat) <0.8 (pat)	2.6
15pter→q11.1–q24	<0.9	
16pter→q11.1	<1.8 (mat) 0 (pat)	
18pter→q11.1–q21	<1.3 (mat) 0 (pat)	
20pter→q11.1	<4.4 (mat) ?0 (pat)	
21pter→q11.1–q22	6.9 (mat)	4.7
22pter→q11.1–q13	<3.5 (mat) ? (pat)	

B. INTERCHANGE TRISOMY		
Chromosome That Would Be Trisomic	**RISK**	
	%	**S.D.**
13	<0.2 (mat) 0 (pat)	
18	<0.2 (mat) <0.3 (pat)	
21	0.5 (mat) <0.6 (pat)	0.5

Notes. Figures are expressed as a percentage of all live births. Risks for maternal transmission (mat) are typically greater than for paternal (pat) in 3:1 segregations. For segments not listed, no specific data recorded in Stengel-Rutkowski et al. (1988).

?, Rare cases have occurred, but data are too few to derive a figure; ?0, Probably no risk.

*The common t(11;22)(q23;q11).

Source: From Stengel-Rutkowski et al. (1988).

(Table 19–6). Liehr (2025a) recorded only eight examples of uniparental disomy (UPD) for chromosome 7, 15, 16, and 20, in the setting of reciprocal (not Robertsonian) translocations. For example, Silver-Russell syndrome due to UPD(7) has been reported just twice in association with a maternal translocation involving chromosome 7 (Behnecke et al. 2012).

A potential risk for UPD following post-zygotic "correction" is noted above. What looks like alternate segregation in the fetus could actually have been 3:1 interchange trisomy, with a post-conceptual loss of the homolog in question. In practice, this appears to be an exceedingly rare outcome (Dupont et al. 2002; Kotzot 2008a; Heidemann et al. 2010). An example is the case in Calounova et al. (2006): A child with Prader-Willi syndrome had the same 46,XX,t(8;15)(q24.1;q21.2) karyotype as her mother, with absence of a paternal chromosome 15, and thus with UPD(15)mat. This much is certain: Any translocation involving chromosome 15 in particular is to be approached very circumspectly.

Phenotype and Survivability

A major degree of dysmorphogenesis, involving several body systems, and globally disordered brain function, is the typical picture in classical viable autosomal imbalance resulting from a parental reciprocal translocation. The physical phenotype is usually less markedly abnormal in imbalances detectable only on molecular karyotyping, and indeed sometimes essentially physically unscathed, although neurocognitive and behavioral difficulty is often of important degree. Many patients will come with the knowledge of the particular phenotype of at least one of the viable segregant outcomes—the proband in their own family. The same imbalance in a future pregnancy would be expected to lead to a similar physical and mental phenotype.[13]

Survivability is less predictable because, for many conditions, there is a fine line between relative robustness and a fragile hold on existence, intrapartum and post-natally. Whether there is a heart defect (a frequent malformation in many chromosomal disorders) may be a major factor in this. As for the phenotype of potentially survivable outcomes other than those already exemplified in the family, reference to the chromosomal catalogs and databases and to the journal literature provides a guide. For imprintable chromosomes, there may be an influence of the parental origin of the aneuploid segment, as noted above.

THE PARENTAL BALANCED TRANSLOCATION IN A FETUS

The conventional wisdom has been that if the same (balanced) karyotype found in the carrier parent is detected at prenatal diagnosis, there is no increased risk for phenotypic abnormality in the child: Like parent, like child. Some have doubted this, and Fryns et al. (1992) measured a 6.4% risk of mental and/or physical defects in the heterozygous children of translocation carriers (this figure including the background risk of 2%–3%). Others remained skeptical and imputed ascertainment bias as the confounding factor (Steinbach 1986). Theoretical mechanisms whereby an ABT could have a deleterious consequence in a child, the parental normality notwithstanding, are discussed above.

[13] Similar may only mean "quite similar, but a little different." Just as trisomy 21 presents quite a range in intellectual capacity, variation may be observed with the identical segment, duplicated or deleted, in different family members. The rest of the (balanced) genome, which will of course differ, may, in (usually) small degree, dictate a relative vulnerability or resistance to the damaging effects of the imbalance.

If an important additional risk due to one or other of the aforementioned scenarios really does exist, it is surely very small, perhaps no more than "a fraction of a percent" that a child with the "balanced" parental karyotype might have a defect of mostly unpredictable severity and extent. In the meantime, it remains true that in the great majority the balanced translocation really is balanced, structurally and functionally, and of itself will have no detrimental effect (beyond an eventual influence upon the child's reproductive health). Thus, in practical terms, it would be appropriate to advise continuing a pregnancy when the fetal karyotype is the same as that of the carrier parent, and with very considerable (if not absolute) confidence of a normal physical and mental outcome.

If the above advice failed to reassure, this presumably tiny residual risk could be addressed, if this facility is available, by selection at preimplantation diagnosis of only those embryos in which a normal 46,XY or 46,XX chromosome constitution has been inherited (Chow et al. 2020; Pei et al. 2022). This would also have the advantage of eliminating the reproductive risk for the next generation. But, as noted above, the small numbers of embryos available with a balanced karyotype may not allow the luxury of choice in that regard.

Infertility and Pregnancy Loss

INFERTILITY

Both male and female translocation carriers may be affected by infertility, as discussed above, and the infertility can be pregestational (failure to conceive) or gestational (pregnancy loss). Assisted conception, with particular reference to ICSI in the male case, may enable some to become parents (Jesus et al. 2019; Cui et al. 2022; Shetty et al. 2022). But of course in any event, the translocation will convey a genetic risk.

MISCARRIAGE

Conceptions with large imbalances will abort. Against the background population risk of 15% for a recognized pregnancy to miscarry,[14] the risk for the translocation carrier is rather greater, in the range of 20%–30% (Stengel-Rutkowski et al. 1988). For a few, the risk is very high, well over 50%. An increasing viability of conceptuses implies a corresponding declining likelihood of pregnancy loss by miscarriage. Not to diminish the distress felt at the loss of a welcomed and wanted pregnancy, patients can perhaps be heartened that miscarriage in this setting is the natural elimination of a severe abnormality, which provides the opportunity to make a fresh, and hopefully a more fortunate, start. For a couple having lost all pregnancies to miscarriage, karyotyping in the previous generation may be helpful. The consultand would, in her- or himself, embody the proof that the heterozygote *can* have a normal child, should one of his or her parents also be a carrier. Optimism has to be muted, however, in the setting of a family history of many miscarriages, which may indicate a propensity for the production of unbalanced gametes.

[14] This figure applies with respect to clinically diagnosable miscarriage, mostly occurring in the period 8 to 16 weeks of gestation. Severely imbalanced forms may be lost as very early or even occult abortions.

Other Issues

OTHER FAMILY MEMBERS WITH THE SAME TRANSLOCATION

It appears to be the case that a translocation studied in one family member will typically display similar meiotic behavior in other carriers in the family; at least this applies to the male, in whom gametic analysis is more readily pursued (Benet et al. 2005; Wiland et al. 2007). Thus, genetic advice can be, in practice, the same for one and all.

ASSOCIATED MENDELIAN CONDITION

Rare translocations are associated with a Mendelian disorder due either to the breakpoint disrupting or influencing a locus, or with coincidental linkage to a mutation near the breakpoint. We note some examples in the earlier section on "Biology." In such families, over and above any risk associated with unbalanced segregants, one should discuss the risk of transmitting the abnormality peculiar to that chromosome.

A BELATED CHROMOSOMAL DIAGNOSIS

Some familial syndromes have turned out to be due to a segregating translocation. Examples include Pitt-Rogers-Danks syndrome, which is actually due to a 4p deletion and thus a form of Wolf-Hirschhorn syndrome, and Ruvalcaba syndrome, due to a del/dup of 2q37.3qter and 5q35.2qter (Boyd et al. 2025).

CANCER RISK

In rare familial translocations, the rearrangement may disrupt or otherwise influence a cancer-associated gene, or promote mitotic malsegregation and thus comprise a "hit" in the cascade of events leading to the cellular phenotype of cancer, over and above any risks to the heterozygote for offspring of theirs. A more detailed treatment is offered in Chapter 25 (p. 780).

Interchromosomal Effect

There had originally been concern that a reciprocal translocation heterozygote might be prone to produce gametes aneuploid for a chromosome not involved in the translocation, specifically in this context, chromosomes 13, 18, 21, or X. And there has been the occasional report of a translocation carrier having offspring with chromosomal imbalance not related to the family's translocation (Couzin et al. 1987). Warburton (1985) reviewed the associations of reciprocal translocations and trisomy 21 from unbiased (amniocentesis) data and found no evidence to support the contention. Uchida and Freeman (1986) and Schinzel et al. (1992) studied families in which a child with trisomy 21 also had a balanced translocation, and while in several the translocation was of paternal origin, in fact the extra chromosome 21 came from the mother.

More directly, numerous sperm karyotyping studies have, for the most part, shown no increase in disomies unrelated to the translocation, although some workers have raised doubts. Pellestor et al. (2001) suggest that carrier males with poor semen indices are the only ones in whom any such effect might exist; in which case, it might be the altered testicular environment, rather than the translocation of itself, that is the cause (Kirkpatrick et al. 2008). Analysis of embryos at preimplantation diagnosis largely supports the view of little or no evidence that there exists an interchromosomal effect due to

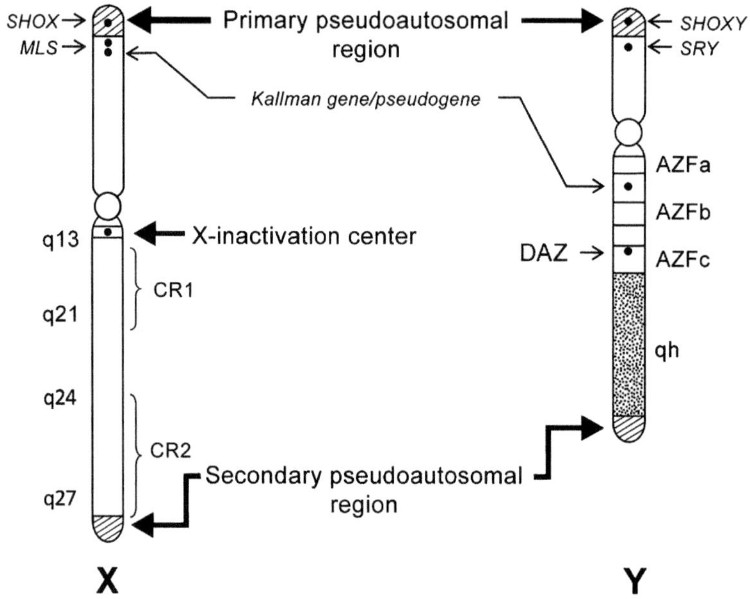

Figure 6–1. Notable regions of the sex chromosomes. AZF, azoöspermia factor regions *a–d.* Dots show specific loci: *DAZ,* deleted in azoöspermia locus; MLS, microöphthalmia with linear skin lesion gene; *SHOX,* short stature homeobox gene (X chromosome); *SHOXY,* short stature homeobox gene (Y chromosome); *SRY,* testis-determining locus. CR1, 2 show Xq critical regions 1 and 2 (p. 156). A more detailed view of the AZF loci is show in Figure 6–19.

every cell of the conceptus is randomly genetically inactivated, such that transcription of most of its genes cannot occur (X chromosome inactivation, XCI). This process of transcriptional silencing is initiated at an X-inactivation center (XIC) in Xq13 (Figure 6–1), and it spreads outwards in both directions along the chromosome. The process is called (after Dr. Mary Lyon) *Lyonization.* In all descendant progeny cells thereafter, the same X chromosomes remain inactive or active, respectively. This "dosage compensation" allows for a necessary functional monosomy of most of the female XX chromosomal genome, analogous to the normal monosomic X state of the XY male: hence, in terms of the expression of genes on the X chromosome, the sexes are, in fact, genetically very similar.

Within the XIC is a gene *XIST* that is cis-acting (that is, it can influence only the chromosome that it is actually on), and *XIST* is transcribed only from the *in*activated X. This transcript—named "XIST" for X (inactive) specific transcript—is not translated into protein, but functions as a long-noncoding RNA molecule (lncRNA). The XIST RNA "coats" the X chromatin and influences the degree of acetylation and other modification of the histones, and this, in turn, prevents the DNA from being transcribed.[4] This

commences with some tissues of the blastocyst, progresses to other lineages thereafter, and is completed embryo-wide by the gastrulation stage, that is, by week 2 to 3 (Khan and Theunissen 2023).

[4] An intriguing suggestion that XIST could have a therapeutic role in trisomic conditions, by inserting an *XIST* transgene into the aneuploid chromosome and thereby "dosage-compensating" the trisomy, is a theoretical concept well beyond the current scope of this book (Gupta et al. 2024).

inactive state is then "locked in" by methylation of CpG islands,[5] and this methylation status thereafter remains in place in the descendant daughter cells of the 46,XX embryo (except for the cells destined to become oögonia, in which the inactive X is subsequently reactivated; Khan and Theunissen 2023). Normal 46,XX women can have ratios of active X^m and inactive X^p chromosomes[6] from fairly even to quite skewed, even more than 90:10; and there can be differences in ratios between different tissues in a woman (Sharp et al. 2000). The inactive X replicates late during the cell cycle; the active X replicates early, along with the autosomes.

But the foregoing is not to say that the female's second X chromosome is unnecessary (a rather obvious statement, considering the difference between 46,XX and 45,X women). This is the reason: not all genes on the second X chromosome are inactivated, and thus some loci are, in the normal female, functionally disomic. This partial functional X disomy is an absolute requirement for normal female development.

Since the major regions in which this active disomy invariably applies are functioning as autosomes do, they are referred to as *pseudoautosomal regions* (PARs). There are two such PARs, a primary and a secondary—PAR1 and PAR2—and, as well as existing on the X, homologous PARs are located on the Y. Thus, the normal 46,XX female has a pair of functioning PAR1s and PAR2s, and likewise so does the normal 46,XY male. These PARs are sited at the terminal segments of each sex chromosome (Figure 6–1). The wave of inactivation, proceeding in either direction along the X chromosome from the XIC, is blocked when it reaches the PARs; thus, both PARs on the X remain genetically active.[7] PAR1 on the X comprises the terminal 2.6 Mb of Xp in band p22.3 and carries at least 25 genes, of which *SHOX*, a gene associated with short stature, is a notable representative.[8] This segment has its homolog on distal Yp. PAR2 extends over 320 kb within distal Xq, holding only four genes and having homology with distal Yq (Mangs and Morris 2007). An obligate recombination event occurs in the PAR1 of the X and the Y chromosome at male meiosis; recombination between the secondary PARs, if it occurs at all, is very infrequent. Otherwise, certain other loci on the X other than in the PARs "escape" inactivation, at least in some tissues, and disomic expression of these genes in the female is normal (Navarro-Cobos et al. 2020). The end result of XCI is that X-linked gene expression between the sexes is near-equalized: each sex has one X, two PAR1s, and two PAR2s, all fully functioning.

Measuring Inactivation Status. Inactivation status can be assessed cytogenetically (replication-banding, or R-banding), which enables, in principle, distinction of the early-replicating (active) and the late-replicating (inactivated) X chromosomes and allows a precise estimate of the ratio of normal-X^{active} to translocation-X^{active} cells. Mostly, however, the analysis is done using molecular methodologies. The androgen receptor locus at Xq13 (quite close to the XIC) is often used as the basis of this test, although results are not informative in all women. There is no consistent cut-off for

[5] Dinucleotide clusters consisting of a cytosine (C) base followed immediately by a guanine (G) base.

[6] Denoting the one from her mother as X^m and the one from her father as X^p.

[7] Similarly, the PARs on the Y are constitutively—in other words, always—active. Thus, both the 46,XX female and the 46,XY male are functionally disomic for PAR1 and PAR2.

[8] *SHOX* deletion leads to a particular skeletal anomaly, Leri-Weill dyschondrosteosis, which includes a distinctive forearm defect, the Madelung deformity. Reflecting the pseudoautosomal nature of this chromatin, the clinical picture is similar between the sexes (Figure 6-2).

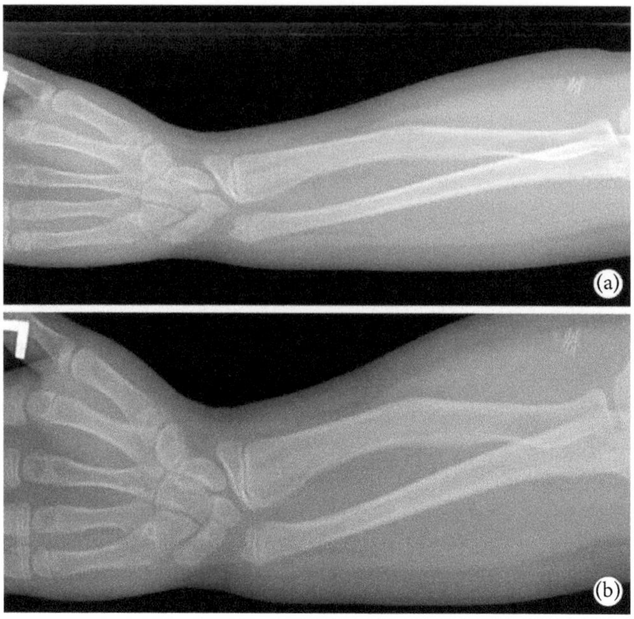

Figure 6–2. The Forearm Skeletal Picture in Males and Females with a *SHOX* Deletion.

Notes: Forearm X-rays of a brother (A) age 13½, and sister (B) age 11, their respective karyotypes 46,Y,del(X)(p22.2) and 46,X,del(X)(p22.2) (the maternal karyotype was not available, but presumably the same deletion). The radius (the upper forearm bone in these images) is short and abnormally curved, and its articulation with the wrist bones is aberrant (Madelung deformity). The notable point is that the degree of the deformity due to Xp *SHOX* deletion is similar between the genders, and if anything, more marked in the female (these siblings also showed other clinical features relating to other loci within the deleted segment).

Source: From E-H Cho et al., A case of 9.7 Mb terminal Xp deletion including OA1 locus associated with contiguous gene syndrome, *J Korean Med Sci* 27:1273–1277, 2012. Courtesy J-K Kim, and with the permission of The Korean Academy of Medical Sciences.

what qualifies as skewing, but a survey of normal adult women identified skewing of >80:20 in 14%, >90:10 in 3.6%, and >95:5 in 1.7% (Sharp et al. 2000). Interestingly, skewing increases with age, at least in blood, and is much less frequent in newborn girls, the corresponding percentages being 4.9%, 0.5%, and 0.2%. In the phenotypically normal heterozygote, the observation of a complete skew of translocation-X^{active} and normal-X^{active} in the representative tissue analyzed would indicate that the same 100:0 proportion applies elsewhere in the soma. Since it is impossible ever to test the entire soma (and in particular the brain), it would have to remain an open question, in a phenotypically abnormal but structurally balanced X-autosome heterozygote, that a more random skewing pattern might apply in some tissues, notwithstanding a complete skew in the peripheral tissue(s) tested. Abnormal individuals may show incomplete inter-tissue concordance of inactivation status, with sometimes quite different ratios in different tissues—for example, 80:20 in blood and 30:70 in skin (Schmidt and Du Sart 1992).

The importance of the foregoing in relation to the X-autosome translocation is this: Transcriptional silencing—inactivation—can spread into the autosomal component of an X-autosome translocation (Cotton et al. 2014). This process can act to mitigate, or equally to exacerbate, an abnormal phenotype.

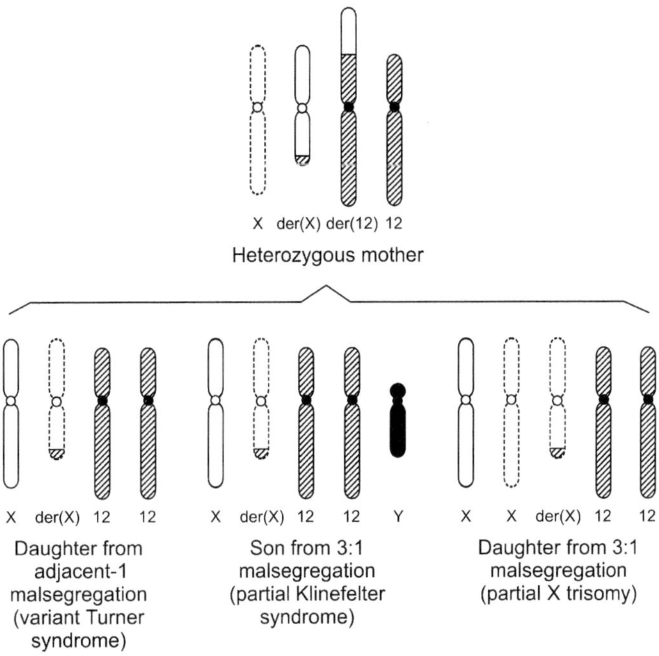

Figure 6–3. Inactivation Patterns.
Mother with a *balanced* X-autosome translocation, showing patterns of inactivation in herself and in her two chromosomally *unbalanced* children with partial Turner and partial Klinefelter syndrome, respectively. Dashed outline indicates inactivated chromosome. The inactivation pattern of a theoretical third child with a partial X trisomy is shown at right. Note that the balanced carrier inactivates her normal X chromosome, while it is the abnormal X which is inactivated in the unbalanced offspring (and, in the third child, one of the additional normal X chromosomes as well). Based on family in Figure 6–11.

THE BALANCED FEMALE X-AUTOSOMAL HETEROZYGOTE

The *phenotypically normal balanced* X-autosome female translocation carrier has two translocation chromosomes, the der(X) and the der(autosome). The X segment in one of these, most commonly the der(X), contains the XIC; and the X segment in the other, usually on the der(autosome), lacks the XIC. The latter segment, having no XIC of its own and being beyond the influence of the XIC on the other derivative, is always active. The only way, then, for the karyotypically balanced female X-autosome heterozygote to achieve a functionally balanced genome is to use, as her active X complement, the two parts of the X in the two translocation chromosomes. Together, they add up to an equivalent whole and functioning X chromosome. The other chromosome, the *normal* X, is inactive. The cartoon karyotype in the 46,X,t(X;12) carrier mother in Figure 6–3 shows the normal X as inactive (dotted outline), and the X-segments of the der(X) and der(12) as active (solid outline).

Probably, the mechanism to bring about this asymmetric inactivation is as follows. Inactivation is initiated at random in each cell, at either one of the XICs. Some cells will be functionally balanced, with the intact X inactive as described above. Others, in which the intact X is active, will have a functional disomy for the X chromosome segment that is translocated to the der(autosome), due to this X segment not being subject to transcriptional silencing and thus genetically active. According to this theory, cell selection then eliminates the cells which are functionally disomic X (Figure 6–4, sequence a→b→c). This mechanism is successful in a fraction of translocation heterozygotes, and aside from a possible gonadal effect or rare position effect (see below), such individuals are phenotypically normal.

The *phenotypically abnormal balanced* X-autosome female translocation carrier will often reflect a failure of the mechanism to achieve a functionally balanced X genome. According to one study, such a failure, and with phenotypic consequence, may affect as many as 25% of apparently balanced female carriers (Schmidt and Du Sart 1992). If some functionally disomic cells should survive and come to comprise part of the soma (Figure 6–4, sequence a→b→d), this would, presumably, have some deleterious effect. The natural prediction is that only cells with small partial disomies would be capable of survival. Thus, in these phenotypically affected carrier females, we might more commonly expect to observe translocation breakpoints in distal Xp or distal Xq (Xp22 and Xq28), which would impart disomy for only a very small segment of either distal X short arm, or distal X long arm. But while this is sometimes so, the pattern is not consistent (Du Sart et al. 1992; Schmidt and Du Sart 1992; Waters et al. 2001; Huang et al. 2023a).

Yuan et al. (2021) give an example of such inconsistency in describing an otherwise normal mother heterozygous for an X-autosome translocation (X;1)(q28;p31.1), but

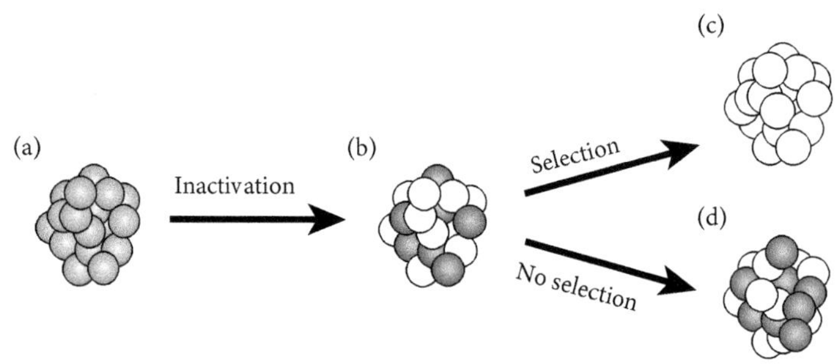

Figure 6–4. Skewing of X Inactivation.

Notes: Skewing or non-skewing of X chromosome inactivation, as a theoretical explanation for the X-autosome carrier being of either normal or abnormal phenotype (and see text). (*a*) Before X-inactivation occurs, both the normal and the der(X) are active in all cells (shown in light gray). (*b*) X-inactivation occurs as a random, cell-autonomous process. Cells shown in white have the der(X) as the active chromosome, and thus the genetic activity of these cells is balanced with respect to X chromosomal output. The cells shown in dark gray have the normal X-active, and in consequence their X chromosomal activity is imbalanced, due to the additional output from the X-segment of the der(autosome). Subsequently in embryonic development: *Either* (*c*) the cells with the normal X-active (dark gray) die out, due to their functional genetic imbalance, leaving only the cells with the der(X) active (white). These latter cells functionally are genetically balanced, and the phenotype is normal. The individual has a skewed X-inactivation pattern. *Or* (*d*) the dark gray cells persist, despite their functional genetic imbalance (the defect is not severe enough to be lethal), and the individual is a mosaic of functionally balanced tissue (white cells) and imbalanced tissue (dark gray cells). In consequence, the phenotype is abnormal.

Source: Adapted from MC Lanasa and WA Hogge, X chromosome defects as an etiology of recurrent spontaneous abortion, *Semin Reprod Med* 18:97–103, 2000.

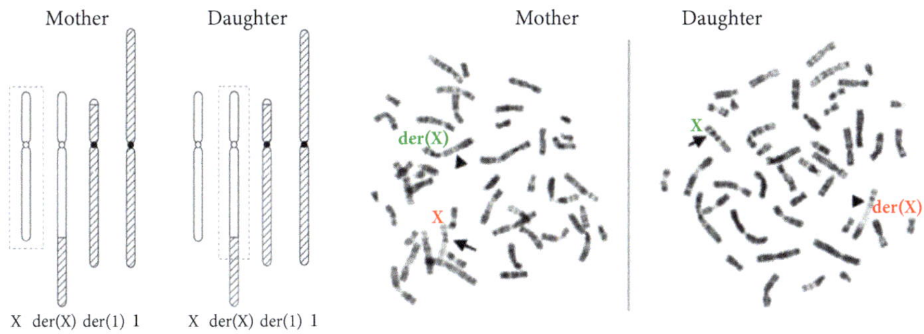

Figure 6–5. The same structurally balanced X-autosome translocation in a normal mother and her abnormal daughter.

Notes: The translocation is (X;1)(q28;p31.1); the Xq breakpoint is right at the qter tip of the chromosome, whereas the 1p breakpoint is about midway along the short arm. The dotted outlines on the cartoon (*left*) indicate inactivation. The karyotypes *(right)* present X-inactivation studies, the inactivated chromosome indicated with red lettering, the active with green; the pale segments of chromatin reveal inactivation. The mother's normal X (arrowed) is (appropriately) preferentially inactivated; but in the daughter, it is the der(X) (arrowhead) which is (inappropriately) inactivated. This inactivation has spread into a small part of the 1p component of the der(X), the segment 1p33-p31.1, effectively determining a functional partial del(1p).

Source: From S Yuan et al., Reproductive risks and preimplantation genetic testing intervention for X-autosome translocation carriers, *Reprod Biomed Online* 43:73–80, 2021. Courtesy F Gong and Y-Q Tan, and with the permission of Elsevier.

whose infant daughter with the same karyotype was of poor developmental status and had a heart and laryngeal defect. Upon X-inactivation studies, while the mother's picture was appropriately skewed toward inactivation of the normal X, in her child it was the der(X)—*not* the normal X—that was preferentially inactivated, and this inactivation had spread into part of the 1p component of the translocation chromosome, the segment 1p33-p31.1. Thus, the child had a partial functional monosomy within this segment of 1p. A tiny distal Xq functional disomy may or may not have contributed to the phenotype (Figure 6–5).[9]

Otherwise, the phenotypically abnormal but apparently balanced carrier may reflect, just as with autosomal rearrangements, disruption of loci at the site of breakpoint (Table 6–1; Figure 6–6). Since her normal X will be preferentially inactivated, the disrupted locus is exposed. An example is seen in Morleo et al. (2008) concerning a girl whose early development was apparently normal, but then regressing with seizure onset (West syndrome) at age 15 months and, at age 12, remaining with no speech. She had a de novo X;20 translocation, which disrupted the *IQSEC2* locus at Xp11.22, this being a known brain-expressed gene. As is typically the case, X-inactivation in this child was extremely skewed, with the der(X) the active and the normal X the inactive; but this attempt at functional balancing could not outweigh the severe effect of the *IQSEC2* mutation, now "exposed" on the active der(X). Molecular analysis of the

[9] "Inappropriately" skewed X-inactivation can be driven by hidden variants on the X chromosome. Ziegler at al. (2024) studied a family in which two females expressed severe hemophilia A with X-inactivation 99.5% skewed. Exome sequencing identified a variant in the gene *VMA21*, located on the opposite X chromosome to the F8 variant, which was predicted to drive skewing by imposing a selective disadvantage on cells expressing the variant.

Table 6–1. Girls with X-linked Mendelian Disorders due to an X-Autosome Translocation

SYNDROME	LOCUS	TRANSLOCATION	REFERENCE
Aarskog	*FGD1*	46,X;t(X;8)(ql3;p21)	Bawle et al. 1984
Duchenne	*DMD*	46,X,t(X;17)(p21.1;q23.2)	Segarra-Casas et al. 2024
Hunter	*IDS*	46,X,t(X;9)(q28;q12)	Lonardo et al. 2014
Lowe	*OCRL*	46,Xt(X;3)(Xq25q27)	Attree et al. 1992
Nance-Horan	*NHS*	46,X,t(X;1)(p22.13;q22)	Gómez-Laguna et al. 2018
Menkes	*ATP7A*	46,X,t(X;2)(ql3;q32.2)	Kapur et al. 1987
OTC deficiency	*OTC*	46,X,t(X;5)(p21.1;q11)	Zenker et al. 2005

Notes: These disorders involve an X breakpoint at a particular well-known Mendelian locus. Several other apparently balanced X-autosome translocations are also seen in girls in whom no Mendelian syndrome diagnosis is made, but whose abnormal phenotypes are probably due to the disruption of a known locus yet to be associated with a named Mendelian syndrome (Morleo et al. 2008 above; Moysés-Oliveira et al. 2015).

apparently balanced translocation may reveal a more complicated picture than initially had been seen (Figure 6–7).

OVARIAN FUNCTION AND THE X "CRITICAL REGIONS"

In the balanced female carrier, breakpoints at certain locations in the X may affect ovarian function (Table 6–2). An Xq critical region spans from Xq13 to Xq27 and is bookended by two smaller segments (at Xq13.1-Xq21.33 and Xq24-Xq27), labeled CR1 and CR2 (critical regions 1 and 2) respectively (Figure 6–1). A breakage and reunion within either of CR1 and CR2 is characteristically associated with premature ovarian insufficiency; these regions are thus also called POI2 and POI1, respectively). CR1/POI2 is the more commonly implicated, as most X-autosome translocations have their breakpoint within Xq21. The deleterious effect upon ovarian function appears not to be due to gene disruption, but rather to a position effect, a "perturbation of the regulatory

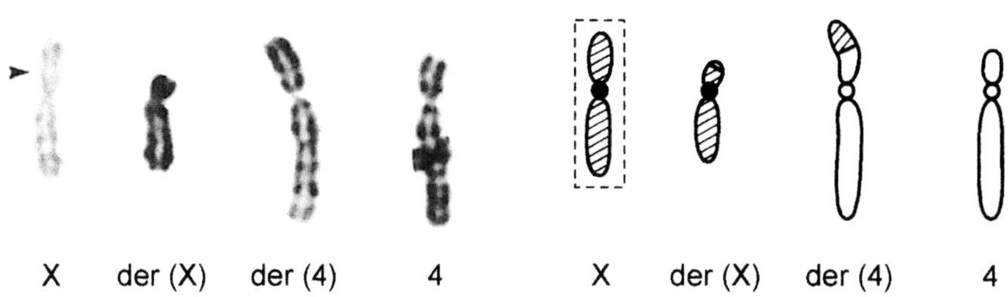

Figure 6–6. Mendelian Disease in the Balanced Carrier.

Notes: A de novo X-autosome translocation 46,X,t(X;4)(p21;p16) in which the *dystrophin* locus at the Xp21 breakpoint is presumed to be disrupted, in a 7-year-old girl. In consequence, very little dystrophin is produced, and the girl has a Becker-like muscular dystrophy. The approximate position of the dystrophin locus is indicated (arrowhead) on the intact X. The intact X is preferentially inactivated, as shown here with replication-banding and indicated in dashed outline on the cartoon karyotype. Early replicating (active) chromatin and the late replicating (inactivated) chromatin stain dark and light, respectively (Case of JA Sullivan).

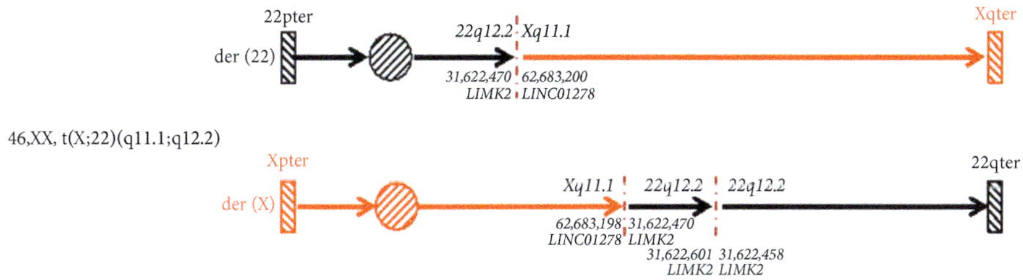

Figure 6–7. Molecular Analysis of an Apparently Balanced X-Autosome Translocation.

Notes: This translocation was initially interpreted as t(X;22)(q13;q13)dn; the corrected karyotype is t(X;22)(q11.1;q12.2). Black = chromosome 22, orange = X chromosome, circles = centromeres, rectangles = telomeres. Red dot-and-dash lines = breakpoints. A very short segment within 22q12.2 is duplicated, and the loci noted (*LIMK2* at 22q12.2 and *LINC01278* at Xq11.1) disrupted. Presumably, the der(X) translocation chromosome would have remained active, since the XIC is distal to *LINC01278*, and thus located on the der(22). The genetic perturbation in consequence of these several factors would lead to phenotypic expression.

Source: From C Redin et al., The genomic landscape of balanced cytogenetic abnormalities associated with human congenital anomalies, *Nat Genet* 49:36–45, 2017. Courtesy ME Talkowski, and with the permission of Springer Nature.

landscape" (Figure 6–8). In one series of 30 women presenting with premature ovarian insufficiency, in whom the cytogenetic findings were reviewed, Devi and Benn (1999) recorded just one to be an X-autosome translocation heterozygote; thus, it is an infrequent cause of this problem.

The Unbalanced Near-Normal Female X-Autosomal Heterozygote

The female carrying an unbalanced translocation may yet be of near-normal phenotype if the inactivation process proceeds favorably. Such a scenario is seen in four women in

Table 6–2. Gonadal Dysgenesis

Occurrence of Gonadal Dysgenesis (Primary or Secondary) in 118 t(X-autosome) Women According to X Chromosome Breakpoint

BREAKPOINT	GONADAL DYSGENESIS	NORMAL GONADAL FUNCTION
Xpter-q12	5	37
q13	4	8
q13-q22	20	1
q22	11	6
q22-q25	7	1
q26	3	5
q27-qter	1	9

Source: From E Therman et al., The critical region on the human Xq, *Hum Genet* 85:455–461, 1990.

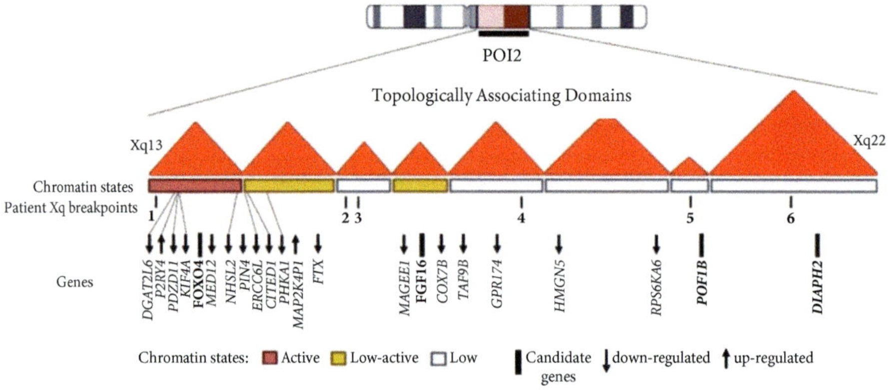

Figure 6–8. The "Regulatory Landscape" of the POI2 Region, Xq13q22.

Notes: Numbers 1–6 refer to the Xq breakpoints in six cases of premature ovarian insufficiency, each woman having a balanced X-autosome translocation. Each red triangle represents a Topologically Associating Domain (TAD), within which several loci interact. Perturbation of this interaction, consequential upon the breakpoint within a TAD, can influence ovarian function accordingly, as loci are inappropriately up- or down-regulated.

Source: From A Di-Battista et al., Premature ovarian insufficiency is associated with global alterations in the regulatory landscape and gene expression in balanced X-autosome translocations, *Epigenetics Chromatin* 16:19, 2023. Courtesy MI Melaragno, and with the permission of Springer Nature.

three generations in the family described in Ciaccio et al. (2020) (Figure 6–9). Each had a genomic imbalance comprising a 23.4 Mb deletion of Xq26.2q28,[10] and an 11.7 Mb autosomal duplication in 7q35q36; and yet the phenotypes were mild, with cognitive capacity within a normal range. The two women in generation II had difficulty conceiving; and autoimmune disease in three of the women may have been an effect of the imbalance. XCI studies in two showed a complete skewing of activation in favor of the normal X.

The Male X-Autosomal Hemizygote

Almost invariably, the *cytogenetically balanced* X-autosomal male hemizygote is, without intervention, infertile due to spermatogenic arrest; disruption of the sex vesicle[11] is the presumed proximate cause of the obstruction (Hwang et al. 2007). In two such men subject to testicular biopsy, Quack et al. (1988) showed germ cell maturation arrest mostly at the pachytene stage of meiosis I, although a few cells managed to make the first, and some even the second, meiotic metaphase, and thus might have become spermatozoa. This outcome of a very modest success might more likely be achieved in those men in whom the breakpoints are more centromerically placed. A man reported in Perrin et al. (2008), hemizygous for a whole-arm translocation (X;18)(q11;p11.1), was subject to

[10] With monosomy for distal Xq, a fragile X test for subfertility in II:2 showed only a single copy of *FRAXA*; the significance of this escaped notice at the time.

[11] The sex vesicle (or sex-body, or XY-body) can be considered as a "peripheral nuclear subdomain" within which the X and Y chromosomes lie, genetically inactivated, during the pachytene stage of meiosis (Turner 2007).

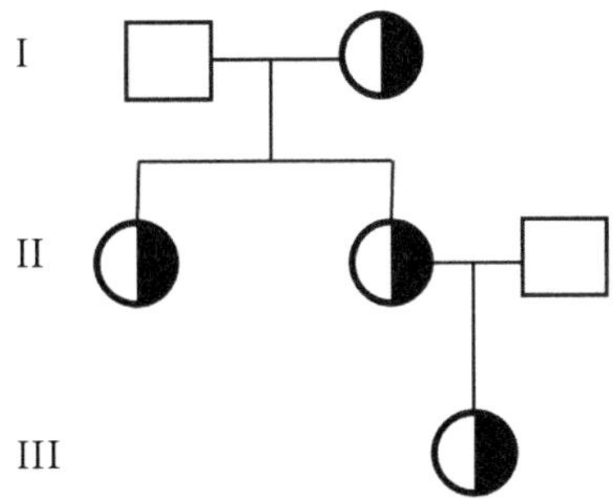

Figure 6–9. An Unbalanced X;Autosome Translocation in a Family with Mild Phenotype.
Source: From the report in C Ciaccio et al., Unbalanced X;Autosome translocations may lead to mild phenotypes and are associated with autoimmune diseases, *Cytogenet Genome Res* 160:80–84, 2020.

sperm chromosomal FISH analysis; he had presented with infertility and "very severe oligoasthenoteratozoöspermia." Analysis showed a range of segregant types in the small number of 447 cells able to be studied: alternate segregation in just over 50% (with half of these normal 23,Y), and adjacent-1, adjacent-2, 3:1, and 4:0 in 8%, 5%, 22%, and 2%, respectively.

If sperm could be retrieved, intracytoplasmic sperm injection (ICSI) may be attempted in order to enable fertility. The man with severe oligoasthenoteratozoöspermia described in Chamayou et al. (2018) had inherited his X;3 translocation from his otherwise normal carrier mother (Figure 6–10). After IVF with ICSI, blastocyst biopsy on 11 embryos showed two 46,XY, two apparently 46,XX (but necessarily X-3 heterozygotes), four with adjacent-2 imbalance, one likely interchange monosomy, and two with other unrelated imbalances.

Patterns of Inactivation in the Unbalanced Offspring

FEMALE OFFSPRING OF THE X-AUTOSOMAL HETEROZYGOTE OR HEMIZYGOTE

As a rule (but one that can be broken), the pattern of inactivation that is observed in the chromosomally unbalanced offspring will be the one that allows the least amount of functional imbalance, as discussed above. This is typically arrived at in the karyotypically unbalanced daughter by inactivation of the *abnormal* chromosome, always supposing that the choice exists (and the choice can exist only if the abnormal chromosome contains an XIC). We may consider these categories: translocations in which the autosomal component is very small; those in which the autosomal component is larger; and those in which the derivative X component lacks an XIC.

The autosomal component is very small. If the abnormal chromosome is a der(X) from an effectively single-segment exchange, containing no autosomal material other than a telomeric tip, it comprises, essentially, a deleted Xp or Xq chromosome. In a girl with the 46,X,der(X) karyotype, preferential inactivation of this

yet have lost functional material (and recalling the extraordinary gene load of this chromosome; Figure 1–4).

The X component of the derivative chromosome lacks an XIC. As with the female child, the male from an X-autosome mother in which the translocated X segment lacks the XIC can suffer a viable functional disomy, if the X segment is "small" (Figure 6–14a). For example, the mother in Giudice-Nairn et al. (2019) carried an Xq;14p translocation, while in her der(14) son, the duplicated distal Xq segment, attached to the short arm of 14, remained active (there would have been no effect of the 14p imbalance). The child was diagnosed with dup *MECP2* syndrome (Chapter 15), and died at age 11 months after a stormy cardiorespiratory course.

DETAILS OF MEIOTIC BEHAVIOR: FEMALE MEIOSIS

In oögenesis, a quadrivalent presumably forms, just as in the two-way translocation between autosomes. 2:2 alternate segregation with the intact X and intact autosome can lead to 46,XX or 46,XY conceptions, while transmission of the translocation in balanced state produces heterozygous or hemizygous conceptions. As for malsegregation, Figures 6–14 and 6–15 set out certain outcomes that may be viable for various categories of single-segment and double-segment translocation, as discussed below. Given the greater survivability of X imbalances due to inactivation, and likewise a possible lessened effect of autosomal imbalance, a greater number of conceptuses are potentially viable than those from the autosome-autosome translocation. The "rules" of segregation (Chapter 5) may not apply; for example, a viable adjacent-2 malsegregation can occur with a derivative chromosome having a large centric segment. The coexistence of tertiary monosomy and adjacent-2 aneuploidy in the family described in Figure 6–17, two otherwise very uncommon segregations, reflects the unique characteristics of the X-autosome translocation.

Categories of Translocation and Modes of Malsegregation

We consider here various chromosomal scenarios that ought to cover the majority of clinical circumstances. Concerning terminology with respect to the size of translocated segments: If one of the translocation breakpoints is at the telomeric tip of either the autosome or the X chromosome, and thus only one of the translocated segments (X or autosomal) comprises an important amount of chromatin, this may be considered an effective "single-segment exchange." If both translocated segments are of significant size, this is a "double-segment exchange."

SINGLE-SEGMENT EXCHANGE, X-TRANSLOCATED SEGMENT

The first two columns in Figure 6–14 and the first column in Figure 6–15, segregations *a*–*c* and segregation *a*, respectively, depict the general form of a translocation in which the single important exchanged segment comprises X chromatin. A particular example

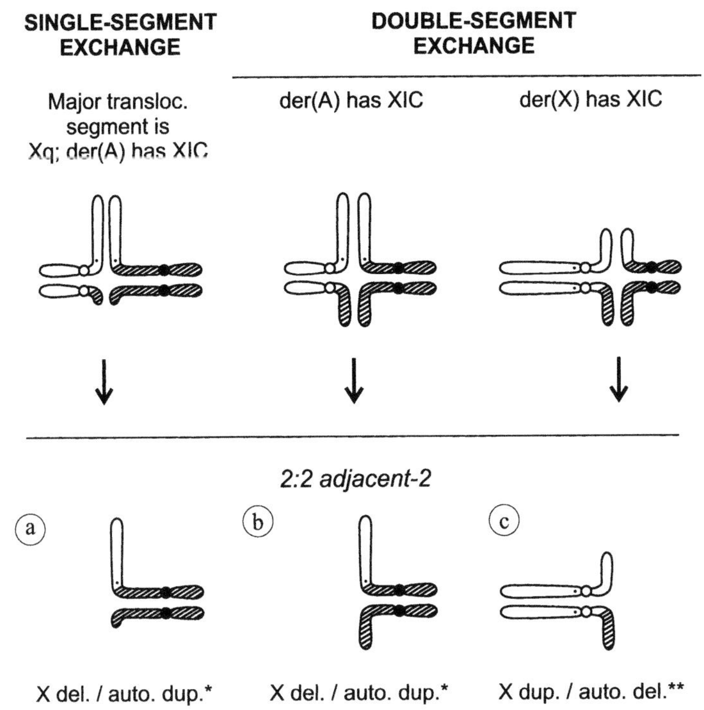

Figure 6–15. Adjacent-2 Malsegregation in the Female X-Autosome Carrier.

Notes: Three categories of adjacent-2 malsegregation in the X-autosome female carrier. The top row shows quadrivalents at maternal meiosis, and the next row various combinations of adjacent-2 segregant products. Note that these potentially viable outcomes occur only in the setting of the transmitted derivative chromosome, be it the der(X) or the der(autosome), having an X-inactivation center (XIC). In the first two columns, the der(autosome) has the XIC; here, the X breakpoint must be in proximal Xq, above the XIC, as depicted. In the third column, in which the der(X) has the XIC, X exchanges can occur either in Xp or in Xq distal to the XIC; only an Xp exchange is shown here. Open, X chromatin; cross-hatched, autosomal chromatin; dot indicates XIC; der(A), der(autosome). Circled letters provide reference points for text comments.

**Effect* of autosomal duplication may be lessened by spreading of transcriptional silencing into the autosomal segment of the der(A).

***Blocking* of spread of inactivation into the autosomal segment of the der(X) may avoid further functional autosomal monosomic effect.

is shown in Figure 6–11, in which the derivative X chromosome is deleted for a large segment of Xq and has only the telomeric tip of 12p in exchange. A child receiving this abnormal "Xq−" in place of a normal X, or as an additional chromosome, could present with a partial form of a sex chromosome aneuploidy syndrome. Thus, a daughter with 46,X,der(X) from adjacent-1 malsegregation (*b* in Figure 6–14) would have a variant form of Turner syndrome. From tertiary trisomy (*c* in Figure 6–14), a son with 47,XY,+der(X) would have incomplete Klinefelter syndrome, and a 47,XX,+der(X) daughter might show the 47,XXX phenotype to a diminished degree.

More severe consequences follow the countertype adjacent-1 segregation: *a* in Figure 6–14. Conceptions with 46,der(12) from adjacent-1 segregation would, in the family in Figure 6–11, be functionally disomic for a large and unsurvivable amount of Xq, and would abort. However, if the translocated X segment is small, the functionally disomic X state may yet be viable. This is shown in Figure 6–13, in which the intellectually disabled and dysmorphic daughter has a 46,XX,der(10) karyotype and is functionally disomic for the small amount of Xp22.31pter.

As for adjacent-2 segregation (Figure 6–15a), such a gamete would, in theory, have viability only if it is the der(autosome) that is transmitted along with the intact autosome *and* if the X segment of the der(autosome) includes the XIC. In that case, inactivation could spread through the autosomal material, at least partially converting a structural autosomal trisomy into a functional autosomal disomy. Of course, there would be a partial X monosomy as well. This scenario is discussed in more detail in the section on "Double-Segment Exchange, Adjacent-2."

> A truly single-segment X-autosome translocation, the translocated segment comprising X material, is recorded in de Vries et al. (1999). A mother had a submicroscopic segment of the PAR1 in distal Xp (p22.31pter) translocated across to the short arm of a chromosome 14—but, as far as could be seen, there was no reciprocal movement back to the X of any 14p material. She transmitted the der(X) to a son, who presented signs interpreted as consistent with nullisomy for certain genes in the distal PAR1: the *SHOX*, *MRX*, *CDPX*, and *STS* genes, their absences responsible respectively and collectively for short stature, short limbs, developmental delay, and ichthyosis.

SINGLE-SEGMENT EXCHANGE, AUTOSOMAL TRANSLOCATED SEGMENT

The single segment being of autosomal origin, with only the telomeric tip of Xp or Xq translocated in exchange, is shown in the middle column of Figure 6–14, segregations *d–g*. The imbalanced conceptions from 2:2 adjacent-1 malsegregation would be partially monosomic or partially trisomic for the autosomal segment: 46,der(autosome) and 46,der(X), respectively (segregations *d* and *e* in Figure 6–14). In the 46 X,der(X) female, the partial autosomal trisomic state may have an attenuated phenotype due to spreading of transcriptional silencing from the XIC of the der(X) into the autosomal segment. The 46,Y,der(X) male conceptus, in which no X-inactivation occurs, would show the undiluted effect of the partial autosomal trisomy. The partially monosomic state—46,XX,der(autosome) or 46,XY,der(autosome)—would be no different than if the other chromosome participating in the translocation had been an autosome instead of an X, and the typical clinical consequence associated with that autosomal deletion would be expected.

DOUBLE-SEGMENT EXCHANGE, ADJACENT-1

In a double-segment exchange with adjacent-1 segregation (right column, Figure 6–14, segregations *h–i*), there may be, in the unbalanced conceptus, effects of a combined X functional disomy and autosomal monosomy, or of X monosomy (or nullisomy) and autosomal trisomy. Such combinations would often be lethal in utero or failing to implant. But in the 46,X,der(X) female (segregation *i*), the effects may be very considerably modified by spreading of inactivation. Consider the t(X;16) illustrated in Figure 6–12. The 46,X,der(X) daughter has both a monosomy for most of Xp, giving a Turner-like phenotype and a structural trisomy for most of 16p. Following spread of inactivation in the der(X) into its autosomal segment in a fraction of cells, the 16p trisomy has been converted in these cells into a functional 16p disomy. However, in 76% of cells (at least in blood) and in the cell illustrated, the inactivation has not extended into the 16p segment. Thus she has, effectively, a functional mosaic 16p trisomy/16p disomy. This same combination with a Y replacing the X as the intact sex chromosome—46,Y,der(X) with nullisomy Xp/trisomy 16p—would not be viable, and thus affected sons are not observed. The other adjacent-1 conceptions with 46,XX,der(16) and 46,XY,der(16) (light arrows in Figure 6–12; *h* in Figure 6–14) would not be similarly "modifiable" and would have a very large functional imbalance, and they would also be expected to abort early in the pregnancy or to fail to implant.

If the translocated segments are small, survival may be possible notwithstanding the inactivation status. Ben-Abdallah-Bouhjar et al. (2012) describe a mother with 46,X,t(X;3)(q27.3;p26.3) whose son, with severe psychomotor delay and a somewhat Prader-Willi-like phenotype, inherited the der(3) in unbalanced adjacent-1 state. The imbalance conveyed a dupX:147.42 Mb-qter (this includes the region of the dup Xq28 syndrome; Chapter 15), and superimposed upon this, a distal 3p monosomy, del chr3:pter-1.42 Mb.

DOUBLE-SEGMENT EXCHANGE, ADJACENT-2

Adjacent-2 segregation typically produces trisomy for much of one chromosome along with monosomy for much of the other, and this is not, in the usual autosome-autosome translocation, remotely viable (e.g., segregation (5) in Figure 5–4). But such an enormous degree of structural imbalance can be accommodated in some X-autosome translocations, in a female conceptus. First, consider the case of the intact autosome and the derivative autosome being transmitted together: 46,X,–X,+der(autosome). Provided the X segment of the der(autosome) includes the XIC (segregation *b* in Figure 6–15), inactivation can spread from the XIC in both directions and into the autosomal segment, counteracting the effect of the autosomal duplication, at least partially. The concomitant partial X monosomy is, of itself, a viable state. The child would be expected to display a partial Turner phenotype, upon which the effect of a variably inactivated partial autosomal trisomy would be added. This is illustrated in Leisti et al. (1975), who record a mother carrying a t(X;9)(q11;q32) and her daughter being 46,X,–X,+der(9). In the daughter, transcriptional silencing spread through much of the autosomal segment which, very substantially although not completely, neutralized the effect of the partial trisomy 9. She had a Turner syndrome picture with superadded microcephaly and intellectual disability. The case in Williams and Dear (1987) is similar, with an intellectually disabled and dysmorphic child having the karyotype 46,X,–X,+der(10),t(X;10)(q11;q25)mat, but in this instance inactivation into the autosomal segment was apparently blocked at the centromere of the der(10). This left the child with an effective duplication of 10p, along with the X deletion (Figure 6–16). Concerning a male conception in this setting, of course, an adjacent-2 conceptus with an X nullisomy could not survive.

Second, viability is also possible in one very rare circumstance of an intact X and the der(X) being transmitted together, with the adjacent-2 karyotype 46,XX,–(autosome),+der(X), segregation *c* in Figure 6–15. The der(X) must contain an XIC; its autosomal segment must comprise a very substantial amount of the chromatin of that autosome; and there must be little or no spread of inactivation beyond the X segment of the translocation chromosome into the autosomal segment. In this way, the autosomal component can maintain sufficient disomic genetic activity to produce a viable phenotype. Only

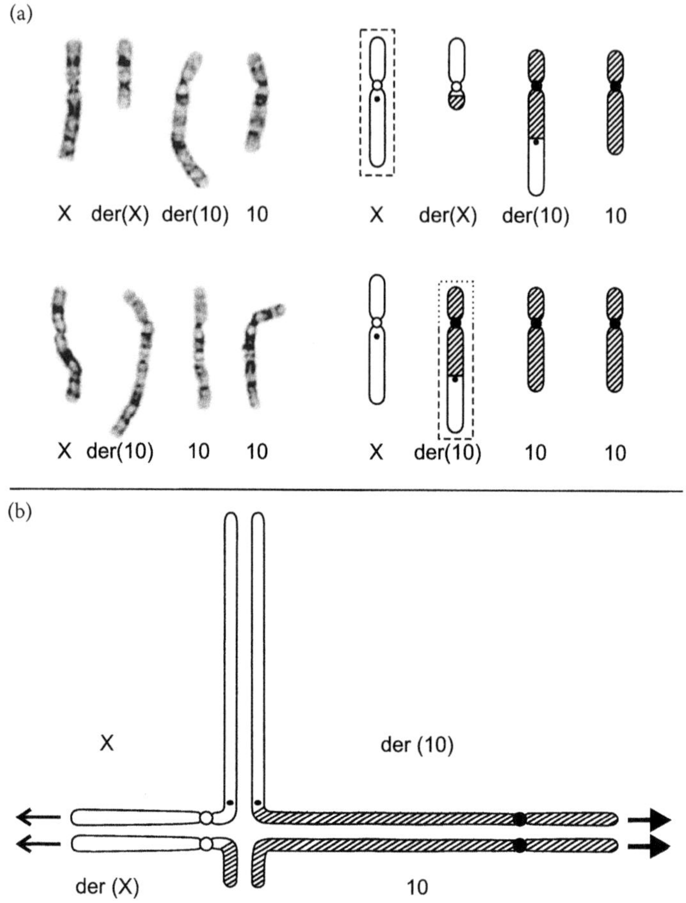

Figure 6–16. Adjacent-2 Segregation.

Notes: (*a*) Mother with balanced X;10 translocation (*above*), and her daughter with a 46,X,–X,+der(10) karyotype (*below*), on G-banding. The translocation is t(X;10)(q11;q25). Replication-banding showed the normal X to be inactivated in all 30 lymphocytes analyzed in the mother (dashed box on cartoon karyotype; dot indicates X-inactivation center). The daughter's der(10) was preferentially inactivated (dashed outline of box) in 50/50 cells, but the inactivation did not continue through to the 10p segment (dotted outline of box). The phenotype is the combined result of the 10p duplication and Xp monosomy. Case of J Williams; in J Williams and PRF Dear, An unbalanced t(X;10) mat translocation in a child with congenital abnormalities, *J Med Genet* 24:633, 1987.

(*b*) The presumed pachytene configuration during gametogenesis in the mother (X chromatin, open; chromosome 10 chromatin, cross-hatched; dot indicates X-inactivation center). Arrows indicate movements of chromosomes to daughter cells in adjacent-2 segregation; heavy arrows show the combination observed in this family. This is segregation *b* in Figure 6–15.

autosomes with "genetically small" short arms could enable these criteria to be met. An example from a maternal t(X;22)(p21.3;q11.21) is shown in Figure 6–17b (daughter with adjacent-2, bottom row). The der(X) comprises most of an X and all, or almost all, of 22q. If its 22q segment were blocked from inactivation, there would be, in effect, a near-normal functional disomy 22 along with a partial XXX syndrome. In fact, this woman had a mild intellectual disability and attended a special school; the relative contributions to her phenotype of the two components of the cytogenetic abnormality are open to speculation.

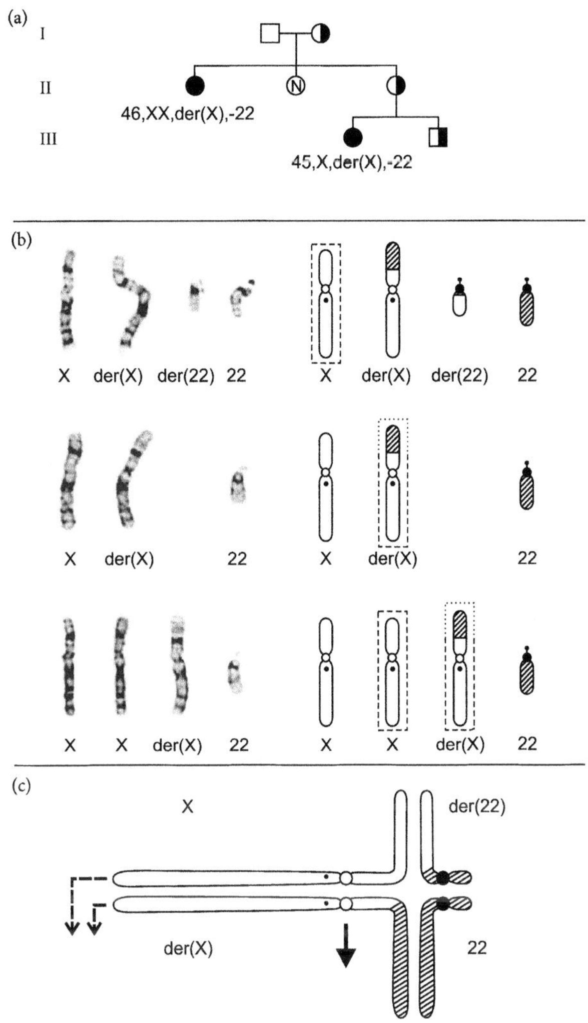

Figure 6–17. Adjacent-2 and 3:1 Segregation.

Notes: 3:1 tertiary monosomy and adjacent-2 segregation both occurring in the same family (and see text).

(a) Pedigree of family segregating a t(X;22)(p21.3;q11.21). Filled symbol, imbalanced state; half-filled symbol, heterozygote/hemizygote; N = 46,XX.

(b) Partial karyotypes of heterozygotes (*top*) and of the two unbalanced states (*lower*). On replication-banding, the normal X is inactivated in all cells analyzed in the heterozygotes, whereas the der(X) is inactivated in the two affected persons (dashed box on cartoon karyotype; dot indicates X-inactivation center). In the affected child in generation III with a 45,X,−X,+der(X),−22 karyotype (middle karyotype), the der(X) was positive for a probe recognizing a sequence in the DiGeorge critical region. The der(X) chromosome showed, in 50/50 cells, apparently no inactivation going through to its 22 component (dotted outline of box), but the clinical picture might suggest otherwise (see text). Her hemizygous brother, III:2, will presumably be infertile. The affected woman II:1 has the adjacent-2 karyotype 46,XX,+der(X),−22 (Case of T Burgess).

(c) The presumed pachytene configuration during gametogenesis in the heterozygote (X chromatin, open; chromosome 22 chromatin, cross-hatched). Heavy arrow indicates movement of the der(X) chromosome to one daughter cell in 3:1 segregation (essentially segregation *k*, Fig. 6–14). Dashed arrows show the movement of chromosomes in the adjacent-2 combination (segregation *c*, Fig. 6–15).

DOUBLE-SEGMENT EXCHANGE, 3:1 SEGREGATION WITH TERTIARY MONOSOMY

The same criteria noted in the preceding paragraph may also obtain in the rare situation of tertiary monosomy being viable (in essence, this is segregation *k* in Figure 6–14). The t(X;22) in Figure 6–17 again provides an example. In the index case in this family having the tertiary monosomy state 45,X,−X,+der(X),−22 (middle row, Figure 6–17b), the der(X) chromosome is preferentially inactivated, but inactivation has not (at least on blood lymphocytes) spread through to the 22q component of the der(X). Thus, a functional 22 disomy is maintained, or nearly so. The important structural imbalance, one might have predicted, could have been limited to the Xp21.3pter deletion (loss of 22p being without effect) with the phenotype confined to a Turner syndrome-like picture. In the event, however, there were minor congenital anomalies, and she was assessed as being intellectually disabled. This does suggest that the pattern of inactivation elsewhere in the soma may have differed from that observed on peripheral blood, and there might have been a degree of functional 22q monosomy in other tissues, including brain.

3:1 SEGREGATION, INTERCHANGE TRISOMY/MONOSOMY

From each of the categories of single- and double-segment exchange, 3:1 interchange trisomy could theoretically produce Klinefelter syndrome or XXX syndrome along with the balanced translocation, and interchange monosomy could produce typical 45,X Turner syndrome. We are aware of only one such outcome from oögenesis: an infertile woman with 47,XX,t(X;12) from her 46,X,t(X;12)(q22;p12) mother, with the imbalance being equivalent to 47,XXX (Madan et al. 1981).

4:0 SEGREGATION

With a trisomically viable autosome, say chromosome 21, as part of an X-autosome translocation, a 48,XX,+der(X),+der(21) karyotype might be equivalent to the potentially viable 48,XXX,+21 state: a combined Down syndrome plus XXX syndrome. But we know of no such report in a liveborn child. At the embryonic stage, however, 4:0 is regularly observed, and this becomes a relevant consideration for the translocation carrier proceeding to IVF with blastocyst biopsy (Zhang et al. 2018).

DETAILS OF MEIOTIC BEHAVIOR: MALE MEIOSIS

Meiosis in the X-autosome hemizygote is typically compromised due to failure of formation of the sex vesicle, and spermatogenesis arrests. Infrequently, some sperm may be made, albeit in small numbers. Perrin et al. (2008) propose formation of a quadrivalent in which the Y chromosome participates with apposition of its PAR1 and PAR2 to the homologous regions on the der(X) and the der(A) (Figure 6–18). As with the female, some malsegregant forms might have viability due to the potential lesser effects of X imbalance. Similarly, according to the principles as set out above for the female but with the additional factor of a Y chromosome to be considered, the reader can determine the range of possibilities in a particular case for this rarely encountered circumstance. The X;3 example of Chamayou et al. (2018) (Figure 6–10) illustrates some of this range: of 11 blastocysts from the male hemizygote presented in this case, two were alternate normal, two were alternate balanced,

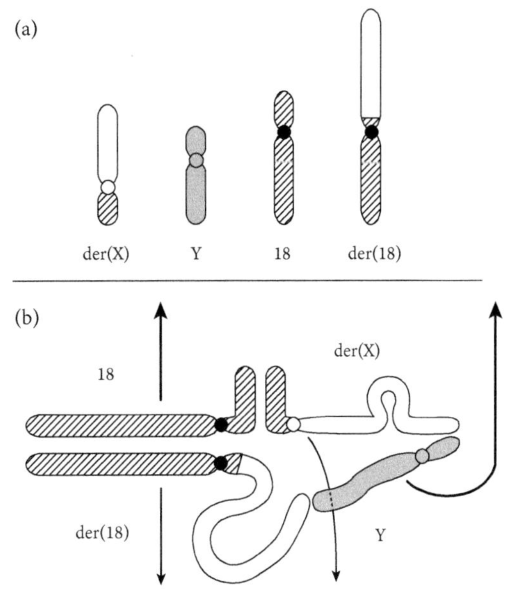

Figure 6–18. Meiosis in the Male X-Autosome Carrier.

Notes: (*a*) Father with balanced X;18 translocation, from whom pregnancy was achieved following in vitro fertilization with intracytoplasmic sperm injection.

(*b*) The presumed pachytene configuration during gametogenesis in the father (X chromatin, open; Y chromatin, gray; chromosome 18 chromatin, cross-hatched). According to this construction, the X segments and the Y align only at the respective pseudoautosomal regions (PARs), and otherwise lie free. Heavy arrows indicate movement of chromosomes to daughter cells in one of the 2:2 alternate segregations, to produce a normal gamete, as observed in the 46,XY son. Light arrows show the other alternate combination, which could lead to a carrier daughter (Drawn after the case in Perrin et al., 2008).

four were adjacent-2, and one was likely 3:1 with monosomy X, along with two having an unrelated aneuploidy.

Y-Autosome Translocations

Y-autosome translocations fall into two major Yq-breakpoint categories, one of which has important clinical implications, and the other of which does not. Certain other rare forms exist. First, some brief comments on the nature of the Y chromosome are in order.

THE ROLE AND BEHAVIOR OF THE Y CHROMOSOME

The particular raison d'être of the Y chromosome is to bring about male development. The testis-determining gene, *SRY*, lies in the euchromatic region on the short arm, just 5 kb proximal to the primary pseudoautosomal (PAR1) boundary. As noted above, and see Figure 6–1, the PAR1s of the Y and X short arm contain homologous loci, and certain other loci elsewhere in the Y have homologs on the X. The secondary pseudoautosomal region (PAR2) is located at distal Yq and distal Xq; its loss from Yq seems to be without phenotypic consequence (Kühl et al. 2001). From the point of view of reproductive health, three "azoöspermia factor regions" on Yq are of importance, named AZF*a*, *b*, and *c*; the internal structure of AZF*b* and *c* includes segments that can be duplicated or deleted (Figure 6–19). Besides sex determination, the Y has certain other, including

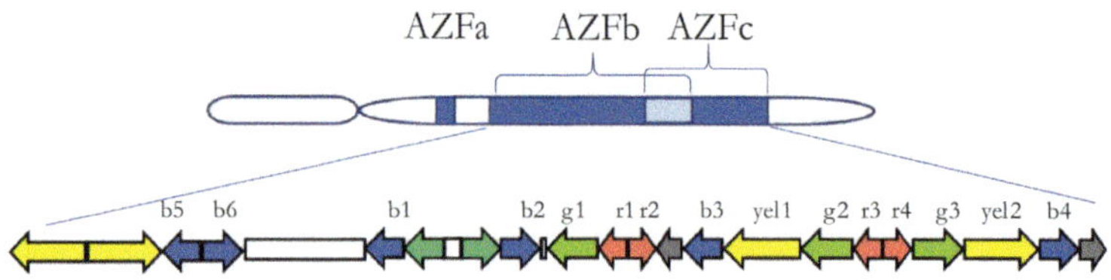

Figure 6–19. The AZF loci on Yq, and Showing the Internal Structure of AZF*b* and *c*.
Source: From R Zhou et al., Identifying novel copy number variants in azoospermia factor regions and evaluating their effects on spermatogenic impairment, *Front Genet* 10:427, 2019. Courtesy Z Xu, and with the permission of Frontiers in Genetics.

immune-related, loci (Maan et al. 2017). Otherwise, half or more of the Y comprises the genetically inert heterochromatic region of the long arm (Yq12), which contains highly repetitive DNA sequences. The Y is the most variable in length of any chromosome, ranging from about 45 to 85 Mb (Hallast et al. 2023).

MEIOSIS

During normal meiosis in the male, the X and Y chromosomes recombine, synapsing at the PAR1 at the tips of Xp and Yp. The two sex chromosomes joined together in this way but otherwise unsynapsed comprise the sex vesicle. A properly formed sex vesicle is necessary for normal spermatogenesis, and anything that interferes with its normal formation—such as the presence of a translocation chromosome—will compromise the process of sperm development.

Y-Autosome Translocation Types

Y LONG-ARM AND ACROCENTRIC SHORT-ARM TRANSLOCATIONS

This essentially harmless rearrangement is the most common form of the Y-autosome translocation, accounting for some two-thirds of all cases. The autosome is one of the acrocentrics, most commonly chromosome 15, der(15)t(Y;15)(q12;p12) (which may be particularly prevalent in an Israeli Ethiopian community; Chen-Shtoyerman et al. 2012), followed by chromosome 22. There is no loss or gain of euchromatin; the result is that one acrocentric carries some phenotypically irrelevant Y heterochromatin, looking rather like (and sometimes mistaken for) a very long short arm (Neumann et al. 1992). The breakpoints are sited in the acrocentric short arm (p11p13) and in the heterochromatin of the Y long arm (Yq12) (Figure 6–20). Males and females can equally be carriers. Neither phenotypic abnormality nor infertility has been associated. Chen et al. (2021b) tested for a theoretical risk of UPD(15) in a prenatally diagnosed case; no such association has actually been reported. The only instance of a possibly related untoward effect is suggested in the case in Rajcan-Separovic et al. (2001), who document the instance of a woman with a Yq;15p chromosome, of older childbearing age, who had had two trisomic 15 pregnancies; no other such cases have since been reported.

The countertype of the common Y;15 is the circumstance in which the other reciprocal product, the der(Y), replaces a normal Y. Hoshi et al. (1998) identified a perfectly normal man, the father of three, who had a 46,X,–Y,t(Y;15)(q12;p13) karyotype. The

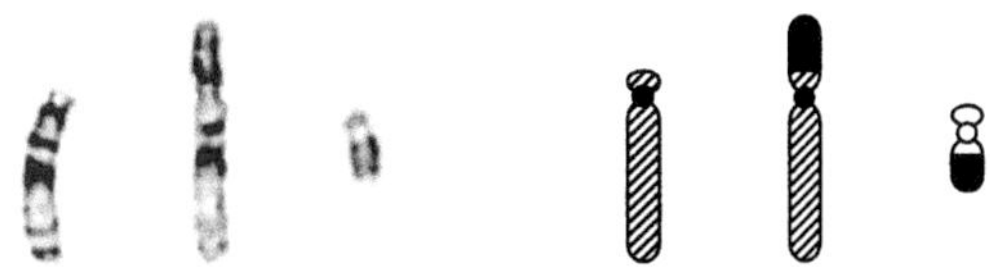

Figure 6–20. A Familial Y-Autosome Translocation.

Notes: An example of the Y-autosome translocation involving an acrocentric autosome, the der(15) depicted here, with the breakpoint in the acrocentric short arm. Normal chromosome 15 and normal Y shown alongside for comparison (chromosome 15 chromatin, cross-hatched; Y heterochromatin, filled; Y euchromatin, open). The translocation chromosome can be carried equally by males and females. The karyotype appears unbalanced, but the phenotype is normal.

der(Y) contained the necessary male-determining and fertility regions. He was only investigated because his sister had had a gonadal tumor of testicular origin, she having the mosaic karyotype 46,X,Y,t(Y;15)/45,X.

BALANCED RECIPROCAL Yq AND AUTOSOME TRANSLOCATION

This translocation is seen only in the male. Reciprocal exchange between the Y long arm and an autosome produces a balanced Y-autosome translocation. In the form being considered here, the Y breakpoint is usually given as q11.2 or q12, and the autosomal breakpoint is anywhere on the autosomal karyotype (other than at an acrocentric short arm, a different entity as discussed in the preceding section) (Braun-Falco et al. 2007). In most, the rearrangement may be truly balanced, with the physical and intellectual phenotype being normal, and male infertility is the usual presenting factor. Given this latter fact, it follows logically enough that the translocation would typically arise as a de novo event, and this is indeed the observation (Pinho et al. 2005). There are associated phenotypic abnormalities in a few individuals, and this may be due to a disruptive effect at the breakpoints or a deletion of autosomal material distal to the breakpoint (Erickson et al. 1995).

Azoöspermia is typical (Kim et al. 2012). Incomplete pairing at meiosis, with failed or abnormal formation of a sex vesicle, may lead to spermatogenic arrest (Figure 6–21). In other cases, loss of the AZF region may explain the infertility (Brisset et al. 2005). But if spermatogenesis is able to proceed, there is a risk for the generation of unbalanced forms, and a few examples are on record. Mademont-Soler et al. (2009) describe a fertile couple, the father having the karyotype 46,X,t(Y;12)(q12;q24.33). The der(12) was deleted for a very small distal segment of chromosome 12 (12q24.33qter), whereas the der(Y) carried this material. In two pregnancies, the two different adjacent-1 segregations were observed: 46,der(12) in one, and 46,der(Y) in the other. Both pregnancies, with thus an autosomal deletion and a duplication respectively, were terminated.

A very few familial cases have been reported with father and son having the same balanced rearrangement. Teyssier et al. (1993) document a man with severe oligoasthenospermia who had a t(Y;1)(q11;q11) and whose father proved to carry the same translocation. Intact fertility is well illustrated in the family described by Sklower Brooks et al. (1998), depicted in Figure 6–22. One son in a sibship of five males and two females, he himself a university graduate, had presented for genetic counseling when his wife had a third miscarriage (they also had a normal daughter). The deceased father must have carried a t(Y;8)(q12;p21.3), with three sons showing the balanced state

sex still retains one copy of the gene, as a heterozygote, on their normal X or Y, respectively. Should a more proximal molecular breakpoint expose a Mendelian "brain gene" such as *CLCN4* mentioned earlier, intellectual disability results. Infertility is almost invariable due to spermatogenic arrest (Gabriel-Robez et al. 1990). The two unkaryotyped fathers in Liu et al. (2023) (Figure 6–26) *may* be exceptions to that rule. Sperm production was documented in a single case, (albeit at a very low level: 125,000 per ml) in a man with the type I karyotype (Morel et al. 2001). He was of normal intelligence, height 165 cm (5 feet 5 inches), with normal external genitalia and normal endocrine indices, and he had presented with infertility. There were equal numbers of 23,der(X) and normal 23,Y sperm, but about 20% of sperm were otherwise abnormal, the most common defect being 24,Y,der(X).

The majority of cases are familial and almost always of matrilineal transmission. Presumably, the X-Y chromosome arose following a reciprocal exchange between the X and Y during spermatogenesis in the man fathering the originating (female) translocation carrier in the family. This event is facilitated by the apposition of X and Y segments having a high degree of homology; for example, a crossover between the Kallmann locus on the X chromosome and a Kallmann-like nonfunctional pseudogene on the Y chromosome long arm (Guioli et al. 1992).

Type III t(X;Y). This is readily recognized cytogenetically with much of a Y chromosome, encompassing some of Yp and the complete q arm, having been attached to distal Xp. The nomenclature *pseudodicentric* refers to the presence of both an X and a Y centromere, with only one of these remaining functional. It is certainly rare. The phenotypic sex relates to the presence or absence of *SRY* within the Yp segment. In the 46,X,psu dic t(X;Y) *SRY*+ case, the t(X;Y) chromosome, containing a near-complete amount of (inactivated) X material, may impose a Klinefelter-like physical phenotype. Mosaicism with a 45,X line may be seen, whether in male, female, or intersex state (Mazen et al. 2013). Fertility is almost unknown (Pavlistova et al. 2016).

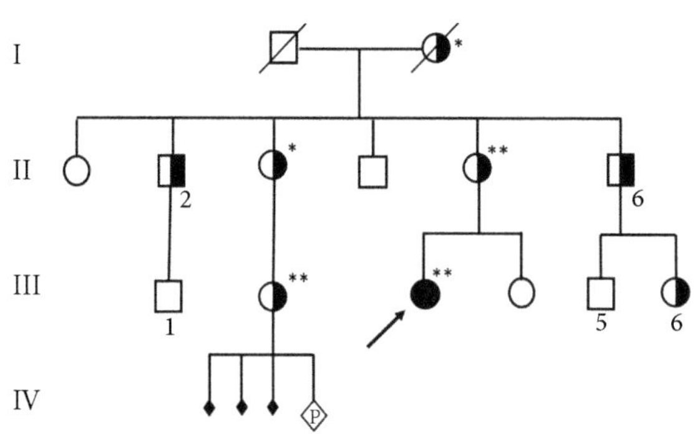

Figure 6–26. Pedigree of a t(X;Y) family.

Notes: The translocation is Liu Type II, 46,X,der(X),t(X;Y)(p22;q11), demonstrated in **some, and presumed in *others. Half-fill symbol = short stature; fill symbol, arrowed = proband with short stature and infertility; open symbol = normal stature; small diamond = biochemical pregnancy; P-in-diamond = 30/40 pregnancy. The deleted Xp segment chrX:251888-1772154 includes *SHOX*. It is possible, but unproven, that the unkaryotyped fathers II:2 and II:6, being of short stature (150 cm), are hemizygotes. If so, their fertility is certainly notable; and it would be consistent that their sons III:1 and III:5 are obligate normal, and the one daughter, III:6, obligate heterozygous.

Source: From S Liu et al., Comprehensive analysis of three female patients with different types of X/Y translocations and literature review, *Mol Cytogenet* 16:7, 2023. Courtesy X Zhang, and with the permission of Springer Nature.

Type IV t(X;Y). This category has been known as the XX male (also as de la Chapelle syndrome) and the 45,X male. In the early days of cytogenetics, a very small translocation of Yp onto Xp could not be discerned, but as technology improved, including in particular the use of FISH probes recognizing Yp material, their true status as X;Y translocations became apparent (Figure 6–24c, d). The translocation arises from an abnormal X-Y recombination during paternal meiosis (Weil et al. 1994). The X breakpoint is within Xp22.3, and the Y breakpoint is in the short arm, proximal to the *SRY* testis-determining gene. The genotypic consequences are loss of the distal region of the X chromosome and the transfer of the *SRY* gene onto an almost intact X chromosome. Thus, the person is typically a male; rare female cases may result from X-inactivation extending into the Yp segment (Liu et al. 2023). This translocation accounts for most supposed XX males and some 45,X males (Y-autosomal forms of 45,X male are discussed above). Almost always, it occurs sporadically, and the affected males are infertile.[12] The extra X in the 46,X,der(X)t(X;Y) case determines a Klinefelter-like physical phenotype. If there is loss of one copy of the *SHOX* gene, Leri-Weill dyschondrosteosis is the expected consequence.

Type V t(X;Y). This rare form comprises a quite small derivative chromosome containing key Yp functional components (including the *SRY* locus) but lacking several Yq loci, and along with the presence of the p arm tip of an X. All cases are male. As an example, the Yq breakpoint of the 46,X,der(Y),t(Y;X)(q11.221;p22.33) azoöspermic man in Bukvic et al. (2013) was at Yq11.221, such that AZF*a* was retained but AZF*b* and *c* lost: this disruption was presumably the basis of the compromised spermatogenic function. These authors perceived a "small reduction of mental capability" in this man, which might possibly have reflected the functionally disomic state of about 8 Mb within Xp22.33pter.[13]

Other Variant Forms. There is a very considerable range of other types of t(X;Y), and Liu et al. (2023) list 22 various rearrangements. The counselor seeing a case not falling within the Types I–V as discussed above but listed in Table 6–4 is referred to the Table in Liu et al. for further detail.

X-X Rearrangements

There are barely double-digit of numbers of reports of this very rare observation. While it is sometimes referred to as an X;X translocation, the expression rea(X) may perhaps be more useful than t(X;X), given that the chromosomal status is always unbalanced, while a lone "t" is often indicative of a balanced-carrier setting. The general karyotype in the heterozygous female is written 46,X,rea(X),t(Xp;Xq), and the resultant imbalance is a dup/del of Xp/Xq, or vice versa. The imbalance can be substantially mitigated due to inactivation of the der(X). Pubertal and/or menstrual abnormality is the usual presentation, and infertility is the rule; a *SHOX* deletion in distal Xp can be the basis of short stature (Reinehr et al. 2001; Tayebi and Khodaei 2011). The de novo rearrangement

[12] A most extraordinary exception, indeed a unique case, is seen in the family reported in Sharp et al. (2004). Two individuals, 46,X,der(X)t(X;Y)(p22.33;p11.2), likely distantly related, presented with an ovotesticular disorder of sex development. One was the child of a 46,X,t(X;Y) mother, and the other was the child of a 46,Y,t(X;Y) father. It may be that *SRY* in the two affected offspring was only partially operating within gonadal tissue, due to a variably penetrant position effect.

[13] And in fact, PAR1 would have been in *trisomic* state: PAR1 from his normal X, PAR1 from the Yp component of the der(Y), and PAR1 from the Xp component of his der(Y).

Table 6–4. Some Recorded X-Y Translocations, Several Being Unique, Having X Breakpoints Elsewhere than at Proximal Xp22

TRANSLOCATION	PHENOTYPIC SEX
46,X,der (X)t(X;Y)(p11.2;q11)dn	F
46,X,psu dic(X;Y)(p11.3;p11.1)	F
46,X,der(X)t(X;Y)(p11.4,p11.2)mat*	F
47,XY,der(Y)t(X;Y)(p21.1;p11.2)	F
46,X,der(Y)t(X;Y)(p21.1;q11)dn	F
46,X,der(Y)t(X;Y)(p21.3;q11.21)	M
46,t(X;Y)(p22.3;p11.2)*	M
46,X,dic(X;Y)(p22.33;p11.32)*	M
46,X,t(X;8)(q13;q11.2)	F
46,X,der(Y)t(X;Y)(q13.1;q11.223)	F
46,X,der(X)t(X;5)(q21;q31)	F
46,X,psu dic(X)t(X;Y)(q22;p11)	F
46,X,der(X)t(X;Y)(q22;q11)dn	F
46,X,der(X)t(X;Y)(q25;q12)	F
46,X,t(X;22)(q25;q11.2)	F
46,Y,t(X;8)(q26;q22)	M
46,Y,t(X;1)(q26;q23)	M
46,Y,t(X;3)(q26;p24)	M
46,X,der(X)t(X;Y)(q26.2;q11.223)mat	F
46,X,der(X)t(X;Y)(q26.3;q11.223)	F
46,der(X)t(X;Y)(q28;p11.2)mat**	F
46,X,der (X)t(X;Y)(q28;q11.2)dn	F
46,X,der(Y)t(X;Y)(q28;q11.23)dn	M

Notes: Translocations are listed in "numerical order" of the Xp and then Xq breakpoints. A few are *mosaic. **The notable case of Politi et al. (2024) concerning the translocation (X;Y)(q28;p11.2) records the extraordinary observation of three generations of phenotypically normal female heterozygotes being *SRY*+, a reflection of very skewed X-inactivation, such that *SRY* function within the Y component of the der(X) was suppressed.

Source: From S Liu et al., Comprehensive analysis of three female patients with different types of X/Y translocations and literature review, *Mol Cytogenet* 16:7, 2023, with the addition of the case in Politi et al., and six cases of Huang et al. (2023).

could have arisen following unequal recombination between the two X chromosomes in the oöcyte. Or, the rearrangement could have occurred within the one X chromosome, folding in upon itself, in which case the origin is more likely paternal (Giglio et al. 2000). Xp11.23 and Xq21.3 are favored as breakpoints, and the translocated del/dup segments may therefore be large.

If female fertility is retained, the rea(X) is transmissible, as is of course the normal X, presumably a 50:50 probability for each. Heterozygous daughters may display a similar phenotype to their mothers, X-inactivation permitting. Viable hemizygous males, in whom the rea(X) is not subject to inactivation, can be severely affected, and especially if the *MECP2* locus is duplicated (Magini et al. 2015; Grams et al. 2016); major fetal malformation may be seen (Lin et al. 2024).

Y Rearrangements

For the sake of completeness, the presumed existence of this very rare circumstance is noted. Similarly to the rea(X;X) just discussed, rea(Y) may be a more useful nomenclature than the sometimes-seen t(Y;Y). A number may in fact have been isodicentric Yq chromosomes (Chapter 15) (Hsu 1994; Hernando et al. 2002).

GENETIC COUNSELING

The X-Autosome Translocation

Fertility is affected in the X-autosome heterozygote and hemizygote. About half of the female carriers and almost all males are likely to be infertile.

The Female Heterozygote

If fertile, the female heterozygote has a substantial risk for having abnormal offspring due to transmitting an imbalanced chromosomal constitution. At one end of the scale, the abnormality might be mild (e.g., partial Klinefelter syndrome) or barely discernible (e.g., partial X trisomy). At the other end, it could be severe (e.g., partial X disomy or autosomal aneuploidy, not modified by inactivation). The counselor should determine the theoretical gametic combinations from the particular category of translocation, with reference to the examples described in the prior section on *Biology*. Adjacent-1 and 3:1 tertiary trisomy are the major malsegregation modes to be considered. Figures 6–14 and 6–15 provide a guide, but each translocation needs to be assessed on its own merits. General comments follow.

1. A "single-segment" translocation (that is, the autosomal segment is very small) with an X segment of *large* size would imply risks, in viable offspring, for partial Turner, partial Klinefelter, and partial XXX syndromes (Figures 6–3 and 6–11; Figure 6–14b, c).
2. A single-segment translocation with an X segment of *small* size would imply a risk not only for one of these three partial gonosomal aneuploidies, albeit in milder form, but also—given the fact of a small segment implying possible viability—for a functional disomy for a small distal Xp or Xq segment. A functional disomy in a child of either sex would have a severe outcome (Figure 6–13*b*, segregation as per heavy arrows; Figure 6–14*a*) (Sanlaville et al. 2005). The other possibility is a nullisomy. While nullisomy in the female would lead only to an attenuated form of Turner syndrome, in the male, for all but the smallest segments, this would be lethal in utero (Figure 6–13*b*, segregation as per light arrows; Figure 6–14*b*). The borderline between viable (but severe) and nonviable Xp deletion in the male may be at Xp22.2, in which about 10 Mb of DNA is removed (Melichar et al. 2007).
3. A single-segment translocation with an autosomal translocated segment of "viable size" (Figures 6–14*d-f*) implies a risk for partial autosomal monosomy or trisomy

rare Yp;13p fusion recorded in Alves et al. (2002), having demonstrated that most sperm had a balanced complement, reassurance could be offered that if pregnancy were achievable, there would be a good chance of producing a normal child in this particular case.

For the infertile man, assisted reproduction may offer the possibility of paternity (Mackie Ogilvie et al. 2010). A sperm count way below the level needed for natural conception may yet allow retrieval of sperm for ICSI. Testicular aspiration may provide sperm even when they are completely absent in the ejaculate. With the need for IVF, PGT becomes attractive because of the probable substantial genetic risk, in most cases, for unbalanced forms, and considering the practical point that the embryo is nicely accessible. Taking the example of the oligospermic man with a 46,X,t(Y;18)(q11.2;q21) karyotype, shown in Figure 6–23, he could, in theory and through IVF, have a 46,XX daughter or a 46,X,t(Y;18) son like himself. The substantial fraction of unbalanced forms that could be viable in this case, out of the 16 total possible conceptions, does becomes a relevant matter at PGT. These issues of IVF and PGT are discussed in more detail in Chapter 23.

THE Yqh-ACROCENTRIC TRANSLOCATION

Probably, these translocations can be regarded as being no more than interesting variant chromosomes, and of no clinical significance. In the case of the t(Yq;15p), a theoretical risk for trisomy 15 with correction to uniparental disomy (White et al. 1998; Rajcan-Separovic et al. 2001) is prudently not to be completely ignored, but certainly not to be overstated.

The "45,X" Yp-Acrocentric Translocation. These chromosomes are probably stable, and not (if fertility is achievable) implying a risk for phenotypically abnormal offspring (Callen et al. 1987).

The Classical X-Y Translocation

The female with the classic Type II X-Y translocation is usually fertile and of normal intelligence. She has a 50% risk for having a child, whether a son or daughter, who would have the translocation. An X-Y translocation son may be abnormal, according to the extent of distal Xp nullisomy and the loci involved. If the mother is short, an X-Y translocation daughter would also be short, likely because of deletion of the *SHOX* locus. As with Turner syndrome, growth hormone treatment may be appropriate for such a child. She would probably be, like her mother, fertile. A child receiving the mother's normal X would of course be normal, 46,XX or 46,XY. Prenatal diagnosis or PGT is appropriately offered.

The male (Type I) X-Y translocation carrier is almost invariably infertile. A sperm chromosome study has been undertaken in only one 46,Y,der(X)t(X;Y) man (Morel et al. 2001, above). He had severe oligozoöspermia and, notably, sex chromosome aneuploidy was recorded in 20% of sperm. Otherwise, 40% of sperm were normal 23,Y, and 40% had the t(X;Y). Conception in such a case could only ever be achieved via IVF. If preimplantation testing were to be attempted, the choice of a 46,XY embryo (the only normal gonosomal possibility) would allow avoiding the genetic risk for the next generation.

Other rare X-Y translocation types (Table 6–4) will need individual assessment.

X-X Translocations

Infertility is the expectation, and a theoretical question of genetic risk will usually be academic. In a small imbalance, fertility may be retained, as in the exceptional examples of Reinehr et al. (2001) and Grams et al. (2016) discussed above. A daughter receiving the X-X translocation would be expected to have a phenotype similar to that of her mother. A male pregnancy would be very likely to miscarry at any early stage, due to an X nullisomy/disomy. If the del/dup segments were very small, viability might be possible, but with probable major phenotypic defect. Children receiving the mother's normal X chromosome would of course be normal, other things being equal. If IVF is proposed, PGT would also be a suitable option.

7

ROBERTSONIAN TRANSLOCATIONS

THE AMERICAN INSECT CYTOGENETICIST WRB Robertson first described translocations of chromosomes resulting from the fusion of two acrocentrics in his study of insect speciation in 1916, and this type of translocation is named Robertsonian[1] (abbreviation *rob*) in his honor. There are five human acrocentric autosomes—chromosomes 13, 14, 15, 21, and 22 (the 13, 14, and 15 are the D group chromosomes, and the 21 and 22 comprise the G group)—and all are capable of participating in this type of translocation. The composite chromosome produced includes the complete long-arm chromatin of the two fusing chromosomes, although it lacks at least some of the short-arm chromatin. Robertsonian translocations are common, with a population frequency of around one in 800 (Poot and Hochstenbach 2021). Historically, the most important are the D;21 and G;21 translocations, which are the basis of most familial translocation Down syndrome. Uniparental disomy is of relevance, although uncommonly so, with respect to the two imprintable acrocentrics, chromosomes 14 and 15.

In this chapter we consider the case of the phenotypically normal person who carries, in balanced form, a Robertsonian translocation, with necessarily a 45-chromosome count. We generally use a short cytogenetic description for the carrier state, thus, 45,XX,rob(14q21q) or simply rob(14q21q), or even just 14;21 when the meaning is clear. The formally correct ICSN designation for a short-arm to short-arm fusion Robertsonian translocation, for example, is 45,XX,der(14;21)(q10;q10) or 45,XX,rob(14;21)(q10;q10).[2]

BIOLOGY

The great majority of balanced Robertsonian translocations involve two different chromosomes (a *heterologous* or *nonhomologous* translocation); those involving the formation of homologs (*homologous* translocation) are rare. Heterologous translocations can be transmitted through many generations of phenotypically normal heterozygotes, whereas the homologous translocation is almost always seen only as a de novo event in the consultand. As Table 7–1 attests, the rob(13q14q) and the rob(14q21q) are the most predominant; these two are the Class I robs, and all the rest are Class II. The rob(13q14q) accounts for about three-quarters of all Robertsonian translocations in unbiased studies, and indeed it is the most common single chromosome translocation in the human race: around one person in 1,000 is a carrier. Karyotypes of the 13q14q and

[1] Many authors continue to write Robertsonian with an uppercase R; the honor accorded Mendel, whose name-related adjective *mendelian* increasingly has a lowercase m, seems not yet to have flowed through to Dr. Robertson.

[2] The reader may have queried this nomenclature, which would seem, *prima facie*, to indicate a chromosome without a centromere. However, given the complexity of formation of this translocation (Figure 7–5), we can simply take this as a pragmatic oversimplification.

Table 7–1. The Relative Frequencies of Robertsonian Translocations in Two Selected Populations

Translocation	Chinese	European	Averages
13;13	1%	0.1%	0.5%
13;14	59%	63%	61%
13;15	4%	3%	3%
13;21	2.5%	1%	2%
13;22	2.5%	1%	2%
14;14	0.7%	0.3%	0.5%
14;15	4%	2.6%	3%
14;21	15%	20%	17%
14;22	2.5%	3%	3%
15;15	1%	0.1%	0.5%
15;21	2.5%	2%	2.5%
15;22	1.5%	2%	2%
21;21	1%	0.3%	0.6%
21;22	2.5%	2%	2%
22;22	0.5%	0.5%	0.5%

Note: Relative frequencies (%) are taken from large studies in Chinese and in European populations based upon diagnostic screening, mostly infertility or childhood abnormality in the former, and cancer diagnoses in the latter. Chinese $n = 583$, European $n = 1{,}987$. The figures are, in essence, very comparable, and thus the averages are likely to apply universally. Fractions greater than 1.0 are rounded.
Source: From Zhao et al. (2015) and Schoemaker et al. (2019).

14q21q carrier states, and of the unbalanced 14q21q state leading to translocation Down syndrome, are shown in Figures 7–1 through 7–3. Balanced carriers for any of the five homologous translocations are of about equal rarity.

Nucleolar Organizing Regions

The nucleolar organizing regions (NORs) of the acrocentric chromosomes have a key role in the formation of the rob translocations. The NORs are located in the short arms of these chromosomes within the p12 band, along with multiple satellite DNA classes and segmental duplications coded at p11 and p13 (Poot and Hochstenbach 2021; McStay 2023) (Figure 7–4). Nucleoli ("little nuclei") have a role in the control of transcription in interphase cells. Only about half of all NORs per cell are actively functioning (van Sluis et al. 2020), and so it is not surprising that a loss of some NORs due to the rob translocation appears to be without consequence.

Formation of the Nonhomologous (Heterologous) Translocation

Pseudo-homologous regions (PHRs) at band p11 in each acrocentric chromosome co-locate in three-dimensional space within the nucleus, due to a mutual attraction between the NORs in p12 (Figure 7–5 *center*). This apposition facilitates meiotic crossing-over

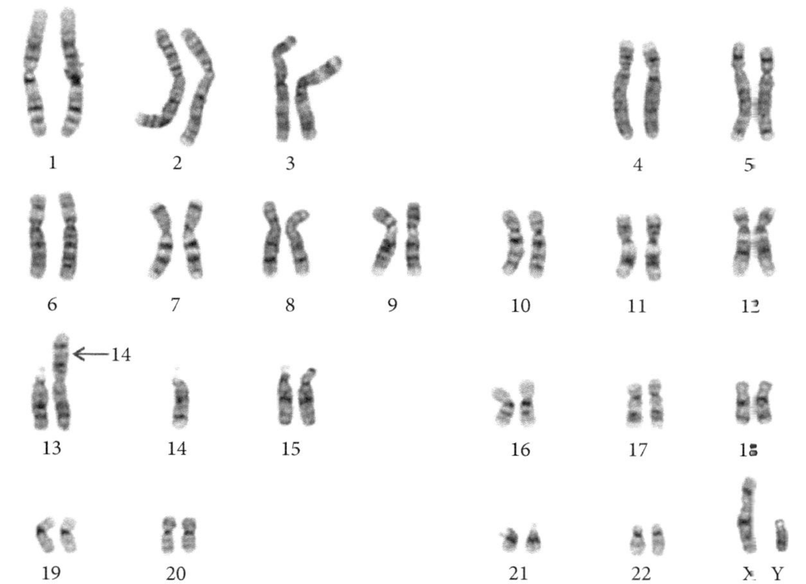

Figure 7–1. The Balanced rob(13q14q) in a Phenotpyically Normal Male.

between non-homologs (Guarracino et al. 2023; de Lima et al. 2025). Uniquely, the PHR of chromosome 14 is inverted (Figure 7–5 *right*), and this leads to its preeminent role (85% of all translocations) within the rob landscape. The common rob(13q14q) and rob(14q21q) translocations are formed predominantly during female meiosis, with

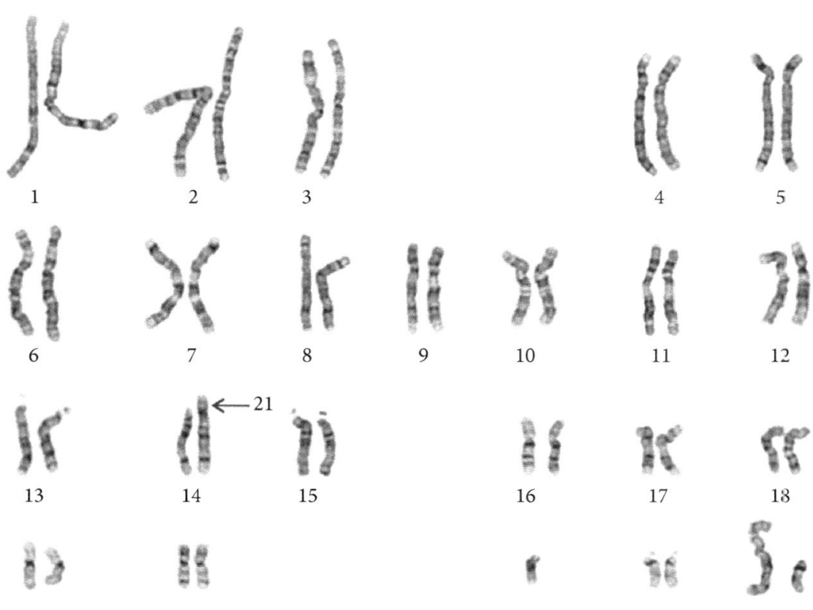

Figure 7–2. The Balanced rob(14q21q) in a Phenotypically Normal Male.

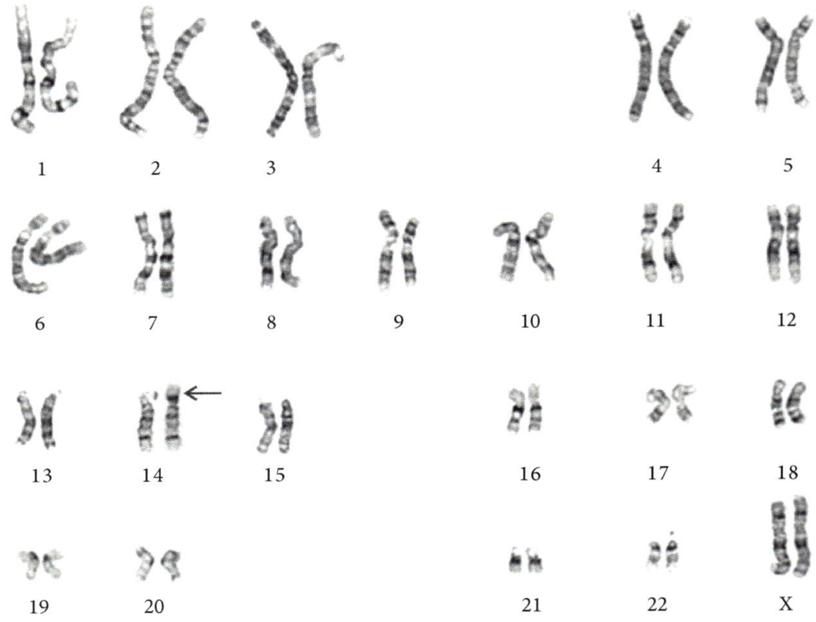

Figure 7–3. The Unbalanced rob(14q21q) in a Girl with Translocation Down Syndrome.

consistent breakpoints at the molecular level (Bandyopadhyay et al. 2002). Variable breakpoints in the Robertsonian uncommon translocations point to a more inconsistent process (Wiland et al. 2020; Poot and Hochstenbach 2021). Rare cases are due to post-zygotic joining together, a point that can be proven when the two component chromosomes can be shown to have come one from one parent, and one from the other (Bandyopadhyay et al. 2003). Just as a Robertsonian translocation can form de novo from the fusion of chromosomes, so can it (very rarely) revert to two separate chromosomes by a "back-mutational" fission (Pflueger et al. 1991) (Chapter 12).

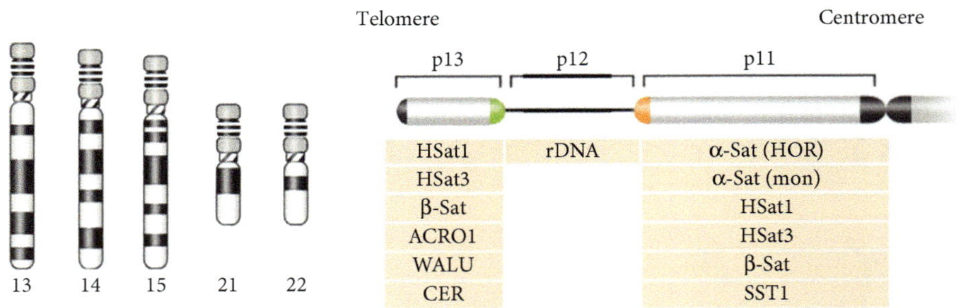

Figure 7–4. The Structure of the Short Arms of the Acrocentric Chromosomes.

Note: rDNA = ribosomal DNA; the other abbreviations refer to satellite (Sat) DNA classes and segmental duplications. The distal and proximal junctions encompassing the rDNA segment are indicated in green and orange, respectively.

Source: Adapted from McStay, The p-arms of human acrocentric chromosomes play by a different set of rules, *Annu Rev Genomics Hum Genet* 24:63–83, 2023. Courtesy B McStay, and with the permission of Annual Reviews of Genomics and Human Genetics.

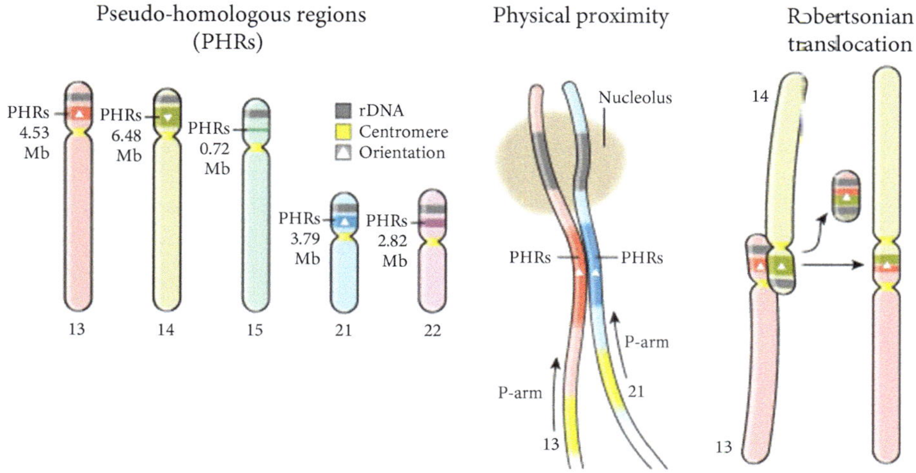

Figure 7–5. Formation of the Non-Homologous Robertsonian Translocation.

Notes: Pseudo-homologous regions (*left*) within each short arm of the acrocentric chromosomes facilitate (*center*) physical proximity of a chromosome pair. Arrowheads show orientation of the segment; note that in no. 14 the segment is inverted cf. nos. 13 and 21. In the case of nos. 13 and 14 (*right*), recombination between the inverted PHR in the no. 14 and the no. 13 PHR leads to formation of the common rob(13q14q). A very small bi-satellited product is sometimes seen (Schmutz and Pinno 1986) as a by-product, and one is depicted here (curly arrow, *right*).

Source: A Guarracino et al., Recombination between heterologous human acrocentric chromosomes, *Nature* 617:335–343, 2023. Courtesy E Garrison, and with the permission of Springer Nature.

Formation of the Homologous Translocation

The rare balanced *homologous* Robertsonian chromosome may arise from fusion in the zygote of the paternal and maternal homologs, in which case it is a true translocation. The site of formation may be at the first mitosis, a conclusion we drew from studying a woman with 45,XX,rob(13q13q), who showed no mosaicism on biopsy samples from a number of different tissues taken during surgery for tubal ligation (Gardner et al. 1974a). Alternatively, it may be an isochromosome, with the stage having been set in meiosis: A nullisomic egg due to a maternal nondisjunction leads to a monosomic conceptus, which is then "rescued" by reduplication of the paternal homolog as an isochromosome, and thus with uniparental disomy for the chromosome in question (discussed below).[3]

THE HETEROLOGOUS ROBERTSONIAN TRANSLOCATION

Details of Meiotic Behavior

This type of Robertsonian translocation chromosome comprises the long-arm elements of two *different* acrocentric chromosomes. At meiosis in the 45-chromosome

[3] Berend et al. (1999) showed a de novo 45,i(13q),upd(13)pat in a normal infant to have complete isozygosity for chromosome 13 markers, indicative of this scenario of post-zygotic monosomy rescue. In another instance, they could show a paternal meiotic origin of the i(13q) in a normal adolescent with 45,i(13q),upd(13)pat. This individual would have had trisomy 13, had it not been for gametic complementation: the mother contributed a nullisomic 13 ovum (she being a rob13;14 heterozygote). These two cases came to attention only through fortuitous discovery at prenatal diagnosis, and subsequently followed up: a maternal-age indication in the former and a rob13;14 family history in the latter.

heterozygote, the translocation chromosome and the two normal acrocentric homologs synapse as a trivalent. Following 2:1 segregation, six types of gamete are produced (Figure 7–6). "Alternate" segregation leads to the production of normal and balanced gametes, and adjacent segregation produces two types of disomic and two types of nullisomic gamete. 3:0 segregation occurs, but it is rare.

In obvious contrast to what happens with the reciprocal translocation, the chromosomally abnormal conceptuses have a complete aneuploidy. Only unbalanced conceptuses that are effectively trisomic for chromosome 13 or 21 can survive substantially through the course of the pregnancy (whether to fetal death in utero, stillbirth, or live birth). Fetal trisomy 14, 15, and 22 are expected to end in miscarriage in the first or early second trimester, and the monosomies would typically abort in early embryogenesis.

Of these six possible outcomes (eight if we include 3:0 segregants), some are much more likely to occur than others. Judging from the outcomes at birth, one might conclude that alternate segregation is favored. From the male heterozygote, translocation Down syndrome (DS) and translocation trisomy 13 are scarcely ever seen in the offspring, and for DS in only a minority (5%–15% of children) from the female (Table 7–2). But of course, as just mentioned, there has been complete prenatal selection against some unbalanced forms, plus a variable prenatal selection against the two potentially viable imbalances, trisomy 13 and trisomy 21.

Gametes. Insight comes from gamete analysis. Sperm and oöcyte studies show considerable fractions, but still a minority, of unbalanced forms. (Naturally, most if not all of the individuals proceeding to gamete testing in these reported studies will have experienced reproductive difficulty, and thus the data from their gametes may not necessarily be applicable to the larger number of carriers with apparently normal fertility.) Zhu et al. (2022a) analyzed nearly a quarter of a million sperm from ten male 13;14 heterozygotes,

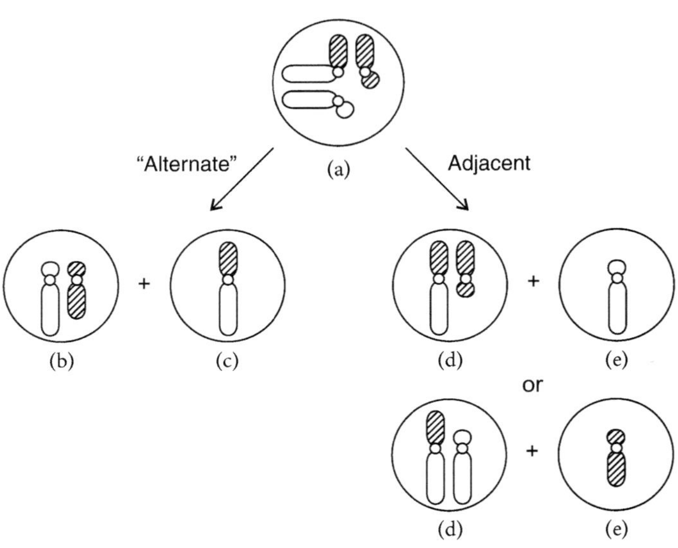

Figure 7–6. Meiotic behavior of the Robertsonian translocation.
(*a*) Trivalent at synapsis. (*b*) Normal and (*c*) carrier gametes from "*alternate*" segregation. (*d*) Disomic and (*e*) nullisomic gametes from *adjacent* segregation. Note that there are six possible combinations (ignoring 3:0 segregation), of which two are normal/balanced, and four are unbalanced.

Table 7–2. Estimates of Risks to Have a Child with Aneuploidy, for the Heterologous rob Carrier

rob	MOTHER	FATHER
13q14q	1%	<1%
13q15q	1%	<1%
13q21q	10%–15%	<1%
13q22q	1%	<1%
14q15q	–	–
14q21q	10%–15%	<1%
14q22q	–	–
15q21q	10%–15%	<1%
15q22q	–	–
21q22q	5%–10%	<1%

Notes: Estimates for the uncommon rob translocations are extrapolated from data for the common robs.

Unbal., unbalanced, with a full aneuploidy for chromosome 13 or 21. The risks for a UPD syndrome from a 14- or 15-containing translocation are uniformly very low (0.06%; Moradkhani et al. 2019).

Sources: From Harris et al. 1979; Ferguson-Smith 1983; Boué and Gallano 1984; Daniel et al. 1989.

showing segregation ratios tilted substantially in favor of balanced forms: an average of 74% of sperm were balanced, ranging from 62% to 85% per subject in this series. Otherwise, an average of 23% of sperm were unbalanced due to adjacent segregation, and just 1.5% with 3:0.

The numbers from pooled series are similar, with a ratio of close to 80%:20%, for balanced:unbalanced in both of the Class I cases, 13;14 and 14;21 (Table 7–3). Across the range of rare Class II rob translocations, Wiland et al. (2020) derived estimates from pooled literature reports, and these data are shown in Table 7-4. The similar picture is graphed in Figure 7–7. What is notable from these data is that the fractions are so similar between all the Class I and Class II rob translocations and that of all imbalanced possibilities in sperm, it is only adjacent segregation that occurs with any substantial frequency.

Ova are somewhat more prone to error. The ingenious approach of FISH analysis on polar bodies allows an inference of what must be the chromosomal constitution of the oöcyte. For example, if a polar body from a 45,XX,rob(14;21) heterozygote has a chromosome 14 but is lacking a number 21 (say, polar body (e) in Figure 7–6), then the 14;21

Table 7–3. Male Meiotic Behavior of rob 13q14q and 14q21q.

Rob	Alternate	Adjacent	3:0/2n	Other
13;14	79%	20%	0.8%	0.2%
14;21	79%	19%	1.4%	0.6%

Note: Shown are segregation patterns in the sperm of carriers of the two common (Class I) rob translocations. Note the substantial bias toward alternate segregations in both cases. 2n = diploidy.

Source: From pooled data in Wiland et al. (2022).

Table 7–4. Male Meiotic Behavior of the Rare Robertsonian Translocations

Rob	Alternate	Adjacent	3:0/2n	Other
13;15	76%	23%	0.9%	0.1%
13;21	89%	11%	0.1%	0.3%
13;22	81%	17%	0.8%	0.3%
14;15	84%	16%	0.4%	0%
14;22	81%	18%	0.7%	0%
15;21	78%	—	—	—
15;22	86%	13%	1%	0%
21;22	80%	19%	0.5%	1%
Averages	82%	17%	0.65%	1%

Notes: Observe the substantial bias, averaging 82%, toward alternate segregations in every case. Note also how closely these percentages match those in the two common rob translocations (Table 7–3). 2n = diploidy.

Source: From pooled data in Wiland et al. (2022).

translocation and a number 21 must be present in its fellow oöcyte (say, gamete (d) in Figure 7–6). Such a gamete would, if fertilized, give rise to the karyotype of translocation DS. Munné et al. (2000) and others have shown that typically, slightly over one-half of oöcytes are balanced; 15% of oöcytes from the 14;21 carrier would potentially be viable (as translocation DS), and from the 13;14 carriers, the corresponding figure is 10% (as translocation trisomy 13) (Table 7–5).

Embryos. The data from analysis of blastocysts at PGT show, as might have been expected, a rather similar spread to that observed in gametes (Table 7–6, Figure 7–8). Alternate segregation with a balanced genotype is the most commonly observed from all categories of the male rob carrier. Alternate segregation is somewhat less seen in the female carrier, but nevertheless, with the exception of the 46,XX,rob(21q22q) case, half

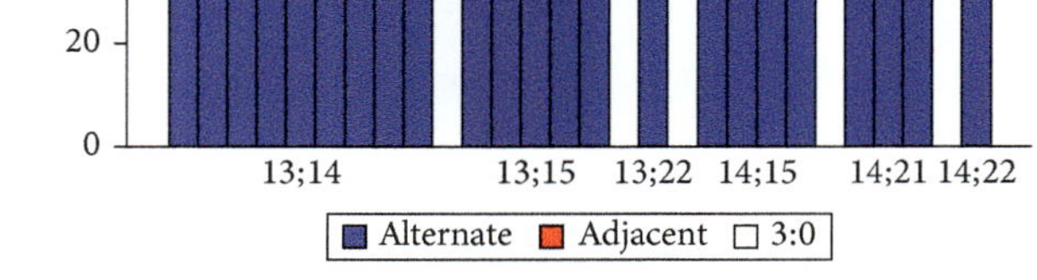

Figure 7–7. Meiotic Segregation in Sperm.

Notes: Each column represents a rob heterozygote. Cases grouped according to the particular rob, *y* axis.

Source: From A Lamotte et al., Is sperm FISH analysis still useful for Robertsonian translocations? Meiotic analysis for 23 patients and review of the literature, *Basic Clin Androl* 28:5, 2018. Courtesy S Hennebicq, and with the permission of Springer Nature.

Table 7–5. Female Meiotic Behavior of rob 13q14q and 14q21q

Rob	2:1 Alternate	2:1 Adjacent	(fractions with the potential viable disomy)
13;14	56%	33%	(10%)
14;21	55%	42%	(15%)
Total	56%	39%	(12%)

Note: These data are derived from oöcyte analysis of 19 13;14 carriers and six 14;21 carriers. Only 2:1 segregants are listed, not 3:0; thus, shortfalls per case from 100% totals are due to 3:0 forms. The potentially viable disomies noted could give rise to trisomy 13 or trisomy 21.

Sources: From Munné et al. (2000), Durban et al. (2001), Pujol et al. (2003), and Molina Gomes et al. (2009).

Table 7–6. The rob 13q14q and 14q21q in Blastocysts

Segregation	Female 13;14	Male 13;14	Female 14;21	Male 14;21
Number of blastocysts	1972	2093	668	403
Alternate	1254	1746	389	316
Adjacent	693	342	267	85
3:0/others	25	5	12	2
Alternate %	64%	83%	58%	78%

Notes: These data are combined from three studies: Zhang et al. 2021a, Dang et al. 2023, and Benn and Merrion 2025.

Source: From P Benn and K Merrion, Chromosome segregation of human nonhomologous Robertsonian translocations: insights from preimplantation genetic testing, *Eur J Hum Genet* 33:711–717, 2025.

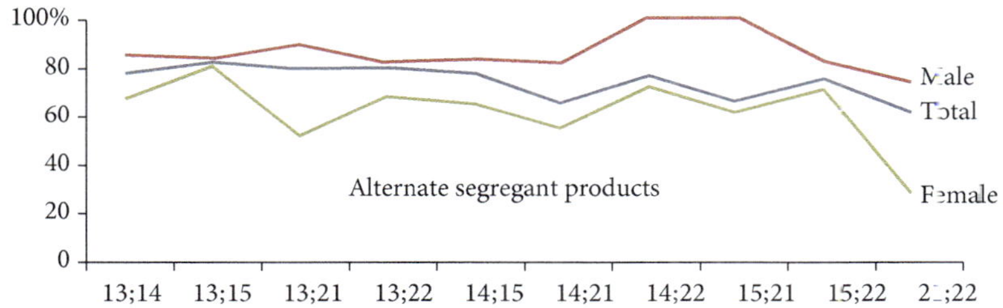

Figure 7–8. The Rates of Alternate Segregant Products in the Blastocysts of Every Category of Heterologous rob Carrier.

Note: In only one type, the rob 21q22q in the female, are balanced segregants in a minority.

Source: From S Zhang et al., Meiotic heterogeneity of trivalent structure and interchromosomal effect in blastocysts with robertsonian translocations, *Front Genet* 12:609563, 2021. Courtesy C Xu and X Sun, and with the permission of Frontiers in Genetics.

to three-quarters of blastocysts result from alternate segregation. Embryos resulting from adjacent segregation will, in the considerable majority, be nonviable, and as noted above, it is only trisomies for 13 and 21 that are potentially viable from this segregant category (and very rare "corrected" uniparental disomies).

Interchromosomal Effect. The concept of an interchromosomal effect (ICE) has been invoked in the setting of the balanced Robertsonian heterozygote. Could a translocation somehow influence the distribution of another chromosome not involved in the rearrangement, with the production of a gamete aneuploid for a chromosome not involved in the translocation? Anecdotal reports of DS children born to 14q22q and 13q14q rob carriers (Farag et al. 1987; Sikkema-Raddatz et al. 1997b) seemed to support this notion. However, formal segregation studies in large numbers of families with a rob(13q14q) or with trisomy 21 showed no apparent excess of trisomic offspring or of parental Robertsonian translocations, respectively (Harris et al. 1979; Lindenbaum et al. 1985). Therman et al. (1989) ascertained no Robertsonian translocation through a trisomic child other than one that included the trisomic chromosome.

Observations in the cleavage-stage embryo suggest that an ICE may apply during the mitoses immediately after the formation of the zygote. Using CGH microarray, Alfarawati et al. (2012) recorded malsegregation of chromosomes not involved in the translocation in 70% of the embryos of Robertsonian translocation carriers, giving 6% over and above the background rate of 64% in controls. As these authors write, "out of every 11 euploid zygotes produced by a Robertsonian translocation carrier, one is expected to become abnormal by the cleavage stage due to an ICE." Zhang et al. (2021a), applying the methodology of single nucleotide polymorphism (SNP) genotyping of whole genome amplification (WGA) products, identified a range of aneuploidies and mosaicisms in 977 blastocysts of rob carriers, showing overall only a very slightly increased risk due to an ICE (Figure 7–9), consistent with Alfarawati et al. (2012) and with other recent studies (Shetty et al. 2022). The practical conclusion to be drawn is that an ICE may indeed exist and is to be taken into account, although in terms of a rob risk, it is a minor player.

Meiotic Drive. Meiotic drive is an influence whereby one of the products at meiosis may be favored and have a better-than-even chance of coming to be in the successful gamete. The Robertsonian translocation provides an example. At the level of the offspring produced, de Villena and Sapienza (2001) demonstrated that children of female carriers of rob translocations have a ratio close to 60:40 for the balanced rob, compared to normal karyotypes. No such effect could be confirmed for the male rob carrier. Daniel (2002) has confirmed these interpretations in a retrospective analysis of prenatal diagnosis data, with rigorous attention to the need to avoid bias, showing a 116:81 ratio in favor of balanced carrier offspring versus normal karyotypes where the mother is the carrier parent, compared to a near unity 42:41 ratio for carrier fathers. Other esoteric differences in ratios are dealt with in Kovaleva (2019).

POST-ZYGOTIC "CORRECTION" AND ASSOCIATED UNIPARENTAL DISOMY

Trisomic Correction. An initially translocation trisomic conception where one parent is a rob carrier may be "corrected" in very early embryonic existence by the mitotic loss of one of the free homologs. If the lineage of this newly produced normal cell is destined to give rise to the inner cell mass, then a chromosomally balanced (albeit rob heterozygous) embryo may result, and the embryo will have uniparental disomy (UPD). UPD has no untoward effect if the chromosome is not subject to imprinting (except for the question

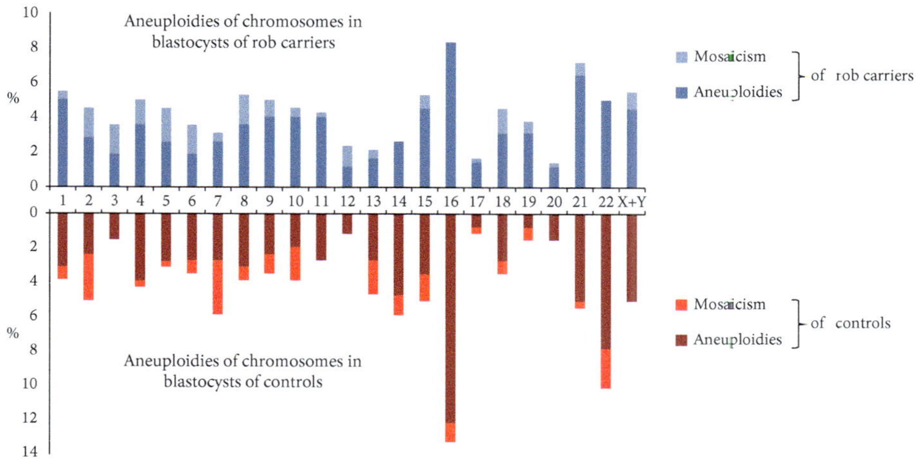

Figure 7–9. Interchromosomal effect, at the level of the blastocyst, from carriers of rob translocations.

Notes: Every type of heterologous rob is represented. The graph shows the range of aneuploidies, and of mosacisms, across the whole karyotype, as seen in 977 blastocysts of rob carrier couples, cf. 785 of control couples. The controls are from blastocysts of couples of quite similar ages (actually, 2-3 years older) at risk for a mendelian condition, and these defined a background rate of aneuploidy affecting any embryo. On simple visual inspection, an increased risk for an ICE in the rob carriers appears, overall, only slightly greater compared with the control group, and only with some chromosomes (no. 16 a spectacular outlier). On formal statistical analysis, the whole group of rob carriers gives an odds ratio of 1.3 cf. controls for an aneuploid embryo due to an ICE. Mosaic and segmental aneuploidies, which are typically of mitotic origin, were not increased in the embryos of rob carriers.

Source: From S Zhang et al., Meiotic heterogeneity of trivalent structure and interchromosomal effect in blastocysts with robertsonian translocations, *Front Genet* 12:609563, 2021. Courtesy C Xu and X Sun, and with the permission of Frontiers in Genetics.

of isozygosity for a recessive gene; see below), and chromosomes 13, 21, and 22 are in this category. But when chromosome 14 or 15 is a partner in a rob translocation, a risk (albeit small) exists for the birth of a child with an imprinting syndrome, chromosomes 14 and 15 being subject to parent-of-origin imprinting (Chapter 19). For example, a presumed mechanism whereby UPD(15) could arise from a rob(13q15q) parent is outlined in Figure 7–10. Essentially, adjacent segregation produces a trisomic 15 conception, and then loss of the chromosome 15 contributed from the *other* parent,[4] at a very early postzygotic stage, "corrects" the quantitative chromosomal content. Observations such as these are very rare.

Liehr (2025a) assembled a total of 40 cases in which a UPD syndrome had been associated with a nonhomologous Robertsonian translocation, comprising 22 cases of UPD(14)mat (Temple syndrome), five of UPD(14)pat (Kagami-Ogata syndrome), seven of UPD(15)mat (Prader-Willi syndrome), and six of UPD(15)pat (Angelman syndrome). Most of these nonhomologous robs had been inherited. Nonetheless, UPD due to a parental rob is extremely rare; the overall risk to have a child with a UPD syndrome, as determined from prenatal diagnosis data where one parent is a heterologous rob carrier, is on the order of only 0.06% (Moradkhani et al. 2019).

[4] Note that with one or other chromosome 15 being the candidate to be lost, the risk for UPD to be generated is 50%. This is in contrast with correction in standard trisomy in which, with three candidate chromosomes, the chances are 1 in 3 for the "wrong" one to be lost.

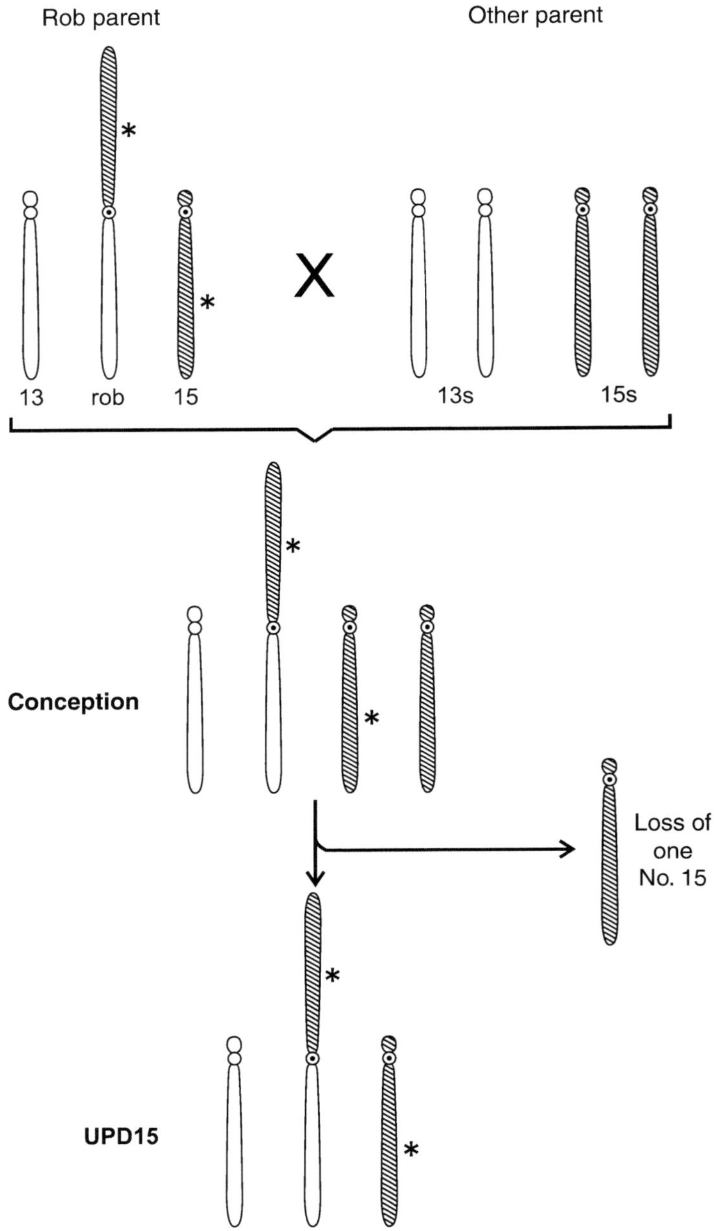

Figure 7–10. Uniparental Disomy.
Uniparental disomy 15 from a rob(13q15q) parent, due to "trisomy rescue." The heterozygous parent produces a malsegregant gamete with the translocation, and with a free chromosome 15. The conception thus has trisomy 15. Subsequently, as a postzygotic event, the chromosome 15 from the other parent is lost. Since most malsegregations will have been of maternal origin, the UPD in this setting will usually be a maternal heterodisomy. (Chromosome 13 elements, white; chromosome 15 elements, cross-hatched. The two chromosome 15 elements from the carrier parent are asterisked.)

Monosomic Correction. Hypothetically, correction may also go the other way—that is, the conversion of a monosomic conceptus, due to a nullisomic gamete from 2:1 adjacent segregation in the rob parent, into a disomic conceptus. This conversion to disomy, or "correction," would be achieved by the replication of the homolog contributed in the (normal) gamete of the other parent. A replicate "free" chromosome might be produced, in which case the karyotype would appear normal. Or, the homolog could replicate as an isochromosome, which would produce the intriguing circumstance of a de novo Robertsonian-like chromosome in the setting of a true Robertsonian parent. This event, whichever one, would take place at a very early post-zygotic stage and would necessarily lead to uniparental isodisomy (Berend et al. 2000). It is, apparently, very rare.

Association with Infertility

Heterozygosity for a rob translocation is an occasionally identified association with infertility in the *male*. Of men with abnormal sperm indices, more particularly oligospermia rather than azoöspermia, the rob carrier rate will be above the population figure, and similarly in those whose partners had suffered recurrent pregnancy loss (Kuroda et al. 2020; Tunç and Ilgaz 2022; Yuan et al. 2023). Estimates of the excess of rob carriers in an infertile population range from three-fold to around ten-fold. In those rob carriers with an abnormal spermiogram, there is an associated increase in levels of aneuploidy in sperm, and the disposition of the individual bivalents at meiosis I may be disturbed due to the presence of a rob trivalent (Solé et al. 2017) (Figure 7–11).

As discussed above, this infertility, if indeed it is a direct consequence of the translocation, could operate at the level of gametogenesis or could be having its effect during very early embryogenesis: pregestational or gestational infertility. In other words, the translocation chromosome may of itself impose an obstructive influence during spermatogenesis, leading to a low sperm count with abnormal forms; or the translocation could, of itself, following a successful fertilization, then compromise the process of chromosome segregation in the cleavage-stage embryo, leading to a lethal imbalance with non-implantation or later miscarriage. And yet, there is the conundrum that a number of infertile rob men will have rob male relatives of normal fertility (Wiland et al. 2020).

It is less straightforward to tease out a causal association concerning *female* rob-related infertility in an individual case, and there is always the fact of a background rate of 1 in 800 women being a rob carrier and many women in the population suffering infertility. In a large Chinese cohort of infertile[5] couples, Yuan et al. (2023) identified 21 female (and 33 male) rob carriers, giving percentages of 0.25% and 0.38% respectively, against the population figure of 0.125%. The doubled rate in the female rob carriers is to be noted, but the numbers studied were small. It remains possible that the infertility in at least some such women might be coincidental. In a review of causes of recurrent pregnancy loss (a different question, in that a conception had occurred), Tunç and Ilgaz (2022) noted in a small fraction (under 1%), one partner is a rob(13q14q) carrier, more usually the female.

[5] Infertility in the sense of infecundity, that is, the inability to achieve a pregnancy.

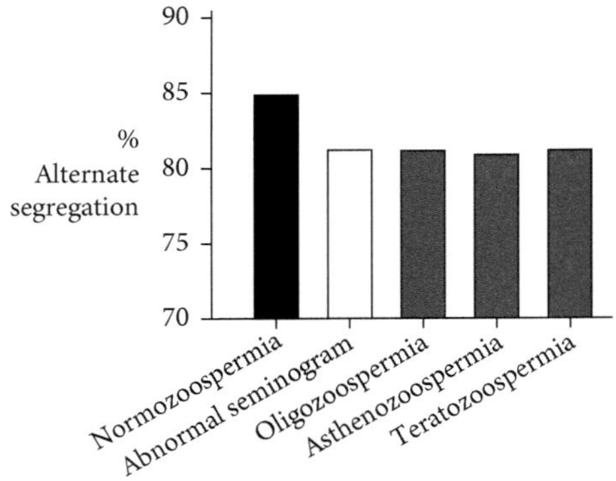

Figure 7–11. Sperm Observations in the rob Carrier.

Notes: The rates of alternate (balanced) segregation in sperm of men heterozygous for a rob, according to findings on semen analysis. Those with abnormal indices, and who may have presented with infertility, have a lesser frequency of normal/balanced forms.

Source: From A Lamotte et al., Is sperm FISH analysis still useful for Robertsonian translocations? Meiotic analysis for 23 patients and review of the literature, *Basic Clin Androl* 28:5, 2018. Courtesy S Hennebicq, and with the permission of Springer Nature.

RARE COMPLEXITIES

Homozygosity for a Robertsonian Translocation Due to Both Parents Being Carriers. An interesting curiosity is the rare case of a union between Robertsonian heterozygotes, usually in the setting of a consanguineous marriage (Figure 7–12). The rob(13q14q) is, unsurprisingly, the most frequently observed—unions of 45,XY,rob(13q14q) × 45,XX,rob(13q14q)—but other robs are also on record in this context (Table 7–7). Thus, the child of a rob(13q14q) × rob(13q14q) union could have all their 13s and 14s in the form of a rob, with the karyotype 44,rob(13q14q)*mat*, rob(13q14q)*pat*. Intriguingly, these $2n = 44$ homozygous individuals have been, for the most part (but not all) of normal phenotype and with intact fertility. The reader may care to construct a hypothetical balanced karyotype with $2n = 41$ and five Robertsonian translocation chromosomes.

Some "carrier couples" have presented with multiple miscarriages, and two have had an aneuploid child: a translocation DS child with 45,XY,rob(14q21q),rob(14q21q),+21mat, from rob(14q21q) × rob(14q21q) parents, and an infant with translocation trisomy 13, from rob(13q15q) × rob(13q15q) parents (Rajangam et al. 1997; Mori et al. (1985). In the latter case, due to a founder effect, this otherwise rare Robertsonian translocation was rather common in their small village in the province of Cuidad Real in Spain, and this couple were surely distantly related, even though they were unaware of any link.

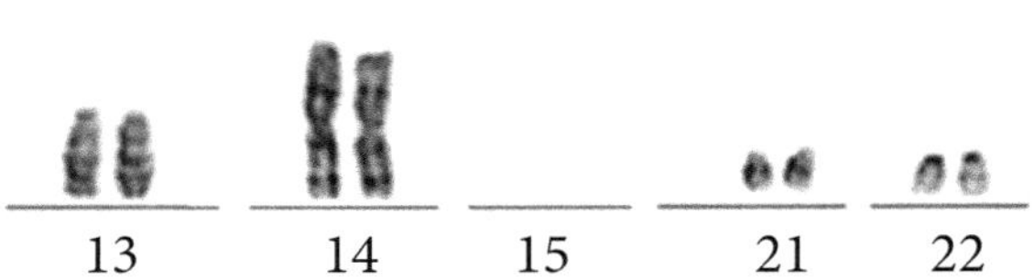

Figure 7–12. Homozygosity for a Robertsonian Translocation.
The karyotype is 44,rob(14;15),rob(14;15). The parents of this case, a phenotypically normal man, were first cousins, and both were rob(14;15) heterozygotes (Song et al. 2016).

Table 7–7. Cases of Homozygosity for a Robertsonian Translocation

Translocation	Number of cases	References
rob (13q14q)	9	Bahçe et al. 1996; O'Neill 2010; Miryounesi et al. 2016
rob(13q15q)	1	Mori et al. 1985
rob(14q15q)	4	Song et al. 2016; Sasi et al. 2020; Sahraeean et al. 2023; Xu et al. 2024b
rob(14q;21q)	3	O'Neill 2010
rob(21q22q)	1	O'Neill 2010

Notes: Most cases listed are from the review in O'Neill (2010); subsequently reported cases are noted individually. The infertile man in Sasi et al. was heterozygous for a rob(13q14q) as well as having the 14q15q homozygosity.

Robertsonian Fission. The Robertsonian translocation arises through a "fusion" of the short-arm sequences. Equally, it can, in somatic tissues, revert to "normality" by fission (Perry et al. 2005). Although the resulting two acrocentric chromosomes would have somewhat truncated short arms that lacked NORs, this appears to be without any clinical consequence.

The Homologous Robertsonian Translocation, or Acrocentric-Derived Isochromosome

This Robertsonian translocation chromosome comprises the long-arm elements of two acrocentric chromosomes that are the *same*. With a 45-chromosome count, the carrier has an essentially balanced genome and is, other things being equal, of normal phenotype. The site of formation is typically postmeiotic (Gardner et al. 1974a; Robinson et al. 1994). If the translocation forms from the fusion of the two parental homologs, then manifestly there is biparental inheritance (Abrams et al. 2001). If, on the other hand, the rearrangement is actually an isochromosome, each long arm is an exact copy of the other, and there will be uniparental isodisomy. Such an isochromosome may have arisen as a "correction" of monosomy in the one-cell zygote, or at a post-zygotic stage (Riegel et al. 2006). A person carrying an isochromosome from this mechanism can be normal, except in the case of iso14q or iso15q (these chromosomes being subject to parent-of-origin imprinting).

DETAILS OF MEIOTIC BEHAVIOR

In principle, only two segregant outcomes are possible at meiosis in the homologous 45,rob heterozygote. Either the gamete will receive the translocation chromosome and be effectively disomic or it will not, and be nullisomic. Essentially, this is 1:0 segregation (or "1+1":0 segregation). No balanced gamete is possible. Thus, if the other gamete is normal, only trisomic or monosomic conceptions are possible. Occasionally, conceptuses with translocation trisomy 13 are viable, and translocation trisomy 21 not infrequently survives to term. None of the other unbalanced possibilities (trisomies 14, 15, and 22, nor any of the monosomies) are viable.

Post-zygotic "trisomic correction" is a mechanism that could, extremely rarely, enable the carrier to have a phenotypically normal child. If, for example, in the case of an

population screening in some jurisdictions (cystic fibrosis, thalassemia, sickle cell disease, Tay-Sachs disease), in fact none has its locus on an acrocentric chromosome.

Risk to Pass on the Balanced Carrier State to Offspring

As noted above, "meiotic drive" applies in gametogenesis of the female rob heterozygote, such that a child is about one-and-a-half times more likely to be him- or herself a carrier than to have a normal karyotype. In the event that PGT is being applied, typically for reasons of infertility, an approach using SNP microarray can distinguish the two states, potentially allowing choice in favor of an embryo of normal karyotype (Zhang et al. 2017).

Infertility and Miscarriage

The Robertsonian translocation involving non-homologs is occasionally associated with repeated spontaneous abortion and with male and (to a lesser extent) female infertility (Table 7–8). The risks for miscarriage are set out in Table 7–9. It may be unclear, in an individual case, whether the association is causal or fortuitous. We can theorize that in some miscarrying couples, there may have been a majority of zygotes with nonviable adjacent segregants; and in some infertile males, the translocation may have disrupted spermatogenesis. Cytogenetic analysis of products of conception and of testicular tissue, respectively, may cast some light. It remains possible that some other cause could underlie the problem. The infertile male usually produces some sperm, and may thus be a candidate for IVF using ICSI, and optionally PGT (Vujisic et al. 2020; Yuan et al. 2023).

THE HOMOLOGOUS ROBERTSONIAN TRANSLOCATION CARRIER

We refer to these rearrangements as "rob," recognizing as discussed above that most such cases do actually involve an acrocentric-derived isochromosome ("rob-iso"). Virtually all conceptions of the 45-chromosome heterozygote result in either trisomy or monosomy. Monosomy results in occult abortion. Trisomy 14 and 15 always, and trisomy 22 virtually always, miscarry. Most trisomic 13 pregnancies miscarry, although some survive until the third trimester, while of course many trisomic 21 pregnancies will proceed through to the birth of a child with Down syndrome. Practically speaking, no normal child could be produced from homologous rob or isochromosome carrier individuals (the scenario of post-zygotic correction, discussed earlier, can scarcely be

Table 7–8. Rates of Robertsonian Translocations Identified in a Large Series of Infertile Couples

Number couples studied	**Number and incidence of rob**	
	In females	**In males**
17,054	21 (0.25%)	33 (0.38%)

Source: J Yuan et al., Detection of chromosome aberrations in 17 054 individuals with fertility problems and their subsequent assisted reproductive technology treatments in Central China. *Hum Reprod* 20;38(Suppl 2):ii34-ii46, 2023.

Table 7–9. Risk of Miscarriage per Pregnancy, and Proportions of Pregnancies that are Trisomic at Prenatal Diagnosis, for the 13q14q and 14q21q Robertsonian Translocations, According to Gender of the Carrier

	rob(13q14q)		rob(14q21q)	
	MISCARRIAGE	TRISOMIC PREGNANCY	MISCARRIAGE	TRISOMIC PREGNANCY
Mother	28%	12%	24%	10%–15%
Father	20%	<1%	33%	1%

Note: The miscarriage rates are to be seen in the context of a background population risk for miscarriage, per pregnancy, of 15%. The rates above that are substantially higher than background might reflect, in part, a maternal-age influence (Cohain et al. 2017) within the rob clinical material.

The risk for a trisomic pregnancy refers to the rate at second trimester prenatal diagnosis.

Source: Table adapted from pooled 14;21 data in Kim et al. (2008) and Shaffer (2002), and 13;14 data in Engels et al. (2008).

raised as a realistic hope). Appropriate advice for these carriers is to use contraception. Alternatively, the use of donor gametes may allow the couple to have a normal child. In the very rarely recognized parental mosaic case, a child may yet be possible, as in the rea(13;13), rea(14;14), and rea(21;21) discussed below.

Specific Translocations

Specific comments relating to the risk for abnormal offspring in each type of rob follow.

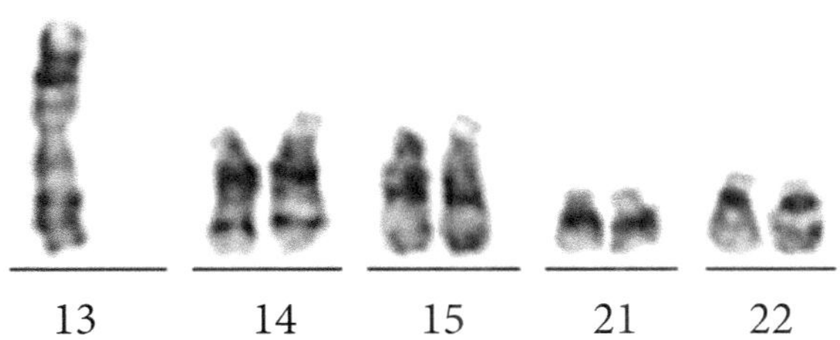

Figure 7–22. rob(13;13).

rob(13q13q). In principle, the carrier parent can produce only monosomic or trisomic 13 conceptions, and these would either miscarry or, in the case of trisomy, produce a very abnormal child (Patau syndrome). Three recorded exceptions to this statement are given in Slater et al. (1994, 1995) and Stallard et al. (1995), of a normal rob(13q13q) parent having a normal child with rob(13q13q). The translocations in the children were probably 13q isochromosomes (and so perhaps we should have written iso(13q) for their karyotypes) arising from post-zygotic correction, and thus the children had uniparental isodisomy. Parental somatic-gonadal mosaicism for a rob(13;13) may leave open the possibility of having a normal child. Bint et al. (2011) report a woman having had a child with translocation trisomy 13, her own karyotype being 45,XX,rob(13;13)[27]/46,XX[33]. At subsequent PGT, a normal embryo was transferred and a normal 46,XX baby born.

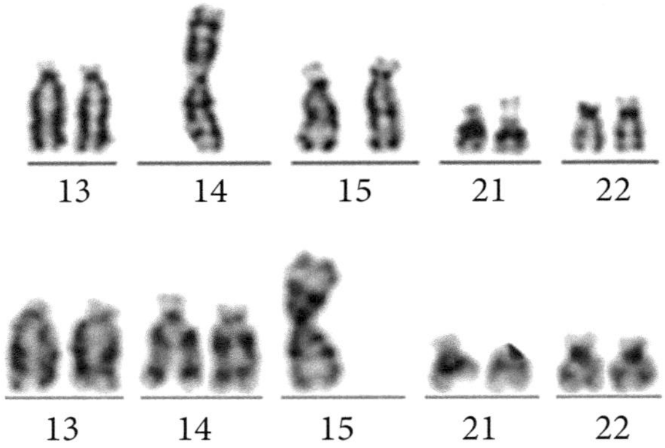

Figure 7–23. rob(14;14) and rob(15;15).

rob(14q14q), rob(15q15q). Trisomies and monosomies for chromosomes 14 and 15 are not viable, and thus all pregnancies of these heterozygotes would be expected to terminate in occult abortion or miscarriage. Proven gonadal (testicular) mosaicism, with a normal cell line in spite of 100% rob(14q14q) on peripheral blood, may allow for having a normal child, but with a risk also for multiple miscarriage (Cinar et al. 2011). Likely confined gonadal (ovarian) mosaicism for a rob(14;14) in the case of Gonzalez et al. (2024) was associated with recurrent pregnancy loss and recurrent failure of embryo implantation. Even if post-zygotic correction did happen, the child would have a UPD syndrome, according to the translocation and the sex of the transmitting parent. Thus it is, in theory and in reality, impossible to have a normal child from any gamete of the heterozygote.

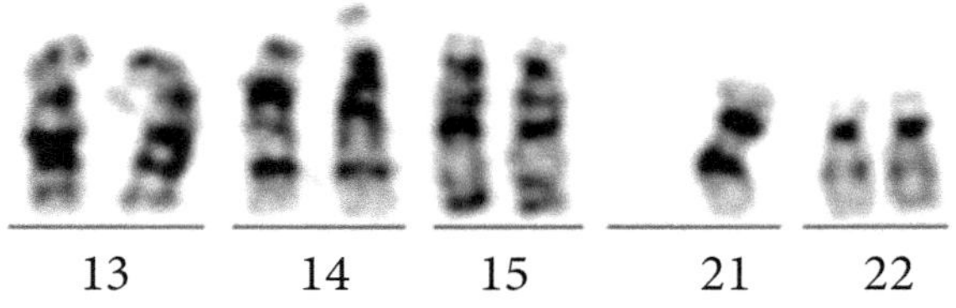

Figure 7–24. rob(21;21).

rob(21q21q), or iso(21q). Although the balanced rob(21q21q) carrier is extremely rare, every counselor knows about this famous translocation. It is a classic example of a risk of (essentially) 100% to have a chromosomally abnormal child: all pregnancies continuing to term can be expected to produce a child with DS. Sudha and Gopinath (1990), for example, report a couple who had 13 pregnancies, with four children proven or presumed to have had DS, and nine miscarriages. The mother was 45,rob(21q21q). Similarly, Kolgeci et al. (2012) describe a 21q;21q mother having had ten miscarriages and two children with DS. The curious case in Yan et al. (2007) of a 45,XY(21;21) father having had a mosaic 46,XX/46,XX(21;21) child is the only such instance on record of an apparent post-zygotic partial correction for this translocation.

Parental mosaicism for this rearrangement, as an isochromosome, is on record and has been associated with the birth of a normal child. Hervé et al. (2015) review the small number of cases. In their own case, a mother of one normal child, herself of 46,XX karyotype on a 1,000-cell count on blood, had had two 46,iso21q pregnancies, thus declaring herself a gonadal, if not somatic, mosaic for the isochromosome. These authors note the importance of distinguishing between a true rob and an isochromosome in the case of parental "45,rob21q," and they comment that "when an i(21q) is detected, extensive cytogenetic analysis of at least 500 cells (from a variety of tissues, if possible) might enable the detection of low-grade parental mosaicism, and thus the provision of appropriate genetic counseling."

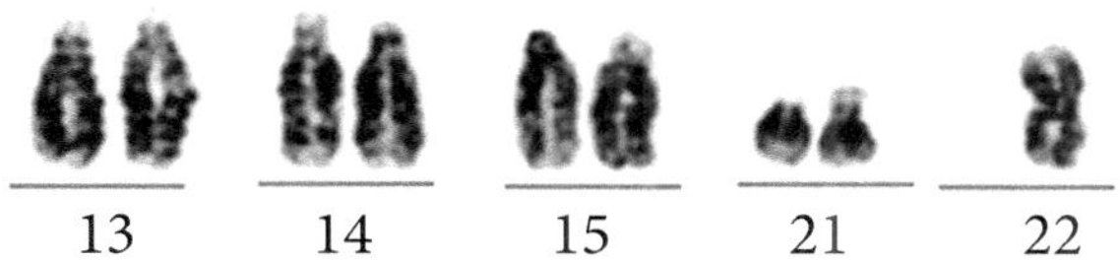

Figure 7–25. rob(22;22).

rob(22q22q). All conceptions would be monosomic or trisomic 22, other things being equal. For example, one carrier woman had 24 miscarriages, but no normal child (Farah et al. 1975). Two cases are mentioned above of post-zygotic correction with the birth of a normal child, but this is not a realistic hope to offer in the individual case. Gamete donation or surrogacy are potential options (Alhalabi et al. 2018).

8
INSERTIONS

INSERTIONS ARE A TYPE OF TRANSLOCATION. Sometimes the expressions *insertional translocation, interstitial translocation*, or *nonreciprocal translocation* are used. In the common, simple insertion, three breaks are required. The first two breaks release an interstitial segment of chromatin, which is then inserted into the gap created by the third break. In the simple one-way *inter*chromosomal insertion, a segment from one chromosome is intercalated into another chromosome. This is the most commonly observed form, at 80% of all insertions (Zhang et al. 2023c). A rarely seen, more complicated four-break rearrangement is the *reciprocal insertion*, whereby two nonhomologous chromosomes exchange intercalary segments. In the *intra*chromosomal insertion, a segment is intercalated into another part of the same chromosome. The segment may be inserted "right way around"—that is, with the same orientation to the centromere as before—this is a direct insertion (dir ins). Or it may be reversed—an inverted insertion (inv ins). Intrachromosomal insertions account for 10% of the total. More complicated scenarios, which may involve both insertional and terminal translocated segments, are more appropriately dealt with in Chapter 10 (Complex Chromosomal Rearrangements). In this chapter, we consider the case of the phenotypically normal heterozygote, in whom the rearrangement is assumed to be balanced.

Insertions are uncommonly recognized rearrangements, but less uncommonly in the molecular age than previously, and Nascimento et al. (2023) propose a carrier frequency for all types of insertion of around one in 4,000 births. All autosomes are on record as having been donor and recipient chromosomes, with no. 11 the most frequently seen donor and no. 22 the most seen recipient chromosome (Zhang et al. 2023c).

THE INTERCHROMOSOMAL INSERTION

BIOLOGY

The formation of the simple *one-way* interchromosomal insertion is depicted in Figure 8–1. The recipient chromosome now carries the insertional segment, and the donor chromosome lacks it. Van Hemel and Eussen (2000) estimated a prevalence, on classical cytogenetics, on the order of one in 80,000 persons; with molecular methodology, the true figure may actually be severalfold this estimate (Nowakowska et al. 2012).

Details of Meiotic Behavior

In theory, two categories of meiotic behavior are possible, according to whether the homologs pair independently or as a quadrivalent.

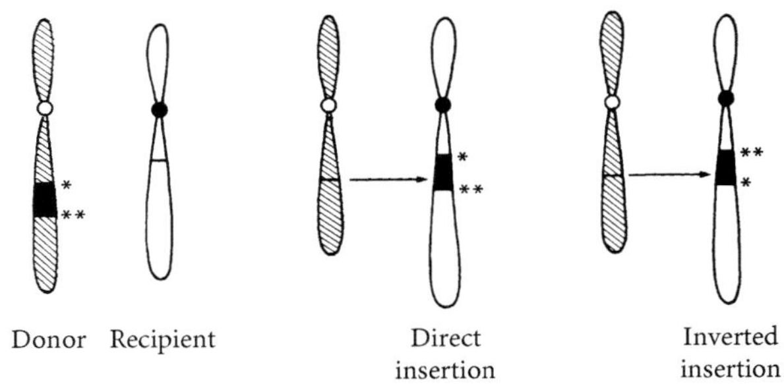

Figure 8–1. The formation of an interchromosomal insertion.

Notes: Single and double asterisks indicate orientation of the insertion segment. The *direct* insertion has the same orientation to the centromere; the *inverted* insertion has the opposite orientation.

Independent Synapsing of Homologous Pairs

Meiosis could proceed in the usual fashion, with homologs pairing independently as bivalents. In essence, we can suppose that the insertional segment is disregarded and that the homologs synapse, with segments matching for as much of their length as they are able. In theory, and perhaps only with larger insertions, the insertional segment could fold out[1] to accommodate this requirement (Figure 8–2, upper). (Some crossing-over will presumably occur between synapsed regions, but this would not alter segregation outcomes.) Alternatively, homologs may pair along their full lengths, which would bring some nonmatching segments "incorrectly" alongside each other ("heterosynapsis").

Then, with normal segregation of the two bivalents, independently of each other, two alternative pairs of gametes are possible. Overall, there would be gametes of four possible segregant types, in the ratio 1:1:1:1. Two of these would have a correct amount of genetic material, and two would not. The former two combinations are 46,N and the balanced insertion carrier. The two unbalanced combinations would produce conceptuses, one with a partial trisomy (duplication), and the other with a partial monosomy (deletion), for the insertional segment (Figure 8–2, lower). As discussed further below, studies of testicular biopsies and sperm have shown that (at least with smaller insertions) the homologs can indeed pair normally as bivalents, and that the expected 1:1:1:1 ratio does hold true. It makes no difference whether the insertion is direct or inverted. The foregoing scenario of independent synapsing is more likely to apply when the insertional segment is of small size. The case illustrated in Figure 8–3 exemplifies this: a small (0.4% of haploid autosomal length, HAL) segment from 8q inserted into 10q, with the duplication and deletion outcomes depicted (this case discussed further below).

Formation of a Quadrivalent

Probably only in exceptional cases, with larger insertional segments, a quadrivalent forms, and this would enable recombination within the insertional segments. In the review of Van Hemel and Eussen (2000), the mean size of the inserted segment in recombining

[1] Described also as ballooning out, looping out, or as translocation loops.

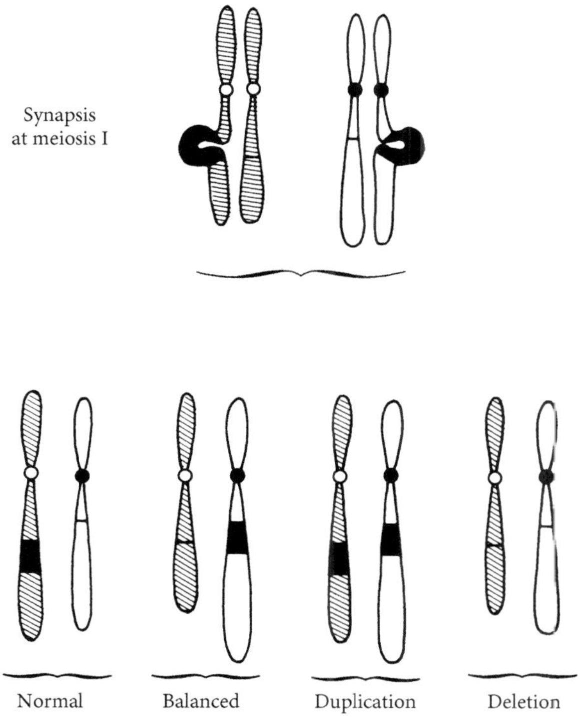

Figure 8–2. Meiosis at independent pairing of the two sets of homologs.
Notes: The insertional segment is shown in black, both in its original and in its translocated positions. The horizontal line marks the site whence came the segment from the donor (cross-hatched) chromosome, and the site of its destination on the recipient (white) chromosome.

cases was 1.5% HAL, compared with 1.0%[2] and 0.5% HAL in non-recombining families in which the imbalances were due, respectively, to duplication and to deletion. With the *direct* insertion, a recombinant chromosome would be monocentric and therefore functional. *Inverted* insertions, on the other hand, could produce dicentric or acentric recombinant chromosomes, with the resulting gametes presumably nonviable.

Consider the large *direct* insertion depicted in Figures 8–4 and 8–5. Most of the material within the chromosome 5 long arm (q11q22) has been removed and inserted within the distal long arm of chromosome 1. A configuration at meiosis I such as that depicted, with the insertional segments thrown into an overlapping loop, would allow for complete synapsis of homologous segments. If no crossover occurred in the insertional loop (and assuming 2:2 disjunction with symmetric segregation of centromeres), the same four outcomes noted in the preceding section would eventuate. The gametic combination [a,c] would produce a del(5)(q11q22), and the combination [b,d] would produce a duplication for this same segment (Jalbert et al. 1975).

But if a crossover did occur, two recombinant chromosomes would be formed, and now three further unbalanced outcomes from symmetric 2:2 disjunction would be possible: gametes [b′,d′], [b′,c], and [a,d′] in Figure 8–4. The duplication/deletion combinations, [b′,c] and [a,d′], are judged to be nonviable, although they might cause miscarriage. The "least imbalanced, least monosomic" combination is the "dup ins" [b′,d′], which

2 1% of HAL equates to approximately 29 Mb of DNA.

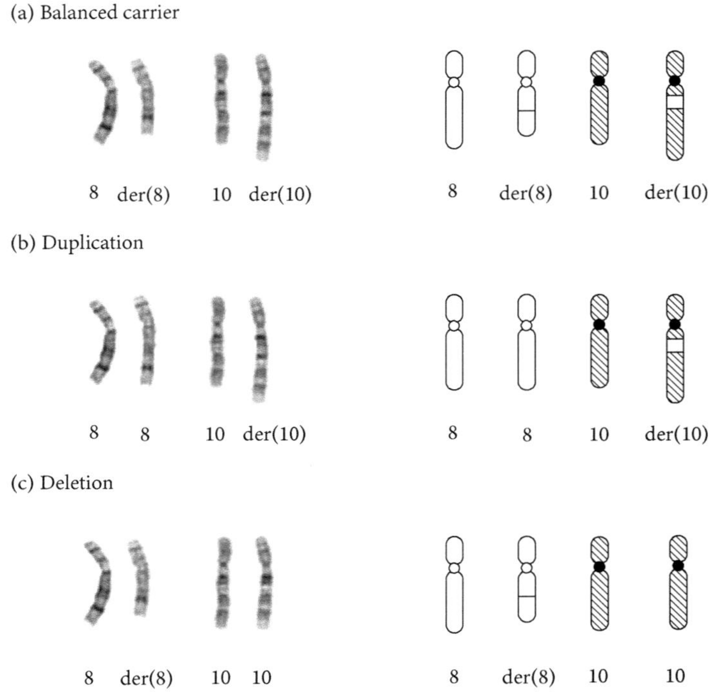

Figure 8–3. An Illustrative Case.

Notes: An insertion from chromosome 8 to chromosome 10, ins(10:8)(q21;q21.2q22), showing (*a*) the balanced carrier, (*b*) the duplication, and (*c*) the deletion states. In this family, the duplication was the only unbalanced form to be observed. Case of PA Bowen; in Bowen et al., Duplication 8q syndrome due to familial chromosome ins(10;8)(q21;q212q22), *Am J Med Genet* 14: 635–646, 1983.

leads to a partial trisomy for the insertional segment, 5q11q22. This was, in fact, the karyotype of the proposita in this family (Figure 8–5). Actually, this karyotype endows the same genetic imbalance as would the non-recombinant [b,d] gamete; so in practical terms, it made no difference that this recombination did happen.

SEGMENT CONTENT AND VIABILITY

The viability of the conceptuses—in other words, the level of risk to the heterozygote of having an abnormal child—depends on the degree of the aneuploid states. Consider the example illustrated in Figure 8–3. A small segment from the middle of chromosome 8 long arm, 8q21.2q22, has been removed and is inserted within the chromosome 10 long arm. This segment comprises about 0.4% of HAL. The heterozygote for this rearrangement could produce two types of unbalanced conceptus: one with a duplication of the segment 8q21.2q22 (Figure 8–3b), and one with this segment deleted (Figure 8–3c). In this family (Figure 8–6), only the duplication was observed. These individuals had mild to moderate intellectual disability and minor physical anomalies (Bowen et al. 1983). A segregation analysis of the family was done, and the segregation ratio was close to 1:1:1:0 for normal:balanced:partial trisomy:partial monosomy. This implies viability for the partially trisomic conceptus, and nonviability for the partially monosomic state.

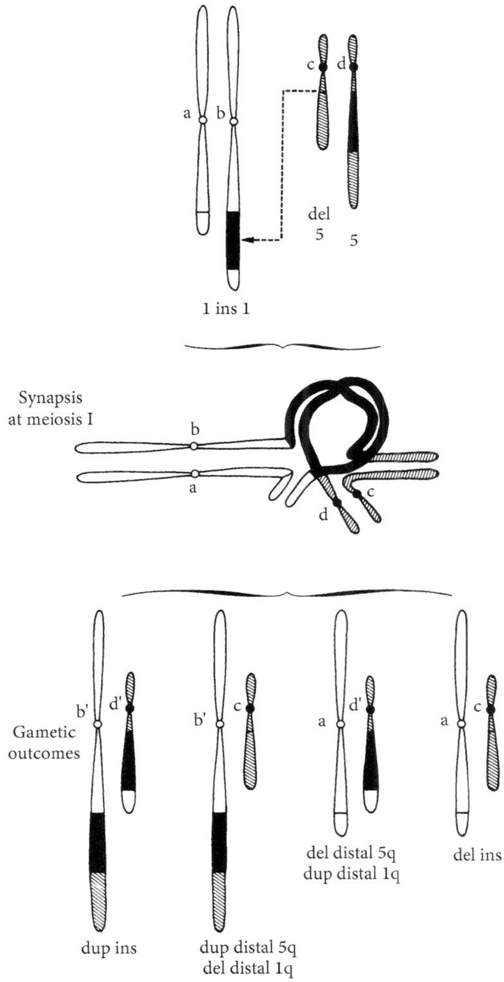

Figure 8–4. Meiosis at Quadrivalent Formation.

Notes: Gamete production following formation of a quadrivalent in the interchromosomal insertion, with a single crossover having occurred in the insertion loop. Only one of each sister chromatid is shown. Recombinant chromosomes noted as b′ and d′. (Based on the case shown in Figure 8–5.)

Thus in this family, the risk for having an aneuploid child is estimated to be 1/1 + 1 + 1 + 0, or 33%. (This assessment is an example of a "private" segregation analysis.)

A genetically smaller insertional segment has the potential to be viable in both the duplicated and deleted states. For example, Doheny et al. (1997) describe two first cousins, one with a duplication of a segment of 10q, the other with a deletion. The connecting relatives carried an ins(12;10)(q15;q21.2q22.1).[3] The insertional segment, 10q21.2q22.1, was small, comprising about 0.5% HAL. The child with the duplication was identified with learning difficulty in first grade, and her IQ measured at 74; the physical phenotype was rather mild. Her cousin with the deletion had considerable lag in neurodevelopmental progress as an infant, which would lead one to anticipate a more

[3] In the ISCN nomenclature, the recipient chromosome is noted first, followed by the donor chromosome.

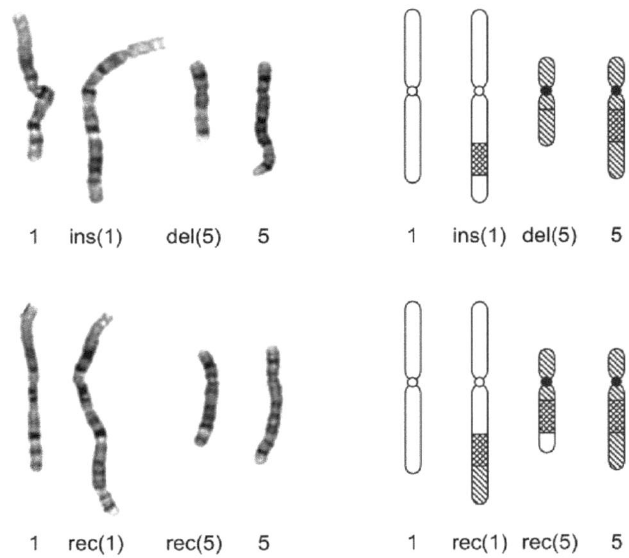

Figure 8–5. Recombinants from an Interchromosomal Insertion.

Notes: Interchromosomal insertion with recombinant chromosomes in phenotypically abnormal offspring. Partial karyotypes of 46,ins(1;5)(q32;q11q22) carrier parent (*above*) and her recombinant child with 46,rec(1)rec(5)dup(5q)ins(1;5)(q32;q11q22) (*below*). The latter is the [b',d'] combination in Figure 8–4. The child is trisomic for the segment 5q11q22. Cartoon karyotype: white, chromosome 1; criss-cross-hatched, 5q11q22; cross-hatched, remainder of 5.

Source: From P Jalbert et al., Partial trisomy for the long arms of chromosome no. 5 due to insertion and further 'aneusomie de recombinaison', *J Med Genet* 12:418–423, 1975.

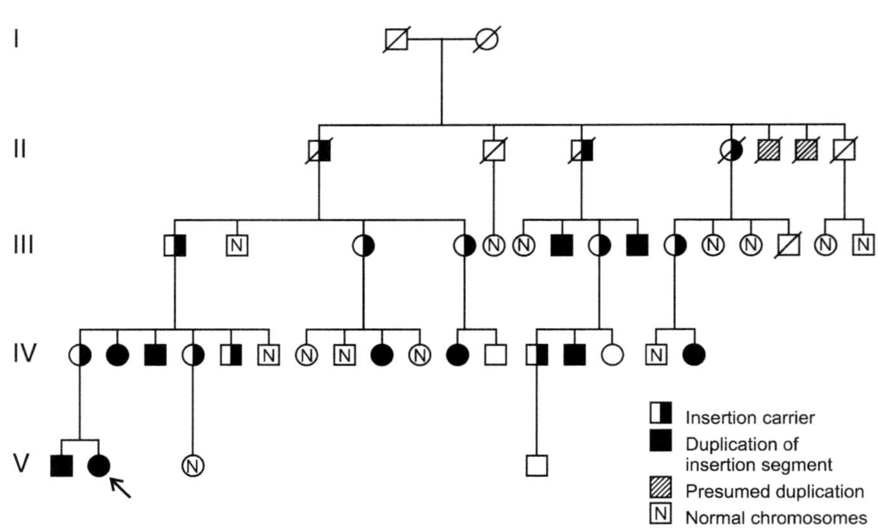

Figure 8–6. An Insertional Translocation Family Tree.

The pedigree of the family in which the insertion illustrated in Figure 8–3 was segregating, quite probably the most extensive on record. Another such is the 4-generation ins pedigree in Arens et al. (2004).

serious intellectual disability at older age, and she had a more obviously dysmorphic appearance. A similar circumstance is illustrated in Arens et al. (2004), who describe a family in which an ins(3;5)(q25.3;q22.1q31.3) is segregating in four generations, with 10 persons having inherited the del or dup state for the 5(q22.1q31.3) segment. Those with the deletion were more markedly affected than those inheriting the duplication state

Insertional segments of smaller size, shading into the measurement lengths associated with copy number variants, may present the remarkable circumstance of pathogenicity due to deletion but normality with the duplication. Such a story is seen in Nowakowska et al. (2012), who describe a family segregating an ins(1;2)(p13q36.3q37.1), the inserted segment 2q36.3q37.1 of size 2.1 Mb. Six family members presented severe intellectual disability and minor dysmorphism, and they each had deletion for the 2q36.3q37.1 segment. But one family member with the duplication was normal, and this observation informed prenatal advice for her carrier nephew.

If an insertional segment coincides with that of a known segmental aneuploidy, the particular syndrome may be observed in the family. Consider the story in Fernández et al. (2016): Two family members, related as uncle and nephew, presented some aspects of the HDR syndrome of hypoparathyroidism, deafness, and renal disease, which is due to monosomy 10p14 (Chapter 14). In this instance, the deletion comprised the segment chr10:2,471,915-14,544,442. The heterozygotes in the family carried a balanced insertion, ins(16;10)(q22;p13p15.2).

The Two-Way Insertion. A two-way reciprocal insertion (a rare observation) has the potential for two different imbalances: a partial monosomy from the segment of one chromosome with the reciprocal partial trisomy of the segment from the other chromosome; or the opposite, with a partial trisomy of one chromosome and a partial monosomy of the other.

Gametogenesis Studies. Gametic analysis has been reported in two male insertion heterozygotes. Goldman and Hultén (1992) examined testicular material from an ins(6;7) heterozygote, and demonstrated independent synapsis of the no. 6 and no. 7 homologous pairs at diakinesis, with the two bivalents occupying quite separate parts of the nucleus. This is a direct demonstration that the segregation scenario set out in Figure 8–2 does happen. Testicular tissue and sperm were studied from one ins(3;10) carrier in whom a very small segment of chromosome 10 (p13p14) was inserted into chromosome 3 at q13.2 (Goldman et al. 1992). In meiosis I, the pairing chromosomes did not loop out the nonhomologous segments; but in fact the normal chromosome 3 appeared to pair fully with the der(3), and likewise the chromosome 10 and the der(10). This is likely heterosynapsis.

Sperm karyotyping from the ins(3;10) carrier in Goldman et al. (1992) showed, as expected from the theoretical considerations noted earlier, similar proportions of gametes with normal, balanced, duplication, and deletion chromosomes. The actual figures were 22%, 32%, 24%, and 22%, respectively. No recombinant forms were seen. This may be the typical meiotic behavior in small insertions. Spermatogenesis may be compromised in some carriers, a conclusion drawn from the observation that only half as many index cases have carrier fathers as they do carrier mothers (Van Hemel and Eussen 2000).

Blastocyst Studies. The segregation ratio with respect to the insertional chromosome, at the level of the blastocyst, essentially reflects the symmetrical balanced:unbalanced ratio as observed in the sperm studies, albeit that unrelated aneuploidies may be

Table 8–1. The Range of Findings at Blastocyst Biopsy from Nine Interchromosomal Insertion Carriers

INSERTION	BLASTOCYSTS BIOPSIED	RESULTS		
		NORMAL	CARRIER	UNBALANCED INVERSION OR ANEUPLOIDY
46,XX,ins(1;2)(q23.1;q31.1q32.2)	17	5	3	9
46,XX,ins(1;13)(p22.1;q22q34)	2	1	0	1
46,XY,ins(3;2)(q27;q22q31)	5	0	0	5
46,XX,ins(4;5)(q21;q13q22)	3	1	1	1
46,XX,ins(5;11)(q33;q24.2q14.2)	8	1	2	5
46,XX,ins(6;5)(q24;q31.1q34)	7	2	0	5
46,XX,ins(6;15)(q24;q22.1q25)	4	0	1	3
46,XY,ins(7;2)(q11.2;q22q34)	2	0	0	2
46,XX,ins(9;18)(q32;q12.3q21.2)	11	2	5	4
TOTALS	59	12	12	35

Notes: These carriers had presented due either to having had a history of miscarriage or to having had a child with an aneuploidy due to the insertion. The lengths of the insertional segments lay between 20 Mb and ~60 Mb, except for the case of the ins(9;18), in which the insertional segment was 12 Mb in length. The fraction of imbalanced embryos is 59%; the "unbalanced" category included aneuploidies. The normal cf. balanced carrier state was distinguished by haplotype phasing. A skewed ratio of female carriers may reflect a degree of infertility in the male.

Source: From S Zhang et al., Comprehensive preimplantation genetic testing for balanced insertional translocation carriers, *J Med Genet*, 61:794-802, 2024.

superadded. In a study of blastocysts from nine couples in S Zhang et al. (2024), 59% were imbalanced (Table 8–1), and in Z Zhang et al. (2023c), 15 couples had, on average, only 30% of blastocysts testing as normal/balanced. In almost all, no insertional crossovers had happened.

Instructive Cases. Because nonreciprocal insertional translocations lead to "pure" single segmental imbalances, they can be helpful in delineating genes or phenotypes, and numerous such cases are on record. One example is an ins(13;11)(q14.1p11.2p12) segregating in a family, in which the deletion individuals had biparietal foramina (skull bone deficiencies), multiple exostoses (bone growths), and developmental delay (Shaffer et al. 1993). The description of this family led to the recognition of other deletion individuals, and eventually to the discovery of genes involved in multiple exostoses and biparietal foramina (Wakui et al. 2005; and see Potocki-Shaffer syndrome, Chapter 14). An insertional translocation involving the critical region for Down syndrome provides an interesting illustration that this small segment is indeed sufficient, of itself, to produce the phenotype. Lee et al. (2005) describe a father with 46,XY,ins(4;21)(q21q22.13q22.2) who had a child with typical Down syndrome, having inherited the paternal ins(4) with the small 21q segment, along with two normal chromosomes 21.

RARE COMPLEXITIES

We may include here mention of insertions which are present in *un*balanced state in the transmitting parent, with the parent's (the mother's) phenotype presumably protected, partially or fully, by X-inactivation. An ins(X;5)(p22.1p13.2p13.2) is described in the family of Walters-Sen et al. (2015). Two brothers had autistic features and mild dysmorphism, and their two sisters had poor language development, one with a major unilateral limb defect. Their mother was of mild physical phenotype and normal development. All five had duplication of the 5p13.2 segment; the mother showed skewed X-inactivation (the X with the 5p segment being preferentially inactivated), while her daughters had random skewing. The inserted segment is chr5:35,669,467-37,010,647(hg19), containing only two genes and indeed, only parts of these genes, *SLC1A3* and *NIPBL*; an abbreviated form of the NIPBL protein might plausibly have been the pathogenic factor.

There can be a link with cancer if a tumor suppressor gene is located in the insertional segment (Barber et al. 1994). An extraordinary case is seen in a father who had had Wilms tumor as a child, and whose daughter had retinoblastoma due to an insertion that was apparently balanced in him and unbalanced in his child. A segment from 13q14 including the retinoblastoma (*RB*) gene was inserted into 11p13, this being the site on chromosome 11 of the *WT1* Wilms tumor locus (Punnett et al. 2003).

Familial dominantly-inherited Alzheimer disease[4] is rarely due to an *APP* duplication. A quite extraordinary case is in Kalfon et al. (2022), in which a small insertional translocation containing *APP* has been transmitted in unbalanced state for at least seven generations, co-segregating with a phenotype of early-onset Alzheimer disease and/or intracerebral hemorrhage. A segment of chromosome 21q21.3 containing the *APP* (and *CYYR1*) locus, along with a segment from chromosome 5, have together been insertionally translocated into chromosome 18. The consequential duplication of *APP* is presumably the proximate cause of the familial disease, although adjunctive roles for the eight chromosome 5 loci, or the disrupted gene within chromosome 18, are also possible.

GENETIC COUNSELING

Insertions are among rearrangements implying the highest reproductive risk. Pooled data from a number of insertion families (Van Hemel and Eussen, 2000) indicate an average risk of having an abnormal child of 32% for the male carrier and 36% for the female. It may reach 50%. Of the phenotypically normal offspring, approximately half will have normal chromosomes and half will be insertion heterozygotes. Broadly speaking, the risk for liveborn unbalanced offspring is greater in the small-segment insertion, and smaller in the large-segment insertion; larger segments will typically be lethal in utero.

Offering prenatal or preimplantation (Table 8–1, Figure 8–7) testing should, in many cases, be the rule given the high risks for either abnormal offspring, or for miscarriage. Zhang et al. (2024) reviewed results in nine interchromosomal insertion carriers undergoing PGT. Of 59 blastocysts, 24 were euploid, and 36 were imbalanced due to malsegregation of the insertion, or otherwise aneuploid. Applying family-based haplotyping, the euploid embryos could be distinguished as balanced or non-carrier, and were seen in equal proportion. Where the choice was available, non-carriers were chosen for transfer to the uterus.

[4] The least rare form is due to the *PSEN1* gene.

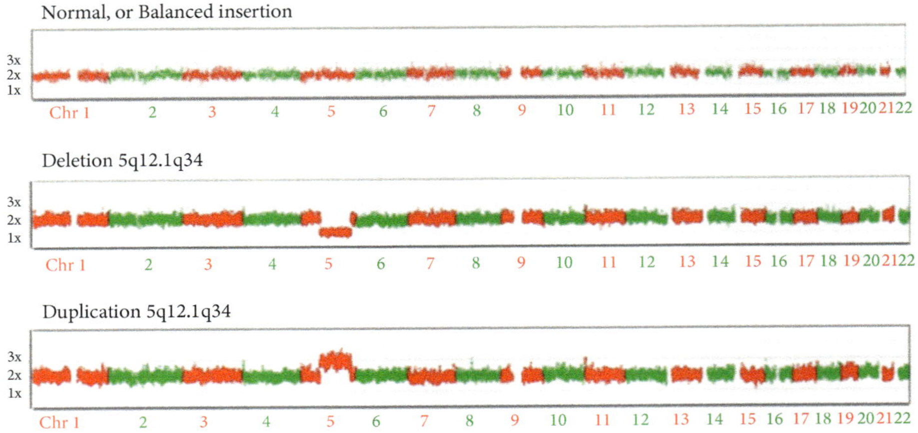

Figure 8–7. Preimplantation genetic testing.

Notes: The mother was heterozygous for an interchromosomal insertion of substantial size, of karyotype 46,XX,ins(13;5)(q32;q12.1q34). Test results in three embryos are shown; the imbalances in the samples of the lower two embryos are clearly seen. The large insertion segment, comprising chr5:61,805,642-162,688,727, would not have been viable in an unbalanced form. The analysis was done on whole genome analysis of trophectoderm cells taken at blastocyst biopsy.

Source: From Z Zhang et al., Clinical outcomes in carriers of insertional translocation: a retrospective analysis of comprehensive chromosome screening results, *F S Rep* 5:55–62, 2023. Courtesy P Xie, and with the permission of Elsevier.

Short Insertion Segment

For the *short* insertion (<1% HAL), the segregation ratio at conception would be expected to be 1:1:1:1 for normal:balanced:duplication:deletion (as discussed above). If the insertional segment is not only short but also genetically "small," both trisomically and monosomically, the maximum risk of having a liveborn aneuploid child would approach 50% (1 + 1/1 + 1 + 1 + 1). The segment 18q11q21 (HAL = 0.8%), for example, meets these criteria, as seen in the insertion family presented in Chudley et al. (1974). Carriers for this insertion had all four karyotypic classes of offspring—insertion heterozygotes, karyotypically normal individuals, individuals with a duplication of a small segment of 18q, and individuals with the same segment deleted—in approximately equal numbers. A similar scenario is seen in Marinescu et al. (1999) with a family segregating an insertion ins(16;5)(q22p14p15.3). Here, the "small" segment comprised 5p14p15.3. In two generations from a heterozygous grandparent, there were two children with 5p–, two with 5p+, four normals, and three carriers. The same level of risk, with a 1:1:1:1 segregation as above, will also apply to the very small insertion that requires molecular karyotyping for its recognition.

If viability is reduced or impossible for the trisomic or monosomic conceptuses, the risk to have an affected liveborn child would be correspondingly less, but the risk increased for miscarriage or for failed embryo transfer. Trisomic lethality presumably increases with an increasing fraction of HAL, with monosomic imbalances being more lethal.

It may not be possible to make a clear judgment based on the literature about the qualitative content of the imbalance, because the insertion involves an interstitial segment of chromosome, whereas most data on record relate to distal segments. A review of the insertional data on record up to the year 2000, taken from nearly 90 families, is provided in Van Hemel and Eussen (2000), and Figure 8–8 is taken from their paper. Any insertion involving the same red bar (deletion) or green bar (duplication) segment, or part thereof, will have a significant risk. Schinzel's (2001) cytogenetic database and the Internet sources DECIPHER and the phenotype tracks of the UCSC genome browser may also be consulted. Of course, any unbalanced child in the counselee's family will provide proof of viability, and an illustration of that particular phenotype. A study of the wider family may provide a guide to the recurrence risk—a "private" segregation analysis, as illustrated above in the "Biology" section. But in any case, the starting point with a patient having a short insertion is that the risk for an abnormal child is high, by which we mean in the range 10%–50%.

Longer Insertion Segment

A *longer* insertion may yet be viable, as the longer green bars (dups) in Figure 8–8 attest, and some of the red bars (dels). Consider these examples. The child in Dittner-Moormann et al. (2020) had deletion of 13q13.3q14, from a paternal insertion 46,XY,ins(12;13)(q21.2;q12.3q14.3), one of the largest ins-related dels (16 Mb) on record, making the point that the nature of the imbalanced segment is key in determining risk. And rather obviously, a risk for viability in the countertype dup form, which would be a partial trisomy 13, must be high, approaching the 1:1:1:1 short-segment risk discussed above. In the family of Jalbert et al. (1975) mentioned above (Figure 8–5), the insertional segment (5q11q22) comprised 2.2% HAL (about 60 Mb), and this duplication did allow survival, although the child was dysmorphic and severely disabled. This case is the sole example of dup(5)(q11q22) in Schinzel's (2001) database. The risk for recurrence in this family, or occurrence in another family, must surely be small, and perhaps x is only a low single-digit number.

Many longer insertions will not imply a risk for an affected liveborn, although the miscarriage risk may be high. In a family such as that in Abuelo et al. (1988), with an insertional segment comprising most of 3p (3p26p13, approximately 75 Mb), one could be rather confident that any imbalanced conception would miscarry. The closest viable segment in Schinzel's database is 3p14pter, and the closest overlapping CNV in DECIPHER is a 43 Mb duplication at 3p24.3p14.2. A risk of "close to 0%" for an abnormal child could be offered. Prenatal diagnosis in cases judged to be of this very low risk category would be discretionary; a normal NIPT result and ultrasonographic fetal anatomy scan would likely be considerably reassuring of itself. As noted above, PGT may be seen as valuable in avoiding the transfer of embryos that would inevitably fail.

With longer insertions, there is theoretically an additional risk for the formation of recombinant duplication and deletion chromosomes. But in fact the deletion for a long segment (whether the result of a non-recombinant or recombinant chromosome) would usually impose a nonviable degree of partial monosomy. The dup/del combinations (see Figure 8–4) are even more unbalanced, leading to spontaneous abortion. Thus, only the duplication (whether non-recombinant or recombinant) is likely to allow for viability. In the great majority of cases, therefore, the segregation ratio for pregnancies going to term is 1:1:x:0 for normal:balanced:partial trisomy:other imbalances, where x is less than 1, and probably very much less than 1. The corollary is that a miscarriage risk will be high, and the attraction of PGT is evident given a likely 1:1:1:1 segregation at the blastocyst stage.

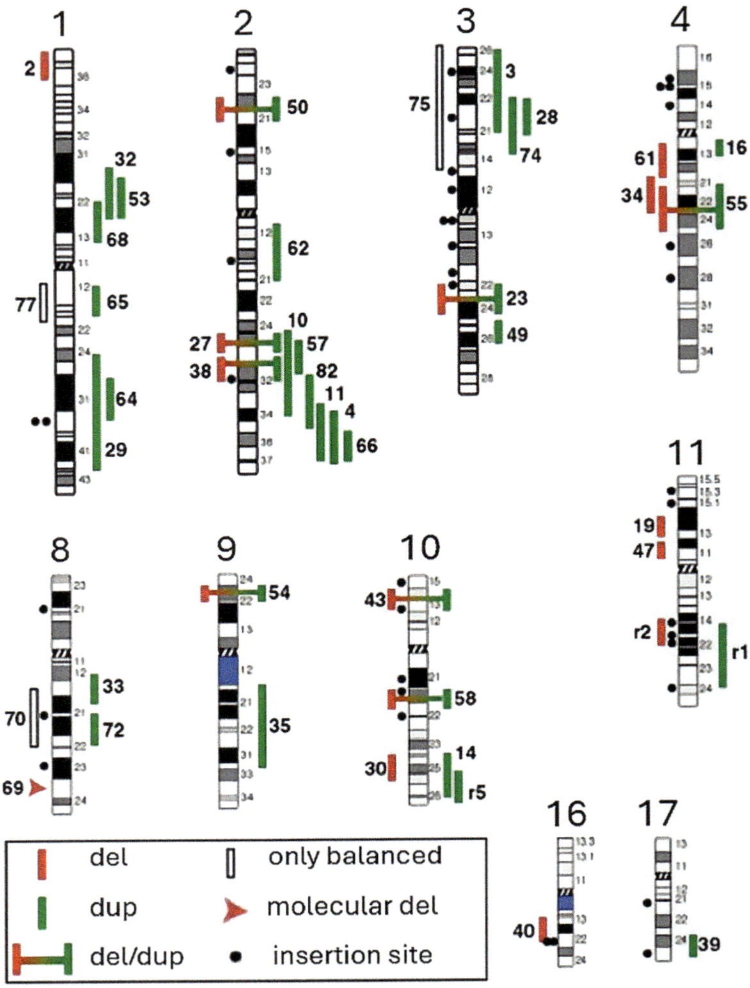

Figure 8–8. Segregations from an Interchromosomal Insertion.
(*Above and opposite*) Presentation of chromosome segments in which recombinant imbalances have been recorded (on classical cytogenetics), in the child of a parent heterozygous for an interchromosomal insertion. Segments seen only as duplications are shown in green, those seen only as deletions in red, and green and red bars connected show segments observed in either state. Insertions seen only in the balanced state are identified with open bars. Numbers alongside bars refer to the numbers of recorded cases. Heterochromatin is in blue.

Source: From JO Van Hemel and HJ Eussen, Interchromosomal insertions: Identification of five cases and a review, *Hum Genet* 107: 415–432, 2000. Courtesy JO Van Hemel, and with the permission of Springer-Verlag.

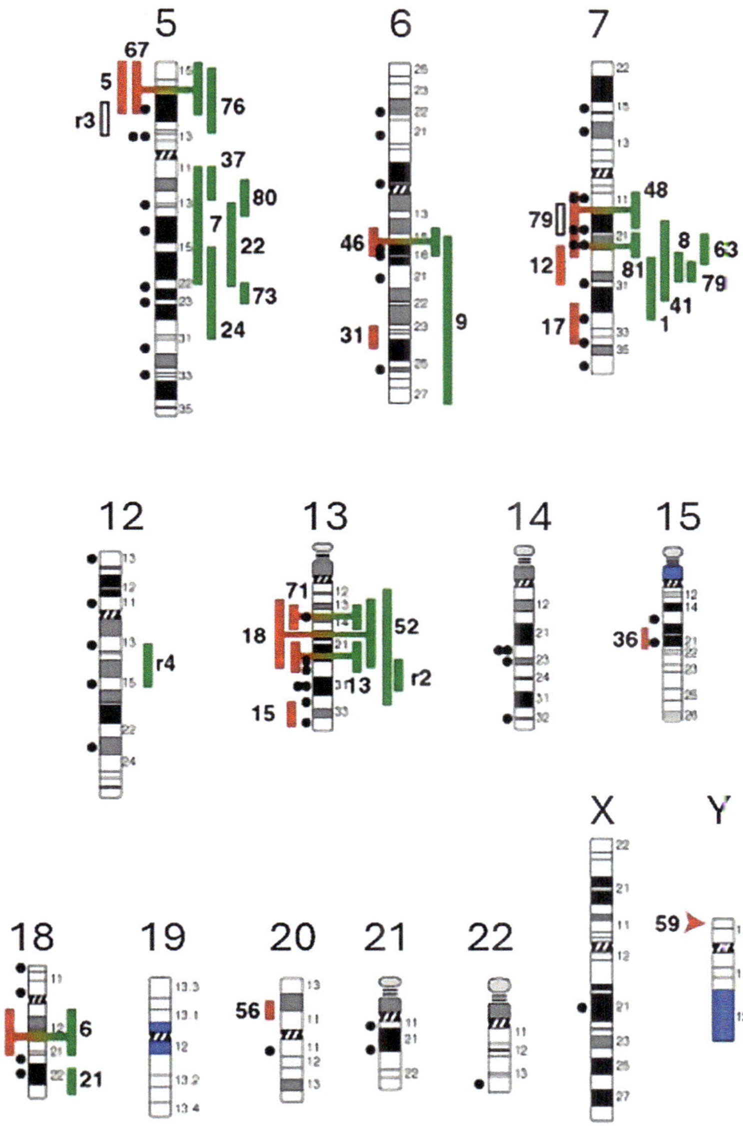

Figure 8–8. Continued.

Intermediate-Length Segment

Intermediate-length segments (1%–1.5% HAL) might imply a risk in the range 5%–10%. But each segment needs to be judged on its merits, both according to the reproductive history in the family and with reference to the cytogenetic databases.

THE INTRACHROMOSOMAL INSERTION

BIOLOGY

Intrachromosomal insertions are rare indeed. These insertions can be between-arm or within-arm (pericentric or paracentric), and direct or inverted. Domínguez et al. (2017), in their literature review, accumulated 70 cases, of which 40 were between-arm and 30 within-arm. Most of these were based upon classical analysis, and the inserted segments were of at least size 5 Mb, and several much larger. The cytogenetic recognition can be difficult, with some having originally been interpreted as paracentric inversions with unbalanced meiotic products (Madan and Nieuwint 2002). The formation of the intrachromosomal insertion is outlined in Figure 8–9, and there may be incomplete or complete synapsis. These differences may have practical reproductive consequences, and it is useful to consider each separately.

The Between-Arm Insertion

The between-arm[5] insertion has a segment of chromatin from one arm inserted into a point in the other arm (Figure 8–9, *right*). If we consider the part of the chromosome containing the centromere as the fixed reference point of a chromosome, we can regard the centromeric segment as "staying still" while the insertion segment shifts from one arm to the other. This somewhat arbitrary point of view allows us to use the term *inserted segment* unambiguously, in the context of the between-arm insertion. Thus, in Figure 8–9, the segment shown in black has moved "up" from the long arm and is inserted into the short arm (rather than the segment containing the centromere moving "down" into the long arm).

Incomplete Synapsis. Perhaps in most cases of the direct between-arm insertion, the inserted segments fold out so as to allow a good degree of synapsis of the bivalent. This synapsis would include that part of the chromosome between the two inserted segments—that is, the centromeric segment. There would be no difference, at least in theory, if the insertion is direct or inverted. One (or any odd number) crossover within the centromeric segment will produce recombinant chromosomes: one with a duplication of the insertion segment, and the other with a deletion (Figure 8–10). The centromeric segment may be quite long as a proportion of the whole chromosome, and provide considerable opportunity for crossover. Thus, the genetic risk is expected to be high, and in theory could approach 50%. In other words, the segregation ratio for the four possible segregant outcomes of normal:balanced insertion:duplication:deletion may be close to 1:1:1:1.

[5] Also called inter-arm, centromere shift, and pericentric insertion.

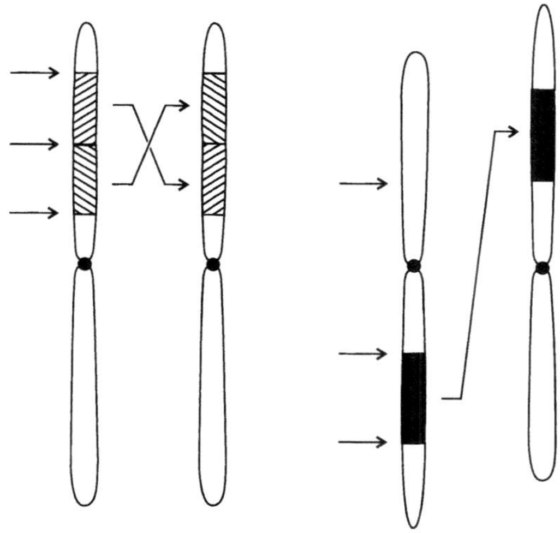

Figure 8–9. The Formation of the Intrachromosomal Insertion.

Left, the within-arm insertion, with the inserted segments cross-hatched. The normal chromosome is on the left, and the insertion chromosome on the right. *Right,* the between-arm insertion, with the inserted segment in black. The normal chromosome is on the left, and the insertion chromosome on the right.

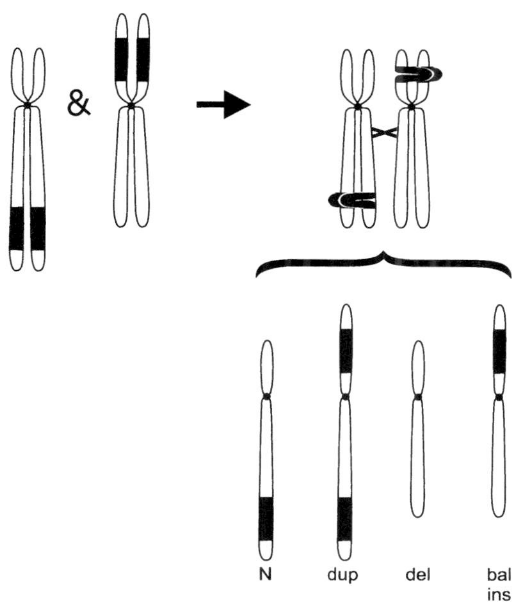

Figure 8–10. Meiosis in the Between-Arm Insertion.

Gamete production following a recombination *between* the sites of rearrangement in the between-arm intrachromosomal insertion. At the top of the figure, the normal chromosome is on the left, and the insertion chromosome on the right. There is incomplete synapsis, with ballooning out. (Cf. the ins(5) shown in Figure 8–13.)

The level of reproductive risk will lie according to the level of in utero genetic compromise imposed by the recombinant duplicated and deleted states, respectively. An insertion segment of substantial size, in either the duplicated or deleted state, may imply a risk only for miscarriage, such as the ins(6)(p24q21q27) reported in Elkarhat et al. (2019). Siblings in Xanthopoulou et al. (2010) with ins(7)(p22q32q31.1) had had two liveborn children and one prenatal diagnosis with the duplication, but no recorded pregnancy from the deletion. Contrariwise, in the family illustrated in Figure 8–11, with a between-arm insertion involving the small Potocki-Shaffer segment (11p11.2), both imbalanced outcomes are observed. Here, it may be the case that with no reduced viability of either imbalanced state in utero, the risk for the carrier to bear liveborn affected children is indeed in the region of the theoretical 50%.

The interpretation can be difficult with a smaller insertion, as Lybæk et al. (2009) discuss in their case of a "19p13-into-19q" insertion, an ins(19)(q13.3p13.2p13.3). A profoundly disabled infant girl with precocious puberty had a distal 19p duplication of 8.9 Mb, and her mother had a rea(19), initially assessed as a pericentric inversion. It took FISH to reveal the true nature of the abnormal chromosome as being due to a between-arm shift.

Complete Synapsis, Direct Between-Arm Insertion. For complete synapsis to be achieved, the insertion and the centromeric segments and their matching segments on the normal homolog would need to loop back and forth into each other, forming a double loop (Figure 8–12, *upper panel*). Crossing-over within the *centromeric* segment will lead

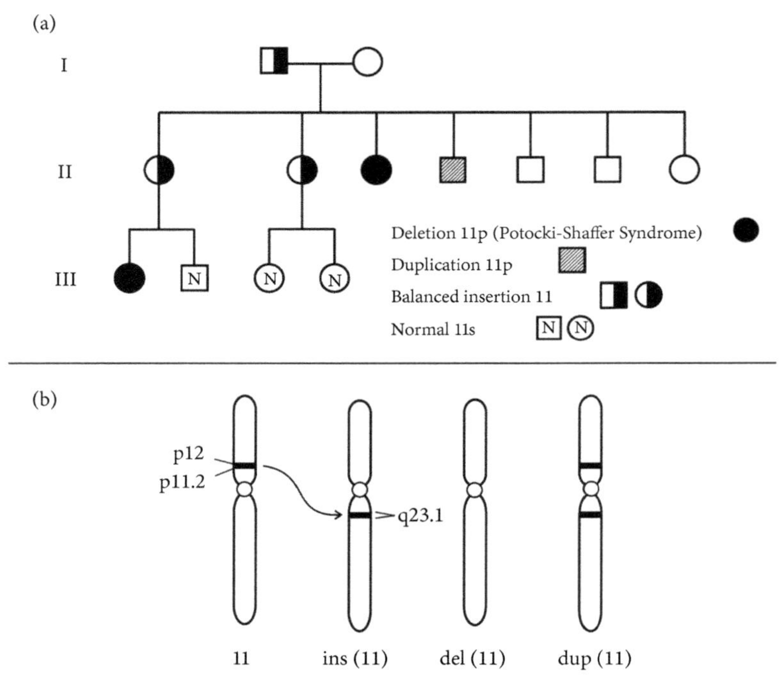

Figure 8–11. Familial Transmission of an Intrachromosomal Insertion.

Family tree (*a*) showing segregation of an intrachromosomal insertion ins(11)(q23.1p11.2p12), with both deletion and duplication observed in the family, and (*b*) cartoon karyotype to show the nature of the rearrangement. The insertional segment is of approximately 2 Mb in length. Half-filled symbol, balanced carrier; filled symbol, 11p deletion (Potocki-Shaffer syndrome); cross-hatched symbol, 11p duplication. The formal karyotypes of the deletion and duplication states are rec(11)del *or* dup(11)(p11.2p12)ins(11)(q23.1p11.2p12). (Case of J Gastier-Foster and C Astbury.) A very similar ins(11) case is reported in Chen et al. (2024d).

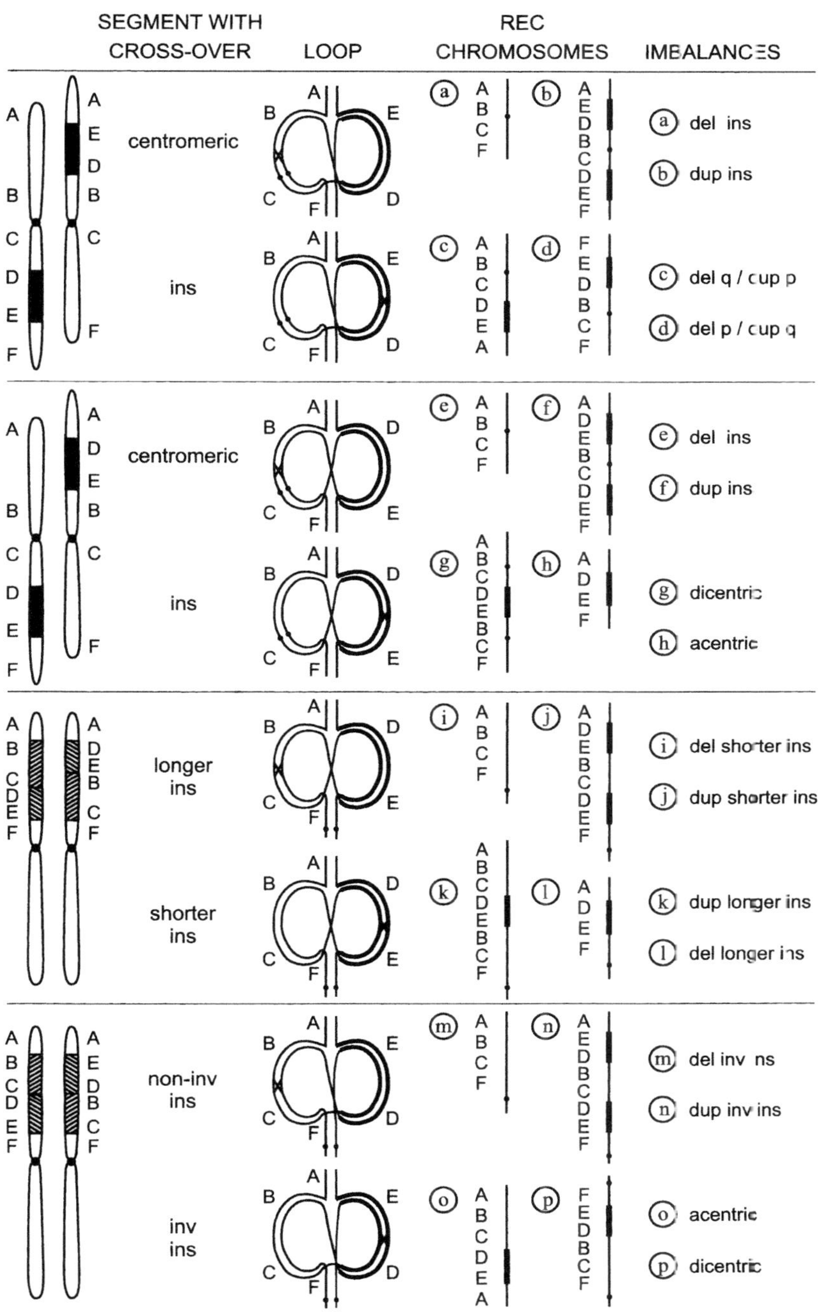

Figure 8–12. The range of possible recombinants from crossing-over in one or other insertion loop following complete synapsis of the intrachromosomal insertion. The four panels show, from above down, the direct between-arm insertion, the inverted between-arm insertion, the direct within-arm insertion, and the inverted within-arm insertion. In the loop diagrams, the dots signify the centromere, and the × shows the point of crossover. The insertion segment DE is shown in thick line in the loop and in the recombinant chromosomes. Circled letters provide reference points for text comments.

Source: Adapted from K Madan and FH Menko, Intrachromosomal insertions: a case report and a review, *Hum Genet* 89:1–9, 1992.

to recombinant chromosomes deficient or duplicated for the inserted segment (Figure 8–12 a, b). If, however, following complete synapsis, there is crossing-over within the *inserted* segment, this will lead to the generation of new recombinant forms: chromosomes that are duplicated for terminal p and deleted for terminal q, or vice versa (Figure 8–12 c, d). A notable such example is illustrated in Ardalan et al. (2005), concerning a mother who carried a dir ins(20)(p13q11.21q13.33) (initially thought to be a pericentric inversion). The "shifted" segment was relatively large, about half the length of the chromosome, and the del qter/dup pter recombinant karyotype conveyed a survivable imbalance.

Complete Synapsis, Inverted Between-Arm Insertion. Recombination in the inverted between-arm insertion, in the setting of complete synapsis, has the same consequences as for the direct insertion as discussed above, when crossovers take place within the *centromeric* segment (Figure 8–12 e, f). The case illustrated in Figure 8–13 demonstrates this. The recombinant child with a dup(5) could equally have arisen from recombination in a partial synapsis (Figure 8–10) or in a complete synapsis (Figure 8–12 f), but in either event, the crossover is within the centromeric segment. The duplication comprises the inverted insertion segment. If, however, the crossover is within the *inserted* segment, dicentric and acentric products will result, and the compromised conceptus will likely degenerate very early and may not even implant (Figure 8–12 g, h).

The Within-Arm Insertion

A shift of chromatin within the same arm is called, logically enough, a within-arm[6] insertion (Figure 8–9, *left*). Since both segments shift, essentially switching positions, each could be called an "inserted segment." If both segments maintain the same orientation toward the centromere, it is a *direct* insertion. If the orientation of one segment is reversed, it is an *inverted* insertion. In the case of the inverted inversion, we can distinguish one segment from the other by referring to respective inverted and noninverted segments. In the direct insertion, the shorter of the two segments can be arbitrarily labeled as the inserted segment, and the longer as the "noninserted" or "interstitial" segment (Madan and Menko 1992; Barber et al. 1994); since they are both really insertion segments, we can also speak of the "shorter inserted" and the "longer inserted" segments.

Incomplete Synapsis. The within-arm shift, in the case of the direct insertion, can have a similar folding out of one inserted segment, and its homolog on the normal chromosome, to enable synapsis of the other inserted segment and its homologous region. In Figure 8–14, we depict the shorter insertion segment folded out, with synapsis of the larger inserted segment; equally, it could have been drawn the other way around, with synapsis involving the smaller inserted segment. Recombination within the *larger* segment will lead, respectively, to duplication or to deletion of the shorter segment in the recombinant products, thus giving rise to the gametocytes. Or, if there is synapsis of the *shorter* inserted segments, followed by recombination, there would be duplication of the larger inserted segment in one gametocyte, and deletion of this segment in the other.

[6] Also called intra-arm, and paracentric insertion.

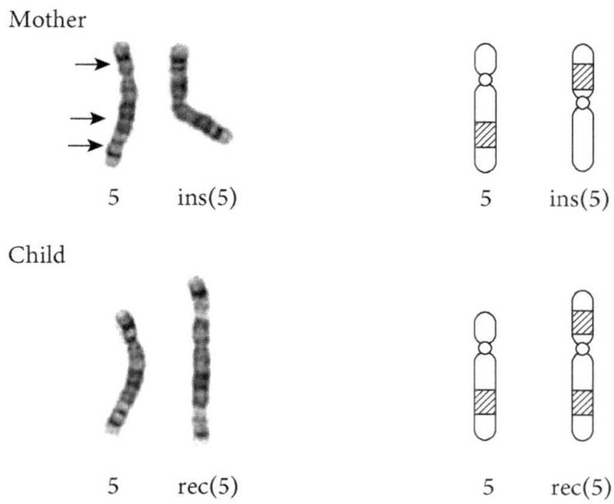

Figure 8–13. Recombination from an inverted between-arm shift.

Partial karyotypes of an insertion heterozygote mother and her recombinant child. The karyotypes are 46,inv ins(5)(p13q22q33), and 46,rec(5)dup(5q)inv ins(5)(p13q22q33). The child is duplicated for 5q22q33 (indicated by the cross-hatched segment). The recombination may have arisen from crossing-over anywhere between 5p13 and 5q22 at either partial synapsis with ballooning out of segments 5q22q33, as in Figure 8–10, or from complete synapsis following double loop formation, as in Figure 8–12*f*. From NJ Martin et al., Duplication 5q(5q22-5q33): from an intrachromosomal insertion, *Am J Med Genet* 20:57–62, 1985.

In theory, the longer the larger segment is, the more likely it is that recombination will happen; but nevertheless, cases are on record of crossing-over taking place in very short inserted segments (Webb et al. 1988; Barber et al. 1994). A molecular example is the following: A girl with a severe intellectual disability, autism, and minor facial dysmorphism had a 3.4 Mb microdeletion at 14q11.2, chr14:19,663,407-23,061,615, and this was interpreted initially as a de novo rearrangement, as a FISH probe for the deleted region hybridized to 14q11.2 in both parents. The family requested that the girl's uncle, a jovial man with mild intellectual disability, be tested—and he proved to have the countertype duplication. It then needed further three-color FISH analysis to reveal the subtlety of the insertion of the 3.4 Mb segment, the whole rearrangement taking place within a single band. The rea in the heterozygote is described broadly (but inadequately) as ins(14)(q11.2q11.2q11.2) (R Beddow and K Gibson, personal communication, 2016).

Complete Synapsis, Direct Within-Arm Insertion. If complete synapsis is achieved in the direct within-arm shift, there is no new category of recombinant form beyond the four that could be generated from incomplete synapsis with folding out of one of the segments (as in Figure 8–14); indeed, distinction between the two processes is not possible. Crossing-over within the longer inserted segment will lead to recombinant chromosomes deficient or duplicated for the shorter inserted segment (Figure 8–12 i, j). Vice versa, crossing-over within the shorter inserted segment will lead to recombinant chromosomes deficient or duplicated for the longer inserted segment (Figure 8–12 k, l). We illustrate such a case from Quinonez et al. (2012), who describe an insertion of 6.33 Mb at 1q21.3q23.3 into 1q42.12, in the mother of two children with multiple malformations, severe intellectual deficit, and anatomic brain abnormalities on imaging. The children were deleted for this 1q21.3q23.3 segment, chr1:153,035,245-159,367,106(hg18). A meiotic crossover within the intervening region (or, within the longer insertion segment) led to gametes deleted for 1q21.3q23.3 (the shorter insertion segment), as per the

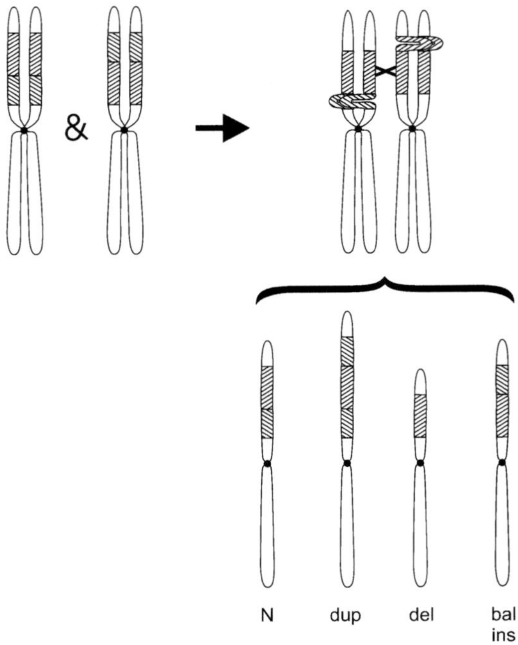

Figure 8–14. Meiosis in the Within-Arm Insertion.

Gamete production following a recombination *within* one of the insertion segments (the longer segments) of a direct within-arm intrachromosomal insertion. The chromosome pair at upper left could be seen as the normal and inverted, respectively; the dotted line indicates the movement of the inverted segment. There is incomplete synapsis, with "ballooning out". There are four possible gametic outcomes. The case in Figure 8–15 exemplifies this scenario, with the segment at 1q21.3q23.3 being removed, and translocating to a position elsewhere on the same arm, at 1q42.12 (in this case, with the same orientation to the centromere, and thus a direct within-arm insertion).

scenarios depicted in Figure 8–14 (del), or Figure 8–12 (imbalance *i*) and as shown in Figure 8–15. FISH was necessary to clarify the picture. (Of interest, this rearrangement had previously been interpreted as a harmless paracentric inversion, and the two affected children's karyotypes as normal.)

Complete Synapsis, Inverted Within-Arm Insertion. Nonviability is the fate of conceptions from crossovers in the inverted within-arm shift, if crossing-over happens within the *inverted* segment (Figure 8–12 o, p). But if crossing-over is in the *noninverted* segment, we see the same imbalances (Figure 8–12 m, n) as in the direct within-arm shift (Figure 8–12 i, j). Thus, Rethoré et al. (1989) describe a child with a duplication for the very short segment 5p13.32p14.2 due to a parental inv ins(5)(p13.31p14.3p15.12) with recombination in the even shorter segment p14.3p15.11, reflecting the scenario set out in either Figure 8–12 n, or Figure 8–14. Offspring with either the deletion or the duplication may be seen, such as Silipigni et al. (2017) show in a kindred segregating a within-arm inverted ins 1q42.13q43.

A notable example of a three-generational inverted within-arm insertion is the inv ins(15)(q15q13q11.2) family described in Collinson et al. (2004). The grandmother, her son and her daughter, and one grandchild were heterozygous for the insertion, with the detailed karyotype written inv ins(15)(pter→q11.2::q13→q15::q13→q1

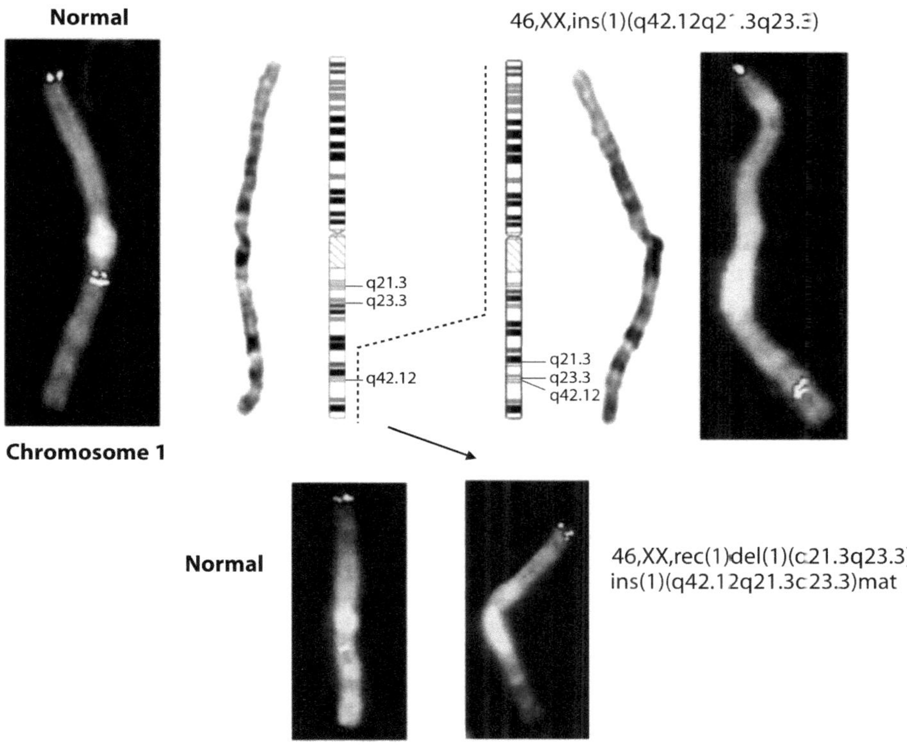

Figure 8–15. Meiosis in the Within-Arm Insertion.

Meiotic recombination from a direct intrachromosomal insertion (within-arm shift). *Above*, chromosomes 1 of a carrier mother, 46,XX,ins(1)(q42.12q21.3q23.3), normal on left, insertion chromosome on right. The segment at 1q21.3q23.3 is inserted into 1q42.12. The zigzag line shows the region of crossover between the normal and the ins(1), in the gametes giving rise to her affected children. *Below*, chromosomes 1 in her affected daughter. FISH with probes for 1q21.3q23.3 shows a normal signal in the normal position on the paternal chromosome 1 (below left), and absence of this signal on the deleted, maternal rec(1) (below right).

Source: From SC Quinonez et al., Maternal intrachromosomal insertional translocation leads to recurrent 1q21.3q23.3 deletion in two siblings, *Am J Med Genet* 158A: 2591–2601, 2012. Courtesy JW Innes, and with the permission of John Wiley & Sons.

1.2::q15→qter). Three grandchildren were abnormal: one with Prader-Willi syndrome (PWS), one with the dup(15)(q11q13) syndrome (p. 428), and the third with Angelman syndrome (AS). As the reader may already have guessed, the AS grandchild was born to the carrier daughter, while the PWS grandchild was fathered by her son: These two grandchildren had each inherited a deletional rearrangement. The grandchild with the dup(15)(q11q13) syndrome, 46,XX,rec(15),dup(15)(q13q11.2) ins(15)(q15q13q11.2)mat, was the carrier daughter's child, having inherited a duplicational rearrangement. The rearrangements would have arisen following either the scenario set out in Figure 8–14 or Figure 8–12 m (the deletion), or Figure 8–12 n (the duplication).

The reader may have discerned a pattern in the various aforementioned constructions. Whichever segment recombination takes place in (the active segment, so to say), it is the *other* (passive) segment that comes to be duplicated or deleted. This is logical.

Chandrasekhar et al. (2024): An inv(X)(p21q21) mother had two sons, half-brothers, each with Duchenne muscular dystrophy and hearing loss: the inversion breakpoints disrupted *dystrophin* in Xp21 and *POU3F4* in Xq21, the latter a deafness-associated gene.

CRYPTIC INVERSIONS

An inversion may not necessarily be detected on routine study, and knowing when to mount a directed search requires clinical acumen. Thus, Yokoyama et al. (1997) discovered an inv(17)(p13.1q25.1) in a father whose child had lissencephaly, a particular type of severe brain malformation. At first sight, the inverted chromosome looked normal. They noted a family history of similarly affected children, suspected a diagnosis of Miller-Dieker syndrome (which is due to 17p13.3 deletion; Chapter 14), and went on to demonstrate the cytogenetic abnormality using FISH with a probe recognizing the Miller-Dieker sequence.

Molecular methodology was needed to clarify in detail the nature of a chromosome 20 inversion in which classical karyotyping had been interpreted as normal, but MLPA and FISH then revealed a del/dup of distal 20p/20q, respectively, in three adult siblings (Stevens et al. 2009). The mother's karyotype was 46,XX,inv(20)(p13q13.33), and the siblings each had the identical rec(20)dup(20q)inv(20)(p13q13.33)mat. The imbalances were molecularly very small, the q duplication being of 2.5 Mb, and the p deletion, 1.1 Mb. Dysmorphology was subtle, but the cognitive/behavioral phenotypes were quite abnormal.

DELETION OR DUPLICATION AT INVERSION BREAKPOINT

A "clean" break and rejoin may not necessarily happen, and rarely, the rearrangement may comprise, or give rise to, an associated deletion or duplication. This is a "complex inversion." Langer-Giedion syndrome (LGS) is due to a deletion at 8q24.11q24.13 (Chapter 14), and Sasaki et al. (1997) studied a child with LGS who had a de novo inv(8)(q13.1q24.11). Molecular analysis revealed a 4 Mb deletion encompassing the LGS region; presumably this segment had been deleted as part of the process that generated the inversion. A familial inv(18)(q21.1q23)—in which a gene for brain myelination and likely some adjacent genes were deleted—led to some features of the 18q− syndrome in a mother and daughter (Keppler-Noreuil et al. 1998). WAGR syndrome (Chapter 14) is due to abnormality of the *PAX6* and *WT1* genes at 11p13, and in the complicated case in Marakhonov et al. (2023) the affected child—presenting with hypospadias, aniridia, and Wilms tumor—had an de novo inv(11)(p12q12), along with a t(10;11)(p15;p13); at 11p13, adjacent genes *PAX6* and *WT1* were both deleted.

"Normal Variant" Heterochromatic Inversions. Inversions having a breakpoint within the heterochromatic regions of chromosomes 1, 9, 16, and Y are frequently seen, and they are to be thought of as normal variants, not abnormal chromosomes. In "the world's largest epidemiological study of the inv(9)", Šípek et al. (2015) found no significant differences in frequencies between the inv(9)(p12q13) and the normal 9 in populations ascertained for various clinical reasons. Male fertility is, as a rule, unaffected, and occasional associations of this inv(9) with reproductive difficulty may simply be coincidental (Ting et al. 2022; Liu et al. 2024c). A single case is recorded of a rearrangement leading to a possibly pathogenic duplication of 9p, from a father with the typical inv(9) (Malinverni et al. 2017). The most common inversion in humans not involving centromeric heterochromatin is the inv(2)(p11.2q13) (Fickelscher et al. 2007); here, just two recorded cases in the world are known of a possibly related pathogenic recombination (see Chapter 18).

Other presumed essentially harmless inversion variants include the following: inv(3)(p11q11) and inv(3)(p11q12), inv(3)(p13q12), inv(5)(p13q13), and inv(10)(p11.2q21.2). The inv(10) has been rather extensively studied by a collaborative group of five laboratories in the United Kingdom that between them had 33 families available for investigation (Collinson et al. 1997). They found no excess of infertility or spontaneous abortion among carriers; of interest, all carriers of the inv(10) may be descendant from the same ancient northern European heterozygote (Gilling et al. 2006).

THE PERICENTRIC INVERSION

BIOLOGY

The Autosomal Pericentric Inversion

Details of Meiotic Behavior. The inversion heterozygote may produce chromosomally unbalanced gametes, and in consequence suffer reproductive pathology. The chromosomal imbalance is a result of the formation of a *recombinant* (rec) chromosome. This is *aneusomie de recombinaison*—aneusomy due to recombination. Recombination occurs if there is, within the inverted segment, crossover between the inversion chromosome and the normal homolog. The risk of this happening is proportional to the length of the inverted segment. Figure 9–3 shows three pericentric inversions, two with a long and one with a shorter inverted segment.

Synapsis and Recombination. Classically, crossing-over follows the reversed loop model (Figures 9–4 and 9–5). This configuration of the bivalent at meiosis allows alignment and pairing of matching segments of the inversion chromosome and its normal homolog (*homosynapsis*) to be as complete as possible. One (or an uneven number of) crossover(s) within the inversion loop, between a chromatid of the normal homolog and a chromatid of the inversion chromosome, leads to the production of two complementary recombinant chromosomes. One of these has a duplication of the distal segment of the short arm, and a deletion of the distal segment of the long arm (chromosome A-A in Figure 9–5), and vice versa in the other rec chromosome (D-D in Figure 9–5). Thus, the conceptuses that result would have both a partial trisomy for one distal segment and a partial monosomy for the other, or vice versa. Typically, only one of these—the least monosomic—is ever viable. Consider the recombinant 7 due to a paternal inversion illustrated in Figure 9–6. There is a duplication of the substantial segment 7p14.2pter, and a deletion of only the tiny segment comprising the distalmost sub-band of 7q (7q36.3qter), this combination being survivable. The countertype conceptus, having a monosomy for 7p14.2pter (and trisomy 7q36.3qter) would, we suppose, fail to implant or would miscarry.

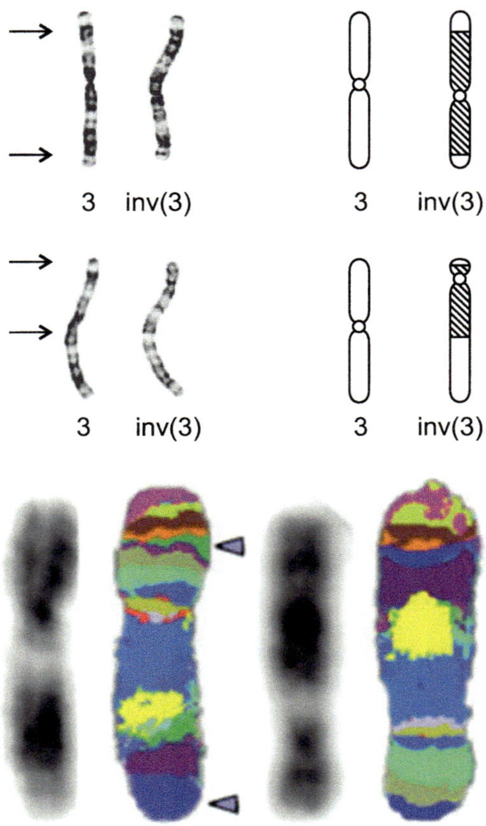

Figure 9–3. Three different pericentric inversions.

Notes: The inverted segments are large in the *upper* inv(3) and in the *lower* inv(11), comprising most of the length of the respective chromosomes, and thus potentially predisposing to recombination. With short noninverted segments, rec forms would likely be viable. In the *middle* inv(3), the inverted segment comprises about half the length of the chromosome, and presumably therefore, with a large noninverted segment, rec forms would be nonviable. The color-staining in the inv(11) (*lower*) very clearly identifies the large inverted segment. The arrows and arrowheads show the breakpoints.

Sources: Cases of NA Adams and LM Columbano-Green; and from T Liehr et al., Recombinant chromosomes resulting from parental pericentric inversions—Two new cases and a review of the literature, *Front Genet* 14;10:1165, 2019. Courtesy T Liehr, and with the permission of *Frontiers in Genetics*.

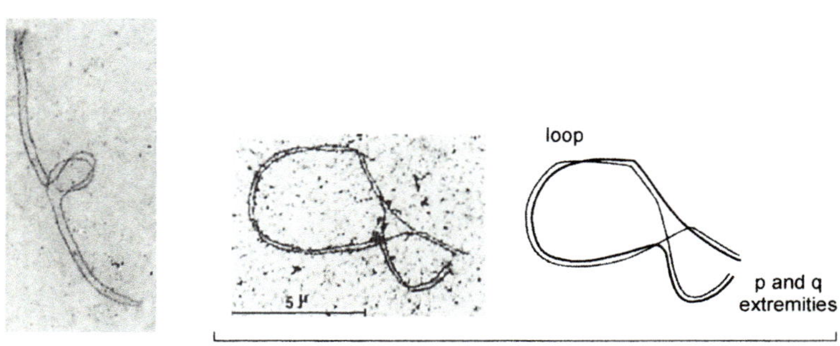

Figure 9–4. Inversion loop in meiosis, direct observation. *Left*, inversion loop in a mouse study. *Right*, spermatocyte study of a man with inv(6)(p22q22.2).

Source: From A de Perdigo et al., Correlation between chromosomal breakpoint positions and synaptic behavior in human males heterozygous for a pericentric inversion, *Hum Genet* 83: 274–276, 1989. Courtesy Y Rumpler, and with the permission of Springer-Verlag.

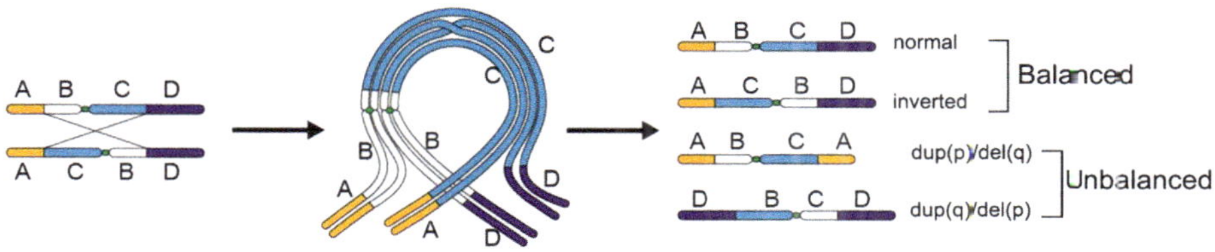

Figure 9–5. Formation of the Inversion Loop.

Notes: Inversion loop in meiosis, theoretical recombinant outcomes (cf. the inv(3) shown in Figure 9–3). Both sister chromatids are shown. The inversion (centromeric) segment is blue and white, the long arm noninverted segment is purple, and the short arm noninverted segment is orange. The four possible gametic outcomes following one crossover within the inversion loop are depicted. Compare with the actual observation in Figure 9–4, right.

Source: From P Xie et al., Retrospective analysis of meiotic segregation pattern and interchromosomal effects in blastocysts from inversion preimplantation genetic testing cycles, *Fertil Steril* 112:336–342.e3, 2019. Courtesy G Lin, and with the permission of Elsevier.

The cytogenetic nomenclature to describe the recombinant karyotype is straightforward. In the above case, for example, we have the following:

- Parent: 46,XY,inv(7)(p14.2q36.3)
- Recombinant offspring (A-A): 46,XY,rec(7)dup(7p) inv(7)(p14.2q36.3)

It is not necessary to put "dup(7p)del(7q)"—the complementary deletion is taken as read (although some may prefer to include both p and q for clarity). More fully, the nomenclature is 46,XY,rec(7)dup(7p)inv(7)(pter→p14.2::q36.3→p14.2::q36.3→qter)pat.

This complex twisting of the chromosomes to form a loop may not necessarily take place. In an inversion with a short inverted segment (Figure 9–7a), a partial pairing may occur. Both distal segments (or sometimes just one) align in homosynapsis. The inverted segment and the corresponding part of the normal homolog either "balloon out" (*asynapsis* of the inversion segment) or lie adjacent but unmatched (*heterosynapsis*) (Gabriel-Robez and Rumpler 1994; Anton et al. 2005). Thus, no crossing-over can happen within the inverted segment, and recombinant products do not form. Conversely, some inversions with long inverted and very short distal segments may undergo synapsis of the inverted segment only, with the distal segments at each end remaining unpaired (Figure 9–7b). Recombination can occur in this setting.

Gamete Studies. Sperm studies in a small number of inversion heterozygotes give an indication of the frequency with which recombination happens, at least in male

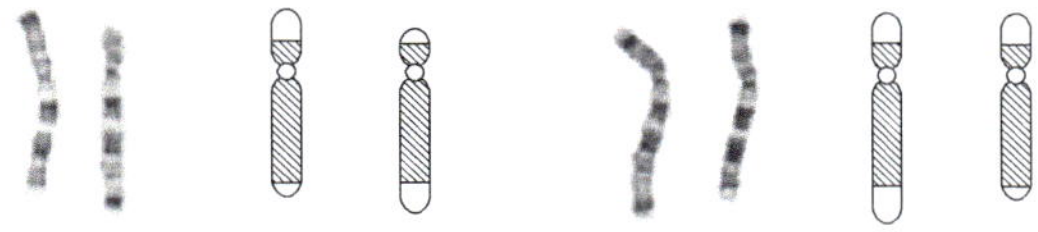

Figure 9–6. Pericentric inversion 7 in the father (*left*) of an abnormal child with a recombinant 7 (*right*). The recombinant chromosome has a duplication of just over half of 7p, and a minuscule deletion involving the distal-most subband of 7q. The child has a triple amount of the segment 7p14.2pter. The karyotypes are 46,inv(7)(p14.2q36.3) and 46,rec(7) dup(7p) inv(7)(p14.2q36.3)pat. (Case of SM White.)

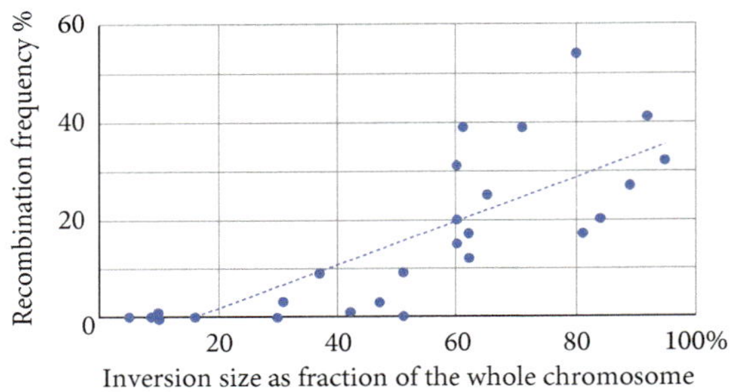

Figure 9–8. Recombinant Sperm from Inversion Carriers.

Note: Graph shows the proportion of gametes (sperm) that are recombinant, compared with the relative size of the inversion. This is graphical representation of the data from Table 9–1; individual data points and the regression line are shown. The clear trend is that the larger the inversion size, the more frequently recombinants are seen.

Source: Adapted from Y Luo et al., Different segregation patterns in five carriers due to a pericentric inversion of chromosome 1, *Syst Biol Reprod Med* 60: 367–372, 2014.

the del(p)/dup(q) state (which is viable) and the dup(p)/del(q) state (which is not), 7% and 6%, respectively.

Morel et al. (2007) offer this rule: A high risk of recombination applies when the inversion segment is over 50% in length; the risk is small when the length is between 30% and 50%; and no recombination appears to take place when the inversion segment comprises less than 30% of the chromosome. Figure 9–8 in essence bears this out. And in any event, even if recombination occurred in a small inversion segment, the recombinant chromosome would have such a large duplication and deletion that the risk of an abnormal live birth would, very probably, be negligible.

Different inversions in the same chromosome can have quite different recombinant fractions, and this relates, as the reader will have surmised, to the length of the inv segment. Luo et al. (2014) studied the sperm chromosomes in carriers of five different inv(1) cases: inv(1)(p11;q12), inv(1)(p32q21), inv(1)(p36.3q21), inv(1)(p32q32), and inv(1)

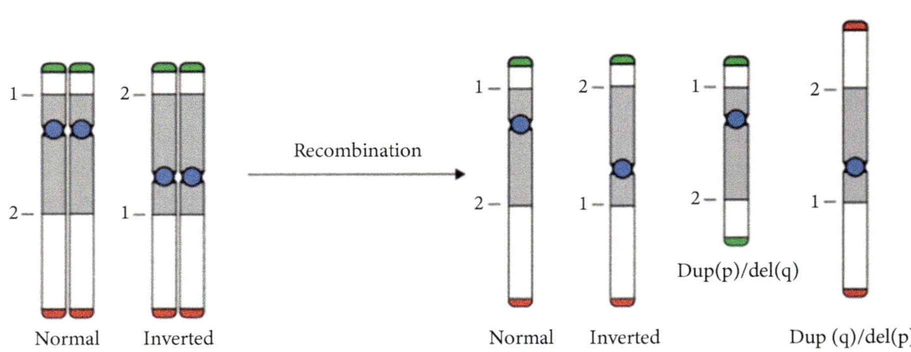

Figure 9–9. Recombinant Sperm in an Inversion Carrier.

Notes: The use of FISH probes to identify rec sperm, from a representative submetacentric inv chromosome. The green probe recognizes the p arm tip, and the red, the q arm (the blue is a centromere probe.) Sperm with a normal or a balanced inv chromosome have one red and one green spot. Rec sperm have both p and q tips of the same color: two green for the dup(p), or two red for the dup(q). The breakpoints *1* and *2* are noted.

Source: From E Anton et al., Sperm studies in heterozygote inversion carriers: a review, *Cytogenet Genome Res* 111:297–304, 2005. Courtesy E Anton, and with the permission of S Karger.

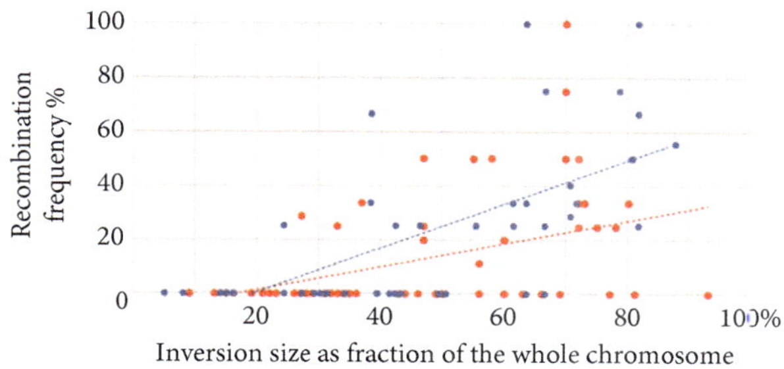

Figure 9–10. Recombinant Blastocysts from Inversion Heterozygotes.

Notes: The correlation between inversion size, as a fraction of the whole chromosome length, and the observed frequency of recombination, in a population of blastocysts from 94 inv carriers. Red, female carrier; blue, male carrier. Note the similarity, with respect to the spread of the data points and the slope of the regression line, compared with the graph of gamete (sperm) data in Figure 9–8.

Source: Adapted from data in P Xie et al., Retrospective analysis of meiotic segregation pattern and interchromosomal effects in blastocysts from inversion preimplantation genetic testing cycles, *Fertil Steril* 112:336–342.e3, 2019.

(p36.2q42), with the size of the inv segments ranging from shortest to longest 9%, 37%, 60%, 62%, and 92% (these men having presented due to infertility or repeated pregnancy loss). The frequencies of recombinant sperm followed accordingly, proportional to segment length: 0% (the shortest inv segment), 9%, 15%, 17%, and 41% (the longest segment).

Concerning the common inv(2)(p11q13), Ferfouri et al. (2009) studied seven men presenting either with infertility or during the course of a family study. Of just over 7,000 sperm, 99.7% were non-recombinant; the rate of aneuploidy otherwise did not differ from a control group. This work is interesting in proving that recombination can occur even with this very short inverted segment; equally, the fact of the very tiny fraction manifesting recombination is to be noted.

Blastocyst Studies. In vitro fertilization provides an insight into the behavior of an inversion chromosome before any selection pressure may have been exerted. From 94 carriers of a pericentric inversion, Xie et al. (2019) analyzed 397 blastocysts, of which 58%[2] were chromosomally balanced (either a normal karyotype, or with the parental inv). The larger chromosomes, nos. 1 to 12 and the X, were the more often seen. As with sperm, blastocysts show recombination to be related to the length of the inverted segment (Figure 9–10). Recombination was infrequent, about 8%, when the inverted segment was less than 57% of the whole chromosome, whereas with a segment above this length, recombination occurred in 43% of male carriers and 24% of female carriers. It is notable that the male figure of 43% is considerably higher than might have been anticipated from the sperm findings outlined above (24% for an inv segment >50%), a sperm cf. blastocyst discrepancy also observed in some cases of the reciprocal translocation (Haapaniemi Kouru et al. 2017). In a blastocyst study focusing on just one chromosome, namely no. 1, Jia and Xue (2023) came up with analogous findings. From 22 carriers, recombination varied from 2% with an inverted segment under 36%, to 33% with a segment of greater extent. Overall, recombination within the inv from a male parent (24%) was twice that (12%) from the female.

[2] Of the remaining 32%, of course, as in any blastocyst study, a considerable fraction of these will be abnormal due to aneuploidy, and unrelated to the inv.

Segment Content and Viability. While a long inversion segment can set the stage for recombination, what determines the viability of the recombinant conceptus is the functional content of the *noninverted* (distal) segments. We speak of a "genetically small" content, if the combined effect of duplication p + deletion q, or of duplication q + deletion p, does not cause lethality during the earlier part of pregnancy but allows development to proceed well through the pregnancy and possibly to live birth. Thus, only those heterozygotes who have inversions with genetically small distal segments will ever have a chromosomally unbalanced, phenotypically abnormal, liveborn child. The inversions shown in Figure 9–3 (upper and lower) and Figure 9–6 illustrate this case. Inversion heterozygotes in whom one or both distal segments are genetically large (e.g., Figure 9–3, middle) cannot have an abnormal recombinant child, although they may well have an increased risk for miscarriage. Any recombinants produced by such a person would impart a degree of imbalance that would be lethal in utero.

Genetic content corresponds fairly well to chromosome length.[3] In inversion families in which recombinant children have been born, the distal (noninverted) p and q segments together add up to a smallish chromosomal burden, whereas in families having no known recombinant offspring, the distal segments together comprise a more substantial load. To put some numbers, in families with rec offspring, on average the distal segments account for just 35% of the total chromosome length, while in those with no rec offspring the figure is almost twice this, at 62% (Kaiser 1988).

A larger potential imbalance can still imply a risk to have a viable recombinant child, if the distal segments comprise "genetically small" material. Consider the inv(13)(p11q14) and inv(13)(p12q13), in which the distal segments comprise as much as 75% of the chromosome length. Although the imbalance in the recombinant is large in terms of haploid autosomal length (HAL), the result in the dup(q) form is, in effect, a partial trisomy 13 (imbalance of 13p acrocentric material, here in monosomic state, being of itself without phenotypic consequence). Partial trisomy 13 is, of course, well known to allow intrauterine and postnatal survival. Likewise, consider the case in Ujfalusi et al. (2020), concerning a mother who carried an inversion 46,XX,inv(22)(p13q13.3)(p13), where one of the breakpoints was in the short arm of an acrocentric chromosome. She had two recombinant children, young adults at the time of study, with full-scale IQs of 72 and 79, one with neuropsychiatric symptomatology and mild facial dysmorphism. Their karyotypes are reported as 46,rec(22)dup(22q13.3)inv(22)(p13q13)mat, and at the molecular level, the q arm imbalance encompassed a short 3.3 Mb of DNA, chr22:47,870,362-51,197,766×3(hg19). This imbalance represented only 6.5% of the genomic content of chromosome 22. Similarly, an inversion in chromosome 18 can have distal segments that may be long relative to a short inversion segment, but they are still small genetically, and the dup(q)+del(p) combination can be viable (Schmutz and Pinno 1986; Ayukawa et al. 1994). With specific reference to chromosome 4, Stipoljev et al. (2002) reviewed 20 reported familial inv cases, and showed that recombinant forms have never been seen in those with smaller inversions, but are seen frequently in the larger ones.

If the deletion of one segment and the duplication of the other are each associated with a clinical phenotype on their own, a combination of both may be seen in the recombinant child. Thus, Putoux et al. (2013) describe a child in whom they saw features

[3] If the reader will forgive this rather crude statement: of course, some larger chromosomes (e.g., no.13) are of relatively sparse genetic content, and no. 19, one of the smallest, is densely packed.

of both Beckwith-Wiedemann syndrome (which can be due to duplication of paternal 11p) and Jacobsen syndrome (which is due to 11q deletion). The father was heterozygous for an inv(11)(p15.3q24.1), and the child had a rec(11)dup(11p)inv(11)(p15.3q24.1)pat.

As noted above, it is typically the case that only one recombinant form is ever viable. This is rather impressively illustrated in Allderdice et al. (1975) in a kindred with the inv(3)(p25q21). Numerous cases of known or suspected dup(3q) children have been born, but none with the countertype del(3q). There is not even an increase in the miscarriage rate, suggesting that the del(3q) is lethal very early post-conception, and either fails to implant or implants only transiently ("occult abortion"). Viability with both recombinant forms from the same inversion, the dup/del and the reciprocal del/dup, is infrequently seen and includes these reported examples: inv(4)(p15.1q35.1), inv(4)(p15.32q35), inv(4)(p16.2q35.1), inv(5)(p13q35), inv(10)(p15.1q26.12), inv(13)(p11q22), inv(18)(p11q21), and inv(20)(p13q13.3) (Kaiser 1984; Hirsch and Baldinger 1993; Dufke et al. 2000; Maurin et al. 2009; DeScipio et al. 2010a,b; Ciuladaite et al. 2014). These instances have this quality in common: The p and q noninverted segments are very short.

It is instructive to consider the inv(4)(p15.32q35) in Hirsch and Baldinger (1993), in which recombinant offspring could be del(4p)/dup(4q) or dup(4p)/del(4q) (Figure 9–11). The four separate segmental imbalances are all well known individually to be viable. Distal 4p is, of course, the basis of the Wolf-Hirschhorn syndrome, and distal 4p trisomy has syndromic, if not eponymic, status. The distal 4q segment is small cytogenetically (0.25% HAL) and functionally, and duplication[4] and deletion are quite well tolerated. So the respective imbalances in the combined states—the del(4p)+dup(4q), and the dup(4p)+del(4q)—remain sufficiently small to be viable, at least much of the time. The index case, with the former imbalance, was a severely disabled child with a Wolf-Hirschhorn phenotype; an aunt, having the latter combination, had rather minor dysmorphism and intellectual disability. The inverted segment is very long: 87% of the total length of chromosome 4. Therefore, crossing-over within the inverted segment is, we assume, very likely to take place. Thus, the genetic risk to heterozygotes for this inv(4) is high. Two other reported families, with slightly different breakpoints (4p16.2, 4q35.1 and 4p15.1, 4q35.1, respectively), also demonstrate a high risk for imbalanced offspring, with both recombinant products observed (Dufke et al. 2000; Maurin et al. 2009).

Likewise, a high risk applies to the inv(13)(p11q22) described in Williamson et al. (1980), in a family with several documented, suspected, or possible recombinant abnormal offspring. Here, the contribution of 13p imbalance to the two recombinant states—the del(13p)+dup(13q) and the dup(13p)+del(13q)—has no phenotypic effect, and the effective "single-segment" imbalances of dup(13)(q22qter) and del(13)(q22qter) are each well known to be viable, as discussed above. Applying the principles of "private segregation analysis" as set out in Chapter 4, the risk for a recombinant form in this family comes to a high 50%. We emphasize again the point that while the length of the inverted segment may influence the likelihood of recombination

[4] Duplication for a considerably longer segment, 4q31.3→qter, comprising 1.15% of HAL, is viable, as the children in the frontispiece photograph illustrate.

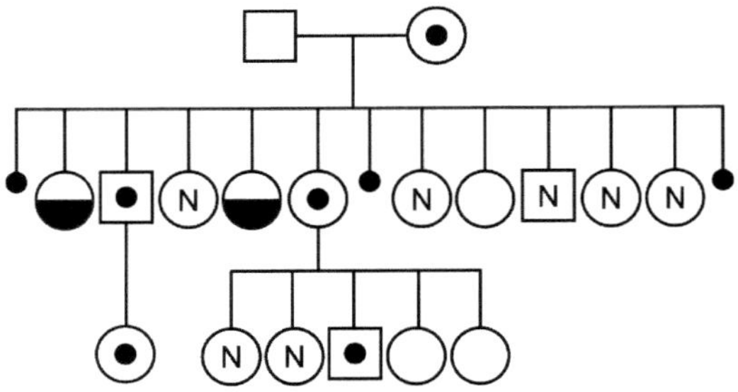

Figure 9–14. Pedigree of a Kindred Segregating an inv(X)(p22q22).

Notes: Carriers have bull's-eye symbol; two women with gonadal dysgenesis and 46,X,rec(X)dup(Xp) inv(X)(p22q22) have half-filled symbol; normal karyotype shown as N; no annotation, not tested; black dot, miscarriage. The fertility of the heterozygous matriarch is very evident.

Source: From Madariaga and Rivera (1997).

had three sons and three daughters—each daughter, of course, an obligate heterozygote. He apparently had no gonadal deficiency, but his two older daughters had menopause at ages 37 and 34 years (the youngest was only 30 years old). There was no family history recorded antecedent to him.

An ovum carrying a recombinant X would have two very different results, depending on whether it is fertilized by an X- or a Y-bearing sperm, as follows.

The 46,X,rec(X) Conceptus. In their review, Madariaga and Rivera (1997) record outcomes in recombinant cases in 10 families. The del(Xq)/dup(Xp) combination is, in female offspring, characterized by normal or tall stature, and ovarian dysgenesis. The countertype, del(Xp)/dup(Xq), is associated with short stature and, in some, intact ovarian function. These phenotypes presumably reflect the loss or gain of stature genes (in particular *SHOX*) located on Xp, and ovarian genes located on Xq, respectively. Any effect of the concomitant duplication is presumably mitigated by selective inactivation of the recombinant X chromosome. There is no obvious effect upon intellect.

Consider the case presented by Buckton et al. (1981) (Figure 9–15). One of the breakpoints is at the tip of the short arm, and the other is in proximal Xq. The recombinant chromosome, with a deficiency of the tip of Xp and a duplication of distal Xq (Figure 9–15, lower right), was in this family associated only with shortness of stature. The partial Xq trisomy made no discernible contribution to the phenotype. A 26-year-old mother with the rec(X) herself had a rec(X) daughter—unarguable evidence that oögenesis had not (at least by age 26 years) been compromised. A more recent case, with the countertype Xp/Xq imbalance and having molecular study, is reported in Kim et al. (2014): a woman with premature ovarian failure who had the karyotype 46,XX,rec(X)dup(Xp)inv(X)(p22.3q27.3) from a maternal inv(X), the Xp duplication involving chrX:pter-8.9 Mb and the Xq deletion, chrX:145.9-qter Mb.

The 46,Y,rec(X) Conceptus. There will be a nullisomy for the deficient X segment. If this segment constitutes any but the tiniest length of chromatin, the conceptus would not be viable. Nullisomy for a tiny telomeric segment may be viable, but with major dysmorphogenesis and severe neurodevelopmental compromise. Furthermore, the concomitant disomy X is functional, not being subject to inactivation, and therefore of itself produces a major deleterious effect. For example, the carrier mother in Chen et al. (2016a), 46,X,inv(X)(p22.3q26.3), had an abnormal ultrasound, and amniocentesis showed

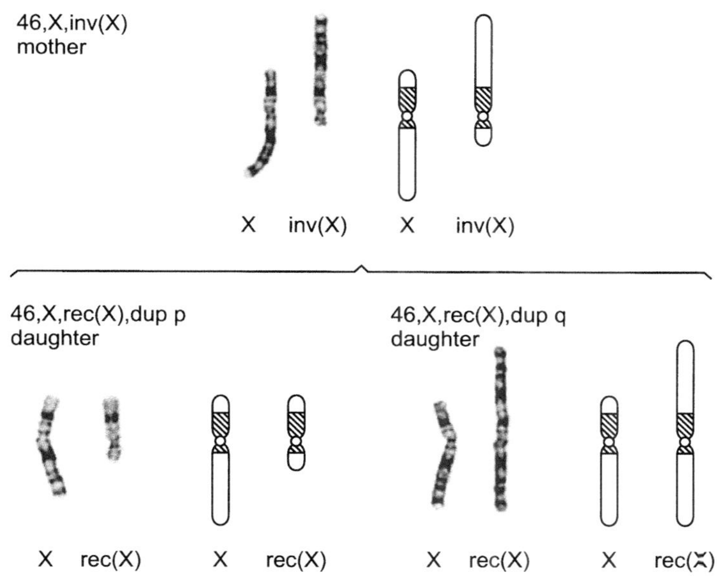

Figure 9–15. X chromosome inversion.

Notes: The mother (*above*) has the karyotype 46,X,inv(X)(p22q13). *Below*, The two possible unbalanced reproductive outcomes in daughters, following recombination within the inverted segment; the normal X on the left in each has been contributed by the father. Each type of daughter would have a variant form of Turner syndrome. Male recombinant conceptuses are not shown: The combination of X nullisomy and functional X disomy in the 46,Y,rec(X) conceptus would in this instance be lethal in utero. (Case of KE Buckton et al. 1981.)

46,Y,rec(X)dup(Xq)inv(X)(p22.3q26.3); at 24-week termination, fetal defects were observed. She had a second pregnancy, amniocentesis showing the inversion in balanced state in a male, 46,Y,inv(X)(p22.3q26.3); the baby boy was born prematurely but did well.

The Male inv(X) Hemizygote

In the male carrier, the rearrangement typically has no apparent effect on phenotype or on reproduction. This is what might have been presumed *a priori*, given that the inv(X) is regarded as being genetically balanced. Meiosis proceeds unperturbed (rather obviously, there can be no recombination within the inverted segment). All his daughters will be heterozygotes. Sons receive his normal Y and their mother's (normal) X chromosome, to become 46,XY. A causal association with infertility may be suspected, although not proven, in those presenting with that particular problem. Thus, in Ge et al. (2020), two brothers inherited an inv(X)(p22.3q22) from their mother, and both had severe oligospermia, with "0–1 spermatozoön per high power field." A role for an effect due to locus disruption at the X breakpoints remains an open question.

THE PERICENTRIC INVERSION Y

A pericentric inversion of the Y, inv(Y)(p11.2q11.23), is not uncommon in the general population (Verma et al. 1982; Tóth et al. 1984). Three major forms are recognized: types I–III, with differing Yq breakpoints, the Yp site being constant (Knebel et al. 2011). Types I and II, inv(Y)(p11.2q11.23) as noted above, typically have no phenotypic effect and imply no risk for having an abnormal child; these may be regarded as normal variants. The Type III, inv(Y)(p11.2q11.223), which splits the *DAZ* and *CDY* fertility gene cluster in *AZFc*, may be associated with infertility. A molecular-level inversion within Yq11.23, known as *r2/r3* and of 1.6 Mb extent, can predispose to partial *AZFc* deletion, with consequential oligo/azoöspermia (Hallast et al. 2021).

UNBALANCED DE NOVO APPARENT RECOMBINANT FROM AN INV
Rivera et al. (2013) studied a number of cases, ascertained either pre- or post-natally, in which a rec-like chromosome—that is, deleted for a p segment and duplicated for a q segment, or vice versa—was found. This might have raised a question of gonadal mosaicism for an inversion in a parent and might thus have implied an important genetic risk. But in fact, they could show that the typical mechanism was that of a nonallelic homologous recombination, which spoke for a sporadic, one-off, meiotic generation.

GENETIC COUNSELING

The Autosomal Pericentric Inversion

Variant Forms. It is important to distinguish between the essentially normal variant inversion, of quite frequent observation, versus the uncommon potentially pathogenic inversion.

The common inv(2)(p11.2q13), a very small pericentric inversion, is regarded as essentially innocuous (Hysert et al. 2006; Ferfouri et al. 2009). Two possible exceptions are on record to belie its reputation: two abnormal children, one with a 2p duplication and the other a 2p deletion, the proximal boundary at or adjacent to 2p11.2, and the fathers being inversion heterozygotes, described as inv(2)(p11.2q12.2) and inv(2)(p11.2q13), respectively (Magee et al. 1998a; Lacbawan et al. 1999). It may be that the configurations adopted by the chromosome 2 homologs led to an unequal crossing-over and hence the duplication or deletion. With only two such observations of recombination in the decades of history of clinical cytogenetics, some circumspection is required, and Lacbawan et al.'s comment is perfectly reasonable that "at this point, it seems premature to recommend prenatal diagnosis of all couples in this situation."

No genetic risks are known to be associated with the other inversion variants noted in the "Biology" section: inversions of 1, 9, 16, and Y heterochromatin, along with the inv(3)(p11-13q11-12), inv(5)(p13q13), and inv(10)(p11.2q21.2). Concerning the inv(10)(p11.2q21.1), Collinson et al. (1997) offer the practical advice that "family investigation of carrier status is not warranted in view of the unnecessary concern this may cause family members." We exclude these inversion variants from the discussion below.

Risks of Having an Abnormal Child

Ascertainment via Recombinant Child. Identification of a family through a recombinant individual proves the viability of at least one of the two recombinant chromosomes. Table 9–2 lists a large number of different inversions for which a carrier is known to have had a recombinant child. There have been various empiric estimates of the overall level of risk to the heterozygote in families ascertained through an abnormal child. From a

Table 9–2. Autosomal Pericentric Inversions Associated with the Birth of a Recombinant Offspring, Listed in "Numerical" Order

CHROMOSOME	INVERSIONS		
1	p36.21q42.13		
2	p25q35	p25.3q33.3	
3	p25q23	p25q25[a]	
4	p13q28	p15.32q35	
5	p13q33	p13q35	p14q35
	p15q32	p15.1q33.3	p15.1q35.1[a]
	p15.3q35		
6	p23q27	p23q25.13	
7	p14.2q36.3	p15q36	p15.1q36
	p22q22		
8	p23q22[a,b]	p23.3q24.1	
9	p24.3q34.1		
10	p11q26	p11.2q25.2[a]	p12q25
	p15q24		
11	p11q25	p13q23.3	p15.3q24.1
12	p13q24.3		
13	p11q21	p11q22	p12q13
	p12q14	p13q21[a]	p13q31
14	p12q31		
16	p13q22	p13.1q22	
17	p11q25	p13.3q25.1	
18	p11q11	p11.2q12.2	p11.2q21.3
19	p13.3q13.33		
20	p11.2q13.3	p12q13.3	p13q13.1
	p13q13.33		
21	p11q21.09	p11.2q22.1	p12q22
22	p11q21	p11.2q13.31	p13q12[a]
	p13q12.2		

Notes: Inversions listed here are from 55 families, published over the period 1981–2012. These comprise the cases reviewed in Ishii et al. (1997); the case illustrated in Figure 9–5; and more recent cases in Lagier-Tourenne et al. (2004), Mehra et al. (2005), Grange et al. (2005), Schluth-Bolard et al. (2008), Tagaya et al. (2008), Stevens et al. (2009), Honeywell et al. (2012), Mundhofir et al. (2012), Putoux et al. (2013), and Sgardioli et al. (2013).

[a]Reported in more than one family.

[b]Associated with San Luis Valley syndrome.

number of studies, a consensus range for the usual risk to have a liveborn abnormal child due to recombination is within the range 5%–15% (Groupe de Cytogénéticiens Français 1986b; Sherman et al. 1986; Stene 1986; Daniel et al. 1989). As a general rule, the longer the inversion segment—and, consequently, the shorter the distal segments—the greater the risk to produce a viable recombinant gamete (Figures 9–8 and 9–10). Very long inversions, such as that in Roberts et al. (1989), an inv(10) that comprised 80% of the whole chromosome, or the inv(20) in Stevens et al. (2009) comprising 94%, would imply

likely well under ½%, and prenatal molecular analysis targeted to the breakpoint regions would not normally be warranted. A question of interchromosomal effect appears not to be an issue.

Preimplantation Genetic Testing. In theory, PGT might be expected to improve reproductive outcomes, and especially so in the case of a parental inversion with a long inverted segment. This view is supported in the work of Xie et al. (2019) noted above, who showed an increased rate of blastocysts with an imbalance, in those in whom the inverted segment comprised above 57% of the chromosomal length (and see Figure 9–10). Jia and Xue (2023) similarly show an increased rate of imbalance with respect to inv(1) cases, the risk according to the inverted segment length (see "Biology" above). Other studies not showing an apparent benefit (Shao et al. 2020b; Tong et al. 2022a) may have been compromised by the inclusion of many cases with low-risk inversions. Thus, in a known (from previous history) or presumed (from the inv characteristics) high-risk scenario, PGT targeting possible rec forms may well have a place.

THE INVERSION X

The female heterozygote could have a premature menopause, if the long arm breakpoint is in the critical region, and if there is a family history of early ovarian failure; pragmatic advice might be to have children sooner rather than later. But normal reproductive function is perfectly possible. Recombination may be less likely than for an autosomal inversion (Pinto Leite and Pinto 2001), although a risk to produce an abnormal daughter with a recombinant X does, certainly, exist. The abnormality is, to some extent, predictable according to the deleted segment, Xp or Xq: Short stature is typically seen in del(Xp), and ovarian failure in del(Xq). Hemizygous sons would be expected to be normal, and reassurance in this respect may be drawn from the observation, if it can be made, of normality in a male relative. For the most part, no practical risk exists for having an abnormal son, because recombinant male conceptuses, having partial X nullisomy and disomy, would be nonviable. Only when the breakpoints are very close to the telomere is male viability possible, and such a child would have major physical abnormalities and intellectual disability, probably severe. Due to this male lethality, the sex ratio of the offspring would, in theory, be 1 male:2 females.

All daughters of the male heterozygote would be inv(X) heterozygotes. Other things being equal, they will be phenotypically normal. If the long arm breakpoint is in the "critical region," and if heterozygous female relatives have had ovarian deficiency (e.g., primary amenorrhea, premature menopause), they may develop the same problem. All sons would have a 46,XY karyotype.

THE INVERSION Y

This inversion—specifically, a macrosopically defined Type I or II inversion, as outlined above—is generally considered a normal population variant of no clinical significance. It is self-evident that all the sons of the inv(Y) carrier will be, themselves, inv(Y) carriers. They are all normal and, other things being equal, have normal gonadal function. All the daughters would be 46,XX. The Type III inv(Y)(p11.2q11.223) may be, but not necessarily so, associated with infertility.

THE PARACENTRIC INVERSION

BIOLOGY

Details of Meiotic Behavior

According to classical theory, the phenotypically normal heterozygote for an *autosomal* paracentric inversion would only have children who are karyotypically normal, or with the same balanced inversion. In theory, they could not have viable unbalanced progeny, for the following reasoning. If a recombinant gamete is formed following a crossover in the inverted segment, the chromosome would be either acentric (lacking a centromere) or dicentric (Figure 9–16). An acentric chromosome is never viable, since it lacks a point of attachment to the spindle fibers. The dicentric is considered a lethal impediment, being attached to spindle fibers pulling in opposite directions, with the chromosome thus suspended between the daughter nuclei at telophase, and excluded from either cell. A minor revision of classical theory is necessary, and a very few cases have proved exceptions (Table 9-3). Three possible mechanisms may conspire to yield a functional gamete that could then produce a viable, although imbalanced, conception. *Firstly*, one centromere of a dicentric rec product might become functionally suppressed, thus allowing the dicentric recombinant to function stably as, in effect, a monocentric (or "pseudodicentric") chromosome. Thus, the rec chromosomes could successfully attach to the spindle

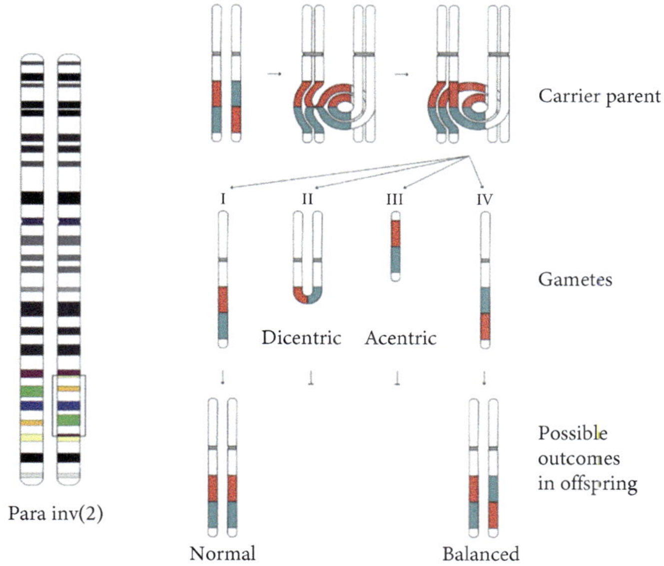

Figure 9–16. Theoretical recombinant products from classical crossover in a paracentric inversion. One is dicentric, and the other acentric.

Notes: The inversion segment is shown in red and blue, and the different colors indicate the parts proximal and distal to the crossover point. This inv(2)(q31.2q33.2) had a possible association with the patient's history of pregnancy loss.

Source: Adapted from J Wincent et al., Genome sequencing differentiates a paracentric inversion from a balanced insertion enabling more accurate preimplantation genetic testing, *Acta Obstet Gynecol Scand* 103:1564–1569, 2024. Courtesy J Wincent, and with the permission of John Wiley & Sons.

Table 9–3. Some Recorded Examples of Parental Paracentric Inversions Associated with the Birth of a Recombinant Child

STUDY	PARENTAL KARYOTYPE	EFFECTIVE IMBALANCE IN THE CHILD
Devillard et al. (2010)	46,XX,inv(2)(q14.2q37.3)	dup 2q14.1q14.2, del 2q37.3**
South et al. (2006)	46,XX,inv(5)(p13.3p15.3)	del 5p14.3**
Hoo et al. (1982)	46,XX,inv(7)(q11.23q22)	dup 7q11.22q11.23
Paskulin et al. (2011)	46,XX,inv(7)(q11.23q33)	del 7q31.32q33
Phelan et al. (1993)	46,XY,inv(9)(p13p24)	dup 9p12p24**
Worsham et al. (1989)	46,XX,inv(9)(q22.1q34.3)	dup 9pter-q22.1, del 9q34.3-qter*
Douglas et al. (2017)	46,XY,inv(13)(q21.2q32.3)	dup 13q21.31q22.3 + 13q32.1q33.3, del 13q33.3qter
Lefort et al. (2002)	46,XX,inv(14)(q13q32.2)	dup 14pter-q13, del 14q32.2qter*
Mules and Stamberg (1984)	46,XX,inv(14)(q24.2q32.3)	dup 14q24.2pter, del 14q32.3qter*
Whiteford et al. (2000)	46,XXinv(15)(q11.2q26.3)	dup 15pter-q11.2, del 15q26.3qter*
Yang et al. (1997)	46,XY,inv(17)(p11.2p13)	del 17p11.2
Anlaş et al. (2023)	46,XX,inv(18)(q11.2q21.3)	dup 18p11.32p11.21 + 18q11.1q11.2, del 18q21.33q23*
Chia et al. (1992)	46,XY,inv(18)(q12.1q23)	dup 18q12.1q21.3, del 9q21.3q23***
Courtens et al. (1998)	46,XX,inv(18)(q21.1q22.3)	dup 18q12.1q21.1, del 18q22.3qter**
McClarren et al. (2006)	46,XX,inv(22)(q11.2q13.3)	del 22q11.2**

Notes: * Dicentric rec chromosome.
** Rupture and reconstitution of rec chromosome.
*** U-loop recombinant chromosome.
See also Madan (1995) and Pettenati et al. (1995), and Warburton and Twersky (1997).

fiber, using just the one centromere. Each product would have a del/dup combination, and the least imbalanced of these could be viable (Madan 1995). *Secondly*, a dicentric recombinant chromosome, pulled in two directions, might rupture, yielding functional monocentric products. *Thirdly*, a crossover within the inversion loop, instead of continuing on in the same direction along the chromatid, could reverse upon itself, known as "U-loop recombination" (Figure 9-17) (Mitchell et al. 1994).

Gamete Studies. Yapan et al. (2014) review the findings from a small number of *sperm* studies, and analyze the extent to which recombination had occurred, showing that the likelihood of recombination is, in considerable part, related to the length of the inv segment. Their own case from a man 46,XY,inv(2)(q21.2q37.3), the largest paracentric inv on record, had the highest level of rec forms, at 28%; presumably, the large size of the inversion, at 103 Mb comprising about three-quarters of 2q, meant that formation of an

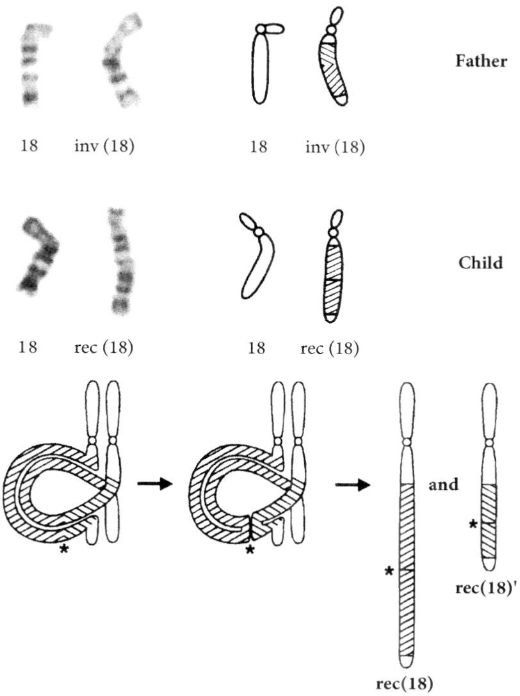

Figure 9–17. Meiotic Behavior of the Paracentric Inversion.

Above, parent with paracentric inversion and child with recombinant ("reunitant") chromosome. Father has paracentric inversion of 18q, inv(18)(q12.1q23). The inverted segment is shown cross-hatched (cross-hatching changes slope at q21.3). Child has duplication of the segment q12.1q21.3 on the reuniting chromosome (shown cross-hatched) and deletion q21.3q23. (Case of NL Chia and LR Bousfield.) *Below,* Proposed mechanism of U-loop exchange depicted; asterisk indicates point of U-loop. The position of the point of exchange within the inversion loop (in this case, q21.3) determines the nature of the imbalance. There is duplication of chromatin proximal to the crossover point (q12.1q21.3), and deletion of distal chromatin (q21.3q23), as in the child's rec(18); and vice versa in the complementary product, rec(18)'. (An alternative interpretation is that the father's rearrangement is a within-arm insertion of 18q, rather than an inversion, in which case the karyotype of the child would have been derived from recombination in the inserted segment.)

inversion loop was not hindered, and recombination was enabled. In contrast, those of shorter inv segments had, in fact, zero rec sperm.

Meiosis in *oögenesis* commences during fetal life, and its direct study therefore requires access to fetal tissue. Cheng et al. (1999) analyzed ovarian tissue from a 19-week termination of pregnancy, in which a de novo inv(7)(q11.23q21.2) had been shown at amniocentesis. By using a FISH probe for the Williams syndrome critical region (WSCR), which is at 7q11.23, they could determine whether the inverted segments were aligned alongside each other (homosynapsis) or not (heterosynapsis). Most cells showed the chromosome 7 homologs lined up side-by-side, but with the WSCR signals off from each other: Thus, the inversion segment was unaligned. A classical inversion loop was seen in only 10% of cells. This single example, concerning a small inversion segment, offers an explanation for the rarity with which recombinant forms are seen, given that the necessary prerequisite of homosynapsis often does not apply.

A mechanism reminiscent of paracentric inversion U-loop reunion may be the cause of some isochromosome Xq Turner syndrome (Wolff et al. 1996). Two zinc-finger

phenotypes of presenting cases is apparent. As Madan comments, there may have been a bias in choosing cases for publication, and editors of journals might not find compelling a paper describing an "uninteresting" inversion discovered incidentally in a normal individual (a series of a dozen or more cases might stand a better chance). In their review, Pettenati et al. (1995) could be confident about a causal association with a specific phenotype only with respect to the paracentric inv(X), and not with any of the autosomal inversions.

The Groupe de Cytogénéticiens Français (1986a) note that the reproductive fitness of heterozygotes in 32 French families was normal. Two quite common inversions seen in a number of families in more than one part of the world are the inv(3)(p13p25) and the inv(11)(q21q23) (Madan 1995). No abnormalities directly attributable to these inversions have been documented. It may be founder effect, or recurring mutation, that is the basis for their frequency.

Interchromosomal Effect. In the series of 197 preimplantation diagnoses from 57 couples, one of whom was a paracentric inversion heterozygote, due to Xie et al. (2019), no interchromosomal effect was discernible, confirming the earlier view of Pettenati et al. (1995) apropos.

Technical Comment. Paracentric inversions are not detected by microarray and can be technically difficult to detect on classical cytogenetics. Gross chromosome morphology is not altered, and unless major landmark bands are shifted, the rearrangement may go unnoticed. Only with the use of good-quality, high-resolution banding are paracentric inversions likely to be detected regularly. Also, for technical reasons, reported cases of recombination in the literature should be regarded with caution; as mentioned above and noted below, some "inversions" are likely actually to be intrachromosomal insertions ("paracentric/within-arm shifts"). The cytogenetic distinction can be difficult to make, especially so for chromosomal regions without distinctive banding patterns, or where the inverted segments are very small (Callen et al. 1985; Madan 1995). For example, the inverted insertion of chromosome 15 described in Collinson et al. (2004), associated with recombinant offspring having Prader-Willi and Angelman syndrome (and see p. 238), had originally been reported, some 10 years prior, as a paracentric inversion. We have seen a family in which the index case seemed to have an unbalanced translocation at distal 4p, but the normal mother and grandfather had the same anomaly, which could then be reinterpreted as the minimum inversion detectable on routine cytogenetics, a one-band paracentric inversion, in this case inv(4)(p15.3p16.3) (Smith et al. 1992).

GENETIC COUNSELING

On practical grounds, the reassuring point to note is that practically all paracentric inversion heterozygotes identified have been discovered incidentally, and not through the birth of a child with an abnormality attributable to the parental inversion (Madan 1995). We agree with Madan: "The vast majority of paracentric inversions are likely to be harmless." Apparently, the genetic risks to offspring are extremely small. In the U.S. collaborative study described in Daniel et al. (1988), there were no unbalanced karyotypes in 30 prenatal diagnoses. The sex chromosomes warrant separate attention, and it may be that some X and Y paracentric inversions have an effect upon gonadal development in the intact (that is, unrecombined) state.

However, a tiny handful of abnormal offspring, and as reviewed at length above, refute a complete harmlessness in the parental paracentric inversion, whether due to classic recombination, or to other forms of rearrangement. Whether this would warrant prenatal diagnosis, when a parent is a carrier of one of these implicated inversions, is a matter for debate. Even where the new chromosome from a classic or U-loop recombinant might on theoretical grounds be viable, the risk for one to be generated, while its exact magnitude is unknown, is surely "extremely small." "Better than 99.9%" might be a fair estimate that there will be no untoward reproductive outcome due to behavior of the inversion. While molecular karyotyping offers the potential to screen, at prenatal diagnosis, for submicroscopic molecular damage associated with a particular apparently balanced inversion, the case for so doing is very modest. Caution—but in realistic perspective—should be exercised during genetic counseling, in that it is prudent never to say "never."

Thus we suggest that in practice, an offer of prenatal diagnosis be discretionary in the case of a fortuitously discovered inversion in the family; and we would regard it as not inappropriate if the offer were declined (or not made). A firmer stance may be appropriate if there has been a previous history of an apparently associated reproductive abnormality. Inversions on record with a demonstrated recombinant (Table 9–3) would oblige the offer of prenatal diagnosis. But again, we return to the expressions used above: "vast majority," and "better than 99.9%" in respect of favorable behavior of the inversion.

As mentioned above, a diagnosis of a paracentric inversion might be incorrect, and the rearrangement is actually a within-arm insertion, which actually carries a high genetic risk (Chapter 8). Since the distinction in the routine laboratory can be difficult, a practical view might be to risk over-interpreting subtle paracentric inversions as potential insertions in those cases where the cytogeneticist is not absolutely certain. The true picture may emerge by determining the order of a number of FISH probes across the relevant region.

The Special Case of the inv dup del(8p)

The inv dup del(8p), noted in the "Biology" section earlier, arises from a maternal cryptic (on classical cytogenetics) paracentric inversion. Yet for a couple who have had this happen, the risk of recurrence is in all likelihood still extremely small. Nevertheless, it would be understandable for a couple having had that experience to seek the reassurance of preimplantation or prenatal diagnosis in a subsequent pregnancy.

The Paracentric Inversion Detected Prenatally

If an apparently balanced paracentric inversion is discovered at prenatal diagnosis, and if the parental karyotypes are normal—in other words, this is a de novo rearrangement—there yet remains a possibility that the rearrangement is not truly balanced, and a risk for abnormality exists (see above, "Mendelian Mechanisms Causing Abnormality"). This question is dealt with in detail in Chapter 22 (p. 702).

10

COMPLEX CHROMOSOMAL REARRANGEMENTS

COMPLEX CHROMOSOMAL REARRANGEMENTS (CCRs) occurring in phenotypically normal persons are rare. In her exhaustive review at the time, Madan (2012) recorded 103 published cases. Three or more chromosomes are involved, and a considerable variety of rearrangements are possible. Translocation may involve distal segments, as in the usual reciprocal translocation, or interstitial segments, as in the insertion. Any chromosome may participate in a CCR. Molecular methodology is revealing more complexity among some classical rearrangements than previously appreciated, and the definition of what actually is a "CCR" could become unwieldy (Poot and Haaf 2015). We here largely limit our discussion to those CCRs that may be seen in balanced form in heterozygotes of otherwise normal health, and who may be at risk of producing abnormal pregnancies.[1]

BIOLOGY

Four Major Categories of Complex Chromosome Rearrangement

Madan (2012) defines CCRs as those involving three or more chromosomes in which there are three or more breaks. This definition excludes the double two-way reciprocal exchange (Chapter 5). She proposes four major categories of CCR, types I–IV, based essentially upon the number of chromosomes versus the number of breaks and whether there are insertions or inversions. In Type I, there is the same number of breaks as there are chromosomes, and the most common is the three-way exchange in which three segments from three different chromosomes break off, translocate, and unite (Figure 10–1). In Type II, there is one more break than the number of involved chromosomes and this is due to one chromosome having an inversion. Some apparent Type I CCRs may turn out, upon molecular dissection, to be Type II (Figure 10–2). Molecular dissection may also be needed to reveal the true state of a "cryptic" CCR karyotype initially interpreted as normal (Figure 10–3). Type III is characterized by translocations having one or more insertions (Figure 10–3). The most complex scenario is seen in Type IV (Figure 10–4), in which one (or more) of the derivative chromosomes comprises segments from three or even more chromosomes. In the discussion below, we group Types II–IV as "exceptional CCRs."

The original CCR in a family typically arises as a single complex event, rather than sequential changes, at a meiosis during male gametogenesis (Grossmann et al. 2010). In the familial CCR, transmission thereafter is much more often seen through the mother,

[1] Most (~90%) apparently balanced CCRs in abnormal individuals prove in fact to be imbalanced on molecular methodology (Feenstra et al. 2011; Plesser Duvdevani et al. 2020).

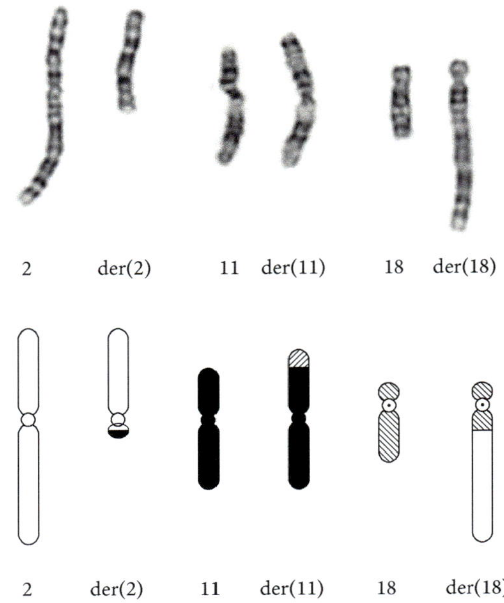

Figure 10–1. A Three-way Complex Chromosome Rearrangement.

Notes: Most of 2q is translocated onto 18q; part of 18q is translocated onto 11p; and the tip of 11p is translocated onto 2q. The formal karyotype is 46,XX,t(2;11;18)(2pter→2q13::11p15.3→11pter;11qter →11p15.3:: 18q21.1→18qter;18pter→18q21.1::2q13→2qter). The woman had presented with multiple miscarriages.

Source: From RJM Gardner et al., A three-way translocation in mother and daughter, *J Med Genet* 23: 90, 1986 and with the permission of the British Medical Association.

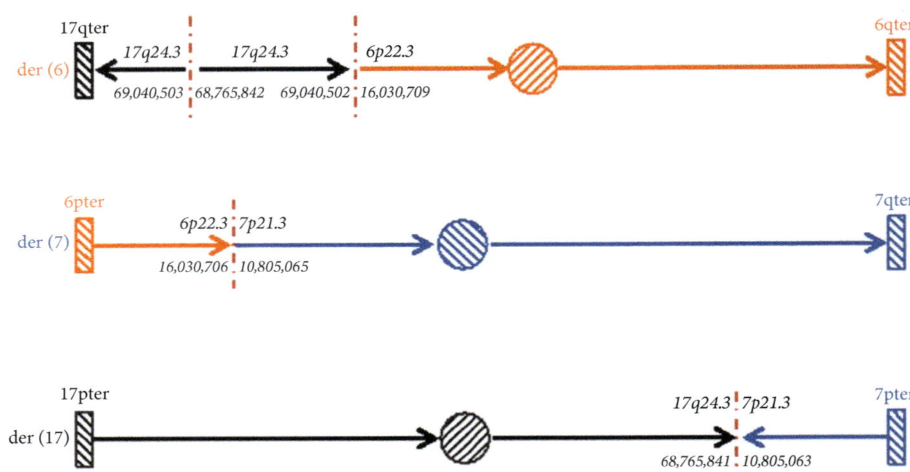

Figure 10–2. A Type I CCR Revealed to be, in fact, Type II.

Notes: This complex chromosome rearrangement was initially interpreted as a simple three-way t(6;7;17)(p23;p22;q25)pat), and thus to be seen as a Type I CCR. As indicated above, on molecular dissection the breakpoints were subsequently refined, and an inverted segment (17q24.3) identified; and the case thus redefined as Type II. Orange = chromosome 6, blue = chromosome 7; black = chromosome 17, circles = centromeres, rectangles = telomeres. Red dot-and-dash lines = breakpoints.

Source: From C Redin et al., The genomic landscape of balanced cytogenetic abnormalities associated with human congenital anomalies, *Nat Genet* 49:36–45, 2017. Courtesy ME Talkowski, and with the permission of Springer Nature.

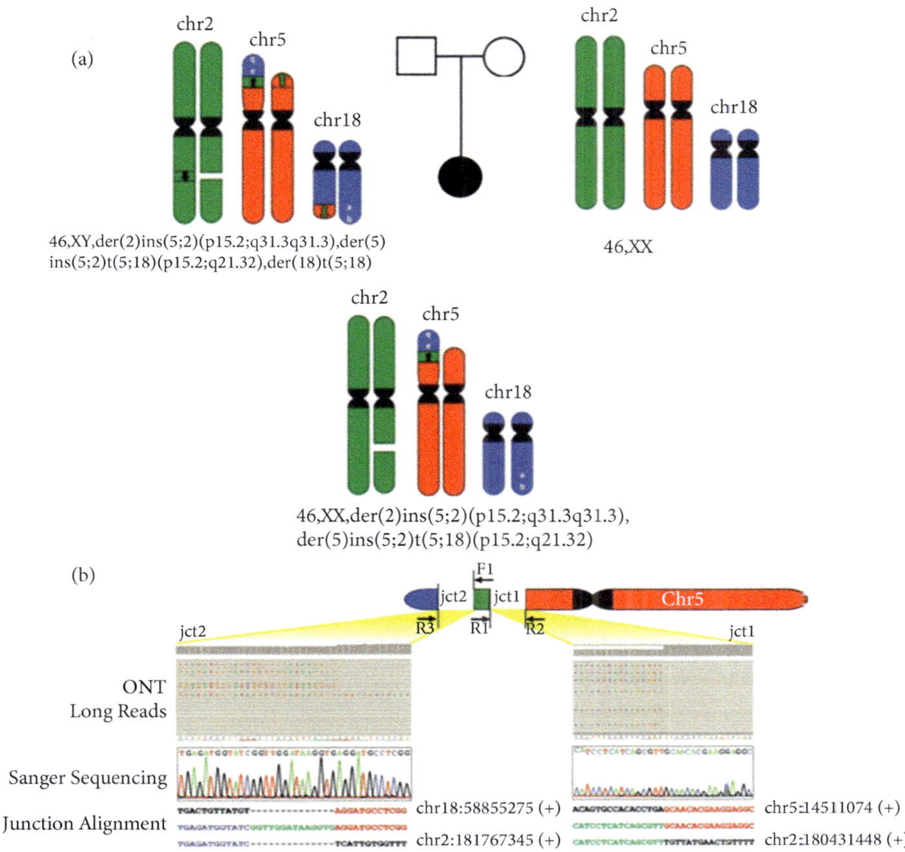

Figure 10–3. Unbalanced Transmission of a CCR.

Notes: Chromosome 2 in green, 5 in red, and 18 in blue. (a) The father's karyotype is balanced. At his daughter's conception, transmitting the der(5) alongside the normal 18 led to imbalance: the der(5) lacks a segment of distal 5p (the red segment with a contained green arrow), and carries additional 18q material (the blue segment annotated a-b). Albeit that the der(5) contains chromosome 2 material (in green), the child is balanced in this respect. The small size of the translocated segments at first misled investigation, and the initial karyotype in the child was 46,XX. The child, with del5p/dup18q, was globally developmentally delayed. (b) The subtleties of the rearrangement within the der(5), revealed by molecular dissection. Jct = breakpoint junction; ONT = Oxford Nanopore Technology.

Source: From Z Dardas et al., Genomic balancing act: deciphering DNA rearrangements in the complex chromosomal aberration involving 5p15.2, 2q31.1, and 18q21.32, *Eur J Hum Genet* 33:231–238, 2025. Courtesy JR Lupski, and with the permission of Springer Nature.

and this is a reflection of the infertility to which the male is often susceptible (although not always so; Figure 10–5). CCRs with up to four breakpoints are more typically familial, and ascertained through the female; those with more breakpoints are usually de novo and discovered through male infertility (Poot and Haaf 2015).

Nomenclature of the CCR, as per the ISCN, is straightforward with the Type I CCR, although it can become rather complicated with exceptional CCRs. In principle, the involved chromosomes and breakpoints are listed in the following order: first, the lowest numbered (or X or Y) chromosome; second, the chromosome that receives

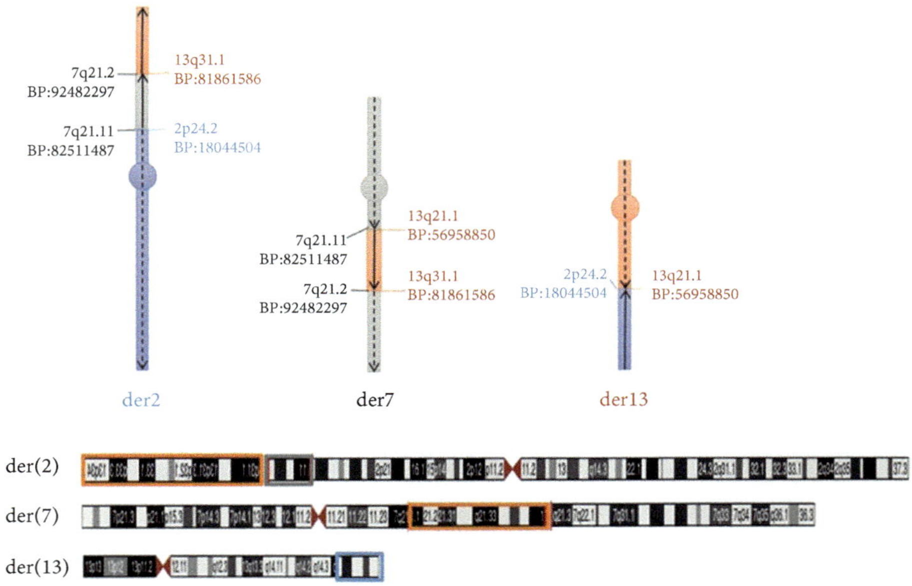

Figure 10–4. The Architecture of a CCR at a Molecular Level.

Note: This CCR was identified in a woman who had had three abnormal pregnancies: two miscarriages, and an induced termination following an amniocentesis result of dup 7q/del 13q. This is an "exceptional CCR" Type IV, with insertions from 7q into 2p, and from 13q into 7q, along with distal exchanges between 2p and 13q.[a] The breakpoints are defined at the level of the base pair.

[a] For the record, the detailed karyotype is 46,XX,der(2)(13qter→13q31.1::7q21.2→7q21.11::2p24.2→2qter), der(7)(7pter→7q21.11::13q21.1 →13q31.1::7q21.2→7qter),der(13)(13pter→13q21.1::2p24.2→2pter).

Source: From L Xing et al., Long-read Oxford nanopore sequencing reveals a de novo case of complex chromosomal rearrangement involving chromosomes 2, 7, and 13, *Mol Genet Genomic Med* 10:e2011, 2022. Courtesy H Liu, and with the permission of John Wiley & Sons.

a segment from the first; and last, the chromosome donating a segment to the first listed chromosome. Thus, in the simplest Type I case, for example, the karyotype of the CCR shown in Figure 10–1 would be written 46,XX,t(2;18;11)(q13;q21.1;p15.3).

Details of Meiotic Behavior

The carrier of a CCR has a risk for an abnormal conception due to malsegregation of the derivative chromosomes (or, rarely observed, due to the generation of a recombinant chromosome). Malsegregation follows the general principles as set forth for the simple translocation, assuming that apposition of homologous segments is able to take place; but if so, naturally the range of unbalanced combinations is greater. The broad categories of malsegregation in the Type I three-way translocation are 3:3 (alternate and adjacent), 4:2, and 5:1 and 6:0; in Types II to IV, the theoretical range is enormous. Unsurprisingly the rates of abnormality are much higher in gametes and embryos than in liveborn children, reflecting the lethality in utero of the many possible unbalanced forms.

The findings from four sperm studies are set out in Table 10–1; from these men, an average of only 17% of sperm were normal or balanced. In those in which different

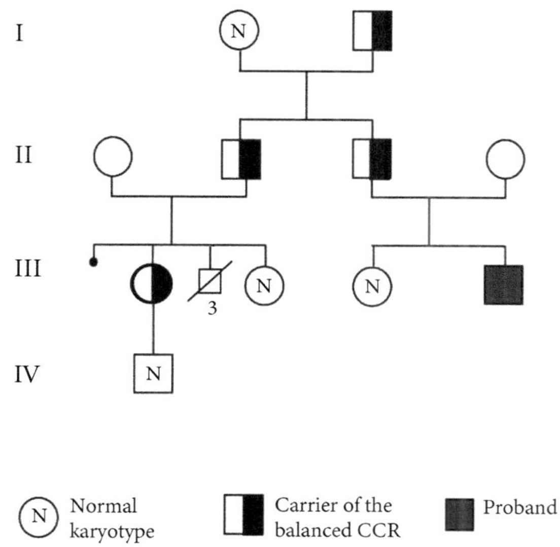

Figure 10–5. Familial Complex Chromosome Rearrangement.

Notes: On initial classic cytogenetics, a CCR with four breakpoints in chromosomes 2, 6, and 18 was diagnosed. Subsequent FISH-based analysis enabled the recognition of eight breakpoints, with five insertional segments.[a] The proband at diagnosis was a dysmorphic and developmentally delayed child, whose imbalance due to missegregation comprised a 6p partial trisomy and an 18q partial monosomy. Case III:3 was an 8-month fetal death in utero, unkaryotyped. Atypically in this family, male fertility is retained.

[a] For the record, 46,XX,der(2)ins(2;6)(q37.2;p22.2p22.2)ins(2;6)(q37.2;p21.1p12.3),der(6)ins(6;18)(p12.3;q21.32q21.32), der(18) inv ins(18;6)(q21.32;p22.2p21.1) ins(18;6)(q21.32;p12.3p12.3).

Source: Drawn after N Gruchy et al., A paternally transmitted complex chromosomal rearrangement (CCR) involving chromosomes 2, 6, and 18 includes eight breakpoints and five insertional translocations (ITs) through three generations, *Am J Med Genet* 152A:185–190, 2010. Courtesy N Gruchy, and with the permission of John Wiley & Sons.

malsegregant forms were identified, a very wide range of possible abnormalities were recorded, apparently close to the theoretical maximum. The sperm study in the case in Loup et al. (2010), for example, showed the following proportions among the unbalanced sperm: 34% from 3:3 malsegregations, 38% from 4:2, and even 5:1 (3.5%) and 6:0 (0.05%, representing one sperm out of 1,822). From PGT studies, the results from 155 embryos, from male and female carriers, are listed in Table 10–2. Again, embryos with a normal or balanced constitution are in a small minority. On these small numbers, the risks appear more marked for the female carrier.

Gorski et al. (1988) proposed a broad-brush risk to the carrier to have an abnormal liveborn child due to an unbalanced form of the CCR to be about 20%, and for a pregnancy to miscarry about 50%. Of the abnormal forms, Madan (2012) noted adjacent-1 to be the most frequently observed malsegregant mode (72%), 4:2 in 25%, and adjacent-2 in only 3%.

Three-Way Complex Chromosome Rearrangement (Type I CCR)

At meiosis in the three-way CCR heterozygote, the expectation is that the chromosomes involved in the rearrangement will come together and form a multivalent (Figure 10–6).

Table 10–1. CCR Sperm Studies

Translocation	Normal/Balanced	Reference
t(2;22;11)(q13;q11.2;q23)	14%	Cifuentes et al. 1998
t(1;19;13)(p31;q13.2;q31)	15%	Loup et al. 2010
t(5;13;14)(q23;q21;q31)	27%	Pellestor et al. 2011
t(1;3;6)(p21.1;q22.1;p21.2)	16%	Hornak et al. 2014
t(4;7;14)(q12;p21;q11.2)	12%	Rossi et al. 2023
Average	17%	

Consider how meiosis would proceed in the rcp(2;18;11) translocation illustrated in Figure 10–1. In theory, a hexavalent configuration would allow full synapsis of homologous segments (Figure 10–7). If disjunction were then 3:3, up to 20 possible gametic combinations could occur. The two arising from alternate segregation (arrows in Figure 10–7) would be the only ones to be balanced; the remaining 18 from adjacent segregation would be unbalanced to a greater or lesser degree. Were 4:2, 5:1, or 6:0 segregation to occur, a great number of extremely unbalanced gametes could result, as Rossi et al. (2023) illustrate.

Table 10–2. Embryos from CCR Carriers

Translocation	Carrier	Normal/ Balanced	Unbalanced	Reference
t(5;13;16)(q35.1;q32.1;q11.1)	F	2	20	Escudero et al. 2008
t(6;11;16)(q16.2;p14.2;q13)	M	0	5	Scriven et al. 2014
t(1;4;14)(p32.3;q23;q13)	M	4	9	*Ibid.*
t(1;9;18)(p13.3;p22;q23)	M	4	13	*Ibid.*
t(1;3;4)(q42.1;q26.2;p15.2)	F	0	8	*Ibid.*
t (3;7;9)(q23;q22;q22)	M	2	14	Frumkin et al. 2017
t(2;3;4)(p13;q13.2;q21)	F	0	2	Hu et al. 2018
t(1;6;3)(p22;q21;p24)	F	0	2	*Ibid.*
t(2;12;4)(p13;p11;q33)	F	1	5	*Ibid.*
t(1;12;21)(q25;q15;q11)	F	1	8	*Ibid.*
t(2;13;9)(p23;q14;p11)	M	0	8	*Ibid.*
t(9;16;12)(p22;q22;q15)	M	0	1	*Ibid.*
t(1;9;15), t(6;8)	F	0	12	*Ibid.*
t(1;4;11)(p31;p16;p22)	M	1	3	Brunet et al. 2018
t(3;13;5)(p14;q21;p14)	M	0	9	*Ibid.*
t(6;11;21)(q21;q21;q13)	F	2	4	*Ibid.*
t(2;4;14)(q21.1;p15.2;q22)	M	0	9	Mas et al. 2018
t(2;6;12)(p21;p25;p13)	F	0	6	Özer et al. 2022
Averages		11%	89%	

Note: Some of the unbalanced embryos had aneuploidies unrelated to the chromosomes of the translocation. M = male, F = female.

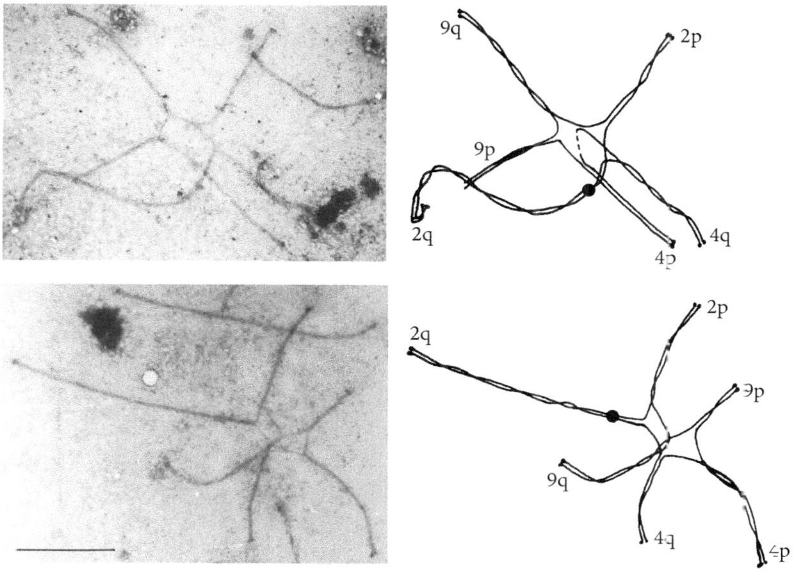

Figure 10–6. A Multivalent at Meiosis I.

Notes: Electron micrograph of a spermatocyte from a testicular biopsy of a man with a type I three-way complex chromosome rearrangement 46,XY,rcp(2;4;9)(p12;q25;p12); line drawing shows component parts of the hexavalent.

Source: From N Saadallah and MA Hultén, A complex three breakpoint translocation involving chromosomes 2, 4, and 9 identified by meiotic investigations of a human male ascertained for subfertility, *Hum Genet* 71:312–320,1985. Courtesy MA Hultén, and with the permission of Springer-Verlag.

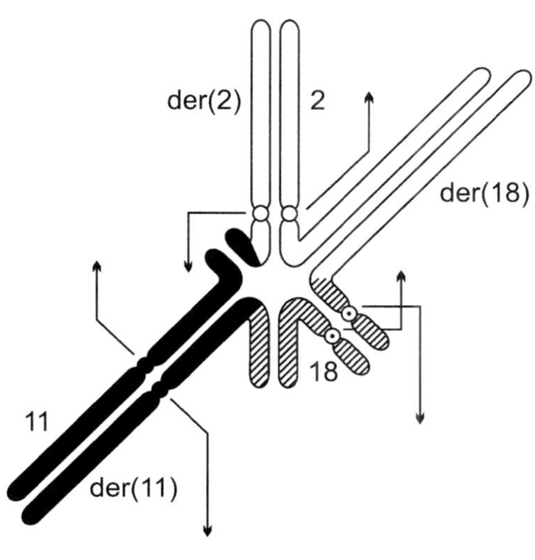

Figure 10–7. A Multivalent at Meiosis I, Diagrammed.

Notes: Diagrammatic representation of the formation of a hexavalent at meiosis in the three-way 2;18;11 translocation depicted in Figure 10–1. The arrows indicate 3:3 alternate segregation. The breakpoint detail is given in Figure 10–1.

Adjacent segregation can be classified as adjacent-1 and adjacent-2, similarly to the principles set forth in the simple reciprocal translocation. Thus, the segregant gamete shown at left in Figure 10–8, having one of each chromosome pair represented (one of each centromere), would reflect adjacent-1 segregation. An example of 3:3 adjacent-2 segregation is given in Xu et al. (1997). A mother had the karyotype 46,XX,t(5;16;22), and cytogenetic analysis of her morphologically abnormal fetus following intrauterine death at 16 weeks gestation showed 46,XY,der(5),der(16),–22,t(5;16;22). In this case, the abnormal ovum would have had one chromosome 5, two chromosome 16s (one normal, one the derivative), and lacked a chromosome 22.

4:2 segregation particularly characterizes CCRs in which chromosomes with "small content" short arms (9, the acrocentrics) are a component. Schwinger et al. (1975) reported a mother of two children with typical Down syndrome, who herself had a three-way t(7;21;11) CCR. The affected children had an interchange trisomy 21, in that they had, in addition to the maternal translocation pattern, a second intact chromosome 21. Fuster et al. (1997) give an example of a 4:2 malsegregant, diagnosed at chorionic villus sampling, from a three-way paternal t(2;22;11) CCR. The fetal karyotype was interpreted as 47,–2,der(2),der(22)t(2;22;11)(q13;q11.2;q23). The parents continued the pregnancy, and the disabled child with multiple anomalies had a double partial trisomy: a duplication of the segments 11q23qter and 22pter-q11.2. The couple had previously had one normal child and three miscarriages.

The risk of having a pregnancy that would go to term but then produce an abnormal child reflects the nature of the rearrangement—that is, the familiar question of whether there are possible chromosomal combinations that would lead to aneuploidy for a survivable amount of genetic material. Thus, considering the preceding rcp(2;18;11) example, three unbalanced combinations—one 3:3 and two 4:2—might be expected to be viable (Figure 10–8). Madan (2012) determined that the criteria applying to simple translocations (Chapter 5) are broadly appropriate for the CCR: If the translocated segments are short, adjacent-1 segregation may lead to liveborn abnormal offspring; and if chromosomes with "small content" short arms (9, the acrocentrics) are involved, 4:2 segregation is usual. Large translocated segments are typically associated only with non-viable products and consequent pregnancy loss. Recombination would add yet further possibility of imbalance, but this is rarely seen.

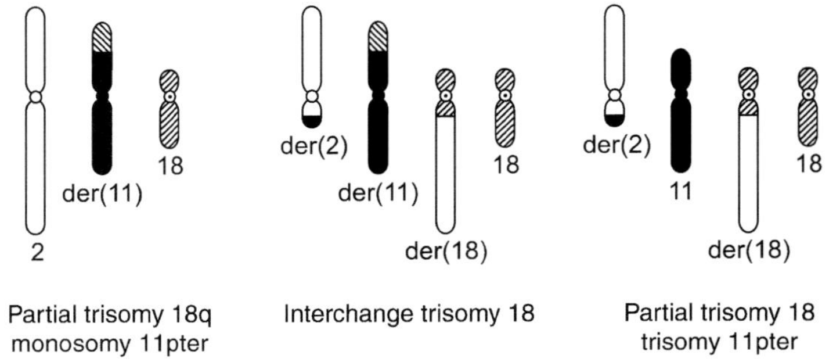

Figure 10–8. Possibly Viable Segregant Outcomes from a CCR.

Notes: Three segregant outcomes of meiosis in the rcp(2;18;11) heterozygote shown in Figure 10–1, that might be expected to produce viable but unbalanced offspring. The 3:3 adjacent-1 gamete on the left may be the one most likely to be observed.

Exceptional Complex Chromosome Rearrangement

More complex rearrangements imply an even greater potential range of abnormal gametes. Kausch et al. (1988) calculated a minimum of 70 possible unbalanced gametes due to 4:4, 5:3, 6:2, and 7:1 segregations from an octavalent, in the case of a woman with a five-breakpoint CCR with translocations of chromosomes 1, 2, 5, and 11, and an inversion of chromosome 1, who had presented with three first-trimester miscarriages. Van der Burgt et al. (1992) report a similarly complex de novo balanced CCR (chromosomes 5, 11, 12, 16; five breakpoints in all) in a mother who had had one miscarriage, one 46,XY child, the index abnormal child, and, as a quite unexpected outcome, a de novo 45,rob(13q14q) at prenatal diagnosis in her fourth pregnancy. The mother with a particularly complex CCR (chromosomes 1, 4, 14, 18)[2] in Campos et al. (2021) had had a normal child and two miscarriages before having her affected son.

One of the more complicated familial CCR scenarios described is the case in Röthlisberger et al. (1999). A father carried a de novo CCR, with eight breakpoints altogether—two in chromosomes 6 and 18, three in 7, and one in 21. Most remarkably, among his three children, three different recombinant forms were passed on: a rec(7), a rec(21), and a rec(18). The child with the rec(21) had a balanced karyotype, and he has become a balanced carrier for a simple translocation, 46,t(7;21)(q21.3;q21.3): a "rebuilt" translocation (see below). The other two have partial trisomies for 6q and 7q. The classical karyotype will often fail to reveal the true nature of an exceptional CCR, as the comparison between the G-banded karyotype and the molecular-based diagram in Figure 10–9 illustrates.

The coming together of several translocation chromosomes during meiosis may set the stage for recombination that Soler et al. (2005) describe as "rebuilding." The CCR shown in Figure 10–10 with six breakpoints in five chromosomes offers useful illustration. The woman who carried this rearrangement had four pregnancies, only one of which miscarried, and two produced offspring with a balanced constitution, though different in each child, and different from their mother! Recombination involving the centric segment of chromosome 1 led to a daughter receiving a rebuilt der(1), with just the 6p segment being translocated, and a son with a different rebuilt der(1) having just the 7q segment. A son and a grandson had unbalanced karyotypes, which were different, but each led to partial 7q trisomy. Readers who relish esoteric puzzles may wish to refer to the original paper.

Effect upon Fertility. In some complex rearrangements, gametogenesis can accommodate itself to the complexity thrust upon it, and the heterozygote may be fertile and have pregnancies that produce phenotypically normal children. Multi-generation transmission is recorded, but is uncommon (Figure 10–5). The rule of the greater vulnerability of spermatogenesis to chromosomal complexity seems to apply particularly in the case of the CCR, and the male heterozygote is often sterile due to spermatogenic arrest (Liang et al. 2022b). Indeed, in Madan's (2012) review of 19 patients presenting with infertility, only one was a woman (and in her case, one of the breakpoints in the CCR being at Xq24, a critical ovarigenesis region, was the likely culprit).

[2] For the record, 46,XX,ins(1) (pter→p22.3:q41→q43orq43→q41:p22.3→q41:q43→qter),t(4;14;18)(4pter→4p15.2:4p14→4qter;14pter→14q24.1:4p15.2→4p14or4p14→4p15.2:18q21.1→18qter;18pter→18q21.1:14q24.1→14qter).

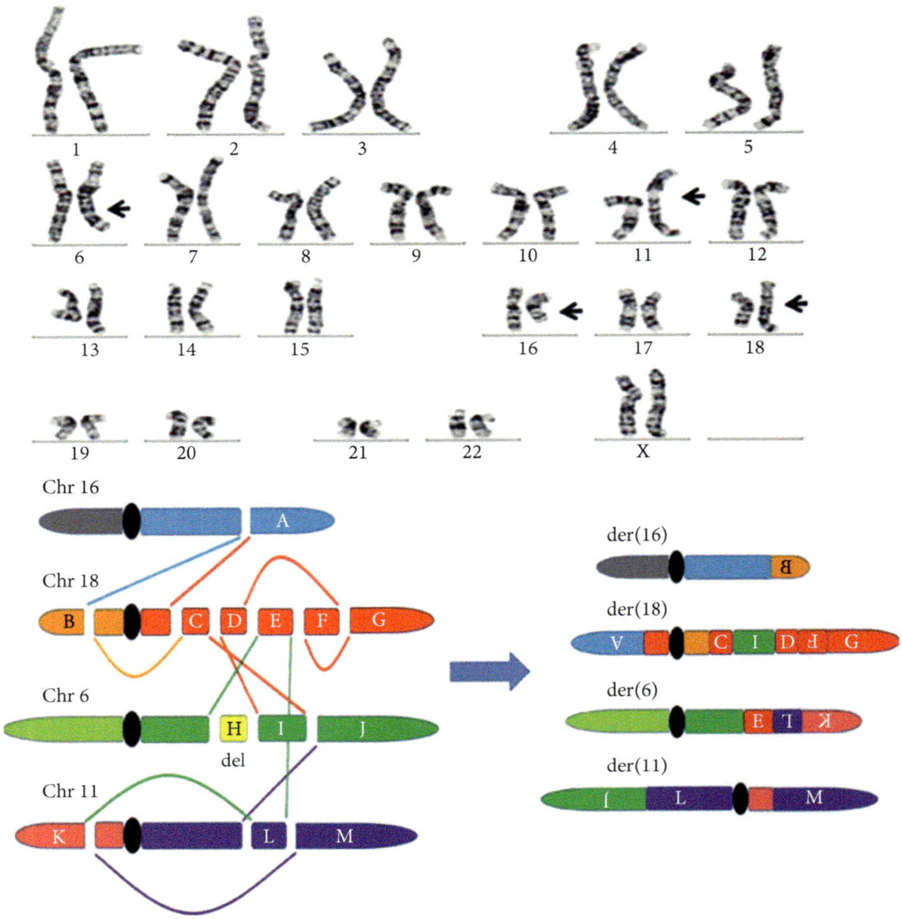

Figure 10–9. Extraordinary Complexity Revealed on Molecular Analysis.

Notes: The classic banded karyotype (above) cannot reveal the full detail of the CCR. Using FISH and WGS, the true nature of the CCR could be determined, and depicted diagrammatically (below). The rearrangement was de novo. The subject had had four miscarriages, and no successful pregnancies. This is an example of chromoanagenesis (p. 320).

Source: From P He et al., Analysis of complex chromosomal rearrangements using a combination of current molecular cytogenetic techniques, *Mol Cytogenet* 15:20, 2022. Courtesy K Lu, and with the permission of Springer Nature.

Wang et al. (2015) undertook testicular biopsy in a man presenting with azoöspermia, with a 46,XY,t(5;7;9;13) karyotype. Germ cells were reduced in number, some undergoing apoptosis; but no sperm or spermatids were present. Meiosis had proceeded part way, and octavalents were identifiable in all pachytene cells, albeit that several of the homologous segments had failed to synapse. A similar story is described in Coco et al. (2004) (Figure 10–11). Attempting fertility treatment with intracytoplasmic sperm injection (ICSI)—provided, of course, that sperm are being produced—is controversial (Joly-Helas et al. 2007; Nguyen et al. 2015). Where conception may have taken place, infertility due to multiple miscarriage is a frequent observation; the basis of this may largely be due to the production of only unbalanced conceptions, from either parental sex (Figure 10–12).

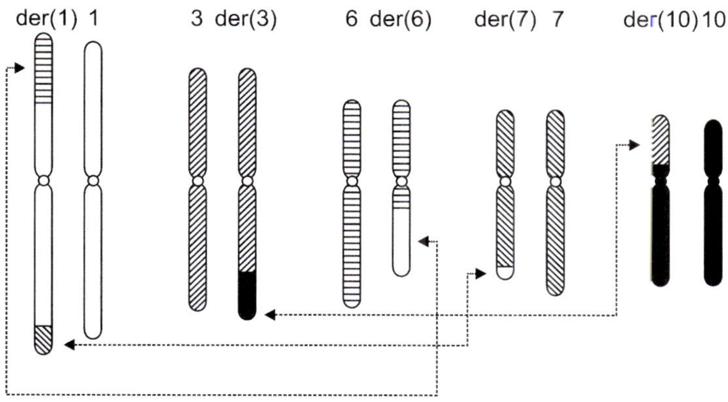

Figure 10–10. A Type IV CCR, with Three Two-Way Exchanges.

Note: There are six breakpoints in five chromosomes.

Source: From HN Bass et al., A family with three independent autosomal translocations associated with 7q32----7qter syndrome, *J Med Genet* 22:59–63, 1985.

GENETIC COUNSELING

For the heterozygote (male or female) who is fertile, or for whom fertility can be achieved, a conceptus having either a normal chromosome constitution or the same balanced CCR as the parent would be expected, other things being equal, to produce a normal child. But a very high proportion of conceptions have an unbalanced karyotype, as PGT has been revealing. The male CCR heterozygote who is not otherwise known to be fertile should have a semen analysis to check whether sperm are being produced. If there is oligospermia, IVF will have to be considered, and PGT would be appropriate.

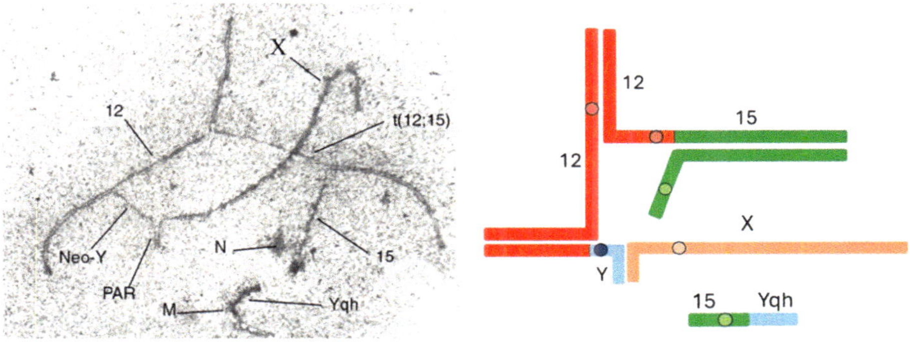

Figure 10–11. Meiotic Arrest in an Infertile Heterozygote.

Notes: This image is from an electron-micrograph of testicular tissue from a man presenting with azoöspermia, and heterozygous for the Type IV CCR t(Y;12;15)t(Y;12)(q11.23;q21.2);t(inv(12);15(p11.2q21.2;q13);t(15;Y)(q13;q11.23). The translocation chromosomes have formed as a pentavalent, and as a small marker. The cartoon karyotype indicates the disposition of the chromosomes, according to this construction. This abnormal configuration was presumed to be the basis of the spermatogenic arrest. Neo Y = euchromatic Y material; PAR = pseudoautosomal region; N = nucleolar mass; M = marker chromosome (the 15;Y element). See also Figure 10–6.

Source: From R Coco et al., A constitutional complex chromosome rearrangement involving meiotic arrest in an azoospermic male: case report, *Hum Reprod* 19:2784–2790, 2004, with the permission of the European Society of Human Reproduction and Embryology.

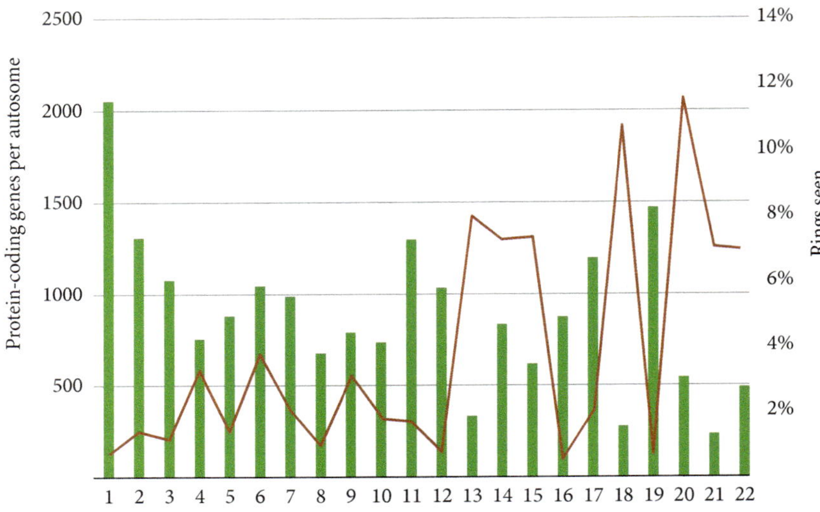

Figure 11–3. The gene-density of chromosomes (green), plotted against the relative frequencies in % of observation (brown) of rings for that chromosome.

Note: Overall, the more gene-dense a chromosome is, the less likely it is that a ring of that chromosome is observed; and vice versa.

Source: From P Li et al., The past, present, and future for constitutional ring chromosomes: A report of the international consortium for human ring chromosomes, *HGG Adv* 3:100139, 2022. Courtesy P Li and T Liehr, and with the permission of Elsevier.

with 1:1 segregation of the ring and the normal homolog (Figure 11–5). Thus, half of the conceptuses would be entirely normal karyotypically, and half would carry the ring. If "dynamic mosaicism" then occurs, these latter may be lethal in utero, or those surviving to term might have phenotypic abnormality. In fact, at least from the male heterozygote in whom some spermatogenic capacity is retained, there may be an intragonadal selection against ring forms, such that production of normal sperm is favored (Nishikawa et al. 2018). Otherwise, in the case of the heterozygote who has mosaicism with a normal cell line on somatic testing, as is occasionally recognized, the fraction of 46(r) conceptuses would in theory be less, according to the fraction of the gonad-containing ring cells.

We list commentaries on the individual ring chromosomes below. In a few, there has been an association with phenotypic normality or near-normality and parenthood, and it is to this category that we pay greater attention. The reader seeking wider and more up-to-date data is directed to the registry websites listed in Li et al. (2022c). Kushwaha et al. (2024) provide a review of considerable number of cases, followed up over some several decades, seen at a single laboratory.

Ring 1, 46,r(1). A ring for the largest chromosome is almost unknown (Gardner et al. 1984; Cutenese et al. 2000).

Ring 2, 46,r(2). Prenatal and post-natal growth retardation and microcephaly are consistent features (Sarri et al. 2015). Lacassie et al. (1999) summarize eight published cases and provide a photographic record of their own patient from birth to age 10 years, a microcephalic child with some mild cognitive and behavioral compromise, and profoundly growth retarded. The format as shown in Figure 11–2a was proven in the case in Severino et al. (2015), whose severely affected patient had, on microarray, a loss at distal 2p of only chr2:1-0.469 Mb, as well as a substantial 2qter deletion comprising chr2:238.7

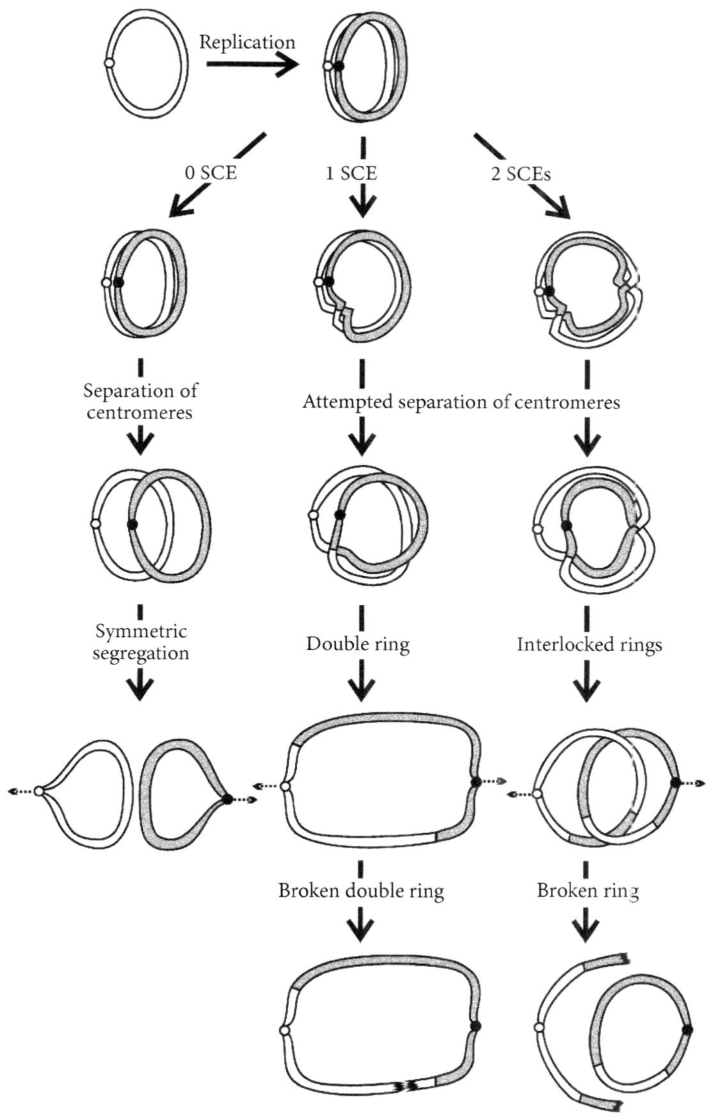

Figure 11–4. Dynamic Mosaicism.

The single-chromatid ring chromosome replicates during interphase. Sister chromatid exchanges (SCEs) may, or may not, take place. At meiosis, if there are no SCEs (*left*), segregation is symmetric (dotted arrows represent spindles drawing homologs to opposite poles). If there is one SCE, a double-sized ring is generated (*middle*). With each centromere being tugged to opposite poles at anaphase (dotted arrows), the chromosome may break. If there are two SCEs, in the same "direction of rotation" (*right*), the two rings become interlocked. Breakage, or other mechanical compromise, is the consequence. A second SCE in the opposite direction of rotation would restore the situation.

Mb-qter. Prenatal diagnosis is recorded (Chen et al. 2012). A single case of parent-to-child transmission is known (Giardino et al. 2002).

Ring 3, 46,r(3). The mechanism of deletion of one arm and fusion with the intact other arm is exemplified in the case in Guilherme et al. (2011), in which there was a 5.7 Mb loss at distal 3p (3p26). The 10-year-old boy was growth retarded, had a mildly

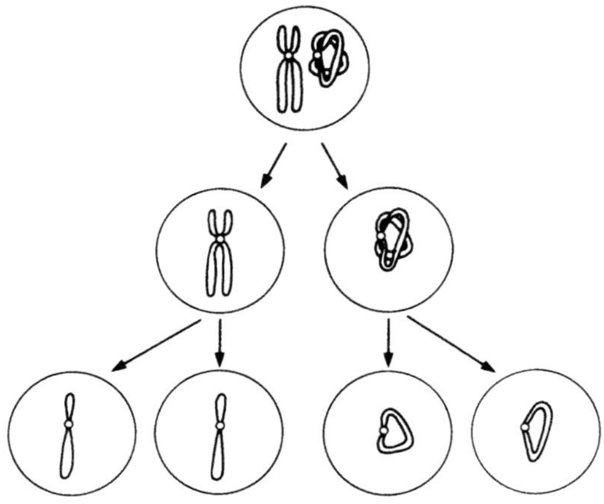

Figure 11–5. Meiosis in the Ring Carrier.
Meiosis with symmetric segregation in the ring heterozygote.

dysmorphic facies, and had a degree of intellectual disability. Barely double figures of this ring are recorded in the review of Zhang et al. (2016b); these authors describe their own r(3) case with a 10 Mb deletion at 3p.

Ring 4, 46,r(4). Sigurdardottir et al. (1999) describe a growth-retarded infant with normal developmental progress and whorled skin areas of hyperpigmentation and hypopigmentation. The r(4) was a true telomere-to-telomere fusion (Figure 11–2b), as demonstrated with FISH. A similar story is told in Burgemeister et al. (2017), who conclude that the concept of the "general ring syndrome" is supported by such cases in which no genetic material is lost. We have seen a man with 46,XY,r(4) manifesting the presumed general ring syndrome: He was considerably shorter than his brothers, and his occupation of warehouse manager compared with the professional qualifications of his siblings. Nevertheless, he could fully appreciate the genetic implications of his condition, and he and his wife chose to have donor insemination. Irregular synapsis of the ring and the normal homolog at meiosis may be the basis of infertility (Figure 11–6). A single case is on record of presumed maternal gonadal mosaicism for a ring 4, a mother having had two children with this ring, with the same p and q arm deleted segments in each (Phillips et al. 2021b).

If the ring formed following terminal deletions, the individual might or might not present a Wolf-Hirschhorn syndrome phenotype, according to the extent of the deletion into 4p (Yao et al. 2014).

Ring 5, 46,r(5). Familial transmission of a r(5) is rare, but recorded in a case of mild phenotype reflecting the general ring syndrome (MacDermot et al. 1990). A ring 5 with a substantial 5p deletion may lead to cri du chat syndrome (Nozawa et al. 2020).

Ring 6, 46,r(6). Urban et al. (2002) and Liu et al. (2018) reviewed 33 published cases. Hydrocephalus was a common observation. At one end of the spectrum, malformations and microcephaly with severe disability are typical (Zhang et al. 2016c). At the other end of the spectrum, a much milder phenotype of growth retardation evokes the general ring syndrome. An example is provided by the case of a young woman with mild dysmorphism and short stature, but normal psychomotor development and intact fertility (her son had a normal karyotype), reported in Höckner et al. (2008). A single case of parental transmission of a r(6) is described in Dong et al. (2022). A small-for-dates child with r(6)

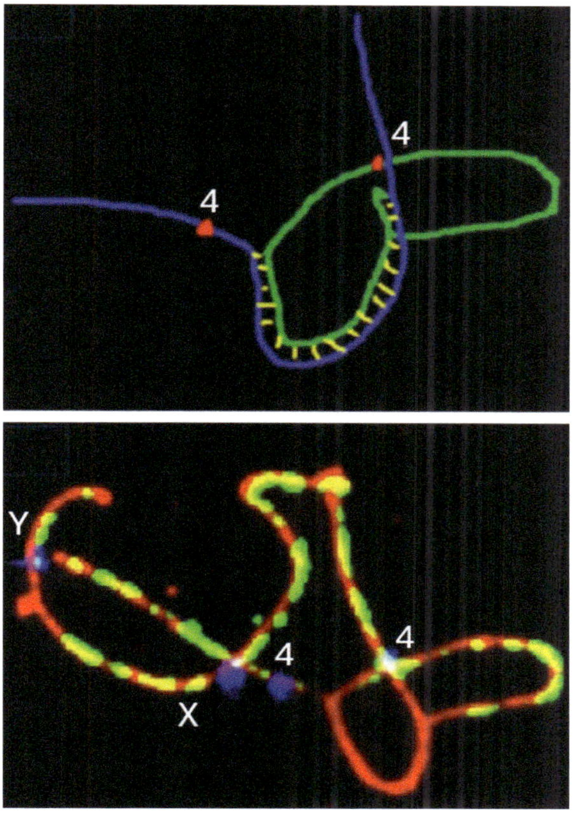

Figure 11–6. Incomplete Synapsis in Meiosis of the Ring 4 and its Homolog.

Notes: This study was made on testicular tissue from a man having presented with severe oligospermia, he showing the mosaic karyotype 46,XY,r(4)(::p16.3→q35.2::)[31]/45,XY,-4[3]. Staining (*below*) with red (SPC3) reveals synaptonemal activity; with green (BRCA1) identifies regions of transcriptional inactivation; and with blue identifies centromeres. The X-Y bivalent is closely associated with the no. 4 bivalent. Diagram (*above*) shows the ring in green, the normal homolog in blue, and the region of synapsing in yellow.

Source: From Q Yao et al., Meiotic prophase I defects in an oligospermic man with Wolf-Hirschhorn syndrome with ring chromosome 4, *Mol Cytogenet* 7:45, 2014. Courtesy Y-X Cui, and with the permission of Springer Nature.

was born to a mother of normal intellect and short stature, she having the mosaic karyotype 46,XX,r(6)[44]/47,XX,r(6),+r(6)[2]/46,XX[15].

Ring 7, 46,r(7). Microcephaly with intellectual disability is a typical presentation. Cleft lip and palate is a common feature (Bangun et al. 2024); Roy et al. (2012) document an association with skin nevi.

Ring 8, 46,r(8). Variable cognitive capacity, including normality, was observed in the family described in Le Caignec et al. (2004), in which the ring 8 chromosome, transmitted from mother to son and likely also carried by grandmother and uncle, was determined to have no loss of euchromatin. No other familial case is on record. A man having a ring 8 with megabase-size deletions at 8pter and 8qter, and whose cognitive impairment was less marked than in most r(8) cases, proved to be mosaic, with a upd(8) pat 46,XY cell line (Gradek et al. 2006). The probable sequence was as follows: 46,r(8) at conception; mitotic loss of the ring to give a 45,−8 cell; and subsequent "rescue" of

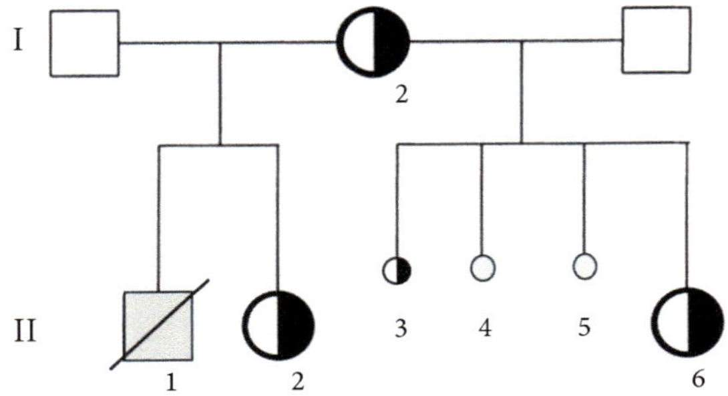

Figure 11–10. Familial Transmission of a Ring 18 Chromosome.

Notes: Half-filled symbols = proven r(18) heterozygosity with mosaicism for monosomy 18; grey symbols = suspected r(18). The mother I:2 was described as manifesting short stature, cleft palate, and mild cognitive impairment, and of karyotype 46,XX,r(18)(p11.3q23)[32]/45,XX,−18[4]. Her child II:1 died at age 2 days. The tested cases II:2, 3, and 6 all showed the r(18) along with monosomy 18 in mosaic state, as in the mother. II:3 was a terminated pregnancy; II:4 and 5 were untested miscarriages.

Source: Redrawn from C Yardin et al., First familial case of ring chromosome 18 and monosomy 18 mosaicism, *Am J Med Genet* 104A:257-259, 2001. Courtesy C Yardin, and with the permission of John Wiley and Sons.

diagnosis from a normal mother with the same very low fraction (4%) of cells with r(19), the ring assessed as being an end-to-end fusion (Figure 11–2 *b* or *c*).

Ring 20, 46,r(20). Two main forms exist: (1) a mosaic karyotype of mitotic origin, with end-to-end fusion of one chromosome 20; and (2) a non-mosaic type, the ring having deletions of p arm or q arm, or of both arms, and having arisen at meiosis (Conlin et al. 2011; Daber et al. 2012). The non-mosaic form presents the more severe picture.

Epilepsy is the notable clinical feature, with the onset of seizures typically at a younger age in the non-mosaic form (Peron et al. 2020; Paprocka et al. 2024). There may be an earlier period of normal mental development, which slows following the onset of epilepsy. In childhood onset, a clinical pointer may be an association with terrifying hallucinations as part of the seizure. The age of onset of epilepsy correlates with the degree of mosaicism: the higher the fraction of r(20) cells, the earlier the onset (Figure 11–11). The electroencephalogram (EEG) has a characteristic pattern, with trains of "theta waves." Any patient with treatment-resistant epilepsy who has long runs of epileptiform activity on the EEG in the non-seizing state (which may or may not be associated with confusion or diminished consciousness) should be tested with this ring chromosome

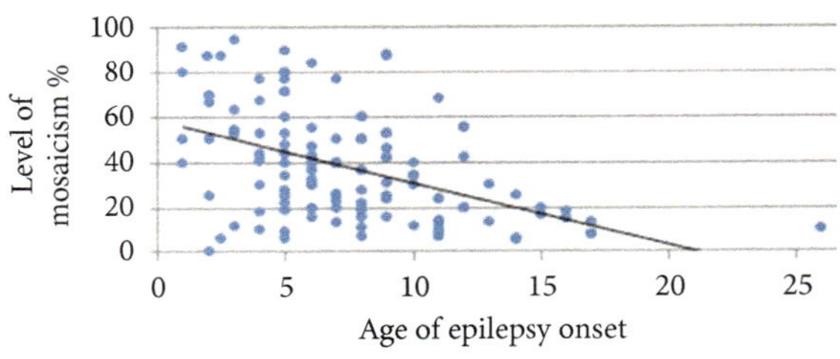

Figure 11–11. The Age of Onset of Epilepsy in Ring 20 Mosaicism.

Notes: The age of onset is shown correlating with the fraction of cells that are r(20).

Source: From A Peron et al., Ring chromosome 20 syndrome: Genetics, clinical characteristics, and overlapping phenotypes, *Front Neurol* 11:613035, 2020. Courtesy A Peron, and with the permission of Frontiers in Neurology.

in mind; James et al. (2024) emphasize the need for a classical cytogenetic study, since molecular methodologies will often not discover a ring. The mechanism whereby the genomic alteration due to the ring causes the susceptibility to epilepsy is yet to be clarified (Myers et al. 2021a).

Familial transmission is recorded (Unterberger et al. 2019). An otherwise unaffected parent with a lower level of mosaicism can have affected children with the ring chromosome in higher proportion (Canevini et al. 1998). Thus, Herrgård et al. (2007) document a mother with 10% r(20) mosaicism, who had an onset of seizures in her mid-20s and who was intellectually normal. Her daughter had epilepsy from age 7 years, and cognitive capacity fell away in subsequent years; her son was always behind in development, showed poor behavior, and had seizures from age 5 years. These children both had 40% of their cells with the r(20).

Ring 21, 46,r(21). The cognitive phenotypes can vary from normal to severe, and the degree of mosaicism for monosomy 21, a frequent concomitant, is likely a major factor in this respect (Ambulkar et al. 2023). A child we followed up into adulthood achieved tertiary education and was a skilled musician; but he was, as can often be the case with the male r(21) heterozygote, infertile, with azoöspermia (Dallapiccola et al. 1986; Gardner et al. 1986b). A sperm study on a ring 21 infertile man with an extremely low sperm count, karyotyping 45,XY,–21[3]/46,XY,r(21)[95]/46,XY[2] on blood and with fairly similar proportions on buccal cells, came up with an interesting result: FISH showed most (92%) of 169 spermatozoa to be normal, 7% with the ring, and 1% disomic with the normal 21 and the ring 21. These authors suggested that the (presumed) small fraction in the gonad of normal spermatogonia were selectively favored at meiosis, leading to the majority of gametes being normal (Hammoud et al. 2009).

Parent-child transmission, and indeed grandparent-parent-child transmission, is well known (Bertini et al. 2008b). Bertini and colleagues describe a mother-daughter, each having the same karyotype on blood, 46,XX,r(21)/45,XX,–21, the ring being the majority species in each (98% and 94%, respectively). In this instance the rearrangement was due to a subtelomeric 21q deletion of 3.4 Mb, and apparently no critical dosage-sensitive genes had been lost. A transmitting father in Papoulidis et al. (2010) had just one cell out of 100 with the ring (discovered after the birth of his child), presumably reflecting a somatic-gonadal mosaicism; the ring 21 child was normal on assessment at 10 months. Counseling in the event of a prenatal diagnosis of non-mosaic r(21), the parent being mosaic for the ring, is challenging (Mazzaschi et al. 2011).

Three-generation kindreds are described in Falik-Borenstein et al. (1992) and Melnyk et al. (1995). In one family, a 46,XX,r(21) heterozygote had had seven pregnancies with four early miscarriages, one normal son, one son with Down syndrome, and one 46,XX,r(21) daughter, the latter herself having a 46,XX,r(21) daughter (Figure 11–12). Most karyotyped cells in these individuals were 46,r(21), but a few were 45,–21, and some had a double-size or multi-size rings. Short stature, but normal IQ/development, accompanied the abnormal karyotype in these females; one male heterozygote may have had a low-normal intelligence. In another family, a 46,XX,r(21) mother had a prenatal diagnosis that showed one 46,XY twin and the other with 46,XX,r(21)/45,XX,–21 mosaicism. Both babies were normal, and the girl's post-natal karyotype was non-mosaic 46,XX,r(21).

The ring 21 might of itself predispose to the generation of a trisomy 21 karyotype, either 47,+r(21) or a recombinant 21 (Kosztolányi et al. 1991; and Figure 11–12). In their review of this circumstance, Muroya et al. (2002) illustrate a reverse picture: a normal

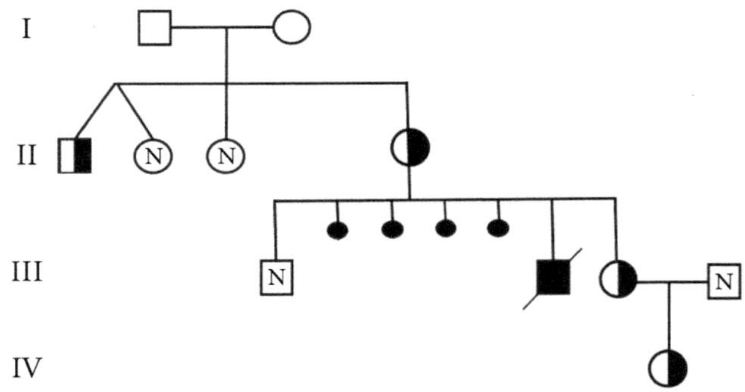

Figure 11–12. Pedigree of a Kindred within which is Segregating a Ring 21 Chromosome.
Note: Half-filled symbol = heterozygote for r(21); N = normal chromosomes; Filled symbol = Down syndrome. Small symbols in generation III refer to miscarriages. The ancestral couple at generation I had not been karyotyped, but presumably one or the other was an obligate heterozygote (or at the very least, a gonadal mosaic).
Source: From TC Falik-Borenstein et al., Stable ring chromosome 21: molecular and clinical definition of the lesion, *Am J Med Genet* 42:22–28, 1992. Courtesy JR Korenberg, and with the permission of John Wiley and Sons.

mother with a rather complex der(21) who had a mildly intellectually disabled son with 46,XY,r(21) and 4/100 cells 45,XY,–21.

Ring 22, 46,r(22). A handful of inherited cases are on record (Teyssier and Moreau 1985; Crusi and Engel 1986; Wenger et al. 2000). In some, the ring was inherited from a phenotypically normal parent to phenotypically normal offspring, and presumably in these no crucial genetic material had been deleted. Male infertility may be a concomitant (Zuccarello et al. 2010; Sha et al. 2012). In other cases, one or more of the family members with the ring have had mental compromise or other clinical features. A parent may be mosaic and the child has inherited the ring in a non-mosaic state, which may substantially explain observed parent-offspring differences in phenotype. In one notable case, the mother's tip-to-tip r(22) underwent change in transmission to her affected child, in whom part of the 22q segment had been deleted (Jobanputra et al. 2009). The r(22) mother in Wenger et al. (2000) had required special education in high school. Her son had bowel and heart defects, with very little language development by age 20 months. (By a strange coincidence he had, on his other chromosome 22, a de novo del 22q11.2.)

Phelan-McDermid Syndrome. Some ring 22s have a more proximal q arm breakpoint and are deleted for the 22q13.33 region, which is the basis of the Phelan-McDermid syndrome (Chapter 14); haploinsufficiency for the *SHANK3* gene is the key pathogenetic factor. The severity of the phenotype is proportional to the length of the deleted segment. The ring formation can be complicated, and Khalifa et al. (2022) describe a child in whom a r(22) carried a concomitant 4.4 Mb deletion at 22q13.31q13.33 and a 3 Mb duplication at 22q13.2q13.31. While a number of loci were present in deleted or duplicated state, the authors concluded that the loss of one *SHANK3* allele in the deleted segment was likely the major contributor to the phenotype, but that imbalance of the other loci would also have had an influence. Koza et al. (2023) propose a recurrence risk for r(22)-associated Phelan-McDermid syndrome of <2% if parental karyotypes are normal, but an increased risk if there is parental mosaicism for the ring, and a 50% risk if a parent is non-mosaic.

A ring 22 may, of itself, function as a "first hit" in the generation of certain tumors. The gene for neurofibromatosis type 2 (NF2) is located at 22q12. The neural crest is the embryonic tissue that gives rise to the investing membranes of nervous system structures. Due to its mitotic instability, a cell line in this tissue might lose the ring and thus become monosomic for 22. Subsequently, a mutation occurring in the *NF2* gene on the remaining intact homolog would be "exposed" and allow the development of a classic NF2 tumor, a schwannoma of the eighth cranial nerve, or a meningioma of the cranial or spinal meninges (Koza et al. 2023). NF2 may be present in as many as 16% of r(22) individuals (Ziats et al. 2020). A similar scenario has been shown with respect to the *SMARCB1* gene, in a child (who also had Phelan-McDermid syndrome) presenting with an atypical teratoid rhabdoid tumor of the brain (Byers et al. 2017).

THE SUPERNUMERARY SMALL RING, 47,+(R)

The small, or very small ring as a 47th chromosome could as well be dealt with under the category "small supernumerary marker chromosome" (sSMC), but we nevertheless record them here, acknowledging their particular ring identity. These rings may have formed as in the 46,(r) story above, with (large) distal deletions and end-to-end fusion; or, the "Barbara McClintock mechanism" involving breaks at the centromere and in one arm, with material from only that arm then represented in the ring (Quinonez et al. 2017a). A supernumerary chromosome implies, naturally, a partial trisomy (but see "Supernumerary Ring with a Balancing Deletion" below). Generally, it is only when the ring chromosome is very small, or when there is mosaicism with a substantial fraction of normal cells—in other words, where the overall load of genetic imbalance is small—that a question of genetic risk for offspring of the heterozygote will be relevant. Post-natally ascertained cases have naturally presented with an abnormal phenotype, and some have been ascertained through (especially male) infertility (Slimani et al. 2020); but a fraction of cases come to attention fortuitously, some being phenotypically normal. The challenge raised at prenatal diagnosis of a small supernumerary ring chromosome is discussed in Joksic et al. (2024).

Mosaicism complicates the interpretation. These very small rings are mitotically unstable, and this is presumably the basis of the frequently observed mosaicism (Spittel et al. 2014). A few cases are known in which a parent with low-level mosaicism has had an abnormal child with a higher proportion of the cells with the ring. The levels of mosaicism as determined from a peripheral blood sample may not necessarily reflect the levels in other tissues, and including brain; and in a number of rings, little correlation is recognized between the degree of mosaicism and the severity of phenotype.

Small supernumerary rings have been reported for almost every autosome. Brief sketches of some of these follow, with particular reference to recorded cases in which a parent with the ring has had offspring. For several of the chromosomes, the genetic content of the rings may vary quite considerably, and thus it is not surprising that often no clearly consistent phenotype is observed between cases due to the same chromosome (and the factor of variable mosaicism, as just mentioned above, also influences the picture).

Ring 1, 47,+r(1). Callen et al. (1999) and Bernardini et al. (2007) presented series of patients with very small supernumerary r(1) chromosomes ranging in phenotype from normal/infertility to abnormal, and showed that the size of the ring was correlated

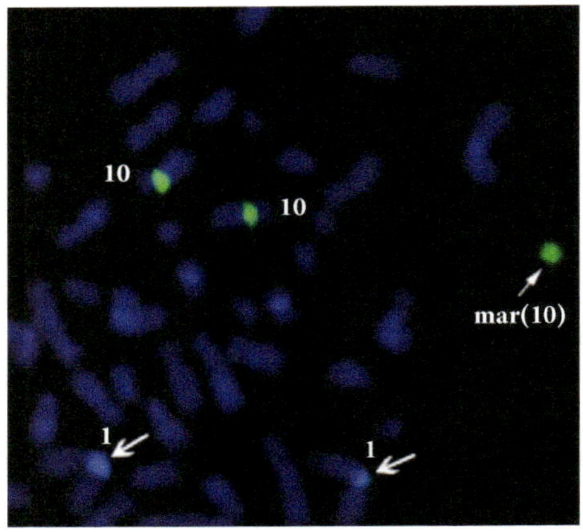

Figure 11–14. A Supernumerary Ring 10 Chromosome.

Notes: This small supernumerary ring 10 chromosome, initially called a marker, was seen following cordocentesis, the indication for the prenatal procedure being fetal nasal bone hypoplasia. Staining with whole chromosome painting confirmed the ring's identity (less intense staining of the centromeric region of chromosome 1qh is also observed). Mosaicism was shown: 47,XX,+r(8)[18]/46,XX[5]. A healthy girl was born at term, and developing normally at age 1 year.

Source: From IN Lebedev et al., Prenatal diagnosis of small supernumerary marker chromosome 10 by array-based comparative genomic hybridization and microdissected chromosome sequencing, *Biomedicines* 9:1030, 2021. Courtesy IN Lebedev, and with the permission of MDPI.

child was apparently normal on assessment at age one year. The identity of the ring in the similar mosaic case of Lebedev et al. (2021) as having been derived from chromosome 10 is shown in Figure 11–14.

Ring 11, 47,+ r(11). The case in Wang et al. (2023b) exemplifies the scenario of a supernumerary ring which is balanced by a concomitant deletion (See "Supernumerary Ring with a Balancing Deletion" below). Otherwise, supernumerary rings of chromosome 11 are almost unknown.

Ring 12, 47,+r(12). No clear clinical phenotype has emerged, other than abnormality in all (Davidsson et al. 2008). Yeung et al. (2009) and Lloveras et al. (2013) document cases in which the supernumerary ring 12 included two copies of 12p, thus determining a Pallister-Killian phenotype (Chapter 14).

Ring 13, 47,+ r(13). Surprisingly, for a "survivable" chromosome, supernumerary ring 13 is scarcely ever reported (Zeng et al. 2019). In the normal mother reported in Sun et al. (2023), whose case came to light following an ambiguous result at NIPT, the supernumerary r(13) was of substantial size, but balanced by a deletion of the same segment in one of the other no. 13 chromosomes.

Ring 14, 47,+r(14). Infertility was the only presenting complaint in a man with a minute ring 14 reported in Stahl et al. (2007). The detailed formation of a r(14) was determined in the case of Castermans et al. (2008), showing the inverted "mirror" nature of the duplicated 14p13 to 14q12 segment.

Ring 15, 47,+r(15). A very small ring 15 may be comparable, in terms of its genetic content, to the relatively common small bisatellited supernumerary chromosome (sSMC) 15 (Chapter 14) (Zou et al. 2006). An exceptional case in Adhvaryu et al. (1998) is that of a sSMC derived from chromosome 15 in grandparent (mosaic) and parent (non-mosaic), evolving into a very small ring 15 in the grandchild. All three, and two other siblings with the sSMC, were normal.

Ring 16, 47,+r(16). In the only reported case (from a prenatal diagnosis), Cignini et al. (2011) note major fetal abnormalities in association with non-mosaic 47,XY,+r(16).

Ring 17, 47,+r(17). A mildly disabled boy with a supernumerary ring 17 is described in Dupont et al. (2003).

Ring 18, 47,+r(18). Jenderny et al. (1993) describe a phenotypically normal mother with 47,XX,+r(18) in only 2/100 cells on blood analysis, the remainder being 46,XX, and who had had a daughter with non-mosaic 47,+r(18). Balci et al. (2014) record another normal mother with ring 18 mosaicism, in her case 47,XX,+r(18)(::p11→q21::)[10]/46,XX[90], who had a disabled son with 46,XY,r(18)[75]/46,XY[25] mosaicism; these authors showed more underlying complexity in the structure and formation of the rings than at first appreciated, in undertaking a SNP-array family study. A man with a VACTERL[4]-like clinical picture, and with a normal intellect, carried at low-level mosaicism a r(18) that endowed "octasomy" for an ~5 Mb segment of pericentromeric chromosome 18 (van der Veken et al. 2010).

Ring 19, 47,+r(19). A few cases are on record, with phenotypes from mild (possibly reflecting mosaicism) through severe (Vaz et al. 1999). A familial case involving twins more likely represents a single affected conception than occult parental transmission (Shahwan et al. 2004). A normal mother with r(19) mosaicism came to attention only because she had had a child with defects probably due to a different, coincidental chromosomal imbalance (Argiropoulos et al. 2011).

Ring 20, 47,+r(20). Guediche et al. (2010) provide a review of 13 cases, eight ascertained post-natally and five prenatally, with psychomotor and growth retardation as frequent but not universal observations. Kitsiou-Tzeli et al. (2009) document prenatal diagnosis following which the child, at age three months, was judged to be essentially normal; in contrast, Callier et al. (2009) describe dysmorphic features in an aborted fetus. The only example of parental transmission is in Pinto et al. (2005). A mother with borderline intelligence and a degree of body asymmetry had a child with dysmorphism and developmental delay. She karyotyped as 47,XX,+r(20)[8]/46,XX[42]; he was 47,XY,+r(20)[25]/46,XY[37].

Ring 21, 47,+r(21). A ring may result from a more complicated process than end-to-end fusions, as Villa et al. (2011) analyze in a child with minor dysmorphism and delay in language development: an initial trisomy 21 at conception gave rise to a large ring, which subsequently "deleted out" a segment, leaving a small ring comprising two non-contiguous regions.

Ring 22, 47,+r(22). Mears et al. (1995) document a family in which a phenotypically normal grandfather and father were mosaic for a tiny ring 22 chromosome, 47,XY,+r(22)/48,XY,+r(22),+r(22). A grandchild, also 47,+r(22)/48,+r(22),+r(22) but whose ring chromosomes had increased in size, had cat eye syndrome (CES) (Chapter 14). These phenotypic differences likely reflect the dosage effect of a CES critical region, with the child having more tissue with a larger ring and/or with two copies of the r(22) of wider body distribution (Figure 11–15).

[4] Vertebral, anal, cardiac, trachea-esophageal, renal, limb association.

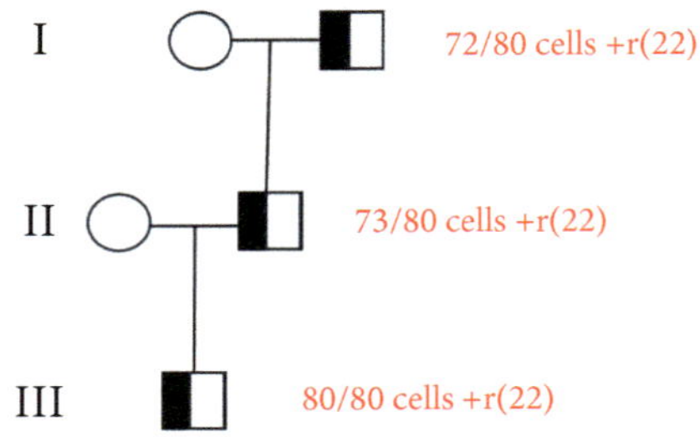

Figure 11–15. Pedigree of a Family in which a Supernumerary Ring 22 Chromosome is Segregating.

Notes: The grandfather and father in generations I and II are phenotypically normal; the child in generation III has cat eye syndrome. Although there are similar fractions, as shown here, on blood karyotyping, of cells with the + r(22), the affected child had more cells with a larger ring, or with two copies of the ring.

Source: From AJ Mears et al., Minute supernumerary ring chromosome 22 associated with cat eye syndrome: further delineation of the critical region, *Am J Hum Genet* 57:667–673, 1995.

RARE COMPLEXITIES

Supernumerary Ring with a Balancing Deletion. If a ring chromosome is derived from a segment of chromosome that has been deleted interstitially from an autosome, and if this newly generated ring contains the centromere (or a neocentromere; see below), it can, in some cases, be transmitted stably at mitosis. If so, the karyotype is balanced (Slimani et al. 2020; Sun et al. 2023), but the carrier can be at high risk to produce unbalanced gametes: the ring might be transmitted as a supernumerary chromosome, to give a partial trisomy; or the deleted chromosome is transmitted, for a partial monosomy. Further, mosaicism might supervene. Mantzouratou et al. (2009) studied embryos from a couple, the wife being 47,XX,del(22),+r(22) and herself normal. They had had two natural pregnancies, both mosaic 47,+r(22)/46, with the first producing an abnormal child and the second terminated after prenatal diagnosis. Following two PGT cycles, none of the embryos had received the normal, intact maternal chromosome 22, and thus none were transferred. Better fortune attended the intellectually normal mother in Wang et al. (2023b) with an ocular anomaly, who was mosaic for a del(11) balanced by a supernumerary r(11): mos 47,XX,del(11)(p14.3p11.2),+r(11)(::p14.3→neo→11.12::)[16]/46,XX,del(11)(p.14.3p11.2)[4]. In her first pregnancy, an abnormal fetus had the del(11) in non-mosaic form. A second pregnancy, enabled through PGT, had the del(11) + r(11) balanced karyotype, and a child born was normal.

If a gene is disrupted in the process of ring formation, the phenotype may be impacted upon, such as Quinonez et al. (2017a) propose in an infertile man with Marfan syndrome, who had an apparently balancing supernumerary ring 15 (the fibrillin-1 gene being located at 15q21).

If the ring is very small, the balancing deletion may be missed on classical cytogenetics, as Baldwin et al. (2008) describe in a mother whose karyotype at first sight was 47,XX,+r(4)/46,XX; but the small r(4) was in fact derived from a deleted segment of 4p on one of her chromosome 4 homologs. She was described as intellectually normal but with unilateral ear anomalies and minor visual deficiencies; this mild phenotype may have reflected a partial 4p monosomy in body tissue with the "46,XX" (but actually del 4p12-cen, chr4:45-50 Mb) karyotype. Her child, who inherited the small ring but not the balancing deleted 4, and thus with dup chr4:45-50 Mb, had a "mild speech delay."

Formation of a Neocentromere. A fragment of a chromosome not containing a centromere would not normally be able to be transmitted during cell division. But if a "neocentromere" is generated on this fragment, its survival may be enabled as a "supernumerary marker chromosome." The supernumerary r(13) seen in the abnormal child in Amor et al. (2005), a chromosome of quite substantial size was studied in detail, and while α-satellite-specific centromere protein CENP-B was absent, the critical histone H3-associated centromere protein CENP-A was present, allowing centromeric function. If the supernumerary ring balances a deletion, the physical phenotype may be normal as noted above, and such as Slater et al. (1999) show in an infertile but otherwise normal man. A segment was deleted from one chromosome 1, and this same segment (1p32p36.1) existed as a tiny supernumerary ring chromosome. This man thus has the karyotype 47,XY,del(1)(p32p26.1)+r(1)(p32p36.1). The ring chromosome was able to activate the formation of certain centromere-binding proteins, which presumably enabled its stable transmission. A similar circumstance is recorded in Knegt et al. (2003), in this case a phenotypically normal woman who had presented with recurrent miscarriage and in whom a tiny ring 13 chromosome was derived from an interstitial deletion of the segment 13q21.31q22.2. Amniocenteses in her fourth and fifth pregnancies demonstrated normal karyotypes. The cases in Wang et al. (2023b) and Quinonez et al. (2017a) described above involved supernumerary rings with a neocentromere.

GENETIC COUNSELING

Parental Karyotype 46,(r), Non-mosaic or Mosaic

The great majority of transmitting parents are 46,XX,(r) mothers, reflecting that most male heterozygotes are infertile. Those offspring inheriting the ring could be expected to present a clinical picture at least similar to, and indeed quite probably more severe than their heterozygous parent. In the review of Kosztolányi et al. (1991), about one-third of familial 46,(r) children were more severely affected mentally than their parent. The 46,(r) parent may be an atypical ring carrier, perhaps having had a fortunate pattern of mitotic disruption, to have reached the level of social phenotype wherein procreation would be likely. The risk is such, certainly for the female carrier, that the attraction of prenatal diagnosis or preimplantation testing is readily apparent. In the case of a male carrier with some retained spermatogenic capacity, and resorting to IVF with ICSI, preliminary data suggests that normal sperm are favored.

In the person who is mosaic on somatic (blood) analysis, with a 46,N/46,(r) karyotype, the mosaicism might extend also into the gonad. This would convey an important risk to have a non-mosaic 46,(r) child—and, even if this might overstate the case, this risk would need to be assumed to exist. Quantifying the risk would be most imprecise: as high as 50%, as low as (almost) zero, but anywhere between.

In the particular case of the 46,r(21) heterozygote, who is often phenotypically normal, there is a small but as yet unquantified risk of having a child with Down syndrome due to an uncommon karyotype: 47,+r(21), 46,rob(21q;21q), or 46,tan dup(21q;21q) (Kosztolányi et al. 1991). If, in prenatal diagnosis for a pregnancy of a r(21) heterozygote parent, the same r(21) karyotype were demonstrated in the fetus, based on the slender evidence thus far available the chance for phenotypic normality would seem to be "substantial," but a (probably mild) degree of abnormality could by no means be excluded. As noted above (Hammoud et al. 2009), gametogenesis (if fertility is retained) in the mosaic 46,N/46,r(21) male may favor the production of chromosomally normal spermatogonia.

> Rings of chromosomes 11, 17, 21, and 22 may predispose to cancer, presumed, in some at least, due to sequential events in susceptible tissue of (1) loss of the ring to produce a cell line with monosomy, and (2) a gene mutation on the remaining homolog within that cell line. Loci known in this respect are *WT1* on chromosome 11 (Wilms tumor), *NF1* on chromosome 17 (neurofibromatosis type 1), chromosome 21 (leukemia), and *SMARCB1* and *NF2* on chromosome 22 (atypical teratoid rhabdoid tumor; neurofibromatosis type 2) (Carella et al. 2010; Zirn et al. 2012; Byers et al. 2017; De John et al. 2023). Tumor surveillance may be considered in persons carrying these rings.

Parental Karyotype 47,+(r)

Each ring needs to be assessed individually. Reference to the brief outlines above will give a sense of the range of outcomes. A non-mosaic parent with a very small ring might be expected to transmit the abnormal chromosome with up to 50% probability, assuming (and this may not necessarily be the case) meiotic and mitotic stability. The parental phenotype would, in principle, predict that of a potential 47,+r child, but could underestimate a likelihood of abnormality (recalling that the ascertainment of a parent of sufficient normality to be seeking genetic counseling is biased).

Mosaicism in the parent, and potential mosaicism in the child, considerably complicate prediction. A higher-grade mosaicism in the child than in the parent, or complete non-mosaicism in the child, would be expected to produce a more severe phenotype and quite possibly cause lethality in utero. Preimplantation testing or prenatal diagnosis is very appropriately offered. Jiang et al. (2024a) document a series of prenatal diagnoses, in most of which transmission of the ring would have been predicted to be pathogenic. Preimplantation testing has been successfully applied in a few cases of parental small supernumerary ring chromosome (Cheng et al. 2019), and the r(11) case in Wang et al. (2023b) is noted above.

Parental Karyotype 47,del(A),+r(A). In the ring with a balancing deletion, normality in an offspring can only be regarded as secure (other things being equal) in the context of the normal homolog (A) having been transmitted from the 47,del(A),+r(A) parent. Even though the carrier parent may be normal, the risk is high that the same balanced karyotype in a conceptus could be followed by post-zygotic misdivision, with the eventual generation of offspring who would be partially trisomic or partially monosomic for the autosome concerned, and thus abnormal. A detailed discussion is offered in Mantzouratou et al. (2009).

Actual PGT data is available only in the case of the r(22), and the findings were not promising (Mantzouratou et al. 2009). A carrier mother in whom a supernumerary r(22) was balanced by a del(22), of karyotype 47,XX,del(22)(p10q12),+r(22)(q10q12) had had one affected r(22) child, 47,XY,+r(22)(p11.2q11.2)/46,XY, and one termination. At IVF, 12 oöcytes were fertilized, but none were normal. Mantzouratou and colleagues propose that the abnormal chromosome compromised the very early mitoses of the embryo.

12
CENTROMERE FISSIONS, COMPLEMENTARY ISOCHROMOSOMES, TELOMERIC FUSIONS, BALANCING SUPERNUMERARY CHROMOSOMES, NEOCENTROMERES, JUMPING TRANSLOCATIONS, CHROMOANAGENESIS, AND MULTIPLE DE NOVO CNVs

THIS CHAPTER PROVIDES a setting for certain very rare abnormalities that cannot readily be accommodated elsewhere. Barely double-digit numbers, if that, are known for most of these. *Centromere fission* results when a metacentric or submetacentric chromosome splits at the centromere, giving rise to two stable telocentric products. In a sense, this is the reverse of what happens in whole-arm translocations. The heterozygote, a phenotypically normal individual, thus has 47 chromosomes. The *Robertsonian fission* reverses the fusion that had originally generated the Robertsonian translocation. *Telomeric fusion* leads to a 45-chromosome count, due to the joining up of two chromosomes tip-to-tip, not unlike the Robertsonian mechanism. The fusion chromosome has two centromeres, but one of these becomes inactivated. With the balanced *complementary isochromosome*, two stable exactly metacentric products are generated. A *balancing small supernumerary marker chromosome* contains material deleted from the normal homolog. A supernumerary chromosome lacking a normal centromere can become stable and functional due to the generation of a *neocentromere*. In *jumping translocations*, a segment can move from one chromosome to two or more recipient chromosomes. *Chromoanagenesis* takes complex rearrangement to a yet more complex level.

BIOLOGY

Centromere Fission

In simple terms, a nonacrocentric chromosome undergoes a horizontal splitting at the centromere (Figure 12–1a), although the true basis may be more complex than this (Rivera and Cantú 1986; Perry et al. 2004). Two new telocentric[1] chromosomes result (Figure 12–2). One comprises the short arm of the original, and the other its long arm. It

[1] The centromere is at the very end of the chromosome.

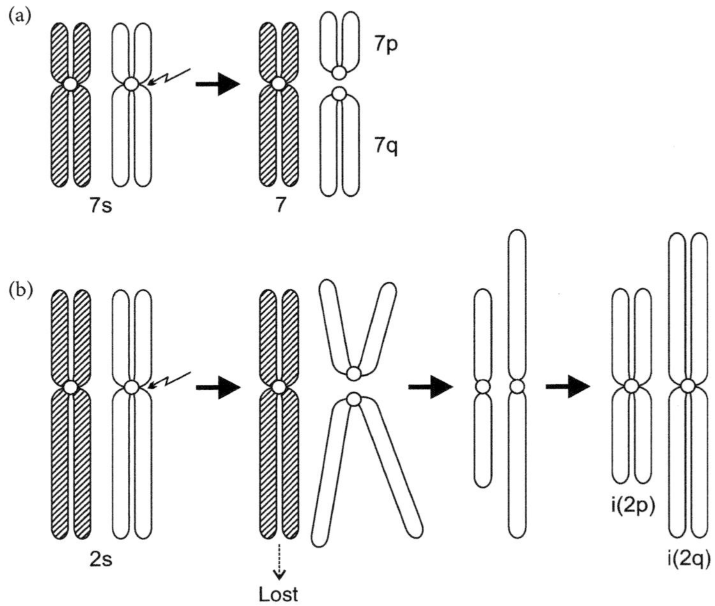

Figure 12–1. Comparing the processes of (*a*) centric fission of chromosome 7 and (*b*) complementary isochromosomes of chromosome 2. The chromosome pairs are to be imagined as existing in the zygote (*left*); they have replicated to give the double-chromatid state. The lightning arrow indicates misdivision of the centromere in one homolog. By the time the cell enters the first mitotic division (*right*), the abnormal states have been generated. Note that according to the proposed mechanisms in (*b*), uniparental disomy would necessarily result. Cross-hatching indicates original homolog from one parent; open indicates original homolog from the other.

is as though the cell ignores the fact that the split happened and continues on normally, treating each part as a properly functioning whole. The other normal homolog remains intact. The heterozygous person (47,cen fis) may have a balanced complement of genetic material and thus be phenotypically normal. Among the very few families on record, just seven chromosomes—4, 7, 9, 10, 11, 12, and 21—have been involved (Shim et al. 2007; Cetin et al. 2011). The karyotype may be written, for example, 47,XX,−4,+fis(4)(p10),+ fis(4)(q10).

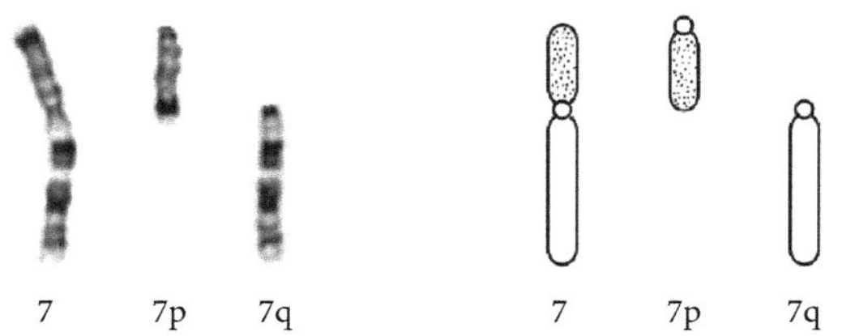

Figure 12–2. Partial karyotype from a case of 47,cen fis(7). One chromosome 7 exists as a normal homolog, and the other homolog is represented by the 7p and the 7q chromosomes.

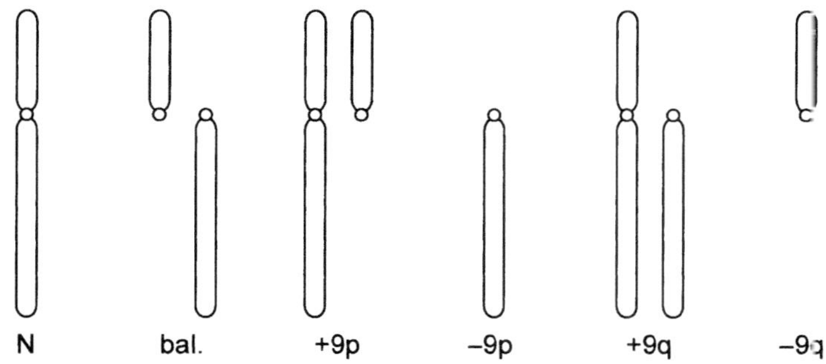

Figure 12–3. The six possible gametes arising from 2:1 segregation in a 47,cen fis(9) heterozygote. Two of these would lead to a normal phenotype, the 46,N and the balanced 47,cen fis(9) states. Of the unbalanced states, only the 48,cen fis(9),+9p, in which the imbalance would be a 9p trisomy, might possibly be viable.

At meiosis in the heterozygote, the centric fission products presumably form a trivalent with the intact homolog, and 2:1 segregation (essentially as in the Robertsonian carrier) then follows. "Alternate" 2:1 segregation produces normal and balanced centric fission gametes, while adjacent 2:1 segregation leads to gametes disomic or nullisomic for either of the fission products (Figure 12–3). Monosomy would likely be associated with occult abortion, and trisomy with miscarriage or, in exceptional cases, with the live birth of an abnormal child. Thus far, consequential viable trisomies are on record only for 4p, 9p, and 12p.

The paucity of data does not allow for a precise assessment of the genetic risk run by the centric fission carrier, other than to suggest that in some, it could be quite high. Dallapiccola et al. (1976) report a chromosome 4 centric fission in a woman who had had two children with trisomy 4p and one normal child. Fryns et al. (1980) describe a man and his normal daughter having a centric fission of chromosome 10. Recurrent miscarriage in the families of Janke (1982) and Shim et al. (2007) may well have been a result of asymmetric segregation of a chromosome 7, and a chromosome 11 centric fission, respectively; in the latter case, the cen fis(11) heterozygous woman then went on to have a normal 46,XX child. Miscarriages and childhood deaths in the family of Del Porto et al. (1984) might have been due to a cen fis 4, which was shown to have been transmitted in balanced state from a mother to her son.

Robertsonian Fission

The Robertsonian translocation is capable of reversing its evolutionary development, and the fused component chromosomes can separate. Perry et al. (2005) studied two families coming to attention due to a known family history of a segregating rob(13;15). They observed fission products in samplings of somatic tissues (chorionic villus, amniocytes, and blood) in 11 individuals or pregnancies, although mostly at single-digit percentage levels. These "new" acrocentric chromosomes were actually telocentric chromosomes 13 and 15, having no visible short-arm material. This phenomenon appeared to be without any clinical consequence. Xu et al. (2024b) report a person from a rob(14;15) family having mosaicism with a normal cell line alongside the 45,rob(14;15).

Chromosome Fusion (Telomeric Fusion)

This is the tip-to-tip fusion of two complete, or practically complete, chromosomes, and the person thus has a 45-chromosome count (Engelen et al. 2000; Lemyre et al. 2001). The fusion occurs at the level of the telomere or the subtelomeric region. All the necessary functional genetic material is "present and correct" (if there is a missing bit, it apparently contains no crucial genes), and the phenotype is normal, other things being equal. The composite chromosome has two centromeres (hence an alternative name of "stable non-Robertsonian dicentric chromosome"), but one of the two centromeres becomes functionally suppressed. The karyotype is written 45,t(A;B), 45,dic(A;B), or 45,tas(A;B), where A and B denote the two chromosomes. The short arm of an acrocentric chromosome is frequently involved, and chromosome 18 is often one of the participating chromosomes. The attachment of an essentially complete long arm of an acrocentric chromosome to the telomeric region of another autosome is a very similar circumstance (Figure 12–4). Ascertainment is typically fortuitous, or through reproductive difficulty (recurrent miscarriage, oligospermia). Familial transmission is recorded.

A normal child could be produced following symmetric, essentially 2:1, segregation. That is, either the two normal homologs are transmitted or the composite chromosome. Asymmetric segregation, were it to happen, would lead to trisomy or monosomy of one of the component chromosomes and, according to the nature of the chromosome, in utero viability would be compromised. If the trisomic state were to be "corrected" by loss of the normal homolog from the other parent, a uniparental disomy would result. The case shown in Figure 12–4 is an example of this.

On sperm analysis from one such man with 45,XY,der(5;15)(q35.3;q10), symmetric segregation was seen in just over one-half, and adjacent in a little under half, along with rare 3:0 segregants (Pylyp et al. 2014). Xie et al. (2021) examined reproductive outcomes in a series of eight carriers of autosome-autosome fusions, male and female, presenting with infertility. At blastocyst biopsy, a little over half showed adjacent segregation, the embryos being trisomic or monosomic for one of the involved autosomes but with most of the remainder being balanced (symmetric segregation), along with a single 3:0

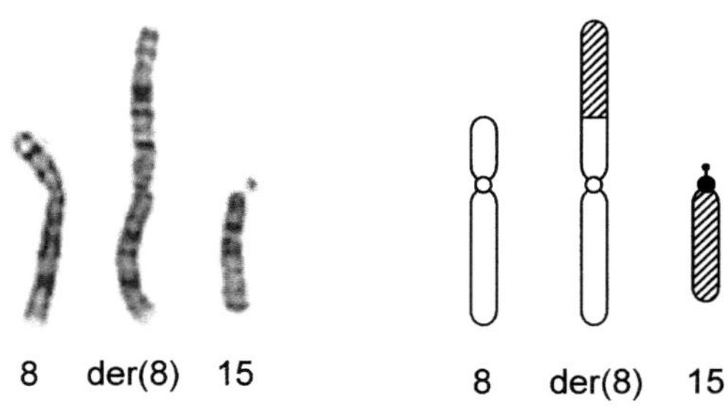

Figure 12–4. A telomeric fusion translocation, 45,XY,t(8;15)(p23.3;q11). The normal father with this karyotype has all the functionally necessary part of chromosome 15 attached to the telomere of a chromosome 8. His child with Angelman syndrome has the same karyotype, but haplotyping with DNA markers showed that both chromosome 15 elements derived from the father, with no chromosome 15 contributed from the mother. Probably, this reflected a "corrected" interchange trisomy.

Source: From A Smith et al., Familial unbalanced translocation t(8;15)(p23.3;q11) with uniparental disomy in Angelman syndrome, *Hum Genet* 93:471–473, 1994.

case. More favorable results were obtained in four carriers of Y-autosomal fusions, with only one of 19 blastocysts showing an unbalanced translocation. Lemyre et al. (2001) document a 45,XX,dic(14;18)(p11.2;p11.3) mother in whose pregnancy intrauterine fetal death was diagnosed at 32 weeks gestation. The fetal pathology examination was consistent with trisomy 18, and the karyotype, 46,XY,+18,dic(14;18)(p11.2;p11.3), confirmed this diagnosis.

An academic fascination in telomeric fusion lies in the theory that such a mechanism may have been a crucial step in the process of human evolution, initiating the separation of *Hominina* from *Pan* (chimpanzees). A fusion of the two ancestral primate chromosomes 2A and 2B, in a single 48-chromosome *Pan* individual, may thus have created the human chromosome 2, around a million years ago (Poszewiecka et al. 2023). It would then have taken inbreeding over some generations to lead to chromosome 2 homozygosity, and this state may then have conferred a survival advantage, ensuring the fixation of a 46-chromosome state in a small population that subsequently, with further genetic change, evolved into *Homo sapiens* (Stankiewicz 2016).

Complementary Isochromosomes

The individual has a full complement of the chromosomal material—and may thus be phenotypically normal—but with the two p arms combined in one chromosome and the two q arms in the other (Figure 12–5). A formal karyotype might be written, for example, as 46,XX,i(2)(p10),i(2)(q10). Chromosomes 1, 2, 4, 5, 7, and 9 have been reported with this picture, and at least four instances are known for chromosome 2 (Bernasconi et al. 1996; Shaffer et al. 1997; Björck et al. 1999; Albrecht et al. 2001; Baumer et al. 2007; Guvendag Guven et al. 2011; He et al. 2019).

The usual mechanism of formation may be that in the zygote, horizontal fission at the centromere of one homologous chromosome produces not two telocentric products (as happened in the fission discussed above), but two mirror-image metacentric chromosomes: an i(p) and an i(q) chromosome (Figure 12–1b). This is followed by segregation of both isochromosomes into one daughter cell. There is loss (if it had ever been there) of the homologous normal chromosome contributed by the other parent (unlike the

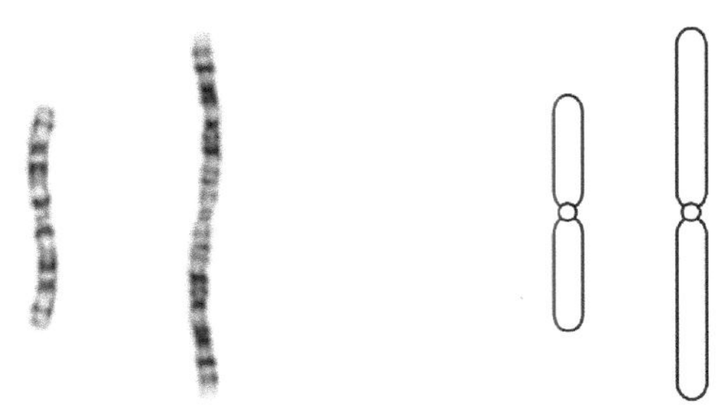

Figure 12–5. Chromosomes from a woman with complementary isochromosomes i(2p) and i(2q) (and see Figure 12–1b). Case of AA Schinzel; in F Bernasconi et al., Normal phenotype with maternal isodisomy in a female with two isochromosomes: i(2p) and i(2q), *Am J Hum Genet* 59:1114-1118, 1996.

centric fission, in which the normal homolog is necessarily retained); thus, this is a form of monosomy rescue that engenders a uniparental disomy, usually maternal. In other cases, one isochromosome may be of paternal origin and the other maternally derived, and this may reflect an initial trisomy rescue followed by post-zygotic isochromosome formation (Albrecht et al. 2001; Kotzot 2001; Baumer et al. 2007).

A typical clinical presentation has been multiple miscarriage in phenotypically normal women. Rather analogous to the rob(21q21q) carrier, it is practically impossible for such a person to have a normal child. Any pregnancies from "symmetric" segregation would be either dup(p)/del(q) or dup(q)/del(p), and thus hugely imbalanced. In the male, infertility may be the presenting feature.

Balancing Supernumerary Chromosomes

If deleted material from a chromosome is then accommodated in a newly formed small supernumerary marker chromosome (sSMC), and if this extra chromosome can be stably transmitted, then the carrier individual can be of normal phenotype but may have a risk to have a child with a deletion, or a duplication, of the material in question (Baldwin et al. 2008; Wang et al. 2023b). Figure 12–6 illustrates such a balance, the sSMC in this case in the form of a small ring.

A most remarkable example is that of a four-generation family in which several persons carried a chromosome 22 with an atypical q11.2 deletion, but this in company with a small supernumerary ring chromosome that comprised the deleted 22q11 material (Nevado et al. 2009). These people had, therefore, a balanced karyotype, and they were phenotypically normal: 47,del(22)(q11.2),+sSMC. On classical karyotyping, the two chromosome 22 homologs had appeared normal, and it required FISH to reveal the deletion on one homolog; thus, the initial impression in this scenario may simply be 47,+sSMC, and the sSMC interpreted as "harmless." In fact, two of these family members had

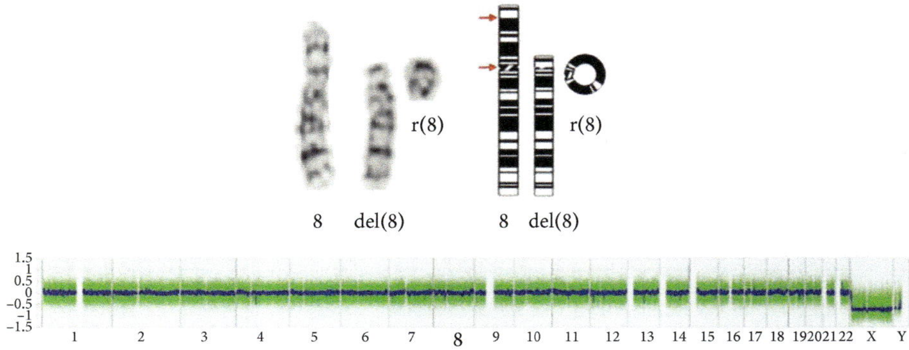

Figure 12–6. A Balancing Supernumerary Chromosome.

Notes: An 8p deletion with an accompanying supernumerary 8p ring chromosome (*above*), identified in a normal man presenting with infertility. The ring balances the deletion, as demonstrated on the SNP array (*below*). At PGT with IVF treatment, four embryos were balanced, two were deleted for 8p, and two duplicated for 8p. A balanced embryo was transferred, and a 46,XY baby born.

Source: From D Cheng et al., Analysis of molecular cytogenetic features and PGT-SR for two infertile patients with small supernumerary marker chromosomes, *J Assist Reprod Genet* 36:2533–2539, 2019. Courtesy Y-Q Tan, and with the permission of Springer.

a child with atypical deletion 22q11.2 syndrome. The deletion had a different proximal breakpoint to the common 22q11.2 deletion, such that the ring chromosome included some alpha satellite from the chromosome 22 centromere. The other potential imbalance, that of dup(22q11) due to a 47,+sSMC karyotype, had not been observed in the family.

Neocentromeres

Neocentromeres are ectopic centromeres that originate occasionally from noncentromeric regions of chromosomes (Amor and Choo 2002; DeBose-Scarlett and Sullivan, 2021). Neocentromeres are determined epigenetically by changes in the chromatin structure, such as the incorporation of the histone H3 variant CENP-A, and lack normal centromeric alpha-satellite DNA. The formation of a neocentromere is nearly always associated with a chromosomal rearrangement that generates a fragment lacking a conventional centromere, and provides a useful reminder of the absolute requirement for chromosomes to have both a centromere and a means of capping the chromosome ends, either with telomeres or by the formation of a ring chromosome. Chromosome rearrangements that are most commonly associated with neocentromere formation include inverted duplications of distal chromosome segments, ring chromosomes derived from deletions within chromosome arms, and, less commonly, deletions of the endogenous centromere. "Centromere repositioning," the formation of a neocentromere in the absence of any chromosome rearrangement, is exceedingly rare (Amor et al. 2004). If material is missing or disrupted from the chromosomal fragment with a neocentromere, pathology may result, such as the man in Quinonez et al. (2017a) with a del(15) and a "balancing" neocentromeric 15-originating sSMC, who had Marfan syndrome due to disruption of the *FBN1* gene at 15q21.1.

Almost all neocentromeres arise de novo, but familial examples are recorded. The mother in Chuang et al. (2005) had the karyotype 46,XX,del(11)(p11.12p11.2), with the deficit corrected by a neocentromere-containing r(11)(p11.12p11.2). Her child inherited only the del(11), and presented with the Potocki-Shaffer syndrome. Other examples, in which the neocentromeric chromosome formed as a ring, are noted in Chapter 11.

Jumping Translocation ("Translocation Sauteuse")

This evocative expression describes a mitotic rearrangement whereby the same piece of one chromosome breaks off, on more than one occasion, and attaches to the tips of other chromosomes. The site of breakage in the donor chromosome is characterized by the presence of an interstitial (internal) telomere, and this region offers the possibility of fusion with the recipient chromosomes (Vermeesch et al. 1997). Jumping translocations are found most commonly in hematological malignancies, but 50 constitutional cases were listed in the review of Reddy (2010).

Levy et al. (2000) identified the phenomenon in two couples, themselves karyotypically normal, presenting with recurrent miscarriage and showing evolving "jumping" cell lines in the cultured products of conception. In one of these, for example, the conceptus was initially 46,XX,der(15)t(1;15)(q10;q10). A second line arose, with the 1q

Chromoanagenesis

If transmission from parent to child is possible (and indeed, cases are on record), the risk for generating further complexity with an associated developmental disorder or miscarriage is likely high. The distinction between a particularly complicated complex rearrangement and a less complicated chromothripsis may be rather subtle.

Multiple De Novo CNVs

The small number of reported cases have all been sporadic, which is consistent with the proposed post-zygotic origin. However, a heritable contribution to the phenotype—in other words, a genetic susceptibility to the generation of these CNVs—is yet to be excluded.

13
DOWN SYNDROME, OTHER FULL ANEUPLOIDIES, POLYPLOIDY, AND THE INFLUENCE OF PARENTAL AGE

IN THIS CHAPTER we consider the circumstances in which there may be an increased risk to have a child, or a pregnancy, with an aneuploidy. First we review the case of parents, themselves karyotypically normal, who have had a child, or a pregnancy that aborted, with a full aneuploidy or a polyploidy. Thus, we include the major trisomies (13, 18, 21) as well as the less commonly seen autosomal aneuploidies. The category of polyploidy is substantially devoted to triploidy. In the great majority, these defects arise from an abnormal event during meiosis or (in some triploidy) at conception. In a few, there is post-zygotic generation of aneuploidy. Only in the case of parental gonadal mosaicism, or in the hypothetical setting of an apparent predisposition to meiotic error, will there apply an increased risk of recurrence of aneuploidy over and above that associated with any parental age effect. Triploidy needs separate consideration.

Second, we touch briefly on the uncommonly encountered circumstance of possible parenthood in (classically cytogenetic) aneuploid persons. Finally, we rehearse the ways in which parental age may influence the risk to conceive a pregnancy, and potentially to have a child, with an aneuploidy.

BIOLOGY

Full aneuploidy is presumed in the great majority to be the result of malsegregation of chromosomes at meiosis. A diminished degree of meiotic recombination is typically observed in aneuploid offspring, and this led Hassold and Sherman (2000) to propose a two-hit sequence, the first hit being a less well-tethered bivalent at meiosis I, and the second hit being a consequential aberrant distribution at meiotic metaphase. Meiotic malsegregation can happen at any parental age, but it is more frequent in older mothers, as we discuss in detail below. Alternatively, an abnormality has arisen in a premeiotic gametocyte, with the parent thus having a "wedge" of gonad that carries the abnormality (gonadal mosaicism). Such a parent would, of course, have an increased risk for only the one karyotypic defect. Finally, a small fraction of apparent full aneuploidy may be due to early mitotic nondisjunction in an initially 46,N conceptus with loss, or restriction to extra-embryonic tissue, of the normal cell line.

were analyzed, and three had a supernumerary chromosome 21.[5] A rather elegant demonstration of maternal gonadal mosaicism is described in Cupisti et al. (2003), who, in the study of a woman presenting for fertility treatment, identified three oöcyte–polar body pairs having one copy of chromosome 21 in the egg, and two copies in the first polar body. As for the male parent, Hixon et al. (1998) analyzed sperm samples from 10 men who had fathered a DS child, the additional chromosome 21 having been demonstrated to be of paternal origin. None showed any increase in the fraction of sperm with disomy 21.

The concept that parental gonadal mosaicism may be a substantial contributor to the occurrence (and recurrence) of aneuploidy, and not merely a matter of small-print interest, is due in particular to Kovaleva (2010), Delhanty (2011), and Hultén et al. (2013). Kovaleva assembled data from the literature and from local records, from 80 families in which one parent was gonadal/gonadal-somatic mosaic for trisomy 21. Where the origin of the trisomy in the mosaic parent could be determined, three-quarters had been due to post-zygotic rescue of a meiosis I error,[6] and one-quarter came from either rescue of a meiosis II error or a post-zygotic mitotic nondisjunction. The sex of the mosaic parent was usually female (61/80 cases), a paucity of mosaic fathers possibly reflecting an impaired spermatogenesis in such men. Kovaleva also proposed a female-specific tendency toward chromosome loss in early embryogenesis (thus allowing trisomy rescue), and suggested that these mosaic females might be not uncommon in the general population. This hypothesis may be supported by observations in the offspring of the mosaic parents. When these parents had non-mosaic DS offspring, the sex ratio was 1.3:1 in favor of males, as observed for DS in the general population. But in the nine instances in which a mosaic DS parent had mosaic DS offspring, in all but one the child was female. The explanation is complex (and unproven), but there may be, first, an intrauterine selection against non-mosaic DS females, and second, a sex-specific tendency for female DS embryos to be converted to the mosaic state by trisomy rescue.

Recurrence Risk Estimates After One Affected Child or Pregnancy. The earliest estimates of risk are due to Penrose (1956),[7] prior to the discovery of the chromosomal basis of DS, and to Stene (1970). Penrose proposed the risk of recurrence to be "doubled, or perhaps nearly trebled" compared to the general population risk, irrespective of maternal age; while Stene derived a figure of 1% for mothers under age 30 years, with no increase in the age-specific risk for those over 30 years at the time of birth of their DS child. More sophisticated analyses were subsequently enabled by the collection of amniocentesis data and from population studies, as we present in the sections on parental age and genetic counseling below. It does remain true that for younger mothers the recurrence risk is, in absolute terms, small.

Recurrence Risk Estimates After Two Affected Children/Pregnancies. When a couple have had two (or more) trisomic 21 conceptions, one has to assume an increased risk applies to a subsequent pregnancy, quite possibly a "substantial" risk. The recurrence may well have been due to gonadal mosaicism, but unfortunate chance always remains a possibility, more particularly if the mother is of older age.

[5] Two of the no. 21 chromosomes had identical haplotypes, indicating that the mother's mosaicism was due to post-zygotic error in an initially normal 46,XX conception (Figure 3–15a).

[6] If gonadal mosaicism is the result of rescue of an initially trisomic conceptus, then advanced *grand*-maternal age is expected to be a risk factor, and this indeed appears to be so (Kovaleva 2010).

[7] His paper was titled "Some Notes on Heredity Counseling," and he also referred to "genetical counseling," one of the first uses of this expression.

Occurrence Risk Estimates with Down Syndrome in a Second- or Third-Degree Relative. More widely in the family, it appears that a history of standard trisomy DS in second- or third-degree relatives does not, in the main, imply an increased risk (Hook 1992; Pangalos et al. 1992b). Berr et al. (1990) assessed 188 families in which a DS child had been born, and there were comparable numbers of DS cases among the second- and third-degree relatives and in the relatives of 185 control families.

MOSAIC DOWN SYNDROME

47,+21/46,N mosaicism accounts for about 2% of individuals with clinically diagnosed DS. With very low-grade mosaicism, an abnormal phenotype may escape recognition. Papavassiliou et al. (2015) provide an exhaustive literature review, from 1961 to 2014, and offer illustrative examples of the milder phenotype. These authors propose that detection of mosaicism can be achieved when present in as little as 1.6%–1.8% of cells using FISH analysis of peripheral blood (1,000 cells scored) and buccal mucosa (500 cells scored).

Mosaicism results from a malsegregation of homologs, or an anaphase lag of one homolog, occurring post-zygotically. Probably the majority of individuals with mosaic DS arise from initially trisomic 21 zygotes, losing one of the chromosomes 21 by anaphase lag as a form of "trisomy rescue" (Figure 3–15c). Others may arise from normal conceptuses, with nondisjunction-producing 45,–21/46,N/47,+21 mosaicism, with the 45,–21 line thereafter lost (Figure 3–15a). Whatever the basis, for practical purposes counseling needs to proceed as though the child has standard trisomy 21, recognizing that this will overestimate the risk in some. Genetic counseling for the mosaic individuals themselves is covered on p. 338.

Isochromosome 21 Down Syndrome. After standard trisomy 21, this is the most common chromosomal category of DS. It has often been called a "21q21q Robertsonian translocation," but in fact it is almost always the case that the two 21q components are identical, from the same parent, and thus *isochromosome* is the more accurate term, and the karyotype is more accurately 46,i(21q) (Kovaleva and Shaffer 2003). An agnostic nomenclature is rea(21;21). Most arise in an early postmeiotic mitosis (Robinson et al. 1994), and so the risk of recurrence is expected to be low. In one series of 112 de novo rea(21q;21q) DS probands, none of 130 full sibs and 34 half-sibs had DS (Steinberg et al. 1984). Nevertheless, three of the parents actually showed a low-grade mosaicism, and presumably their having had an affected child reflected that the 21q21q cell line had arisen in a premeiotic mitosis and was included in the gonad.

Indeed, a few examples of recurrence in subsequently born siblings are recorded, and parental gonadal mosaicism is the presumed or proven basis of such recurrence (Hervé et al. 2015). For example, Mark et al. (1977) studied a woman having had sequential pregnancies with the karyotype 46,i(21q), and she herself typed 46,XX,i(21q)/46,XX on ovarian fibroblast analysis (but 46,XX on blood). Hall (1985) offers the cautionary story of a mother given a low risk of recurrence, who went on to have a second affected child from a second marriage (on resampling of her, a single 46,XX,i(21q) cell was found in 100 cells analyzed). An i(21q) is a recognized cause of a false-negative cfDNA prenatal screening result for DS, this observation attributed to post-zygotic isochromosome formation leading to placental mosaicism (Huijsdens-van Amsterdam et al. 2018).

the phenotype ranged from clinically normal to delayed motor and intellectual development, with mild dysmorphic signs and asymmetry. In two of the five cases, a trisomy 20 cell line was also detected, suggesting origin in a post-zygotic mitotic nondisjunction; and in one, the monosomy 20 was seen only in urine cells.

Monosomy 21. This is the most common full monosomy, and Viana et al. (2022) summarized data from nine mosaic and nine non-mosaic cases. Their own case, a 13-year-old boy, was the oldest surviving patient with mosaic monosomy 21. He presented with microcephaly, low weight, facial dysmorphisms, and severe intellectual disability; monosomy 21 was seen in 81% of lymphocytes. A similar phenotype has been described in other cases. When non-mosaic, monosomy 21 typically results in miscarriage or neonatal death, and is likely incompatible with life. In some reported cases, there may have been undetected mosaicism for a tissue-limited cryptic cell line. Burgess et al. (2014b) emphasize this point in their description of a growth-retarded and dysmorphic neonate, who karyotyped full monosomy 21 on blood and buccal swab, but fibroblast study revealed a cryptic ring chromosome karyotype 45,XX,-21[8]/46,XX,r(21)[42].

Monosomy 22. Pinto-Escalante et al. (1998) reported a dysmorphic and malformed infant, delivered at 30 weeks gestation and who died from septicemia on day 11; 15% of lymphocytes were monosomic. The authors reviewed six other literature cases, noting recurrent observations of growth retardation, microcephaly, facial dysmorphism, joint abnormalities, and cardiac defects. Early death was usual, although two children were alive at age two years. In three cases, 100% of lymphocytes and fibroblasts were monosomic, yet the phenotype was not obviously more severe. Cryptic mosaicism for a normal cell line may have been present.

POLYPLOIDY

Triploidy

The chromosome count in triploidy is $3n = 69$, with a double ($2n$) chromosomal contribution to the conceptus from one or other parent (Figure 13–6). Triploidy can reflect di-*andry* or di-*gyny*, with the double contribution coming from the father or mother, respectively (Figure 13–7). The very great majority of triploid conceptions abort during the first or early second trimester. Increasing maternal age does not increase the risk for triploidy.

The Two Distinct Forms of Triploidy. *Diandry* is usually the consequence of dispermy—that is, two sperm simultaneously fertilizing the ovum (Zaragoza et al. 2000; McFadden et al. 2002).[9] A shorthand description is P1 P2M. The fundamental basis in this instance may lie in the "zona reaction," which is the response of the investing shell of the ovum, the zona pellucida, to prevent further sperm entering after the first has penetrated.

Digyny is most commonly due to a diploid egg, which may be the result of nondisjunction of the entire chromosome set at either the first or the second meiotic division in oögenesis, meiosis II being the more vulnerable—or, a polar body may fail to be

[9] Dispermy could be deduced simply from the cytogenetic analysis in the case reported in Lim et al. (2003), the man carrying a translocation 46,XY,t(2;6)(p12; q24). The 69,XXY mole had both the balanced translocation and one unbalanced form, reflecting fertilization with one sperm from alternate segregation and the other from adjacent-1. A dispermic mole, at the center of a criminal case, posed a challenge to the assigning of paternity (Budowle et al. 2017).

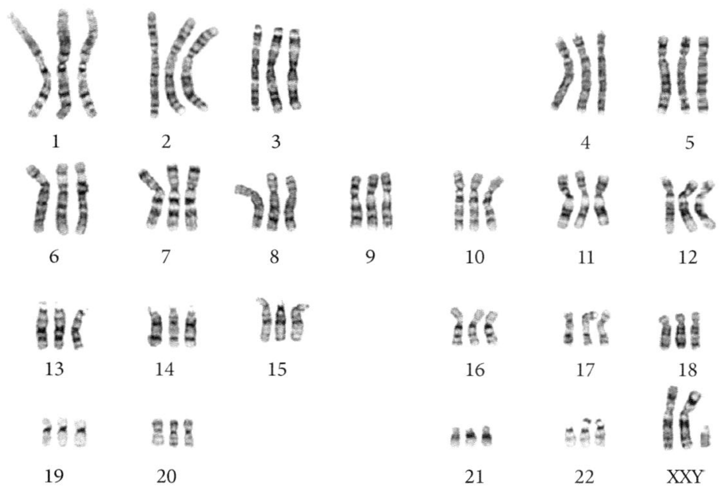

Figure 13-6. Triploidy.
Note: The 69,XXY karyotype of a triploid embryo (the embryo shown in Figure 20-18).

extruded (Filges et al. 2015). An individual susceptibility may exist, as discussed below. A very rare cause may be the fusion of two eggs (whimsically called "dieggy"). Diploidy can be presumed to exist in the "giant binucleate oöcyte," and these visibly abnormal gametes have actually been shown at IVF to lead to a triploid embryo (Balakier et al. 2002; Rosenbusch et al. 2002).

Natural History. Triploidy is not uncommon in early pregnancy (~1% of recognized conceptions and 10% of recognized miscarriages), but about 99.99% are lost as first-trimester miscarriage or second-trimester fetal death in utero. Of those aborting at the embryonic stage, most are digynic, while in contrast, most fetal losses reflect a diandric state (McFadden and Robinson 2006). The appearances on morphological examination at the stage of the embryo do not differ according to a digynic versus diandric origin,

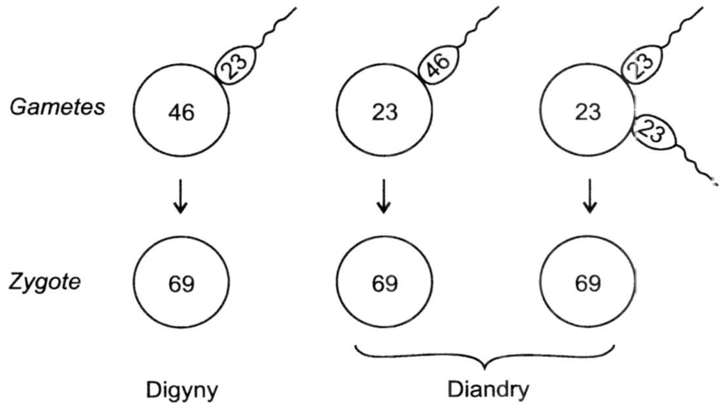

Figure 13-7. Triploidy Origins.
Notes: The three major routes whereby triploidy may arise. A complete failure of a meiotic division produces a diploid egg (*left*) or sperm (*middle*). Simultaneous fertilization by two sperm is dispermy (*right*).

whereas the clinical presentations are readily distinguishable by the time of the fetal stage of development, as follows:

Diandric triploids mostly abort in the first or early second trimester, presenting as hydatidiform mole (Scholz et al. 2015). The very few diandric triploid pregnancies that survive to the second trimester typically show partial hydatidiform mole; growth retardation of the fetus is usual but not invariable (Daniel et al. 2001).

Dygynic triploids are non-molar, and mostly abort early (mean 10 weeks), although those exceptional few that remain are able to continue through to the third trimester. These surviving digynic triploids develop as a severely growth-retarded fetus with marked head-body disproportion, the head being relatively large, and with an abnormally small and non-molar placenta (McFadden and Langlois 2000; Daniel et al. 2001). In one case of a digynic 69,XXX triploid coexisting with a normal 46,XY twin, survival to 20 weeks (when selective feticide was done) may have been supported by the normal fetus (Gassner et al. 2003). Intrauterine survival may also be promoted if there is fetal-placental karyotypic discordance, with the placenta being diploid (Kennerknecht et al. 1993a). Survival through to the third trimester progresses almost invariably to perinatal death. Of those liveborn, hardly any digynic triploids survive for more than a month; there is one extraordinary instance of death not until 312 days (Sherard et al. 1986; Hasegawa et al. 1999).

From Hawaiian data, of 38 recognized triploid pregnancies over the period 1986–1999, ~40% were XXX, 60% XXY, and a single case of XYY. Most (80%) aborted early, a few (10%) presented as fetal deaths in utero, and 10% were electively terminated (Forrester and Merz 2003a). In a large Danish series, 84% of triploids were diandric. Of the diandric cases, 69,XXX, 69,XXY, and 69,XYY karyotypes were seen in the proportions 7:8½:1. Of the digynic cases, XXX and XXY cases were of similar frequency (Joergensen et al. 2014). Of all 16-week pregnancies, only one in 30,000 are estimated to be triploid, and at 20 weeks only one in 250,000 (Snijders et al. 1995).

RECURRENCE

Given that triploidy affects 1% of recognized pregnancies, most recurrence is a chance event, and after one digynic triploid pregnancy the risk of a second is no greater than the background figure. Nonetheless, the question remains whether specific risks might apply to a small subset of women, including those having had three (Huang et al. 2004; Brancati et al. 2003) or even four (Khawajkie et al. 2017) triploid pregnancies. Filges et al. (2015) make the case for a failure of maternal meiosis II as a common basis for this predisposition.

There may be a genetic basis for some of these recurrences. In the study of an extraordinary mother-daughter pair, both of whom had had multiple miscarriages known or likely due to recurrent triploidy, Filges et al. analyzed a number of candidate genes. One was *PLCD4*, for which mother and daughter were both heterozygous for a predicted pathogenic mutation; and this gene may have a role in the extrusion of the second polar body. Two other candidate genes, each with a role in maternal meiosis, have since been identified in single consanguineous families: Liang et al. (2024) identified a homozygous truncating variant in *HORMAD2* in a woman with recurrent digynic triploid miscarriage, and Fatemi et al. (2021) identified a homozygous missense variant in *CCNB3* in two sisters who both had recurrent pregnancy losses, two of which were confirmed as digynic triploidy. Confirmation of the role of these loci awaits the identification of additional families.

Recurrence of diandric triploidy with partial hydatidiform mole is also well reported, although in the series of Nguyen et al. (2018), none of eight patients had more than two. In a registry study of partial hydatidiform mole, 0.3% of women had a recurrence in a subsequent pregnancy, including one woman with three confirmed dispermic triploid pregnancies (Eagles et al. 2015). Recurrent diandric triploidy is to be distinguished from the autosomal recessive form of recurrent hydatidiform mole, which occurs in the setting of a diploid biparental genome in which the cause is biallelic variants in the oöcytes, the major causal genes being *NLRP7* and *KHDC3L* (Slim et al. 2022) (p. 619).

Coincidence is the most likely explanation for the occurrence of triploidy of both digynic and diandric etiologies to the one couple, and for the occurrence of both partial hydatidiform mole (due to diandric triploidy) and complete mole (the rare type associated with biparental disomy) to the same couple (Kircheisen et al. 1991; Deveault et al. 2009).

The risk of a triploidy is lower in IVF pregnancies, first because intracytoplasmic sperm injection can ensure the ovum is fertilized by only one sperm, and second by excluding embryos with three pronuclei (5% of all embryos) (Nickkho-Amiry et al. 2019). Having made that point, Capalbo et al. (2024) note that pronuclei number is a poor predictor of embryo ploidy, and that PGT can provide a more accurate ploidy assessment (Caroselli et al. 2023).

The prevention of chromosomal pathology, as a direct exercise, largely involves secondary prevention: in essence, the selective termination of pregnancies in which a chromosomal abnormality has been identified, or the discarding of abnormal embryos following PGT. Primary prevention is indirect, and encouraging a younger maternal age may be the only feasible approach absent any clear understanding of environmental factors that might compromise the chromosomal integrity of gamete or zygote. But one remarkable exception to this state of affairs concerns the actual correction of a chromosomally abnormal zygote; this involves the diandric triploid zygote, otherwise destined to undergo implantation failure or, in the minority that actually implant, to proceed to a severe fetal defect. A triploid zygote due to dispermy will possess three pronuclei. In vitro removal of one pronucleus at IVF would restore normality. In the case of dispermy, this would have to be one of the paternal pronuclei, thus leaving one maternal and one paternal pronucleus. Escribá et al. (2006) applied this approach to tripronuclear embryos in the research laboratory, removing the pronucleus farthest from the second polar body (the one closest to the polar body being very likely maternal), and followed the embryo through to the blastocyst stage. They were able to confirm restoration of diploidy and could also observe that these corrected embryos showed normal development at day 5, unlike the uncorrected embryos in which no inner cell mass was seen to form. And in the first ever example of "chromosomal cure" of a child-to-be, Kattera and Chen (2003) corrected a tripronuclear zygote, implanted the embryo, and a normal 46,XY boy was subsequently born. These authors comment, cautiously, that this approach should be used "only as a last resort."

Diploid/Triploid Mosaicism. Van de Laar et al. (2002) accumulated 25 cases from the literature, and reported three of their own. These three came from a population catchment of 15 million over a 20-year period, attesting to the rarity of the condition. Characteristic features include learning difficulties, seizures, short stature, truncal obesity, syndactyly, and body asymmetry. Phenotypic overlap with imprinting disorders is

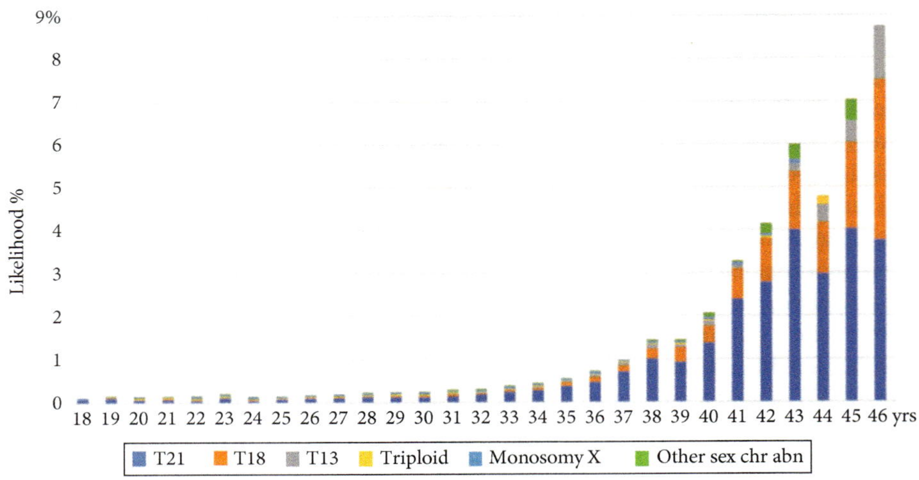

Figure 13–8. The Likelihood of a Survivable Aneuploidy according to Maternal Age.

Notes: These data are based on a whole population cohort in Denmark, and record pregnancies in which trisomy 21, 18, or 13, triploidy, or monosomy X were diagnosed. Mothers in the age group 30-34 had a small increased risk (Odds Ratio, OR, of 1.7) above the baseline of 20 to 29-year-olds, to have a pregnancy with one of these aneuploidies; those in the 35-39 age group had an OR of 4.7; 40 to 44-year-olds had a 16-fold risk; while the oldest group, 45 and older, had a 36-fold increased likelihood.

Source: From L Elmerdahl Frederiksen et al., Maternal age and the risk of fetal aneuploidy: A nationwide cohort study of more than 500 000 singleton pregnancies in Denmark from 2008 to 2017, *Acta Obstet Gynecol Scand* 103:351–359, 2024. Courtesy CK Ekelund, and with the permission of John Wiley and Sons.

The oöcyte being the key player, studies have been directed to this gamete. Segregation errors within female meiosis fall into three categories (Franasiak et al. 2014; Gruhn et al. 2019): (1) meiosis I nondisjunction (NDJ); (2) precocious separation of the sister chromatids (PSSC); and (3) reverse segregation (RS) (sister chromatids separate at meiosis I and homologs separate at meiosis II). These are illustrated in Figure 13–9.

The relative contribution of these three mechanisms varies according to the chromosome involved, and with maternal age. Oöcytes from young girls and women are more vulnerable to meiosis I NDJ events that particularly affect the largest chromosomes

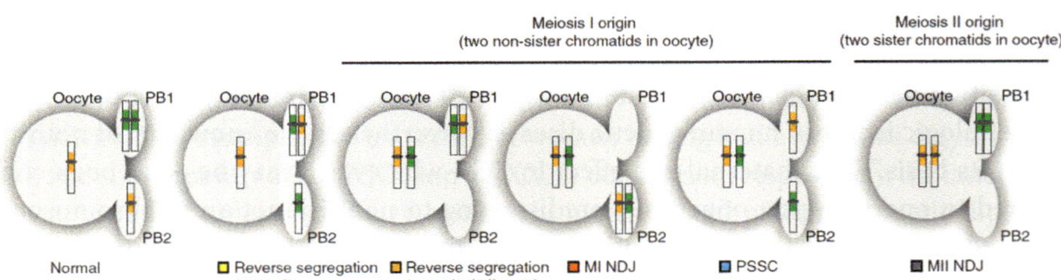

Figure 13–9. Segregation Patterns in Female Meiosis Leading to a Trisomic Conceptus.

Notes: Pericentromeric haplotypes shown in orange and green. MI NDJ, meiosis I nondisjunction; PSSC, precocious separation of sister chromatids; MII NDJ, meiosis II nondisjunction.

Source: From CS Ottolini et al., Genome-wide maps of recombination and chromosome segregation in human oocytes and embryos show selection for maternal recombination rates, *Nat Genet* 47:727–735, 2015. Courtesy CS Ottolini, and with the permission of Springer Nature.

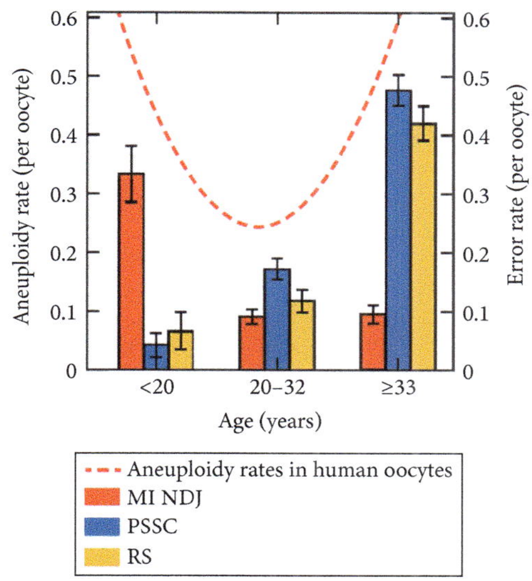

Figure 13–10. Chromosome Missegregation Patterns across the Lifespan.

Notes: Aneuploidy rates in human oöcytes (*dashed red line*) peak in both young girls (<20 years) and in women of older maternal age (≥33 years). This increase at either end of the age spectrum reflects a combination of three different chromosome missegregation patterns, with young oöcytes being affected primarily by MI NDJ (*red*), and advanced maternal age oöcytes impacted by PSSC (*blue*) and RS (*yellow*).

Source: From JR Gruhn and ER Hoffman, Errors of the egg: The establishment and progression of human aneuploidy research in the maternal germline, *Annu Rev Genet* 56:369–390, 2022. Courtesy ER Hoffmann, and with the permission of Annual Reviews.

(chromosomes 1 to 5).[10] In contrast, oöcytes from older women are more likely to be affected by PSSC and RS errors of the smaller acrocentric chromosomes (Gruhn et al. 2019). These findings explain the "U-curve" of aneuploidy against maternal age, with peaks at both ends of the age spectrum, and the lowest chance of aneuploidy corresponding to maternal age 27.5 years (Figure 13–10). The age-dependent increase in PSSC and RS likely relates to the prolonged oöcyte arrest and potential protein deterioration over time, with degradation of cohesin proteins and proteins involved in spindle function contributing to aneuploidy formation.

Paternal age generally does not usefully enter the equation, at least with respect to the numerical full aneuploidies (Donate et al. 2016).[11] Fathers of DS children are older than average, but simply because couples are usually of similar ages, a point determined by Penrose in 1934. On meta-analysis, a paternal age >40 years was associated with a relative risk of 1.13 for Down syndrome compared to paternal age <40 years, a difference that was just statistically significant (Oldereid et al. 2018). In contrast, Steiner et al. (2015) made the surprising observation of a subtle but definite effect of younger age of the father (Figure 13–11), the proposed explanation being that of a reduced intrauterine survival for the trisomic pregnancy from older fathers.

[10] Trisomies of these chromosomes will seldom result in recognized pregnancies, therefore the main consequence of these aneuploidies will be reduced fertility in girls and young women, possibly having provided an evolutionary advantage in prehistoric times.

[11] As for structural rearrangements, a true paternal-age effect is considered to exist, albeit at an order of magnitude less than the maternal/aneuploidy association (Sloter et al. 2004).

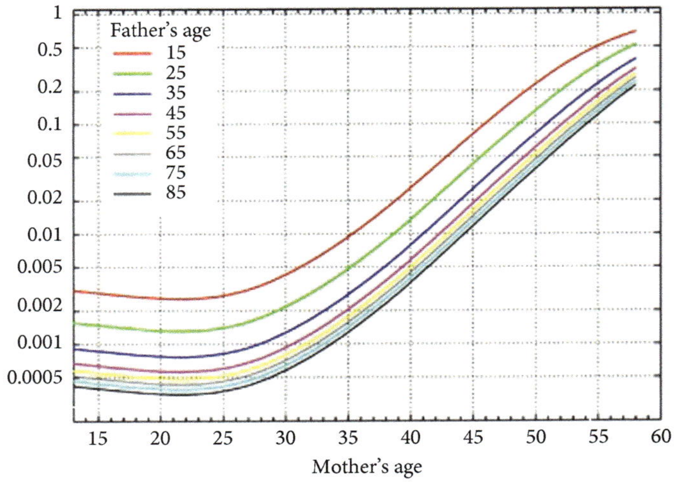

Figure 13–11. Parental Age and Down Syndrome.

Notes: Parental ages compared to risk to have a child with Down syndrome. Note that *younger* paternal age is a slight risk factor, against the well-known and marked older maternal age effect.

Source: From B Steiner et al., An unexpected finding: Younger fathers have a higher risk for offspring with chromosomal aneuploidies, *Eur J Hum Genet* 23: 466–472, 2015. Courtesy B Steiner and A Schinzel, and with the permission of Springer Nature.

Concerning gametic studies in older men, numerous sperm analyses have been done, with somewhat conflicting findings (Robbins et al. 1997; Shi and Martin 2000; Eskenazi et al. 2002; Shi et al. 2002; Iwarsson et al. 2015). Some have shown slight increases in some autosomal disomies, and some have shown increases in sex chromosome disomies, with XY disomy being more consistently noted. Other studies report no significant differences in at least autosomal abnormalities comparing older and younger men (one group even using testicular sperm from men in their 80s; Guttenbach et al. 2000). Given that trisomy 21 is of paternal origin in only 5% to 10% of cases, it is unlikely that a small increase in sperm disomy from older fathers, even if real, would lead to a measurable increase in birth prevalence for DS, if paternal age profiles should increase. Dviri et al. (2021) reviewed evidence from embryos derived from young oöcyte donors, to minimize maternal-age effects, and concluded that advanced paternal age is not associated with higher rates of aneuploidy in PGT-tested embryos.

Risk Figures According to Maternal Age

How old is "older," and what is "advanced" maternal age at childbearing? Conventionally, the mid- to late thirties is taken as the boundary. The risk curve for DS, the major condition of concern, begins to steepen during this period, although there is no sudden jump. Risk figures for individual ages with respect to this and other aneuploidies have been collected in various jurisdictions, and estimates refined according to certain statistical assumptions, and the information from these studies has long been used as the basis of preconceptional and prenatal genetic counseling. These data are also useful in screening programs for fetal trisomy (Chapter 21), the woman's age-related risk being an important datum to be included, along with the various laboratory test results, in order to derive her overall risk estimate.

For trisomies 13, 18, and 21, spontaneous abortion is more likely than for a normal conceptus. Thus, the prevalence of chromosome abnormality is greater at the time of prenatal diagnosis than at term, and we need access to stage-specific figures. Looking through these different windows of observation—at CVS and noninvasive prenatal testing (10 or 11 weeks), at amniocentesis (about 15–17 weeks), at screen-triggered amniocentesis (may be closer to 20 weeks), and at term—the frequency of chromosomal abnormality for a particular maternal age progressively reduces. For trisomy 21, it is estimated that about one-third of all pregnancies existing at the time of CVS spontaneously abort between then and term, and one-quarter abort during the period from amniocentesis to term (Table 13–5 and Figure 13–12). Trisomies 13 and 18 (and monosomy X) have high rates of fetal lethality, with the majority of pregnancies aborting. For XXX and XXY, in contrast, there appears to be very little if any selective loss in the latter part of pregnancy.

These matters may be of particular importance to those women who, having had an abnormal result, nevertheless decide to continue a pregnancy. How likely is it that they will have a liveborn baby with the trisomy in question, or that fetal death in utero will supervene? Won et al. (2005) reviewed 392 women who had continued a trisomy 21 pregnancy, and 106 with trisomy 18; the diagnoses had been given somewhat later than might be usual, because these women had entered a public maternal serum screening program at gestations ranging from 15 weeks to 20 weeks, with amniocentesis then offered to those who returned an increased risk result. For trisomy 21, fetal demise occurred in 10%, and for trisomy 18, 32%. About one-third of the trisomy 21 losses happened before the stage of viability (i.e., 24 weeks), the comparable figure in trisomy 18 being 15%. In those pregnancies proceeding beyond 24 weeks, the losses were evenly spread according to duration. More recent figures for trisomies 13 and 18 are due to Cavadino and Morris (2017), derived from a whole-population study in England and Wales. From their work, a surprisingly high 50% of fetuses diagnosed at 12 weeks with trisomy 13 will survive to term, and for trisomy 18, the figure is 30%. These authors discuss possible reasons for the very considerable differences between studies. It is their more recent data that we use in Table 13–5.

Table 13–5. Natural Fetal Loss Rates from Early Pregnancy Through to Term, Estimated for the Three Major Autosomal Trisomies and X Monosomy

	ESTIMATED AVERAGE NATURAL PREGNANCY LOSS RATE (%)		
CHROMOSOME ABNORMALITY	FROM 9–14 WEEKS TO BIRTH	FROM 15–20 WEEKS TO BIRTH	FROM >20 WEEKS TO BIRTH
Trisomy 13	50	44	40
Trisomy 18	70	65	64
Trisomy 21	32	25	10
Monosomy X	65	52	

Note: 9–15 and 15–20 weeks approximate to the stages at which CVS and amniocentesis are performed.
Sources: From Snijders et al. (1995), Won et al. (2005), Savva et al. (2006), and Cavadino and Morris (2017).

ETHNICITY

Systematic calculations from other than Caucasian ethnic groups have come from Nigeria, China, Japan, South America, and Hawaii. Adeyokunnu (1982) showed no difference in incidence of trisomy 21 in Nigeria compared with Europeans; and in a study encompassing nine South American countries, Carothers et al. (2001) demonstrated incidence data and maternal-age correlations very similar to those recorded from other jurisdictions. In Japan, Yaegashi et al. (1998) collected data from four clinics, comprising, in all, 5,484 pregnancies of women aged 35 years or older. The risks for trisomy 21 (and for aneuploidies) overall were, on the face of it, somewhat less than in a European population. The raw figures did, however, fluctuate somewhat, with rather small numbers of affected fetuses at each age category. A question might be raised whether some cases could have escaped ascertainment by earlier screening and not otherwise recorded. It may be premature to suppose that aneuploidy rates could differ to any important degree between Japanese and other ethnic groups, a view that is supported by the observation otherwise of no significant differences in a Hong Kong population (Lau et al. 1998); but bearing in mind also data from Hawaii suggesting that at older maternal ages, the DS rate *may* be somewhat less in a Pacific Island population (Forrester and Merz 2003b). Within the US population, the birth prevalence of DS is highest among the Hispanic population and lowest among blacks, with whites having an intermediate prevalence (Mai et al. 2019); these data differences likely reflect social and cultural rather than genetic factors.

Taking a more fundamental viewpoint, Ghosh et al. (2009) demonstrated that rates of meiotic recombination in families with a DS child in India were essentially the same as in a US population, pointing to a basic identity of nondisjunctional mechanism across these populations. And taking a refined view of ethnicity (by genotyping of "ancestry informative markers"), Franasiak et al. (2016) saw no differences among patients attending an IVF clinic, and whose embryos had been tested for aneuploidy, among those of European, African, East Asian, or Central/South Asian ancestry.

GENETIC COUNSELING

Down Syndrome

The central requirement for accurate genetic advice in DS is knowledge of the chromosomal form in the affected family member. If a child diagnosed as having DS has died and no chromosome studies were performed—and more so in a case of younger maternal age—it may be reasonable to check for the possibility of a familial translocation in the consultand.

PREVIOUS CHILD WITH STANDARD TRISOMY 21 (INCLUDING MOSAICISM)

If the child has standard trisomy 21, or is a 47,+21/46 mosaic, it is unnecessary routinely to study the parents' chromosomes.[12] One can assume with considerable confidence that they will type as 46,XX and 46,XY. The risk of recurrence of trisomy 21 (homotrisomy),

[12] But parental chromosome studies should be considered following the prenatal diagnosis of trisomy 21 by microarray, since microarray cannot distinguish translocation DS from standard trisomy 21.

or occurrence of a different aneuploidy (heterotrisomy), is typically small, but above that of a same-age maternal population. Broad-brush estimates of increased risk are listed in Table 13–11. More precise data are shown in Table 13–12. Small differences between these estimates may relate to simple statistical variation, but note also that Table 13–11 refers to risk for the birth of an affected child, whereas Table 13–12 relates to the risk at the time of amniocentesis.

In any event, regardless of the exact figure, the practical point is that the risk for a recurrence of DS is comfortingly low, only approaching the 1% mark by the mid-30s of maternal age. Nevertheless, most couples seek the reassurance of prenatal diagnosis in pregnancies after having had a child with DS. Many may choose the option of noninvasive prenatal diagnosis, which relieves the couple of having to balance the risk of recurrence against the risk of a procedure-related pregnancy loss. Elkins et al. (1986b) observe that some of these parents declare they would not abort a trisomy 21 fetus, and the counselor needs to be sensitive to possible ambivalent feelings of the parents in this setting.

TWO PREVIOUS TRISOMIC 21 CONCEPTIONS

One can only offer an educated guess that the risk for a third trisomic conception will be "substantial." A skin biopsy study of a parent would be largely academic. If gonadal mosaicism (rather than de novo recurrence) is the cause, a considerable fraction of whichever gonad it is must be involved, since two separate samplings have already come from this

Table 13–11. Risk after Previous Trisomy
Increases in Recurrence Risk, Given as Multiples Compared with the Maternal Age–Related Baseline, for Women Who Have Had a Previous Trisomic Pregnancy

	FOLD INCREASED RISK OF RECURRENCE FOR:	
PREVIOUS ABNORMAL PREGNANCY	SAME TRISOMY	OTHER VIABLE TRISOMY
Trisomy 21 at maternal age <30, current maternal age <30	8.2×	2.4×
Trisomy 21 at maternal age <30, current maternal age ≥30	2.2×	2.4×
Trisomy 21 at maternal age <35	3.5×	1.3×
Trisomy 21 at maternal age ≥30	1.6×	1.7×
Trisomy 21 at maternal age ≥35	1.7×	1.5×
Trisomy 13 overall	8.6–9.5×	1.5×
Trisomy 18 overall	1.7–3.1×	1×
Trisomy 13 or 18 at maternal age <35	7.8×	1.6×
Trisomy 13 or 18 at maternal age ≥35	2.2×	1×
Trisomies 13, 18, XXX and XXY	2.3×	1.6×
Nonviable trisomy in spontaneous abortion*		1.8×

Notes: The above figures relate to the *probability of trisomy at livebirth*. Separate figures are given for the risk of recurrence of the same trisomy (homotrisomy) or of a different trisomy (heterotrisomy). If wished, the appropriate multiple for a particular case can be applied to the woman's current age-related risk, as listed in Tables 13–6 to 13–9, in order to generate an adjusted recurrence risk figure. Figures are from the prenatal data of Warburton et al. (2004) and pre- and post-natal data of De Souza et al. (2009), and they are grouped in various ways according to the formats of these papers. Specific age-related figures for previous trisomy 21 are also given in Table 13–12, column B.

*But cf. Robinson et al. (2001), who discerned no increased risk following an aneuploid miscarriage.

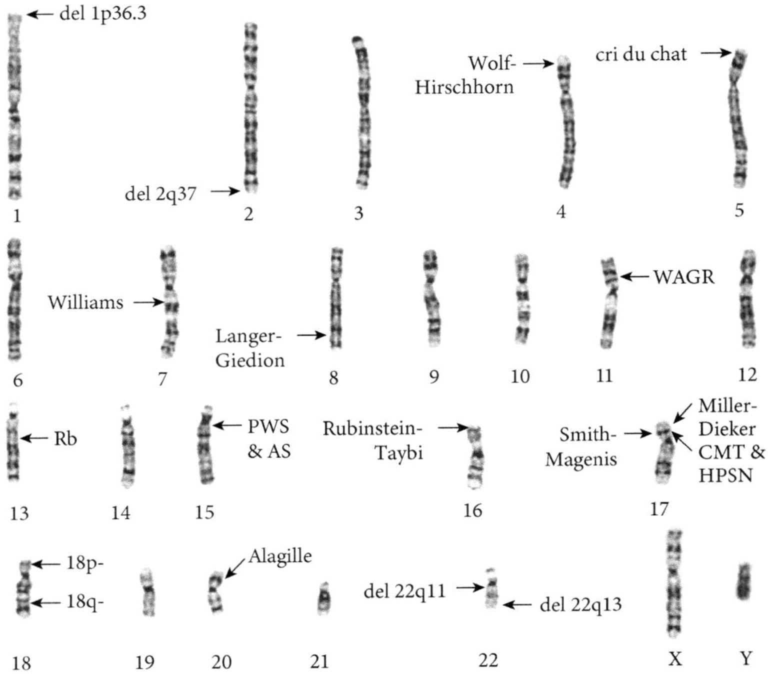

Figure 14–1. "Composite Karyotype" of the Classical Deletion/Duplication Syndromes. "Composite karyotype" showing the site of the cytogenetic defect in some of the classic syndromes. AS, Angelman syndrome; CMT, Charcot-Marie-Tooth neuropathy; HPSN, hereditary pressure-sensitive neuropathy; PWS, Prader-Willi syndrome; Rb, retinoblastoma plus other features; WAGR, Wilms tumor, aniridia, genital defects, retardation syndrome.

form is hardly ever seen in the classical cytogenetic rearrangement syndrome; but in contrast, familial transmission is quite often the case in molecular-demonstrable imbalances, and parental normality or near-normality can complicate interpretation of the imbalance.

In the majority of molecular-demonstrable del/dups of small size, for which the expression copy number variant[2] (CNV) is often applied, the transmission is simple Mendelian. The considerably more difficult questions relate to penetrance (Appendix C) and expressivity of the particular imbalance, and in some of smaller size, making a distinction from the CNV being a potentially harmless "variant of unknown significance" (VUS). Every chromosome is represented, some more often than others, and the experience of Colombian researchers is typical (Figure 14–2). The ways in which these structural rearrangements may arise are outlined in Chapter 3.

A rearrangement might be more complicated than a simple del or dup. Many examples are on record whereby terminal deletions, apparently simple on light microscopy, upon molecular investigation prove to be complex rearrangements with submicroscopic duplications, triplications, and inversions, in addition to the deletions. Zuffardi

[2] Since many of the conditions we discuss here typically present an abnormal phenotype, the usual CNV nomenclature would be "known pathogenic CNV." It may be less confusing to use the alternative nomenclature of microdeletion and microduplication, in which the inference of phenotypic abnormality is a given. See also the discussion in Chapter 18.

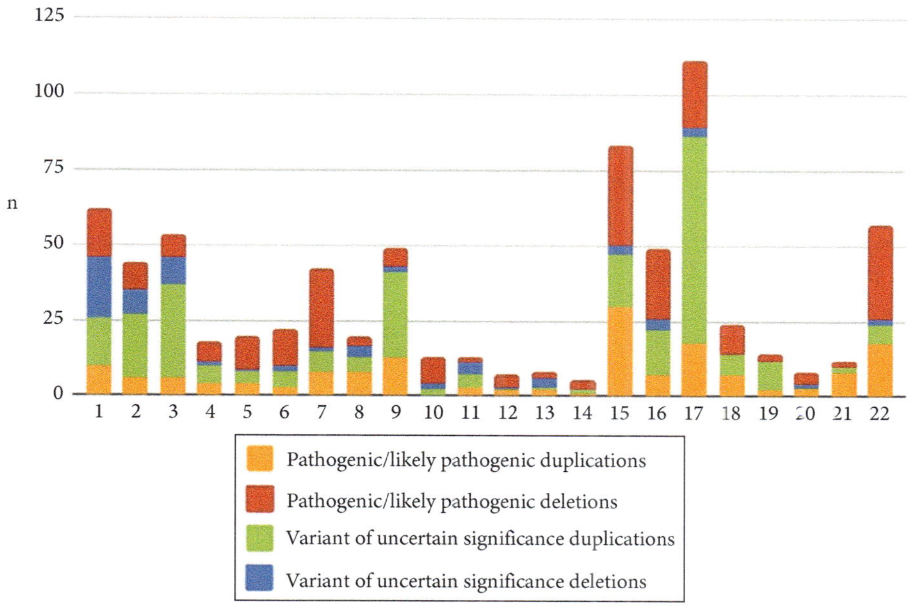

Figure 14–2. The Spread of 686 Autosomal Duplications and Deletions in a Cohort of 3,380 Cases Studied by Chromosomal Microarray over the Period 2016–2021 in Colombia.

Notes: The cases studied had presented due to the typical reasons for ordering a chromosome study, mostly neurodevelopmental delay, intellectual disability, autism spectrum disorder, short stature, and dysmorphisms. Not shown here are an additional 87 cases with sex chromosomal dup/dels.

Source: From YD Carrillo et al., Diagnostic yield of chromosomal microarray in the largest Latino clinical cohort, *Am J Med Genet* 194A:218–225, 2024. Courtesy JJ López-Rivera, and with the permission of John Wiley & Sons.

et al. (2009) propose that many "deletions" according to cytogenetic analysis are actually inverted duplications contiguous with terminal deletions.

> Some patients, indeed quite a number, previously testing normal on classical karyotyping have since been revealed on molecular testing as having a chromosomal imbalance. This belated discovery may make no real difference to management, but it is often a source of considerable relief to the parents to have, finally, a definite explanation for the problem. And of course, precise genetic advice can now be offered to others in the family.

CONTIGUOUS GENE SYNDROME

Recollect that loci are arranged in linear order along a chromosome. Some neighboring loci may be functionally related, but in others the contiguity is mere happenstance. The non-significance of two loci being adjacent has been likened to the unimportance one would attach to "Appalachian Mountains" being next to "apple" in an encyclopedia. Our genome differs from an encyclopedia in that about one-third of all the entries relate to one topic: the development and functioning of the brain—unsurprisingly so, this organ being, as it is said, the most complex structure in the known universe. Many of the other entries (loci) relate to the control of morphogenesis during embryonic life.

If a length of chromosome is deleted or duplicated, a sequence of adjacent (contiguous) genes will be lost or gained, and so the phenotype resulting from this imbalance can be described as a contiguous gene syndrome (Schmickel 1986; Tommerup 1993). In almost any deletion or duplication detectable cytogenetically, some of the loci deleted or in excess will be brain loci, while others could be for anything, but likely including some morphogenesis loci. Thus, we have the classic clinical picture in del/dup syndromes of intellectual deficit of some degree, dysmorphism, and in some, organ malformation. The deletion produces a monosomy—or "haploinsufficiency"—for the region of the chromosome that has been removed, and the outflow of genetic information is halved. Duplication causes a trisomy for the additional segment: a "triplo-excess" with a 150% amount of genetic information.

PHENOTYPES

While our focus in this book is substantially upon genetic risk, of course we must make reference to the clinical pictures observed in the setting of the several chromosomal aberrations we consider. Some of the deletions and duplications occur sufficiently frequently and/or present a sufficiently distinctive phenotype that they have acquired eponymic status, and the reader will be familiar with such names as Wolf, Hirschhorn, Williams, and cri du chat. The classical route whereby a chromosomal syndrome came to be established followed the recognition of a group of patients with a very similar clinical picture, often with a characteristic dysmorphology: the "phenotype-first" approach. Subsequent cytogenetic studies revealed the underlying chromosomal basis in common. Williams syndrome is a typical example: The facies and the cardiovascular malformation added up to a distinctive picture, recognized in 1961; but it was not until decades later, 1993, that the chromosomal basis was discovered.

Nowadays, taking the molecular approach, the typical path is "genotype-first," or "reverse dysmorphology." Subtle deletions and duplications may not present a distinctive enough phenotype that would allow the clinician to "call" a syndrome. But in the laboratory, data on recurrent rearrangements—whether seen in-house or often in collaboration with other cytogenetic services, nationally or internationally—can be collected. It is then up to the clinicians to draw together the observations from the patients thus identified and to construct the core features of the new syndrome. This approach of identifying the chromosomal abnormality first-up can reveal the natural clinical variation of the genomic rearrangements, which might scarcely have been possible with the traditional phenotype-first approach.

The brain is the organ exquisitely vulnerable to the effect of a genomic imbalance, and the phenotypes observed reflect this. The affected phenotype due to a small imbalance may be confined to a neurocognitive or behavioral disability; and many of the del/dups listed below include autism as a clinical manifestation (and see Figure 25–2). In some of the smaller-size del/dups detectable on molecular karyotyping, the natural clinical variation may include a brain-functional phenotype well within the range of essential normality. Otherwise, epilepsy, also a brain-functional trait, is a concomitant of several of the del and dup syndromes (Figure 25–7).

Some of the loci whose haploinsufficiency/triplo-excess contributes to the phenotype in the various deletion syndromes are being defined. It seems likely that many such genes will have their untoward outcome not in a simple one-to-one relationship with a single gene product, but rather in a complex layering and interlacing of consequential effects (Figure 3–21). As yet, however, it is mostly just the simple case that we can understand quite well: such as, for example, the brain white matter abnormality of the 18q− syndrome, which is presumably a direct consequence of the loss of one structural myelin gene, *MBP*, on 18q (Lammert et al. 2019). As molecular karyotyping defines del/dups of very small extent, only a few genes may be located within the particular segment, and the counselor blessed with a scientific curiosity has the opportunity to check which genes these are, and perhaps to make an informed speculation (which some parents might find helpful) as to which of these might have contributed to a child's phenotype.

If two or more Mendelian disorders coexist in the one person, a contiguous gene deletion is a strong possibility. In order to prove the point, molecular methodology can be brought to bear; or a direct chromosomal test using FISH offers an immediate visual demonstration of the deletion. We have, for example, seen a young woman presenting with a history of recurrent bacterial infections since childhood, and night blindness and diminishing peripheral vision since teen age, leading to diagnoses of, respectively, chronic granulomatous disease and retinitis pigmentosa (Coman et al. 2010b). The X-linked forms of these conditions being very closely linked, a contiguous gene deletion suggested itself, and a FISH probe targeted to a DNA sequence between the two loci was generated. Its non-hybridization to one X chromosome confirmed the supposition of a deletion. Furthermore, this led the way to another diagnosis, that of a partial protein intolerance, due to deletion of the *OTC* (ornithine transcarbamylase) gene that lies in the same Xp region.

BIOLOGY

Origin Intra-, Pre-, or Post-Meiosis

The "recurrent" category of de novo deletion or duplication is considered typically to reflect an origin during *meiosis*. Thus, for a number of deletion syndromes involving a recurrent segment—such as Williams, Prader-Willi, and Smith-Magenis syndromes, along with several others—a risk of recurrence is taken to be very low, because typically only the particular gamete from that particular parental meiosis carried the defect (Giglio et al. 2001; Saitta et al. 2004). These cases arise anew—"de novo"—with the affected child. On the other hand, imbalances which are single observations (or which are of a group involving a cytoband or bands in common, but with relatively distant breakpoints) are "non-recurrent," and knowledge about the likely origin for these may be scant. Some may indeed have been of meiotic origin, and therefore without increased risk of recurrence.

But, alternatively, a non-recurrent imbalance could have originated in a *premeiotic mitosis*. In that case, the abnormal cell line is confined to a "wedge" of the parental gonad (gonadal mosaicism), and the parent will have a normal phenotype and (on routine tissue sampling) a normal chromosome analysis (Figure 14–3). If, however, the abnormal cell line is present in the parental gonad and also in non-gonadal tissues (somatic-gonadal mosaicism), the parent may have an (often very subtly) abnormal phenotype, and the imbalance may be detectable, in a mosaic form, in parental blood. In either scenario, there is risk of the imbalance being passed to a child (in whom it would

2000s–2010s definition, reflecting the widespread application of molecular karyotyping in the early 21st century. All those del/dups listed in the ClinGen Curation of Recurrent CNVs, current at the time of writing, are included and noted with an asterisk (*), and penetrance data for recurrent CNVs is provided in Appendix C. Nucleotide numbers are mostly expressed in build hg38, but some in hg 19. Each chromosomal section is seen with a banded ideogram, taken from ISCN (2004), with particular segments subject to recurrent deletion/duplication indicated along with a selected relevant gene (or other identifier) located within that segment, as a useful "landmark." Longer or "busier" chromosomes have of necessity been divided into p and q arms. Some are illustrated with a display of the del/dup range against a karyotype, not merely for decoration but to familiarize the reader with this way of demonstrating these abnormalities. Only "pure" imbalances are considered; it is not feasible to include here those due to combination del/dups of different chromosomes.

We comment in greater or lesser length upon the genetics of each and, to the extent that knowledge allows, on recurrence risks; those in which recurrence has been recorded are given a more generous hearing. Clinical comments are mostly synoptic and selective, and "intellectual deficiency and facial dysmorphism" very frequently mentioned. Uncommon or distinctive or otherwise interesting phenotypic traits rate particular mentions. More perspectives on recurrent copy number variants are given in Chapter 18. The essays in *Cassidy and Allanson's* Management of Genetic Syndromes (2020) offer detailed commentaries for some of the more common of these syndromes. The UNIQUE website (rarechromo.org) has excellent quite detailed descriptions for some of the more common (or less rare) conditions.

Chromosome 1

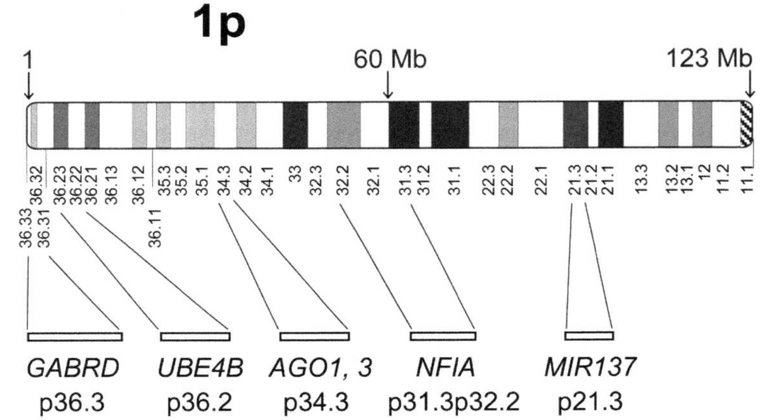

Figure 14–4.

1p21.3

Deletions. This microdeletion is rare (case reports barely in double figures; Willemsen et al. 2011b; D'Angelo et al. 2015), but it is of particular interest in that the reduced amount of a microRNA may be a key factor in determining the clinical picture of intellectual deficit of borderline/mild/moderate degree and abnormal behavior. For the most part, deletions are non-recurrent and of variable sizes. The smallest region of overlap, of 1 Mb in extent, runs from chr1:97.5-98.5 Mb, and including the sequence coding for *MIR137*. This microRNA is particularly expressed in certain brain regions, and it influences the functioning of client genes; its reduced activity has been correlated with psychiatric disease and with obesity (Strazisar et al. 2015; Tucci et al. 2016). Three of the cases in Willemsen et al. were siblings; their deceased parents were known to have been of low cognitive ability, and rather probably one of them had the same 1p21.3 deletion.

1p31.3p32.2

Deletion. This syndrome includes a functional neurocognitive and epileptic phenotype associated with brain malformation, commonly including agenesis of the corpus callosum along with limb and urinary tract defects. Labonne et al. (2016) provide a review and describe in detail their case of a young woman, first diagnosed on classical karyotyping as a 10-year-old. Moyamoya disease (narrowed arteries causing stroke) is associated (Pires de Oliveira-Sobrinho et al. 2024). Most arise de novo, but familial cases are on record. The syndrome could essentially have the alternative name of *NFIA* deletion (Revah-Politi et al. 2017; Bertini et al. 2022) (Figure 14–5).

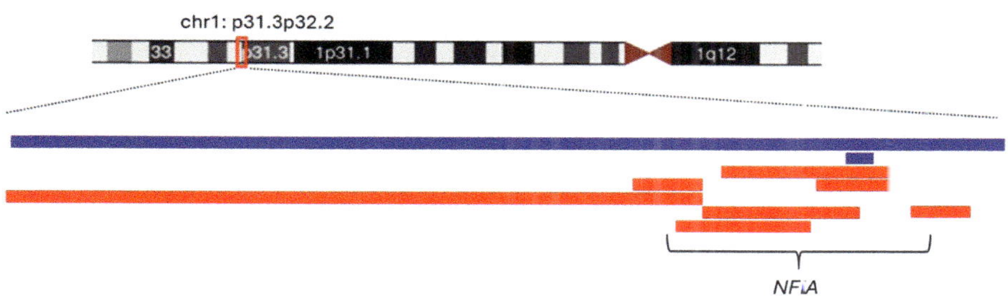

Figure 14–5. 1p31.3p32.2 Deletions and Duplication.

Notes: Deletions in red, duplication in blue. All encompass the *NFIA* gene.

Source: From V Bertini et al., Phenotypic spectrum of *NFIA* haploinsufficiency: Two additional cases and review of the literature, *Genes (Basel)* 13:2249, 2022. Courtesy A Orsini, and with the permission of MDPI.

1p34.3

Deletions in this cytoband, similarly to del 1p21.3 above, may also have their pathogenic effect through a perturbation of the microRNA system. Tokita et al. (2015) describe deletions of sizes 1.1 Mb–3.1 Mb, with *AGO1* and *AGO3* (at chr1:36.3 Mb) resident in the 290 kb segment in common. These are "argonaute" genes, whose products direct the process of post-transcriptional gene silencing (that is, RNA interference); their removal may be the basis of the observed phenotype of hypotonia, moderate intellectual disability, and subtle facial dysmorphism. Galesi et al. (2022) analyze in detail the behavioral traits of their patient, a 9⅔-year-old boy, who had particular deficits in hyperactivity and inattention components of ADHD at the 95th–98th percentile, and restlessness/impulsivity at the 95th–98th percentile. A de novo origin has been observed in all tested cases.

1p36.11

Duplication including the *ARID1A* gene is the basis of this rare, but recurrent condition, albeit that the breakpoints are heterogeneous (Bidart et al. 2017). Microcephaly is common.

1p36.22p36.21

Duplication. The physical phenotype is that of "focal facial dermal hypoplasia type 3," also known as Setleis syndrome, characterized by atrophic facial lesions and otherwise facial dysmorphism, and aberrant hair growth. Duplications (and triplications) are non-recurrent and of varying extents; a set of four duplicated genes are seen in common (Oh et al. 2023). Of the few cases thus far reported, developmental delay has been a feature in most, but an example is also on record of an intellectually normal man with Setleis syndrome, who had inherited the duplication from his phenotypically normal (and non-mosaic) carrier father (Lee et al. 2015).

1p36.3

Deletion. This is one of the more common deletion syndromes, seen in from one in 5,000 to 10,000 births. We may speak of a distal "classical" (Group A) deletion and a more proximal (Group B) deletion. Within these broad categories, Jacquin et al. (2023) delineate four subgroups, clustering around common regions of overlap (Figure 14–6).

The most usually encountered is the *distal "classical"* deletion. *GABRD* is proposed to be an important pheno-critical locus. The facies is variably dysmorphic, with deep-set eyes and midface retrusion a particular observation, and several minor physical anomalies may be observed (Shimada et al. 2014; Jordan et al. 2015). The intellectual disability is usually severe; an unsurprising observation given that perisylvian polymicrogyria, a major brain malformation is seen in some, and it is plausible that in others, anatomic defect might be beyond MRI resolution. Also, defects in white matter are common (Õiglane-Shlik et al. 2014). A milder phenotype is seen in the mosaic case (Shimada et al. 2014). A phenotypic overlap with Angelman syndrome and Rett syndrome has been noted.

In the review of Jacquin et al. (2023), inheritance data was available in 54 cases. Of these 50 (93%) were de novo. The deletion was seen in three parents (mosaic in one) and from a translocation in one. Other rare examples of familial transmission are known, including due to presumed parental gonadal mosaicism (Di Donato et al. 2014; Nistico' et al. 2020).

1q12q31

Duplication. A very large 50 Mb duplication, ~40% of the length of the long arm, is reported in Sifakis et al. (2014) concerning a fetus of 23 weeks gestation with multiple malformations. They review a very heterogeneous prenatally diagnosed dup(1q) series from the literature; termination had been chosen in almost all, while survival was mostly measured in minutes or days in the pregnancies going to live birth. The even larger duplication described as 1q21qter, a length of fully 100 Mb, causes multiple severe, lethal malformations (Machlitt et al. 2005).

*1q21.1**

Deletion. Two recurrent deletions reside within this segment (Figure 14–8), each flanked by numbered breakpoint low-copy repeat regions (BPs 2 to 4) that dictate a susceptibility to rearrangement due to unequal crossing-over (Edwards et al. 2021; Pang et al. 2020; Bourgois et al. 2024). Both deletions are characterized by incomplete penetrance, and may thus be discovered when phenotypically normal parents of an affected child are karyotyped. A larger 2.15 Mb recurrent deletion encompasses both smaller deletions.

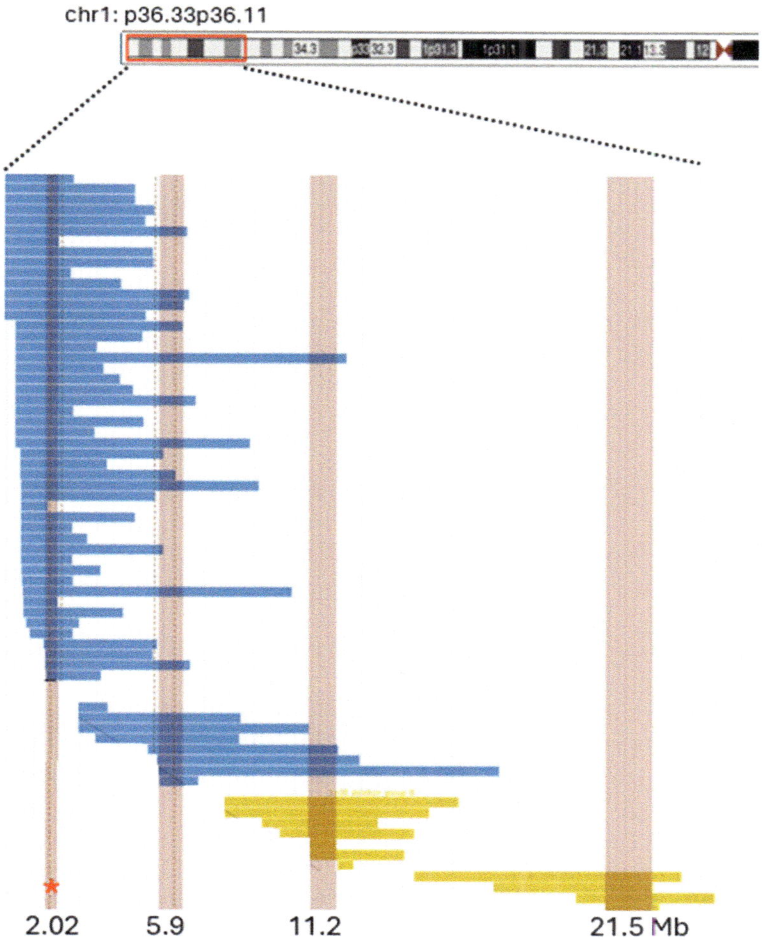

Figure 14–6. The Different Categories of 1p36 Deletions.

Notes: There are two major critical regions, seen in patients from Groups A and B respectively: a more common "classic" distal deletion (cases in blue bars), and a proximal deletion (orange bars). The minimal regions of overlap (MRO) that characterize four subgroups within the major grouping are shown as the pink shading. Red asterisk = *GABRD* site.

Source: Adapted from C Jacquin et al., 1p36 deletion syndrome: Review and mapping with further characterization of the phenotype, a new cohort of 86 patients, *Am J Med Genet* 191A:445–458, 2023. Courtesy C Jacquin, and with the permission of John Wiley & Sons.

Duplication. The typical recurrent duplication at 1q21.1 involves the same segment as the distal region in the countertype deletion (Figure 14–9). The phenotype of this duplication includes intellectual disability (or at least borderline cognitive functioning) and autism. As the deletion leads to microcephaly, so does the duplication cause macrocephaly; brain scanning may show reduced white matter volume. Dolcetti et al. (2013) document an increased risk for schizophrenia. A range of heart defects are seen (tetralogy of Fallot having a particular association), likely relating to a triplo-excess of *GJA5* (Soemedi et al. 2012; Digilio et al. 2013). In the review of Bernier et al (2016), of those patients whose parents were studied, all but one were familial cases. It is true to

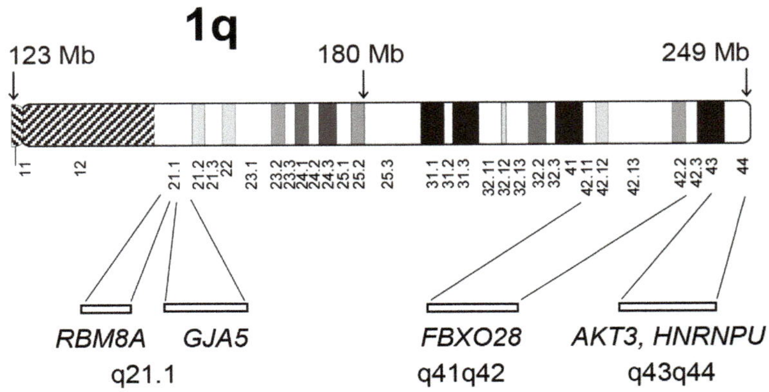

Figure 14–7.

say that incomplete penetrance and variable expressivity complicate interpretation and counseling; an important factor here is likely the role of CNVs elsewhere in the genome (Qiao et al. 2017). Triplication of 1q21.1 is described in Van Dijck et al. (2015).

*1q21.1 (proximal)**

Deletion. The smaller proximal deletion at BP 2-3 is 0.3 Mb in size and includes *RBM8A* (Figure 14–8). The 1q21.1 proximal deletion has the particular interest of being a susceptibility factor for thrombocytopenia-absent radius (TAR) syndrome (Strauss et al. 2023). The majority of TAR, 90% or more, is due to having a 1q21.1 deletion on one chromosome and a hypomorphic *RBM8A* variant (in 3% of European populations) on

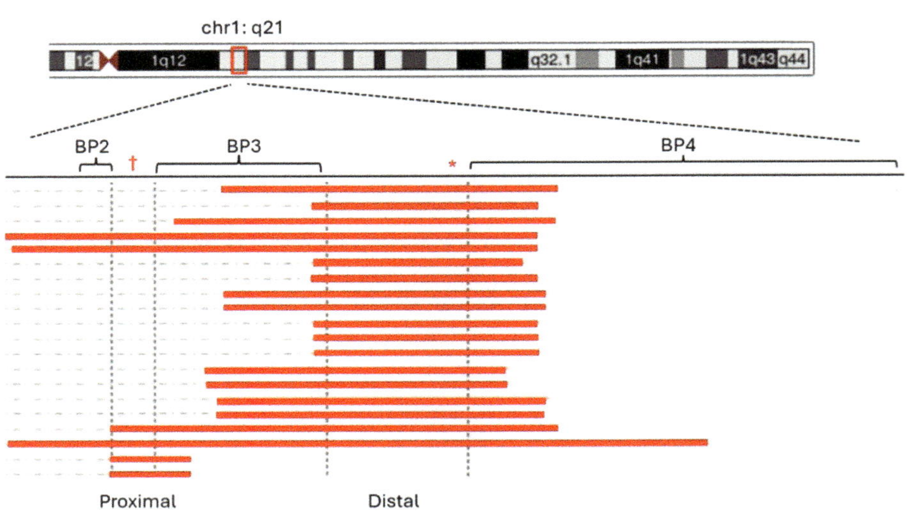

Figure 14–8. The Range of Deletions at 1q21.1.

Notes: The sequences labelled BP (breakpoint) 2 to 4 comprise low-copy repeats, which promote unequal recombination between them. Imbalances can involve the proximal region (between BP2-3), the distal region (between BP3-4), or can span both regions. †Position of *RBM8A*, *position of *GJA5.*

Source: From H Pang et al., Disorders associated with diverse, recurrent deletions and duplications at 1q21.1, *Front Genet* 11:577, 2020. Courtesy S Li and H Gu, and with the permission of Frontiers in Genetics.

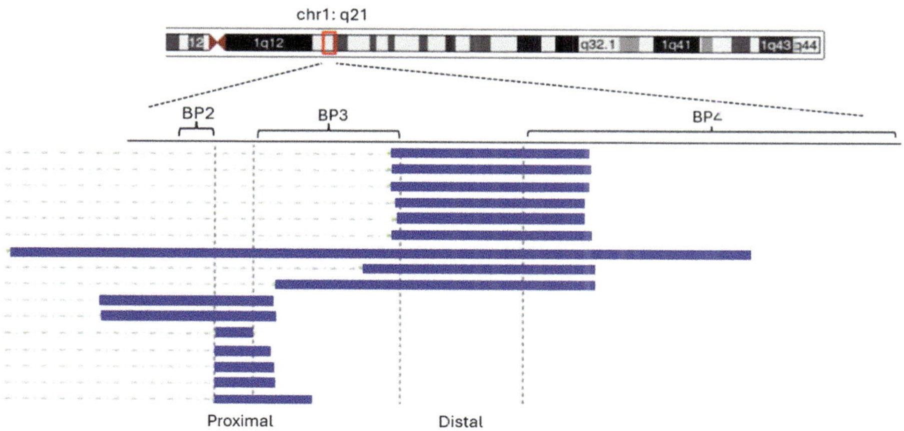

Figure 14–9. The Range of Duplications at 1q21.1.

Notes: The sequences labelled BP (breakpoint) 2 to 4 comprise low-copy repeats, which promote unequal recombination between them. Imbalances can involve the proximal region (between BP2-3), the distal region (between BP3-4), or can span both regions.

Source: From H Pang et al., Disorders associated with diverse, recurrent deletions and duplications at 1q21.1, *Front Genet* 11:577, 2020. Courtesy S Li and H Gu, and with the permission of Frontiers in Genetics.

the other. The deletion is usually (75%) familial, but may be de novo. Where one parent is heterozygous for the deletion and the other carries one or other of the *RBM8A* SNPs, the pattern of inheritance of TAR mimics that of autosomal recessive disease, with its attendant recurrence risk. Goh et al. (2025) calculate a penetrance for proximal 1q21.1 deletion of 18%, but it remains unclear to what extent this penetrance includes neurodevelopmental disability in addition to TAR syndrome.

Duplication. The countertype duplication of the proximal 1q21.1 segment (Figure 14–9) may be a susceptibility variant of incomplete penetrance contributing to a largely neurobehavioral but also malformative phenotype in several, although with normality in some carriers (Levy et al. 2023). Goh et al. (2025) calculate a penetrance of 9%. Maternal transmission appears to be more harmful than from the father. Familial epilepsy co-segregating with dup(1)q21.1 is recorded in Fanciulli et al. (2014).

*1q21.1 (distal)**

Deletion. The distal 1q21.1 microdeletion (*GJA5*) at BP 3-4 (Figure 14–8) is one of the more common CNVs observed in clinical cohorts. The clinical picture includes cognitive impairment, autism, seizures, cardiac defects, cataract, and minor dysmorphic features. The 1q21.1 distal CNV has a large effect on head circumference, with a high prevalence of microcephaly in deletion carriers and macrocephaly in duplication carriers (Sønderby et al. 2021). Some are de novo cases, some familial with a (usually mildly) affected parent, and some are familial from an apparently unaffected parent; penetrance in Goh et al. (2025) is 30%.

A detailed study in Bernier et al. (2016) documents the phenotypic range, with a particular focus on neurocognitive/psychological/behavioral traits. They note that while IQ might "officially" be in a normal range—that is, above 70—the average was about one standard deviation below the mean. Phonological processing, the ability to distinguish the meanings of words, is notably impaired. Digilio et al. (2013) describe a family in which a brother had pulmonary valve stenosis and an IQ of 87; his sister had learning difficulties, with an IQ of 58; and the daughter of this sister had moderate intellectual disability (IQ of 48) and difficult behavior, absence seizures, a complex heart defect, and some dysmorphic features. Each had the same 1q21.1 deletion. As can apply in the generality of microimbalances, loci elsewhere, if variant, may exacerbate the clinical phenotype (and indeed bring to medical attention a family that might otherwise have escaped notice).

Duplication. Distal 1q21.1 duplication (Figure 14–9) has a nonspecific phenotype comprising mild to moderate cognitive impairment and neuropsychiatric and behavioral findings, along with macrocephaly (Sønderby et al. 2021). There is an increased risk of cardiac disease and diabetes. The duplication is usually inherited, with penetrance of 19% (Goh et al. 2025).

A larger, 5 Mb duplication 1q21.1q21.2 in Brisset et al. (2015) was in company with a 16p11.2 deletion, and the phenotype in the child more severe than a simple "sum of the parts"—a multiplicative two-hit. The dup 1q21 had come from the father, and the del 16p11.2 from the mother; the father suffered from psychopathy and mild intellectual disability, and the mother from depression. A yet larger duplication, 1q21.1q44, is recorded in mosaic state in brain tissue from a non-dysmorphic child suffering from intractable epilepsy, who had had surgical resection of a part of one frontal lobe (Conti et al. 2015). On imaging, and subsequently on histopathology, the cerebral cortex was dysplastic. Triplo-excess of *AKT3* (see dup 1q43q44, below) may have led to the brain defect. The duplication was not seen in blood or saliva; the abnormality likely arose at a post-zygotic mitosis in neuroectodermal tissue at an early stage of embryonic development, and was confined to this lineage.

1q21.3

Deletion. The few cases on record of this small deletion have involved different breakpoints, but all including these disease-associated loci: *GATAD2B*, *TPM3*, and *HAX1*, of which *GATAD2B* is likely to have the major role in determining the phenotype, which includes an intellectual disability and a characteristic facies (Tim-Aroon et al. 2017).

1q23.3

Duplication. A familial dup 1q23.3 is described in Speevak and Farrell (2013), a presumed benign copy number variant including two genes, *MPZ* and *SDHC*, seen in three generations: a grandfather, father, and one child. But in a second child, the duplication was itself duplicated, to give a 1q23.3 "quadruplication." This infant presented with a severe form of Charcot-Marie-Tooth (CMT) neuropathy due to the excess dosage of the *MPZ* gene (mutation in which is the usual basis of CMT type 1B). The quadruplication may represent a second nonallelic homologous recombination (NAHR) event on this no. 1 chromosome in the family, the first having occurred one cannot say how many generations ago.

1q32.1q44

Duplication. These distal long arm duplications are of substantial size, up to 42 Mb, and thus readily detectable on classical cytogenetics; the proximal breakpoint is variable (Balasubramanian et al. 2009). The clinical picture is one of a distinctive facial dysmorphism, due in particular to craniofacial bone maldevelopment along with developmental delay. Whether an association with myelodysplastic syndrome in one dup 1q41qter case is causal or coincidental remains to be established (Morokawa et al. 2018).

1q41q42

Deletion. This syndrome is to be numbered among those with an Angelman resemblance. Intellectual disability and seizures are observed. Loci *FBXO28* and *WDR26* are proposed as key pheno-contributory factors (Yanagishita et al. 2019; Bi et al. 2023); the characteristic facies is notably similar to cases with a point mutation at the *WDR26* locus (Skraban-Deardorff syndrome). All cases have been de novo, except for the small (63 kb) deletion in Bi et al., which had been transmitted from a phenotypically unaffected father.

1q43q44

Deletion. There is considerable variation in the extent of these deletions (Figure 14–10). Microcephaly may be due to the *AKT3* haploinsufficiency; agenesis of the corpus callosum might be consequential upon deletion of the regulatory factor *ZNF238*, while seizures could inhere in the *HNRNPU* gene in those in whom these loci are lost (Ballif et al. 2012; Depienne et al. 2017; Pelle et al. 2020). The ways in which these and other genes within the segment may interact and impact upon head size are rehearsed in Raun et al. (2017). We have seen a young woman—originally and not unreasonably diagnosed as Rett syndrome—with severe epilepsy, but normal on *MECP2* mutation study in the early 1990s; microarray some 20 years later showed a microdeletion chr1:244.4-245.3 Mb (hg19) (R Beddow, personal communication, 2012). *HNRNPU* was the only one of the above-mentioned three genes included in this segment; very similar deletions are reported in Thierry et al. (2012).

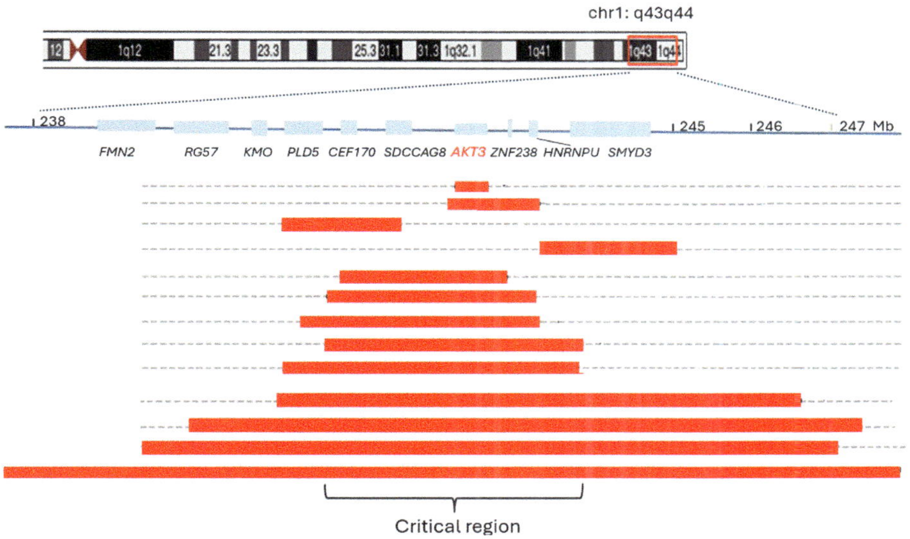

Figure 14–10. Deletions of 1q43q44.

Notes: Loci within the broad range of deletions, and within the critical region, shown; the pheno-critical locus is proposed to be *AKT3*. Scale is in hg38.

Source: Adapted from B Khadija et al., Clinical and molecular characterization of 1q43q44 deletion and corpus callosum malformations: 2 new cases and literature review, *Mol Cytogenet* 15:42, 2022. Courtesy B Khadija and S Mougou-Zerelli, and with the permission of Springer Nature.

De novo inheritance is the norm, but very rare familial cases are recognized (Ballif et al. 2012). Gai et al. (2015) describe a normal father and his microcephalic son, both carrying a 1q44 deletion removing just the *AKT3* gene. Parental very-low-level (3.4% on blood) somatic and inferentially gonadal mosaicism has been demonstrated (Campbell et al. 2014).

Duplication, triplication, and quadruplication of 1q43q44 are on record (Lopes et al. 2019). The interest here is the proposed role of the *AKT3* gene, which is a component of the important PI3K growth control pathway. The macrocephaly typically associated has its counterpart in the microcephaly due to the deletion. A single instance of parental transmission concerns a father and son with a 1 Mb quadruplication.

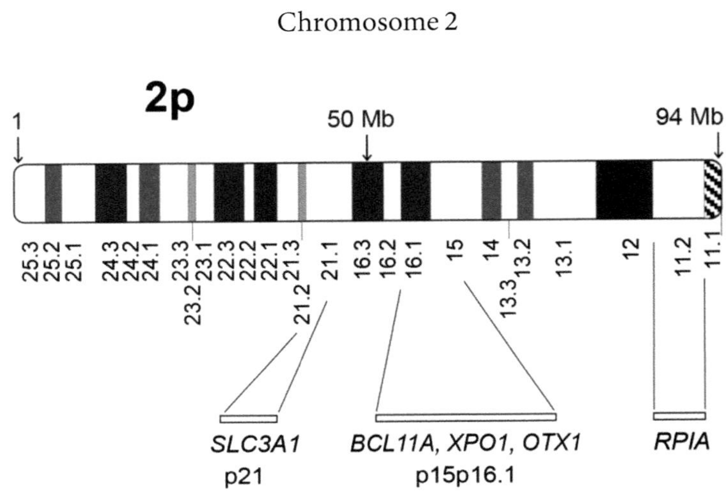

Figure 14–11.

*2p11.2**

Deletion. Ferrario et al. (2023) review the 10 cases then reported. Key loci are taken to be *EIF2AK3* and *RPIA*. The phenotype encompasses an intellectual disability of borderline to moderate degree and, in some, a functional neurological disorder. A single case is known of parental transmission, from a father who had had only surgery for hypoacusia, to an affected daughter who had unilateral microtia and atresia of the external auditory canal; Ferrario and colleagues propose triplo-excess of *FOXI3* to be responsible for this latter trait.

2p16.1p15

Deletions of up to 10 Mb within this region are non-recurrent, and all have been de novo. Miceli et al. (2023) determined shortest regions of overlap of the deletion in a review of 38 cases, identifying those including the landmark genes *BCL11A* alone, *USP34/XPO1* alone, and both *BCL11A* and *USP34/XPO1*, the phenotypes differing accordingly (Figure 14–12). Fannemel et al. (2014) describe a man having the smallest recorded deletion (230 kb), removing the *USP34/XPO1* gene, who was mildly dysmorphic and intellectually affected but able to have sheltered employment.

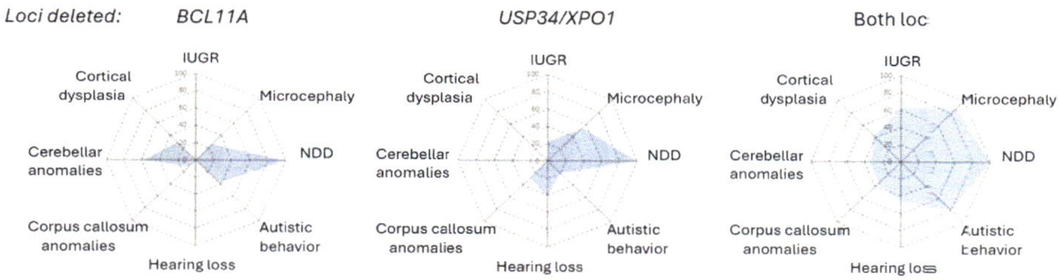

Figure 14–12. Phenotypic Variation in 2p15p16.1 Deletions, According to the Two Key Loci Lost.

Notes: These "radar plots" give a visual indication of how severe a particular trait is, according to its distance from the central 0 point, in relation to which loci have been deleted (*BCL11A* alone, *USP34/XPO1* alone, or both). By eye, severity with both loci deleted is cumulative. IUGR, intrauterine growth retardation; NDD, neurodevelopmental delay.

Source: From M Miceli et al., Trait-driven analysis of the 2p15p16.1 microdeletion syndrome suggests a complex pattern of interactions between candidate genes, *Genes Genomics* 45:491–505, 2023. Courtesy M Fichera, and with the permission of Springer.

Duplication. Twelve cases of dup2p15p16.1 in which the duplication includes *BCL11A* and *PIX13* are listed in Wang et al. (2023a), and another two in which *PEX13* was the only gene in common. Little clinical information was available for some of these cases (from the DECIPHER and ISCA databases); the child in Mimouni-Bloch et al. (2015) had a mild developmental delay, attention deficit and oppositional behavior, and mild dysmorphism. The macrocephaly seen in some cases is a countertype to the microcephaly observed with the deletion. *BCL11A*, in those cases duplicated for this gene, bids fair as a pheno-critical candidate. All those in whom parental studies were noted were of de novo generation.

2p16.3

Deletion. Non-recurrent deletions of *NRXN1*, at 2p16.3, cause a range of neurodevelopmental phenotypes including intellectual disability, autism, epilepsy, and schizophrenia. The *NRXN1* gene is large and generates hundreds of splicing isoforms, complicating the interpretation of exonic deletions (Montalbano et al. 2024). Goh et al. (2025) estimated penetrance of 37% for deletions that include at least one exon of *NRXN1*, but this may vary with the size of the deletion and exons involved.

2p21

Deletion. This extremely rare syndrome is unusual in being seen in only the homozygous state (Bartholdi et al. 2013), and thus displaying an autosomal recessive mode of inheritance. The loci implicated are *PPM1B, SLC3A1, PREPL,* and *CAMKMT. SLC3A1* is the basis of the cystinuria seen in the syndrome (a smaller deletion including just *SLC3A1* and *PREPL* leads to the hypotonia-cystinuria syndrome). Seizures, intellectual disability, and a Prader-Willi-like facial dysmorphism are observed.

2p22.3-p22.2

Deletion. Quiñones-Pérez et al. (2018) report a 3-generation family in which some members had a clinical picture reminiscent of Marfan or Loeys-Dietz syndrome. The transmission of a 2p22.3p22.2 segment, within which 11 loci were accommodated and of

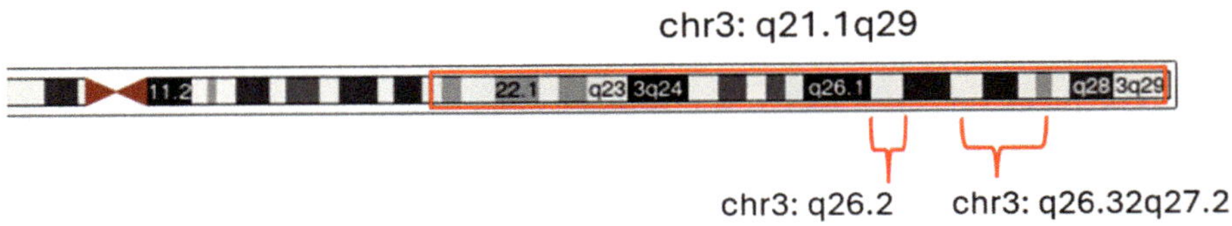

Figure 14–19. Duplication Regions of 3q, Common Segments Indicated.
Notes: A wide range of duplication within this very large segment are on record, a few encompassing over half of the entire segment (Molck et al. 2018).

Prader-Willi phenotype. Both had a mild pervasive developmental disorder. At least the larger duplication was confirmed de novo; it is likely both were.

3q22.3q25

Deletion. According to the extent of deletion within this chromosomal region, the phenotype may include features of blepharophimosis-epicanthus inversus syndrome (BPES),[7] the Dandy-Walker cerebellar malformation, and the Wisconsin syndrome. Ferraris et al. (2013) define three critical regions within which the deletions of the observed cases have fallen. Deletions that remove *FOXL2* (at q22.3) produce BPES; loss of *ZIC1* and *ZIC4* (q24) likely contributes to the cerebellar defect (but this component of incomplete penetrance); and deletions extending into 3q25.2 may lead to Wisconsin syndrome. Thus, a child described in Ferraris et al. who carried a large 3q22.1q25.1 deletion, 19.2 Mb in length and which removed the *FOXL2, ZIC1*, and *ZIC4* genes, had both BPES and Dandy-Walker malformation as part of the overall complicated clinical picture. The Wisconsin syndrome, characterized by a distinctive facial gestalt, may reside more distally, with the loci *MBNL1* and *WWTR1* plausibly key factors (Okano et al. 2022).

3q22.2q29

Duplications within this segment are of considerable length and can be 60 Mb or more. This is large enough that the condition—named the "dup(3q) syndrome"—was detectable on classical cytogenetics as early as 1966 by Falek et al. (1966). The clinical phenotype is notable in a resemblance to Cornelia de Lange syndrome (and indeed this dup(3q) misled early efforts to locate the gene).

3q26.32q28

Deletion. This rare syndrome is due to deletion of variable (2 to 8.4 Mb) extent (Robilliard and Caylan 2020), and in some is more accurately described as del 3q26.3q27.2. A distinctive facies, intellectual disability, and severe growth retardation characterize the clinical picture. Where studied, cases have been of de novo origin.

Duplication. Two regions declare themselves as recurrent: dups which include 3q26.2, and those including 3q26.32q27.2 (Figure 14–19). There may be complex dysmorphology; the frequent observation of caudal abnormalities in the latter duplication may lie in the loss of *DVL3* and/or *EPHB3* at 3q27.1 (Pavone et al. 2016; Dworschak et al. 2017). A pheno-contributory role for *TBL1XR1* is proposed in Riehmer et al. (2017), who studied a familial case in which a mother and two offspring were duplicated for a very small segment of 521

[7] Isolated BPES may be due to a translocation having one breakpoint in this region, but distant from the actual gene—a laboratory diagnosis that might be missed unless a karyotype is preformed (Yang et al. 2014).

kb, at 3q26.32. Most of these duplications have arisen following a parental malsegregation of a translocation involving chromosome 3; pure cases are less frequent.

3q27.3

Deletion. This syndrome gained definition through interrogation of the DECIPHER database. Thevenon et al. (2014) collected recorded patients with variable non-recurrent deletions, in whom two shortest regions of overlap (SRO) were identified. A slender and gloomy facial appearance is very distinctive (Castori et al. 2015). The *SST* gene (within SRO1) may be responsible for the neuropsychiatric picture ranging from autism to psychosis, and the *AHSG* gene (in SRO2, which extends into q27.2) for the somewhat Marfanoid skeletal phenotype. Most arise de novo, but parental transmission is known.

*3q29**

Deletion. This recurrent 1.6 Mb deletion encompasses the neighboring *DLG1* and *BDH* loci (Città et al. 2013). Variable behavioral traits, mild to moderate intellectual disability with microcephaly, and mild facial dysmorphism are core features of the phenotype; the facies is sufficiently distinctive that a phenotyping algorithm (Face2Gene) can recognize it (Mak et al. 2021). Some, in addition, have clefting and genitourinary malformation. The deletion predisposes very significantly to schizophrenia, indeed a 41-fold increased risk (Mulle 2015). Glassford et al. (2016) were able to recruit a cohort of 44 cases and documented neuropsychiatric traits including anxiety disorder, panic attacks, depression, and bipolar disorder, as well as schizophrenia. These psychiatric traits reflect, in part at least, a hypoplasia of the cerebellum (Figure 14–20); genes influencing cerebellar formation within 3q29, such as *BDH1* and *DLG1*, may be instrumental in this respect (Sefik et al. 2024).

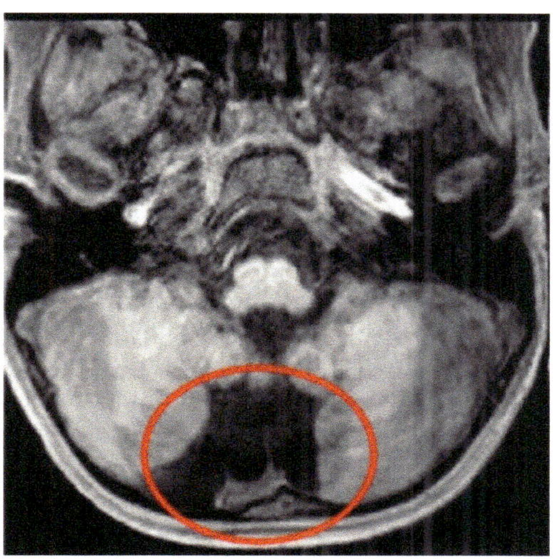

Figure 14–20. The Cerebellum in 3q29 Deletion.

Notes: The red circle shows near-complete absence (hypoplasia) of brain tissue in the midline, between the cerebellar hemispheres. The cerebellum has a major role in cognition and liability for psychopathology, along with its classic role in motor control.

Source: From E Sefik et al., Structural deviations of the posterior fossa and the cerebellum and their cognitive links in a neurodevelopmental deletion syndrome, *Mol Psychiatry* 29:3395–3411, 2024. Courtesy JG Mulle and S Shultz, and with the permission of Springer Nature.

2024). The cri[9] in the newborn is characteristic, and may even allow the diagnosis to be suspected, sight unseen, as one enters the neonatal nursery. Van Buggenhout et al. (2000) document in quite some detail, with several photographs, the phenotypes in seven older individuals, teenagers and adults; and Nguyen et al. (2015) provide detail collected from a support group (the 5p Minus Family Database). Cognitive compromise is typically mild/moderate in more distal small (5p15.31pter) deletions, moderate to severe with deletions from 5pter to 5p14.1, and profound in those extending into 5p13.2p13.3 (Marignier et al. 2012).

While most cases are sporadic, about 10% are due to a familial translocation, and this possibility should be checked for in each case; a rare cause is a large parental inversion (Ohnuki et al. 2010). Cases of recurrence of del(5) attest to the reality of parental gonadal mosaicism (Hajianpour et al. 1991; Alkaya et al. 2020). Very seldom, in milder cases, parental transmission may be seen; here, a more distal deletion is common. These transmitting parents typically display a compromised cognitive and behavioral phenotype. Almeida et al. (2024) report a mildly intellectually affected mother and her two moderately affected children, in whom the 6.2 Mb deletion did not include *CTNND2*. Both children had a high-pitched cry as babies. Remarkably, Zhang et al. (2016a) describe one del(5p) father who had had a cat-like cry as a baby, learning difficulty at school, and who was yet able to graduate with a bachelor's degree in computer science. The deletion had been transmitted through three generations of his family.

More proximal deletions, outside of the core cri du chat region, may not necessarily impose a phenotype. Papoulidis et al. (2013) report a man (a physician) presenting only with infertility, who carried a de novo interstitial 15.5 Mb deletion at 5p13.3p14.3, this segment being described as somewhat of a "gene desert."

5q11.2

Deletion. This rare disorder has the interest of an associated immunodeficiency, presenting as recurrent infections, along with a learning disorder and mild dysmorphism. Deletions are non-recurrent. A key locus may be *DHX29*, while the immunodeficiency may reside in loss of *IL6ST* (Arora et al. 2019; Bayat et al. 2021). All cases have occurred de novo.

5q14

Deletion. This condition has some resemblance to Rett syndrome. The severe intellectual disability is associated with the brain malformation, microcephaly with simplified gyral pattern. Most but not all involve the deletion of *MEF2C* at 5q14.3 (Fernández Hernández et al. 2021). In some, deletions may be small enough that only *MEF2C* is removed.

Duplication. As with the 5q14 deletion, the neurocognitive phenotype of this rare imbalance inheres in the *MEF2C* locus. Duplications are of varying size. Cesaretti et al. (2016) documented, at the level of macroscopic fetal neuropathology, partial agenesis of the corpus callosum. All cases have been de novo.

5q22q23

Deletion: Polyposis Plus Syndrome. A minor degree of facial dysmorphism and mild to moderate intellectual disability are nonspecific features seen in these deletions; the

[9] The name of the syndrome was whimsically given by nurses at Hôpital Enfants-Malades, Paris.

unique feature is adenomatous polyposis of the bowel, and indeed it was such a deletion that led to discovery of the *APC* (adenomatous polyposis coli) gene (Hockey et al. 1989). Absence of one *APC* allele of itself allows polyps to develop, and any subsequent mutation/loss of the allele on the intact chromosome 5 then leads to loss of the tumor suppressor function of this gene. If mental capacity is only mildly affected, parenthood is achievable, but of course with a risk of transmission (Tanabe et al. 2024).

Duplication. The large 5q22.1q23.2 duplication, of variable extent and obvious on classical cytogenetics, is associated with a clinical picture of variable intellectual disability, typically microcephaly, minor facial dysmorphism, and short stature. In the cases reported in Schmidt et al. (2013) of an affected mother and her two children, the (inverted tandem) duplication extended approximately from the *CAMK4* to the *ZNF608* loci, encompassing a little over 14 Mb in length.

5q31

Deletion. The clinical picture in this rare 5q31.2q31.3 deletion syndrome is predominantly neurodevelopmental, with severe intellectual disability, marked hypotonia, apneic episodes, and poor feeding. A particular observation is abnormal movements in the neonatal period resembling a seizure, but with no epileptic activity on the electroencephalogram. Brain MRI shows poor frontal lobe structure (Brown et al. 2013). Bonaglia et al. (2015) record the life history of the oldest known patient, who survived to age 26 years. Deletion sizes range from approximately 1 Mb to 5 Mb, and *PURA* and *LRRTM2* are proposed as key loci (Kleffmann et al. 2012). We may need to consider that two "subsyndromes" exist: one defined by loss of *PURA*, in which epilepsy is a feature (Kofoed et al. 2024), and another by loss of *LRRTM2*, although most del 5q31.2q31.3 deletions combine the two. All cases have been de novo.

*5q35**

Deletion: Sotos Syndrome. The central locus in this overgrowth syndrome is *NSD1*. An alternative name is cerebral gigantism, and macrocephaly is essentially invariable: brain imaging shows cortical malformation in most (Neeman et al. 2024). Mild-to-severe intellectual impairment is universal. A curious observation in the genetics of Sotos syndrome is an ethnic difference: about half of Japanese cases are due to microdeletion 5q35.2q35.3, but only 10% of a UK population (the remainders having an *NSD1* point mutation). Furthermore, deletion lengths varied quite considerably in UK cases, from 0.5 Mb to 5.0 Mb; but in the Japanese, most had a recurrent 1.9 Mb deletion, chr5:176.1-178.0 Mb. A similar picture is seen in Korean patients (Sohn et al. 2013). These differences likely reflect an ethnic heterogeneity of "genomic architecture," and specifically the nature of flanking low-copy repeats, which may predispose to rearrangement (Tatton-Brown et al. 2005; Mochizuki et al. 2008). A large majority of deletions occur de novo on the paternal chromosome.

Duplication. The dup (5)(q35.2q35.3) is the countertype of the deletion, and growth is in the opposite direction to Sotos syndrome: length and head circumference are typically more than two standard deviations below the mean, and bone age is delayed. Parental transmission has been recorded, although the majority represent de novo cases. Van der Lugt et al. (2023) report a minimally affected mother and her markedly affected son, raising the matter of a considerable intra-familial variability. A duplication of somewhat greater distal extent, typically to 5qter, is referred to as Hunter-McAlpine syndrome (Jamsheer et al. 2013; Žilina et al. 2013).

Chromosome 6

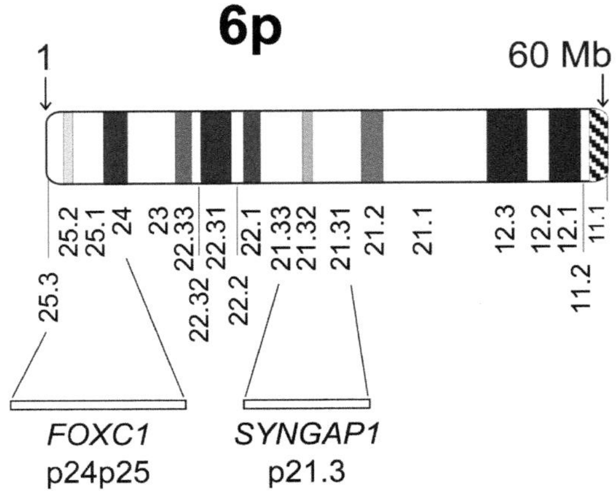

Figure 14–25.

6p21.1p12.3

Duplication. Savarese et al. (2013) report duplication for a 13.8 Mb segment at 6p21.31p12.3 transmitted from a mildly disabled mother to her daughter; these two bear a most striking facial resemblance to each other. Contained within this segment is band 6p21.1, and Varvagiannis et al. (2013) focus on the syndrome confined to dup(6)(p21.1), noting that the most remarkable feature was a craniosynostosis and proposing that an additional dose of *RUNX2* (the gene for cleidocranial dysplasia) may be the basis of this. The duplication may be due to a 6p-containing de novo translocation (Sivasankaran et al. 2017; Türkyılmaz et al. 2023).

6p25p24

Deletion. Terminal deletions at 6p25 may involve just that band, or extend into 6p24 or further (Qi et al. 2015) (Figure 14–26). The "deleted region in common" includes the *FOXC1* gene. Eye defects are common (Le et al. 2023). Brain imaging can show a cerebellar malformation and variable leukoencephalopathy (Cellini et al. 2012; Delahaye et al. 2012). Prenatal diagnosis, following ultrasonographic demonstration of multiple anomalies, is recorded (Ergin et al. 2015). Vernon et al. (2013) report an adult, of normal intelligence (certainly an atypical observation), with a CADASIL-like[10] leukoencephalopathy, who showed a del 6p25.3p25.2 (chr6:0.2-2.7 Mb) karyotype, *FOXC1* included in the deleted segment.

A notable familial case is described in Qi et al. (2015): A mother mosaic del(6p)/dup(6p)/normal for the interstitial segment 6p25.1p24.3 (chr6:4.74-10.38 Mb, R3-8 in Figure 14–26) had a del(6p) daughter with mild speech delay and minor dysmorphism, and a dup(6p) son of normal development and the softest of soft dysmorphic signs. The mother's chromosomal state likely arose from an unequal sister chromatid exchange in early embryogenesis.

Duplication. We note above (Qi et al. 2015) the dup(6p) child of normal development and of soft dysmorphology.

[10] CADASIL = cerebral autosomal dominant arteriopathy with subcortical infarcts and leukoencephalopathy.

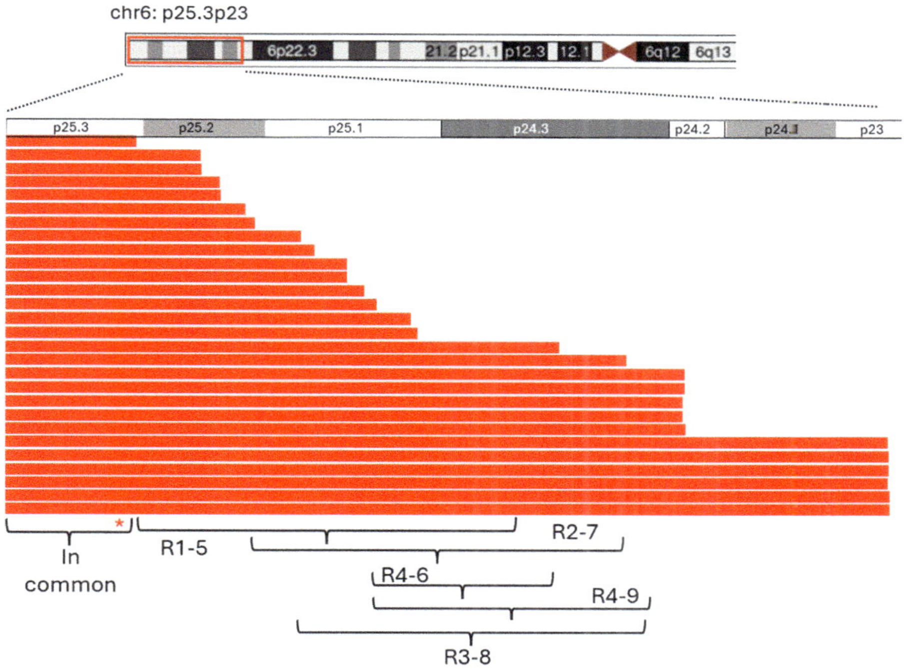

Figure 14–26. Distal 6p Deletions.

Notes: Some recorded deletions of chromosome 6 distal short arm. Interstitial deletions occurring within the bracketed regions enabled a division into nine subregions (R1–R9). The red asterisk pinpoints the position of *FOXC1*.

Source: From Qi et al., Haploinsufficiency and triploinsensitivity of the same 6p25.1p24.3 region in a family, *BMC Med Genom* 8: 38, 2015. Courtesy J Yu, and with the permission of Springer Nature.

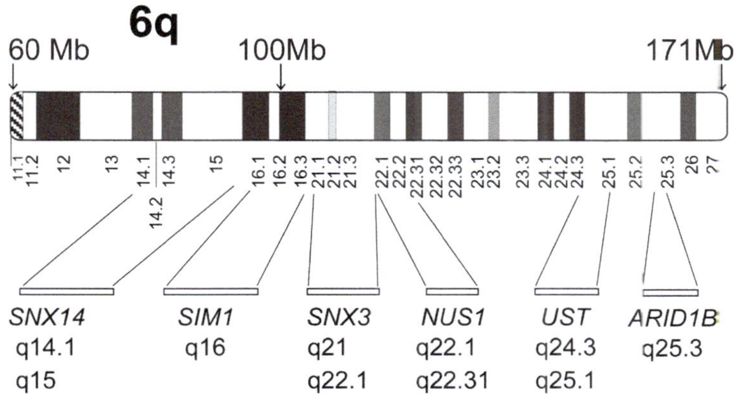

Figure 14–27.

6q14.1q15

Deletion of 6q14.1q15 can determine a clinical picture of dysmorphic features, congenital malformation, and neurobehavioral difficulty—but within these bounds, quite some variation is seen (Quintela et al. 2015). Body habitus has been described with the opposite observations of a resemblance to Marfan or Prader-Willi syndrome (Lowry et al. 2013). All are intellectually affected. A 5 Mb segment including *SNX14* in 6q14.2q14.3 appears to comprise the pheno-critical component of the syndrome. No familial case is known.

6q16

Deletion. Two very closely linked loci, *POU3F2* at 6q16.2 and *SIM1* at 6q16.3, determine two factors involved in an appetite pathway (the leptin → melanocortin → SIM1 → oxytocin pathway) (El Khattabi et al. 2015; Kasher et al. 2016) (Figure 14–28). A deletion including just one, just the other, or indeed both of these two genes, leads to a syndrome in which obesity associated with hyperphagia is a cardinal observation, along with cognitive compromise; the condition has been called Prader-Willi-like. The breakpoints are almost all non-recurrent.

Most cases are de novo, but very rare familial transmission of a ~1 Mb *POU3F2*-containing deletion is recorded. The penetrance point estimate from Goh et al. (2025) is 17%, but the confidence interval spans 0% to 100%.

6q21q22.1

Deletion. The lengths of deletion cover a wide range (Figure 14–29), but almost all include the segment contained between loci *MARCKS* and *HDAC2*, these loci straddling the interface of 6q21 and 6q22.1; several other deletions include *CDC40*. Structural brain abnormalities are commonly revealed upon imaging.

In the review of Minotti et al. (2024), in only one case had there been transmission from a similarly affected parent; every other case in which the information was known had arisen de novo.

6q22.1q22.31

Deletion. Epilepsy and tremors are the notable clinical observations in this deletion; dysmorphology is borderline or essentially absent. Intellectual disability is moderate or severe. Deletion sizes range from 0.2 Mb to 16 Mb; the loci *NUS1* and *SLC35F1* in particular are implicated (Szafranski et al. 2015).

Duplication. A very few cases of duplication involving the 6q22 segment are recorded. The clinical picture is rather nonspecific, with mild to moderate intellectual disability, growth deficiency, and facial dysmorphism (Pazooki et al. 2007). In some, it has been interpreted as a benign variant, or possibly as a variant of incomplete penetrance (Srebniak et al. 2016). *LAMA4* is a landmark locus.

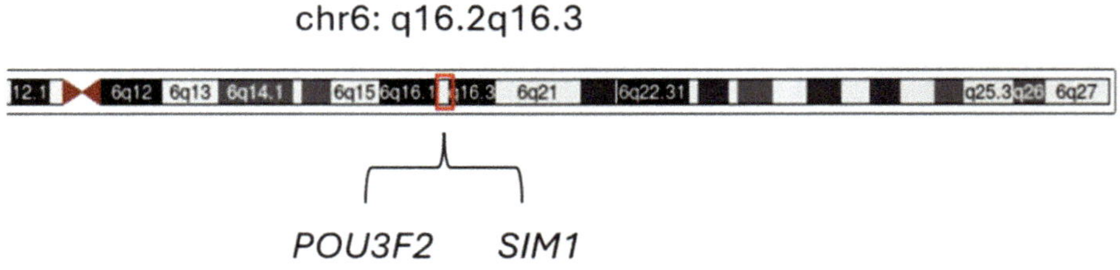

Figure 14–28. An Obesity-associated Deletion on 6q.

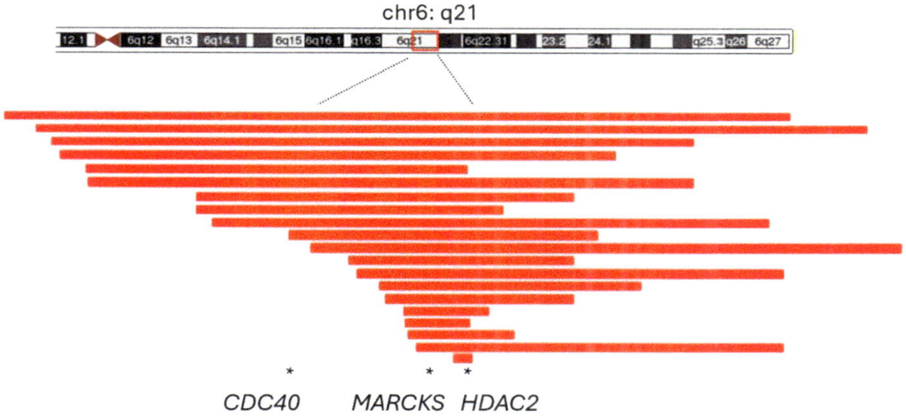

Figure 14–29. Deletions at 6q21q22.1.

Notes: Asterisks show the positions of three loci. The *HDAC2* gene is deleted in all, and *MARCKS* in all but one.

Source: From C Minotti et al., Case report: A new de novo 6q21q22.1 interstitial deletion case in a girl with cerebellar vermis hypoplasia and developmental delay and literature review, *Front Genet* 14:1315291, 2024. Courtesy C Minotti, and with the permission of Frontiers in Genetics.

6q23.2q24.2

Deletion. Only one case is on record, but this is worth noting, given the clinical picture. A 3-year-old girl del(6)(q23.2q24.2), whose development was "completely normal to advanced," and who had only been karyotyped as a newborn because of low birth weight (Kumar et al. 1999). While the facies was distinctive, she was said to resemble her family. One might imagine that this particular segment contains no critical brain loci.

Duplication. The remarkable trait in duplications of the segment 6q24 is transient neonatal diabetes. This reflects an overactivity of a triple dose of loci in this region that are normally subject to parent-of-origin imprinting (Chapter 19). *PLAGL1* at 6q24.2 is a suspect gene (Hassan et al. 2024).

6q24.3q25.1

Deletion at the distal long arm, 6q24.3q25.1, is well recognized, albeit that most cases are non-recurrent (Salpietro et al. 2015). A very few cases extend into q24.2 or q25.2, or, as in Stagi et al. (2015), into both. The condition has a resemblance to Noonan syndrome. Notable traits are a joint hypermobility reminiscent of Ehlers-Danlos syndrome, and heart disease, in particular mitral valve disease and cardiomyopathy (Engwerda et al. 2021). Mild to moderate developmental delay is typical. *TAB2* is the key locus

6q25.3

Deletion. The *ARID1B* gene (mutation in which causes Coffin-Siris syndrome) is the important basis of this syndrome (Paulraj et al. 2018). Deletions are of variable extent, falling within the wide range of 6q24.3 to 6q27 (and thus some having overlap with the del(6)(q24.3q25.1) described above), but nevertheless there are some breakpoints in common. The clinical picture includes intellectual disability, dysmorphism, dysgenesis of the corpus callosum, and hearing loss. An instance of inheritance has been described due to a parental acrocentric translocation (Domínguez et al. 2020).

impairment, and neurobehavioral disorder (Birca and Myers 2022). The key locus is *HIP1*, with possibly a contribution from *YWHAG* in some having a slightly larger deletion. It is typically a de novo event, but familial transmission is on record.

7q21.3

Deletion DLX6 and *DLX5* are limb development genes under the control of enhancer *DYNC1I1*; the *SGCE* gene codes for epsilon sarcoglycan. Loss of these neighboring two loci contained within 7q21.3 can lead to a split hand/foot malformation and myoclonus-dystonia, respectively; deletion of adjacent loci contributes to a broader phenotype. Deletion of *DYNC1I1* alone, *DLX6* and *DLX5* being intact, may nevertheless also lead to the hand-foot defect in some, this reflecting a loss of the influence of *DYNC1I1* over its client loci (Ambrosetti et al. 2023) (Figure 14–35).

Duplication. As with the deletion, the split hand-foot malformation is associated (Velinov et al. 2012).

7q21qter

Duplication. The q arm of chromosome 7 is long, comprising some 82 Mb of DNA, and yet a partial trisomy of more than half of 7q is viable. Presumably, rather like 13q, which is of similar length, the gene content is such that the qualitative functional imbalance over many loci is nevertheless tolerable, at least in terms of enabling survival through to live birth. Paththinige et al. (2018) report the longest survival, a child of 2⅓ years, in whom the 7q22.1qter duplication encompassed fully 58 Mb. Their case, and six others in their review, had resulted from the transmission of a parental translocation, with imbalances of 7q22qter to 7q21qter. One, a child surviving to 11½ months, carried a der(7q21.2;15p) and therefore represented an essentially "pure" partial 7q trisomy (the 15p segment being without phenotypic effect).

7q31

Deletion. The notable feature of this syndrome is poor speech development, presumed due to haploinsufficiency of *FOXP2*, a well-known speech apraxia gene. Nagy et al. (2021) report a family segregating a deletion, in which the heterozygotes had an expressive speech disability along with minor dysmorphism. In one notable family, a mother carrying a de novo 4.7 Mb del 7q31.2q31.31 inherited by two children of hers—and all three with impaired speech production and poor language comprehension—*FOXP2*

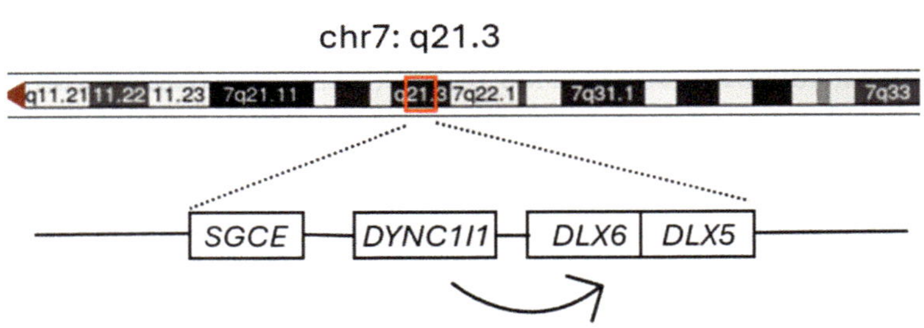

Figure 14–35. Gene Interaction at the 7q21.3 Deletion.

Notes: Loss of *DLX6* and *DLX5* causes a hand-foot malformation. Loss of *DYNC1I1* may in some cases (in other words, with reduced penetrance) perturb the function of the (intact) *DLX* loci, and lead also to the limb defect.

was intact, but its very close proximity to the deletion suggested a possible position effect (Rieger et al. 2020).

7q33q35

Deletion. There is a wide range of deletion (Kale and Philip 2016). A gene in this region, which will otherwise be familiar to the counselor, is *BRAF;*[12] whether this gene is contributory to the phenotype in the 7q33q35 deletion is an open question. The typical phenotype is of intellectual disability, dysmorphism, epilepsy, and susceptibility to infection.

One case of extraordinary interest concerns the IVF clinic (Chalas et al. 2020). Four couples had received sperm from the same donor, with simultaneous ongoing pregnancies. In one, fetal abnormalities were seen at ultrasound, and on amniocentesis, a 7q32.1q33 deletion was found, with termination chosen. Amniocenteses (presumably done with all dispatch) in two of the other couples gave a normal result, and normal babies were born. But upon sperm analysis from the donor, the same 7q deletion was identified in 12% of spermatozoa, attesting to the reality of gonadal mosaicism.

7q36qter

Deletion. Terminal 7q deletions can involve as much as q33qter, but are more usually of q36q26 to qter (Ayub et al. 2016). The classic clinical correlate is holoprosencephaly, a developmental brain defect that can vary from devastatingly severe to rather mild. The pheno-critical locus in this deletion is *SHH*, albeit that penetrance for holoprosencephaly is incomplete. De novo deletion is the rule, but inherited holoprosencephaly has been recorded in the setting of a familial 7q36 translocation (Hatziioannou et al. 1991). The phenotype overall is typically severe (Aneja and Krishnan 2024).

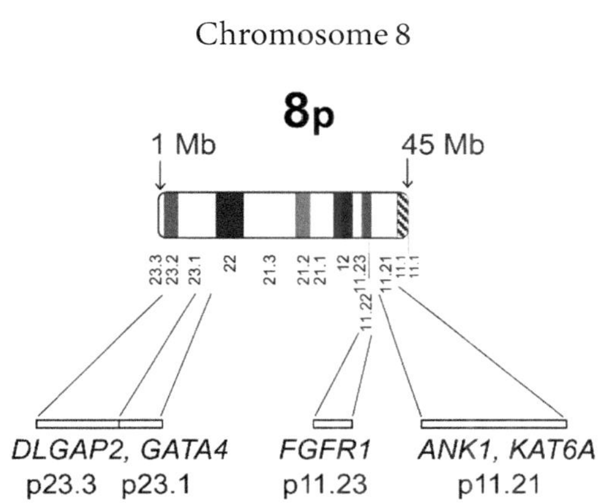

Figure 14–36.

8p11

Deletion. Notable loci within proximal 8p that can be pathogenic in the event of haploinsufficiency include *FGFR1* at 8p11.23 and *KAT6A* at 8p11.21. Loss (or mutation) of one

[12] In the germline, activating missense *BRAF* mutations cause cardiofaciocutaneous syndrome; somatically, mutations occur in certain "cancer cascades."

8q24.13q24.3

Deletion. If this deletion includes a segment containing *KCNQ3*, a neurofunctional syndrome typically results. Small deletions either side of this segment appear to be benign (Maya et al. 2021).

Chromosome 9

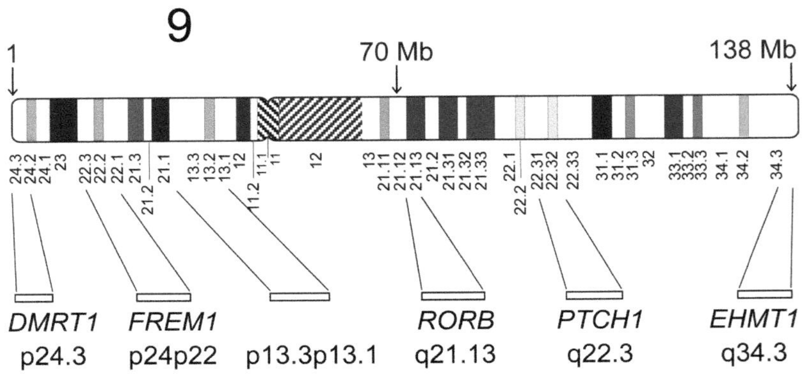

Figure 14–39.

9p24p22

Deletion: Alfi Syndrome. A number of 9p deletion cases involving the p22p24 region are recorded, more than 700, and they present a characteristic phenotype (Sams et al. 2021). Most breakpoints occur in bands 9p22 and 9p24. In about two-thirds, the deletion is terminal; in some, the deletion is accompanied by a duplication elsewhere. Trigonocephaly is a classic craniofacial malformation, and this may relate to loss of *FREM1* at 9q22.3. The brain is abnormal, and a curious imaging observation is a widening of the Sylvian fissure, the major cerebral sulcus. Other traits inhere in other regions (Starosta et al. 2024). The deletion is equally likely to have happened on the paternal or maternal chromosome 9. If the deletion extends into 9p24.3, a gonadal phenotype may be seen, as noted in the section below.

Most del(9p) arises de novo, but recurrences in a family due to a segregating translocation are on record (Abreu et al. 2014).

9p24.3cen

Duplication: Trisomy 9p Syndrome. This is one of the more common partial trisomies, indeed said to be fourth in frequency after the three major full trisomies and known since 1970 (Guilherme et al. 2014). In many, the duplication extends into the 9qh heterochromatic region, 9q11q12, and occasionally as far as q21.11. A paucity of dosage-sensitive loci within 9p, and a concentration of repeat sequences within the pericentromeric region, are the basis, respectively, of its viability and frequency. The craniofacies is characteristic. Intellectual disability is typical, and Martínez-Jacobo et al. (2015) report in addition psychotic behavior; brain abnormality is often seen on imaging. However, Bouhjar et al. (2011) record a few cases, mostly with smaller 9p duplications, in whom intelligence was within a normal range.

Most cases in fact occur in the setting of a rearrangement with another chromosome (in these, the recurrence risk relates to the parental carrier status; Figure 5–14), but isolated examples are well recorded.

Triplication. Tetrasomy 9p typically exists in the form of an isodicentric or pseudodicentric iso(9p). In those who survive, it is seen in the mosaic state (Süleyman et al. 2022).

9p24.3

Deletion. These deletions occur distal to the 9p deletion syndrome core region, and remove the *DMRT1* gene. This is the most conserved of any known sex-determining gene, and it is actually on the Z chromosome (the homogametic chromosome) of birds. Its expression is normally greater in the male than in the female embryo, and this dosage is the basis of its testis-inducing action. Loss of one *DMRT1* allele in the deleted segment brings the amount of product down below this threshold, thus potentially leading to a disorder of sex differentiation of varying form (hypospadias through to gonadal dysgenesis or male-to-female "sex reversal") in the 46,*XY*,del(9)(p24.3) person. This observed variable expressivity—but also, in some, a non-penetrance such that normal male development is seen—may reflect that other loci are intact or absent; that is, a second-hit scenario may apply (Quinonez et al. 2013). Concerning the 46,*XX*,del(9)(p24.3) female, Bartels et al. (2013) report primary ovarian dysfunction proceeding to menopause in young adulthood, and suggest that this may be a reflection of the *DMRT1* haploinsufficiency.

9q22.3

Deletion. A notable feature of this deletion syndrome is the involvement of the *PTCH1* gene in 9q22.32, and thus the Gorlin basal cell nevus syndrome is a component of the phenotype (Muller et al. 2012). Deletions are mostly within the range chr9:95-97 Mb, but can extend further into adjacent bands. Other aspects include craniosynostosis with trigonocephaly, hydrocephalus, overgrowth, facial dysmorphism of no consistent character, and intellectual disability. Ewing et al. (2021) describe a curious case of a teenager with a small deletion (0.4 Mb), and yet with an atypically severe phenotype. De novo generation is the rule.

9q34.3

Deletion: Kleefstra Syndrome. This subtelomeric microdeletion syndrome of intellectual disability typically of severe degree, difficult behavior, distinctive facies, and multiple malformation may be, after 1q36 and 22q13, the third most frequent of the subtelomeric deletion syndromes. Haploinsufficiency of (and also point mutation in) the gene *EHMT1*, the penultimate gene on chromosome 9, determines the core phenotype, and varying degrees of the extent of deletion may impose further compromise (Morison et al. 2024; Figure 14–40). The protein encoded by this gene, Eu-HMTase1, has a role in maintaining the integrity of histones that comprise a key component of the architecture of the chromosome; this syndrome can thus be considered as a disorder of chromatin remodeling.

Parental somatic-gonadal mosaicism with recurrence in offspring has been recognized, but the large majority represent a de novo occurrence (Willemsen et al. 2011a).

Duplication of the 9q34.3 locus encompassing *EHMT1* is associated with mild developmental delay, mild intellectual disability, autism spectrum disorder, and behavioral

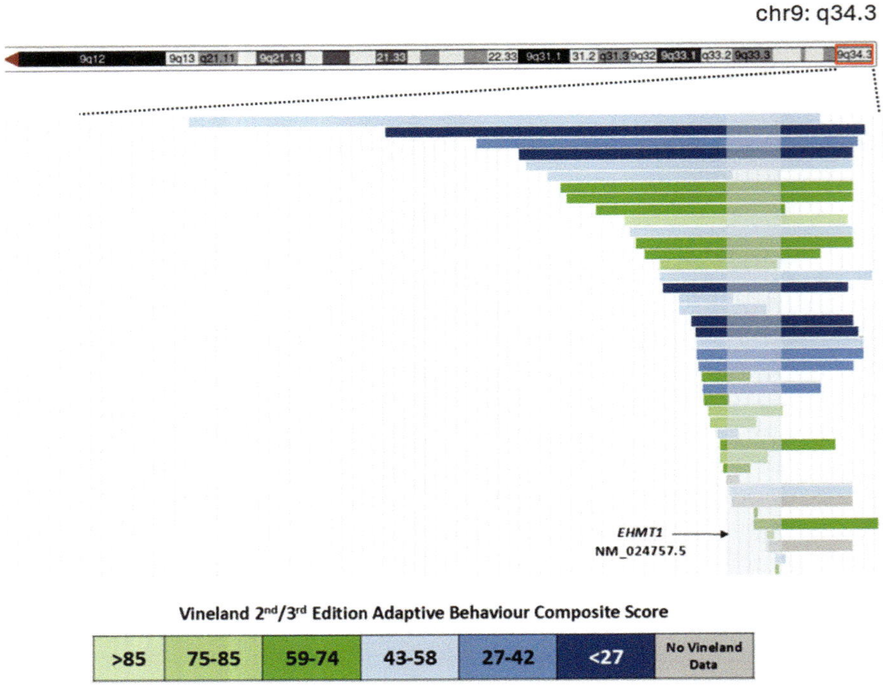

Figure 14–40. Deletions and the Adaptive Behavior Phenotype in Kleefstra Syndrome.

Notes: The color coding denotes the severity of adaptive behavior in 103 individuals, from the mildest in pale green, progressively darkening through to the most severely affected in dark blue. No information was available in those with gray bars. The assessment was done using the Vineland II/III ABC scale, ranging from >85 in the green, through to <27 in the blue (the mean for a normal population is 100, SD 15). The pale vertical column reflects the position of the *EHMT1* gene.

Source: Adapted from LD Morison et al., Expanding the phenotype of Kleefstra syndrome: speech, language and cognition in 103 individuals, *J Med Genet* 61:578–585, 2024. Courtesy A Morgan.

difficulty (Rots et al. 2024). The penetrance estimate in Goh et al. (2025) is 100%. As with the deletion, there are varying lengths of the duplicated segment. It is often inherited from a mildly affected parent, or can be de novo.

Chromosome 10

10p12.1p11.23

Deletion. All deletions have been of differing extents and lengths (0.5–10 Mb), but analysis of overlapping segments has allowed proposition of a probable 1.1 Mb critical region at p12.1 (Mroczkowski et al. 2014). Within this, two subregions may determine the phenotypic components of cryptorchidism (*MKX* the likely culprit) and craniofacial malformation (*BAMBI* the possible basis). A very specific segment further upstream at 27.1 Mb is associated with familial thrombocytopenia, probably due to *MASTL* in this region having a role in platelet production (Manohar et al. 2024). The variable pattern of dysmorphism presumably reflects specific deleted regions. Developmental delay in survivors has been universal.

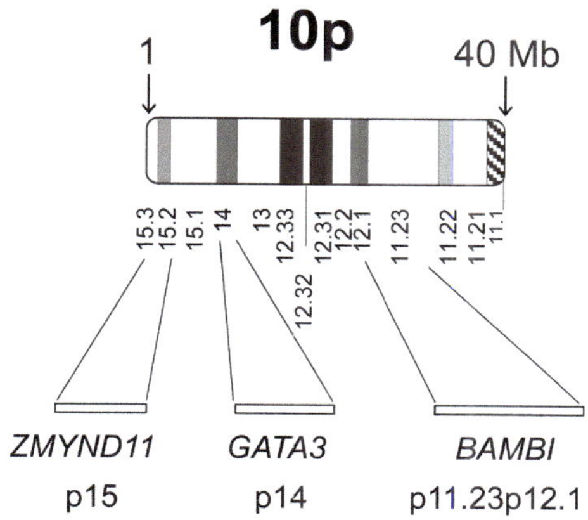

Figure 14–41.

10p14

Deletion: "HDR" Syndrome, Barakat Syndrome. All three components of this syndrome—hypoparathyroidism, deafness, and renal dysplasia (HDR)—inhere in deletion (or point mutation) of *GATA3*. Haploinsufficiency of adjacent genes leads to a broader phenotype, with typically severe intellectual disability; the deletion can extend proximally within p14 or further, and likewise distally within p14 or further—indeed, as far as pter (and thus overlapping with the deletion of the following entry). Centromerically extending deletions may remove a segment within 10p14, which has been labeled the critical region for a DiGeorge-like syndrome, DGS2, although no specific genes have been implicated. But this distinction may not be entirely clear; a DGS-like phenotype is not consistently observed (Benetti et al. 2009; Melis et al. 2012). Sporadic occurrence is typical in 10p14 deletions (but see Chapter 8, familial HDR due to a segregating insertional translocation).

10p15

Deletion: DeScipio Syndrome. Deletions may be confined to subtelomeric p15.3 (which contains only two genes, *ZMYND11* and *DIP2C*) or may extend further into the short

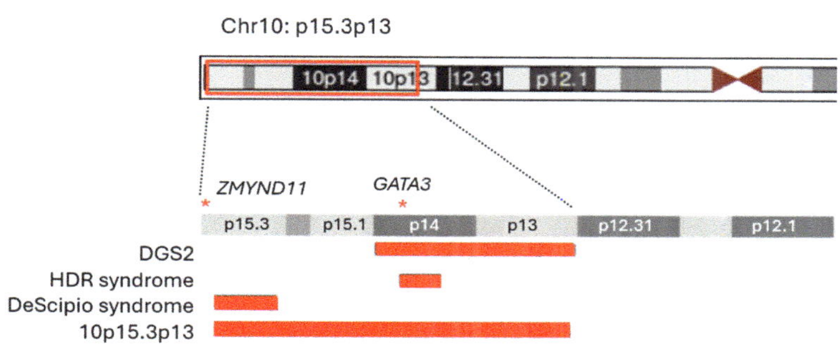

Figure 14–42. 10p Deletions.

Notes: Deletions declare themselves of two categories: a proximal segment, wherein *GATA3* is located; and a distal segment, which includes *ZMYND11*. The proximal segment is associated with Barakat syndrome and DiGeorge syndrome type 2; deletion of the distal segment leads to DeScipio syndrome.

Source: From YQ Pan and JH Fu, Case report: Clinical description of a patient carrying a 12.48 Mb microdeletion involving the 10p13-15.3 region, *Front Pediatr* 25;9:603666, 2021. Courtesy J-H Fu, and with the permission of Frontiers in Pediatrics.

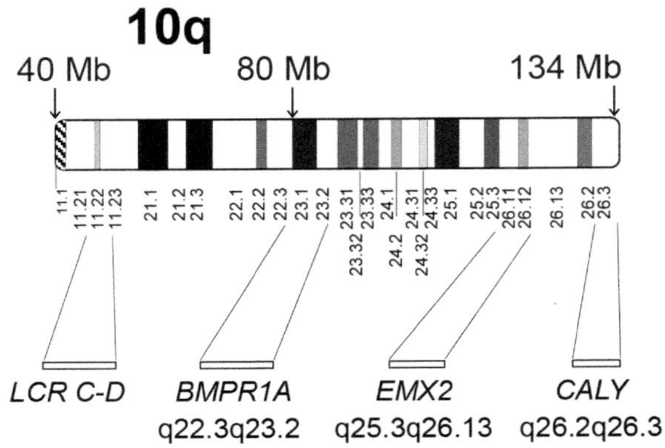

Figure 14–43.

arm of the chromosome. The important clinical aspect is typically a severe neurocognitive compromise, often with dystonic cerebral palsy, associated with cortical abnormality identifiable on brain imaging (Poluha et al. 2017). Surprisingly, there is little difference clinically between those with the smaller and those with the larger deletions; this supports the view that the *ZMYND11* and *DIP2C* genes are the likely key phenocritical factors (Eggert et al. 2016).

Almost all cases have been de novo, but two known or assumed transmitting mothers are on record.

10q11.21q11.22

Duplication. A recurrent duplication in 10q11.21q11.22 reflects the agency of low-copy repeats (LCR) C and D (Figure 14–43). There is some controversy concerning the pathogenicity, or not, of this segment. It has been associated with cases of autism, but normal children also have been seen, followed up into early infancy after detection of the duplication at prenatal diagnosis (Ouyang et al. 2024).

*10q22.3q23.2**

Deletion. This recurrent deletion arises due to flanking low-copy repeats LCR3 in 10q22.3 and LCR4 in 10q23.2. The clinical phenotype is fairly nonspecific, with facial dysmorphism and, in most, delayed language development (but in one case, as an infant, language development was judged to lie within normal limits; Petrova et al. 2014). Juvenile polyposis may arise (Lecoquierre et al. 2020). The *BMPR1A* gene at 10q23.2 is proposed to be pheno-critical. If the deletion extends more distally into 10q23.2 and removes *PTEN*, the gene for Cowden syndrome, the result is a severe gastrointestinal syndrome of infantile onset pan-enteric polyposis (an overlap of juvenile polyposis syndrome and Cowden syndrome); treatment with mTOR inhibitors may improve the symptomatology (Taylor et al. 2021).

Most del q22.3q23.2 cases have arisen de novo, but inherited cases are known (van Bon et al. 2011). Based on deletion size and gene content, penetrance is likely to be complete (Goh et al. 2025)

Duplication 10q22.3q23.2. This is one of several microduplications that raises a dilemma when seen at prenatal diagnosis, due to its incomplete penetrance and a paucity of recorded information. Goh et al. (2025) propose a penetrance of 27% with respect to a neurodevelopmental phenotype. Kong et al. (2016) describe prenatally diagnosed cases, in the context of one parent being a carrier, and with a causal link between genotype and (variable) phenotype being uncertain. One case concerned a (presumably monozygous) twin pregnancy, both twins heterozygous for a dup 10q22.3q23.2. While the index fetus was growth-retarded and had ventriculomegaly, the "internal control" twin and the carrier mother were considered to be phenotypically normal. This illustrates the point that phenotypic abnormality is often the basis of ascertainment, and thus subject to bias. With this, and with so many other of the del/dups of uncertain significance, the collection of family data beyond the proband, and this being available internationally, is a desideratum of high degree.

10q24.3

Duplication: Split Hand Foot Malformation Syndrome Type 3. Duplications of small (kb size) extent in the 10q24.3 region are associated with this malformation syndrome; dysregulation of the *BTRC* and *SHFM3* genes at 10q24.32 (chr10:101.4 and 101.6 Mb, respectively) may be the key factor (Sowińska-Seidler et al. 2014). Neurocognitive functioning is typically intact, and familial transmission in an autosomal dominant pattern is common (Dai et al. 2013).

Sibship recurrence due to maternal somatic-gonadal mosaicism is on record (Dimitrov et al. 2010; Filho et al. 2011); we have seen 30% mosaicism in an unaffected father of a child with split hand foot malformation.

10q25.1q25.3

Duplication: Distal 10q Trisomy Syndrome. Large duplications of distal 10q involving most or all of 10q25, have been known for some time, the first reports appearing in the 1970s (Al-Sarraj et al. 2014). The clinical picture includes intellectual disability, microcephaly, facial dysmorphism (often with blepharophimosis), and distal limb defects.

Most cases have been due to the malsegregation of a parental translocation, but some have reflected a de novo event, the duplication being in that case "pure."

10q25.3q26.12

Deletion. If *EMX2* at10q26.11 is involved, this syndrome is associated very notably with a disorder of sex development, and the XY male may present with genital ambiguity. Piard et al. (2014) describe micropenis, dysgenetic testes, and a "Mullerian recessus" (a uterine rudiment) entering the urethra in a non-dysmorphic child with developmental delay including failure of acquisition of language.

10q26.2q26.3

Deletion. Terminal deletions in distal 10q may comprise loss within only bands 10q26.2q26.3; or, they may be of larger extent and include the segment 10q25.3q26.13 as described in the section above; or, they may involve more proximal segments, such as were identifiable on classic cytogenetics and called the 10q− syndrome. Focusing on those deletions confined to the terminal bands 10q26.2q26.3, the clinical picture is one of moderate intellectual disability, growth retardation, and mild facial dysmorphism. The neurobehavioral phenotype is variable, with some exhibiting attention deficit and hyperactivity; the *CALY* gene (the seventh-last gene on the chromosome) may be

13q12.12*

Deletion. Three loci determining neuromuscular disorders lie closely together within 13q12.12: *SACS*, for autosomal recessive spastic ataxia of Charlevoix and Saguenay (ARSACS); *SGCG*, for autosomal recessive limb-girdle muscular dystrophy type 5; and *MIPEP*, for a syndrome of left ventricular non-compaction, developmental delay, seizures, and severe hypotonia. A deletion within 13q12.12 may be harmless unless there happens to be, on the other homolog, a recessive mutation in one of these three loci "unmasking" the heterozygosity. We have seen a woman with ataxia and a Charcot-Marie-Tooth-like neuropathy inheriting a (normally non-pathogenic) paternal 0.2 Mb CNV deletion, which removed *SACS*, and an accompanying maternal *SACS* mutation on the other homolog, thus enabling a diagnosis of ARSACS. Other such cases are on record (Liu et al. 2016; Eldomery et al. 2016; Dougherty et al. 2018).

13q

Deletion. The "13q− syndrome" was first described in detail by Allderdice et al. (1969), and the association with retinoblastoma recorded in the days of "solid-stain" cytogenetics. The no. 13 chromosomes were distinguished from the others of the D group on the basis that no. 13 was later replicating during the cell cycle, using the (long-since discarded) methodology of treating cells in culture with tritiated thymidine (autoradiography). In 1993, Brown et al. reviewed the syndrome in light of the sophisticated cytogenetics of the day, and they proposed three main categories: Group 1 within q12.2q31, with a phenotype of minor abnormalities, mild or moderate intellectual disability, and susceptibility to retinoblastoma; Group 2 within q12.2q32, with particular reference to band q32 in cases with major malformation and severe intellectual disability; and Group 3, comprising those with deletion of the distal segment q33q34, with severe mental compromise but typically without major malformation. The risk for retinoblastoma lay in the *RB1* gene in q14, loss of which by deletion comprises a classic first-hit of carcinogenesis, as initially proposed by Knudson (1971).

A review in Ballarati et al. (2007) noted that the grouping as above did not always hold true. Mitter et al. (2011) offered an updated and more molecular categorization for deletions which included *RB1*-containing 13q14: small deletions within q14 of less than 6 Mb; medium deletions within q12.3q21.2 and of size 6–20 Mb; and large deletions within q12q31.2, of greater than 20 Mb in extent (Figure 14–50). The foregoing assessments inform the following entries. (For the record, possibly the largest constitutional deletion ever reported may be del(13)(q13.3qter), encompassing 75.7 Mb, in a fetus diagnosed at 16 weeks gestation with cerebellar hypoplasia; Ballarati et al. 2007.)

Duplication. Partial trisomy 13, of large segments, is often viable—an unsurprising fact given observations in the full trisomy. With the availability of G-banding from the 1970s, a number of cases of partial trisomy 13 came to light, and the conclusions from that period quite considerably hold today (Rogers 1984). Duplications are grouped broadly into proximal and distal, with bands 13q14q22 as the dividing region (Figure 14–49). Those of substantial size are invariably associated with psychomotor retardation. Certain features are peculiar to the segment; thus, polydactyly is seen only in the distal duplication.

Most cases are due to a parental rearrangement, while some are de novo; and of these, several involve the attachment of a 13q segment to another chromosome as an "add."

13q14.2q14.3

Deletion. Small (less than 6 Mb, and as low as 0.15 Mb) deletions lead to a syndrome of mild or only borderline intellectual disability, with language acquisition in particular affected and a mild, "soft" facial dysmorphism. As noted above, loss of one *RB1* gene predisposes to a very high risk for retinoblastoma, 50% or more (Figure 14–50).

The considerable majority of deletions arise de novo, but familial cases are recorded, such as a father and two sons with a 3.33 Mb deletion, and an aunt and nephew with a 1.17 Mb deletion, recounted in Mitter et al. (2011). Of these, the father had a retinal scar, likely a spontaneously regressed tumor; one son had a unilateral and the other a bilateral retinoblastoma; and the aunt and nephew both had a unilateral tumor. A parental insertional translocation may be the basis of some familial cases (Punnett et al. 2003).

13q12.3q21.2

Deletions of 6 Mb–20 Mb extent within these chromosomal bands are (as in the entry foregoing, which this larger segment encompasses) at very high risk for retinoblastoma (Figure 14–50). Delayed motor and speech development are the rule, as is growth retardation. Physical features include a distinctive facies. Almost all cases are of de novo origin.

13q12q31.2

Deletions of large size, above 20 Mb, generally produce a more marked phenotype in comparison to the above entry in terms of the neurodevelopmental compromise, and

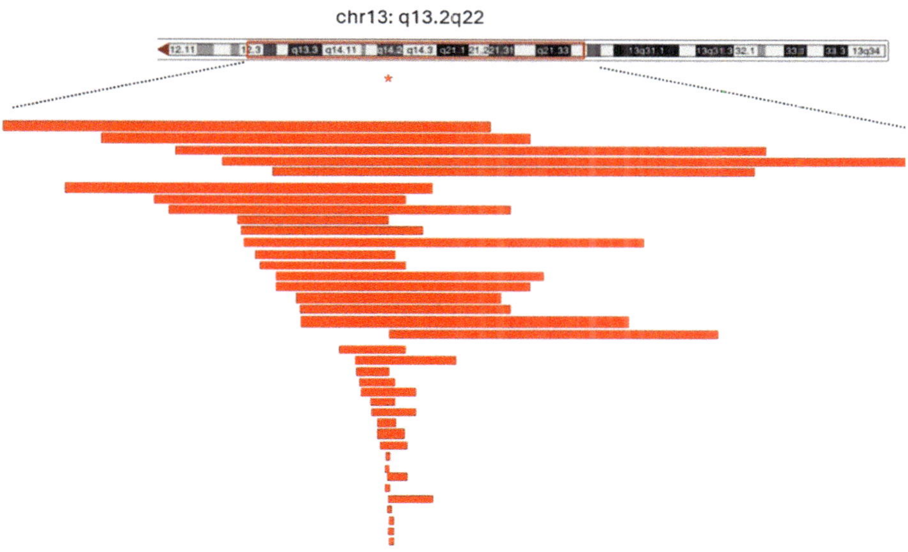

Figure 14–50. 13q Deletions in Retinoblastoma.

Notes: Shown here is the range of 13q deletions including the *RB1* locus in band 13q14.2 (its position asterisked), from a cohort of retinoblastoma patients. These are divided into large (>20 Mb), medium (6–20 Mb), and small (<6 Mb) sizes. Note that deletions are not recurrent, suggesting nonhomologous end-joining as the generative mechanism.

Source: From D Mitter et al., Genotype-phenotype correlations in patients with retinoblastoma and interstitial 13q deletions, *Eur J Hum Genet* 19:947–958, 2011. Courtesy D Mitter, and with the permission of Macmillan Publishers Ltd.

a more notable facial dysmorphism. Microcephaly is seen in some. Those deletions removing the *EDNRB* locus at q22.3 are associated with variable signs of Waardenburg-Shah syndrome[13] (Tüysüz et al. 2009). Again, the high risk for retinoblastoma applies. Practically all are de novo.

13q32

Deletions that include this cytoband, and however extensive otherwise, typically present a severe neurodevelopmental picture with major brain malformation. The presumed key loci in this respect are *ZIC2* and *ZIC5* in sub-band q32.3, with holoprosencephaly and cerebellar dysgenesis the respective concomitants (Mimaki et al. 2015). Other loci determine other aspects of the malformative phenotype (Kotani et al. 2022).

Duplication. Jobanputra et al. (2012) observed clinical normality in an infant with a de novo dup 13q32.2; these authors conclude that the *ZIC2* gene resident within this segment does not lead, in the dup state, to holoprosencephaly.

13q33q34

Deletion. These distal 13q deletions can be interstitial or terminal. Microcephaly and intellectual disability are typical in those encompassing both cytobands (Sagi-Dain et al. 2019). Genital malformation is often seen in the male, and a considerable resemblance to the VACTERL[14] syndrome has been observed (Dworschak et al. 2013). Smaller deletions, restricted to 13q34, may present a different picture, such as the child in Yang et al. (2013), a boy with a borderline IQ of 71, four-limb hexadactyly, and heart disease (a single atrium), who had a 1 Mb terminal deletion. The case in Myers et al. (2017) was due to recombination from a maternal inversion 13.

Chromosome 14

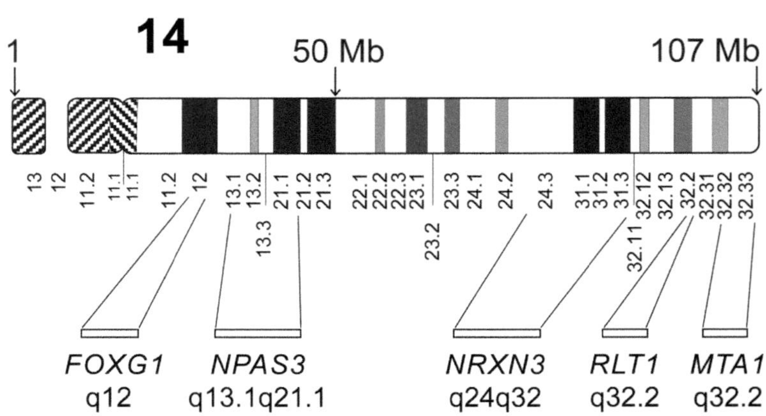

Figure 14–51.

14q12

Deletions: FOXG1 Syndrome. Cytoband 14q12 contains the *FOXG1* locus, and loss of this gene as part of a typically 0.4 Mb–4.0 Mb microdeletion leads to the "*FOXG1*

[13] Waardenburg-Shah syndrome: deafness; hypopigmented skin, hair, and irides; and Hirschsprung disease.
[14] Vertebral, anal, cardiac, trachea-esophageal, renal, limb association

syndrome" of marked post natal microcephaly (head circumference with a standard deviation of −4 to −6), severe intellectual disability, and absent or near-absent language acquisition; a resemblance to Rett syndrome is noted (Brimble et al. 2023; Ellaway et al. 2013). The facies is unremarkable. Epilepsy is frequent. Bertossi et al. (2014) speak of a "dyskinetic encephalopathy of infancy," a movement disorder which may include jerks, athetosis, chorea, and dystonia. The clinical picture is very similar in 14q12 deletions not actually removing *FOXG1*, and a dysregulation of the *FOXG1* pathway, due to loss of a nearby *cis*-acting regulatory element, may lead to the same end result of a *FOXG1* functional haploinsufficiency.

Duplication. A syndrome of epilepsy, cognitive impairment, and dysmorphism, but not microcephaly accompanies a 14q12 duplication that includes the *FOXG1* locus (Hettige and Ernst 2019). De novo inheritance is the rule, but malsegregation from a parental translocation is on record.

del 14q24q32

Deletions within q24q32 can vary in size from 4 Mb to 20 Mb (Nicita et al. 2015; Stokman et al. 2016). A phenotype of intellectual disability is typical, and brain scans can show structural defects. The facies is abnormal. The region in common between most reported cases includes *NRXN3*, a "brain gene" (Figure 14–52). The deletion in Stokman et al. (2016) does not quite extend this far; these authors postulate *IFT43* as another pheno-contributory gene. Inheritance is typically de novo.

14q32.2

Deletion: Kagami-Ogata Syndrome, Temple Syndrome. See Chapter 19.

14q32.11

Deletion. This new syndrome imposes a neurodevelopmental phenotype, along with mild dysmorphisms (Eno et al. 2021). One child with autism was "good at math." Transmission from a very mildly affected mother is known. It may be more common than initially supposed.

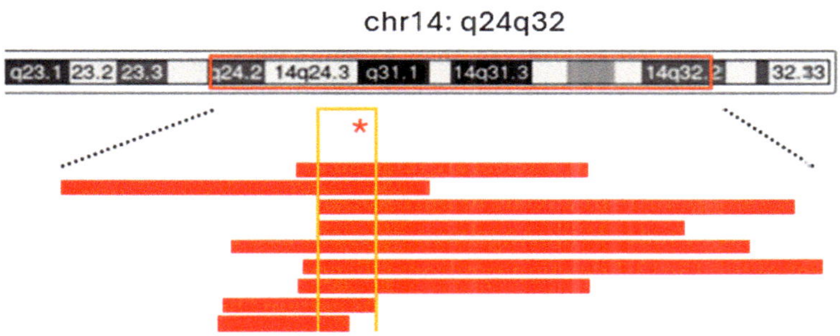

Figure 14–52. A Series of Deletions within 14q24q32.

Notes: These cases are from a series of eight, and another single report. The position of the key locus *NRXN3* is asterisked; it lies within the common region outlined. The single case (lowest bar) did not include *NRXN3*.

Sources: From F Nicita et al., Neurological features of 14q24-q32 interstitial deletion: report of a new case, *Mol Cytogenet* 8:93, 2015; with the additional case from MF Stokman et al., De novo 14q24.2q24.3 microdeletion including IFT43 is associated with intellectual disability, skeletal anomalies, cardiac anomalies, and myopia, *Am J Med Genet* 170A:1566–1569, 2016, and with the permission of Springer Nature.

NIPA2,[15] *CYFIP1*, and *TUBGCP5*. While the deletion can vary in size (from 0.25 Mb to 1.5 Mb, most commonly 0.5 Mb), only these four loci are ever lost; Butler (2023) discusses potential roles for each of these. The background population carrier rate may be as high as 0.25% (1 person in 400), and about double that, 0.57%, in a cohort of those of neurobehavioral phenotype (Cafferkey et al. 2014). It is the single most common chromosome finding in large cohorts of those presenting with neurodevelopmental disability and/or autism (Butler 2023).

The clinical picture is very largely confined to a neurocognitive/behavioral/psychiatric/autism phenotype (Cox and Butler 2015). Learning is affected, especially with respect to reading and writing. Attention deficit and hyperactivity are commonly seen, as also may be oppositional defiant disorder. Schizophrenia is a risk.

This chromosome imbalance is a classic example of the incompletely penetrant microdeletion/CNV. It is typically an inherited deletion (in 80%–85%), but often (50%) the parent is reportedly unaffected; the remaining cases are of de novo origin (Vanlerberghe et al. 2015). A penetrance estimate of 10% (Goh et al. 2025) might be slightly low, and it would likely vary according to the stringency of phenotypic assessment of carriers. In other words, if microsigns of neurobehavioral disorder in parents were sought, the penetrance could well be higher.

Duplication. A similar pattern of neuropsychiatric traits is reported in the BP1–BP2 duplication (Meossi et al. 2023), but the penetrance for overt manifestation, at 5%, is no greater than the background risk, arguing against pathogenicity (Goh et al. 2025).

*15q11.2q13.1 BP2-BP3**

Deletion: Prader-Willi Syndrome, Angelman Syndrome. See Chapter 19.

Duplication for the segment 15q11.2q13.1 BP2-BP3 may, but not necessarily will, lead to a syndrome of neuropsychiatric dysfunction; Goh et al. (2025) propose a penetrance figure of 77%. The imbalance can also exist as a triplication, or even as a hexasomy, due to a supernumerary chromosome (inv dup or isodicentric 15) (Chan et al. 2025). The intellectual impairment ranges from borderline to severe ("pervasive developmental disorder"), with autism often a prominent feature (Battaglia 2008; Hogart et al. 2010). Epilepsy is recognized, and gastrointestinal symptoms are common (Coppola et al. 2013; Shaaya et al. 2015).

Most (80%) are inherited, and more often recognized from the mother (Bisba et al. 2024). An unaffected parent can transmit the duplication, with children then affected, as Bonuccelli et al. (2017) show in a three-generational pedigree and as Han et al. (2021) report with respect to a sibship of three, two with autism and one with schizophrenia, from their normal mother.

Of particular interest is the susceptibility to schizophrenia due to the duplication. Almost exclusively, it is in those in whom the duplication is of maternal origin that this psychiatric disease is seen (Figure 14–55). The penetrance for schizophrenia in the maternally inherited dup15(BP2-BP3) is 12%, compared to only 1%—practically the population figure—in paternal transmission (Isles et al. 2016). Thus it is that the condition is sometimes referred to as "Maternal 15q11.2q13.1 duplication syndrome" (Colijn et al. 2024). The penetrance with respect to developmental disability, autism spectrum disorder, and multiple congenital anomaly also shows a bias, but less markedly so, toward

[15] The naming of these two *NIPA* genes is of interest, according to what they are *not*: "not imprinted in Prader-Willi or Angelman."

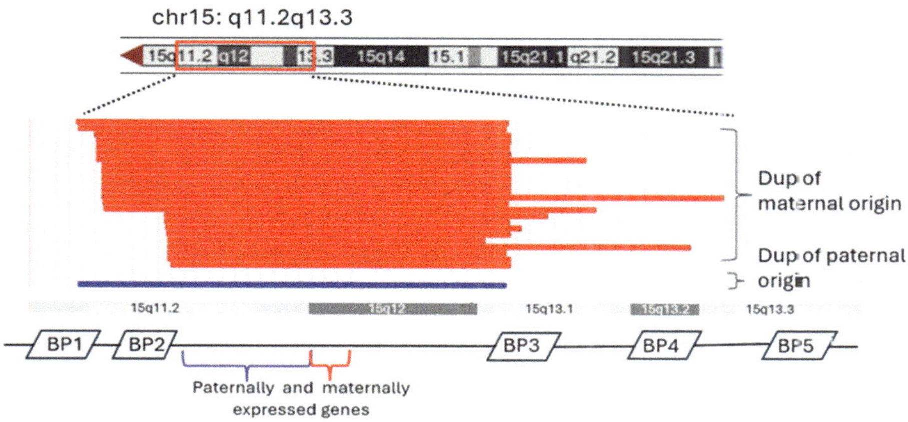

Figure 14–55. Duplications at 15q11.2q13.3 Causing Schizophrenia.

Notes: Duplications comprise segments BP1-BP3, BP2-BP3, BP1-BP4, and BP2-BP4. All include *NIPA1, NIPA2, CYFIP1*, and *TUBGCP5*, which lie within BP2-BP3. The very considerable majority of duplications are of maternal origin, presumably an effect of the imprinted status of the contained loci.

Source: From AR Isles et al., Parental origin of interstitial duplications at 15q11.2-q13.3 in schizophrenia and neurodevelopmental disorders, *PLoS Genet* 12: e1005993, 2016. Courtesy MJ Owen and G Kirov, and with the permission of the Public Library of Science.

maternal transmission. The respective parental penetrances with respect to these traits are 50% (mat) and 20% (pat). These differences presumably reflect the differing roles of imprinted genes with the segment.

*15q13 BP3-BP4**

Deletion. This deletion may be a rare cause of familial autism; imbalance of *APBA2* is proposed as the crucial factor (Babatz et al. 2009).

Duplication. Peycheva et al. (2018) describe the three-generation transmission of a dup15q13.1, the heterozygotes having histories of intellectual compromise, psychopathy, and epilepsy. *APBA2* is known of itself to have an association with autism and schizophrenia.

*15q13.3 BP4-BP5**

Deletion. This 1.5 Mb deletion lies between BP4 and BP5. Uncommonly, larger ~4 Mb deletions can encompass BP3–BP5, or smaller deletions can be "nested" within BP4 and BP5. The associated phenotype is essentially one of neuropsychiatric expression, and Lowther et al. (2015) determined these fractions, corrected for ascertainment: intellectual disability in 58%, epilepsy in 28%, poor speech development in 16%, autism spectrum disorder in 11%, schizophrenia in 10%, mood disorder in 10%, and attention deficit hyperactivity disorder in 7%. A similar inference comes from Torres et al. (2016), who determined high odds ratios for epilepsy, intellectual disability, autism, and schizophrenia. The average nonverbal IQ in the series of Ziats et al. (2016) was 60, and one-third of cases met criteria for a diagnosis of autism spectrum disorder. Galantamine (an acetylcholinesterase inhibitor) may offer some hope as a treatment in order to improve the behavioral component of the phenotype (Casas-Alba et al. 2021).

About 85% of cases are inherited, and in 62 transmitting parents studied by Lowther et al. (2015), half had been diagnosed with a neuropsychiatric condition, although none had schizophrenia; those with schizophrenia in their study had all been probands in their own right. Thus, we have a further example of a molecular chromosomal imbalance of incomplete penetrance and variable expressivity; however, the fact that Lowther and colleagues found no cases in 23,838 adult controls suggests that penetrance is, in fact, high. Penetrance in Goh et al. (2025) is 54%. The crucial factor, in terms of the phenotype, is haploinsufficiency for one or both of the genes *CHRNA7* and *OTUD7A*, which are located within the deleted segments of both the 1.5 Mb deletion and the smaller nested 0.44 Mb deletion (Unda et al. 2023).

Duplication of 15q13.3 BP4-BP5 is one of the most frequently seen of the microduplications; triplication is also known (Soler-Alfonso et al. 2014). It is seen with developmental delay and intellectual disability, poor speech, autism, and subtle dysmorphism (Budisteanu et al. 2021); however, penetrance is quite low, at 8% for the 1.5 Mb duplication and just 3% for the nested 0.44 Mb duplication (Goh et al. 2025). Counseling is complicated by this incomplete penetrance and by the variable expressivity of this genomic disorder (Miller et al. 2009; van Bon et al. 2009).

*15q24**

Deletion. The breakpoints of this imbalance are for the most part founded upon a series of four low-copy repeats, breakpoints (BPs) A through D, which can promote nonallelic homologous recombination, a 3.1 Mb deletion at BP A–D being the most frequently observed (Mefford et al. 2012). This genomic variation matches a variable but fully penetrant phenotype. Speech development is severely affected in many, some being nonverbal, and some show attention deficit hyperactivity. The BP C–D region, wherein lies *SIN3A*, may be central to the pathogenesis (the SIN3A protein interacts with the Rett syndrome protein, MeCP2; Witteveen et al. 2016). Facial dysmorphism is mild or "soft," with a large forehead a common observation. No familial case is known.

Duplication. Duplication of 15q24 may cause developmental delay, with or without mild dysmorphism (El-Hattab et al. 2010). Goh et al. (2025) estimate a penetrance of 37%, but with wide confidence intervals. Evidence supports pathogenicity of the larger [A-D] duplication, but is borderline for the smaller [A-B] duplication.

15q24.2q24.3

Deletion. This recurrent but rare 2.2 Mb deletion includes 15 protein coding genes, including *FBXO22* and *TSPAN3*. Goh et al. (2025) calculated a penetrance of 69%, with wide confidence intervals.

Duplication. The corresponding 15q24.2q24.3 duplication has a penetrance estimate of 73% (Goh et al. 2025).

*15q25.2 and 15q25.2q25.3**

Deletion. Low-copy repeat sequences B, C, and D generate recurrent B–C, C–D, and B–D deletions. The 1.5 Mb deletion B–C, at 15q25.2, is proximal; and deletion C–D, at 15q25.2q25.3, is distal. Others, B–D, take in both segments (Figure 14–56). Phenotypic features in the proximal deletion include intellectual disability or developmental delay, short stature, and craniofacial abnormalities. Penetrance is 100% (Goh et al. 2025). Of several plausible candidate genes within the B–C segment, *CPEB1* is one that might have a role in the neurocognitive phenotype (Burgess et al. 2014a); *HOMER2* is another candidate. The proximal deletion has been implicated in premature ovarian insufficiency; the locus of relevance may be *BCN1* (Hyon et al. 2016; Chen et al. 2020d). *RPS17* is

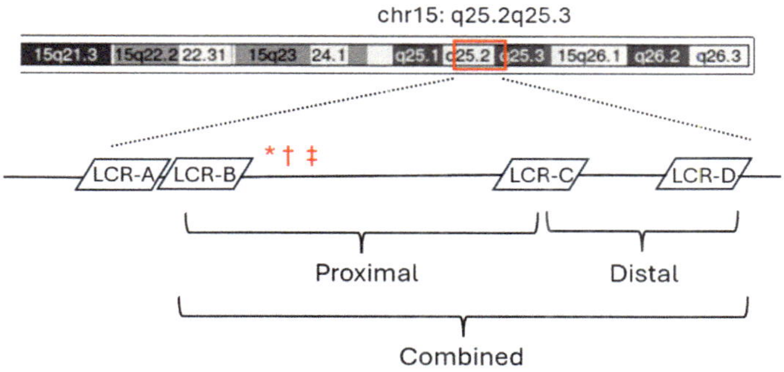

Figure 14–56. Proximal and Distal Deletions at 15q25.2q25.3.

Notes: Low copy repeats generate adjacent deletions, B-C and C-D. The deletion B-D takes in both segments. The relative position of *CPEB1* is asterisked; the dagger indicates *HOMER2*; the double dagger indicates *BNC1*.

within this segment, and its haploinsufficiency causes Diamond-Blackfan anemia. The distal deletion may represent a "susceptibility locus" for neurodevelopmental dysfunction (Doelken et al. 2012), but data apropos are few.

Duplication. No consistent phenotype is seen in the proximal 15q25.2 duplication. Goh et al. (2025) provide a penetrance figure of 71%, with wide confidence intervals due to small sample size.

15q26.3

Deletion. A particular phenotypic feature of this terminal deletion, which can be of variable extent, is growth retardation, with height and weight often 2 to 4 SD below the mean (Jezela-Stanek et al. 2012). This reflects loss of the *IGF1R* growth factor gene (as also in the ring 15, p. 300). The intellectual impairment ranges from borderline to severe ("pervasive developmental disorder"), with autism often a prominent feature (Battaglia 2008; Hogart et al. 2010). Facial dysmorphism and genital abnormality are concomitants. The considerable majority of probands are of de novo generation.

Duplications at the terminal band 15q26.3 are associated with overgrowth, an *IGF1R* effect (Tatton-Brown et al. 2009; Cannarella et al. 2017). Intellectual disability and facial dysmorphism are observed. These duplications are often the result of malsegregation of a parental translocation or inversion, but de novo examples exist (Chen et al. 2011a; Kim et al. 2011; Burada et al. 2021).

Chromosome 16

Rearrangements in chromosome 16p are among the more often seen in the genetic clinic. As with proximal 15q, the proximal short arm of 16 is of evolutionary interest, being a site of particularly active rearrangement in primate speciation and accumulating, in the time of *H. sapiens*, loci having putative roles in autism. This region has come to command a major role among CNVs associated with intellectual disability and psychosis. There is also a link with growth as measured by body mass index, and head circumference. There are five listed breakpoint (BP) regions within 16p11.2p12.2, numbering 1–5 from telomeric to centromeric (distal to proximal), enabling classification of different

elsewhere in the genome. They propose that "monosomy for 16p13.3 unmasks the effects of other variants genome-wide"; in other words, the variable expressivity of this deletion syndrome may relate more to loci on other chromosomes than in the del 16p13.3 itself. The only consistent observation is that of the thalassemia.

De novo occurrence is often so, but parental rearrangements are not infrequent and should always be sought. Of the 41 cases in Babbs et al., 20 were familial, from five families.

(2) *del 16p13.3: Rubinstein-Taybi Syndrome.* The Rubinstein-Taybi syndrome[18] (RTS) has a distinctive phenotype, and the facies and the broad thumbs are very characteristic. Most cases are due to point mutation in the *CREBBP* gene, but around 10%–25% have a small (1 kb–15 kb) deletion that removes part or all of *CREBBP* (Wójcik et al. 2010). There is no obvious clinical distinction between those RTS patients with or without the microdeletion, suggesting closely adjacent genes may not be dosage-sensitive (Rusconi et al. 2015). The range of observed severity presumably reflects a variable expressivity of the abnormal genotype, and the case of monozygous twins with RTS having rather different neurobehavioral phenotypes supports this suggestion (Preis and Majewski 1995). The oldest putative case, from 500 AD–900 AD, is that of a skeleton excavated at the Yokem site in Illinois (Wilbur 2000); some kind of record would be set were this case ever to yield to a paleocytomolecular genetic analysis!

Duplications in 16p13.3 are the "countertypes" of the Rubinstein-Taybi deletion, include the key *CREBBP* locus, and are of similarly variable sizes. In the smallest kilobase-size duplications, *CREBBP* may be the only gene involved (Mattina et al. 2012). Intellectual disability with poor speech, mild periorbital dysmorphism, micrognathia, and proximally implanted thumbs are notable features (Demeer et al. 2013; Li et al. 2013).

De novo inheritance is almost always the case, but non-penetrance has been observed in two parents who had "followed normal schooling, function normally in society, and do not present the typical face" (Thienpont et al. 2010). Inheritance from an affected parent is reported in Lee et al. (2016).

16q21q22.1

Deletion. Yamamoto et al. (2008) reported a series of 14 cases, including some of classical cytogenetic description; and Genesio et al. (2013) reviewed six examples of a precise molecular definition. Pre- and post-natal growth retardation, microcephaly with psychomotor retardation, and facial dysmorphism are observed. Loss of *HSD11B2* within 16q22.1, consistently observed, might be the basis of the growth retardation. Notably, a partially overlapping region just centromeric of *HSD11B2* can be deleted without any effect upon the phenotype; this is a "euchromatic variant," reflecting a very low gene density in this segment of 16q21 (p. 511).

16q24

Deletion. Three separate or overlapping syndromes involve band 16q24.

First, the *del 16q24.1* syndrome, as well as implying neurocognitive deficit may also predict certain organ malformations, according to the regions of deletion: the severe and

[18] A similar condition due to mutation in the *EP300* gene, a paralog of *CREBBP*, has been called RTS type 2 (Hamilton et al. 2016).

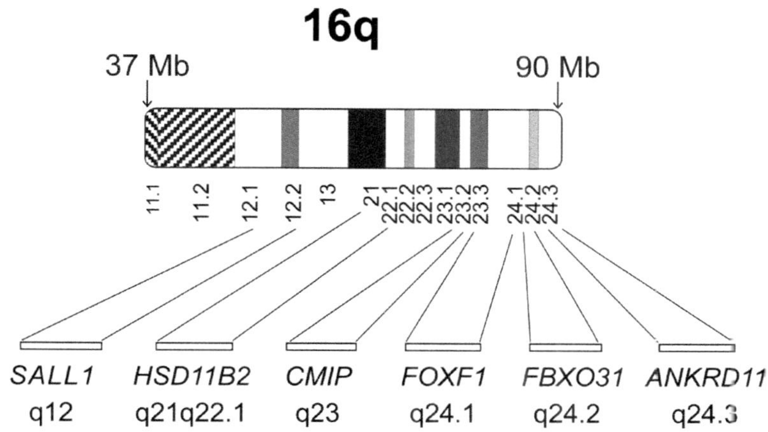

Figure 14–63.

usually lethal lung disorder, alveolar capillary dysplasia; bilateral hydronephrosis, likely consequential upon urinary tract obstruction; and heart and gut defects (Stankiewicz et al. 2009). Deletions are non-recurrent and of variable size. *FOXF1* is a key phenocritical candidate in many.

> This syndrome provides an example of a phenotype which can be due not to haploinsufficiency of a gene, but rather to haploinsufficiency of a distant enhancer of a gene. Thus, Szafranski et al. (2016) show that deletion removing an upstream enhancer of *FOXF1* (a long non-protein coding RNA, *LINC01081*) while the *FOXF1* gene itself, some 272 kb away, remains intact, can nevertheless lead to a functional non-expression of the gene and in consequence, the typical lung disease.

Second, *del 16q24.2* is associated with autism and intellectual disability, often of severe degree, and minor craniofacial dysmorphism (Handrigan et al. 2013). Deletions range from 27 kb to 2.7 Mb in size. One of the contained genes, *FBXO31*, is plausibly a key factor in the neurobehavioral phenotype. Parental transmission is quite frequently observed, with the deletion size in these being less than 1 Mb; an instance of maternal mosaicism for the deletion is known.

Third, *deletion of 16q24.3* leads to a syndrome in which intellectual disability, minor facial anomalies, macrodontia, and short stature are typical observations (Kim et al. 2015). Deletions range up to about 2 Mb in size. Loss of *ANKRD11* (the gene responsible for KBG syndrome), is the central factor; loss of neighboring genes extends the phenotype (Novara et al. 2017). Familial transmission is recorded, including from a mosaic mother (Sacharow et al. 2012; Khalifa et al. 2013).

16q12qter

Duplication. Extensive 16q duplications involving nearly all of the long arm are on record, typically in the context of the concomitant monosomy of another chromosome from a parental translocation. Most are lethal in infancy, but a few "pure" partial trisomies are described, with associated ongoing survival and considerable morbidity (Manor et al. 2021).

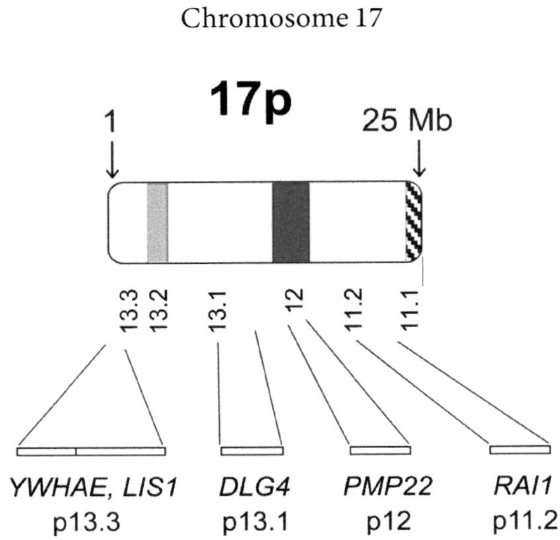

Figure 14–64.

Chromosome 17 short arm has remarkably high density of segmental duplications, and about a quarter of its DNA consists of low-copy repeats (Blazejewski et al. 2018). Thus it is that a number of del/dup conditions due to nonallelic homologous recombination reside in 17p.

*17p11.2**

Deletion, Smith-Magenis Syndrome. This classic syndrome comprises a picture of dysmorphology, intellectual disability, and fractious behavior. Speech and hearing are substantially affected (Brennan et al. 2024). Brain anatomy may be abnormal (Maya et al. 2014). Sleep disturbance is a characteristic feature (associated in most cases with a reversal of the normal circadian pattern of melatonin secretion); and a habit of self-mutilation and markedly diminished pain sensitivity can manifest as "onychotillomania" (pulling out nails). To the practiced eye, the facies may be distinctive (Allanson et al. 1999).

Most (>90%) patients have an ~3.8 Mb deletion, arising by NAHR between low-copy repeats; a larger deletion may be associated with a more complicated phenotype (Park et al. 2002; Vieira et al. 2012). The crucial locus within the deleted segment is *RAI1* (Figure 14–64), and the syndrome may result from mutation within this gene alone. Haploinsufficiency of *RAI1* may compromise the activity of a number of downstream genes, and each of these, thus compromised, then contribute to a component of the syndrome.

Recurrence is very rare, but one case is recorded due to low-level (25% on blood) parental somatic, and inferentially gonadal, mosaicism (Campbell et al. 2014). Otherwise, familial transmission may result from a balanced parental rearrangement.

Duplication: Potocki-Lupski Syndrome. This condition was predicted to exist as the reciprocal recombination product of the Smith-Magenis syndrome (SMS) deletion (Potocki et al. 2000). The clinical picture is largely that of a neurobehavioral and neuropsychiatric syndrome; the contrasting phenotypes of Potocki-Lupski syndrome and

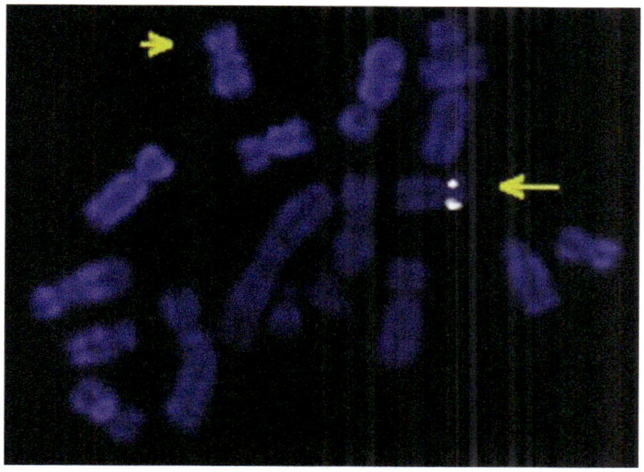

Figure 14–65. The 17p12 Deletion Causing Hereditary Pressure-Sensitive Neuropathy.
Notes: This FISH demonstration, using a probe that recognizes the *PMP22* gene, shows normal hybridization (arrow) to one no. 17, but not the other (arrowhead). This reflects the absence of the p12 segment on the deleted chromosome.

SMS are outlined in Neira-Fresneda and Potocki (2015). As with SMS, the key locus is *RAI1*. Parent-to-child transmission is known (Kolbasin et al. 2024).

*17p12**

Deletion: Hereditary Pressure-Sensitive Neuropathy. A recurrent 1.4 Mb deletion at 17p12 is the typical basis of hereditary pressure-sensitive neuropathy (HPSN), which has the alternative names of hereditary neuropathy with liability to pressure palsies (HNPP) and tomaculous neuropathy (Chance 2006). The deletion of a particular "nerve gene," the *PMP22* or peripheral myelin protein 22 gene, leads to abnormal myelination of the peripheral nerves, and this compromises their function. A typical presentation is the backpacker who complains of numbness (sensory nerves) and weakness (motor nerves) in the arms after a day's hiking, and these symptoms are due to the pressure of the shoulder straps on the nerves in the armpit. The former mainstay of cytogenetic diagnosis was by FISH, using a probe that hybridized to the region; Figure 14–65 is still useful in giving a direct pictorial demonstration of the deletion. The deletion can arise de novo or, as is more usual, can be transmitted from an affected parent, in which case the risk to transmit the disease is 50%.

Duplication: Charcot-Marie-Tooth Neuropathy. The most common form, by far (two-thirds or more), of all Charcot-Marie-Tooth neuropathy, CMT1A, is due to the recurrent duplication of 1.4 Mb in 17p12, which encompasses the *PMP22* (peripheral myelin protein 22) gene (Salpietro et al. 2018).[19] It is the reciprocal duplication of the deletion described above which causes pressure-sensitive neuropathy.[20] FISH was a formerly used diagnostic method (Figure 14–66). The duplication leads to the production of a 150% amount of the PMP22 protein, and this excess mars the capacity for proper

[19] The duplicated segment of chromosome 17 is some 1.7 Mb in size, but it is "gene-sparse." The very few other genes contained therein appear to imply no phenotypic consequence, due to their being in imbalanced state.

[20] An extraordinary coincidence is for one no. 17 chromosome to carry a *PMP22* deletion and the other a *PMP22* duplication, and thus a balanced genome and the person free of either neuropathy (Hirt et al. 2015).

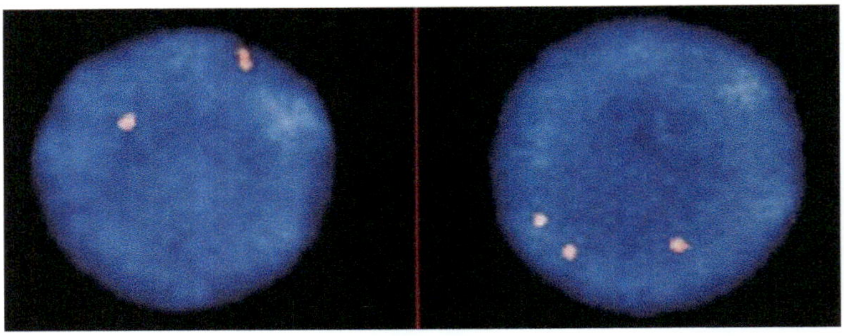

Figure 14–66. FISH Demonstration of the Charcot-Marie-Tooth Duplication.

Notes: These two images are of interphase blood cells from a patient with CMT neuropathy. The probe (pink) recognizes the *PMP22* gene. At *left*, the duplication can be seen at 1 o'clock with two juxtaposed signals, almost overlapping. At *right*, the signals from the dup(17) at 8 o'clock are somewhat more separated.

Source: From H Slater et al., Improved testing for CMT1A and HNPP using multiplex ligation-dependent probe amplification (MLPA) with rapid DNA preparations: comparison with the interphase FISH method, *Hum Mutat* 24:164–171, 2004. Courtesy KHA Choo, and with the permission of John Wiley and Sons.

functioning of the peripheral nerve. The sensory nerves are affected, but the major functional effect is on the motor nerves, and weakness is the important consequence. The nerves to the peroneal muscles (on the outside of the leg, with tendons passing around the ankle to the foot) are particularly vulnerable, and an alternative name for the condition is peroneal muscular atrophy. A rare circumstance is that of homozygosity for the duplication, effectively a partial 17p tetrasomy, which leads to a more severe manifestation of the neurological phenotype (Pareyson et al. 2003).

About 80% of CMT1A is familial, inherited as an autosomal dominant trait. Of the 20% arising de novo, the considerable majority arose in male gametogenesis, in most cases due to a rearrangement between non-sister chromatids (Lee et al. 2020). Preimplantation testing is appropriately offered to the person with the condition planning a family (Zou et al. 2024).

17p11.2p12

Duplication encompassing both *RAI1* and *PMP22* produces a syndrome showing features of both Potocki-Lupski syndrome and Charcot-Marie-Tooth type 1A neuropathy (Yuan et al. 2015). Segmental lengths range from 3.2 Mb to 19.7 Mb. These duplications are non-recurrent, and all tested cases have been of de novo origin.

17p13.1

Deletions of 17p13.1 are of differing extents, but typically under 1 Mb in size. Microcephaly with profound intellectual disability is typical, and these children are nonverbal. Carvalho et al. (2014) propose an "oligogenic" model, whereby the microcephaly flows from a perturbed epistatic interaction between five critical genes within the deletion segment (*ASGR1, ACADVL, DVL2, DLG4*, and *GABARAP*) rather than an independent effect of each locus (Figure 3–21). In all studied cases, inheritance has been de novo.

Duplication encompasses the same critical region as in the deletion. Very few cases are on record, but all include the critical region (Leka-Emiri et al. 2019). Intellectual disability, of varying degree, is seen in common. Almost all cases studied have been de novo, but maternal transmission is recorded.

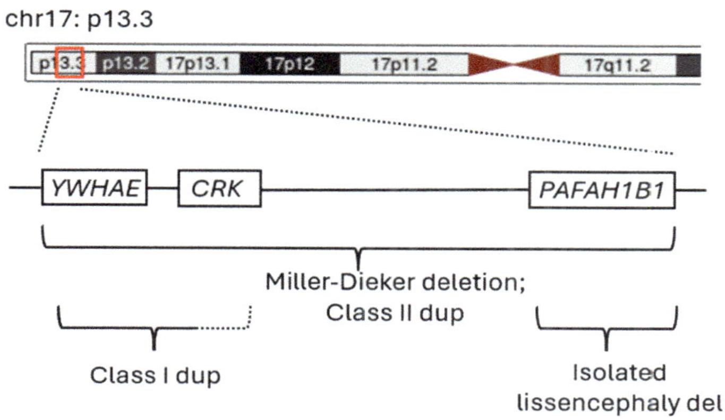

Figure 14–67. Deletions and Duplication at 17p13.3.

Notes: The extents of deletions and duplications, with respect to the different syndromes, are shown. The Class I duplication can sometimes extend to include *CRK* (dotted bracket). *PAFAH1B1* was formerly known as *LIS1*.

17p13.3

Deletion. A proneness to rearrangement in 17p13.3 reflects a local richness in *Alu* sequences (Gu et al. 2015), and deletions of variable extents, interstitial or terminal, may remove some or all of these loci. Three loci of particular note are *YWHAE, CRK*, and *PAFAH1B1* (*PAFAH1B1* shown as *LIS1* in Figure 14–64). According to the pattern of deletion, different syndromes arise (Figure 14–67). In the well-known Miller-Dieker syndrome (MDS) of "lissencephaly plus," all three genes are deleted. MDS is not uncommonly diagnosed following prenatal ultrasonography (Figure 14–68); it is usually fatal in early childhood. Loss of *PAFAH1B1* alone causes isolated lissencephaly, associated with cognitive incapacity, epilepsy, and motor impairment (Cardoso et al. 2003). Deletion of *YWHAE* and *CRK*, but not *PAFAH1B1*, lead to neurodevelopmental compromise, structural brain abnormalities, and epilepsy (Romano et al. 2020). A series of representative del/dups from Liang et al. (2022a) is depicted in Figure 14–69. Most 17p13.3 deletions arise de novo, but a parental balanced rearrangement is occasionally recognized.

Duplication of 17p13.3 is divided into a milder Class I and a more severe Class II, based on the absence or presence of *PAFAH1B1* in the duplicated segment; both classes include *YWHAE* (Blazejewski et al. 2018). Intellectual disability and behavioral abnormality—in some diagnosed as autism, speech and motor delay, and subtle facial dysmorphism—characterize Class I. Some have IQs in the normal range, and indeed Liang et al. (2022a) raise a question that this duplication (e.g., the short blue bar in Figure 14–69) might be a variant of uncertain significance. Penetrance in Goh et al. (2025) is 41%. The phenotype in Class II includes microcephaly and other brain abnormality, such as the hypoplasia of the corpus callosum and mild cerebellar volume loss (Curry et al. 2013). The penetrance for duplications that include *PAFAH1B* in Goh et al. (2025) is 79%.

The Class I condition may be familial. Affected parents are typically less affected than their (proband) child; somatic-gonadal and (presumed) confined gonadal mosaicism, with normal parents, are both recorded.

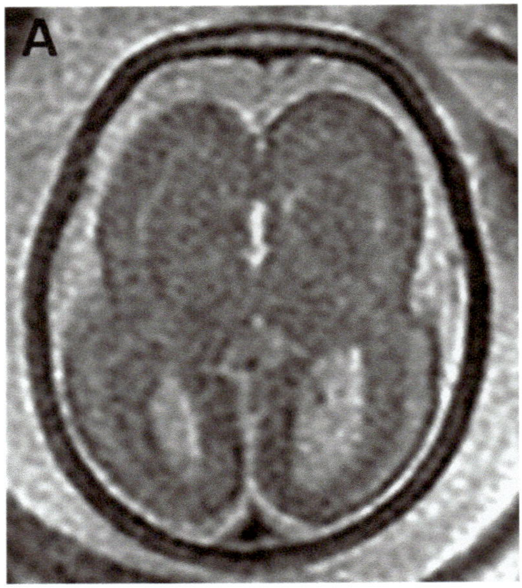

Figure 14–68. The Lissencephaly of Miller-Dieker Syndrome.

Notes: Prenatal brain MRI shows lissencephaly ("smooth brain") in Miller-Dieker syndrome. This was a 31-week fetus with a de novo del 17p13.3. Frontal lobe in upper part of image, occiput in lower. The surface of the brain (the cortex) is smooth, lacking the normal furrowed appearance at this gestation. The occipital ventricles are mildly enlarged, reflecting a reduction in brain parenchyma.

Source: From C-P Chen et al., Chromosome 17p13.3 deletion syndrome: aCGH characterization, prenatal findings and diagnosis, and literature review, *Gene* 532: 152–159, 2013. Courtesy C-P Chen, and with the permission of Elsevier.

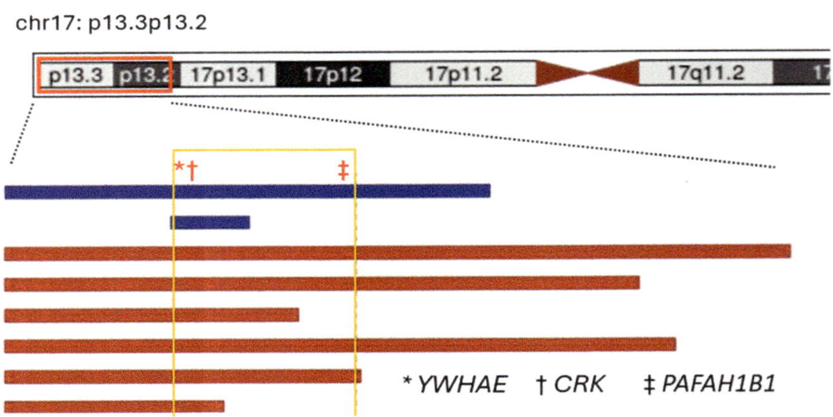

Figure 14–69. A Representative Series of 17p13.3 Deletions and Duplications.

Notes: Deletions are in red, duplications are in blue. The Miller-Dieker region is outlined. The relative positions of the three key loci noted are indicated. In one duplication and two deletion cases, *PAFAH1B1* remained intact. The duplication case was a prenatal diagnosis, an increased nuchal translucency. The child has since developed normally, and his healthy mother, who had received an undergraduate education, was shown to carry the same duplication. Of the deletion cases with *PAFAH1B1* intact, one comprised a fetus with IUGR and a brain cortical anomaly; and the other was a child with intellectual disability and severe motor delay.

Source: From B Liang et al., Clinical findings and genetic analysis of patients with copy number variants involving 17p13.3 using a single nucleotide polymorphism array: a single-center experience, *BMC Med Genomics* 15:268, 2022. Courtesy N Lin, H Huang, and L Xu, and with the permission of Springer Nature.

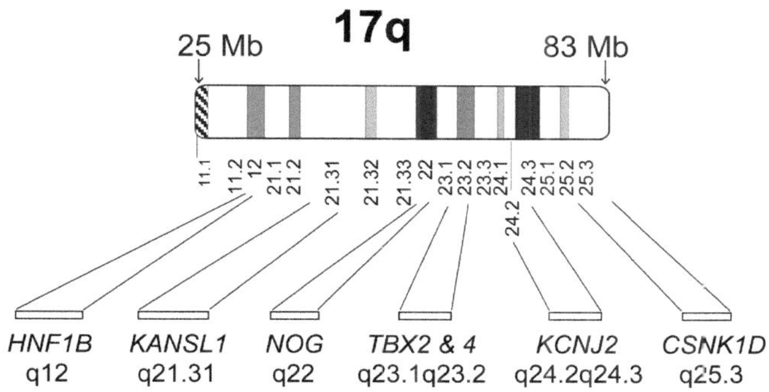

Figure 14–70.

*17q11.2**

Deletion. About 5%–10% of all neurofibromatosis type 1 (NF1) is due to a recurrent 1.4 Mb deletion at 17q11.2, which includes the *NF1* gene. The clinical picture is typically more severe than in NF1 due to point mutation. Tritto et al. (2024) hypothesize that the deletion might lead to changes in the 3D chromatin structure in the 17q11.2 region, thus influencing the phenotype for the worse.

Duplication. The 17q11.2 microduplication syndrome, reciprocal to the deletion, includes intellectual disability and dysmorphism as the only clinical features in common (Tassano et al. 2017). NF1 signs are not seen. Penetrance in Goh et al. (2025) is 74%.

*17q12**

Deletion. A key observation is that of renal cystic disease progressing to chronic renal dysfunction (Buffin-Meyer et al. 2024). At fetal ultrasonography, hyperechogenic kidneys may be detected (Zhou et al. 2021). Developmental delay is usually of mild degree, but autism is a possibility. Facial dysmorphism may be moderate, "soft," or essentially absent. Pancreatic, liver, and genital abnormality may be seen, and some are diabetic, with MODY-5[21] (Xin and Zhang 2023). The crucial gene is *HNF1B* (Figure 14–70) which, as a Mendelian mutation, is responsible for the renal cysts and diabetes (RCAD) syndrome. Mother-to-child transmission is recorded. Goh et al. (2025) calculate a penetrance of 63%, but caution that some with RCAD are likely undiagnosed, affecting the validity of this figure.

Duplication. Rare 17q12 duplications encompassing *HNF1B* have been associated with gastrointestinal pathology such as tracheo-esophageal fistula, and choledochal cyst presenting as neonatal cholestatic jaundice. Intellect may be normal, but variable cognitive impairment, difficult behavior, and occasionally epilepsy are observed. Second-hit CNVs elsewhere in the genome may exacerbate the phenotype. Renal function is, as with the deletion, affected; in contrast, diabetes is not over-represented in the duplication (Cannon et al. 2023). Penetrance in Goh et al. (2025) is a low 20%. Inheritance from a normal mother has been seen (Kotalova et al. 2018).

*17q21.31**

Deletion: Koolen-de Vries Syndrome. This is a condition that could, in retrospect, have been seen as a syndrome, but in which the collection of features did not impress

[21] Maturity-onset diabetes of the young type 5.

sufficiently that recognition was likely to have been achieved ahead of the laboratory discovery ("genotype-first") of this recurrent deletion (Tan et al. 2009). Having made that point, features of the facies are sufficiently distinct that "next-generation phenotyping," in which facial photographs are assessed by computer, was able to identify a case (Brand et al. 2022). Poor speech development, epilepsy, and "hypersocial behavior" may be seen as having a resemblance to Angelman syndrome. *KANSL1* is the relevant gene (point mutation can also produce the syndrome); a 990 kb inversion polymorphism spanning 17q21.31 is a necessary predisposing element (Koolen et al. 2016).

Recurrence is very rare. One case is known of mother-to-child transmission (Rendeiro et al. 2016). Koolen et al. (2012) studied two instances of recurrence due to low-grade maternal mosaicism. One mother had 0.5 Mb deletion in 8% of buccal mucosal cells, and in the other mother there was an essentially similar deletion in 3% of peripheral lymphocytes. In the de novo case, Koolen et al. calculate a risk of recurrence of 1/9,446 (0.01%), which is about twice the baseline population risk of 1/16,000. This overall calculation is based upon the separate risks according to the parental genotypes for the inversion polymorphism mentioned above; the interested reader is referred to p. 78 for a fuller exposition.

Duplication. The reciprocal duplication of the 17q21.31 deletion is unusual in that the remarkable abnormal phenotype, a dementia, does not emerge until middle age, mean onset at 50 years with a disease duration then of 10 years. In childhood, there may be a mild neurodevelopmental phenotype of borderline cognitive and behavioral capacity (Gregor et al. 2012). Later neurodegeneration is due to duplication of the *MAPT* gene (adjacent to *KANSL1*; Figure 14–71), there is abnormal accumulation of tau within certain brain regions, and the disorder can be called a primary tauopathy (Wallon et al. 2021). The typical onset is of an amnestic syndrome, that is, a loss in memory; the condition can evolve to affect other functional neurological domains. Penetrance is high, possibly 100% (Goh et al. 2025). Since the dup can be transmitted, the counseling issues rather reflect those of other adult-onset neurodegenerative conditions such as dominantly inherited Alzheimer disease. Its unanticipated discovery at chromosome analysis would raise an ethical question (p. 810).

17q22

Deletion of the *NOG* locus is the basis of this syndrome (Carlson et al. 2021). The limbs and the ears are vulnerable anatomy. Symphalangism (fusion of joints of fingers and

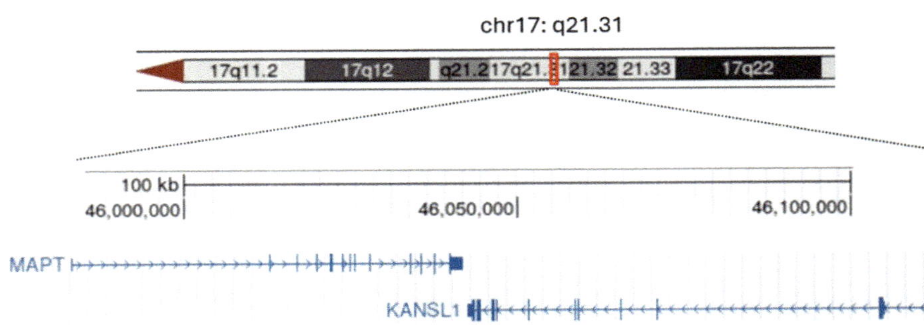

Figure 14–71. The Adjacent Loci *MAPT* and *KANSL1* at 17q21.31.

Notes: MAPT is the relevant locus in the dup17q21q31, while *KANSL1* is the important factor in the deletion. Loss of *MAPT* in the deletion, and gain of *KANSL1* in the duplication, seem without evident effect.

Source: Drawn after the UCSC genome browser entry for chr17:45,962,338-46,172,143 (hg38).

toes) and other digital defects, joint contractures developing through childhood, and conductive hearing loss are typical. Intellectual disability associated with microcephaly and a distinctive facial dysmorphism are also noted. De novo inheritance is more usual, but parent-to-child transmission is known.

*17q23.1q23.2**

Deletion. An inconsistency of phenotype mirrors the considerable range of deletions within this region, although a mild to moderate developmental delay, particularly affecting speech, is frequent. In those in whom the deletion removes the adjacent transcription factor genes *TBX2* and *TBX4*, heart and limb defects are characteristic (Ballif et al. 2010). All cases have been de novo. Penetrance in Goh et al. (2025) is complete.

Duplication. A phenotype is yet to be established for this rare recurrent duplication, but if a phenotype exists, it is likely to be mild and incompletely penetrant (Goh et al. 2025).

Chromosome 18

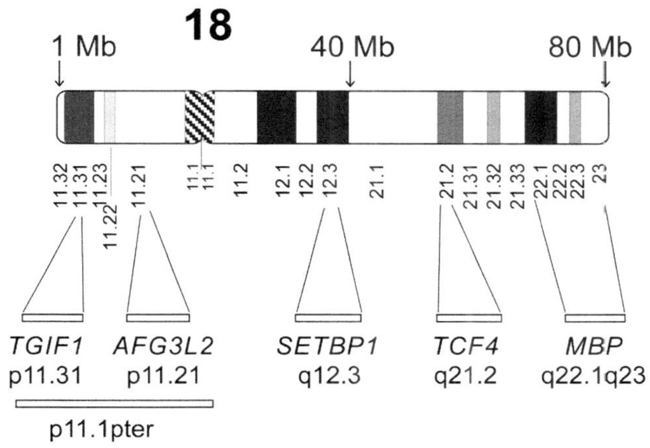

Figure 14–72.

18p

Deletion: de Grouchy Syndrome. The most frequent form of 18p deletion involves a whole-arm loss, the breakpoint at the centromere (thus "centromeric 18p– syndrome") seen in almost one-half of del 18p cases (Sebold et al. 2015). *TGIF1* and *AFG3L2* (Figure 14–72) are two of several genes reviewed in Hasi-Zogaj et al. (2015) that may be contributory to the phenotype. Albeit that this is a homogeneous cytogenetic material, the clinical picture can vary quite considerably. Intellectual impairment may be relatively mild, with an IQ range around 50–100, an average of 70 (Hasi-Zogaj et al. 2015). Soileau et al. (2015) provide very detailed data concerning short (and long) arm 18 deletions. Coping with everyday life is difficult. Many will die before adult age.

Partial 18p deletion breakpoints are recorded along the whole length of the short arm, very few of which are recurrent. In principle, the milder the phenotype the less the degree of 18p loss. Most cases occur de novo, but there are rare instances of parental transmission. Certainly, in any 18p deletion, parental rearrangement is prudently to be excluded.

20p13

Deletion. This deletion is sited near the telomere. Fang et al. (2019) define the phenotype as comprising motor and language delay, minor dysmorphic features, and epilepsy; Landau-Kleffner syndrome (loss of speech recognition, nocturnal seizures) is reported. Some achieve an IQ formally within a normal range. Deletions are terminal, and most are non-recurrent, typically from kilobase to 1–2 Mb in extent. The subtelomeric genes *NRSN2* and *SOX12* are proposed to be pheno-critical. Where tested, de novo inheritance has been universal.

20q11.22q11.23

Deletions that reside within the segment 20q11.22q11.23 determine a heterogeneous range. Clinical presentation typically includes growth retardation, intractable feeding difficulties with gastroesophageal reflux, hypotonia, and psychomotor developmental delay. Bensaid et al. (2024) propose two critical regions, one defined by the locus *GDF5*, at 20q11.22, and the other by *TOP1* at 20q12.

> One of a pair of non-identical monozygous twins in Meredith et al. (2017) had the smallest recorded deletion, likely in constitutional mosaic state, with only *GDF5* deleted of the three genes just named; intriguingly, his phenotypically normal co-twin also showed mosaicism for the deletion, presumably as a consequence of chimerism confined to blood, reflecting that the two had shared a placenta. A mitotic origin of the deletion in one twin, after the splitting of the conceptus, is a probable basis of the abnormality.

Duplication. Avila et al. (2013) and Goetzinger et al. (2021) delineate the syndrome due to dup 20q11.22q11.23. A notable clinical feature is trigonocephaly (if *ASXL1* is within the deleted segment) with ridging of the metopic suture along with psychomotor delay, poor speech acquisition, and short hands and feet. *GDF5* is a plausible pheno-contributory locus. The duplication may exist as an insertional segment into another chromosome. All cases have been of de novo generation.

20q13.33

Deletion. Epilepsy is a particular feature of the phenotype due to this deletion, which might or might not coexist with a neurocognitive component (Okumura et al. 2015; Lewis et al. 2018). A 20q terminal deletion might remove only the last two genes on the chromosome (*MYT1* and *PCMTD2*), or if of wider extent, genes of possible epileptic susceptibility (*KCNQ2* and *CHRNA4*) could be included (Mefford et al. 2012).

Chromosome 21

21q21.3

Duplication of 21q21.3 alone, containing the *APP* (amyloid precursor protein) gene, is of itself a determinant of early-onset dementia (Figure 14–79, 80). Kalfon et al. (2022) report a segregating rea(18) which included the segment dup21q21.3 carrying *APP* and just one other 21q gene (*CYYR1*). In this seven-generation family, the heterozygous women had presented with dementia and the men with intracerebral bleeds. Kasri et al. (2024) demonstrate accumulation of amyloid β peptide (Aβ; the product of

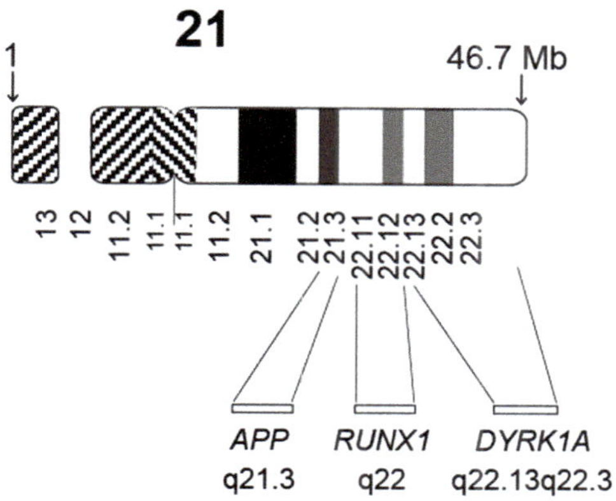

Figure 14–78.

proteolytic processing of APP) in the brains of dup 21q21.3 carriers (Figure 14–80). As with the17q21.31 duplication (above), counseling will need to follow the norms established for other adult-onset neurodegenerative disease.

21q22.12

Deletion: Braddock-Carey Syndrome. Clinical observations include neurocognitive compromise typically of severe degree, agenesis of the corpus callosum, the Pierre Robin sequence, facial dysmorphism, heart malformation, and in some, congenital thrombocytopenia (Braddock et al. 2016). This latter trait is due to loss of the *RUNX1* gene (Figure 14–78); in Braddock-Carey syndrome in which this gene is intact, platelet production is normal. All cases of this syndrome have been of de novo generation.

21q22.13

Deletion. The locus of particular interest within 21q22.13 is *DYRK1A*, a gene of note with respect to the Down syndrome neurocognitive phenotype. This deletion is close by, but distinct from, the Braddock-Carey deletion. Ji et al. (2015) define a *DYRK1A* deletion syndrome characterized by growth retardation, microcephaly

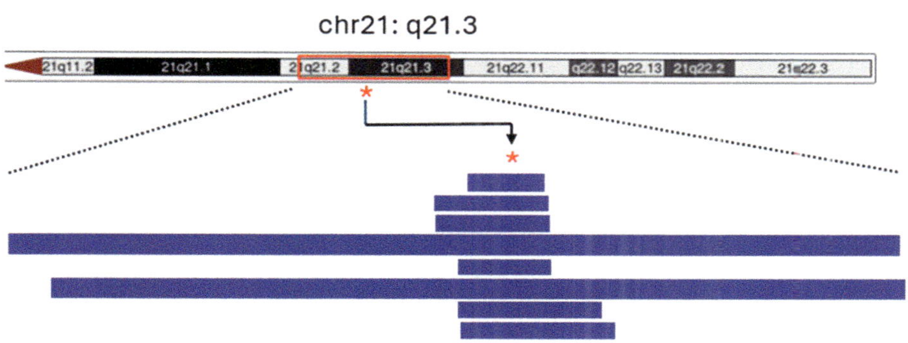

Figure 14–79. Duplications at 21q21.3 that Included *APP*.

Notes: These data are from Kalfon et al. (2022) and Kasri et al. (2024). The relative position of the *APP* gene is asterisked. The smaller duplications included only *APP* and one other gene (either *GABPA* on the centromeric side, or *CYYR1* telomerically).

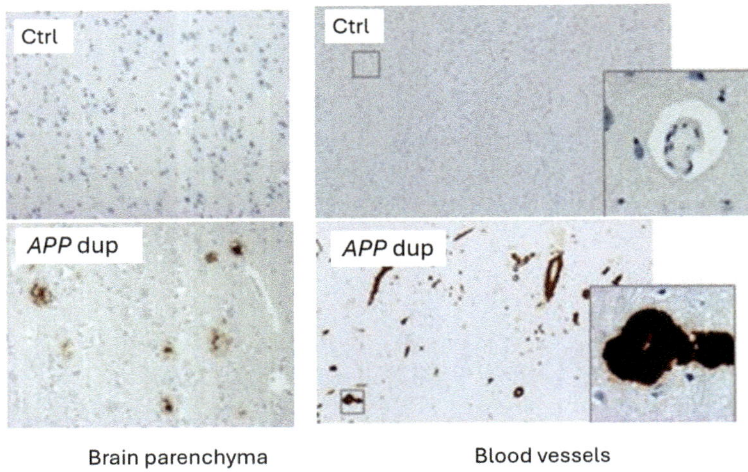

Figure 14–80. Amyloid Accumulation in the Brain in dup21q21.3.

Notes: This brain biopsy, of frontal lobe cortex, was taken at post mortem from a person who had suffered dementia, and who was a dup21q21.3 heterozygote, the duplicated segment including the *APP* gene. The scattered islands of brown staining in brain parenchyma (*left*) show amyloid β peptide (Aβ) accumulation; none such is to be seen in the control sample. Deposits of Aβ in blood vessels are shown at *right*. The high-magnified images show a vessel, the lumen patent in the control, but occluded in the dup case.

Source: From A Kasri et al., Amyloid-β peptide signature associated with cerebral amyloid angiopathy in familial Alzheimer's disease with APPdup and Down syndrome, *Acta Neuropathol* 148:8, 2024. Courtesy H Zetterberg and M-C Potier, and with the permission of Springer.

with various types of brain malformation on imaging, global neurofunctional compromise, epilepsy, and a distinctive facial gestalt. Deletions are mostly in the range 0.5 Mb–10 Mb. Sibship recurrence due to a maternal insertional translocation is recorded in Ji et al.

Duplication. Broadly speaking, a duplication containing this segment, and more so if it includes *DYRK1A*, leads to a Down syndrome picture (Schnabel et al. 2018).

Chromosome 22

22q11.1q11.21

Duplication, Triplication: Cat Eye Syndrome, Schmid-Fraccaro Syndrome. The cytogenetics of this imbalance varies, and it can be seen typically as a supernumerary inv dup(22)(q11.21) or der(22)(q11.1q11.21) but also as an intrachromosomal duplication or triplication. The eponymous eye sign is iris coloboma; developmental delay, ear tags, renal and anal anomaly, and occasionally the severe cardiovascular malformation, and total anomalous pulmonary venous return are variably associated. The landmark locus is *CECR2.* Both the intrachromosomal and supernumerary forms can be familial, and it would be obligatory to offer parental testing (Jedraszak et al. 2024). Mosaicism is common. One mother had 4.5% mosaicism in blood, while her two affected sons had levels of 85% and 70%; and reproductive study in one mosaic man, the father of three mosaic children, showed 50% of sperm to carry the inv dup(22) (Kvarnung et al. 2012).

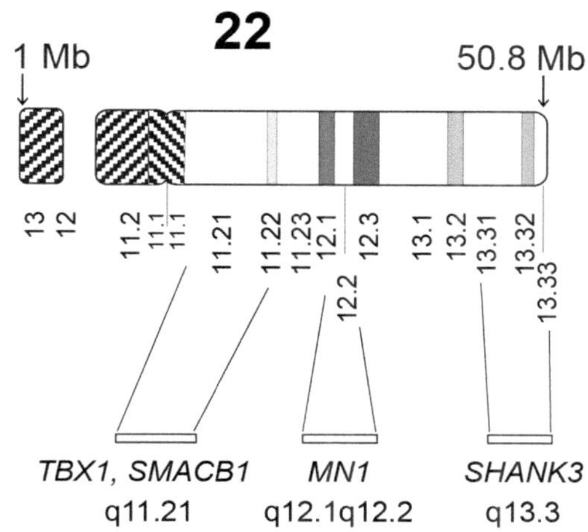

Figure 14–81.

*22q11.21**

Deletion. Before their common cytogenetic basis was understood, the 22q11 deletion clinical presentations had a number of labels, including DiGeorge syndrome (DGS), velocardiofacial (VCF) syndrome, and Shprintzen syndrome.[22] DGS was the name typically applied to a child with heart defect, parathyroid abnormality, and immunodeficiency; in Shprintzen syndrome a cleft or deficient palate was the notable feature, while VCF syndrome emphasized the facial appearance along with palatal ("velo") clefting and a heart defect, typically including a malformation of the great vessels of the outflow tract. Kousseff syndrome and Cayler syndrome were names given to variants with a neural tube defect, and asymmetric crying facies plus cardiac outflow defect, respectively.

The intellect is affected; median full-scale IQ is 76 (Campbell et al. 2015). The variable expressivity with respect to IQ is in large part explainable on the basis of the parental IQ levels (Klaassen et al. 2016). Difficulty in social interaction may relate mostly to the degree of intellectual disability. A psychiatric/behavioral component is frequent, with susceptibility to psychosis including schizophrenia (Van et al. 2024). Those in whom the cognitive impairment is more marked have a greater tendency to develop a psychotic disorder (Vorstman et al. 2015). If other features are absent, the chromosomal diagnosis may be delayed until adolescence or adulthood (Furuya et al. 2015; Fonseca-Pedrero et al. 2016). The evolution of the *tout ensemble* phenotype in the adult, with whom neuropsychiatric disease is the main cause for concern, presents its own challenges (Fung et al. 2015).

With a birth incidence of about one in 4,000 (estimates vary), this is the most common human site of deletion, and this vulnerability resides in the existence of LCRs and palindromic AT-rich repeats in the 22q11.21 region (Vervoort et al. 2025). The most frequently observed (~90%) deletion, of 2.54 Mb, lies between LCR A–D (Figure 14–82). Otherwise, 8% span the ~1.5 Mb segment LCR A–B, and rare deletions occur at other sites, including LCRs E through H. *TBX1* is the locus seen as key to the cardiac defects,

[22] In true acknowledgment of the first definition of the syndrome in the Czechoslovakian literature in 1955, Sedlácková syndrome may be the most fitting name (Turnpenny and Pigott 2001).

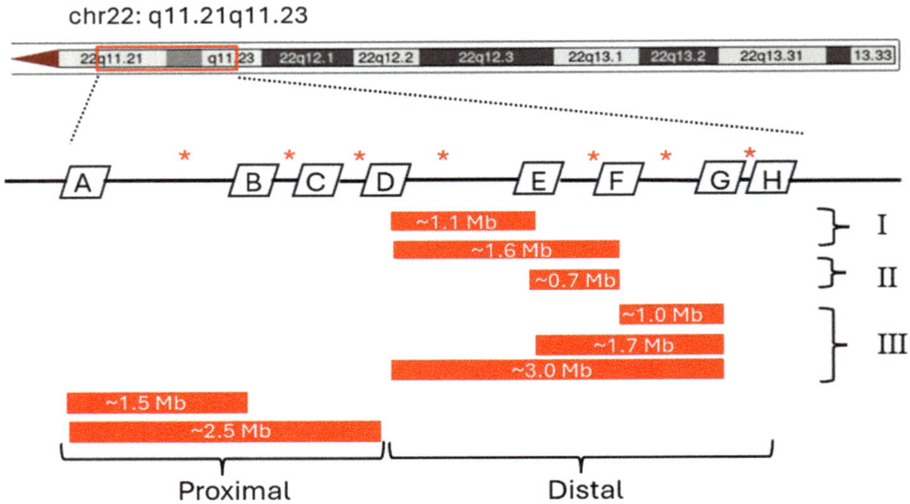

Figure 14–82. Deletion and Duplication at 22q11.21q11.23.

Notes: Deletions and duplications arise due to recombination between Low Copy Repeats A through H, and are grouped as proximal (A-D) and distal (E-H) imbalances. The considerable majority, 90%, are due to del/dup of LCR A-D within 22q11.21. The distal del/dups are subdivided into Classes I to III, according to the pattern of imbalance. Within the segments between each of the LCRs, a key locus is identified, and their relative positions are shown as the asterisks. In order from centromere to telomere, these loci are *TBX1, SCARF2, SNAP29, MAPK1, BCR, SMARCB1,* and *UBP1.*

and possibly also contributory to the psychopathy (Hiramoto et al. 2011); this gene lies between LCRs A and B (Figure 14–82). An uncommon deletion LCR B–D associated with a clinical picture of immune dysregulation can point to a likely causative role of the immune locus *CRKL* within this segment (Lin et al. 2021b).

Incomplete penetrance for components of the syndrome, and variable expressivity for those that are present, is very much the rule. The overall penetrance estimate in Goh et al. (2025) is 86%, but this would likely increase to near 100% with thorough phenotyping. Monozygous twins are often discordant (Singh et al. 2002b). In the familial case, a parent can, for example, show mild features of the condition or have a predominantly Shprintzen facial and palatal phenotype, with a child showing a characteristic DGS cardiac and endocrine phenotype (Devriendt et al. 1997). Hart et al. (2016) rehearse issues in sensitively raising with parents the risk for psychosis. The condition is typically more severe in second-generation subjects, although ascertainment bias is a likely explanation[23] (Cirillo et al. 2014). Variable expressivity with respect to facial appearance is compounded due to ethnic differences, and Kruszka et al. (2017) propose that digital facial analysis technology is a more accurate "observer" than a clinician.

In advising about recurrence risk, genetic counseling must take account of the possibilities of a parent being so mildly affected that the condition had not been recognized, and thus parental chromosomal analysis is appropriately offered. Most cases are de novo, but about 10% may be inherited. Gonadal and somatic-gonadal mosaicism are rarely reported but nevertheless have been seen; and a "very small" risk of recurrence,

[23] Another is "positive assortative mating." The de novo case is likely to have arisen from normal parents. But in the next generation, an affected person is more likely to have a partner of a similar level of intellectual capacity, compounding the effect in children of theirs.

following a de novo case, is to be acknowledged (Sandrin-Garcia et al. 2002; Chen et al. 2019). Vergés et al. (2014), in a study of fathers of children with the de novo 22q11 deletion, found two of nine fathers with levels of del(22q11) sperm that were approximately threefold higher than those of controls.

Clearly, the recurrence risk from a heterozygous parent will be 50%. Earlier estimates of a larger fraction of affected parents may have been biased due to studying more remarkable families (Swillen et al. 1998). Indeed, Smith and Robson (1999) report only 5% of parents to have had the deletion in an Australian series of 59 cases. However, in the case of the "nested deletions" LCR-B to LCR-D, and LCR-C to LCR-D, a majority, 60%, are familial (Campbell et al. 2018). Rare familial cases can result from a translocation (Peter et al. 2021).

The deletion is detectable on maternal blood screening, NIPT (Blagowidow et al. 2023), which could be offered to a whole pregnant population or targeted to couples with a previously affected child or to increased-risk mothers (e.g., heart defect seen on ultrasound).

Duplication. The dup22q11.21 most often involves breakpoints LCR-A to LCR-D (Figure 14–82). Curiously, it may be more common than the deletion (Olsen et al. 2018). The clinical picture is quite diverse, ranging from overt normality in many to a degree of neurocognitive compromise. IQ overlaps substantially with the lower fraction of a normal population; one-fifth have a mild intellectual disability, and language acquisition is affected (Lin et al. 2020; Verbesselt et al. 2022, 2023). Penetrance in Goh et al. (2025) is 19%. Congenital anomalies are not infrequent (Bartik et al. 2022). Susceptibility to autism is, to a small degree, increased (Drmic et al. 2022). In perhaps a first for a chromosomal imbalance, dup heterozygotes may have, in at least one respect, *better* mental health than a general population: There may be a protective effect against schizophrenia (Lin et al. 2020).

Familial examples are well recorded, and indeed comprise a majority of cases (Verbesselt et al. 2022; Jiang et al. 2024b); and there is one notable report of a three-generation family in which eight individuals had the dup(22), evincing a range of fairly minor malformation and neurobehavioral phenotypic effects (Yu et al. 2008). This frequent familial observation has enabled a comparison of the phenotype in probands versus non-probands, and unsurprisingly the clinical picture is milder and more often merging into a normal range in those in whom the diagnosis was made only after a proband had brought the family to notice (an example of ascertainment bias, favoring the recognition of a more severe manifestation) (Drmic et al. 2022). This very wide range of expressivity, and merging into non-penetrance, makes for challenging counseling (Dupont et al. 2015); the coexistence of CNVs elsewhere in the genome may be the basis, in part at least, of this phenotypic variation.

Recurrence from chromosomally normal parents presenting with a de novo case has not as yet been reported, but a theoretical risk exists due to parental gonadal mosaicism. Demaerel et al. (2016) report siblings of normal parents, one with dup 22q11 the other with del 22q11, both coming from the mother.

A smaller, less often seen nested 22q11.21 duplication encompasses the segment bounded by LCR-B and LCR-D (Figure 14–83). Woodward et al. (2019) documented a phenotype of intellectual disability and autism, along with normality in several. *PIK4A*, located between LCRs C and D, may have an important contributory role to the phenotype. Distal duplication, extending into LCR-E or further (and which, if beyond LCR-F, may include the *SMARCB1* locus), is uncommon (Egger et al. 2023).

precisely, and in recurring examples, a specific syndromal status may be assigned (Jafari-Ghahfarokhi et al. 2015). Most are derived from an acrocentric chromosome. A number have been listed above: the 11p11.2 neocentromeric sSMC; the inv dup or isodicentric 15 (pathogenic and non-pathogenic); the 18p sSMC, whose centromere is of 13/21 material; and the inv dup(22)(q11.21) or der(22)(q11.21) sSMC of cat eye syndrome. Some small isochromosomes (next section) have been referred to as sSMCs.

If the parental blood karyotypes are normal, parental mosaicism is unlikely but not completely excluded. The load in gametes may be less than seen on peripheral blood, at least in the case of the male (Cotter et al. 2000; Oracova et al. 2009). The dup(22)(q11.21) of cat eye syndrome (above) is exceptional in that mosaicism, which can be familial, is commonly observed.

ISOCHROMOSOMES (NON-ACROCENTRIC)

We deal in detail with isochromosomes in relation to their discovery at prenatal diagnosis in Chapter 22, and including the following derived from a non-acrocentric[26] chromosome: 47,+i(5p), 47,+i(8p), 47,+i(9p), 47,+i(10p), 47,+i(12p), 47,+i(18p), 47,+i(18q), and 46,i(20q). A couple having had a child with an isochromosome, for a chromosome other than an acrocentric, can generally be given encouraging advice, especially if the child is mosaic. The major mechanisms of generation are considered to operate either at meiosis II or post-zygotically, and in either case no discernibly increased risk of recurrence would be implied, albeit that a premeiotic mechanism may apply in some (de Ravel et al. 2004; Rittinger et al. 2015). Very rare exceptions exist: for example, the history in Boyle et al. (2001) of two half-sisters both with 47,XX,i(18p), their mother an inferred gonadal mosaic.

[26] As for the acrocentric-derived isochromosome (Chapter 7), a post-zygotic mechanism may be the rule, and thus of optimistic outlook for a subsequent pregnancy (Riegel et al. 2006).

15
SEX CHROMOSOME ANEUPLOIDY AND STRUCTURAL REARRANGEMENT

THERE ARE FOUR MAJOR sex chromosome abnormalities[1] due to *complete aneuploidy*. Otherwise unassisted, infertility is practically inevitable in XXY Klinefelter syndrome (KS) and 45,X Turner syndrome (TS). The other two conditions, XXX and XYY, apparently have little effect on fertility; furthermore, they are not discernibly associated with any increased risk for chromosomally abnormal offspring. Mosaic forms need to be considered on their own merits, albeit that infertility is often the case with Klinefelter and Turner mosaicism, at least in those cases coming to clinical attention. As for recurrence, to parents who have had a child with one of these aneuploidies, typically the risks are low.

Structural rearrangement of X or Y leads to a partial imbalance. This may involve a large amount of chromatin, such as in substantial deletions, a ring, or an isochromosome. Or, deletion or duplication may involve only a small segment (of kilobase or a few megabases in extent). Some of the latter may have little effect upon fertility, and reproductive risk assessment becomes of practical importance. The recurrence risks vary.

BIOLOGY

We need briefly to consider why X chromosome aneuploidy can be associated with so little phenotypic abnormality, compared with autosomal imbalance. The important factor is dosage compensation. Only one X in each cell needs to be fully active. Thus, potentially detrimental effects of an X chromosomal imbalance are mitigated (although not exactly canceled out) by *in*activating a supernumerary or abnormal X, or by *not* inactivating a sole remaining X, as the case may be.

The conceptus with an X chromosome complement in excess of the normal 46,XX or 46,XY accommodates to this imbalance by inactivating any additional X chromosome—or, as Migeon (2007) emphasizes, by maintaining just one X in the active state in each cell. This is nearly successful in the 47,XXX female and the 47,XXY male, in each of whom there is apparently normal in utero survival and a relatively mild post-natal phenotype. The fact that some loci are not subject to inactivation and may therefore continue to function in the X disomic (XXY), trisomic (XXX), or even quintasomic (49,XXXXX) states, is presumably the predominant reason for the phenotypic abnormalities associated with these karyotypes.

[1] The student of history will enjoy Malcolm Ferguson-Smith's tribute to Victor McKusick, the founding Father of Medical Genetics, on the occasion of the centenary of his birth, which relates some of the early history of cytogenetics in the 1950s and 60s, and with a particular focus on the sex chromosome disorders (Ferguson-Smith, 2021).

In females with abnormal X chromosomes, the pattern of X-inactivation is usually nonrandom,[2] particularly when the imbalance due to the abnormality is "large." In the 46,X,abn(X) karyotype, with one normal X and one abnormal X—an "abn(X)," as we write it here—the abnormal X is characteristically the inactive one. However, if the abnormality is a small deletion or duplication, the inactivation pattern can be random. In the case of the X-autosome balanced translocation heterozygote, the normal X is usually, although not invariably, inactive (Chapter 6).

Laboratory Test for X-Inactivation. Analyzing the pattern of X chromosome methylation with molecular methodology shows whether inactivation is random or nonrandom. A useful assay is methylation-specific polymerase chain reaction based on the androgen receptor gene, located at Xq13 (or any other gene with a convenient polymorphism). A highly skewed pattern, with one X mostly methylated and the other mostly not, is indicative of nonrandom inactivation (Kubota et al. 1999). While this test is performed routinely on a blood sample, there are grounds for believing that the assay result may, at least to some extent, fairly represent the state in other body tissues (Bittel et al. 2008). The former tests of Barr body and late-labeling BrdU analysis are of historic interest; both assays still provide a nice visual illustration of the concept of X-inactivation (Figures 15–1 and 15–2).

Y chromosome imbalance is similarly mild in its effects, but for a quite different reason, namely the very low gene carriage of this chromosome and the very narrow scope of activity—male gonadal development—of most of these genes. As discussed elsewhere, the *SRY* gene on the Y short arm has the critical role of directing the gonad to form as a testis; other loci, most notably the *DAZ* family of genes within the AZFc region on the long arm, determine aspects of spermatogenesis (Krausz and Casamonti 2017).

Complete Aneuploidy

DETAILS OF MEIOTIC BEHAVIOR

Meiosis proceeds differently in persons with each of the various sex chromosome abnormalities, and each warrants separate consideration.

XXX

On theoretical grounds, one might have expected the three X chromosomes to display 2:1 segregation, with the production of equal numbers of X and XX ova. But this is not the case. No discernible increased risk for chromosomally abnormal offspring of these women has been demonstrated. In the extensive review of Otter et al. (2010), only one case had ever been reported of an XXX mother having had an XXX daughter. Apparently only normal ova with a single X are regularly produced. It may be that the extra X is lost before meiosis occurs (Neri 1984), with meiosis then proceeding as in the normal XX female. Fertility may, however, be affected, due to premature ovarian insufficiency (Tartaglia et al. 2010).

[2] Or, more accurately, random X-inactivation is followed by selection against cells expressing the abnormal X.

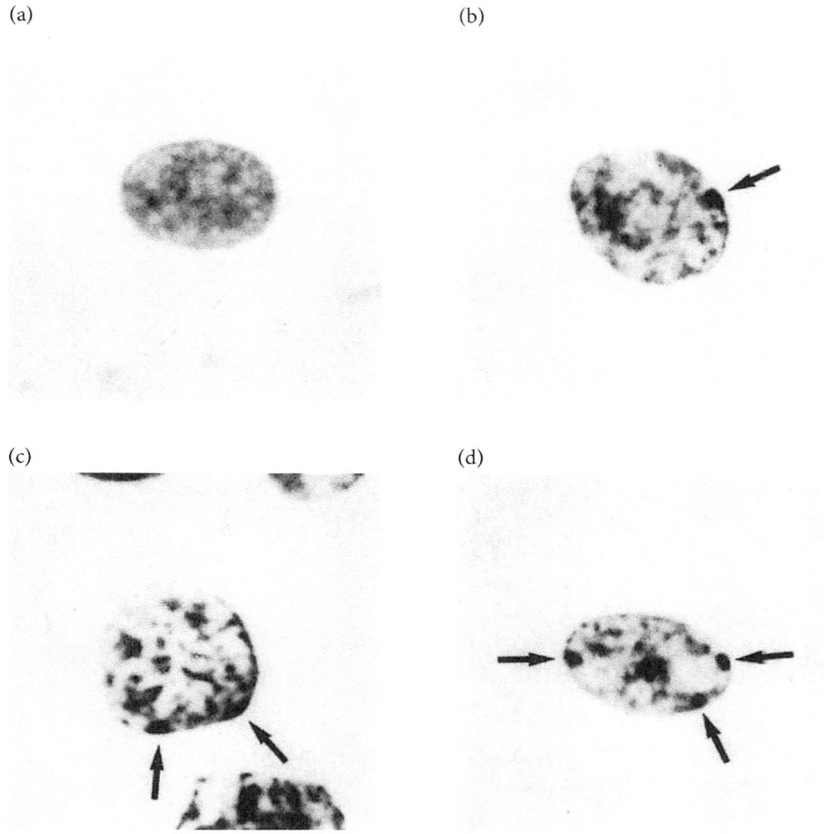

Figure 15–1. Buccal mucosal cells from (*a*) a 45,X female, with no Barr body present; (*b*) a 46,XX female showing the inactive X as a Barr body; (*c*) a 47,XXX female showing two Barr bodies; and (*d*) a 48,XXXX female with three Barr bodies.

XXY AND XXY MOSAIC STATES

In the germ cells of the XXY fetus, the second X chromosome escapes X-inactivation, and the consequent dysregulation of X-linked gene dosage leads to arrest of germ cells at an early stage (Lu et al. 2024). When present, all spermatogonia in non-mosaic KS patients have a 46,XY karyotype, suggesting that these germ cells have lost the extra X chromosome during embryonic, fetal, or neonatal life (Gül et al. 2024). Barring medical intervention, infertility is almost inevitable in non-mosaic Klinefelter syndrome, although some remarkable exceptions exist (Terzoli et al. 1992); undetected XY/XXY mosaicism could account for some of these cases. Van Saen et al. (2012) list three subgroups of adult men with KS, according to findings on testicular biopsy: one group in which mature spermatozoa can be retrieved by testicular extraction, a group with no testicular spermatozoa but in which germ cells are present, and a third group with no germ cells at all.

Several workers have karyotyped sperm from XXY men, and all find an excess, albeit not a large one, of 24,XX and 24,XY sperm. Possibly, the abnormal gonadal environment may of itself predispose to gonosomal nondisjunction in the XY tissue; and from that stance, autosomal segregation may also be vulnerable, as indeed sperm studies indicate. There is a higher rate of disomy 21 on sperm studies from KS men, 6.2% versus

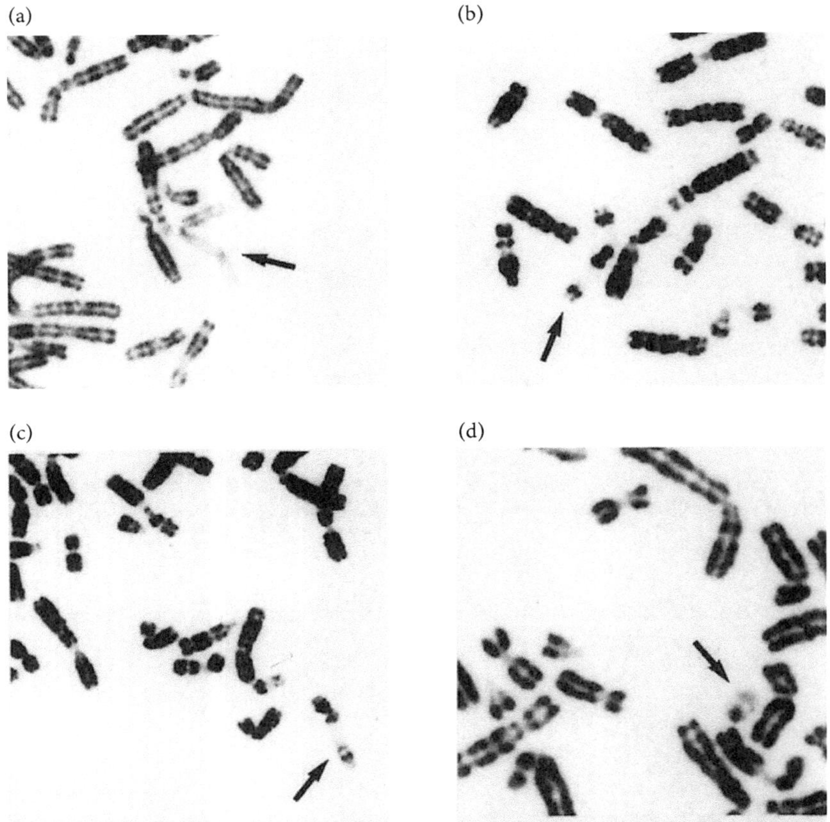

Figure 15–2. Partial metaphases showing X-inactivation: (*a*) a normal X chromosome, (*b*) an isochromosome of X long arm, (*c*) an X with a short arm deletion, and (*d*) a ring X. BrdU had been added for the last 6 hours of culturing. The inactive chromosomes, replicating at this late time in the cell cycle, incorporate BrdU extensively, and thus are palely stained. The active X stains darkly.

0.4% in controls (Hennebicq et al. 2001; Bergère et al. 2002). As for XY/XXY mosaicism, Samplaski et al. (2014) showed better androgenization on a number of criteria in these men, including a higher rate of men having sperm in the ejaculate (half, compared to only 4% in non-mosaic XXY).

XYY

The clinical observation is that XYY men have no discernible increase in risk to have children with a sex chromosome aneuploidy (and XYY or XXY would have been the theoretical risk outcomes from an XYY trivalent at meiosis), and in the UK Biobank study, men with XYY appeared to have normal reproductive function (Zhao et al. 2022). A true increased risk of a fraction of a percent could be distinguished only with great difficulty, when the background population risk is of a similar order of magnitude. The proposed model is that the additional Y chromosome is randomly lost in a germ line precursor, followed by selection in favor of euploid clones due to these having a proliferative advantage (Evans et al. 1970). On laboratory study, XYY spermatocytes proceeding through meiosis encounter checkpoints that may lead to elimination of most of the abnormal forms (Milazzo et al. 2006), but nevertheless, some men may have a small increased fraction of 24,YY and 24,XY spermatozoa in the ejaculate and in some, also of autosomal disomies.

A distinction may be drawn between XYY men presenting with infertility and those whose fertility is intact, with the sperm aneuploidy rate somewhat higher in the former. Rodrigo et al. (2010) studied the cytogenetics of the preimplantation embryo from five infertile XYY men having had IVF, and identified a significant increase in chromosomally abnormal embryos compared to those of fertile XY controls; however, when compared to embryos of XY males with abnormal spermatogenesis, the proportion of aneuploid embryos was similar. Therefore, the increase in aneuploidy may be a nonspecific feature of abnormal spermatogenesis rather than a direct consequence of the XYY state per se.

A unifying mechanism for infertility in XYY men is yet to be identified. In one man with azoöspermia having come to testicular biopsy, both Y chromosomes were present and in synapsis in all meiotic spermatocytes, and in association with—but not synapsing with—the X chromosome; this configuration may possibly have been the cause of spermatogenic arrest (Wu et al. 2016). A different picture was evident in the azoöspermic XYY man studied by Sciurano et al. (2019): At testicular biopsy, 98% of primary spermatocytes were XY, and the authors hypothesized that the XYY Sertoli cells may have contributed to spermatogenesis failure. It may be that in some cases the XYY is an incidental finding, and the male infertility has an alternative explanation.

NON-MOSAIC 45,X TURNER SYNDROME

Turner syndrome is not uncommon. From a US-wide study 2000–2017, the prevalence was ascertained to be 3.2 per 10,000 female livebirths, or 1 in 3,125 girl babies[3] (Martin-Giacalone et al. 2023); and when diagnoses after the first year of life are included, the prevalence increases to 1 in 2,000 (Gravholt et al. 2024). The great majority of women with 45,X TS are infertile and do not spontaneously menstruate or develop secondary sexual characteristics. The ovaries initially appear to be normal but typically begin to degenerate in mid–fetal life. Oöcytes undergo apoptosis and disappear at an accelerated rate and, in most cases, are gone by the age of two years: "The menopause occurs before the menarche" (Federman 1987; Modi et al. 2003). It may be that a 45,X oöcyte could not proceed through meiosis I, given that the sex chromosome has no homolog with which to pair. In one series of 18 45,X girls, none had ovarian follicles on biopsy in childhood or teen age (Borgström et al. 2009).

Completed pregnancy in women with an apparent 45,X karyotype is very rare. In a Danish study based on a national TS register, none of 200 45,X women achieved a natural pregnancy (one had twins by ovum donation) (Birkebaek et al. 2002). In a large French study, coming from seven endocrine units nationwide, 480 adult women with TS were recruited (Bernard et al. 2016). Of the 181 with monosomy X, only two had achieved pregnancy, although presumably not all had been attempting motherhood (Table 15–1; other chromosomal forms of TS also listed here). Sybert (2005) was able to record a total of 18 45,X women having had 42 pregnancies, and observed that the

[3] The most commonly observed congenital malformation in this cohort was coarctation of the aorta; and the 5-year survivability (excluding cases with hypoplastic left heart syndrome) was 95%.

Table 15–1. Turner Syndrome Reproductive Outcomes

CHARACTERISTICS	PREGNANT TS PATIENTS (*N* = 27)	NON-PREGNANT TS PATIENTS (*N* = 453)
Age at diagnosis*	20 (0–45)	10 (0–64)
45,X	2/27 (7%)	179/453 (40%)
45,X/46,XX	19/27 (70%)	111/453 (25%)
Mosaicism with Y	1/27 (4%)	20/453 (4%)
Mosaicism with ring X	2/27 (7%)	30/453 (7%)
Isochromosome X	1/27 (4%)	27/453 (6%)
Other	2/27 (7%)	86/453 (19%)
Spontaneous menarche	25/27 (93%)	70/453 (15%)
Age at first pregnancy (years)	27.5 (18–38)	n/a
Delay to conceive (months)	6 (0–84)	n/a

Notes: These data are from 480 adult women with Turner Syndrome. *Years, median and range. n/a = not applicable. TS = Turner syndrome.

Source: From V Bernard et al., Spontaneous fertility and pregnancy outcomes amongst 480 women with Turner syndrome, *Hum Reprod* 31:782–788, 2016.

risks for spontaneous abortion, sex chromosome aneuploidy, and trisomy 21 were all elevated. Only 17 of the pregnancies proceeded to live birth, including two cases of 45,X and one of trisomy 21.

What is the explanation for fertility in these rare cases? An obvious point to consider is gonadal mosaicism, with a 46,XX cell line in the ovary. This has often been suggested, but rarely proven (Birkebaek et al. 2002). Jacobs et al. (1997) undertook a systematic search in 84 subjects with TS whose standard blood karyotype was 45,X with molecular testing of blood and of a second tissue (buccal cells), and found only two cases of X/XX mosaicism. One very thorough study is that reported in Magee et al. (1998b) concerning a 45,X woman who had had seven pregnancies: five miscarrying, one producing a healthy male, and the last terminated following demonstration of fetal cystic hygroma and a 45,X karyotype on amniocentesis. Biopsies of skin, uterus, and ovary at subsequent gynecological surgery all gave a 45,X karyotype, but molecular testing showed two alleles in ovarian DNA, indicating the presence of occult 46,XX tissue. A similar investigation is reported in Sugawara et al. (2013) of a woman 45,X on standard blood karyotype, but other XX and XXX cell lines seen when 500 cells were analyzed and skin and cumulus tissue studied (and inexplicably, even 4/260 cumulus cells were XY). It is difficult to know, but fair to consider, whether such subtly occult mosaicism might be the explanation for the very rare instances of true natural fertility in (apparently) non-mosaic 45,X TS.

X/XX, X/XX/XXX, AND X/XXX MOSAICISM TURNER SYNDROME

The relative fractions of the various karyotypes—at least as may be judged on standard peripheral blood analysis—are listed in Tables 15–2 and 15–3 and illustrated in Figure 15–3. In the X/XX state, some gonadal function is likely to be retained if the 46,XX fraction reaches 10%, as evidenced by a spontaneous menarche (Castronovo et al. 2014). Among the TS categories, the X/XX karyotype is associated with the best chance for pregnancy, natural or IVF-assisted. In the cohort of Calanchini et al. (2020) 11/23

Table 15–2. Sex Chromosomal Karyotypes, Associated and Not Associated, with Turner Syndrome

	FREQUENCY (%)	DESCRIPTION
KARYOTYPES ASSOCIATED WITH TURNER SYNDROME		
45,X	40%–50%	Monosomy X
45,X/46,XX*	15%–25%	Mosaicism with 46,XX
45,X/47,XXX 45,X/46,XX/47,XXX	3	Mosaicism with 47,XXX
45,X/46,XY	10%–12%	Mosaicism with 46,XY
45,X/46,X(r)X	Rare	Ring X chromosome
46, X,i(Xq) 46,X,idic(Xp)	15%	Isochromosome Xq Isodicentric Xp
46,XX,del(p11)		Proximal deletion of Xp
X-autosome translocation, unbalanced	Rare	Various
KARYOTYPES NOT ASSOCIATED WITH TURNER SYNDROME		
46,XX,del(p22.3)		Distal deletion Xp22.3 (SHOX)
46,XX,del(q24)		Premature ovarian insufficiency
46,X,idic(X)(q24)		Isodicentric Xq24

Notes: *A diagnosis of Turner syndrome is usually not considered in women with less than 5% 45,X cells.

Source: From CH Gravholt et al., Clinical practice guidelines for the care of girls and women with Turner syndrome. *Eur J Endocrinol* 190:G53–G151, 2024.

Table 15–3. Karyotype-Phenotype Associations in Turner Syndrome

KARYOTYPE	PHENOTYPE
45,X	Higher frequency of comorbidities and a higher mortality compared to individuals with other TS karyotypes.
45,X/46,XX	Milder phenotype with left-sided congenital heart defects, obesity, and hypertension being less frequent, age at menarche being near-normal, more likely to experience spontaneous menarche and pregnancies.
45,X/47,XXX	Milder external and cardiovascular phenotype compared to 45,X, but neurodevelopmental disabilities and mental health domains remaining a concern.
i(Xq)	Intermediate severity of left-sided congenital heart defects and spontaneous menarche, and a lower incidence of aortic coarctation.
45,X/46,XY	Lowest incidence of autoimmune thyroid disease and severe hearing loss, and a low incidence of aortic coarctation.
(r)X	*Without functional loss of XIST,* possible increased risk of metabolic syndrome, low risk of bicuspid aortic valve. *With functional loss of XIST*, a more severe cognitive phenotype.

Source: From CH Gravholt et al. (2024) as above.

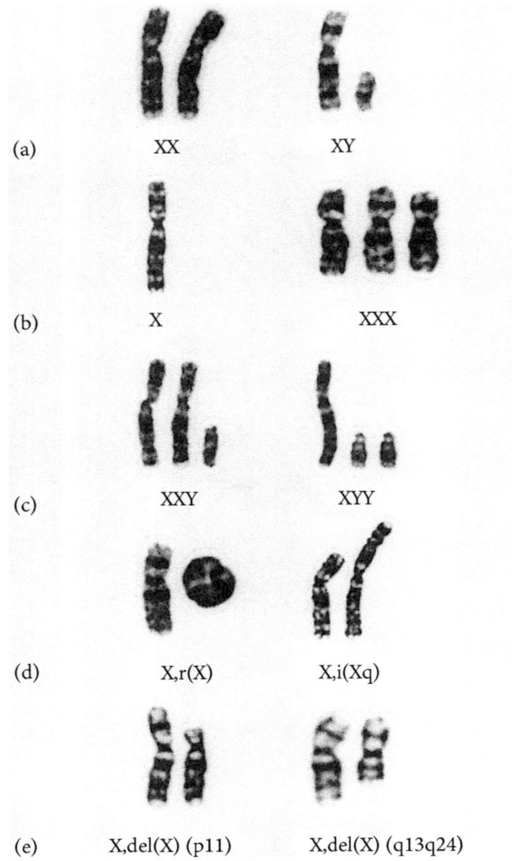

Figure 15–3. Some sex chromosome complements: (*a*) normal female XX and normal male XY; (*b*) X and XXX females; (*c*) XXY and XYY males; (*d* and *e*) abnormal chromosomes from females with a ring X, an isochromosome of X long arm, an X short arm deletion, and an X long arm deletion.

women with 45,X mosaicism achieved a spontaneous pregnancy[4] compared to just 2/62 45,X women. Across both categories, all women who achieved spontaneous pregnancy had a history of spontaneous menarche and regular menstruation. Most oöcytes appear to have arisen from 46,XX cells: in the series of Peek et al. (2019), 91% of oöcytes had two X chromosomes despite supporting granulosa cells being 45,X.

The survival of 45,X cells in the gonad may be enabled by support from surrounding 46,XX oögonia; such a 45,X cell might, in theory, be able to produce a nullisomic X egg, if its sole X is sequestered to the polar body at meiosis I. This could be the basis of the observation in Uehara et al. (1999b) of a woman with 45,X/46,XX having had three monosomic X pregnancies, all showing fetal hydrops; she also had a normal son. Pubertal development may often be apparently normal in the 45,X/47,XXX case (Lim et al. 2017a). The X/XXX patient in Bouchlariotou et al. (2011) had two normal children, and one (unkaryotyped) deceased, severely growth-retarded baby, while Sahinturk et al.

[4] In contrast, fertility appears to be minimally impacted in 45,X/46,XX women ascertained from the general population with <20% of 45,X cells (Tuke et al. 2019).

(2015) report a woman with 45,X[8]/47,XXX[12] who had had five miscarriages and one healthy 46,XX daughter.

XY/X MOSAICISM TURNER SYNDROME

Approximately 10% of women with TS have a mosaic karyotype containing Y chromosome material. The clinical spectrum of patients with 45,X/46,XY mosaicism is wide and includes women with TS, patients with ambiguous genitalia, and infertile males (Guzewicz et al. 2021). These individuals are at risk of gonadoblastoma, a benign tumor that arises in dysgenetic gonads and is subject to malignant transformation. Karila et al. (2022) studied 70 women with 45,X/46,XY TS and identified nine with gonadoblastoma (13%), of which two had undergone malignant transformation. A recommendation for gonadectomy depends upon the nature of the Y: whether it is an intact, or a structurally abnormal chromosome. If intact, gonad removal is advised; if a rearranged Y, careful monitoring can reasonably be offered.

The variability of phenotype according to the degree of mosaicism is well illustrated in the report of Lespinasse et al. (1998), who studied monozygous (but not identical) triplets with 45,X/46,XX mosaicism. One child with typical TS had only 6% 45,X cells on blood karyotyping but 99% on fibroblast analysis. One sister with only mild features to suggest TS had 43% of fibroblasts with 45,X, and the third triplet, of normal phenotype, had just 3%. Presumably, the mosaicism existed from a very early stage, and the three-way division of the 45,X/46,XX early conceptus happened to cut across an asymmetric disposition of normal/monosomic cells.

MOSAIC LOSS OF THE X CHROMOSOME (MLOX) IN PHENOTYPICALLY NORMAL WOMEN

This category is to be distinguished from that of TS due to 45,X/46,XX mosaicism discussed above, and it is supposed to be without reproductive consequence. Advice from the European Cytogeneticists Association a propos is presented on p. 614. Mosaic loss of the X chromosome (mLOX) to give an occasional 45,X cell is a normal characteristic of aging in the 46,XX female (Ziętkiewicz et al. 2009). The phenomenon may reflect variation in a number of cell-cycle factors, similarly to but less markedly than the male equivalent, mosaic loss of the Y, as discussed below (Wright et al. 2017). Russell et al. (2007) reviewed data from a large number of women having had a peripheral blood cytogenetic analysis, and correlated the degree of mLOX with age, documenting a clear association. Up to age 30 years, 1% or less of cells showed mLOX, but rising to an average 2%, 3%, and 5% at median ages of 40, 50, and 65 years respectively.

Liu et al. (2024a) analyzed genomic data from ~ 900,000 women participating in various biobanks and detected mLOX in 12%, with a median mLOX fraction of 2%. The frequency of mLOX increased with age, being 3% below 40 years and 35% after 80 years (Figure 15–4). Interestingly, smokers overall had no increased risk of mLOX, but among those who did have mLOX, smokers had a greater proportion of affected cells. mLOX fractions of >10% were associated with a near twofold increased risk of leukemia. Liu et al. propose that mLOX is a polygenic trait, the genes thus implicated being involved in chromosome segregation and cancer predisposition.

45,X/46,XY AND 45,X/47,XYY MOSAICISM IN THE MALE

X/XY mosaicism may be diagnosed at birth due to genital abnormality, or be detected later in life in males presenting with hypogonadism and infertility with oligo/azoöspermia; in

Parents Having Had a Child with a Sex Chromosome Aneuploidy

XXX, XXY, XYY, 45,X, AND OTHER SEX CHROMOSOME ANEUPLOIDY

There is no firm evidence that a recurrence risk above the age-specific figure exists, and indeed in respect of XXX and XXY, no recurrences of either homotrisomy or heterotrisomy were observed in the study of Warburton et al. (2004). NIPT could be offered for additional reassurance.

Structural Rearrangement

As in the preceding chapter on autosomal rearrangements, we are dealing here with a *segment* of a chromosome existing in an imbalanced state, mostly with respect to the X but with the Y chromosome making a small appearance. Broadly, we may consider two categories: large rearrangements that have been known from the early days of cytogenetics; and microrearrangements, originally detected on G-banding and now including deletions and duplications seen only with molecular karyotyping. Typically so, the large rearrangements are associated with disorders of gonadal development, and variant forms of TS predominate among these. Here, X-inactivation enables an otherwise massive genetic imbalance to become functionally viable. The viability of large Y imbalances reflects the very small component of active genes on this chromosome. Contrariwise, microimbalances of the X chromosome in the female are not necessarily subject to "correction" by inactivation, and they may be damaging but not necessarily lethal in the male. Thus, in some respects the implications may be similar to the autosomal microimbalance.

We list here selected deletions and duplications of the X and Y chromosomes. As for the X, for the most part we categorize (as commented above) according to (1) large "classic" rearrangements and (2) microdeletions and microduplications. Y abnormalities, although so few, follow suit. Deletions of the X and Y with a particular association with infertility are summarized in Figure 15–6.

LARGER X DELETIONS

del Xp Turner Variant. Substantial Xp terminal deletions, many of which had been seen on the solid-stain analysis of the early days of cytogenetics, typically lead to variant or incomplete "formes frustes" of TS (Figure 15–3e). These deletions can remove up to most or even all of the short arm. X-inactivation is markedly skewed toward the abnormal X. Short stature is largely due to haploinsufficiency of the *SHOX* growth control gene in the pseudoautosomal region.

Ovarian function may be retained, in part at least, with the more distal Xp deletions, but is typically absent in proximal deletions (Lachlan et al. 2006). In those women who achieve fertility—and numerous examples of transmission of a del(Xp) are on record (Periquito et al. 2016)—presumably a partial synapsis occurs at meiosis in the 46,X,abn(X) oöcytes, with the intact segment of the abnormal X pairing with the homologous region of the normal X. A segregation ratio of 1:1 would be expected, with equal frequencies of gametes carrying either the normal X, or the abnormal X from that part of the gonad tissue containing the abn(X).

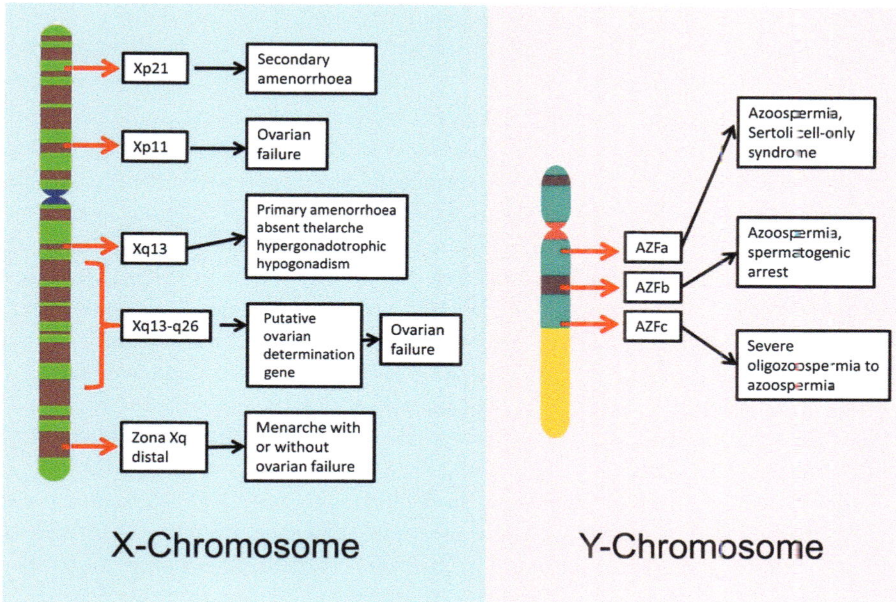

Figure 15–6. Regions of the Sex Chromosomes in which Deletions are Associated with Infertility.

Source: From A García-Rodríguez et al., DNA damage and repair in human reproductive cells, *Int J Mol Sci* 20:31, 2018. Courtesy R Roy and S Johnston, and with the permission of MDPI.

Not infrequently, mosaicism is recognized. Palka et al. (1994) describe an apparently non-mosaic 45,X woman who had had an abnormal child with an interstitial Xp deletion, del(X)(p22.2p11.3). Upon restudy, the mother herself had one 46,X,del(X) out of 450 cells, allowing the presumption of a somatic-gonadal mosaicism. In a more direct demonstration of gonadal mosaicism, Varela et al. (1991) studied a woman with TS and normal menstruation and who had had a 46,X,del(X)(p21) daughter. They showed 5/100 cells with 46,X,del(X)(p21) in one ovary, while all cells from the other ovary, fibroblasts, and lymphocytes were 45,X. Gonadal function can vary in a family, as Zinn et al. (1997) show for a familial del(X)(p21.2). The 45,X/46,X,del(X) mother had had three pregnancies, including one miscarriage, and had normal menses till age 39 years. Her two daughters were both 46,X,del(X). The elder was amenorrheic at age 15 years, while the younger had spontaneous menarche at age 14½ years, with regular cycles one year later. A very similar family is on record in Adachi et al. (2000).

An Xp deletion might coexist with an Xq duplication, the consequence of recombination within an inversion chromosome. Stoklasova et al. (2016) report a four-generation family—clearly, fertility was retained—of women with the karyotype 46,X,rec(X) inv(p21.1q27.3). A great-great-grandparent may have been the heterozygote in whom the recombinant arose.

del Xp22.12pter. This deletion, and others of lesser extent, may be associated in the female with only the short stature component of TS, this segment including the *SHOX* gene. Cho et al. (2012b) report a deletion Xp22.12pter, which had been passed from a mother to her two daughters. The mother's height was just a little above the range seen in classic TS at 149 cm (−3.3 SD); her young daughters plotted somewhat higher, on −2.1 and −1.8 SD, respectively, at their ages of close to 9 and 12 years. The mother's pubertal development had been normal.

del Xq Turner Variant. Deletions may be of very substantial size, up to 74 Mb, or approximately three-fourths of the q arm length. Mercer et al. (2013) reviewed the clinical picture in a series of 10 del(Xq) cases, of whom eight were non-mosaic (two had a concomitant 45,X cell line). Of the non-mosaic cases, six had terminal deletions, with proximal breakpoints from Xq21.1 to Xq25; where parental testing had been done, all were de novo. The clinical presentations had been due to primary amenorrhea, premature ovarian insufficiency, infertility, and in one child, short stature; few other features characteristic of TS were present. If puberty commences naturally, it remains the case that premature ovarian insufficiency is likely; and it is practical advice that childbearing—if wished, and of course other things being equal—should be embarked upon sooner rather than later. Assuming 1:1 segregation (a fair assumption), the deleted X would be transmitted in 50% of ova.

Ring Turner Variants. The imbalance in the classic 46,X,r(X) TS is essentially due to distal Xp and Xq deletion, the deletions of variable extent. In the series of Cameron-Pimblett et al. (2017), 58% experienced primary amenorrhea. Rare reports of fertility exist. Blumenthal and Allanson (1997) record a woman with mosaic ring X TS, 45,X/46,X,r(X), who had been amenorrheic until being given hormone replacement therapy. She had three pregnancies: a healthy 46,XY son, a 12-week miscarriage, and a healthy daughter with the same 45,X/46,r(X) karyotype. The latter was presumably 46,X,r(X) at conception, with post-zygotic loss of the r(X) in some tissue. Other such cases are known (Sybert 2005). A rather different example is that in Matsuo et al. (2000), in which a mother and daughter were 45,X/46,X,r(X)(p22.3q28), the ratios of X:X,r(X) being 97:3 in the mother and 73:27 in the daughter. The ring comprised an almost complete X, but small distal Xp and Xq segments were deleted. The two X chromosomes were randomly inactivated, and presumably in consequence some "brain genes" would have been functionally nullisomic in those cells having the normal X-inactivated. Thus, cognitive function in the mother, and more so in the daughter, was compromised. A male with r(X) is almost unknown, but Ellison et al. (2002) describe transmission from a non-mosaic 46,X,r(X) mother to her non-mosaic 46,Y,r(X) son, mother and son both short-statured. The breakpoints were very distal, within and beyond the Xp and Xq pseudoautosomal regions respectively.

The "*tiny ring X syndrome*" with the karyotype 45,X/46,X,r(X), is a quite different entity. There may be a functional X disomy due to the ring lacking the *XIST* locus and thus not undergoing inactivation. The syndrome is typically, but not universally, seen with a severe phenotype of physical and intellectual disability, in some resembling Kabuki syndrome. In others, the clinical picture may merely be that of TS (Rodríguez et al. 2008). Similarly, in the male with the tiny ring as a supernumerary chromosome, usually as 46,XY/47,XY,+r(X) mosaicism, the clinical picture is typically abnormal, and in some severely so (Baker et al. 2010). Chen et al. (2006d) report a notable exception from the prenatal diagnosis at amniocentesis of 46,XY[17]/47,XY,+mar[6], the marker chromosome turning out to be a very small *XIST*-negative r(X). The infant boy, on whose blood the proportions of the two cell lines were similar to the amniocentesis findings, was normal physically and developmentally on follow-up to one year of age. These various phenotypic differences in male and female may reflect the composition, proportion, distribution, and activation status of the abnormal chromosome.

LARGER X DUPLICATIONS

Isochromosome Xq Turner Variant. The imbalance in i(Xq) TS is a monosomy of Xp and a trisomy of Xq. Outcomes closely match those seen in 45,X TS, other than a lower incidence of congenital heart disease (Cameron-Pimblett et al. 2017). The condition is almost invariably associated with infertility.

Isochromosome Xq Klinefelter Variant. In this rare form of KS, 47,X,i(Xq),Y, there is a monosomy of Xp and trisomy of Xq (as with i(Xq) TS), along with a normal Y complement. Compared to XXY KS, isochromosome Xq KS has been associated with normal height, intelligence, and secondary sexual characteristics (Simsek et al. 2019), and at least in terms of height, this can be attributed to the lack of duplication of Xp. Infertility is usual, but rare fertility with recourse to IVF is on record (Sabbaghian et al. 2011).

dup Xq21q26. Large duplications of (and microduplications within) this segment are noted below. A functional disomy can influence the clinical picture, according to the pattern of X chromosome inactivation (Armstrong et al. 2003).

LARGER Y REARRANGEMENTS

Y Isochromosome, Isodicentric Y. The inactivation of one of the two centromeres allows this chromosome to be mitotically functional. The distinction here is between Yp and Yq isochromosomes—or, since typically there are two copies of the centromere, they are usually called Yp and Yq isodicentric chromosomes, thus i(Y)(p) and i(Y)(q), or idic(Y)(p) and idic(Y)(q). Or, more fully, for example, idic(Y)(pter→q11.22::q11.22→pter); note the identical palindromic sequences on either side of the :: breakpoint. Note also that the Yp or Yq designation refers to the site of breakpoint, and that the idic(Y)(*p*) has two complete Y*q* copies, while the idic(Y)(*q*) has two complete copies of Y*p*.[7] There is considerable heterogeneity of size, according to the site of breakpoint (Figure 15–7). An idic(Y)(p) with a breakpoint at distal Yp, with mirror copies of the remainder of the Y, would comprise almost a double copy of the whole chromosome (Figure 15–7a). An idic(Y)(q11.223) would convey a double copy of Yp and a double copy of the proximal long arm (Figure 15–7c). A breakpoint at Yq11.1 would give an idic(Y)(q), with a double copy of only the short arm and absence of long-arm material (Figure 15–7d). Generation is de novo, typically in (obviously) paternal gametogenesis and reflecting a vulnerability due to the apposition of similar Y sequences; uncommon cases may be due to a post-zygotic event.

Mosaicism very frequently accompanies as a post-zygotic event, with 45,X and a second abn(Y) the usual additional cell lineages. The clinical presentations range from a majority with male infertility (e.g., the idic(Y)(*p*11.3) in Figure 15–8), male with mild cognitive impairment, through ovotesticular disorder of sex development (DSD) or mixed gonadal dysgenesis with genital ambiguity, to TS. The gonadal phenotype is presumably directed in keeping with the regional presence or absence of *SRY*. In a series of 14 cases in Kalantari et al. (2014), all with idic(Y)(*q*11.22), 13 were men with azoöspermia (note that this chromosome would lack the *b* and *c* AZF spermatogenic factors). Most had a concomitant 45,X cell line. Immature germ cells in the ejaculate were, overall, of fairly similar fractions of haploid 23,X and 23,idic(Y) karyotypes indicating

[7] This can sometimes lead to muddling of nomenclature. Beaulieu Bergeron et al. (2011) note that "when referring to an idic with unspecified breakpoints, some authors use idicY(p) or idic(Yp) when two copies of the short arm are present, and idicY(q) or idic(Yq) when two copies of the long arm are present, therefore creating some confusion among readers." ISCN (2024) does not adjudicate.

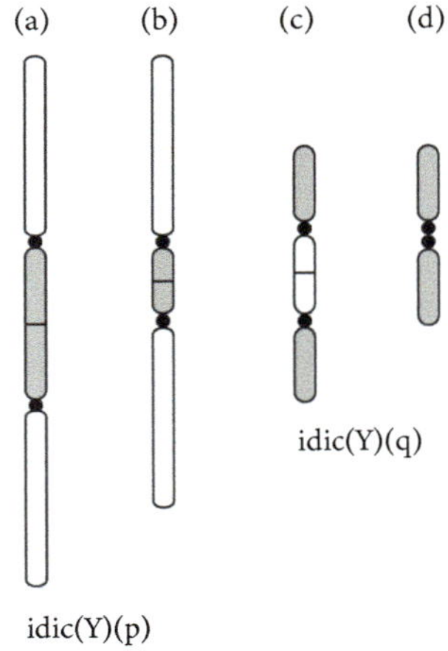

Figure 15–7. Formation of the isodicentric Y chromosome (Yp chromatin, gray; Yq chromatin, white). The idic(Y)(p) has mirror copies around a distal (*a*) or mid (*b*) Yp breakpoint, whereas the idic(Y)(q) has mirror copies around a Yq breakpoint (*c*) or practically at the centromere, Yq11.1 (*d*). Thus, heterogeneity of chromosome length relates to a heterogeneity of breakpoint site.

that the first stage of meiosis (division of the primary spermatocyte) had been entered. In the series of Abur et al. (2022), sperm were retrieved from 4/12 men with idic(Y), but no pregnancies were achieved.

In the 14 cases reported by Kalantari and colleagues the only woman had a TS-like clinical picture, and about half of cells on blood were 45,X; in comparison, in the series of Beaulieu Bergeron et al. (2011), four women all had gonadal dysgenesis. Ambiguous genitalia with ovotesticular DSD/mixed gonadal dysgenesis was the presenting sign in

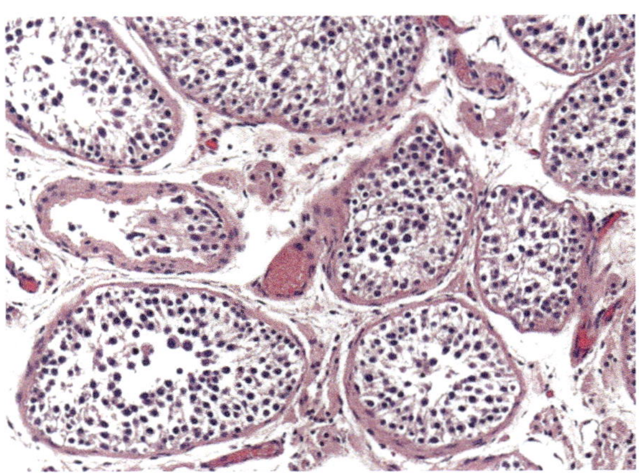

Figure 15–8. Testicular histology in an infertile man with 45,X[9]/46,X,mar[3]/46,X,idic(Y)(p11.3)[33]. There is a maturation arrest at the level of the primary spermatocyte, reflected in the azoöspermia of this man. The idic(Y) had the format as in Figure 15–5a.

Source: From KJ Lehmann et al., Isodicentric Yq mosaicism presenting as infertility and maturation arrest without altered SRY and AZF regions, *J Assist Reprod Genet* 29: 939–942, 2012. Courtesy MA Fischer, and with the permission of Springer.

three children in Mekkawy et al. (2012) and in the infant in Becker and Akhavan (2016). The Y isochromosomes were idic(Y)(*p*11.32) in two and idic(Y)(*q*11.222) in two; all were mosaic for at least 45,X, and two with an additional idic(Y)(p11.32)×2 line.

Ring Y. The usual case is of 46,X,r(Y)/45,X mosaicism, although it is likely that the 45,X line had arisen secondarily following post-zygotic loss of the ring. Double and interlocked rings are occasionally seen as late mitotic events. Retention of the *SRY* locus determines a male phenotype and provided that cells within gonadal tissue retain the r(Y); nevertheless, testicular gametic function is compromised. Loss of loci in the AZF regions in Yq11.23, if the ring breakpoint in Yq is proximal to these loci, adds further insult to gametogenic potential. Short stature is common, and loss of *SHOX* in the pseudoautosomal region is the presumed basis of this. If the gonad is 45,X, a TS-like phenotype is seen; or, if the gonad comprises both 45,X and 46,X,r(Y) lineages, a mixed gonadal dysgenesis, possibly with a genital ambiguity, may be the consequence (Milenkovic et al. 2011). A TS-like habitus, albeit in a male, may in any event arise if the ring is very small and lacks any Yq material (Tzancheva et al. 1999).

In the ring Y man, azoöspermia is usual, and less than 1% of cases have been inherited from a ring Y father (Arnedo et al. 2005). In the rare event of spermatogenesis proceeding, almost always fertility could only ever be achieved through IVF. In theory, and since only the 46,X,r(Y) gametocytes are "meiotically competent" (Blanco et al. 2003), sperm would be equally 23,X and 23,r(Y). Thus, normal 46,XX daughters and (probably mosaic) ring(Y) sons would be the predicted outcomes, although a 45,X cell line arising in the latter could potentially lead to a disorder of sex development. PGT would have an obvious place (Spinner et al. 2008).

X;Y Translocation. See Chapter 6.

Inversion Y. This normal variant is mentioned in Chapter 9.

GENETIC COUNSELING

Larger Rearrangements

TURNER SYNDROME VARIANTS

Lachlan et al. (2006) reviewed their own experience and the published literature, and they noted fertility with respect to these terminal Xp deletions: p11.4, p21, p21.1, p22.1, p22.12, and p22. Presumably, the risk to transmit the del(Xp) is 50:50. The implications for offspring differ according to the gender of the child. The limit of viability for the hemizygous deletion male is defined by the cases studied in Melichar et al. (2007), with the maximum survivable loss being ~10 Mb. The phenotype is very abnormal and includes severe intellectual disability, Léri-Weill syndrome, chondrodysplasia punctata, ichthyosis, Kallmann syndrome, and ocular albinism. Periquito et al. (2016) describe a woman with 45,X/46,Xdel(Xp) TS, who had been advised that she would be infertile but who went on to have two (non-mosaic) 46,X,del(X)(p11.4) daughters and a 46,XY son.

Fertility in women with a terminal Xq deletion is rare but reported. In the series of Mercer et al. (2013), three out of 20 women had pregnancies, for two live births and one miscarriage. As with the del(Xp), the risk of transmission is presumed to be 50:50, but the outcome is dependent upon the gender of the child. A male pregnancy with a degree of nullisomy Xq is presumed to be nonviable. Fertility with a ring X is known. An r(X) mother can have chromosomally normal children or an r(X) daughter. As for pregnancy in the isochromosome X, we know only of the single report in the series of Bernard et al. (2016).

KLINEFELTER SYNDROME VARIANTS

Infertility is the rule. In one example, normal daughters were born to a man with the karyotype 47,X,i(Xq),Y, following IVF with ICSI (Stabile et al. 2008).

Deletions and Duplications

Chromosome X

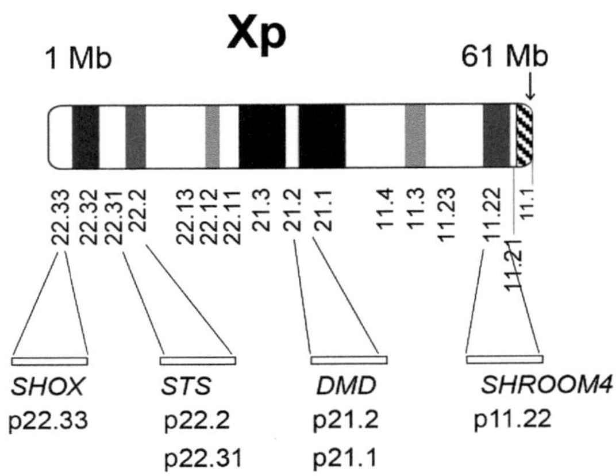

Figure 15–9.

Xp11.22

Duplication. A distal duplication at Xp11.22 includes the genes *SHROOM4* and, in most, also *DGKK* (Figure 15–10) (Grams et al. 2016). Some recurrent breakpoints are observed, sited at points of long terminal repeats. Males show a phenotype essentially the same as with the female. This may reflect that disomy of the chrX:48.4-52.6 Mb segment expresses the same in the male as in the female (in whom, curiously, the abnormal X is preferentially active, as mentioned below); of course, the male's single X is active. Intellectual disability ranges from mild to severe degree, with language in particular impaired; in one case the IQ, at 86, was within a normal range. Autistic behavior and epilepsy (or at least an abnormal electroencephalographic pattern) are recorded. Brain scan can show minor anomalies or, in one case, actual cortical atrophy. Early puberty is observed. Facial dysmorphism is of mild or subtle degree.

All inherited cases of this duplication have come from a carrier mother. In these, the inheritance pattern could be described, in essence, as X-linked dominant. Most cases, however, have been de novo, and in these, the abnormal X has consistently been of paternal derivation. In female de novo cases, X-inactivation, where measured, has been nonrandom and markedly skewed toward the *normal* X—a most remarkable observation (Di-Battista et al. 2016). Thus, the *abnormal* X is preferentially activated, and loci within the duplicated segment may express a functional and therefore potentially damaging disomy.

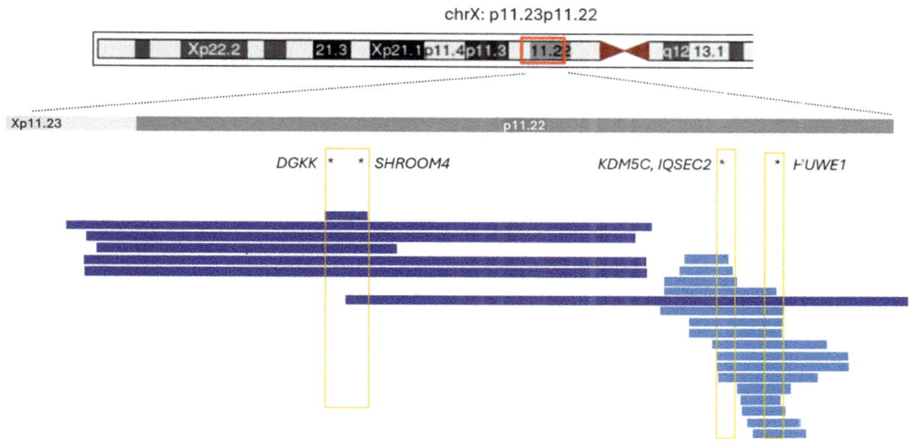

Figure 15–10. Duplications at Xp11.22.

Notes: While there is some overlap, duplications largely sort themselves into a distal and a proximal group. The distal group are defined by the particular involvement of *SHROOM4*, and some extending into Xp11.23, while the proximal group are further subdivided into groups in which *KDM5C* and *IQSEC2*, or *HUWE1*, are the defining loci.

Sources: From data in SE Grams et al., Genotype-phenotype characterization in 13 individuals with chromosome Xp11.22 duplications, *Am J Med Genet* 170A:967–977, 2016; and C Moey et al., Xp11.2 microduplications including *IQSEC2, TSPYL2* and *KDM5C* genes in patients with neurodevelopmental disorders, *Eur J Hum Genet* 24:373–380, 2016. Dark blue data are due to Grams et al., and light blue to Moey et al. Courtesy SE Grams and C Shoubridge, and with the permission of John Wiley and Sons, and Springer Nature.

Duplication. Proximal duplications within Xp11.22 are to be distinguished from the distal ones; overlap is rare (Figure 15–11). Within this group, further distinction is made upon the basis of the loci duplicated, with particular reference to *IQSEC2* and *HUWE1* (Moey et al. 2016). The observed phenotype in the affected male is one of intellectual disability and attention deficit/hyperactivity; mild facial dysmorphism is noted. In contrast to the distal duplication, epilepsy is not a feature. All cases in Moey et al. were maternally inherited. One child had two affected male cousins, these boys being the sons of three carrier sisters; one of the maternal grandparents was likely a mosaic hemizygote or heterozygote.

Xp11.4

Deletion. We have seen a young woman with retinitis pigmentosa, chronic granulomatous disease, and ornithine transcarbamylase (OTC) deficiency, having an Xp deletion

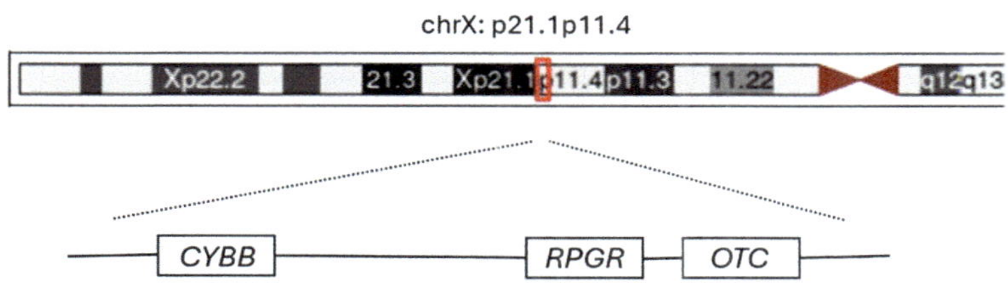

Figure 15–11. A Contiguous Gene Deletion at Xp11.4.

Notes: The key three loci removed in this deletion are *CYBB*, the basis of chronic granulomatous disease; *RPGR*, the basis of one form of retinitis pigmentosa; and *OTC*, the gene for ornithine transcarbamylase deficiency.

which removed these neighboring loci (Figure 15–11). She suffered recurrent upper respiratory tract infections and had a history of surgery for mastoid osteomyelitis and lung abscess. Her peripheral vision was poor, and she unconsciously self-managed the OTC deficiency by avoiding high-protein foods. X-inactivation was random. She came to prenatal diagnosis and elected to terminate a male pregnancy with the deletion, the predicted phenotype being severe (Coman et al. 2010b).

Xp21

Deletion. Cytogeneticists can claim some credit for the initial location of the gene for Duchenne muscular dystrophy (DMD) at Xp21.1p21.2 (Lindenbaum et al. 1979), and at least for that historical reason we include a mention of deletion in this region. Loss of neighboring loci in the hemizygous male leads to a contiguous gene syndrome, sometimes referred to simply as the "Xp21 deletion syndrome" (Figure 15–12). According to the extent of the deletion, these conditions may comprise the syndrome: DMD, adrenal hypoplasia, and hyperglycerolemia, along with developmental delay. The condition is often familial; while the carrier mother is typically unaffected, rare cases of clinically affected girls with a de novo deletion are reported (Heide et al. 2015).

Duplication. A locus of important effect in this duplicated state is *NR0B1*, which may lead to sex reversal in the 46,dup(X),Y genetic male (in the deleted state, *NR0B1* is the basis of the adrenal hypoplasia noted above). Small (<1 Mb) duplications including *NR0B1* are associated with sex reversal and isolated gonadal dysgenesis of differing forms, while larger duplications impose a broader phenotype with some dysmorphism and neurodevelopmental compromise (Zheng et al. 2024). Penetrance of the sex-reversal phenotype is incomplete (Veyt et al. 2024). The 46,X,dup(X)(p21) female carrier is normal (seven carriers in the six-generation kindred in Barbaro et al. 2007), and X-inactivation is random.

Xp22.31

Deletion of *STS* in this Xp22.31 causes the skin disorder X-linked ichthyosis. The nature of any additional neurocognitive phenotype is yet to be resolved, but the fact of *STS* being expressed in the brain raises that question. In the UK Biobank, Brcic et al. (2020) identified STS deletion in 86 males and 312 carrier females and found them to have slightly poorer performance on the Fluid Intelligence Test compared to controls, although not apparently affecting academic achievement. Male deletion carriers had an increased rate of depressive and anxiety-related traits, but which "may feasibly be related to having to live with a potentially stigmatizing lifelong skin condition." An increased risk of atrial fibrillation might relate to altered steroid hormone levels. Larger deletions

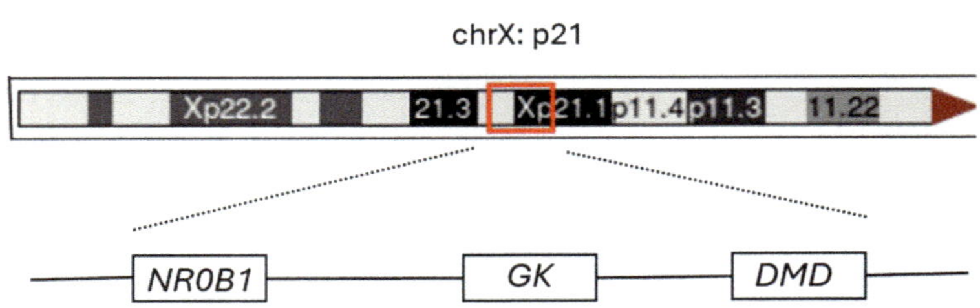

Figure 15–12. The Contiguous Gene Deletion of the Xp21 Syndrome.

Notes: The three loci shown here are *NR0B1*, *GK* (glycerol kinase), and *DMD* (Duchenne muscular dystrophy).

that include the gene *NLGN4* have the additional phenotypes of autism and intellectual disability.

Duplication of the *STS* region in Xp22.31 has been reported in patients with a wide range of phenotypes, but is likely to be an incidental finding. STS duplications are common in the general population (0.3%–0.4%) and are not enriched within the clinical population. From 414 male and 938 female carriers in the UK Biobank, health, cognitive function, and academic achievement did not differ from the general population (Gubb et al. 2020). An intriguing finding was of greater happiness among those with the duplication; the authors postulate that this might be the result of STS duplication causing elevated steroid hormone levels.

Xp22.2

Deletion. Some deletions in the 46,X,del(Xp) female which include this segment, either as an interstitial or as a terminal deletion, lead to the syndrome of microphthalmia and linear skin defects (MLS). In 90% of cases MLS is caused by deletions that include the *HCCS* gene, this gene directing a component of the mitochondrial respiratory chain (Morleo et al. 2018).[8] The intriguing question is this: Why is MLS seen in only some deletions of Xp22.2? Unfavorable X-inactivation is the reasonable explanation and in theory, inactivation of the normal X could lead to a functional nullizygosity of *HCCS*. Thus, in tissue derived from neural crest destined to contribute to skin and eye, mitochondrial failure could lead to cell death and hence the MLS phenotype. Favorable inactivation, skewed toward the del(Xp), could see the normal X hold sway. If there is mosaicism with a 45,X cell line, this may be protective by virtue of retained activity of *HCCS* when the gene is present on a single, active X. Wimplinger et al. (2007) suggest this to be the basis of a mildly affected mosaic 45,X/46,X,del(X)(p22.2) mother with MLS having a more severely affected non-mosaic 46,X,del(X)(p22.2) daughter.

> Another example of mother-daughter difference is seen in Margari et al. (2014), in this case with a large (and apparently non-mosaic) Xp22.2pter deletion. The mother was of short stature, and she had had one eye removed in infancy; the daughter was blind due to bilateral eye involvement, short, dysmorphic, had lost language ability and developed signs of autism. Both showed, at least on blood, preferential inactivation of the del(Xp) of ratios 10:90 in daughter and 15:85 in mother. The smallest deletion (of ~200 kb), removing only *HCCS* and part of one other gene (*ARHGAP6*), is described in Vergult et al. (2013) and concerned a mother and daughter, both of normal intellect, each with only one eye affected, and skin lesions only in the mother; X-inactivation was completely skewed in both.

It is presumed that an Xp22.2 deletion in a male conceptus would lead to inevitable early abortion. Thus, the risk to the female carrier to have a living affected child is one-third, the segregation ratio of 1:1:1 applying to normal female:affected female:normal male.

Duplication. Sismani et al. (2011) describe a family in which a mother heterozygous for a 9 Mb duplication Xp22.2p22.13 had four intellectually disabled sons, three of whom died in childhood. She herself and her carrier daughter were of short stature but normal

[8] A small minority, MLS is due to other X-borne loci, *COX7B* at Xq21.1 and *NDUFB11* at Xp11.3, which, like *HCCS*, code for components of mitochondrial function (Indrieri et al. 2012; Van Rahden et al. 2015). Thus far, *COX7B* and *NDUFB11* cases have been due to point mutation or intragenic deletion, not X chromosomal microdeletion.

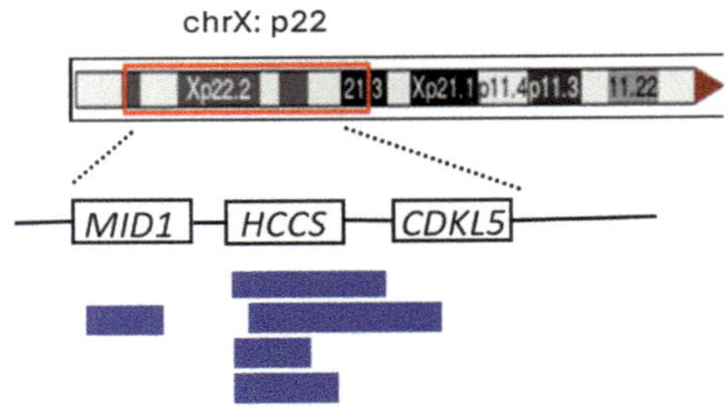

Figure 15–13. Duplications at Xp22.

Notes: Within the full segment Xp21.3 to Xp22.32 outlined, there are seven known X-linked intellectual disability loci, including the three shown.

Source: From data in C Sismani et al., 9 Mb familial duplication in chromosome band Xp22.2-22.13 associated with mental retardation, hypotonia and developmental delay, scoliosis, cardiovascular problems and mild dysmorphic facial features, *Eur J Med Genet* 54:e510–515, 2011.

intelligence. These authors compare two similar duplications within the region Xp22.11 to Xp22.2, each with different breakpoints but encompassing in common seven known X-linked intellectual disability loci (Figure 15–13).

Xq12q13.3

Duplication. Three families (one a five-generational pedigree) are on record segregating very similar duplications, with the gene *MED12* in common (Apacik et al. 1996; Kaya et al. 2012; Prontera et al. 2012). The affected males are microcephalic with marked intellectual disability, and in Apacik et al. (with a slightly more extensive duplication) multiple malformations were associated with death in early infancy. Female carriers are phenotypically normal but with completely skewed inactivation of the dup(X); the inheritance pattern is essentially that of an X-linked recessive disorder. A locus of particular interest within this segment is *XIST*, the X-inactivation center.

Xq21.1q21.2

Deletion. Smaller Xq21.2 deletions that include *POU3F4* cause the Xq21 deletion syndrome in males, the key phenotypic features being choroideremia (CHM), deafness, and intellectual disability (Bonati et al. 2024). Female carriers are generally asymptomatic, but they may show mild signs of choroideremia and rarely, mild hearing loss.

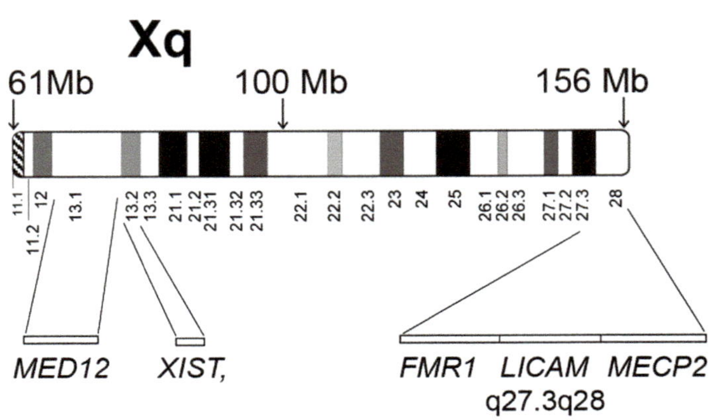

Figure 15–14.

Xq21.1q21.3

Duplication. Gabbett et al. (2008) describe a boy with poor motor and language development who became a "food seeker" as an infant, and who is described as presenting a Prader-Willi phenocopy, in whom a dup(X)(q21.1q21.31) was identified. His mother, who had had "learning difficulties" at school, proved (on blood analysis) to be a mosaic carrier of the duplication, with a random pattern of X-inactivation. A similar duplication (chrX: 83.6-87.6 Mb) and phenotype in brothers was reported by Sherlaw-Sturrock et al. (2022). Chromosomally adjacent to this case (but not overlapping), Basit et al. (2016) report a family in which five mild to moderately intellectually disabled brothers were the offspring of a consanguineous couple, but in fact a 3.95 Mb dup(X)(q21.31q21.32) proved to be the causative factor. Some displayed a facial dysmorphism; one was epileptic. Hyperphagia with obesity, dry skin, and self-mutilation were further observations. The phenotypically normal carrier mother and one sister showed markedly skewed X-inactivation with respect to the abnormal X. Of the three genes within the duplicated segment, *PCDH11X* bids fair to be a pheno-critical locus; the other two are *TGIF2LX* and *PABPC5*.

Yet, some microduplications in this region are not to be over-interpreted: they may in fact be harmless, that is to say a benign copy number variant. Maurin et al. (2017) make this point in their report of a 3.6 Mb microduplication at Xq21.33, discovered incidentally at prenatal diagnosis, and inherited through the mother from a normal grandfather. The fact of this being a gene-sparse region—only two loci resident therein, *DIAPH2* and *RPA4*—is the likely basis of the non-pathogenicity, with these genes tolerating duplication. This principle applies more widely: a large CNV is not necessarily pathogenic.

Xq21q26

Large Duplications. A number of dup(Xq) cases have been reported, of varying lengths, within this large (~60 Mb) Xq segment. Some are extensive and readily detectable on classical cytogenetics, while others (see below) warrant the appellation of microduplication. Both genders are seen; the clinical picture in the female, more so in the larger duplication, is often mitigated by skewed X-inactivation. One of the largest in a *female* is a de novo dup(X)(q21.1q25) initially diagnosed prenatally due to intrauterine growth retardation, in a girl whose circumstance at age two years remained one of a substantial physical and neurodevelopmental disability (Tachdjian et al. 2004). These authors list reports of a variety of relatively large Xq duplications in affected females. Cheng et al. (2005) review a number of reports of *male* cases of large duplication and present their own patient with 46,Y,dup(X)(q21.32q35), a profoundly disabled 2-year-old boy. Mostly, these are inherited from a heterozygous mother; grandpaternal meiosis may be the usual origin of the duplication.

Xq22.1

Deletions that include the *TIMM8A* and *BTK* loci at chrX:101.3 Mb cause a contiguous gene deletion syndrome in males comprising deafness and dystonia, and X-linked agammaglobulinemia due, respectively, to loss of these two loci (Rendtorff et al. 2022).

Xq22.1q22.3

Deletions of ~3 Mb in Xq22.1q22.3 are seen only in the heterozygous female, and the non-observation of males points to a lethality of the nullizygous state. The resultant "early-onset neurological disease trait" in 46,XX females comprises neonatal hypotonia, outcome. Inference from prenatal X-inactivation analysis, in abn(X) cases, may be fraught with uncertainty.

Sex Chromosome Deletions and Duplications

Del(X), dup(X). If the female del(X) or dup(X) carrier is fertile, the risk to transmit the abnormal chromosome will presumably reflect symmetric segregation, 1:1. If passed from a 46,X,del(X) mother to a *daughter*, the daughter's phenotype may be the same as that of the mother (which may well be quite normal). But a firm statement cannot be made. If the rule of selective Lyonization holds, the abn(X) is consistently the inactivated one, and normality might, in theory, be expected. If the rule fails, random inactivation could, in the case of the duplication, lead to an attenuated functional partial disomy with phenotypic abnormality, such as may be seen in the *MECP2* syndrome due to dupXq28.

If a del(X) is passed from a 46,X,del(X) mother to a 46,Y,del(X) *male* conceptus, the hemizygous male fetus will be nullisomic for loci within the compass of the deletion. Viability may be possible, but the absence of loci will lead to a "contiguous gene syndrome." A classic example is the variable combination of Duchenne muscular dystrophy, adrenal hypoplasia, glycerol kinase deficiency, and intellectual disability, due to deletion within Xp21. Larger microdeletions will often be lethal in utero due to nullisomy for the segment concerned.

Fertility is usually an academic question in the male hemizygote for a del(X) or dup(X) (but the reader will well understand that were his Y chromosome to be passed on, the child would, other things being equal, be normal).

Del(Y), dup(Y), r(Y). Fertility is achievable, with medical assistance, in some rea(Y) hemizygotes. In these cases, a 50:50 segregation with respect to the X and the rea(Y) chromosomes is to be assumed. A son inheriting the rea(Y) would very likely recapitulate his father's reproductive phenotype. IVF may enable fertility in those few males with extractable sperm, but with a high risk to offspring (in principle 50%) and with post-zygotic karyotypic evolution unpredictable, as per the phenotypic range outlined elsewhere (Chapter 20).

16
CHROMOSOME INSTABILITY SYNDROMES

A DEFECT OF DNA repair is the factor underlying the chromosome instability syndromes, also known as chromosome breakage syndromes (Taylor et al. 2019). The "instability" refers to the predisposition of the chromosomes to undergo rearrangement or to display other abnormal cytogenetic behavior. Their inclusion in this book is warranted in that special cytogenetic techniques may be useful in clinical diagnosis and prenatal diagnosis, albeit that direct molecular analysis now usually has the major role, as more is learned of the mutational basis of these syndromes.

The classic chromosome instability syndromes are Fanconi pancytopenia syndrome, Bloom syndrome, Nijmegen breakage syndrome, and ataxia-telangiectasia. The main cytogenetic features are listed in Table 16–1. They are Mendelian conditions, and in each the mode of inheritance is autosomal recessive. There is genetic heterogeneity in Fanconi syndrome, with cells homozygous for one mutation able to correct in vitro cells homozygous for another mutation ("complementation"). We briefly note two other rare mutagen-hypersensitivity syndromes: the immunodeficiency, centromeric instability, facial anomalies (ICF) syndrome, and Seckel syndrome. Proneness to cancer is a common concomitant of several of the breakage syndromes (Duker 2002), and for many even a single hypomorphic allele can be sufficient to increase cancer risk (Taylor et al. 2019). Some of these genes have in common their interaction with the breast cancer susceptibility gene *BRCA1*, their protein products forming a "BRCA1-associated genome surveillance complex" (Futaki and Liu 2001).

Rare or even unique families with various clinical presentations have been associated with chromosomal instability, and some representatives are mentioned in this chapter. Chromosome instability has been reported as an occasional observation in quite a number of known conditions. This list includes, among others, the Cockayne/cerebro-oculo-facial-skeletal syndrome spectrum, xeroderma pigmentosum, Rothmund-Thomson syndrome, Werner syndrome, Dubowitz syndrome, and Riyadh chromosome breakage syndrome. But in several the associations are not clear, the relevance for genetic counseling is uncertain (other than in supporting a diagnosis), and we do not consider them here. Likewise, chromosome instability is a feature of many cancers, and it may indeed be a crucial factor in the process of carcinogenesis; but this is a somatically acquired attribute and not of relevance in the present context.

A different cytogenetic observation is that of premature sister chromatid separation. This is a feature of Roberts syndrome, Cornelia de Lange syndrome, variegated aneuploidy syndrome, Warsaw breakage syndrome, and the chronic atrial and intestinal dysrhythmia syndrome; and we make brief mention of these conditions. The genes underlying these disorders code for cohesins, which contribute to the control of sister chromatid segregation at cell division and thus are dubbed "cohesinopathies." Cohesins are one component of the "structural maintenance of chromosomes" (SMC) complexes,

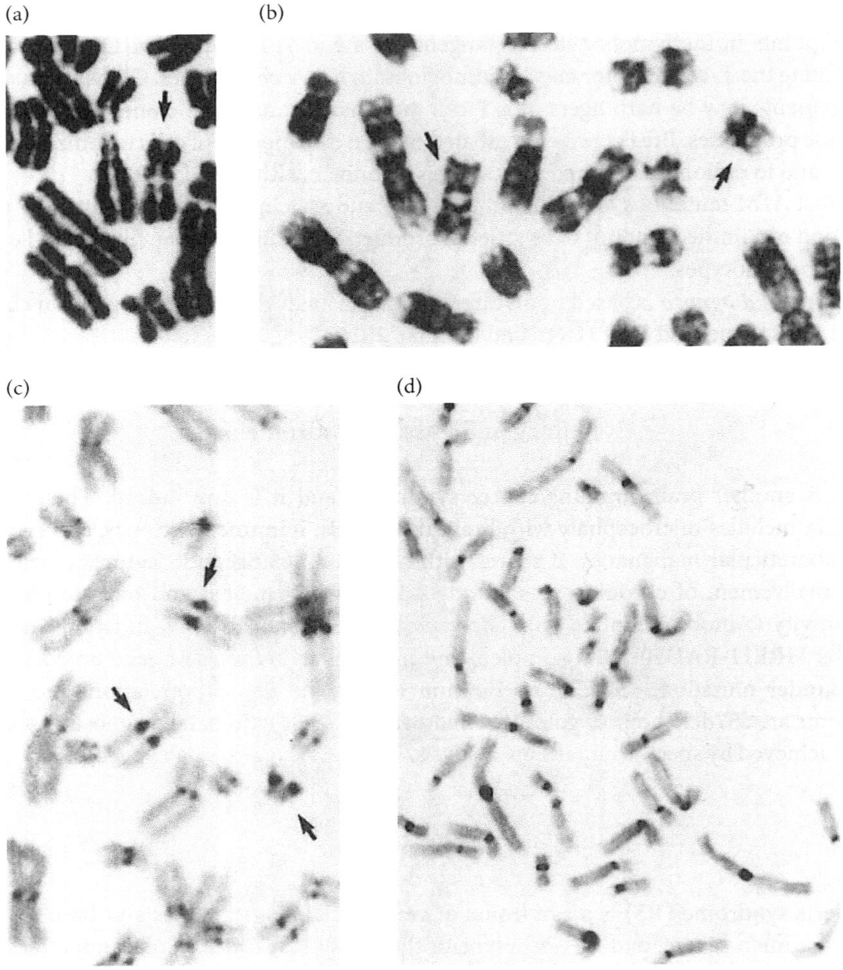

Figure 16–4. Unusual appearance of the chromosomes in Roberts syndrome: puffing at the centromeres (*a* and *b*); a C-banded preparation showing separation of the heterochromatic segments (*c*) is compared with a C-banded preparation from a control showing the normal centromere appearance (*d*).

Source: From NP Mann et al., Roberts syndrome: Clinical and cytogenetic aspects, *J Med Genet* 19:116–119, 1982, with the permission of the British Medical Association.

Cornelia de Lange Syndrome

The clinical phenotype of Cornelia de Lange Syndrome (CdLS) is, in the classic case, very distinctive. Five causative genes are known: *NIPBL* (the most frequently seen); *SMC1A*, *RAD21*, and *BRD4* cause autosomal dominant CdLS, typically due to de novo mutations; and mutations in *SMC3* and *HDAC8* are the basis of X-linked CdLS (Avagliano et al. 2020). The cytogenetic phenotype is PCS, and thus CdLS is another cohesinopathy. Be that as it may, testing for PCS is not useful in the diagnosis of CdLS, with one study showing it to be no more frequent in CdLS patients than in controls (Castronovo et al. 2009).

Very Rare Syndromes

ICF (Immunodeficiency, Centromeric Instability, Facial Anomalies) Syndrome. The ICF syndrome is characterized by immunodeficiency, an unusual facies, and growth and developmental retardation, together with a most remarkable tendency of chromosomes 1, 9, and 16 to form "windmill" multiradials by interchange within heterochromatic regions (Figure 16–5). This instability of the pericentromeric heterochromatin reflects hypomethylation of satellites II and III, which are important components of its structure. Hagleitner et al. (2008) document the variability of the phenotypic range. The phenotype, physical and cytogenetic, can be considered to be secondary to a failure of methylation. Five genes have been reported in ICF patients, but most cases are due to autosomal recessive mutations in either DNA methyltransferase 3B (*DNMT3B*, ICF1), or *ZBTB24* (ICF2) (van den Boogaard et al. 2017).

Mosaic Variegated Aneuploidy. The core phenotype of this recessively inherited syndrome comprises microcephaly with functional neurological abnormality, growth retardation, and susceptibility to childhood malignancy, with most of the lymphocytes and about half of skin fibroblasts showing premature chromatid separation. Many cells are aneuploid, with trisomies, double trisomies, and monosomies with almost every chromosome represented (Bohers et al. 2008; García-Castillo et al. 2008). In mosaic variegated aneuploidy (MVA) type 1, the underlying defect in the cell cycle involves one of the checkpoint proteins (BUB1B) that control progression through the mitotic process, maintaining an alert for chromosome malsegregation. The *BUB1B* heterozygote may display the tendency in a proportion of lymphocytes, and some mitotic cells may present the striking observation of a 92-chromosome count. At least five other MVA loci have been identified. Prenatal diagnosis has been reported based on conventional cytogenetics, the abnormalities being very obvious (Plaja et al. 2003; Chen et al. 2004b). If the molecular basis is known, preimplantation testing would be applicable.

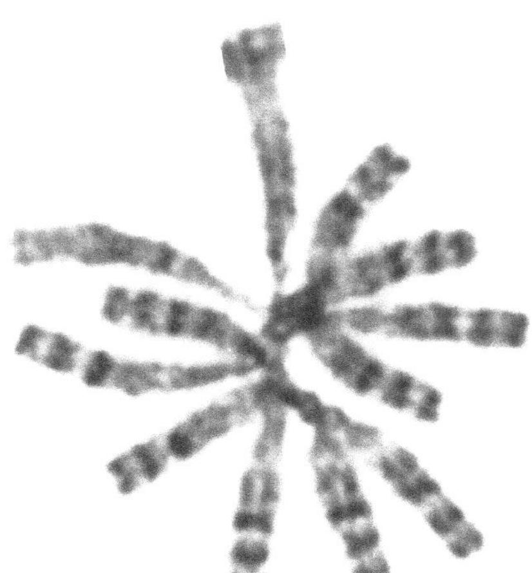

Figure 16–5. A "windmill" or "starburst" multiradial chromosome 1 in the ICF syndrome.
Source: From JR Sawyer et al., Chromosome instability in ICF syndrome: Formation of micronuclei from multibranched chromosomes 1 demonstrated by fluorescence in situ hybridization, *Am J Med Genet* 56: 203–209, 1995. Courtesy JR Sawyer, and with the permission of Wiley-Liss.

adjacent to the centromeres of each chromosome (hence, the C), substantially comprising alpha-satellite DNA consisting of hundreds of thousands of copies of a 171 base pair repeat. Certain chromosomes show quite marked differences in their C-band pattern, particularly chromosomes 1, 9, 16, and the Y, and the large blocks of heterochromatin thus stained are labeled 1qh, 9qh, 16qh, and Yqh.[2] They are of no phenotypic effect.[3]

Acrocentric Short Arms

The short arms of the acrocentric chromosomes (13, 14, 15, 21, and 22) can vary quite considerably in their lengths. Indeed, some p arms are apparently completely absent, and others are several times the typical length. This reflects variation in the three components of the short arm: the centromeric heterochromatin, the satellite stalk, and the satellite material, identified as bands p11, p12, and p13, respectively (Figure 7–4). Band p12 contains multiple copies of genes coding for ribosomal RNA; because the nucleolus of the cell is formed by an aggregation of rRNA, this region is also called the nucleolar organizing region (NOR). Acrocentric short arm variation appears to be without any phenotypic effect.

Banding Pattern: Euchromatin

Most of a chromosome consists of euchromatin, which contains the active genetic material, resident in greater amount in G-light bands (pale-staining on Giemsa banding) than in G-dark bands. The light microscope cannot reliably enable detection of alterations of less than 3 Mb–5 Mb, and most deletions and duplications of more than this size can be presumed to have phenotypic consequences. Exceptions to this rule include first, euchromatic variants that involve common copy-number variable regions that become visible when copy number is high enough, or when the size of the copy-number variable tract is large enough. Second, there are chromosomal segments whose deletion or duplication has no phenotypic consequence.

Euchromatic Variants

Euchromatic variants (EVs) due to copy-number variable tracts (Table 17–1) can be considered, in a sense, as extreme forms of CNVs, either because their copy number is at the high end or higher than the normal range, or because their size is greater than 3 Mb (at which point they are excluded from the Database of Genomic Variants; see below). Thus, EVs and the molecular CNVs (Chapter 18) essentially form a continuum, with no fundamental genetic distinction. For example, Tyson et al. (2014) analyzed the *REXO1L1* gene and pseudogene cluster that resides within a 12 kb tandem repeat in band 8q21.2, and of which the diploid copy number ranges from approximately 100 to

[2] Variation in the size of Yqh in an extended Canadian kindred could inferentially be traced back over three centuries, allowing Genest (1973, 1981) to claim that it was "the oldest known chromosome aberration."

[3] This has been the prevailing, if not universal view, for quite some time. Reproduction may, however, be a vulnerable sphere; and Tempest and Simpson (2017) review the reported associations with infertility and unfavorable reproductive outcomes.

Table 17–1. Euchromatic Variants Due to Copy-Number Variable Tracts

EUCHROMATIC VARIANT (EV)	REPEAT/SEGMENT SIZE	CONTROL COPY NUMBER	EV COPY NUMBER
dup 8p23.2	2.5 Mb	2	3
amp 8p23.1	>260 kb	2-9	8–12
amp 8q21.2	12 kb	97–277	265–270
amp 9p12	~1 Mb	1–3	7–12
del/dup 9p11.2p13.1	~5 Mb	4	3–5
dup/trp/ins 9q12	~5 Mb	4	5–6
del/dup/trp/amp 9q13q21.1	~5 Mb	4	3–8
amp 15q11.2	~1 Mb	IGVH 1–3; NF1 1–4	IGVH 4–9; NF1 5–10
amp 16p11.2	692–945 kb	3–8	8–10

Abbreviations: amp = amplification; dup = duplication; EV = euchromatic variant; ins = insertion; IGVH = immunoglobulin variable heavy chain; NF1 = neurofibromatosis 1; trp, triplication.

Source: From Tyson et al. (2014)

200. This repeat may account for almost half of band 8q21.2 and, at the upper end of this range, additional G-light material is discernible (Figure 17–1). While D'Apice et al. (2015) proposed that deletion of this segment (but with several copies yet remaining) could be the basis of a new microdeletion syndrome, Barber et al. (2016) argue that more likely, it may typically be a benign EV. The same interpretation of innocuousness likely applies to the other EVs listed in Table 17–1.

Some of these EVs may have been confused, on classical karyotyping, with pathogenic imbalances. On microarray analysis, however, the distinction should be clear; and in fact many microarrays exclude the repetitive regions that EVs involve.

Imbalances of Chromosomal Segments with No Apparent Phenotypic Effect

In a review in 2005, Barber found only 23 examples of families with directly transmitted autosomal segmental imbalance in which two or more carriers were unaffected, and a few have since been published (Table 17–2). These cases were often ascertained for incidental reasons, such as prenatal diagnosis for maternal age. The gene content is often lower than the genome average, and the lack of phenotype is attributed to the absence of dosage-sensitive genes, or to dosage compensation by related genes. Similar imbalances with no phenotypic consequence are recorded in more than one family for the gene-poor G-dark bands 2p12, 5p14, 13q21, and 16q21. Most of the families listed in Table 17–2 remain as isolated examples, and may yet turn out to reflect segmental incomplete penetrance. This may apply, for example, to the distal 3p cases, as other families with similar deletions are more often phenotypically affected. This question of penetrance in these few cases of cytogenetically visible imbalances is somewhat of a harbinger of the immense challenge that came to be presented by the flood of CNVs of 21st-century molecular analysis, as we discuss at length in Chapter 18.

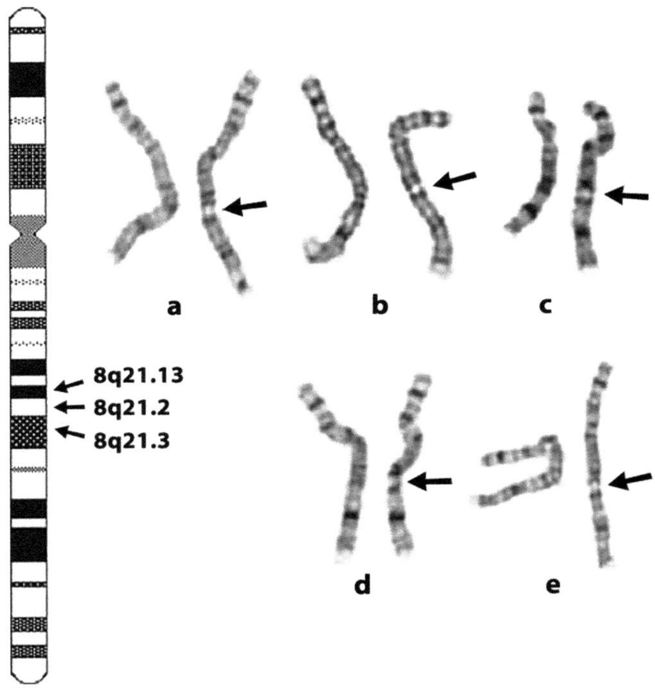

Figure 17–1. The likely benign euchromatic variant at 8q21.3, which reflects copy number variation of the *REXO1L1* gene and pseudogene cluster. This observation could be viewed, in a sense, as an intermediary between classical and molecular cytogenetic variation.

Source: From C Tyson et al., Expansion of a 12-kb VNTR containing the *REXO1L1* gene cluster underlies the microscopically visible euchromatic variant of 8q21.2, *Eur J Hum Genet* 22: 458–463. 2014. Courtesy JCK Barber and C Tyson, and with the permission of Springer Nature.

Inversions. We mention normal variant inversions seen in certain chromosomes (1, 2, 3, 5, 9, 10, 16, and Y) in Chapter 9.

Fragile Sites. Under certain stressed culturing conditions some, indeed most, chromosomes show apparent rupture in one, or less commonly both chromatids (Sutherland 2003; Mirceta et al. 2022). This is almost always without phenotypic implication. The spectacular exception is the fragile site FRAXA at Xq27, and indeed this laboratory observation lent its name to the well-known fragile X syndrome, originally referred to as a "marker" X (Lubs 1969). The fragile site observed by the microscopist reflected the trinucleotide expansion within the *FMR1* gene. Three other sites in the same region are FRAXB, FRAXD, and FRAXE, of which only the latter is pathogenic.

Otherwise, only two fragile sites may be of clinical import. FRA11B, at 11q23.3, is possibly the basis of some (not all) Jacobsen syndrome 11q deletions (Michaelis et al. 1998; and see p. 419). In the case in Clang and LaBaere (2023), neither parent of an affected child showed the fragile site. A single case of a man with 46,XY,fra(16)(q22.1), the fragile site classed FRA16B/C, in whom 1% of sperm and two out of 10 PGT embryos showed chromosome 16 imbalance, is to be noted (Martorell et al. 2014). We mention the fragile site FRA10A at 10q23, which may or may not be relevant at prenatal diagnosis, on p. 699. The full range of fragile sites is presented in Mirceta et al. (2022).

Table 17–2. Euchromatic Duplications and Deletions

CHROMOSOME	Del	Dup	qdp
1		p21-p31	
		q31.1-q32	
2	p12-p12 (x2)		
	q13-q14.1		
3	p25.3-pter (×2)	q28-q29	
4	q34.1-q34.3	p16.1-p16.1	q12q13.1
5	p14.1-p14.3 (×2)		
6	q22.31-q23.1		
7		p22.3-pter (×2)	
8	p23.1/2-pter	p22-p22	
	q24.13-q24.22	p23.1-p23.3	
9	p21.2-p22.1	p12-p21.3	
10	q11.2-q21.2	p11.1-q11.22	
		p13-p14	
11	p12-p12	11p15.3p15.1	
	q14.3-q22.1		
12		q21.31-q22	
13	q14.3-q21.33	q13-q14.3	
	q21-q21	q14-q21	
	q21.1-q21.31		
	q21.1-q21.33		
16	q13q22 (×4)		
18	p11.31-pter	p11.2-pter	
		q11.2-q12.2	
22	q11.21-pter		

Notes: These del/dups (and one quadruplication) are detectable by microscope cytogenetics and without phenotypic effect, as inferred from the observation of transmission from phenotypically normal parent to normal child.

The estimated sizes of the deletions and duplications range from 4.2 Mb to 16.0 Mb (del) and from 3.4 Mb to 31.3 Mb (dup). The numbers of studied families, where more than one, are shown in parentheses.

Source: From JCK Barber, Directly transmitted unbalanced chromosome abnormalities and euchromatic variants, *J Med Genet* 42:609–629, 2005, and the Chromosome Anomaly Collection website at http://www.ngrl.org.uk/wessex/collection (updated information is posted in the "What's New" section). Additional material due to Chen et al. (2011b), Coussement et al. (2011), Kowalczyk et al. (2013), Liehr et al. (2009), and Singer et al. (2021).

GENETIC COUNSELING

A person carrying a classical chromosome variant has, practically by definition, no increased risk for having abnormal offspring, pregnancy loss, or any other reproductive problem. Some view it as at best pointless and at worst counterproductive even to mention to the individual that a variant chromosome has been found; others feel obliged to pass on the observation. If it is discussed, it must be made clear that it is a normal finding—perhaps interesting but of no practical importance. For the heterochromatic size variants (C-band and NOR) and euchromatic variants, the point can simply be made that some chromosomes come in short, medium, and long forms, and where a chromosome happens to fit in this continuum is without significance. For segmental imbalances ascertained in apparently unaffected individuals, careful clinical assessment should be made, if practicable, of carriers from the same family; incomplete penetrance and variable expressivity should be borne in mind in assessing innocuousness, or not, of the variant. Fragile sites are practically always normal findings. The primacy of molecular karyotyping in the 21st century in fact means that discovery of variants such as these will be rather infrequent events.

There is considerable potential for iatrogenic anxiety, whereas in reality the biology of the supposed anomaly has no pathogenic implication. The counselor may thoroughly understand the presumed harmlessness of a variant chromosome, but the person in whose family it has been discovered may react "non-scientifically." To put a stark setting on it, the worst possible response might be for a couple to choose to terminate a pregnancy because of an overinterpreted variant chromosome, as has actually happened with the 16p11.2 euchromatic variant (López Pajares et al. 2006). *Primum non nocere*: First do no harm.

18
COPY NUMBER VARIANTS

The molecular lens, when it began to be applied from the late 20th century, came up with a somewhat surprising observation: Short genomic segments could exist in deleted or duplicated state, invisible on routine classical cytogenetics, among individuals in the general, normal population. These segments acquired the name Copy Number Variants (CNVs) and were to be distinguished from pathogenic, relatively larger microdeletions and microduplications. They are certainly common, indeed universal: every person has, on average, 31 CNVs of >5 kb size (18 deletions and 13 duplications) compared to a reference genome, with an average size of 430 kb for deletions and of 900 kb for duplications (Hujoel et al. 2022). Some CNVs are "recurrent" with identical breakpoints driven by low copy repeats at specific chromosome locations, but most are novel, confined to a particular individual or family. Many of these CNVs contribute, often subtly, to complex human traits; others may be of no phenotypic effect. Less commonly, individual CNVs may be the basis of a monogenic disorder. If the phenotypic contribution of a CNV is unknown, another expression may be applied: Variant of Uncertain Significance (VUS).

> The word "variant" has gained considerable currency in the genetic lexicon of this century (Richards et al. 2015), and is the "V" in CNV and VUS. Molecular laboratories may issue reports concerning a Mendelian gene, referring to a "pathogenic variant" in preference to the formerly favored expression "mutation." The word *variant* does allow, in principle, for a nuanced interpretation, and conventionally the gamut runs a sliding scale from pathogenic, through likely pathogenic, of uncertain significance,[1] likely benign, to benign/nonpathogenic (Figure 18–1). The matter is further complicated by variation within a variant: It may be harmless in one setting and pathogenic in another. Using the word *variant* can allow for agnosticism in terms of pathogenicity; adjectives and adjectival qualifiers can be added accordingly as the interpretation unfolds, and a descriptive classification conferred.

Had it been possible to make a clear distinction between all "CNVs" consistently harmless and all those consistently pathogenic, the discussions in this chapter and in the chapters on autosomal and sex chromosomal microdeletions and microduplications (Chapters 14 and 15) could have been quite self-contained. But that is not the case, at least as of the present writing.

What is the actual basis of the variation? A short segment of chromatin—a "copy"—would normally exist on a chromosome in single state, and thus with one copy on each chromosome. Variation lies in the presence of these copies in absent or double (sometimes triple or quadruple or higher) states on a chromosome; hence the expression

[1] Fowler and Rehm (2024) comment that dealing with so many variants of uncertain significance (VUS) is a major challenge to the practice of precision genomic medicine; yet, they express optimism that many of these uncertainties will be resolved by 2030, and that ultimate elimination of all VUS is an achievable goal.

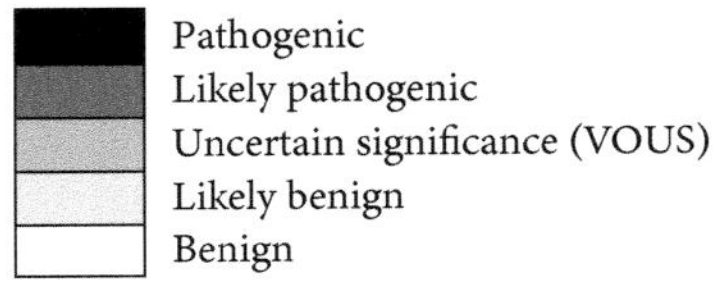

Figure 18–1. CNV Gradations.

copy number variant. The copy size can vary from 50 bp[2] to ~3 Mb (MacDonald et al. 2014).[3] Some segments are in "gene deserts"; others contain known genes. If there is an observation that no untoward effect exists in the presence of a single, triple, or higher multiple amount of these genes, this then allows the inference that these genes are not dosage-sensitive.

The difficulty lies in determining that a CNV is indeed a normal variant and of no phenotypic import (Hehir-Kwa et al. 2013). The harmlessness of many CNVs is attested by their segregation within a family in which only the proband (through whom the CNV was ascertained) may have been of abnormal phenotype. In these, the CNV can usually be taken as benign/nonpathogenic, and its discovery merely coincidental. The finding of a de novo change may more reasonably be considered as likely causative; but the gene content of this genomic segment should be considered in the context of the patient's phenotype, and not losing sight of the fact that de novo CNVs are seen in one in 50 healthy individuals (Itsara et al. 2010). Interpretation may need to account for ethnicity: the frequencies of some CNVs vary depending on the background of the individuals tested (Figure 18–2).

The five-part classification is not necessarily as clear-cut as the grayscale above might imply. With what confidence can a CNV be called indeed pathogenic, or benign? The bar is high: Only those "practically certain" to be so, can be called so. How likely is "likely"? In the similar setting of Mendelian variants, an expert group[4] views 90% as a suitable cutoff (Richards et al. 2015). That leaves another 80% or so in the "variant of uncertain significance" (VUS) territory. Every counselor can expect to encounter and to deal with VUSs.

The genic content of a CNV would seem, intuitively, to be a key—probably *the* key—factor determining pathogenicity or not. This "common-sense" viewpoint is given formal support in Rice and McLysaght (2017), who determined that a pathogenic CNV is more likely to contain a gene or genes that are dosage-sensitive, that have a role in embryonic development, or that are evolutionarily conserved. This information is now available to the counselor through publicly available databases, as outlined below, enabling a more precise interpretation of which CNVs are of clinical significance.

We mentioned in Chapter 14 the concept of a deletion "unmasking heterozygosity" of a recessive allele coincidentally on the other chromosome. The similar scenario may obtain with an otherwise benign deletion CNV if a locus therein happens to code for a Mendelian recessive disease. Thus, Liu et al. (2016) diagnosed autosomal recessive

[2] Elements below 50 bp are known as insertions or deletions, or "indels."

[3] The DGV database uses an arbitrary cutoff of 3 Mb; this could be seen as a pragmatic border between the euchromatic segmental variants described above and the CNVs as discussed here.

[4] American College of Medical Genetics and Genomics and the Association for Molecular Pathology.

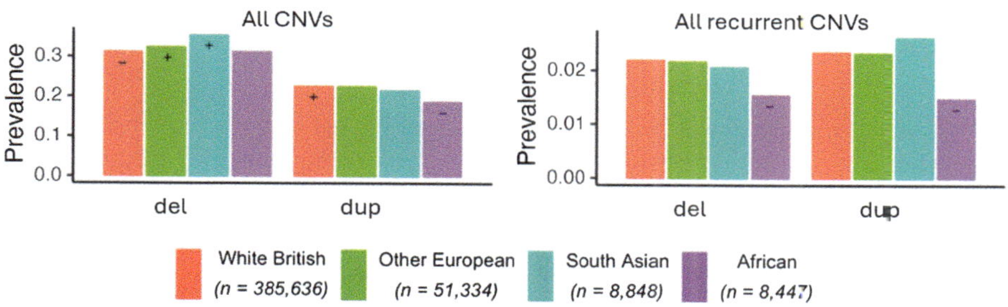

Figure 18–2. CNV Carrier Frequency by Ancestry Group.

Notes: These data are taken from the UK Biobank. Deletion (del) carrier prevalence (*left*) is significantly higher than expected (+) for the South Asian ancestry group, and duplication (dup) carrier prevalence is lower than expected (-) for the African ancestry group. When considering only recurrent CNVs (*right*), there were fewer (-) African del and dup carriers than expected.

Source: From LM Schultz et al., Copy-number variants differ in frequency across genetic ancestry groups, *HGG Adv* 5:100340, 2024. Courtesy LM Schultz and L Almasy, and with the permission of Elsevier.

spastic ataxia of Charlevoix and Saguenay (ARSACS) in a patient with a *SACS* mutation at 13q12.12 on one chromosome, and a 1.33 Mb CNV deletion encompassing the *SACS* locus on the other. We have seen a very similar case in a woman with ataxia and a Charcot-Marie-Tooth-like neuropathy inheriting a (normally nonpathogenic) paternal 0.2 Mb CNV deletion which removed *SACS*, and an accompanying maternal *SACS* mutation on the other homolog, thus enabling a diagnosis of ARSACS.

DATABASES

The counselor dealing with a family in which a CNV has been shown has formidable resources to which to appeal. Collaborative efforts from around the world bring together data, and repositories are assembled to which enquiry may be made.

DECIPHER. This name comes from *D*atabase of *C*hromosomal *I*mbalance and *P*henotype in *H*umans Using *E*nsembl *R*esources. It lists known or possibly pathogenic variants and VUSs. The Internet link is http://deciphergenomics.org. A panel displays CNVs that either match or overlap with a segment of interest. Duplications are shown in blue, and deletions are shown in red. The distinction between pathogenic variants and VUSs is indicated by the differing color intensity (the darker, the more likely to be pathogenic). The user will note that many cases show DDD as the data source: This is the database *D*eciphering *D*evelopmental *D*isorders. The DECIPHER browser also includes CNV data from gnomAD, DGV, ClinVar, and pHaplo/pTriplo scores.

ClinGen. This is a "National Institutes of Health–funded resource dedicated to building an authoritative central resource that defines the clinical relevance of genes and variants for use in precision medicine and research." It provides a comprehensive evaluation of dosage sensitivity at the levels both of the gene and of the genomic region, based on data from the published literature and public and internal databases. Each gene and genomic region evaluated receives a separate haploinsufficiency (HI) score and triplosensitivity (TS) score, according to whether copy number loss (HI) or copy number gain (TS) results in a clinical phenotype. Within each category, a score of "3" denotes sufficient evidence for dosage sensitivity; "2" denotes emerging evidence; "1" is equivalent to little evidence; and "0" means no evidence for dosage sensitivity (Riggs et al. 2020).[5] Each listed variant has a thumbnail sketch of condition and available evidence alongside; the link is http://clinicalgenome.org.

Genome-Wide Dosage Sensitivity. Collins et al. (2022) analyzed several large genomic datasets in order to predict the probabilities of haploinsufficiency (pHaplo) and triplosensitivity (pTriplo). A score of 0 indicates a low probability of dosage sensitivity, whereas a score of 1 indicates a high probability of dosage sensitivity. Applying this scoring to all human genes, including those not yet associated with a phenotype, they identified 2,987 as haploinsufficient (corresponding to pHaplo ≥ 0.86) and 1,559 as triplosensitive (pTriplo ≥0.94). Of note, 648 genes were uniquely triplosensitive. pHaplo and pTriplo scores are provided in the DECIPHER browser.

DGV. A more encyclopedic collection, including the smallest normal variants, is that due to the *D*atabase of *G*enomic *V*ariants, which is curated at The Center for Applied Genomics at the Hospital for Sick Children, Toronto. The Center records "genomic alterations that involve segments of DNA that are larger than 50 bp. . . . The content of the database only represents structural variation identified in *healthy control samples*." The data derive from upwards of eight million entries from worldwide populations (MacDonald et al. 2014; Zarrei et al. 2015). The database is accessed directly at http://dgv.tcag.ca/dgv/app/home. Continual refining and addition of sequence-based CNV data leads to increasing accuracy and confidence, and a special track within the DGV lists "gold standard structural variants" (GSSVs).

UCSC Genome Browser. The *U*niversity of *C*alifornia, *S*anta *C*ruz genome browser site at http://genome.ucsc.edu can be configured to display information from DECIPHER, ClinGen, OMIM, RefSeq genes, GeneReviews, gnomAD, and other useful datasets. It can include the Copy Number Variation Morbidity Map of Developmental Delay, a dataset which displays CNVs ascertained from nearly 30,000 children with various developmental disabilities, derived from Cooper et al. (2011) and Coe et al. (2014). Comparison data from nearly 20,000 controls allows the user to assess whether a particular CNV is enriched in the clinically ascertained population.

Gene Constraint Metrics. "Constraint scores" are epidemiological measures of genetic fitness in human populations, without consideration of gene function. Intolerant genes are those for which loss of a single copy has been reproductively disadvantageous over human history, either due to lethality or reduced reproductive fitness. Constraint metrics are features of the gnomAD database [https://gnomad.broadinstitute.org/] and can be used to interpret the clinical significance of copy number variants; they are also available in the UCSC browser. The key metrics for CNV interpretation are those that measure "intolerance to haploinsufficiency": that is, the extent to which loss-of-function (LoF) variants in a given gene are depleted in the general population.[6] LoF constraint is measured by two different scores. The "probability of being loss-of-function intolerant" (pLI) score divides genes into those that are intolerant to LoF (pLI >0.9) and those that are tolerant to LoF (pLI ≤0.9) (Lek et al. 2016). The "Loss-of-function Observed/Expected Upper bound Fraction" (LOEUF) is a continuous metric that reflects the full spectrum of intolerance to pLoF. LOEUF ranges from 0 to 2, with values below 0.35 suggestive of intolerance (Karczewski et al. 2020).

[5] Following Riggs et al. (2020), the suggested corresponding clinical classification is: 3, Pathogenic; 2, Likely Pathogenic; 1, Variant of Uncertain Significance (VUS); 0, VUS or Likely Benign.

[6] Constraint metrics are also available for missense and synonymous variants, but these are seldom relevant for assessing the pathogenicity of CNVs.

COPY NUMBER VARIANTS AND THE BRAIN

The most complex organ, the brain, is the most susceptible to CNV imbalance, typically presenting as cognitive/behavioral/psychological dysfunction (Molloy et al. 2023; Mollon et al. 2023a); indeed, in most CNV imbalances there is no observable physical phenotypic abnormality. In a large study of children with intellectual disability/developmental delay, an excess of those with a CNV compared to controls emerged significantly at a CNV size of 400 kb and became more evident at 1.5 Mb (Cooper et al. 2011). At least some of these CNVs, therefore, would have been pathogenic. Again unsurprisingly, larger (>1.5 Mb) CNVs were overrepresented in de novo cases; presumably this reflects a reduced reproductive fitness of those with larger, and pathogenic, CNVs.

Similar conclusions are reached in Coe et al. (2014). McCormack et al. (2016) recorded frequencies of benign versus pathogenic CNVs in an abnormal population (Figure 18–3). A subtler study was performed in Estonia (Männik et al. 2015); in this study, the CNV status of a large population was shown to correlate with educational attainment (Table 18–1). These subjects had been selected due to attendance at a general medical practice, and could be considered as quite close to a true random population sampling. Of the CNVs analyzed in these subjects, only smaller (0.25–1 Mb) duplications appeared to be consistently benign.

In considering clinical outcomes relating to brain function, the effects of CNVs do not fit neatly into a "pathogenic vs benign" binary, but rather are quantitative. The study of genotypes in large, well-phenotyped population cohorts has shed light on the subtler manifestations of CNVs that may not be immediately apparent in the clinic.

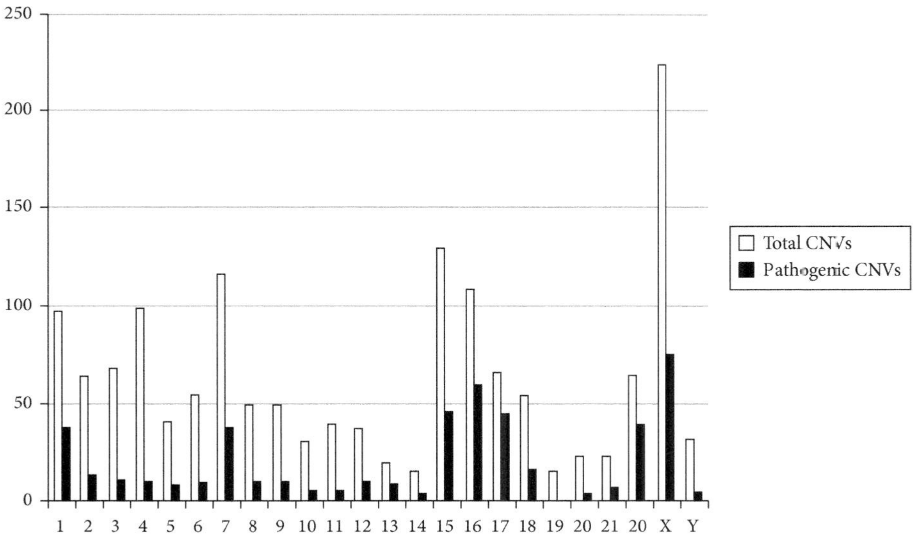

Figure 18–3. Population Frequencies of CNVs.

Notes: Total number of pathogenic CNVs, compared to total CNV frequencies, in an abnormal population. These data derive from a series of 5,369 postnatal (single or multiple congenital abnormalities, neurodevelopmental delay with or without neuropsychiatric disorders) and prenatal (two or more abnormalities detected on ultrasound) samples.

Source: From A McCormack et al., Microarray testing in clinical diagnosis: An analysis of 5,300 New Zealand patients, *Mol Cytogenet* 9: 29, 2016. Courtesy DR Love and AM George, and with the permission of BioMed Central.

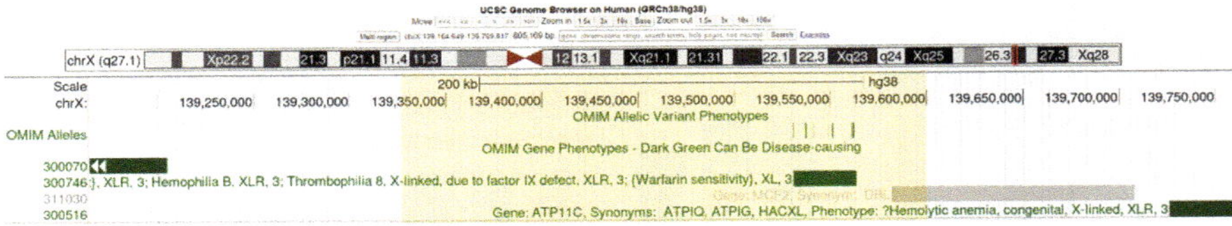

Figure 18–9. The UCSC Browser.

Notes: An example of a CNV display using the UCSC (University of California, Santa Cruz) browser, based on the trpX:139,332,751-139,601,714 bp described in the text. The Factor IX gene (*F9*, green) is completely contained within the segment; the *MCF2* gene (grey) is partially included (Case of J Watt). Green denotes an OMIM gene, grey is a gene not yet linked to a phenotype.

trp(X) under discussion is shown in Figure 18–11. Checking the DGVa link[11] mentioned above, and entering the coordinates of the trp(X)(q27.1), the CNVs contained therein are displayed (Figure 18–12). The largest is a 316,901 bp duplication, and smaller dels and dups are listed. But these, by definition in DGVa, are normal variants and can therefore be dismissed as pheno-contributory.

The important next step is a family study, if feasible. In the example just given, it transpired that the brother and mother both had the same trp(X) *and* were both normal intellectually. But interestingly, they had both suffered thrombotic episodes with elevated levels of Factor IX. The conclusion to be drawn is that the neurological compromise[12] in the presenting child is likely coincidental. A genetic diagnosis yet awaits, if indeed there is one. (The reader may well have similar stories to tell.)

GENETIC COUNSELING

The data from the laboratory which, as described above, can be rather sophisticated, needs to be clearly conveyed to those for whom the report is intended, which will very often be the genetic counselor, and through the counselor to parents and patients themselves.

Novel CNVs

The distinction between harmful and harmless variants can be a subtle exercise in the case of novel CNVs. As outlined above, interrogating databases such as UCSC browser, DECIPHER, and DGVa may be a first court of appeal. If a parent or other family member has the same variant and is of normal phenotype, the CNV may be adjudged a "likely benign" variant; or, other data—and especially pedigree data in the public domain—may be sufficiently powerful to indicate indeed a nonpathogenic CNV. A qualitative assessment of the genic content, as discussed above, may well be valuable. A de novo CNV may

[11] Or, if a segment is identified in the University of California Santa Cruz (UCSC) browser, and the track "DGV Struct Var" under the Variation category is chosen, the region will be displayed and segments of deletion (red) and duplication (blue) within the vicinity indicated. Clicking on to a CNV within the segment of interest will link to the DGV database.

[12] Brain imaging was normal, and there was no evidence that cerebral vascular thromboses could have been the basis of her abnormality.

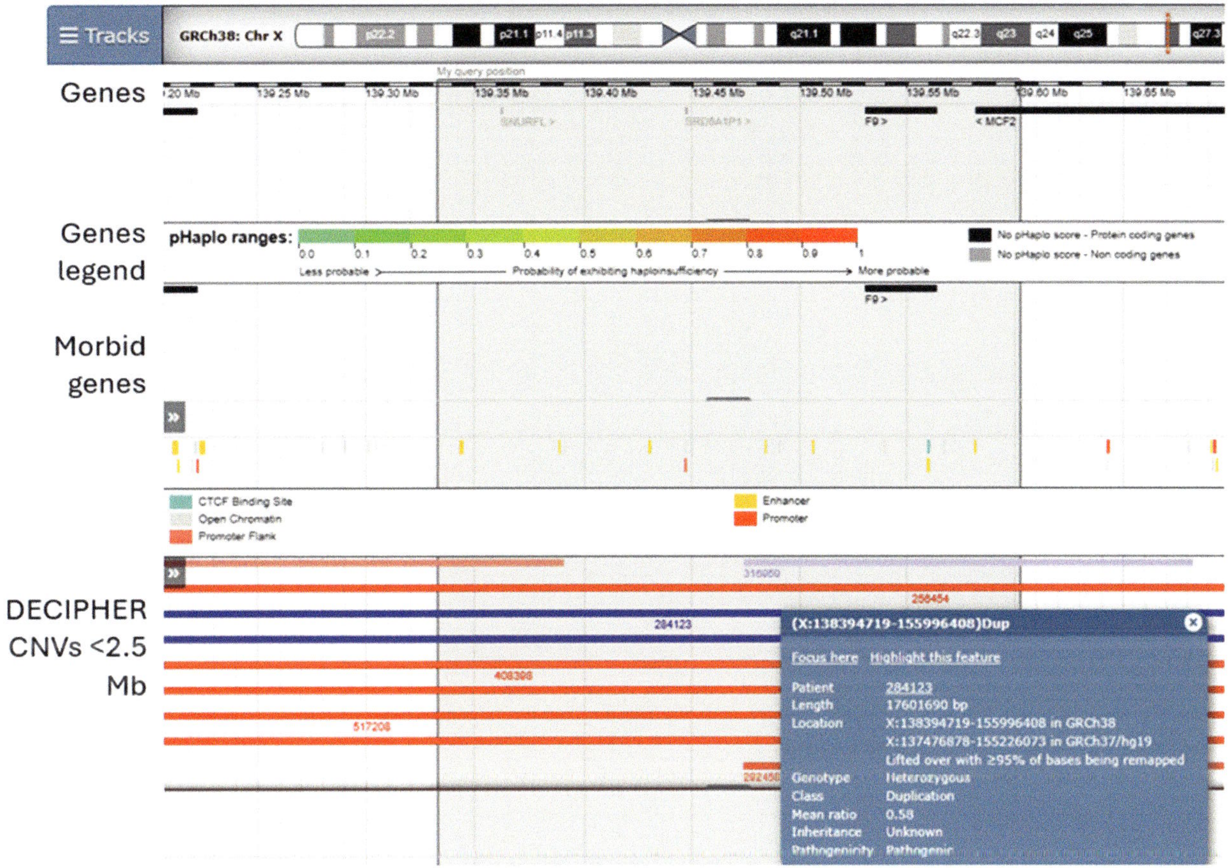

Figure 18–10. DECIPHER.

Notes: An example of an interrogation using the DECIPHER database, based on the [hg38]trpX:139,332,751-139,601,714 bp described in the text. Entering these coordinates, and then scrolling through a list of cases that DECIPHER presents with some degree of overlap, and looking at duplications (the blue lines), the closest variant is Patient 284123 who has [hg38] dupX:138394719-155996408. Clicking on this bar gives a dialog box with detailed information. In this example, the imbalance in the DECIPHER case is too large to usefully apply to the case in question.

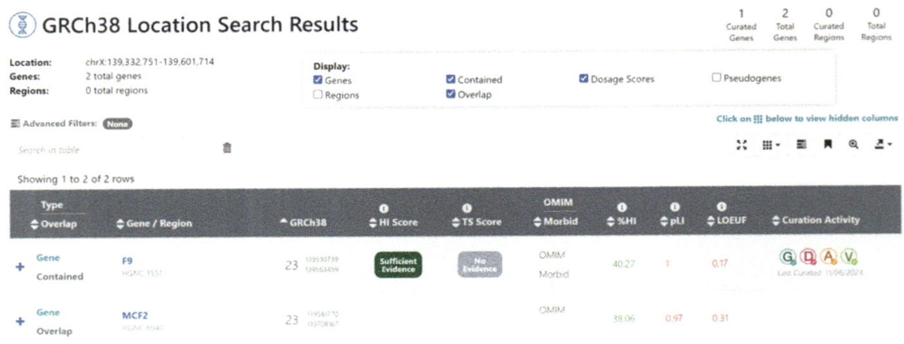

Figure 18–11. ClinGen.

Notes: The display according to the ClinGen database, of the [hg38] trpX:139,332,751-139,601,714 described in the text. The display highlights F9 as an OMIM Morbid gene contained within the region, and MCF2 as a non-OMIM morbid gene that is overlapping the region. ClinGen dosage sensitivity scores indicate evidence for haploinsufficiency, and no evidence for triplosensitivity. DECIPHER haploinsufficiency score and gnomAD pLI and LOEUF scores are consistent with known pathogenicity of factor IX deficiency, but do not provide information about the effect of duplication (or triplication). Links within the table take the reader to synoptic data about each locus.

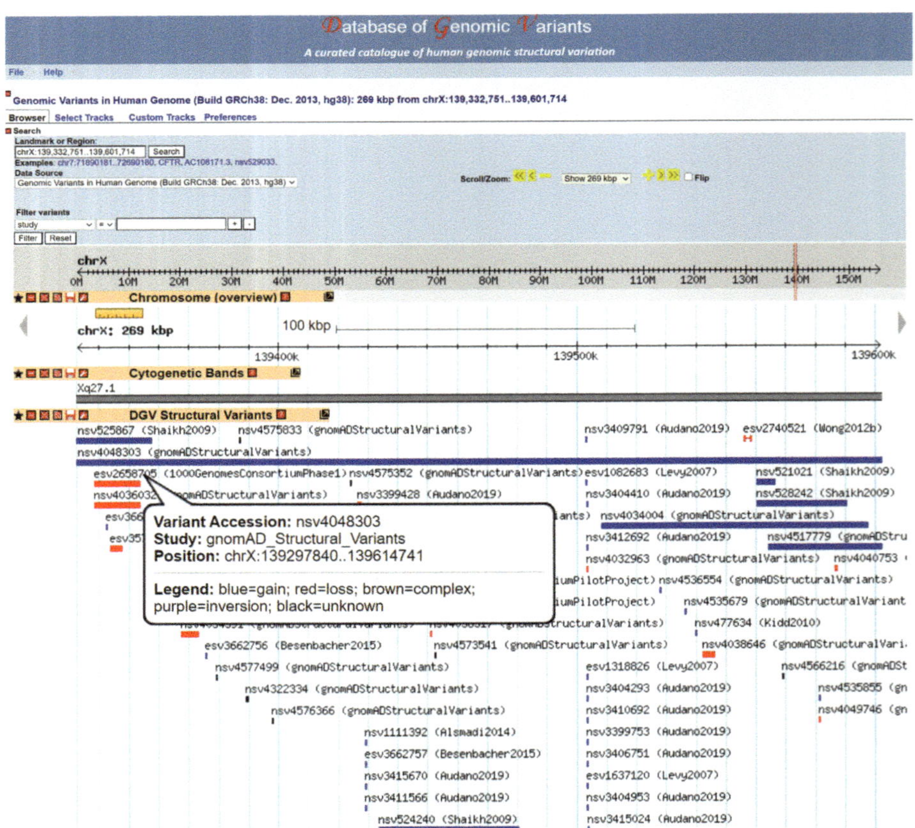

Figure 18–12. Database of Genomic Variants (DGVa).

Notes: An example of an interrogation using the Database of Genomic Variants (DGVa) based on the trpX:139,332,751-139,601,714 bp described in the text. The website is accessed at http://dgv.tcag.ca/gb2/gbrowse/dgv2_hg38. Nucleotide numbers are entered according to the appropriate "build" chosen (here, hg38). Duplicated CNV segments (blue) and deleted CNV segments (red) are presented. These are mostly labeled *nsv* and *esv* (*sv*, structural variant, archived and accessioned by dbVAR and DGVa, respectively). The largest duplication is nsv4048303, with breakpoints very similar to the triplication investigated in the example case. Clicking on each entry links to detail about the variant, including the lengths.

need to be considered as "likely pathogenic" unless there is solid evidence otherwise; a data resource in this respect is the website http://denovo-db.gs.washington.edu (Turner et al. 2017).

A detailed format for the practical assessment of a CNV is outlined in Di Gregorio et al. (2017), who assessed a little over 1,000 individuals with developmental delay/intellectual disability (Figure 18–13). These variants were classified into CNVs of size greater than 3 Mb (which we might equally call microdeletion/duplications); del/dups associated with known syndromes; CNVs spanning known Mendelian disease genes; likely pathogenic CNVs, and noting the genes contained within them; and VUSs/likely benign. These authors referred to the databases of a number of publicly available sources, in order to judge the possible pathogenicity of abnormal copy number of the loci contained within CNVs. In some, a diagnosis was clear enough at the outset, with a number of known syndromes seen. In others, it required a detailed weighing of the nature of the loci and appealing to information from the several sources. The reader wishing further demonstration of the rationale in CNV assessment is referred to this paper.

The question of non-penetrance, or at least reduced expressivity of a CNV, is a challenging one. Attempting to dissect out "micro-phenotypes" in a parent may prove rather fraught. Adding to this is the problem of "second-hit" CNVs and the degree to which they may modify or exacerbate a phenotype. In the meantime, in advising about the risk to a future child, the counselor will need to consult current sources and to seek expert advice. A problem of long familiarity in genetic counseling, that of dealing with uncertainty, certainly applies here (Wilkins et al. 2016). Conveying the information about a novel CNV to counselees is an exercise to which genetic counselors are becoming more accustomed, which is not to say that they find it straightforward. Finally, a question of well-considered clinical judgment, and of which the answer might differ between

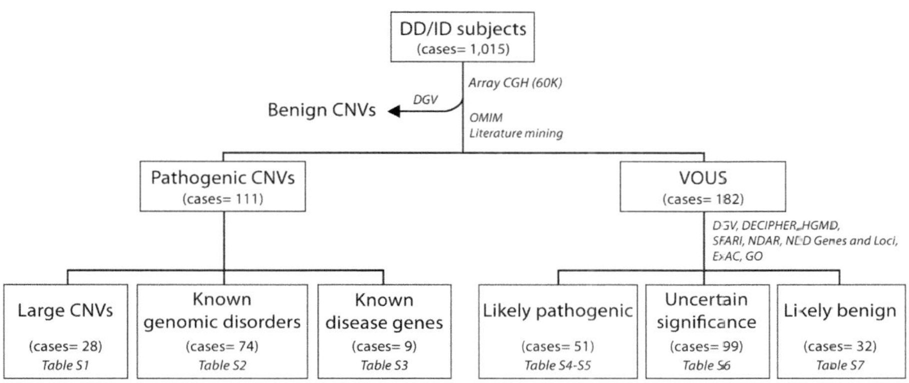

Figure 18–13. A schema for the analysis of copy number variants.

Notes: The data from a series of 1,015 cases of developmental delay/intellectual disability were assessed, and in 10%, a pathogenic CNV was identified. The criteria by which the CNVs were judged are set out in fine detail in the Tables S1-S7 in the original paper. Sources referred to: DGV, DECIPHER as noted above; OMIM, Online Mendelian Inheritance in Man; HGMD, Human Gene Mutation Database; SFARI, Simons Foundation Autism Research Initiative; NDAR, National Database for Autism Research; NDD, neurodevelopmental disorders; ExAC, Exome Aggregation Consortium; GO, Gene Ontology Consortium; VOUS, Variant of Uncertain Significance.

Source: From Di Gregorio et al., Copy number variants analysis in a cohort of isolated and syndromic developmental delay/intellectual disability reveals novel genomic disorders, position effects and candidate disease genes, *Clin Genet* 92: 415–422, 2017. Courtesy A Brusco and GB Ferrero, and with the permission of John Wiley & Sons.

families: Having discovered a CNV that would qualify as a VUS, would it, or might it not, be helpful to pursue a family study?

Recurrent CNVs

Many recurrent CNVs are known, and the counselor has access to considerable resources to assist with interpretation. Information about individual recurrent CNVs is provided in Chapter 14, and pooled penetrance data from Goh et al. (2025) are in Appendix C. And yet, the concept of incomplete penetrance for a range of continuous neurodevelopmental and neuropsychiatric phenotypes muddles accurate interpretation and complicates communication of the data. At the level of the individual patient, our understanding of the complex genetic factors contributing to neurodevelopmental phenotypes remains well short of complete.

Counseling will necessarily be tailored to the means of ascertainment. After the incidental detection of a recurrent CNV at prenatal diagnosis, a parent is likely to ask, "What does this mean for my child, and will they have a disability?" Whereas the identical CNV detected in a disabled child will prompt the question, "Does this explain my child's developmental delay?" For the clinician, attribution (or not) of pathogenicity has additional implications for deciding whether to offer further genomic testing, and for laboratories whether to report certain CNV findings, particularly in the prenatal setting.

A useful starting point is to consider the reported penetrance of the specific recurrent CNV for the phenotype of intellectual disability, over and above the background likelihood of intellectual disability in the general population. Using this stringent definition, and a background prevalence of intellectual disability of 1.1%,[13] Goh et al. (2025) provide penetrance estimates for recurrent CNVs, noting that many are close to 0% and most are <20%. These are presented in full in Appendix C. A more nuanced question is whether a recurrent CNV might contribute to a range of neurodevelopmental phenotypes such as attention deficit hyperactivity disorder, motor disorders, and mild autism, but will fall short of the severity threshold required for a diagnosis of intellectual disability. Additional considerations relate to the risk of congenital malformations and, in later life, the question of risk of psychiatric and medical diagnoses. For many recurrent CNVs, the answer to at least some of these questions will be yes, but with the qualification that magnitude of the effect is often small, such that it may not be apparent at the level of the individual. The counselor will need to keep abreast of evidence available for the specific CNV and have forefront in mind the individual concerns of the counselee.

[13] Note that other several authors have used prevalences in the range 1%–5%.

PART FOUR

DISORDERS ASSOCIATED WITH ABERRANT GENOMIC IMPRINTING

19

UNIPARENTAL DISOMY AND DISORDERS OF IMPRINTING

UNIPARENTAL DISOMY IS A FASCINATING and important pathogenetic mechanism, albeit that it is the basis of only a small number of well-defined clinical conditions. Table 19–1 lists the 10 described uniparental disomy (UPD)[1] syndromes, representing chromosomes 6, 7, 11, 14, 15, and 20.[2] Some of these syndromes can be due to genetic causes other than uniparental disomy, the two main categories being cytogenetic alterations (namely, CNVs affecting imprinted loci), and altered imprint in the absence of UPD or cytogenetic abnormality. For convenience we also include a discussion of the other causes in this chapter. In a category by itself, UPD can be the cause of homozygosity for an autosomal recessive gene. Nevertheless, the fact remains that most UPDs appear to be without any phenotypic consequence, and a number of syndromes that had originally seemed fair candidates turned out, in fact, not to be due to UPD (Kotzot 2002). A distinction is to be made between UPD where both chromosomes are identical (uniparental *iso*disomy, UPID) and where they are different (uniparental *hetero*disomy, UPHD) (Figure 19–1a). Both forms can coexist: meiotic recombination can lead to a UPD with both isodisomic and heterodisomic parts (see also Figure 19–16). A third category, segmental UPD, arises via mitotic recombination, possibly a consequence of an attempted rescue of a deletion or pathogenic variant. UPD is normally demonstrable only at the molecular level.

Typically, although not invariably, the UPD pair of chromosomes are cytogenetically normal, and the (classical) karyotype appears normal, 46,XX or 46,XY. The pattern of polymorphic DNA markers shows that both chromosomes have the same haplotype as just one of the chromosomes from one of the parents (isodisomy); or, the two chromosomes have the same haplotypes as the chromosome pair from one of the parents (heterodisomy). For example, the chromosome 1 haplotypes from parents and child set out in Figure 19–1b show that the child has two identical copies of one of the father's chromosomes: thus, paternal uniparental isodisomy. This UPD had been discovered fortuitously, when the child was investigated for a clinical diagnosis of congenital insensitivity to pain, an autosomal recessive disorder (Miura et al. 2000). He proved to be homozygous for a mutation in the appropriate gene (*TRKA*, located at 1q21q22), and his father

[1] As a general rule, abbreviations for "uniparental disomy" are in uppercase (UPD, UPHD, UPID) when making broad reference to the concept of uniparental disomy/heterodisomy/isodisomy, and in lowercase (upd, uphd, upid) according to the rules of cytogenetic nomenclature, when attention is more focused upon a specific case.

[2] Another imprinting syndrome, but one without an association with UPD, is Birk-Barel syndrome, caused by gain-of-function variants in the paternally imprinted gene *KCNK9* at 8q24. The phenotype of intellectual disability and dysmorphism is expressed only when the variant is transmitted from a mother (Cousin et al. 2022).

Table 19–1. Imprinting Disorders due to UPD or Copy Number Variants

IMPRINTING DISORDER	LOCUS	UPD	DEL / DUP
Transient neonatal diabetes	6q24	pat	dup(6q)(pat)
Silver-Russell syndrome	7	mat	dup(mat)
	11p15.5	mat	dup(11p)(mat)
Beckwith-Wiedemann syndrome	11p15.5	pat	dup(11p)(mat)
Temple syndrome*	14q32	mat	del(14q)(pat)
Kagami syndrome	14q32	pat	del(14q)(mat)
Prader-Willi syndrome**	15q11q13	mat	del(15q)(pat)
Angelman syndrome	15q11q13	pat	del(15q)(mat)
Pseudohypoparathyroidism type 1B	20q13	pat	del(20q)(mat)
Mulchandani-Bhoj-Conlin syndrome	20q11q13	mat	

*Paternally inherited loss-of-function variants in the *DLK1* gene at 14q32.2 cause central precocious puberty (Dauber et al. 2017).
**Maternally inherited loss-of-function variants in the *MAGEL2* gene at 15q11.2 cause Schaaf-Yang syndrome

carried the mutation but his mother did not. This scenario—a child with a recessive disorder for which only one parent is heterozygous—is commonly the circumstance behind the discovery of UPIDs that would otherwise have been without clinical effect, and it is sometimes referred to as the "unmasking" of a recessive gene. The other typical route to recognition of harmless UPDs is through the incidental discovery of long continuous/contiguous stretches of homozygosity on single nucleotide polymorphism (SNP) microarray or genomic sequencing.

The state of iso- or heterodisomy can allow an inference as to the site of the initial chromosomal error. Isodisomy for an entire chromosome typically reflects a meiosis II nondisjunction (in the absence of recombination) or a mitotic error (including monosomy rescue). In contrast, heterodisomy for an entire chromosome is due to nondisjunction at meiosis I. More commonly, recombination at meiosis I results in the coexistence of partial heterodisomy and partial isodisomy for the same chromosome pair. For example, a crossover at meiosis I in the distal long arm, followed by meiosis I nondisjunction, could lead to a disomic gamete isodisomic for distal long arm and heterodisomic for proximal long arm (Figure 19–1a, lower right). If the nondisjunction were at meiosis II, the isodisomy and heterodisomy would be the other way around, involving the proximal and distal segments, respectively (Figure 19–1a, lower left). Recognizing some forms of UPD can be achieved on SNP array, and we discuss this below.

EPIGENETICS AND IMPRINTING

In epigenetic variation, a core consideration is that a phenotype may differ according to whether a DNA sequence is active, or inactive but with the DNA sequence itself remaining unchanged. Our focus is on the activity or non-activity of a gene (or

(a)

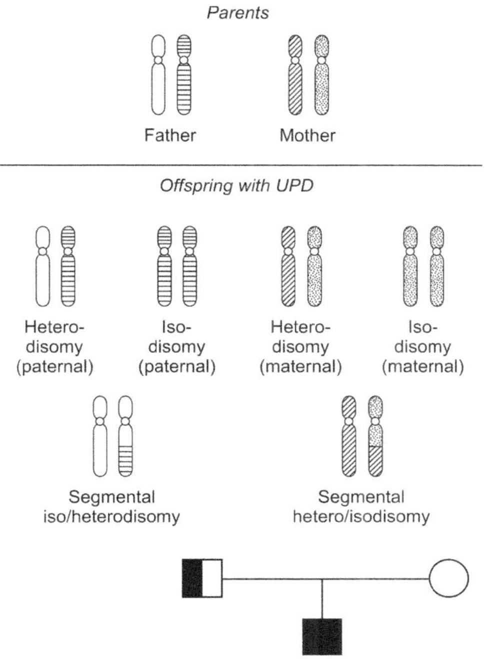

(b)

Marker	Father		Child		Mother	
D1S468	1	1	1	1	1	3
D1S214	3	2	3	3	1	3
* D1S450	4	4	4	4	5	6
* D1S2667	4	4	4	4	1	3
D1S2697	3	2	3	3	3	3
* D1S199	4	4	4	4	1	5
* D1S234	6	2	6	6	1	5
D1S255	4	1	4	4	2	4
* D1S2797	3	5	3	3	4	7
* D1S2890	4	2	4	4	2	2
* D1S230	2	4	2	2	4	4
D1S2841	4	2	4	4	1	4
* D1S207	1	5	1	1	2	4
D1S2868	1	2	1	1	1	2
* D1S206	2	1	2	2	4	5
* D1S2726	3	2	3	3	1	4
* D1S252	5	5	5	5	2	6
D1S498	2	3	2	2	2	3
→ * D1S484	4	3	4	4	1	2
D1S2878	2	2	2	2	2	5
D1S196	3	2	3	3	3	3
* D1S218	2	5	2	2	1	4
* D1S238	1	2	1	1	3	3
* D1S413	3	2	3	3	1	2
D1S249	2	7	2	2	2	7
* D1S425	1	2	1	1	2	3
* D1S213	4	6	4	4	2	5
D1S2800	2	1	2	2	1	2
D1S2785	4	5	4	4	1	4
D1S2842	3	3	3	3	3	3
* D1S2836	1	5	1	1	3	3

Figure 19–1. Uniparental Heterodisomy and Uniparental Isodisomy.

(a) The distinction between uniparental heterodisomy and uniparental isodisomy. The four parental homologs are shown in different patterns. In the child with *hetero* disomy, the two homologs are different. In *iso* disomy, they are identical. Meiotic crossing-over can lead to segmental iso/heterodisomy, and the pattern can reveal whether the initial nondisjunction had been at meiosis I or II (see text). *(b)* The molecular picture of a child with paternal uniparental isodisomy 1. The markers run from D1S468 at the top of chromosome 1 down to D1S2836 at the bottom. Both the child's chromosome 1 haplotypes are the same, and the same as one of his father's no. 1 chromosomes. He has no chromosome 1 from his mother. (The arrow points to the position of the *TRKA* locus. Homozygosity for an abnormal *TRKA* allele was the cause of his having the recessive condition congenital insensitivity to pain, which had led to his ascertainment.)

Source: From Y Miura et al., Complete paternal uniparental isodisomy for chromosome 1 revealed by mutation analyses of the *TRKA* (*NTRK1*) gene encoding a receptor tyrosine kinase for nerve growth factor in a patient with congenital insensitivity to pain with anhidrosis, *Hum Genet* 107: 205–209, 2000. Courtesy Y Indo, and with the permission of Springer-Verlag.

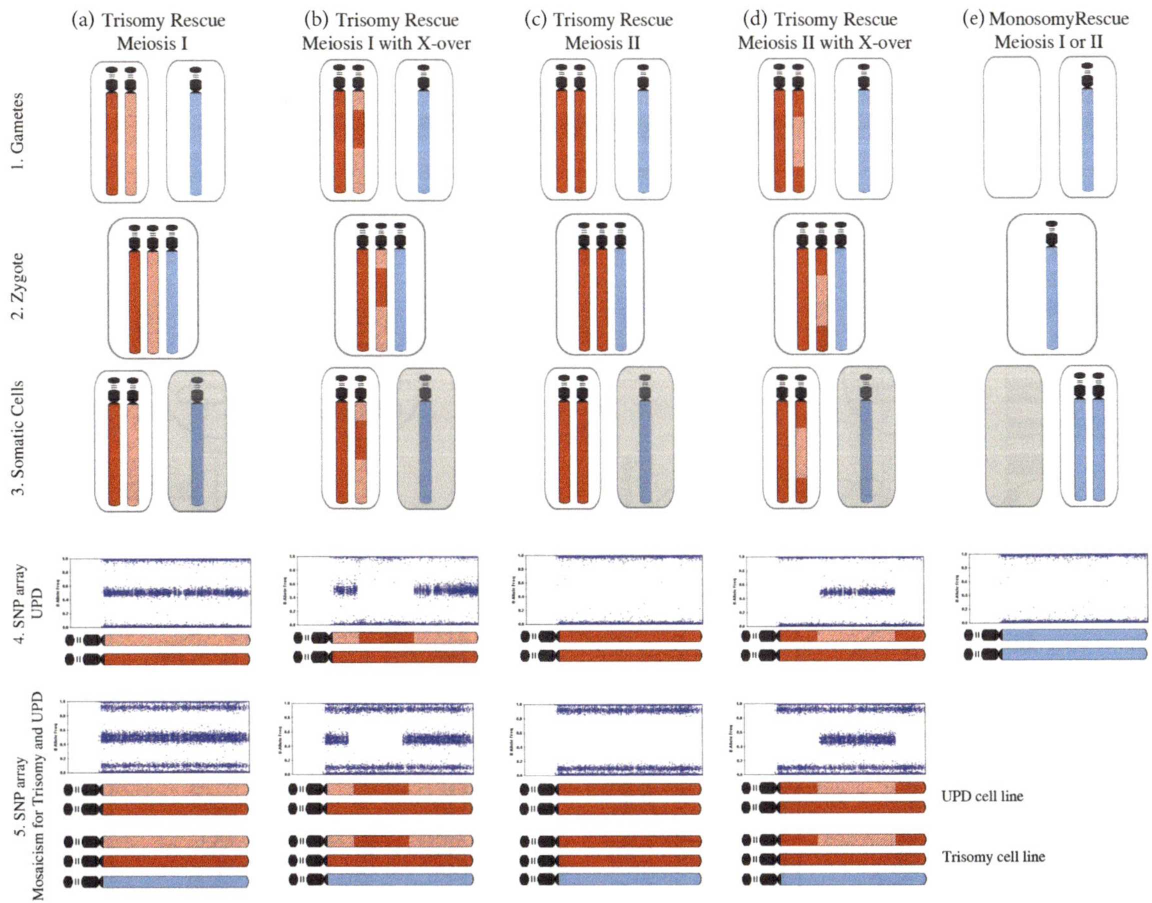

Figure 19–5. Ways in which UPD Arises.

The several routes by which UPD may arise (rows 1–3), and the observations on SNP array that may inform interpretation (rows 4–5). (*A* and *B*) Meiosis 1 nondisjunction with postzygotic trisomy rescue: UPD with centromeric heterodisomy ± distal isodisomy. (*C* and *D*) Meiosis 2 nondisjunction with postzygotic rescue: UPD with centromeric isodisomy ± distal heterodisomy. (*E*) Postzygotic monosomy rescue: complete isodisomy.[4]

Source: From HM Kearney et al., Diagnostic implications of excessive homozygosity detected by SNP-based microarrays: Consanguinity, uniparental disomy, and recessive single-gene mutations, *Clin Lab Med* 31:595–613, 2011. Courtesy HM Kearney and LK Conlin, and with the permission of Elsevier.

contradictory statement can be appreciated upon considering the mechanism of monosomic rescue after mostly maternal nondisjunction, this being the usual initiating cause of paternal UPD.

Rare mechanisms to generate complete UPD include the following:

- Correction of interchange trisomy
- Correction of interchange monosomy
- Isochromosome formation
- Correction of imbalance due to small marker chromosome

If one parent carries a reciprocal translocation, asymmetric segregation of the chromosomes may lead to an interchange trisomy (p. 113) at conception, in which the translocation chromosomes, plus one of the normal homologs, are transmitted. Post-zygotic correction by the loss of one homolog restores disomy, but if it is the other parent's chromosome that is lost, UPD is the consequence. Or, if a nullisomic gamete meets a normal gamete (interchange monosomy), the normal gamete may replicate the homolog in question to restore disomy (just as in monosomy rescue, mentioned above).

Liehr (2025a) records more than 100 examples of UPD associated with a Robertsonian translocation, involving UPDs for chromosomes 13, 14, 15, 21, and 22.[6] In the case of a parent with a Robertsonian translocation, the most common mechanism leading to UPD is a trisomy rescue after nondisjunction. A monosomic acrocentric chromosome, after nondisjunction from a Robertsonian translocation parent and fertilization with a normal gamete, could replicate as an isochromosome in a monosomy rescue (Berend et al. 2000; McGowan et al. 2002).

Complementary isochromosomes (p. 317), of which scarcely a double-digit number have ever been described, can even allow the circumstance of "contraposed UPD": that is, there may be UPD of the p arm from one parent and UPD of the q arm from the other. Finally, in the setting of a supernumerary small marker chromosome (SMC) there may be a coexisting UPD for the same chromosome from which the SMC was derived (James et al. 1995; Liehr 2025b).

SEGMENTAL UNIPARENTAL DISOMY

Segmental UPD may be acquired as the consequence of a post-zygotic somatic recombination between the maternal and paternal homolog (Figure 19–6), and in that case it will necessarily be an isodisomy (Kotzot 2008a). An assessment of "long contiguous stretches of homozygosity" may prove a useful means to demonstrate the state (Papenhausen et al. 2011). The UPD segment lies distally, the rest of the chromosome pair having a normal biparental disomy. The classical karyotype is normal.

Segmental UPD can have an effect if the particular chromosomal segment incorporates loci subject to imprinting. If the recombination occurs in a cell after the formation of the inner cell mass (which gives rise to the embryo), the segmental UPD will involve only some cells; in other words, there is *mosaic segmental UPD*. Beckwith-Wiedemann syndrome, Russell-Silver syndrome, UPDs for chromosome 14, and transient neonatal

[6] These data include both inherited and de novo Robertsonian translocations, as well as homologous Robertsonian translocations (acrocentric-derived isochromosomes).

MLID is characterized by disruptions at multiple loci across the genome including, but not limited to, those associated with known imprinting disorders. Most people with MLIDs have clinical features of BWS, Silver-Russell syndrome, or TNDM. Eggerman et al. (2022) review candidate genes for which variants in the maternal genome may contribute to this phenotype. These include hypomorphic variants in *NLRP7*, a gene of particular interest because women with biallelic inactivating *NLRP7* variants are affected by recurrent hydatidiform mole (p. 623).

No consistent phenotype otherwise has been associated with UPD(6)mat, although intrauterine growth retardation and prematurity have been noted in the majority of reported cases, and post-natal short stature in about half (Li et al. 2024a). In keeping with this observation, Mackay et al. (2022) identified UPD(6)mat in 7/4721 referrals for Silver-Russell syndrome testing.

Chromosome 7. Silver-Russell syndrome (SRS) has as its major feature intrauterine and post-natal growth retardation, often with a concomitant limb asymmetry. Genetic causes include maternal UPD(7) (~7%–10%), and 11p15 epimutation and structural 11p aberrations (see "Chromosome 11" below); SRS due to UPD(7)mat presents with more speech and language difficulty but less incidence of congenital abnormality (Wakeling et al. 2010; Lin et al. 2021a). Executive function appears to be spared, with one small study finding a mean full-scale IQ of 101 in three individuals with SRS due to UPD(7)mat (Burgevin et al. 2023). The specific loci responsible for UPD(7) imprinting have not been identified, but one or more genes in the *MEST* imprinted region at 7q32.2 are strongly implicated[12] (Carrera et al. 2016). There is a maternal-age association: Mean maternal age is five years older in SRS due to UPD(7)mat than 11p15 epimutation (Lin et al. 2021a); most are consequential upon "trisomy rescue" from an initial maternal meiotic nondisjunction (Chantot-Bastaraud et al. 2017). Two cases are recorded of SRS in the setting of a maternal reciprocal translocation involving chromosome 7 (Dupont et al. 2002; Behnecke et al. 2012). In both instances, the conception was probably an interchange trisomy, with subsequent loss of the paternal chromosome 7 producing the balanced state but with a maternal UPHD 7.

As for paternal UPID 7, Liehr et al. (2025a) collated five cases that were identified following a diagnosis of cystic fibrosis (CF). We have seen a similar example, which was in fact the only instance of a child being born with CF from more than 10,000 women who had screened negative for CF carrier status (Archibald et al. 2014). Another such case was a woman of normal linear growth and a normal intellect, and it was only because she had a recessive condition with its locus on chromosome 7 (congenital chloride diarrhea) that she had been investigated (Höglund et al. 1994). Apart from unmasking of recessive genes, there does not appear to be a phenotype associated with paternal UPD(7).

Chromosome 8. More than 25 cases of UPD(8) have been reported. UPD(8)pat is apparently without any phenotypic effect, and one may suppose that this reflects a lack of imprinted genes on this chromosome. Yu et al. (2022) diagnosed a fetus with paternal UPD(8) after an NIPT result showing high probability of trisomy 8. The pregnancy continued after amniocentesis showed paternal UPD(8) with a normal karyotype, and the resultant child was healthy at three-year follow-up. Benlian et al. (1996) had made the fortuitous discovery in an otherwise normal child with lipoprotein lipase deficiency, a

[12] Microdeletions of 7q32.2 on the paternal allele involving *MEST* also cause a Silver-Russell syndrome-like phenotype (Vincent et al. 2022).

recessive condition for which the locus maps to 8p22. Karanjawala et al. (2000) discovered maternal isodisomy 8 by chance in a man participating in a research study.

Chromosome 9. UPD(9) has been reported in over 15 cases, most ascertained through the diagnosis of recessive diseases. Maternal UPD(9) itself appears to be without effect, as evidenced by its identification in a healthy woman who presented with recurrent miscarriage and was found to have a karyotype 46,XX,i(9)(p10),i(9)(q10) (Björck et al. 1999). Homozygosity due to upid(9) at these loci has been reported in children with the corresponding recessive disease: *SURF-1* with Leigh syndrome, and *FOXE* with syndromic congenital hypothyroidism (Tiranti et al. 1999; Castanet et al. 2010).

Chromosome 10. A little over 10 cases of UPD(10) are on record. Maternal UPD(10) appears to be without effect of itself, and it is only pathogenic when a recessive disease is unmasked, the latter including familial lymphophagocytic histiocytosis and mitochondrial DNA depletion syndrome (Jones et al. 1995; Al-Jasmi et al. 2008; Nogueira et al. 2013). Jones et al. (1995) detected uphd(10)mat in a healthy 8-month-old infant ascertained after the prenatal diagnosis of confined placental mosaicism for trisomy 10. In one case of uphd(10)mat with concomitant trisomy 10 mosaicism, it was presumably the trisomy rather than the UPD that caused a severe phenotype (Hahnemann et al. 2005).

Chromosome 11. There are growth regulation loci in 11p15 that are expressed monoallelically according to the parent of origin of the allele (Figure 19–9). These include the paternally expressed genes *IGF2* and *KCNQ1OT1*, and the maternally expressed genes *H19* and *CDKN1C*. *IGF2* and *H19* are located within one of two "differentially methylated regions"[13] (DMR1), such that *IGF2* is only expressed from the paternal allele and *H19* only from the maternal allele. Similarly, *KCNQ1OT1* (paternal expression) and *CDKN1C* (maternal expression) are under the control of the second region, DMR2 (Manipalviratn et al. 2009; Weksberg et al. 2010). Perturbation of these regions and genes can lead to two syndromes of opposite growth disorder: BWS, of which overgrowth and hemi*hyper*plasia are characteristic, and SRS, in which growth retardation and hemi*hypo*plasia are key features. UPD(11), either segmental or for the whole chromosome, has been reported only in a mosaic form.

Beckwith-Wiedemann Syndrome. In BWS, the striking clinical picture is that of overgrowth of tissues and organs. Mosaic segmental UPD(11p15)pat is the basis of ~20% of sporadically occurring BWS. Thus, in UPD(11p)pat, *IGF2* and *KCNQ1OT1* are expressed biallelically, and *H19* and *CDKN1C* are silenced ("nulliallelic"). That BWS patients with paternal UPD always show mosaicism[14] indicates a mitotic origin and suggests that non-mosaic paternal UPD(11) is an embryonic lethal. Brioude et al. (2018) provide an international consensus statement outlining an approach to clinical and molecular diagnosis of BWS, along with tumor surveillance targeted by molecular subgroup. BWS due to 11p15 epimutation, affecting in particular the DMR2, has a particular association with in vitro fertilization (IVF) (Amor and Halliday 2008; Carli et al. 2022).

The UPD(11p) subtype of BWS (UPD for the whole 11 short arm) carries a high risk of Wilms tumor and hepatoblastoma, and smaller risk of exomphalos (Brioude et al.

[13] There is a multiplicity of nomenclature of these regions. DMR1 and DMR2 may be referred to as Imprinting Control Regions 1 and 2, ICR1 and ICR2, or simply as Imprinting Centre 1 and 2, IC1 and IC2. DMR1 is also known as H19 DMR, and the telomeric cluster; and DMR2 is also known as KvDMR1, KCNQ1OT1 DMR, LIT1 DMR, and the centromeric cluster.

[14] Using diagnostic SNP array, we have detected mosaic segmental UPD(11p)pat in individuals with no clinical features of BWS. We presume that in these cases the mosaic UPD(11p) is restricted to tissues that do not contribute to the BWS phenotype.

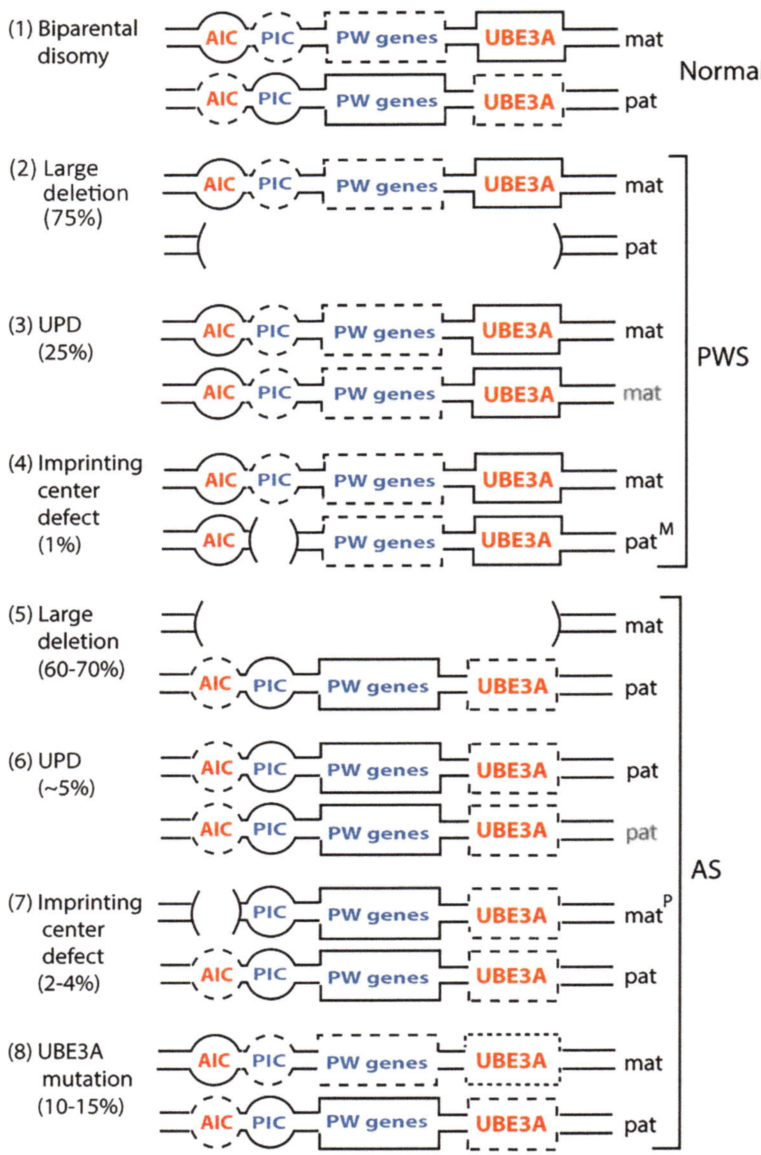

Figure 19–13. An outline of the different genetic forms of Prader-Willi syndrome (PWS) and Angelman syndrome (AS).

Notes: The PWS/AS critical region of chromosome 15 is depicted. A bipartite imprinting center with AS and PWS components (AIC and PIC) controls, in *cis*, the activity of a set of PWS genes and the *UBE3A* gene. A switched-on IC and an actively functioning gene are shown in unbroken line; a switched-off IC and an inactivated gene are shown in dashed outline. A mutated *UBE3A* gene is shown starred and with a dotted outline. (1) Normally, the *UBE3A* gene is transcribed only from the maternal chromosome (mat), and the PWS genes only from the paternal chromosome (pat), with each chromosome thus functioning appropriately for its parent of origin. In PWS there is nonfunctioning of the PWS genes because: (2) the PWS genes have been removed by a typical large deletion from the paternal chromosome; (3) both chromosomes are of maternal origin; (4) a microdeletion of, or mutation in, the PIC has fixed a maternal imprint status on the paternal chromosome. In AS there is nonfunctioning of the *UBE3A* gene because: (5) the *UBE3A* gene has been removed by a typical large deletion from the maternal chromosome; (6) both chromosomes are of paternal origin; (7) a microdeletion of, or mutation in, the AIC has fixed a paternal imprint status on the maternal chromosome; (8) there is a mutation in the *UBE3A* gene on the maternal chromosome. A further category (9) is not shown, comprising the 10%–15% in which no genetic defect can be shown. Approximate percentages of each PWS/AS category are indicated; in another ~10% of AS, no genetic defect can be identified. pat^{M}, a maternally functioning chromosome of paternal origin; mat^{P}, a paternally functioning chromosome of maternal origin.

Table 19–3. Categories of Prader-Willi and Angelman Syndromes

		DELETION ON MICROARRAY	LOH ON SNP MICROARRAY	METHYLATION PATTERN OF NO. 15s	PARENTAL ORIGINS OF NO. 15s	*UBE3A* GENE
Prader-Willi syndrome	Classical deletion	+	+	Mat	Bi	
	UPD(15)mat	N	±	Mat	Mat	
	Imprinting defect	N	N	Mat	Bi	
	Imprinting center microdeletion*	N	N	Mat	Bi	
Angelman syndrome	Classical deletion	+	+	Pat	Bi	Deleted
	UPD(15)pat	N	±	Pat	Pat	Intact
	Imprinting defect	N	N	Pat	Bi	Intact
	Imprinting center microdeletion*	N	N	Pat	Bi	Intact
	UBE3A variant	N	N	Bi	Bi	Mutated

Notes: The assessment of genetic category of Prader-Willi and Angelman syndromes according to results of molecular testing.
*Detection of imprinting center microdeletion requires specialized testing, most commonly the methylation-sensitive multiplex ligation-dependent probe amplification (MS-MLPA) kit from MRC Holland.

LOH = loss of heterozygosity. A normal chromosome microarray result is indicated by N, an abnormal result by +. An inconsistent result is shown as ± (LOH will be seen in all UPD due to meiosis II error or UPD of post-zygotic origin, but will only be seen in UPD due to meiosis I error when there has also been recombination). Bi = biparental; Mat = maternal; Pat = paternal. "Intact" means that the DNA sequence of the gene is normal, but its function is epigenetically compromised.

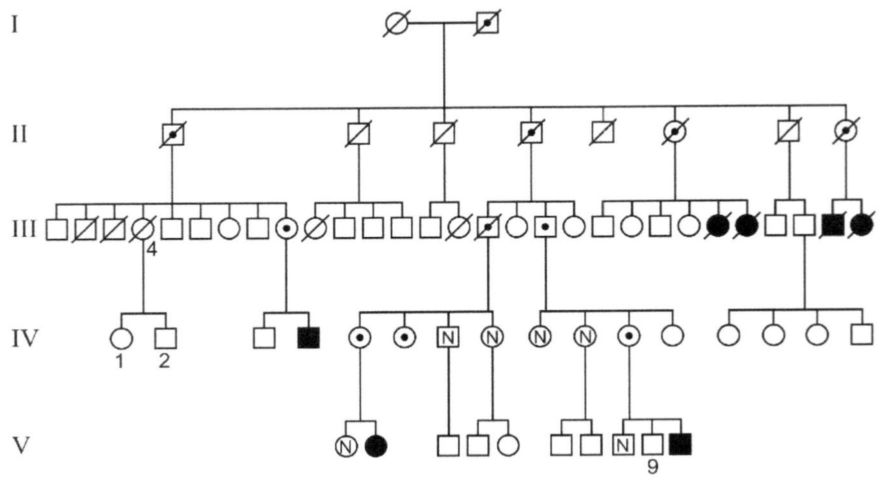

Figure 19–14. Familial Angelman Syndrome.

Notes: A family with inherited Angelman syndrome, due to a *UBE3A* mutation, reported in Moncla et al. (1999). Filled symbol, Angelman syndrome; bull's-eye symbol, mutation carrier, demonstrated or inferred; N, demonstrated noncarrier. Note that all the affected children are born to carrier *mothers*, but that these mothers are related to each other through the *male* line. Some normal children have been proven to be noncarriers with molecular testing (N in symbol), but the reader can also determine that any unaffected child of a potential carrier mother, such as IV:1 and 2, the children of III:4, or V:9, the sibling of an affected child, cannot be carriers. An inherited imprinting center mutation could present a similar pedigree.

Angelman Syndrome with No Deletion, No Uniparental Disomy, No Imprinting Defect, and No UBE3A Variant. In some 10%–15% of AS, no genetic defect can be found (Beygo et al. 2019). There is a normal karyotype with no deletion demonstrable on FISH, normal methylation analysis (at least on the sampled tissues), biparental inheritance, and an apparently intact *UBE3A* gene. There may be an epigenetic influence whereby a normal *UBE3A* gene on the maternal chromosome fails to activate normally during embryogenesis. Or there may be some other AS genetic basis, as yet unknown.

Chromosome 16. This is one of the more commonly seen UPDs, and it is almost always due to correction of trisomy 16 of maternal meiotic origin. Thus, it is typically a *maternal* UPHD or UPHID. It has been difficult to separate out the effects of the UPD and of a placental insufficiency due to confined placental mosaicism for trisomy 16, this typically being the route by which the UPD comes to be recognized following chorionic villus sampling; and in addition, a possible residual occult fetal trisomy mosaicism always remains as a potential confounder.

Opinions differ. Yong et al. (2003) showed in a large series of mosaic trisomy 16 discovered at prenatal diagnosis that the degree of fetal growth restriction, and probably the malformation rate, was greater in those with UPD(16)mat than in those with biparental inheritance, thus suggesting a role of the UPD per se. Imprinting of the *ZNF597* locus at 16p13.3 has been proposed as a mechanism underpinning some phenotypic features of UPD(16)mat (Yamazawa et al. 2021). Phenotypic overlap with Silver-Russell syndrome may be seen, and Inoue et al. (2019) found two patients with upd(16)mat in a series of 94 patients who met diagnostic criteria for SRS. On the other hand, Scheuvens et al. (2017) suggest that UPD(16)mat is of itself without phenotype, and may serve merely as a biomarker for an underlying trisomy 16 mosaicism. As for *paternal* UPD(16), it seems probable that it has no clinical consequences (Zhang et al. 2021b).

The usual rare risk from isozygosity for a recessive gene applies, as exemplified in Wattanasirichaigoon et al. (2008), who report a child with hydrops fetalis due to hemoglobin Bart's, consequential upon UPD(16)mat. Hamvas et al. (2009) reported three infants with paternal isodisomy 16 resulting in surfactant deficiency due to *ABCA3* mutation, but none of whom exhibited a non-pulmonary phenotype.

Chromosome 17. Several cases of complete UPD(17)mat have been described. One 46,XY child was normal, ascertainment having been via the discovery of trisomy 17 mosaicism at amniocentesis (Genuardi et al. 1999). A recessive etiology was suspected in a girl with developmental delay, microcephaly, and seizures, in whom upd(17)mat was identified by exome sequencing, although no definite causative mutation was found (King et al. 2014). UPD(17)pat has been seen in the setting of a number of the recessive phenotypes. Lebre et al. (2009) identified the UPD in an infant with cystinosis, a recessively inherited multi-organ storage disease, the locus of which is on chromosome 17p and this segment being in isodisomic state in the child. Similarly, Natsuga et al. (2010) and Verebi et al. (2023) have seen cases of junctional epidermolysis bullosa and of limb-girdle muscular dystrophy (the respective genes on no. 17) due to UPD(17)pat.

Chromosome 18. Given the frequency of trisomy 18 at conception, it is surprising that UPD for the entire chromosome 18 is so rare. Paternal UPD(18) has been unmasked through the diagnoses of autosomal recessive deafness due to *LOXHD1* variants (Morgan et al. 2018) and Dyggve-Melchior-Clausen syndrome, a rare recessive syndrome of skeletal dysplasia and intellectual disability (López-Garrido et al. 2022). Kariminejad et al. (2011) present an extraordinary example of segmental maternal UPD of 18p and segmental paternal UPD of 18q in a girl whose consanguineous parents both carried a pericentric inversion inv(18)(p11.31q21.33). The healthy child received two recombinant chromosomes 18—from the mother a derivative chromosome 18 with dup(18p)/del(18q), and from the father a derivative chromosome 18 with dup(18q)/del(18p).

Chromosome 19. It took until 2018 for the first cases of UPD(19) to be identified. Paternal isodisomy for chromosome 19 was reported in a pair of monochorionic diamniotic twins who presented with dysmorphic feature, hypotonia, and global developmental delay (Yeung et al. 2018). Loss of imprinting for known imprinted genes on chromosome 19 was detected, and this was the probable cause of the phenotype. The second report of UPD(19)pat was a 17-month-old boy in whom upid(19)pat was detected after he had presented with a homozygous variant in the gene *EXOSC5*, leading to an autosomal recessive disorder of cerebellar ataxia brain abnormalities and cardiac conduction defects (Slavotinek et al. 2020). Apart from developmental delay, his phenotype was not a strong match for the twins described by Yeung et al., and the possible delineation of a UPD(19) syndrome will require the ascertainment of additional cases. UPD(19)mat is yet to be reported, with or without a phenotype.

Chromosome 20. Eggermann et al. (2001) reviewed three reported cases of UPD(20), one paternal and two maternal, with a major malformation phenotype in the former and growth retardation the common observation in the latter two. But it took until 2016 for *maternal* UPD(20) to be confirmed as a bona fide imprinting syndrome, following the diagnosis of eight new cases due in large part to improved ascertainment via SNP microarray (Mulchandani et al. 2016). The condition has since been referred to as Mulchandani-Bhoj-Conlin syndrome. There is phenotypic overlap with Silver-Russell syndrome, and UPD(20)mat has been detected in about 0.2% of children referred for SRS molecular testing (Hjortshøj et al. 2020; Mackay et al. 2022). Neverthelss, Hjortshøj and colleagues note that while individuals with UPD(20)mat share with SRS the features of pre- and post-natal growth retardation and prominent feeding difficulties, they do not fulfill the consensus SRS criteria. Dysmorphic features are common but without consistent pattern, and hypotonia and developmental delay are present in about half of cases. The predominant mechanism is trisomy rescue after maternal meiosis II nondisjunction.

Pseudohypoparathyroidism type 1b (PHP1b) is caused by imprinting defects in *GNAS*, which, in certain tissues such as renal proximal tubules, is predominantly expressed from the maternal allele. Hence, symptoms of PHP1b would be expected to accompany *paternal* UPD(20), and indeed ~20%[23] of patients with sporadic PHP1b have UPD(20)pat, either involving the whole chromosome, or more commonly as a segmental mitotic error (Fernández-Rebollo et al. 2010; Bastepe et al. 2011). Colson et al. (2019) suggest that early-onset obesity, resolving after six years, may be an additional UPD(20)pat feature. More commonly, PHP1b follows an autosomal dominant pattern of inheritance, and these cases are caused by deletions that disrupt imprinting the *GNAS* DMRs on the maternal allele.

Chromosome 21. UPD(21), maternal and paternal, have been ascertained in healthy individuals and appears to be without effect (Engel and Antonarakis 2002). Both UPDs have been described in individuals with a der(21;21)(q10;q10).

Chromosome 22. More than 25 cases of UPD(22) have been reported, in most cases unmasking autosomal recessive diseases. Maternal UPD(22) has generally not, of itself, been causally associated with any defect (Kotzot 1999; Engel and Antonarakis 2002). Intrauterine growth retardation, if present, may more likely reflect the influence of a trisomic 22 placenta or low-level "occult" mosaicism of the fetus (Balmer et al. 1999; Bryan et al. 2002). A der(22;22)(q10;10q) has been reported in association with both maternal and paternal UPD(22), typically having presented with recurrent miscarriage in otherwise healthy individuals (Liehr et al. 2025a), and Ouldim et al. (2008) report the unexpected transmission of a der(22;22)(q10;10q) from a father to (normal) son (and see p. 208). An instance of homozygosity for a *PLA2G6* mutation, leading to neurodegeneration with brain iron accumulation in monozygous twins from an IVF conception, was due to paternal UPD(22) (Tello et al. 2017).

Chromosome X. Neither UPD(X)mat nor UPD(X)pat appears to have any consequence in the 46,XX person, with the usual exception of homozygosity for a recessive mutation. An example is a 3-year-old girl with a typical fragile X phenotype, homozygous for a fully expanded *FMR1* allele (288 CGG repeats) due to maternal UPID of the X chromosome, her mother carrying a pre-mutation allele (Kim et al. 2020). However, there may be a subtly different neuropsychological phenotype according to the parent of origin in monosomy X (self-evidently a uniparental condition). In a British study, 80 girls with Turner syndrome underwent behavioral evaluation, 55 of whom were $45,X^{M}$ and 25 were $45,X^{P}$. The $45,X^{P}$ girls were more socially adept and more articulate than the $45,X^{M}$ girls. Speculatively, this may represent the effect of an imprintable X-borne "locus for social cognition" that is functional on the X chromosome transmitted from a father, and nonfunctional on the X from a mother (Skuse et al. 1997). Autism, which is a male-susceptible condition, is associated with $45,X^{M}$ in the case of autistic girls with Turner

[23] The other 80% of cases of sporadic PHP1b have a *GNAS* methylation defect without underlying genetic cause (epimutation).

syndrome (Donnelly et al. 2000). In terms of response to growth hormone, it makes no difference whether the child is 45,X^M or 45,X^P (Tsezou et al. 1999).

UPD(X)pat offers the intriguing scenario of father-to-son transmission of an X-linked gene. A 24,XY gamete from a hemizygous father could produce a 47,XXY zygote, which could subsequently lose the maternally contributed X; or the ovum could be nullisomic X, with sex chromosomal complementation producing 46,XY. Either mechanism could explain the observations in a family with the X-linked form of ectodermal dysplasia, as presented in Ferrier et al. (2009).

Chromosome Y. Self-evidently, all karyotypes 47,XYY are UPD(Y)pat.

UNIPARENTAL DISOMY FOR THE ENTIRE CHROMOSOMAL COMPLEMENT

Non-mosaic paternal uniparental disomy (UPDpat) for the full diploid complement—all 46 chromosomes are of paternal origin—produces the placental disorder of complete hydatidiform mole. When, in addition to a double set of paternally derived chromosomes, there is also a haploid maternal set (triploidy, with a total chromosome count of 69), a partial hydatidiform mole results. Hydatidiform mole is discussed in more detail in Chapter 20.

Complete UPDmat of an oöcyte following failure of a premeiotic or of a meiotic cell division leads to benign cystic ovarian teratoma, an unusual tumor of the ovary in which several embryonic tissues may be represented (Miura et al. 1999).

Mosaicism for Genome-Wide Uniparental Disomy. Abnormal cytogenetic events around the time of fertilization—such as two sperm entering an ovum to produce a zygote with three pronuclei, or an ovum undergoing a mitosis and then cell lines of different (but diploid) genetic constitution being produced—can be the basis of a mosaicism for genome-wide UPD. This can be UPDmat/biparental or UPDpat/biparental mosaicism, and it may be confined to the placenta or also involve the fetus.

Complete UPDpat/normal mosaicism in the placenta (androgenetic/biparental mosaicism) leads to the histological phenotype of mesenchymal dysplasia (p. 673). If the UPDpat line also involves the fetus, a complex clinical picture may be observed, comprising features of different paternal UPD syndromes such as BWS, AS, and transient neonatal diabetes. About 20 such cases have been reported (Jawahir-Schönauer et al. 2022). Malignant and nonmalignant cystic lesions, and a cystic placenta, are frequently present (Inbar-Feigenberg et al. 2013; Christesen et al. 2020); and there is the additional possibility of unmasking an autosomal recessive disease carried by the father (Ohtsuka et al. 2015). The *tout ensemble* of observation presumably reflects the cellular distribution of the UPD tissue. Darcy et al. (2015) reported a 6-month-old girl who was mosaic for a complete UPDpat cell line and a Down syndrome cell line, her phenotype comprising features of both conditions. Complete UPDmat/normal mosaicism is very rare, with only three cases reported (Bens et al. 2017). A consistent phenotype is yet to emerge, but might be expected to comprise mixed features of SRS, Temple syndrome, PWS, and UPD(20)mat syndrome.

Two unique cases cast light on how aberrant chromosomal behavior in the perizygotic period can lead to UPD-related pathology. A 46,XX/46,XY male child described in

2005), and so non-demonstration (on blood) of the mutation in the mother does not necessarily exclude a genetic risk. It may be appropriate to track the mutation through the patrilineal family in order to be able to offer genetic counseling to female cousins who might be carriers. The reader should study the illustrative pedigree in Figure 19–14.

No Genetic Defect Demonstrable. In a small fraction of AS, ~10%, no cytogenetic or molecular defect, nor *UBE3A* mutation, is demonstrable. Most of these cases will be phenocopies, and an alternative diagnosis should be sought; but some could conceivably reflect a mutation that has not been able to be detected. The family history, if positive, may compel the assumption of a mutation and thus imply a high recurrence risk. A negative family history might support the inference of a low risk, but it would not allow a definite assumption. If a normal sibling carried the same 15q11q13 haplotype on molecular study, a low-risk scenario would be probable. Expert advice should be sought.

Uncommon Cytogenetically Detectable Rearrangement. The nature of the rearrangement, and the parental karyotypes, will determine the recurrence risk in each type. The rare circumstance of UPD associated with a parental Robertsonian translocation is noted on p. 213.

A Simplification for Angelman Syndrome

Some parents will not find it easy to come to grips with these various possible causes for their child's condition even if, in the end, they need only consider the category that applies to themselves. It may be helpful to discuss AS, and the risks of recurrence, in the following terms.[26] Let us say that AS is due simply to a lack of the UBE3A protein, a very important protein that is necessary for the brain to grow normally. The gene for *UBE3A* works only on the chromosome 15 from the mother, while the gene on the father's chromosome is dormant. There is a switch on the mother's chromosome that makes this gene work.

- If the bit of the maternal chromosome that contains this gene is missing (deletion), or if the mother's chromosome is replaced by another one from the father (UPD), no UBE3A protein can be made. These two types happen as one-off events.
- If the switch fails on the mother's chromosome, then the gene remains dormant and no protein is made (imprinting center fault). This type can happen one-off, as though the switch "gets stuck" for reasons that we do not well understand. Or, there may be a genetic fault in the actual switch, and in this case the defect could be passed to a subsequent child.
- If the *UBE3A* gene itself is faulty on the mother's chromosome (mutation), no protein is made, or only an abnormal protein that cannot function. The genetic risk depends on whether the faulty gene started with the child (no increased risk) or if the mother is a carrier (high risk). Note that the mother can be a carrier and still be perfectly normal, since the faulty gene would be the one she got from her father, and so in any event it would have been switched off.
- Sometimes the *UBE3A* gene fails to work, even though the maternal chromosome is normal and has a normal switch. We do not know why this happens (there has been a suggestion that one cause *may* be if there had been difficulty achieving the pregnancy, either naturally or with IVF). This type is a one-off event.

[26] See also the *European Journal of Human Genetics* Clinical Utility Card (Buiting et al. 2015).

A common question parents have is whether their normal children might, in the next generation, have an AS child. Or the aunts and uncles of an AS child might want advice about risks to their future children or to their grandchildren. The answers are as follows:

- The normal siblings of an AS child have no increased risk for any genetic category, with the possible exception of a familial translocation. Even if the AS child has (or had) a potentially heritable type of *UBE3A* genetic defect, the fact that the sibs themselves are normal self-evidently declares that they cannot have received it. If they had got the abnormal gene, they would have AS; since they do not have AS, they cannot have the gene. The sex of the siblings is immaterial.
- Aunts and uncles have an increased risk for children or grandchildren of theirs only if a heritable type of AS is involved (imprinting center defect, *UBE3A* mutation). In that case, an uncle could be a carrier, but his children would not be at risk, since the *UBE3A* gene would be dormant anyway. Daughters of his, however, could have an AS child. A carrier aunt would have a high risk (50%) to have an AS child. But her grandchildren, through her normal sons and daughters, would have no increased risk. Her normal children would have declared themselves, by their very normality, not to have inherited the genetic defect.

Uniparental Disomy for the Entire Chromosomal Complement

UPD for the entire *paternal* chromosome set (hydatidiform mole) is associated with an increased recurrence risk; this is discussed in detail in Chapter 20. There is no discernibly increased risk for the recurrence of UPD for the entire *maternal* chromosome set (ovarian teratoma).

Diagnostic Testing for Uniparental Disomy

Guidelines from the American College of Genetics and Genomics summarize the indications for diagnostic testing for UPD (Del Gaudio et al. 2020; Table 19–5). SNP microarray is the mainstay. Much UPD (between 50% and 100%, depending on origin of UPD) is detectable by microarray of the index case via the detection of homozygosity. However, a normal SNP in an individual cannot detect UPD originating in meiosis I when there has been no meiotic recombination—these cases can only be detected using patient-parent trios. UPD can also be detected using data from exome or genome sequencing (Yauy et al. 2020; Dong et al. 2021).

As for prenatal diagnosis, two scenarios warrant specific mention. First, a small risk[27] of UPD applies for non-Robertsonian translocations if one or both chromosomes carry imprinted genes, specifically when there is a risk of 3:1 nondisjunction and where trisomy or monosomy rescue or gamete complementation could occur. Reports of this (very rare) occurrence are listed in Table 19–6.

[27] Using data from UPD risk in the setting of Robertsonian translocations (Moradkhani et al. 2019) and data showing segregation in PGT embryos (Zhang et al. 2018; Jia et al. 2023) we estimate this risk to be approximately 1 in 5,000.

20
REPRODUCTIVE FAILURE

HUMAN CONCEPTION and pregnancy is both a vulnerable and a robust process. Vulnerable in that a remarkably large proportion of all conceptions are chromosomally abnormal, with the great majority of such pregnancies aborting.[1] Robust in that ~99% of the time, a term pregnancy results in a chromosomally normal baby; unbalanced chromosomal abnormalities are seen in only ~1% of newborns (Table 1–2). But the cost to society of chromosomally abnormal conceptions is not horrendous; it is measured largely in terms of miscarriage, seen or unseen. The occasional chromosomally abnormal child is, relatively speaking, an exceptional outcome—the tip of an iceberg (Figure 20–1).

Much of this chromosomal vulnerability lies in the process of producing sperm, and in particular, eggs. Meiosis hangs, literally and figuratively, upon "tender filaments,"[2] and often the meiotic chromosomes are incorrectly distributed to the daughter cells. The small group who are exceptionally likely to produce abnormal gametes are carriers of balanced chromosome rearrangements, and much of this book is devoted to that fact.

"Reproductive failure" is an all-encompassing term and includes infertility, subfertility, infecundity and sterility, along with pregnancy loss, miscarriage, spontaneous abortion, blighted ovum, implantation failure, and perinatal death. Reproductive failure may be primary (no successful pregnancies) or secondary (previous pregnancy success). The language in this setting is not always as precise as one might wish (Gurunath et al. 2011). The terms *infertility*, *infecundity*, and *sterility*[3] are sometimes used more or less interchangeably. The duration in terms of years, before lack of success in "trying for a baby" can be called *infertility*, has been variably defined. Estimates of the prevalence of infertility, at least in the latter 20th century among women in the fertile age group, have varied quite widely from 4% to 14%, and the lifetime prevalence from 13% to 33% (Schmidt and Münster 1995); a global decline in fertility is discussed in Aitken (2024). We will bypass these controversies and confine ourselves to making the distinction between the following:

1. reproductive failure operating at the level of the gamete, with failure to conceive;
2. reproductive failure when an embryo from in vitro fertilization (IVF) does not implant in the uterus;

[1] Dorothy Warburton suggested that this error rate conveyed an evolutionary advantage in former times: Miscarriage due to aneuploidy led to a wider spacing of offspring, allowing a woman to devote scarce resources to a more manageable number of children, more of whom would survive to contribute their genes to the following generation. What was beneficial in a prehistoric society has been quite the opposite for many women, now hostage to their biology in the present century (a concept not without several other examples).

[2] "I that have examined the parts of man, and know upon what tender filaments that fabric hangs." –Thos. Browne MD, *Religio Medici*, 1642.

[3] Broadly speaking, "fecundity" is the biological capacity for reproduction, while "fertility" is the actual production of offspring (Davies et al. 2005). Thus, some see fecundity as referring to the capacity to achieve a conception and fertility as the capacity to carry this through to childbirth. "Sterility" may carry, for some, an implication of irreversibility.

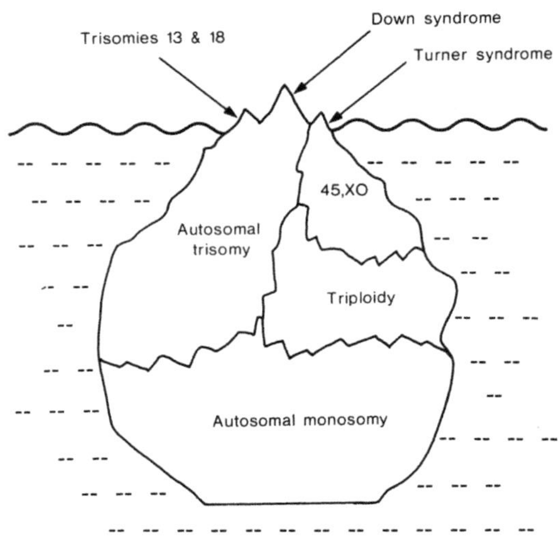

Figure 20–1. The Iceberg of Chromosomal Pregnancy Loss.

3. reproductive failure following the natural loss, by miscarriage, of a confirmed pregnancy; and
4. reproductive failure due to fetal death in later pregnancy.

BIOLOGY

Embryology

A knowledge of embryology underpins an understanding of certain processes of chromosomal pathology, and the counselor should be familiar with some basic terms. While not every detail of anatomy of the embryo is requisite knowledge, it is a minimum requirement to appreciate the different roles of the inner cell mass/embryoblast, and of trophoblast/chorionic villi, in their separate paths of development giving rise to the embryo proper and to the placenta, respectively. The counselor should understand the evolution of gametes → zygote → cleavage-stage embryo → morula → blastocyst → embryo → fetus, according to the following broad stages and as illustrated in Figures 20–2 and 20–3.[4]

- The *zygote* is the cell that arises from fertilization of an egg by a sperm, and this cell can be called a *conceptus* ("that which is conceived"). This cell then undergoes a series of cell divisions, and this cell mass, by day 2–3, is the *cleavage-stage embryo*; the expression conceptus can continue to be applied. The bunch of cells at day 4 is a *morula*.

[4] Strictly speaking, in utero life is divided into three periods: *pre-embryonic* (the first 2 weeks after conception), up to formation of the primitive streak; *embryonic* (to the end of the 8th week) when the body forms and organs are largely constructed; and *fetal* (from 8 weeks to term), characterized by growth and changes in proportion rather than the appearance of new features. In clinical and everyday parlance, pregnancy timing is dated from the last menstrual period, and so, with conception usually happening mid-cycle, the first 2 weeks of a 40-week pregnancy are "non-pregnant," and a normal pregnancy is really only of 8½ months.

- At days 5 to 12 post-conception, the conceptus is a *blastocyst*. The "cyst" in that name refers to the fluid-filled cavity within a sphere of cells (Figure 20–2 left, Day 6), this outer layer of cells comprising the *trophoblast*,[5] which will eventually develop into *chorionic villi*, forming the placenta. A group of cells within the cyst, attached to the inner surface of the sphere, is the *inner cell mass/embryoblast*, and it is from these cells that the actual embryo will arise. During about day 7, *implantation* occurs: that is, the attachment of the conceptus to the lining of the uterus.
- After implantation, the embryonic tissue types (ectoderm, endoderm, mesoderm) differentiate from the epiblast (Figure 20–2 *right*, Germ layers), and then the basic body and organ formation is laid down, through to the 8-week mark.
- From 8 weeks to birth is the fetal stage.

Gametic Cytogenetics

The logical starting point in an assessment of fertility is the gamete, and from a chromosomal point of view it is the process of meiosis, the final act of gametogenesis, to which we address our main focus. Many more sperm are made than eggs, by orders of magnitude, and one might have expected a higher standard of meiotic fidelity in the scarcer gamete (Hunt and Hassold 2002); but in fact, it is the other way round, and so it is the egg that commands most of our attention in terms of the practical relevance of gametic chromosomal pathology.

OÖCYTES AND POLAR BODIES

In vitro fertilization (IVF) is widely applied in the management of infertility, and one consequential benefit of this has been the access afforded to study of the oöcyte and its minor partner, the polar body. Many eggs sampled at IVF prove to be surplus to the requirements of the couple, and they are often willingly donated for research. Several studies addressing the chromosomal status of oöcytes of 46,XX women have shown that a remarkably substantial fraction of these gametes are aneuploid, and the rate is markedly related to the woman's age (Samura et al. 2023). Comparing euploidy rates to age gives an inverted U-shaped curve, with aneuploidies seen more in the very young and in older women, and euploidy peaking at 75% in the late 20s (Figure 20–4). In women in their mid-30s, about a half of eggs are disomic or nullisomic, whereas by around age 40 the fraction rises to a remarkable three-quarters, and with an astonishing high of up to 90% in the mid-40s. These rates are influenced by the woman's ovarian reserve, as measured by the anti-Müllerian hormone levels: the higher the level, the better the odds for euploidy (La Marca et al. 2022).

The typical frequencies of aneuploidies per individual chromosome in the eggs of women of older childbearing age[6] are depicted in Figure 20–5. It is the smaller chromosomes that are the more vulnerable to error, as the tail to the right of the graph attests. In the data of Tschare et al. (2023), analyzing oöcytes from women of age range 25 to 42, the chromosomes most often seen in aneuploid state were, by a substantial margin, numbers 15, 16, 21, and 22. The molecular basis of the maternal age link—and knowing

[5] This is also the tissue—*trophectoderm*—that is taken at the time of preimplantation genetic testing (PGT) biopsy, typically on day 5–6.

[6] Older women are more likely to seek IVF, and so this is where most data have come from.

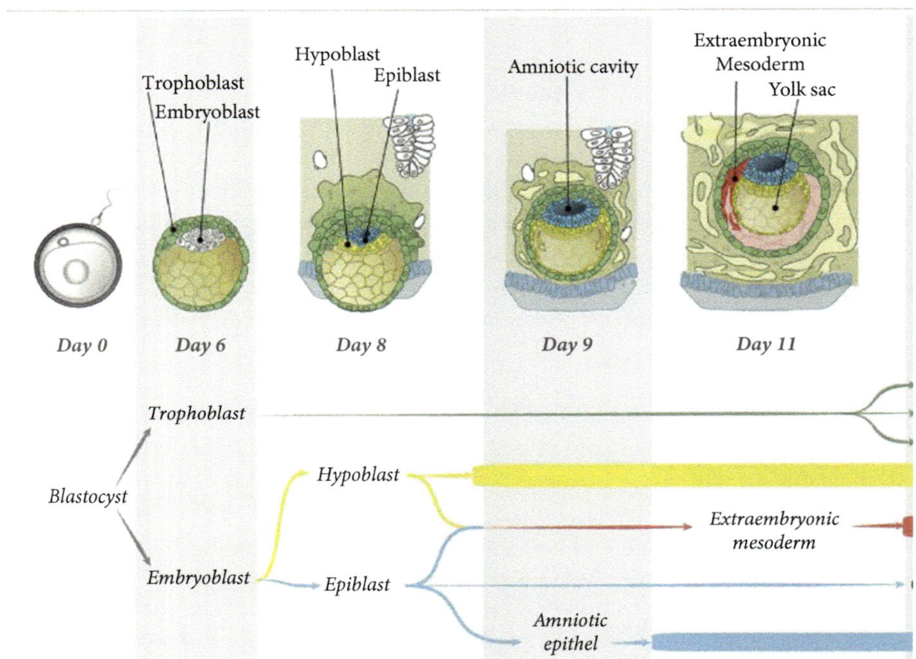

Figure 20–2. The timeline of embryogenesis, and the development of the different tissues.

Note: "Embryoblast" (day 6) is synonymous with Inner Cell Mass, and these cells will give rise to the actual embryo. The unlabeled black and white cells shown at days 8 and 9 (upper right in each panel) represent decidua placentalis.

Source: From R Essers et al., Prevalence of chromosomal alterations in first-trimester spontaneous pregnancy loss, *Nat Med* 29:3233–3242, 2023. Courtesy A Salumets and MZ Esteki, and with the permission of Nature Medicine.

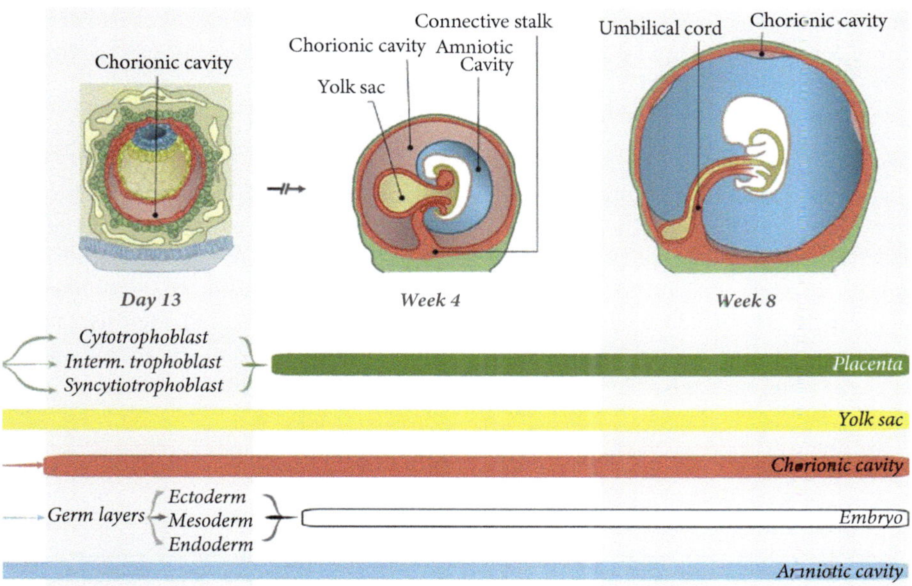

Figure 20–2. Continued.

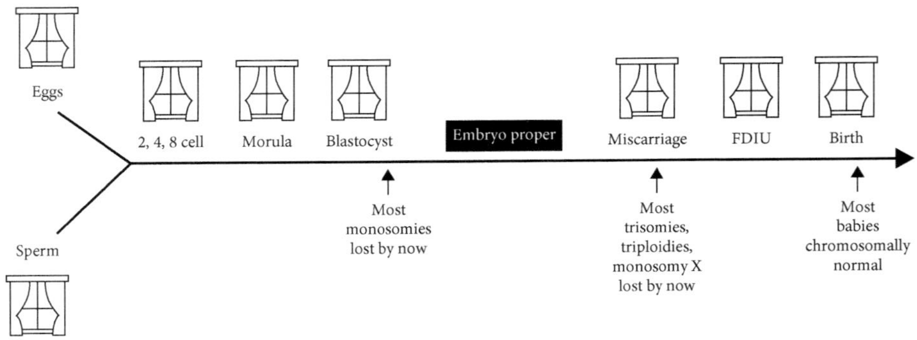

Figure 20–3. The windows of observation available to the researcher, along the timeline of chromosomal interest from gametes to child. Only the 3-8 week embryonic period remains substantially unstudied.

Note: Evidently, time on the *x* axis is depicted asymmetrically. FDIU, fetal death in utero.

that the first meiotic division remains in a "holding pattern" for decades, from birth to ovulation—may lie in a vulnerability of, inter alia, the aging kinetochore and the spindle mechanism (Zielinska et al. 2019; Mikwar et al. 2020). This is strikingly illustrated in the work of Battaglia et al. (1996): their images of oöcytes show how the structural integrity of the meiotic apparatus declines as a woman gets older (Figure 20–6). Meiosis is under genetic control, and ~20 known Mendelian conditions are associated with mutation in relevant genes that cause oöcyte maturation arrest (Sang et al., 2021; Zhang et al. 2022; Zhang et al. 2024b; Lin et al. 2025).

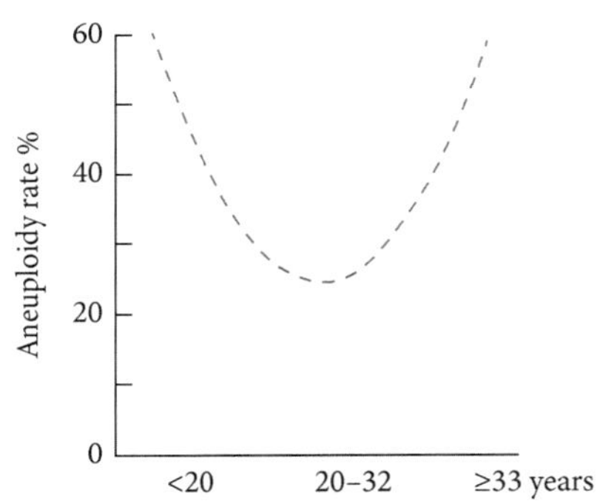

Figure 20–4. Aneuploidy Rates in Oöcytes by Age.

Note: These data were derived from ovarian tissue taken from girls and women at the time of "fertility-insurance" storage, ahead of their undergoing potentially damaging chemotherapy; and from eggs donated from patients attending an IVF clinic. Note that the best chance for euploidy is seen in the late twenties. See also Figure 13-10 for more detail.

Source: Adapted from JR Gruhn and ER Hoffman, Errors of the egg: The establishment and progression of human aneuploidy research in the maternal germline, *Annu Rev Genet* 56:369–390, 2022. Courtesy ER Hoffmann, and with the permission of Annual Reviews.

SPERM

The gamete whose chromosomes are more readily accessible to analysis is the spermatozöon, and very large numbers can be analyzed. In most men, 1%–2% of sperm are chromosomally imbalanced (Bell et al. 2020) (Figure 20–7). In general, there is no

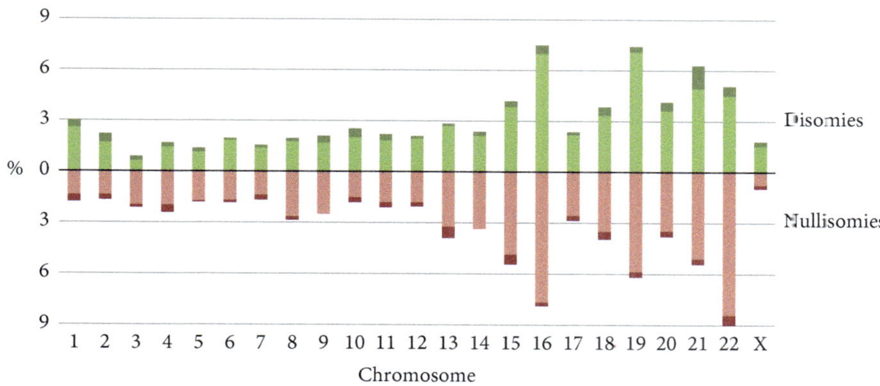

Figure 20–5. Aneuploidies in oöcytes of women of ages 36-40. Disomies per chromosome are shown above the 0% baseline, nullisomies below.

Note: The mirror-like appearance, above and below the line, reflects the agency of meiotic error, with essentially equal likelihoods of the missegregating chromosome going to the egg (for disomy), or to the polar body (for nullisomy); the similar observation of equal numbers of disomies and nullisomies is seen also in Oberle et al. (2024). The smaller chromosomes are the more susceptible to aneuploidy. Light green = chromatid gain, darker green = 2-chromatid chromosome gain; Light red = chromatid loss, darker red = 2-chromatid chromosome loss. These findings are based on inferences from the analysis of the first and second polar bodies in 676 oöcytes, from women undergoing PGT-A (PGT for aneuploidy).

Source: From P Verdyck et al., Aneuploidy in oocytes from women of advanced maternal age: analysis of the causal meiotic errors and impact on embryo development, *Hum Reprod* 38:2526–2535, 2023. Courtesy P Verdyck, and with the permission of Oxford University Press, and the European Society of Human Reproduction and Embryology.

discernible correlation of either full aneuploidy or deletion with paternal age (Bonus et al. 2022; Samarasekera et al. 2023). As with the egg, a number of Mendelian loci are known, mutation at which leads to meiotic arrest and non-obstructive spermatogenic failure (Kasak and Laan 2021; Xie et al. 2022).

It might have been thought that fathers of aneuploid children, in whom the aneuploidy had been of paternal origin, could have represented a group with a particular susceptibility to producing aneuploid sperm, but in fact this appears usually not to be the case (Hixon et al. 1998; Blanco et al. 1998). Nevertheless, at least in the case of *some* fathers of Down syndrome or Turner syndrome children, a propensity to produce aneuploid or disomic sperm has been noted, and it may be that that a minority of normally fertile men are predisposed to meiotic errors at spermatogenesis, whether generalized or restricted to one chromosome (Martin 2008). A case is proposed for chromosome 9 heteromorphism as a susceptibility factor (Mottola et al. 2023), but not supported in Hernandez-Nieto et al. (2021).

Cytogenetics of the Preimplantation and Embryonic Periods

An aneuploid gamete (nullisomic or disomic) will lead to an aneuploid conceptus (monosomic or trisomic). A diploid gamete combining with a normal gamete will give rise to a triploid conceptus. With many oöcytes and some sperm aneuploid, and simplistically supposing equal fertilizing/fertilizable capacity, the expectation is for a very

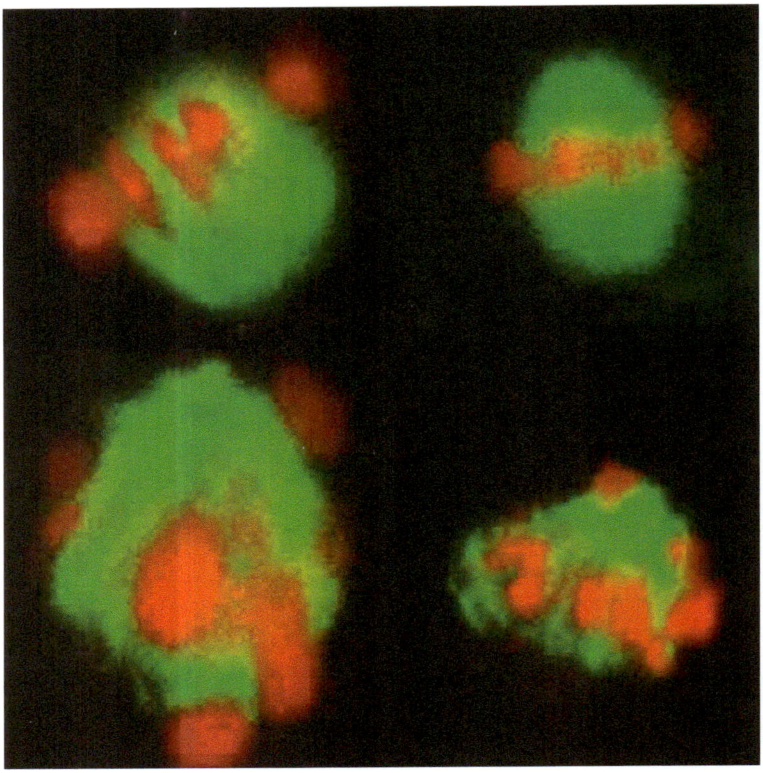

Figure 20–6. Eggs of Younger and Older Women at Meiosis II.

Notes: Shown here is the disposition of the chromosomes at meiosis II in the oöcytes from younger and older women, illustrating what may be the physical basis of the maternal age effect. The microtubules of the spindle stain green, and the chromosomes stain orange. The chromosomes are well organized at the metaphase plate at the equator of the cells in the younger women (the 22-year-old's oöcyte, on the upper left, is viewed on a tilt). In contrast, the 40-year-old's oöcyte shows the chromosomes in disarray. The 42-year-old woman's oöcyte has one chromosome, at the top, dislocated from the metaphase plate, and the disposition of the other chromosomes at the equator is not as regular as in the younger women.

Source: From Battaglia et al., Influence of maternal age on meiotic spindle assembly in oöcytes from naturally cycling women, *Hum Reprod* 11: 2217–2222, 1996. Courtesy DE Battaglia, and with the permission of Oxford University Press, and the European Society of Human Reproduction and Embryology.

considerable fraction of conceptions to be chromosomally unbalanced. On top of this, dispermy (two sperm fertilizing the one ovum) can cause triploidy. An abnormal post-zygotic cell division can give rise to mosaicism, and this is a common happening. These several possibilities all add up to a substantial potential for chromosome abnormality in the very early conceptus, in the first days (even hours) of existence.

NON-IMPLANTATION AND "OCCULT ABORTION"

Although the natural in vivo circumstance might differ from the extrapolated observations in vitro, it is nevertheless a fair assumption that unbeknown, a substantial fraction of all human conceptions have a lethal chromosomal burden and will not implant. Transient implantation may be associated with little or no perturbation of the menstrual cycle, although the woman may fleetingly feel pregnant as a hormonal response is briefly elicited. This is "occult abortion". It becomes a semantic question whether the existence

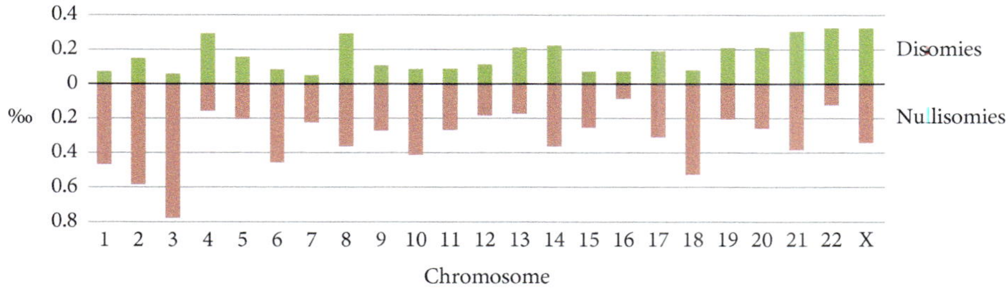

Figure 20–7. The Relative Frequencies of Aneuploidy per Chromosome in Sperm.

Notes: Disomies per chromosome are shown above the 0‰ baseline, nullisomies below. In most sperm, there is a single abnormality; some may have more than one. Overall, around 0.3% of sperm in this study were nullisomic, and 0.2% disomic; this excess of nullisomy over disomy is also seen in other such studies (García-Mengual et al. 2019). Additionally, 0.4% of sperm were diploid. 99% were normal haploid. No readily discernible pattern presents itself (cf. eggs, Figure 20-5 above). Note the orders of magnitude difference in the *y* axis measurements of eggs (Figure 20-5) cf. sperm: the egg data is shown in whole numbers %, vs. the sperm data in fractions ‰ (per thousand). These data are derived from ten normozoöspermic men, from whom near a quarter-million sperm were analyzed.

Source: Drawn from data in Table 3 in S Zhu et al., Comprehensive chromosome FISH assessment of sperm aneuploidy in normozoospermic males, *J Assist Reprod Genet* 39:1887–1900, 2022.

of a non-implanting conceptus could be described as a pregnancy and whether its loss could be considered an abortion.

THE CLEAVAGE EMBRYO ("PRE-EMBRYO") (DAYS 1–3)

In the first three days of existence, the conceptus is a simple sphere, a number of cells contained within an outer shell (the zona pellucida) (Figure 20–8 *a* to *c*). The population background rate of abnormality of the day 1–3 embryo can be assessed in the study of those whose fertility is not in question, namely in couples, one of whom is a heterozygote for an X-linked Mendelian condition, presenting at IVF for PGT for specific mutation testing. Pellicer et al. (1999), assessing some or all of chromosomes 13, 16, 18, 21, 22, X, and Y, studied 16 Mendelian heterozygous women, 10 of whom were of age range 30–36 years and six of 37–41 years. The younger women had a total of 12 chromosomally abnormal embryos out of 62 tested (19%), but a considerably higher figure (46%) was observed in the older mothers. Similar findings, from larger numbers, are due to Rubio et al. (2003; Table 20–1). These FISH-based studies did not include data on the remaining 17 chromosomes and are thus necessarily underestimates, and substantially so, of the total abnormal burden.

The "atypical" group of patients otherwise presenting to the IVF clinic are of course a population of clinical interest, and thus the observations gained from study of them, however unrepresentative they might possibly be of the general population, are very germane to the agenda of the counselor. Demko et al. (2016) studied more than 22,000 day-3 embryos tested using SNP microarray (thus looking at all 24 chromosomes) and found that the proportion of aneuploid embryos remained fairly constant at 65% between maternal ages 24 and 35 years, but increased markedly at older ages. With similar numbers studied, Matorras et al. (2024) observed 86% of day-3 embryos to be aneuploid from mothers of age above 35 years.

Mosaicism of the very early embryo (Figure 20–9) has been one of the more startling discoveries to emerge from the laboratory, and it is fair to imagine a similar picture may apply in vivo. Many IVF embryos are aneuploid or diploid/aneuploid mosaics,

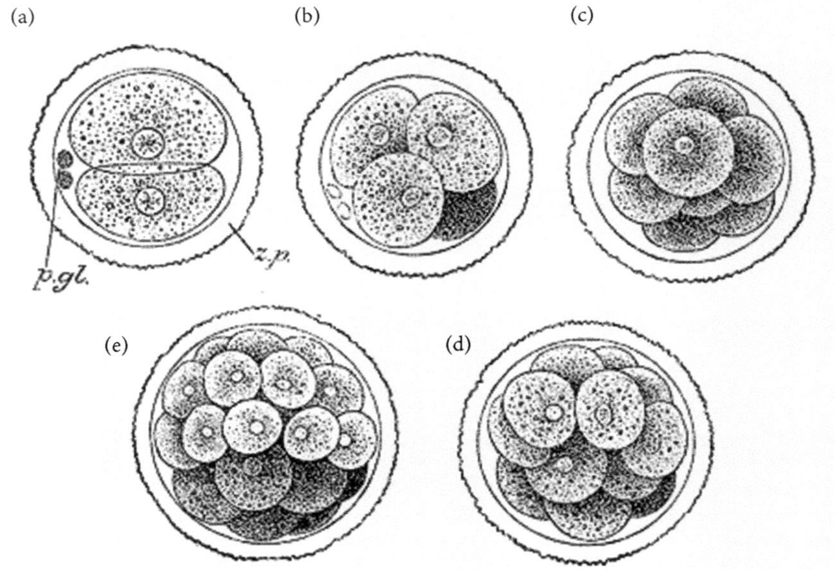

Figure 20–8. The cleavage-stage embryo and morula. Days 1 to 3, *a* to *c*, the 2-cell, 4-cell, and 8-cell cleavage stages. Day 4 to 5, *d* and *e*, morula.
Notes: z.p., zone pellucida; p.gl., polar bodies.
Source: H Gray, Anatomy of the Human Body, 1918.

reflecting the fact that the first few post-zygotic divisions are particularly susceptible to errors in chromosomal distribution[7] (Voullaire et al. 2000b; Currie et al. 2022; McCoy et al. 2023). At younger maternal ages, mosaicism may surpass maternal meiosis as a type of day-3 abnormality (Figure 20–10). The main mechanism may be chromosome loss due to anaphase lag,[8] but chromosome gain is also frequent; mitotic nondisjunction (inferred from observing different cells with the corresponding monosomy and trisomy) occurs in a small minority (Daphnis et al. 2008). When the mosaicism is extensive, exhibiting several different karyotypes, these embryos may be referred to as being chromosomally "chaotic." Blennow et al. (2001), studying embryos from translocation carriers that had been diagnosed as aneuploid on PGT, demonstrated in some that every cell could be different: the absolute maximum mosaicism. However, lesser degrees of mosaicism might not necessarily predestine the embryo to failure, and the aneuploid cells may be "sequestered off" from those that will become the inner cell mass, these being the cells that will give rise to the embryo proper (Liñán et al. 2018; Griffin et al. 2023).

THE MORULA AND BLASTOCYST (DAYS 4–5)

IVF methodology has largely moved on to the slightly later timeframe of the blastocyst (day 5–6), and the more extensive data now available from this period may be of more current relevance. The short period (days 4 to 5) during which the cleavage embryo

[7] The very earliest cause of failure of the embryo may apply at the very earliest mitoses, from as early as mitosis number 1 (Bell et al. 2020). These initial mitoses require integrity of, among others, the *TLE6* and *PADI6* genes; mutation in these genes leads to embryonic arrest at this stage (Maddirevula et al. 2017).
[8] Anaphase lag at mitosis no. 1 is dramatically illustrated in time-lapse photography in Currie et al. (2022).

Table 20–1. Frequencies (%) of Aneuploidies for Certain Chromosomes in the Day-3 Embryos of a Cohort of 28 Presumed Normally Fertile Women, According to Maternal Age

CHROMOSOME	<37 YEARS	≥37 YEARS
13	7	21
16	7	16
18	5	15
21	9	30
22	5	14
X,Y	7	15

Notes: Figures are percentages, based upon an analysis of 215 embryos. In addition to these aneuploidies, small numbers (3%) of haploid and polyploid embryos were observed, too few to allow a useful age comparison. The cohort comprised women having preimplantation genetic testing for an X-linked Mendelian condition.

Source: From C Rubio et al., Chromosomal abnormalities and embryo development in recurrent miscarriage couples, *Hum Reprod* 18:182–188, 2003.

advances through the morula stage (Figure 20–8, d to e) and into the blastocyst may be an important hurdle at which the development of many chromosomally abnormal pre-embryos can arrest. Not all may fall at the hurdle: some mosaic aneuploid day-3 embryos may have converted, by day 5, into euploidy (discussed below).

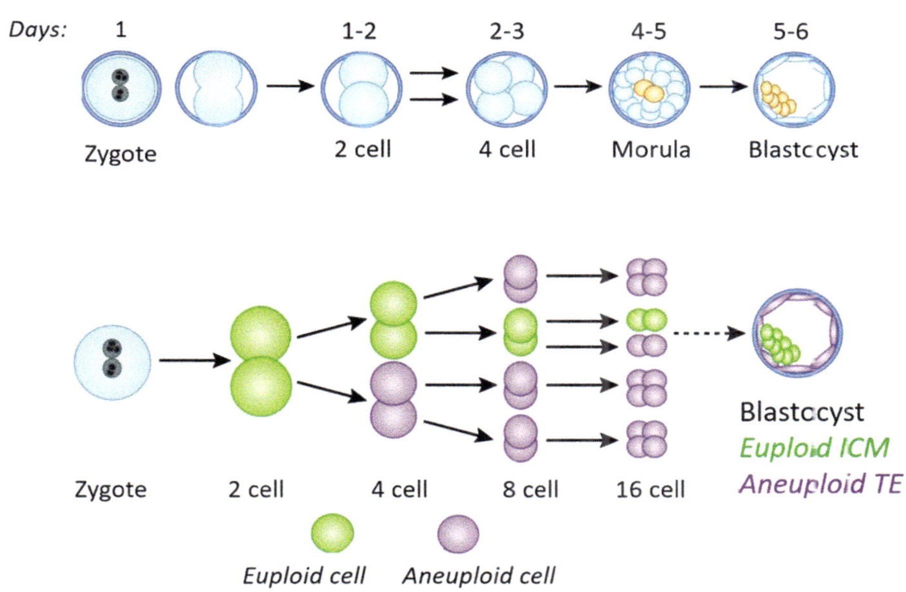

Figure 20–9. Scenarios whereby Mosaicism may Arise.

Note: In these examples, (*above*) a mitotic error at the morula stage produces aneuploid cells (orange), which then go on to involve the inner cell mass (ICM), but the trophectoderm (TE) (in blue) is normal. (*Below*) a newly aneuploid lineage (purple) arises at the 4-cell stage, following error during the second round of mitosis, and this lineage generates the TE, while the ICM (green), the presumptive embryo, is euploid.

Source: A Lee and AA Kiessling, Early human embryos are naturally aneuploid—can that be corrected? *J Assist Reprod Genet* 34:15–21, 2017. Courtesy AA Kiessling, and with the permission of Springer Nature.

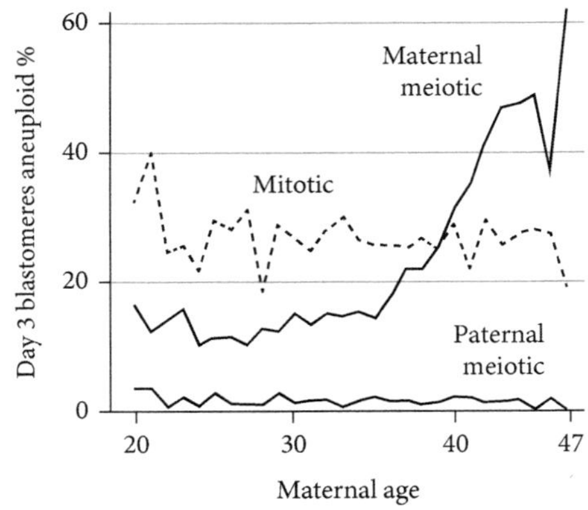

Figure 20–10. Meiotic cf. Mitotic Mosaicism in Day-3 Embryos.

Notes: If the dotted line were smoothed, mitotic abnormality could be seen as being practically constant, at a little under half of all blastomeres, irrespective of maternal age. The abrupt take-off during the mid 30s in the maternal meiotic data is very evident (the dip at 45-46 may reflect smaller numbers at this age). The paternal meiotic data would probably, in actuality, reduce to a near-straight line barely lifting above the baseline, at 1%–2%. These data are derived from an analysis of single blastomeres.

Source: Drawn after RC McCoy, Mosaicism in preimplantation human embryos: When chromosomal abnormalities are the norm. *Trends Genet* 33:448–463, 2017. Courtesy RC McCoy, and with the permission of Elsevier.

A very substantial fraction of blastocysts are aneuploid. Franasiak et al. (2014), for example, analyzed more than 15,000 blastocysts of parents presenting at IVF/PGT for biopsy for a variety of reasons, using 24-chromosome methodology, and could thus derive rather precise estimates of aneuploidies according to maternal age. A small increase above baseline is seen in the youngest mothers; the least rate was in the 25- to 34-year-old age group, progressively increasing steeply from age 35 years and then into the mid-40s (as the graph in Figure 20–11 attests) when well over a half, and finally up to 80%–90% at age 43–45 are aneuploid. The shape of this graph reflects the similar tendency to aneuploidy in the oöcyte (Figure 20–4). The reader will note also that the aneuploidy graphs in Figures 20–5 (oöcytes) and 20–12 (blastocysts) quite closely overlap, at least with respect to the trisomies.[9]

This observation of somewhat equivalent fractions per chromosome, of trisomy and monosomy in oöcytes and blastocysts, is consistent with the following interpretations: that meiotic nondisjunction in oöcytes produces essentially equal numbers of disomic and nullisomic gametes, which have equal chances of fertilizing/being fertilized; and that most trisomies and monosomies can survive through to the morula (day 4) stage. As the morula morphs into a blastocyst (days 4–5) a lethality begins to operate, and the aneuploidy rate overall falls (Matorras et al. 2024). This is most notable in the monosomies, at least for the larger chromosomes, and monosomies are mostly seen in slightly lesser fractions than are the trisomies (Figure 20–12, upper). A day or so later, when implantation would normally happen, almost all autosomal monosomies will have succumbed (De Munck et al. 2021).

[9] A notable exception is trisomy 3, one of the more common aneuploidies at oögenesis, but infrequent in the blastocyst and rare at miscarriage (cf. Figure 20–22). And monosomy 3 is scarcely observed. Presumably, this chromosome is gene-dense with respect to very early-developmental critical loci.

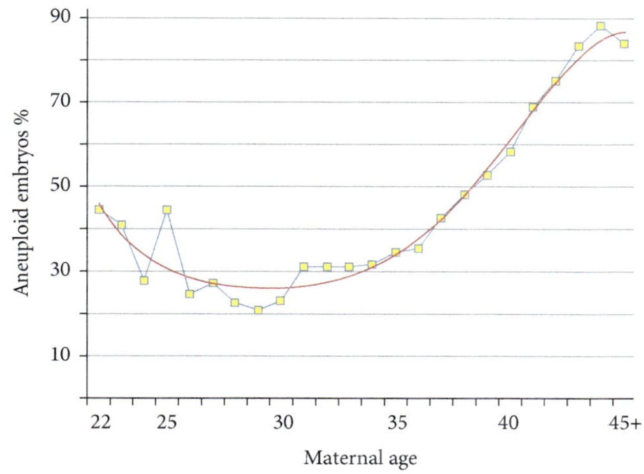

Figure 20–11. Aneuploidy Rates in Blastocysts, According to Maternal Age.

Notes: The regression curve (red) is derived from the actual data points. Note how this curve closely reflects that of oöcyte data (Figure 20–4 above).

Source: From JM Franasiak et al., The nature of aneuploidy with increasing age of the female partner: A review of 15,169 consecutive trophectoderm biopsies evaluated with comprehensive chromosomal screening, *Fertil Steril* 101: 656–663.e1, 2014. Courtesy JM Franasiak, and with the permission of Elsevier.

Mosaicism of the blastocyst of various categories is very commonly seen, and this is necessarily of mitotic origin (Figures 20–9, 20–13, and 20–14). Making a diagnosis of mosaicism in clinical practice will naturally depend upon how closely the sampled tissue (trophectoderm) is representative of the whole embryo, and what fraction of cells are abnormal. True mosaicism of the embryo, studied at biopsy of trophectoderm, will likely be missed if the level of mosaicism in the biopsied tissue is less than about 20% (Figure 20–15).

If it is a relatively simple mosaicism (e.g., a single trisomy; the diploid-aneuploid mosaic in Figure 20–13), and with the coexistence of a normal euploid lineage, there may often be an optimistic outlook as the blastocyst stage proceeds. Similarly as with the day-3 embryo discussed above, Chavli et al. (2024) describe how abnormal cells may be "sequestered off" to the trophectoderm and become a part of the placenta, or fall by the wayside. Such aneuploid mosaic embryos may thus undergo progressive normalization that can then, in due course, go on to produce a euploid fetus and a normal child (Greco et al. 2015; Liñán et al. 2018). And yet, exceptions are on record: for example, Greco et al. (2023) report two cases of mosaicism of the blastocyst—one for trisomy 21 and the other for a segmental loss of 1p36—going on to the same mosaicism being identified at follow-up prenatal diagnosis.

THE "EMBRYO PROPER" (WEEKS 3–8)

The embryo proper, in the sense that the body plan is beginning to be laid out, takes form from about the middle of the third week post-conception and is barely 1½ mm long; by the end of the eighth week post-conception (10 weeks by maternal dates[4]), it will be 3 cm. (To the embryologist, this is Carnegie stages 8 through 23.) This is a timeframe, now well beyond the gaze of the IVF laboratory, that is not easily studied (Figure 20–3). First, this appears to be a period during which the threshold for natural abortion is relatively

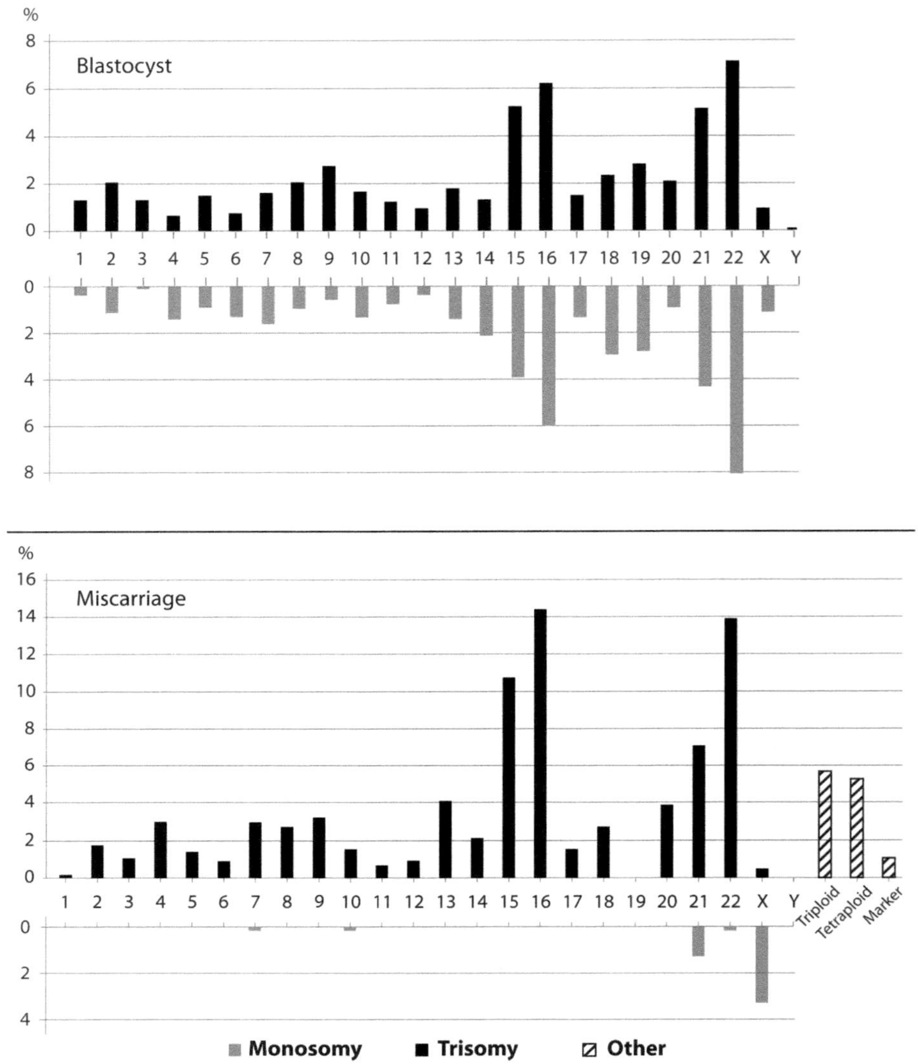

Figure 20–12. Aneuploidies in Day 5 Blastocysts.

Notes: (*Upper*) The range of aneuploidies observed in day 5–6 blastocysts, and their frequencies as a percentage of all aneuploidies. Note that trisomy and monosomy for each chromosome rather closely mirror their relative frequencies. Note also the broad similarity with the spread of data in oöcytes (Figure 20–5). Here, as in other studies, chromosomes 16 and 22 are seen to be the most susceptible to aneuploidy. (*Lower*) Comparing the distributions of aneuploidies in Miscarriage vis a vis Blastocysts. The spread of trisomies is fairly similar, whereas the autosomal monosomies have all but disappeared, attesting to the differential early pregnancy survival of the two aneuploidy classes.

Source: From J Rodriguez-Purata et al., Embryo selection versus natural selection: How do outcomes of comprehensive chromosome screening of blastocysts compare with the analysis of products of conception from early pregnancy loss (dilation and curettage) among an assisted reproductive technology population? *Fertil Steril* 104:1460–1466, 2015. Courtesy J Rodriguez-Purata, and with the permission of Elsevier.

high, and many abnormal embryos seem able to maintain existence (however imperfect that existence might be). Second, the practicalities of collecting intact embryos from very early spontaneous miscarriage present obvious drawbacks: the embryos are scarcely or not at all discernible among the products of conception otherwise (chorionic

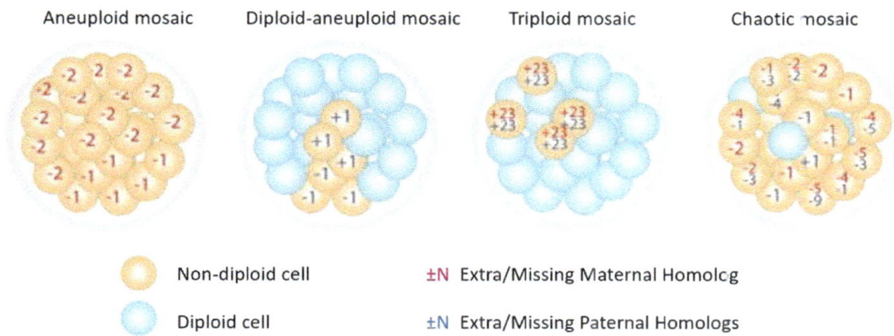

Figure 20–13. Categories of Mosaicism of the Embryo.

Notes: The aneuploid mosaic has monosomic (-1), and doubly monosomic (-2) cells. The diploid-aneuploid mosaic has normal (clear) and trisomic (+1) cells. The ploidy mosaic has normal and triploid (+23) cells. The chaotic mosaic has several different monosomies, and a few normal cells.

Source: From RC McCoy, Mosaicism in preimplantation human embryos: When chromosomal abnormalities are the norm. *Trends Genet* 33:448–463, 2017. Courtesy RC McCoy, and with the permission of Elsevier.

villi the main component). Nevertheless, a very few studies are on record concerning observations at therapeutic abortion, at "missed abortion," and at early first-trimester miscarriage.

Observation at *induced abortion* offers the earliest window to this period. An example is the day-25 trisomy 8 embryo illustrated in Figure 20–16, showing a gross distortion of

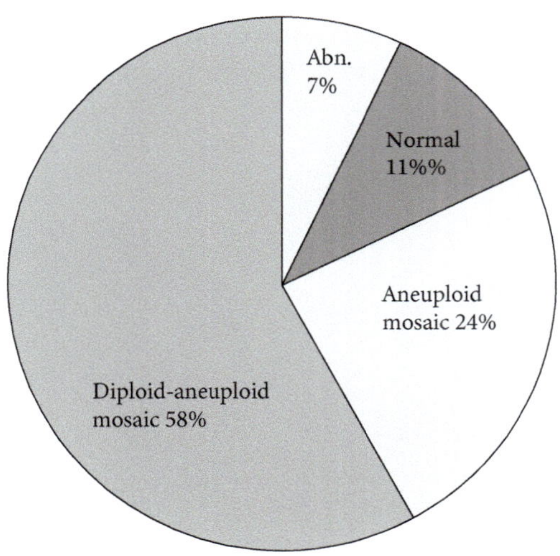

Figure 20–14. Mosaicism in Day-5 Blastocysts.

Notes: The normal figure of only 11% might seem disconcerting, but several of the diploid-aneuploid mosaics could subsequently "self-correct", and become euploid.

Abn., uniformly abnormal. The material comprised 55 cleavage-stage embryos or morulae, cultured in vitro through to the blastocyst stage, from donors of median maternal age 34 (range 22-42), and analyzed by single-cell sequencing.

Source: Drawn after EA Chavli et al., Single-cell DNA sequencing reveals a high incidence of chromosomal abnormalities in human blastocysts, *J Clin Invest* 2024:e174483, 2024. Courtesy EB Baart, and with the permission of the American Society for Clinical Investigation.

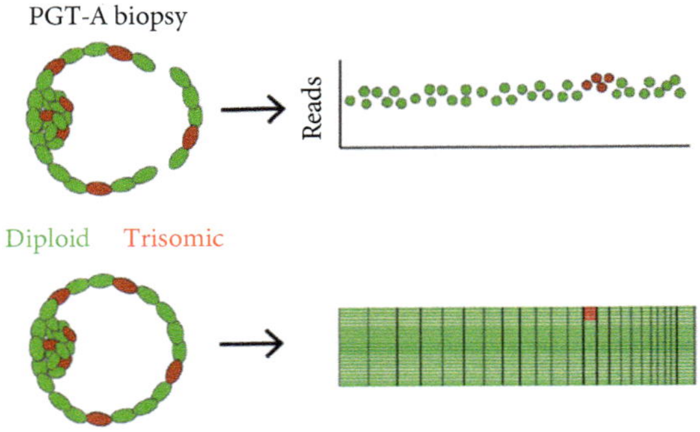

Figure 20–15. Mosaicism of the Embryo.

Notes: The detection of mosaicism will depend upon the fraction of trisomic cells, and their distribution within the biopsied trophectoderm. In the lower image, only four cells are trisomic, out of 529; such a low level could well be missed at routine PGT.

Source: From EA Chavli et al., Single-cell DNA sequencing reveals a high incidence of chromosomal abnormalities in human blastocysts, *J Clin Invest* 2024:e174483, 2024. Courtesy EB Baart, and with the permission of the American Society for Clinical Investigation.

normal anatomy, as can be appreciated alongside the photograph of a normal embryo of similar gestation. It is a fair assumption that some other trisomies, particularly of chromosomes containing crucial early-developmental genes, may be of similarly devasting effect and lead to very early natural miscarriage. *Missed abortion* refers to embryonic death without expulsion of the products of conception. Philipp et al. (2003, 2004) were able to study by endoscopy the anatomy of embryos in women prior to uterine evacuation for missed abortion. Some embryos showed no recognizable external structures (e.g. trisomy 3; Figure 20–17), while in some an outline embryonic form could be

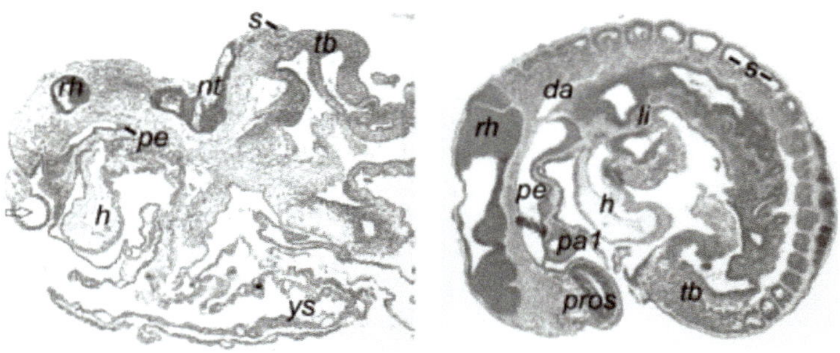

Figure 20–16. Trisomy 8 in a Very Early Embryo.

Notes: Midline sagittal section of a day-25 embryo with non-mosaic trisomy 8 (*left*), due to meiotic I nondisjunction. A normal embryo is shown (*right*) for comparison. The trisomic embryo is devastatingly malformed. Normal brain structure, the prosencephalon (pros) and rhombencephalon (rh), and regular somite (s) development are clear to see in the normal embryo, compared with the gross deformity in the trisomic embryo. da, dorsal aorta; h, heart; nt, neural tube; pa1, first pharyngeal arch; pe, pharyngeal endoderm; tb, tail bud; ys, yolk sac.

Source: From C Golzio et al., Cytogenetic and histological features of a human embryo with homogeneous chromosome 8 trisomy, *Prenat Diagn* 26:1201–1205, 2006. Courtesy HC Etchevers, and with the permission of Wiley-Blackwell.

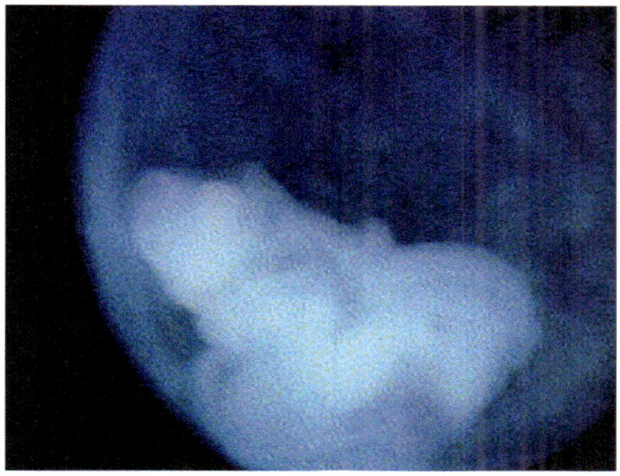

Figure 20–17. Trisomy 3 in an Embryo at Missed Abortion.

Notes: View by hysteroscopy prior to evacuation of products of conception. No normal anatomic structures are discernible, only an irregular tissue mass.

Source: From T Philipp et al., Abnormal embryonic development diagnosed embryoscopically in early intrauterine deaths after in vitro fertilization: a preliminary report of 23 cases, *Fertil Steril* 82:1337–1342, 2004. Courtesy T Philipp, and with the permission of the American Society for Reproductive Medicine and Elsevier.

recognized (e.g. trisomies 4 and 7). We have seen a triploid embryo from a missed abortion (Figure 20–18). In a Thai study of *early first trimester abortion*, based upon chorionic villus analysis and which included a fraction of losses happening during weeks 5 to 7^{+6}—in other words, within the embryonic period—these workers were able to chromosomally analyze 17 cases, of which 9 were aneuploid, with trisomies of 15, 18, 19, 20, 21, and 22 (Parinayok et al. 2022).

The practice of noninvasive cell-free DNA prenatal screening, now becoming widespread, has given clearer insight into the chromosomal picture of early pregnancy, at the time at which the blood sample would have been drawn (usually at the 10-week by-dates mark, or shortly thereafter, as the embryonic period segues into the fetal stage). Pertile et al. (2017) analyzed findings due to just under 90,000 samples from ongoing pregnancies, mostly from late first trimester, with a minority from second, thus representing in particular the transition from the embryo into the early fetal developmental stage. Some would have presented due to advanced maternal age, but ascertainment in the majority was, in all likelihood, essentially unbiased. Of these, 306 (0.34%) had a "rare autosomal trisomy"; that is, a trisomy of other than 13, 18, 21, or sex chromosomal. And while the spread of abnormality was somewhat comparable to that seen at miscarriage, with trisomies 15, 16, and 22 prominent, the largest single contributor was actually trisomy 7. These pregnancies, if left alone, would surely have gone on to later miscarriage or intrauterine fetal death.

Cytogenetics of Very Early Pregnancy Failure

RECURRENT IMPLANTATION FAILURE AT IVF

Couples 46,XX and 46,XY. A failure of implantation following natural (in vivo) fertilization cannot be recognized as such; but in vitro, the whole process can be followed. In

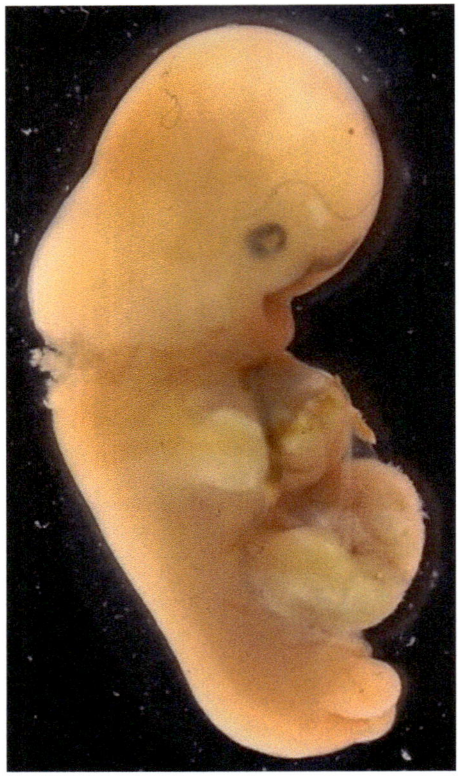

Figure 20–18. A Triploid (69,XXY) Embryo.

Notes: The face has no landmarks other than eyes and a single opening. The anterior trunk is open, with the heart and liver visible. The disrupted tissue at the neck was the site of biopsy for the cytogenetic analysis.

the case of recurrent implantation failure (RIF[10]) following IVF, more than one cause may apply, and a distinction is to be made between maternal ("uterine receptivity") and embryo-related characteristics. Maternal causes notwithstanding, a substantial fraction of RIF is due to chromosomal abnormality of the embryo (Ma et al. 2022). Matorras et al. (2024) observed that women having had more previous aneuploidies at embryo biopsy, and proceeding to subsequent IVF, had fewer embryos that were euploid compared with women whose embryos at previous PGT had mostly been euploid (Figure 20–19). Xi et al. (2022) applied the methodology of noninvasive chromosome screening (NICS) of the embryo in IVF patients presenting with previous RIF: those having had NICS achieved a clinical pregnancy rate of 47%, compared with 29% in those in whom choice of embryo transfer was judged purely on blastocyst morphology. Observations such as these lead to the assumption that, in at least a considerable number of cases, recurring errors at cell division may be the basis of the RIF.

[10] The European Society of Human Reproduction and Embryology defines RIF thus: RIF describes the scenario in which the transfer of embryos considered to be viable has failed to result in a positive pregnancy test sufficiently often in a specific patient to warrant consideration of further investigations and/or interventions (ESHRE Working Group on Recurrent Implantation Failure, 2023).

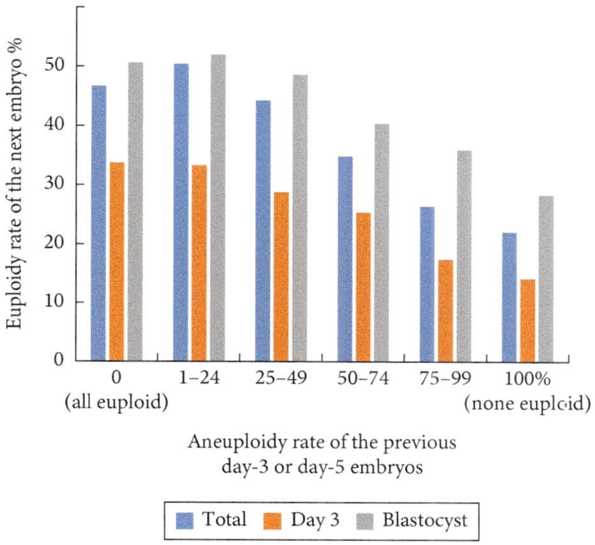

Figure 20–19. The Likelihood of Euploidy According to History of Previous Embryos.
Note: A history of previous aneuploid embryos portends a higher subsequent risk for aneuploidy.
Source: From R Matorras et al., Lessons learned from 64,071 embryos subjected to PGT for aneuploidies: results, recurrence pattern and indications analysis, *Reprod Biomed Online* 49:103979, 2024. Courtesy R Matorras, and with the permission of Elsevier.

A question: at which cell division? A vulnerability might in fact lie as much in very early mitosis rather than at meiosis. Voullaire et al. (2007) compared the frequency of aneuploidy at PGT in embryos from women with RIF and without such history and found a higher rate of complex chromosome abnormality, which they defined as aneuploidy of three or more chromosomes, in the RIF group. McCoy et al. (2015) studied large numbers of day-3 embryos and day-5 blastocysts, and identified previous IVF failure to be associated slightly, but nevertheless significantly, with mosaicism due to mitotic error. Kort et al. (2018), analyzing blastocyst data, calculated an odds ratio of 1.36 cf. fertile controls, that a couple having suffered RIF might have yet another failure due to aneuploidy, independent of maternal age. In their review, Kim et al. (2024) determined that PGT-A (PGT for aneuploidy) improved the implantation rate (42% cf. 22% in those not having had PGT-A) and livebirth rate (47% cf. 29%) in women having suffered previous RIF, notwithstanding that the PGT-A group were a little older (average 38) than the non–PGT-A group (35).

Thus it may be that in at least some of these RIF couples, mitosis rather than meiosis presents the more hazardous stumbling block (McCoy et al. 2015). An underlying susceptibly may obtain, in embryos of theirs, to undergo post-zygotic chromosomal error during the first two or three rounds of mitosis—an effect that might relate to either maternal or paternally inherited factors and be unrelated to parental age (Figure 20–10). Recurrent meiotic error may be marginally less contributory.

Translocation Carrier Couples. As for the small category of those with heterozygosity for an autosomal translocation, in one series of 65 women who had had ≥15 failed transfers, 8% were translocation carriers, two being sisters with the same translocation (Raziel et al. 2002). On somewhat larger numbers, Stern et al. (1999) noted the rate of balanced rcp and rob carriers to be 3% in 219 couples (both partners tested) who had failed more than 10 embryo transfers, but 9% in 130 couples who had three or more consecutive first-trimester abortions.

Cytogenetics of Spontaneous Abortion and Later Pregnancy Failure

CLINICAL MISCARRIAGE

Most (80%) miscarriages happen in the first 12 weeks of pregnancy, and mostly in weeks 8 through 12. By this stage, tissue from "products of conception" is often obtainable and analyzable. Of all recognized pregnancies (recognized in the traditional way, that is), ~15% end in natural miscarriage, also referred to as spontaneous abortion (Quenby et al. 2021).[11]

If the products of conception (POC) are successfully karyotyped, a majority of abortuses are shown to have a chromosome abnormality (Finley et al. 2022; Essers et al. 2023; Kutteh et al. 2024; Xu et al. 2024a). Finley and colleagues studied 24,900 POC samples by SNP microarray methodology, and the abnormalities documented are set out in Figure 20–20; similarly, Kutteh and colleagues analyzed 65,333 POC samples, classifying by maternal age (Figure 20–21). A clinically significant chromosome abnormality was seen in these studies in ~60% of samples, and in practically all, this would have been the cause of the miscarriage. Thus, most miscarriages reflect "biology in action": the natural elimination of an unsurvivable abnormality.

Trisomies account for about two-thirds of all cytogenetic abnormalities identified at spontaneous abortion, and the full range of trisomies and their relative frequencies are depicted in Figures 20–20 and 22. The most commonly seen abnormal karyotypes are trisomy 16, monosomy X, and triploidy. Indeed, as many as 1% of all human conceptions may have trisomy 16 (Benn 1998); monosomy X and triploidy account each for approximately 10% of all abnormalities. Double trisomy (trisomy for two chromosomes) is infrequent, and triple trisomy is rarely seen. Pathogenic CNVs and unbalanced structural rearrangements constitute much of the remainder (Dai et al. 2024).

> The origin of the abnormality is, in most, an error at maternal meiosis I, and this includes most of the major trisomies: trisomies 13, 14, 16, 21, and 22, with trisomy 18 a possible exception. Robinson et al. (1999) analyzed the originating status of certain of the less studied karyotypes: trisomies for chromosomes 2, 4–10, 12, 15, 17, and 20. Around three-fourths showed three alleles for the trisomic chromosome,

[11] The distinction between an embryo and a fetus (and see footnote 2) in this setting is not necessarily straightforward. Embryonic development may have arrested, and spontaneous abortion will be inevitable, but the pregnancy may continue for one or a few weeks ("missed abortion") and using apparent gestational age would give a misleading impression. In this case, it is more useful to consider the developmental stage of the embryo in judging the effects of a particular aneuploidy (Philipp et al. 2003). For example, the triploid embryo (not fetus) shown in Figure 20–18 was retained in the uterus until 18 weeks, but development had arrested at the 7–8 week mark.

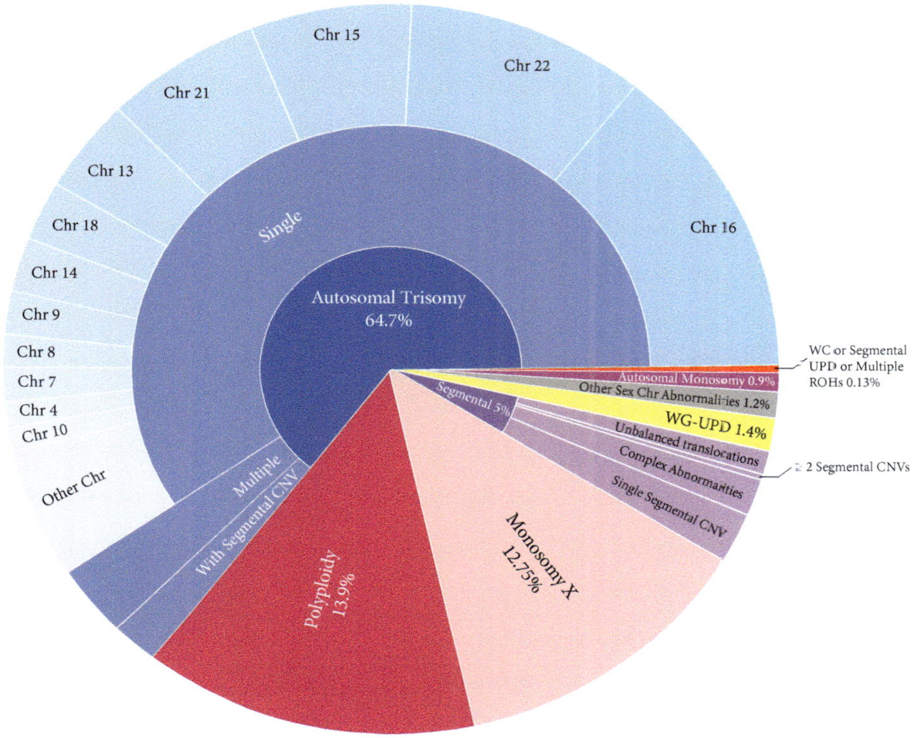

Figure 20–20. Chromosomal Findings in Products of Conception from Spontaneous Abortions.

Notes: These abnormal cases comprised 54% of the total of 24,900 analyzed POCs. "Single" refers to trisomy for a single chromosome, with those chromosomes more frequently represented individually indicated by number. Note the substantial involvement of trisomies 16 and 22, reflecting their high frequencies at oögenesis and blastogenesis (see above), and their presumed relatively low critical-gene content, that has allowed them to survive through to at least this stage of pregnancy. Polyploidy and monosomy X are also prominent. Chr = chromosome; ROHs = regions of homozygosity; WC = whole chromosome; WG-UPD = whole-genome uniparental disomy.

Source: From J Finley et al., The genomic basis of sporadic and recurrent pregnancy loss: a comprehensive in-depth analysis of 24,900 miscarriages, *Reprod Biomed Online* 45:125–134, 2022. Courtesy T Sahoo, and with the permission of Elsevier.

thus confirming a meiotic origin. Most of the remainder are presumed to have been due to somatic errors; some might have been mosaic but not detected as such. Trisomy 8 is notable in that all cases were due to a meiotic error, which stands in contrast to somatic errors being almost entirely the basis of the mosaic trisomy 8 syndrome (Warkany syndrome, p. 687) that is diagnosed post-natally. Uniparental disomy appears not to be an important causative factor in miscarriage (Xu et al. 2024a).

There is a striking maternal-age effect in the risk, per pregnancy, for a miscarriage, increasing tenfold from late teens to 40s—an effect presumably due in large part to a chromosomal basis (Nybo Andersen et al. 2000; Cohain et al. 2017;

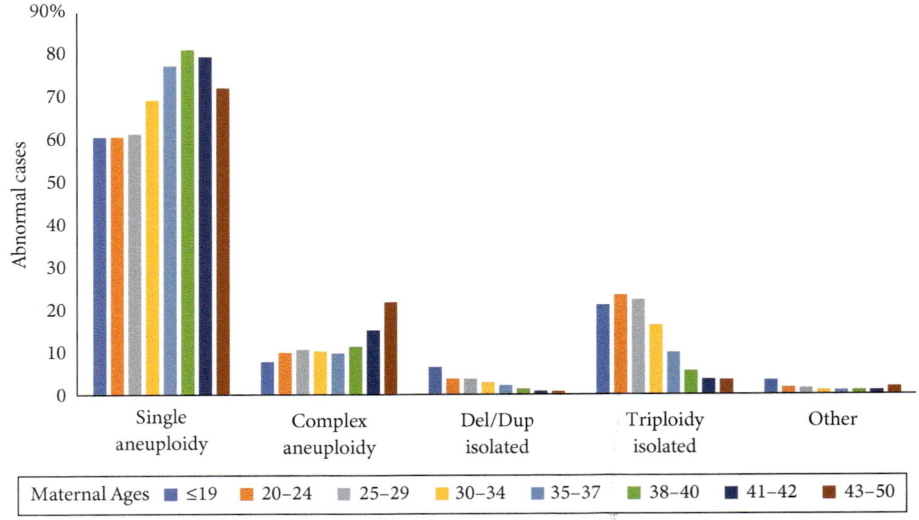

Figure 20–21. Chromosomal Findings in Products of Conception from Spontaneous Abortions, According to Maternal Age.

Note: The maternal age effects are opposite in aneuploidies (essentially increasing with maternal age) cf. del/dups and triploidy (falling with increasing age).

Source: From WH Kutteh et al., Role of genetic analysis of products of conception and PGT in managing early pregnancy loss, *Reprod Biomed Online* 49:103738, 2024. Courtesy WH Kutteh, and with the permission of Elsevier.

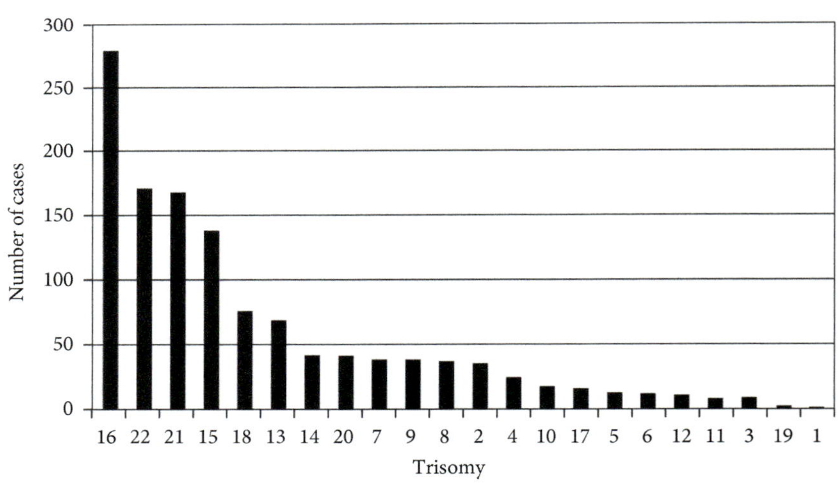

Figure 20–22. The Relative Frequencies of Trisomies Observed in Products of Conception.

Notes: The frequencies descend from the most often seen (trisomy 16) to the least (trisomy 1). These data are from the 1,872 abnormal results of a series of 5,457 consecutive samples of products of conception, on G-banding analysis. The curious pre-eminence of trisomy 16 is noted, and yet this aneuploidy, as a non-mosaic abnormality, never survives through to term (Peng et al. 2021). Unsurprisingly, the largest chromosome, no. 1, is the least represented, attesting to its extreme lethality in the trisomic state; but notably, one of the smallest, no. 19, is the second-most lethal, presumably reflecting its very high gene load (Table 1-1). The findings here are very similar to those of Rodriguez-Purata et al. shown in Figure 20–12, and near identical to those of Gu et al. (2021).

Source: From BT Wang et al., Abnormalities in spontaneous abortions detected by G-banding and chromosomal microarray analysis (CMA) at a national reference laboratory, *Mol Cytogenet* 7:33, 2014. Courtesy BT Wang, and with the permission of Springer Nature.

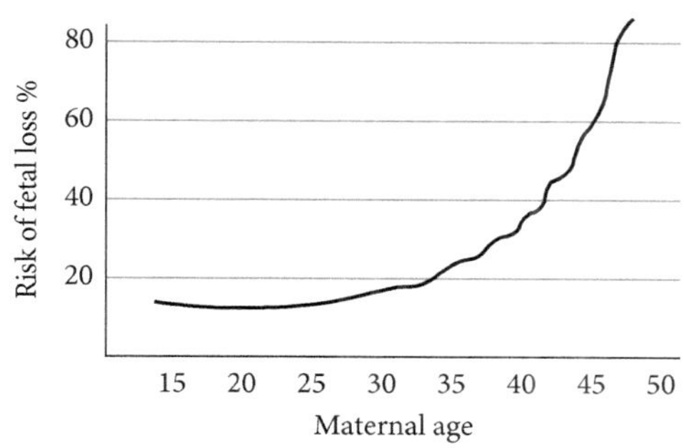

Figure 20–23. The Effect of Maternal Age upon Pregnancy Loss.

Notes: These data are derived from over a million Danish women intending carrying to term in 1978-1992, according to their age. The maternal age effect is very evident.

Source: Drawn after AM Nybo Andersen et al., Maternal age and fetal loss: population based register linkage study, *BMJ* 320:1708–1712, 2000.

Figure 20–23). The influence of a slight paternal-age effect is open to argument (du Fossé et al. 2020).

Twinning. If an abnormal twin dies, the normal twin may ensure continuation of the pregnancy, with only a parchment-like vestige (*fetus papyraceus*) remaining, preserved in the uterus along with the normal twin. A "vanishing twin" is plausibly proposed in the circumstance of two cell lines being identified at chorion villus sampling, 46,XX and 47,XY,+autosome, and a normal singleton baby subsequently born (Falik-Borenstein et al. 1994).

A very rare observation is the trisomy that would otherwise lead inevitably to early miscarriage, but in which a monozygous euploid co-twin allows some ongoing in utero survival. These cases may result from a very early post-zygotic event that generates a trisomic cell line (or which generates a normal cell line from a trisomic conceptus), and the trisomic co-twin, among other grossly devastating defects, fails to form a heart (acardius). The normal euploid co-twin provides the blood circulation to the abnormal fetus (twin reverse arterial perfusion). This scenario has been reported with trisomies 2 and 11 (Blaicher et al. 2000; Mihci et al. 2009), and we have seen one case due to trisomy 3 (Figure 20–24).

RECURRENT PREGNANCY LOSS

Couples 46,XX and 46,XY. More than two miscarriages is the criterion for "recurrent pregnancy loss"[12] (RPL). In principle, the causal error could have been with the sperm, with the egg, with the embryo, or with the mother (Klimczak et al. 2021). For those who are karyotypically normal, do some couples miscarry due to a predisposition to produce aneuploid conceptions? Or is the basis in a maternal rather than an embryonic cause: do certain factors influence uterine carrying capacity? Or, could recurrent aneuploid miscarriage, in the setting of a high background rate of aneuploidy in humans,

[12] Definition from the American Society for Reproductive Medicine (2008): "Recurrent pregnancy loss is a disease distinct from infertility, defined by two or more failed pregnancies. When the cause is unknown, each pregnancy loss merits careful review to determine whether specific evaluation may be appropriate. After three or more losses, a thorough evaluation is warranted."

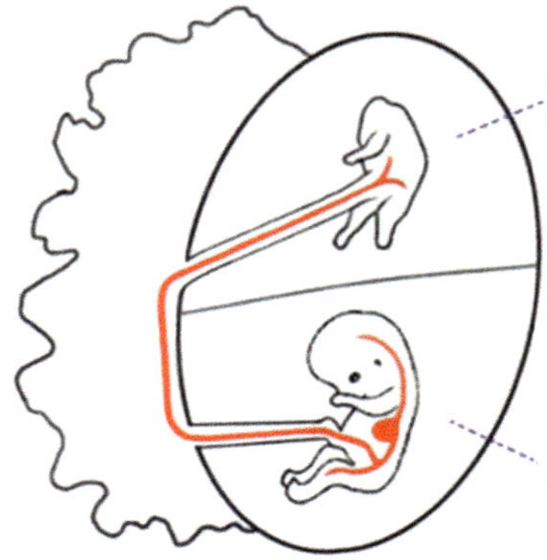

Figure 20–24. Trisomic Co-Twin Survival.

Notes: The euploid twin enabled survival of the trisomy 3 monozygous co-twin. The abnormal co-twin, identified at mid-trimester ultrasonography, was anencephalic and acardiac, but survived to that stage due to a shared circulation from the "pump twin". A likely scenario is that a mitotic error in an initially normal conceptus at a very early stage, perhaps the second or third mitosis, led to the generation of a trisomic 3 cell line, with the embryo then splitting along a plane of separation between the euploid and aneuploid tissue. Case of G McGillivray et al. (2004).

simply reflect random biology, with increasing maternal age the only clear predisposing factor? A common event is common, and not uncommonly it may happen more than once.

In fact, the major contributors may be these: uterine receptivity; and random biology, maternal-age related. Van den Berg et al. (2012) determined, on a review of the literature at that time, that the aneuploidy rate in products of conception following previous RPL (39%) was slightly *less* compared to the background rate of 45% in sporadic, one-time miscarriage. The more broadly focused (including del/dup) categories of chromosomal abnormality due to Li et al. (2024c) are listed in Table 20–2. In this dataset, from a younger (average age 30) cohort, chromosomal imbalances of all types occurred in a substantial fraction (59%) of pregnancies of those having had previous RPL. Narrowing the viewpoint to autosomal trisomies, and with the mechanism of recurrent single-chromosome meiotic error in mind, these, at 33%, contributed rather less to the overall POC chromosomal abnormality (albeit the largest single category). In other words, there appears not to be a particular maternal propensity to produce aneuploid eggs, as a cause of RPL.

A comparative viewpoint is afforded in Ozawa et al. (2019), who studied aneuploidy rates in women of mostly an older maternal age (into their late 30s and 40s) and comparing those who had had just one, with those having had two or more miscarriages. Table 20–3 sets out the individual trisomies as identified in the notable fraction of 61% of POCs from those who had previously suffered multiple miscarriages, but this high proportion is still *less* than in those having had only one previous miscarriage, with an aneuploidy rate of 72%.

The points emerging from the foregoing is that aneuploidy of the POC is *less* often observed in couples who have had a large number of miscarriages, sometimes into double figures, than among those who have had fewer; and that maternal age is a major factor behind much RPL. Returning to Li et al. (2024c), these workers followed prospectively women with an RPL history, having had one tested ("index") POC: and those women whose index POC was euploid had a slightly lower eventual live birth outcome

Table 20–2. Range of Abnormalities in Products of Conceptions, from Women Having Suffered Previous Recurrent Loss

CATEGORY (The abnormality in an "index POC"; see Notes)	%	%
Single aneuploidy		41
Autosomal trisomy	33	
Autosomal monosomy	0.5	
Monosomy X	7	
Sex chromosome trisomy	0.2	
Multiple aneuploidy		2.5
Polyploidy		8
Triploidy	6	
Hypotriploidy	0.7	
Hypertriploidy	0.8	
Tetraploidy	0.3	
Partial aneuploidy (large CNVs)		5
Terminal deletion/duplication	1	
Interstitial deletion/duplication	0.3	
Terminal deletion + terminal duplication (suggestive of unbalanced translocation)	1.5	
Multiple deletions and/or duplications	2	
Pathogenic microdeletion/duplication		1.5
Terminal microdeletion/duplication	0.5	
Interstitial microdeletion/duplication	1	
Multiple microdeletions and/or duplications	0.1	
UPD (whole-genome)		1
Total % Abnormal		59
Total % Normal		40

Notes: These data come from a cohort of 830 couples having had previous recurrent miscarriage, the mean number of previous miscarriages being 2.4, at mean gestational age 9.8 weeks. The average maternal age was 30. These couples went on to have a further miscarriage, the "index POC," which was tested by CMA (chromosome microarray analysis) as in the data above, the figures shown as percentages (note that a majority of the POCs, 59%, were chromosomally abnormal). At follow-up for at least two years, 627 went on to have a live birth. Those having had a chromosomally abnormal index POC had a slightly higher livebirth rate than the euploid POC group (72% cf. 67%,) and a slightly lesser miscarriage rate (23% cf. 27%).

Source: From Y Li et al., Reproductive outcomes in couples with recurrent pregnancy loss after embryonic chromosomal microarray analysis, *J Assist Reprod Genet* 41:161–170, 2024.

(67%) compared with the aneuploid POC group (72%), and a marginally higher miscarriage rate (27% cf. 23%). As well as the ploidy status of the index miscarriage, the rates of subsequent live birth were notably related to the number of previous miscarriages, as follows: those with two, three, or four or more previous miscarriages, the index miscarriage being *euploid*, had subsequent livebirth rates of 76%, 56%, and 44% respectively, these percentages quite markedly falling away with increasing numbers of miscarriages. The comparable figure for those in whom the index miscarriage was *aneuploid* were 74%, 71%, and 63%, these percentages showing a lesser decline (Figure 20–25).

Table 20-3. Autosomal Trisomies in Products of Conception, Following Previous Recurrent Pregnancy Loss (RPL) or a Previous Single Miscarriage

Trisomy	Previous RPL (N, out of 175)	Previous single miscarriage (N, out of 189)	Trisomy	Previous RPL (N, out of 175)	Previous single miscarriage (N, out of 189)
1	0	0	15	14	20
2	2	2	16	10	22
3	0	1	17	2	1
4	4	0	18	4	7
5	1	4	19	0	0
6	0	3	20	3	4
7	2	1	21	11	29
8	1	4	22	25	16
9	2	3	Triploid	7	9
10	2	0	Mono X	3	10
11	1	0	Double	10	4
12	1	1	Complex	9	3
13	4	6	Other	11	9
14	7	5			

Notes: A total of 175 and 189 POCs had been analyzed, from women having had previous multiple losses (RPL), or a single miscarriage, respectively. Overall, 146 (87%) of POCs in the RPL cohort and 164 (78%) of POCs in the single cohort had a chromosomal abnormality. This 9% difference is substantially accounted for by a lesser fraction of viable trisomies in the RPL group, 11%, cf. 22% in the single miscarriage group; there was little difference (44% cf. 46%) in the rates of non-viable trisomy. The excess of monosomy X in the single group, and an excess of trisomy 22 in the RPL group, is also to be noted, although the denominators are small. The maternal-age profile in this cohort was substantially skewed towards older age: a minority were <35 (87), 160 were 35–39, and 117 were 40 and over. Miscarriage happened prior to 12 weeks gestation.

Source: From data in N Ozawa et al., Maternal age, history of miscarriage, and embryonic/fetal size are associated with cytogenetic results of spontaneous early miscarriages, *J Assist Reprod Genet* 36:749–757, 2019.

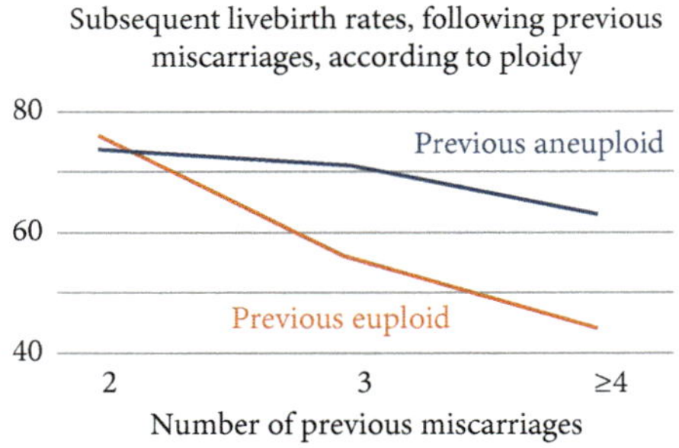

Figure 20-25. A Comparison of Livebirth Rates Following Previous Miscarriage, According to Ploidy Status of the POCs.

Source: From data in Y Li et al., Reproductive outcomes in couples with recurrent pregnancy loss after embryonic chromosomal microarray analysis, *J Assist Reprod Genet* 41:161–170, 2024.

In other words, euploidy of a POC implies a worse outlook for a future pregnancy than does aneuploidy; and in that circumstance, an "inhospitable endometrium" may be the probable basis. For these women, a detailed endocrine and immunological[13] work-up may be indicated (Kuroda 2024). If no cause is then shown, Eliwa et al. (2024) refer to these couples as having "truly unexplained RPL." Otherwise, a combination of certain genetic factors may predispose to a risk for euploid miscarriage (Aminbeidokhti et al. 2024). These researchers speak of an "intolerome": genes and variants that are subjects of biological intolerance and natural selection.

Nevertheless, some couples might have a particular proneness to produce aneuploid gametes, and indeed, from the recurrence data with respect to the three viable autosomal trisomies discussed elsewhere (Chapter 13), this might seem, *prima facie*, logical. But the question: Is this indeed so? (Mumusoglu et al. 2025). Kort et al. (2018) found that women with a history of RPL were 1.3 times more likely to produce aneuploid embryos compared to fertile controls who had undergone PGT for sex selection. This increase applied to both meiotic and mitotic errors. Similarly, Liu et al. (2020) found that in women <35 years old with a history of RPL, 49% of embryos were aneuploid, compared to 37% aneuploidy rate in a control group having PGT for monogenic disorders.

But these findings are not consistently seen: several other studies have found that a woman's prior reproductive history, including previous miscarriage, shows no association with rate of euploidy in her embryos (Kornfield et al. 2022; Turgut et al. 2023; Cimadomo et al. 2021). What we may distill from these contradictory conclusions is that if there is indeed a susceptibility, it must be small and likely affecting only a minority.

Couples with Abnormal Karyotypes. For the small group of people who are heterozygous for a chromosomal rearrangement, RPL may of course occur with a much higher frequency, and this briefly stated fact is the basis of much of what is written in this book. The more usually seen rearrangement is the reciprocal translocation, and this is the observation in around 2%–3% of all couples suffering loss of two or more pregnancies before 20 weeks' gestation. Smaller fractions are due to Robertsonian translocations and inversions. Unsurprisingly, the rates are similar in whichever part of the world studies have been done (Elkarhat et al. 2019).

These chromosomal rearrangements are usually of sufficient size to be readily detectable at standard karyotyping, and typically of sufficient size that the imbalanced combinations will very frequently lead to inevitable miscarriage. But the application of molecular methodology can sometimes discover a subtle parental rearrangement that previously would have passed muster—a possibility especially to be pursued in the event of recurrence of the same structural abnormality (Li et al. 2024b). Chapters 5 to 9 set out particular circumstances.

The large study due to Park et al. (2022), based upon 19,000 couples presenting with recurrent spontaneous abortion, is representative. These researchers document a long list of chromosome abnormalities seen in 844 of these couples, and Figure 20–26 shows the broad distribution of abnormalities. Among these 844, balanced reciprocal translocation was the most common abnormality, in almost one-half. Otherwise, Robertsonian

[13] "It is a wonder of pregnancy that the fetus is not rejected by the mother's immune system," as Kent (2009) comments. One genetic factor proposed to be central to this process is HLA-G, which "plays a mysterious role in the mechanism of maternal-fetal immune-tolerance" (Zhuang et al. 2021).

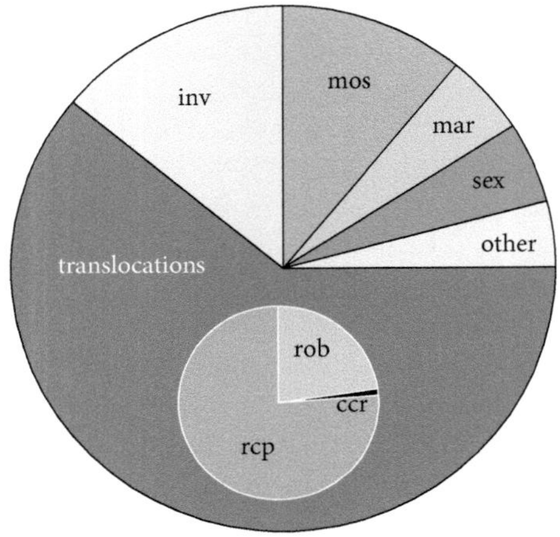

Figure 20–26. Chromosome Abnormalities carried by Couples who have had Recurrent Pregnancy Loss.

Notes: These data come from a survey of 844 couples, they comprising 4.4% of a cohort of 19,000 couples presenting with recurrent pregnancy loss. Translocations (61%) are clearly the predominant category, and the relative proportions of the three different categories of translocation are shown in the "pie-within-pie". *Inv*, inversions (14%); *mos*, mosaicisms (11%); *mar*, marker chromosomes (5%); *sex*, non-mosaic sex chromosome aneuploidy (5%); *others* (4%); *rob*, Robertsonian (14%); *ccr;* balanced complex chromosome rearrangement (0.6%); *rcp*; reciprocal translocations (47%).

Source: Redrawn from SJ Park et al., Chromosomal abnormalities of 19,000 couples with recurrent spontaneous abortions: a multicenter study, *Fertil Steril* 117:1015–1025, 2022, with the permission of Elsevier.

translocations were seen in 14%, and inversions also in 14%. Sex chromosome aneuploidies comprised most of the rest, including Turner syndrome variants, Klinefelter syndrome and variants, 47,XXX and mosaic forms, 47,XYY and mosaic forms, and X deletions and duplications.

Fetal Death In Utero, Stillbirth, and Perinatal Death

Fetal Death in Utero. This expression, abbreviated FDIU (and also "in utero fetal demise" or "second-trimester fetal demise"), refers to fetal death occurring after the usual time of clinical miscarriage (c. 13 weeks) through to the time of potential viability (c. 26 weeks). A classical chromosomal abnormality is typically seen in 5%–10%. Gawron et al. (2013) studied 118 such cases, many with concomitant malformations, finding these aneuploidies: trisomies 13, 18, and 21, triploidy, monosomy X, and "rare chromosomal aberrations." Others have found similarly, in small-for-gestational-age fetuses (Pasquini et al. 2023).

Stillbirth and Perinatal Death. A stillbirth refers to fetal death occurring after the time of viability (c. 26 weeks) or, in lay parlance, "the birth of an infant that has died in the womb." Some use 28 weeks as the cut-off, others ≥20 weeks. A perinatal death occurs from 28 weeks through to the first seven days of life, and thus includes stillbirth. From Irish data, malformations are seen in about one-third of such cases, and half of these (thus ~10% of all) are chromosomally related (Power et al. 2020). Similarly to FDIU, it is trisomy 21, trisomy 18, trisomy 13, and monosomy X that are most often seen, along with an occasional rare pathogenic del or dup (Reddy et al. 2012).[14] A role for CNVs and other genetic variation in the etiology of stillbirth is the subject of ongoing research (Ernst et al. 2015; Stanley et al. 2020). Chromosomal microarray yields a result more often than does classical karyotyping, in which the nature of tissue sampled at postmortem can lead to culture failure (Giordano and Wapner 2024).

Among liveborn babies, only 1 in 250 has an unbalanced chromosome abnormality on standard, classical karyotyping. Thus, there has been a very effective selection, at several stages along the prenatal developmental pathway, against those conceptions that were abnormal.

Cytogenetics of Infertility

Infertility is defined thus in the American Society for Reproductive Medicine (2012): "A disease, defined by the failure to achieve pregnancy after 12 months or more of regular unprotected intercourse." Certainly it is common, affecting at least 15% of couples, and increases with increasing age (Figure 20–27). Of the many causes of infertility, a chromosomal basis is seen in a small minority, 1%–2% (Figures 20–28 and 20–29). The frequency of karyotypic abnormality in couples with infertility depends upon the criteria of ascertainment and the threshold for determining abnormality, and quite wide ranges of figures have been produced (Table 20–4).

Sex chromosomal abnormalities include XXY and XXY/XY in the male, and Turner syndrome and its variants in the female. AZF deletions on the Y chromosome are common; the "XX male" and XY female are rare (Chapter 24). *Autosomal* rearrangements as a cause of infertility are noted in several chapters. The reciprocal translocation (especially when an acrocentric is involved) and the inversion may be associated, though

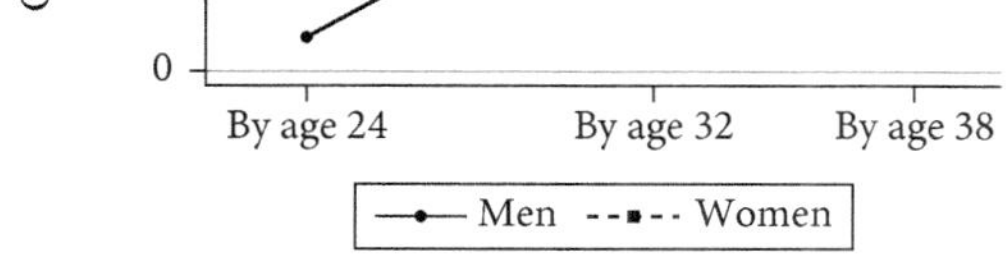

Figure 20–27. The Rates of Infertility According to Age.

Notes: The fractions represent the proportions of persons by sex and age to have ever tried for 12 months or more to conceive, or to have sought fertility advice. These data were derived from a whole population study, the Dunedin Multidisciplinary Health and Development Study.

Source: From T Van Roode et al., Cumulative incidence of infertility in a New Zealand birth cohort to age 38 by sex and the relationship with family formation, *Fertil Steril* 103:1053–1058.e2, 2015. Courtesy WR Gillett, and with the permission of Elsevier.

[14] Data from the post prenatal-diagnosis era will presumably have been influenced by the practice of elective abortion.

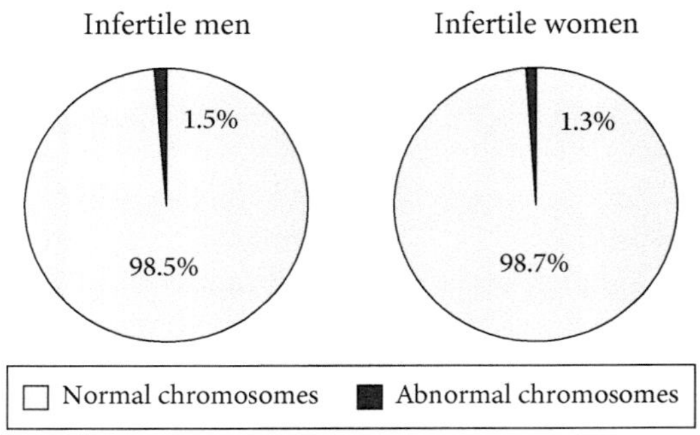

Figure 20–28. The Fractions of Male and Female Infertility having a Chromosomal Basis.

Note: These data were derived from couples attending fertility clinics, and who went on to take advantage of assisted reproductive technology (IUI, IVF, ICSI). The fractions in men and women in this study (2,646 men, 2,620 women) are remarkably similar, 1.5% cf. 1.3%.

Source: From the data in A Riccaboni et al., Genetic screening in 2,710 infertile candidate couples for assisted reproductive techniques: results of application of Italian guidelines for the appropriate use of genetic tests, *Fertil Steril* 89:800–808, 2008.

infrequently, with moderate to severe oligospermia (Chapters 5 and 9). Robertsonian translocations are occasionally associated with infertility in the male, or less often the female (Chapter 7). Translocation between a sex chromosome and an autosome is a rarely identified cause of infertility (Chapter 6). Complex rearrangements (Chapter 10) and rings (Chapter 11) usually present an insurmountable obstacle to cell division in the spermatocyte, resulting in azoöspermia; oögenesis is typically more robust.

An association of infertility with chromosomal polymorphism is controversial. In a Hungarian study from Andó et al. (2022), the common inv(9)(p11q12)/inv(9)(p11q13) proved to be *less* frequent among infertile males, and no different among

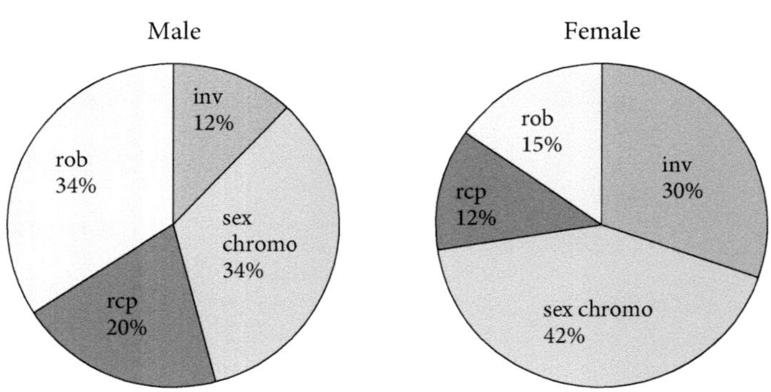

Figure 20–29. The Categories of Chromosomal Abnormality seen in Male and Female Infertility.

Note: This study included 40 men and 34 women (representing the "wedges" in Figure 20–28 above). inv = inversion, rcp = reciprocal translocation, rob = Robertsonian translocation. It is notable that Robertsonian translocations were seen twice as often in the male, and inversions twice as often in the female. The sex chromosomal abnormalities were, in the male, mostly Klinefelter syndrome, and in the female, X mosaic states; in some women, low-level X mosaicism may or may not have been relevant.

Source: From the data in A Riccaboni et al., Genetic screening in 2,710 infertile candidate couples for assisted reproductive techniques: results of application of Italian guidelines for the appropriate use of genetic tests, *Fertil Steril* 89:800–808, 2008.

Table 20–4. An Overview of the Frequencies (%) of Chromosomal Abnormalities Associated with Couple Infertility

			Male	Female	All
Chromosome aberration			2.5	1.6	2.0
Autosomal			1.1	1.1	1.1
	Translocation		1.0	0.9	1.0
		Reciprocal	0.6	0.7	0.7
		Robertsonian	0.4	0.3	0.3
	Inversion		0.1	0.1	0.1
	Other		0.03	0.04	0.04
Sex chromosome			1.1	0.1	0.6
	Numerical		1.0	0.1	0.5
	Structural		0.1	0.05	0.1
Mosaicism			0.1	0.3	0.2
Marker chromosome			0.03	0.6	0.5

Notes: Percentages are rounded. Karyotyping was performed in 17,054 patients affected by infertility, which was defined as not being able to conceive a pregnancy after at least 12 months of unprotected intercourse. This study did not include analysis for Yq *AZF* deletion.

Source: From J Yuan et al., Detection of chromosome aberrations in 17 054 individuals with fertility problems and their subsequent assisted reproductive technology treatments in Central China, *Hum Reprod* 38(Suppl ii):34–46, 2023.

females, than in a control population. Yet, in Yuan et al. (2023), an abnormal sperm morphology was more often seen among inv(9) heterozygotes.

INFERTILITY: CHROMOSOMAL FACTORS IN THE FEMALE

Fertility in the 46,XX female begins to fall in the mid-30s as the ovarian reserve dwindles. The average maximum number (but a wide range) of 300,000 ovarian follicles is reached in mid-fetal life, reducing thereafter to less than 1,000 remaining at the age of menopause (Figure 20–30). A diminishing ovarian reserve, as indicated by a low level of anti-Müllerian hormone, may point to an increasing risk for aneuploidy (Gat et al. 2017). An important age-related factor may be a decline in the functional competence of the meiotic spindle, compromising chromosomal distribution and leading to the generation of aneuploid gametes (Figure 20–6). Premature ovarian insufficiency (POI), also referred to as premature ovarian failure (POF), can be primary or secondary, associated with primary or secondary amenorrhea. Several genes have been implicated (França and Mendonca 2022; Fan et al. 2023a); our focus here is limited to the chromosomal.

X Chromosome. Classical and variant forms of Turner syndrome account for a number of cases of female infertility (Table 15–1). The variant forms include mosaic states which involve a 45,X cell line, and which may be in the company of a normal 46,XX cell line, a 47,XXX cell line, an isochromosome of the X long arm, or a ring of the X chromosome. In a Malaysian study, Ten et al. (1990) karyotyped 117 women with *primary* amenorrhea who had previously been investigated for other causes, and one-third had a sex chromosome abnormality. They were classified as follows: X aneuploidies (8%),

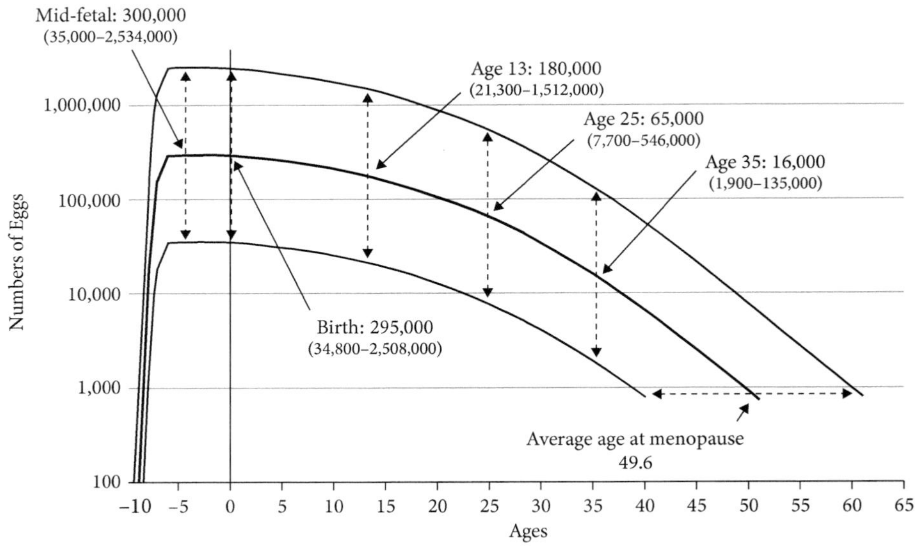

Figure 20–30. The Natural Fall-off in Oöcyte Reserve with Increasing Age.

Notes: Numbers of egg cells (non-growing follicles) are shown at different ages. 95% prediction intervals are shown in brackets, and as the two outer limits of the graph. Ages are in months, prior to birth (0); ages after birth in years. Mid-fetal refers to 18-22 weeks post conception. The *y* axis is a logarithmic scale.

Source: Redrawn from WHB Wallace and TW Kelsey, Human ovarian reserve from conception to the menopause, *PLoS One* 5:e8772, 2010. Courtesy WHB Wallace, and with the permission of the Public Library of Science.

X structural abnormalities (7%), presence of a Y (14%), and presence of a gonosomal marker chromosome (2%). Six women were mosaic, all having a 45,X cell line. Similar findings from India, although of a lesser frequency (16%) overall, are due to Chandel et al. (2023) (Table 20–5). As for *secondary* infertility, Devi and Benn (1999) studied 30 women with unexplained secondary amenorrhea under the age of 40 years. Four (13%) had chromosomal abnormalities: an Xq isochromosome, Turner syndrome mosaicism (45,X/46,XX), an X-Y translocation, and an X-autosome translocation.

Low-level X aneuploidy may or may not matter. The conundrum of how to interpret low-level X aneuploidy—for example, just one or two 47,XXX or 45,X cells[15]—is addressed in a newsletter from the European Cytogeneticsts Association (Madan and Lundberg 2015). The salient points listed in this article are worth noting:

- The frequency of low-level X aneuploidy is correlated with age and gender but not with reproductive history.
- There is no significant difference in the number of aneuploid cells between women with recurrent abortions (1.64%) and age-matched controls (1.78%).
- Approximately 16% of women of reproductive age show X aneuploidy in 2%–10% of blood cells.
- The finding of low-level X aneuploidy in peripheral blood of a mother is not a predictor of fetal aneuploidy.
- Low-level X aneuploidy is found in blood but not in skin or bone marrow.

[15] See also Mosaic loss of the X, p. 471.

Table 20–5. Chromosomal Observations (%) in a Population of 470 Women presenting with Primary Amenorrhea

Numerical		
	46,XX	84%
	45,X	4.3
	46,XY (sex reversal)	3.4
Mosaicisms, numerical		
	45,X/46,XX/47,XXX and 45,X/46,XX	1.3
	45,X/46,XY and 45,X/47,XXY and 46,XX/46,XY	0.6
Structural		
	Del Xp and del Xq	0.9
	Inv X	0.2
	Autosomal rcp	0.2
Mosaicisms, structural		
	45,X/del X	0.9
	45,X/iso X	0.9
	45,X/46,X+mar and 47,XX+mar	0.9
	45,X/46,derX from an X-X translocation	0.2

Note: Those abnormalities listed as 0.2% were seen in only single cases.

Source: From D Chandel et al., Clinical profile and cytogenetic correlations in females with primary amenorrhea, *Clin Exp Reprod Med* 50:192–199, 2023.

Autosomal Translocation Carriers. Of the many possible causes of POI, an uncommon finding is an autosomal structural anomaly, mostly rcp or rob, accounting for only 2% of POI cases (Vichinsartvichai 2016; Chen et al. 2023e) and with only a single representative of such a case, 46,XX,der(10)t(10;15)(p15;q22.1), in Table 20–5.

A most remarkable coincidence leading to infertility in a young woman is described in Kuechler et al. (2010). Her father was heterozygous for a mutation in the *FSHR* (follicle-stimulating hormone receptor) gene, which is located at 2p16.3; and her mother carried an apparently balanced translocation, t(2;8)(p16.3;p23.1), but which in fact had a microdeletion at the 2p16.3 breakpoint demonstrable on microarray. This microdeletion removed two exons of the *FSHR* gene. The daughter inherited this translocation, plus the paternal mutation, and in consequence the former "unmasked" the latter; no normal FSHR was produced, and folliculogenesis was arrested.

INFERTILITY: CHROMOSOMAL FACTORS IN THE MALE

Much couple infertility is associated with inadequate (quantitative and qualitative[16]) sperm production in the male partner, and a fraction of this, in particular where

[16] Quantitative: A normal number of sperm must be produced, namely, 15–200 million per ml of semen. Oligospermia ("few sperm") may be mild (10–15 million), moderate (5–10 million), or severe (<5 million). A complete absence of sperm is azoöspermia. Qualitative: Sperm should have a normal appearance and normal motility. Teratozoöspermia refers to an abnormal appearance of sperm: asthenozoöspermia is a lack of "swimming" capacity.

material is not routinely done, and so chromosomal normality or abnormality cannot usually be demonstrated (Stephenson et al. 2002 speak of "this unfortunate omission" compromising the management of couples presenting with recurrent miscarriage.) Analysis of products of conception can be useful in offering clearer advice to these women (Papas and Kutteh 2021), and the Royal College of Obstetricians and Gynaecologists (RCOG) advise that "Cytogenetic analysis should be offered on pregnancy tissue of the third and subsequent miscarriage(s) and in any second-trimester miscarriage" (Regan et al. 2023). Kutteh et al. (2024) advise that if the work-up proposed by the American Society of Reproductive Medicine is applied (including a search for autoimmune, endocrine, and uterine anatomical factors), alongside a chromosome study, an explanation for RPL may be forthcoming in a substantial majority of cases (Figure 20–32).

Trisomy of the conceptus is a common underlying cause, more so in women of older maternal age, but recurring euploid miscarriage may also be observed and if so, imply a less promising outlook (Figure 20–25). Euploidy of the POC likely reflects an underlying maternal factor that would apply to all pregnancies, whereas aneuploidy at least offers the hope that better fortune might attend the next ovulation. Past history of having had a child is relevant: Cohain et al. (2017) advise that "parous women until their late 30s, who have experienced multiple miscarriages, can be counseled that if they keep trying, they will likely carry a pregnancy to term . . . but she should act expediently".

PGT in a subsequent pregnancy would be discretionary, and while we acknowledge the policy of the RCOG that "There are currently insufficient data to support the routine use of PGT for aneuploidies (PGT-A) for couples with [otherwise] unexplained recurrent miscarriage, while the treatment may carry a significant cost and potential risk," we note also the belief of Kutteh et al. (2024) that "there is a clear role for PGT-A in RPL, especially in cases with recurrent POC aneuploidy." Liang et al. (2023) rehearse various factors that may influence the aneuploidy recurrence risk: maternal age, number of previous pregnancy losses, the estradiol level on the ovulation trigger day, and the blastocyst formation rate.

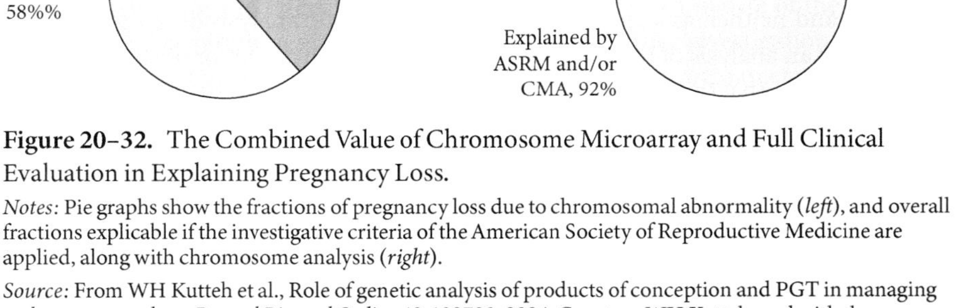

Figure 20–32. The Combined Value of Chromosome Microarray and Full Clinical Evaluation in Explaining Pregnancy Loss.

Notes: Pie graphs show the fractions of pregnancy loss due to chromosomal abnormality (*left*), and overall fractions explicable if the investigative criteria of the American Society of Reproductive Medicine are applied, along with chromosome analysis (*right*).

Source: From WH Kutteh et al., Role of genetic analysis of products of conception and PGT in managing early pregnancy loss, *Reprod Biomed Online* 49:103738, 2024. Courtesy WH Kutteh, and with the permission of Elsevier.

Chromosome Abnormality in the Couple. If a chromosomal rearrangement in one of the couple is identified, this will very probably be the underlying cause, but the possibility of a fortuitous discovery is not to be discounted. The precise nature of the rearrangement (consult the appropriate chapter), the reproductive history of any others in the family who have it, and the presence or absence of gynecological pathology allow one to make a judgment of its role in the etiology of the abortions. An offer of PGT at IVF, at a future planned pregnancy, may be very appropriate in order to reduce the likelihood of another miscarriage (Li et al. 2024c).

Recurrent Implantation Failure

A "failed embryo transfer" following IVF may be considered as a form of pregnancy loss not unlike that of the natural miscarriage of a wanted pregnancy. A distinction needs to be made between a parental versus an embryonic cause. A detailed format is offered by the European Society of Human Reproduction and Embryology (2023), which includes advice on immune, endocrine, hematologic, and other factors in the couple. Concerning the chromosomal question, while there is some controversy, this expert group nevertheless comments that " . . . where embryo testing is conducted by either array comparative genomic hybridization or NGS approaches on blastocyst biopsies . . . PGT for aneuploidies could be considered a good strategy for women with RIF, as a reduced number of embryo transfers [may be] required to achieve pregnancy and live birth"—a conclusion broadly supported in Mei et al. (2024). In other words, PGT is discretionary and potentially helpful, but with some reservation (Liu et al. 2024d).

Fetal Death In Utero, Stillbirth

Microarray analysis is useful in identifying a chromosomal cause (Martinez-Portilla et al. 2019). If such is discovered, appropriate genetic counseling can be provided according to the nature of the chromosomal finding.

Hydatidiform Mole

Having had one *complete mole*, the recurrence risk is 1%. But having had a second mole, the risk then rises to 1 in 4 (Eagles et al. 2015). Those suffering a second or third mole will often represent the rare category of a genetic predisposition due to maternal homozygosity for one of two known genes, *NLRP7* and *KHDC3L* (Rath et al. 2023). This latter group is recognized by every pregnancy being molar (Kalogiannidis et al. 2018). These repeating cases typically show biparental inheritance, in contradistinction to the androgenetic basis of the majority of moles. Ovum donation offers the best chance for parenthood.

The risk for recurrence of a *partial mole* is much less: "having a partial mole does not appear to significantly increase the risk of further hydatidiform mole in later pregnancies" (Eagles et al. 2015). If there is a recurrence, it will more likely be of the same type. In essence, the risk is largely that of a recurrent triploidy. Very rare exceptions with multiple recurrence exist, and presumably reflecting a different, yet to be clarified genetic basis (Filges et al. 2015; Guha Sarkar et al. 2022; Salima et al. 2023).

21
PRENATAL TESTING PROCEDURES

THE MEANS TO DIAGNOSE the fetal karyotype provides medical cytogenetics with one of its major areas of application. The discovery of an abnormality allows the option of termination of the pregnancy or, later in gestation, a more suitable obstetric management. The main indications for prenatal cytogenetic diagnosis are the following: (1) fetal anomaly detected on ultrasonography; (2) increased risk on maternal screening test; (3) parental heterozygosity for a chromosome rearrangement; (4) the birth of a previous child with a chromosome defect; (5) in the absence of other screening, the pregnant woman being of older childbearing age; and (6) opportunistic testing when prenatal sampling has occurred for single gene testing.

PRENATAL LABORATORY DIAGNOSTIC PROCEDURES

Prenatal diagnosis (PND) of chromosome disorders began in the early 1970s by the culturing of amniotic fluid cells obtained from amniocentesis at about 16 weeks of pregnancy, and analyzed according to classical methodology. A number of other approaches to PND have since been developed, ranging from preimplantation genetic testing (following in vitro fertilization) through chorion villus sampling (CVS), to the testing of cell-free DNA in maternal plasma.

Naturally, parents-to-be are anxious to have results as early as possible. A desire for an early result needs to be balanced against a number of considerations, which can include complexity of the procedure, both clinically and in the laboratory; procedural complication; reliability of results; cost; and the prior risk for a fetal abnormality. Four particular analytical procedures have enabled a faster return of results for common aneuploidies, compared with classical cytogenetics, namely FISH, QF-PCR, MLPA, and microarray analysis (and see also Chapter 2).

Fluorescence In Situ Hybridization

Fluorescence in situ hybridization (FISH) using multiple colored probes and targeting the chromosomes most prone to survivable aneuploidy (13, 18, 21, X, and Y) bypasses the need for culture, whether the cells are from amniotic fluid or CVS, and the result can be given within the space of one working day (Morris et al. 1999). By way of example, Feldman et al. (2000) applied amniotic fluid cell FISH to high-risk pregnancies (that is, with ultrasonographic abnormalities). They detected 14 cases of trisomy 21, 10 of trisomy 18, three of trisomy 13, four of monosomy X, and one triploid, in 4,193 samples over the period 1996–1998, for a total abnormality rate of 11%, and at a 24-hour turnaround.

Low Pass-Genome Sequencing

Low pass-genome sequencing (LP-GS) refers to genome sequencing performed at a lower average depth of coverage, specifically below 15× (Raca et al. 2023). LP-GS can be used to detect chromosome deletions and duplications with a resolution at least equivalent to microarray (Wang et al. 2020a), and with advantages in terms of workflow efficiency and scalability (Mighton et al. 2024). Importantly, the use of genomic sequencing for copy number detection provides the opportunity for a single streamlined platform for the detection of a broad range of genetic variants.

PRENATAL DIAGNOSTIC CLINICAL PROCEDURES

Chorionic Villus Sampling

Chorionic villus sampling (CVS) is typically a first-trimester procedure, the usual time being at 10–11 weeks gestation. The normal approach is transabdominal (transvaginal CVS was formerly used). The operator inserts a needle through the lower abdominal wall, under ultrasound guidance, to penetrate to the placental tissue; with gentle negative pressure on the syringe, a small amount of chorionic villus tissue is aspirated. (The expression "placental biopsy" could also be applied, although in practice this term is used when the testing is done in later pregnancy; see below). Compared with amniocentesis, the earlier period of diagnosis permitted by CVS may be seen as more useful in the setting of a higher genetic risk. If a genetic abnormality is identified and abortion is chosen prior to 14 weeks, this can be a more private matter, and the termination procedure is an operative intervention (curettage or suction evacuation of the uterus) (Verp et al. 1988). There is potential in CVS for diagnostic difficulty due to the occasional detection of confined placental mosaicism (which may, for some chromosomes, carry a risk also for uniparental disomy). Non-mosaic results for the common aneuploidies are, however, highly reliable (Smith et al. 1999). In experienced hands, there is a high degree of safety: A meta-analysis concluded that the risk of procedure-related miscarriage in women who had undergone CVS was only 0.22%, about 1 in 500 procedures (Akolekar et al. 2015).

Direct, Short-Term, and Long-Term Chorionic Villus Sampling. Chorionic villi can be analyzed directly (same day), after short-term culture (next day or two), or after long-term (a week or so) culture. For microarray analysis, DNA extracted from whole villi (uncultured cells) are typically used as the source of DNA, but "backup" cultures can be established that are available if the microarray fails, or if a microarray finding requires additional confirmation. For karyotype analysis, most laboratories offer only long-term CVS in which the mesenchymal core of the villus is the source of the analyzed cells. Trophoblast is the source of the cell population studied at direct and short-term CVS culture; these cells are no longer extant after the first few days in culture. DNA from uncultured CVS is likely to be derived from both cytotrophoblast and mesenchyme, and if mosaicism is detected in these samples, confirmation on cultured cells or amniocentesis should be considered.

In the early 1990s, there were disconcerting reports of an increased incidence of transverse limb deficiencies and tongue and jaw defects—"oromandibular-limb hypogenesis"—following early CVS (before 10 weeks, and especially up to 8 weeks). The association appeared likely to be causal, and one line of circumstantial evidence was that the rate of anomalies fell with increasing gestational stage from 9 to 11 weeks (Firth 1997). Various mechanisms were proposed: oligohydramnios, bradycardia, hypovolemia, thromboembolism, vasoconstriction, antibody-mediated reaction, and increased apoptosis following disruption of end arteries (Luijsterburg et al. 1997). Given these observations, it became normal practice for CVS not to be done earlier than 10 weeks.

Amniocentesis

Transabdominal amniocentesis from 15 weeks' gestation onwards, with culture of cells for chromosome analysis, has been the standard cytogenetic prenatal diagnostic procedure since the 1970s. It has a high degree of safety to both mother and fetus: Maternal complications or fetal injury due to direct trauma are practically unknown. The risk for maternal Rhesus immunization (Rh-negative mother, Rh-positive fetus) can be circumvented by administering an antibody injection. In their meta-analysis, Akolekar et al. (2015) concluded that the risk of procedure-related miscarriage in women who had undergone amniocentesis was 0.11%, about 1 in 1,000 procedures. The cytogenetic results are very reliable. The biological sources of error are, first, that maternal rather than fetal cells, or a mixture of both, are sampled. In practical terms, this rarely causes a problem. Second, fetal mosaicism may go undetected, since only a limited number of cells can feasibly be examined. Very few examples of this error are recorded.

Amniotic fluid culture has a high success rate. If amniotic cells fail to grow for no obvious reason, there may be a substantial risk for fetal aneuploidy. Reid et al. (1996) followed up 42 failures (1%) among 4,134 amniocenteses. Complete information could be obtained on all but one of these 42 cases. Karyotyping was ultimately done in most (78%) of these failed cases, and of these, 19% revealed an abnormality (compared with a 4% abnormality rate in the whole material). The clear lesson from these studies is that women having had a failed amniocentesis culture should be offered careful review and retesting. Prior cell culture is not necessary for microarray analysis but, as with CVS, "backup" cultures may be established for use only if the microarray fails or if an abnormal microarray result requires confirmation or additional analysis. As with CVS, DNA from uncultured cells may provide a more accurate picture than from cultured cells, due to chromosomally abnormal cells being selected-against in vitro or being more prone to fail in culture.

The obvious disadvantage of amniocentesis is that the results are not available until about 16–18 weeks. If the reason for the amniocentesis had been an abnormality on second-trimester ultrasound, the procedure may not be done until 18–20 weeks, aggravating this difficulty. The outlook for the long-term health of the child does not differ between CVS and amniocentesis (Schaap et al. 2002).

Noninvasive Prenatal Testing Using Cell-Free DNA from Maternal Blood

Noninvasive prenatal testing (NIPT) for fetal aneuploidy detection, using cell-free DNA from maternal blood, has been used in the clinical setting since 2012. Although in reality

NIPT is a screening test (some write NIPS) rather than a diagnostic test, in practical terms it is such a good test that we are considering it separately from other screening modalities.

Cell-free DNA (cfDNA) testing takes advantage of the fact that everyone has free DNA (i.e., not within the nucleus of cells) circulating in the bloodstream, and in pregnant women a proportion of that DNA is derived from the fetus. Or more specifically, it is derived from the placenta, and in fact from apoptosing cells of the cytotrophoblast. This is the "fetal fraction" of the maternal sample which, in the late first trimester of pregnancy, typically comprises approximately 10% of the whole (Becking et al. 2024). cfDNA can be analyzed by short-read sequencing, using either whole-genome analysis or by methods that target specific chromosomes, and can also be quantified by microarray (Stokowski et al. 2015). Although it is possible to distinguish fetal DNA from maternal DNA through single nucleotide polymorphisms (SNPs) within the cfDNA sample, most methodologies simply measure the total amount of DNA (i.e., maternal and fetal contribution) derived from each chromosome, and compare each chromosome with other chromosomes within the sample.

For example, in a euploid pregnancy with fetal fraction of 10%, for each chromosome the total amount of DNA is 90% maternal and 10% fetal. In the setting of a Down syndrome pregnancy, the fetal contribution from chromosome 21 increases by 50%, as there are now three copies of fetal chromosome 21 instead of the normal two. The relative excess in chromosome 21 cfDNA fragments will be $(0.9 \times 2) + (0.1 \times 3) = 2.1$, compared with the normal for a euploid fetus of $(0.9 \times 2) + (0.1 \times 2) = 2.0$. The relative increase in the number of chromosome 21 counts is therefore only 5% ($2.1/2.0 = 1.05$). The fact that such a small difference can be measured accurately is testament to the power of short-read sequencers as a molecular counting tool.

NIPT for the Common Trisomies. NIPT using cfDNA for trisomies 21, 13, and 18 has very high sensitivity and specificity (Table 21–1). A related and possibly more relevant measure of test accuracy is the positive predictive value (PPV), which equates to the proportion of women with an abnormal result who actually do have an aneuploid fetus. The PPV incorporates the pretest likelihood that the aneuploidy is present, and therefore increases with maternal age. Even when an NIPT test has very high sensitivity and specificity, in a young woman with low pretest risk of having an aneuploid fetus, the PPV for a rare aneuploidy such as trisomy 13 will be low. Estimates of PPV for common aneuploidies detected by NIPT at different maternal ages are presented in Table 21–2, and they serve as a useful reminder that high-risk NIPT results should always be followed up

Table 21–1. Sensitivity and Specificity of NIPT for Common Aneuploidies

ANEUPLOIDY	SENSITIVITY (%)	SPECIFICITY (%)
Trisomy 21	99.4	99.9
Trisomy 18	97.7	99.9
Trisomy 13	90.6	100

Source: The meta-analysis of A Mackie, Using cell-free fetal DNA as a diagnostic and screening test: current understanding and uncertainties, *BJOG* 124:47, 2017.

Table 21–2. Positive Predictive Values of NIPT Results at Different Maternal Ages

	PPV (%) AT MATERNAL AGES			
ANEUPLOIDY	25 YEARS	30 YEARS	35 YEARS	40 YEARS
Trisomy 13	7	10	21	50
Trisomy 18	15	21	39	69
Trisomy 21	51	61	79	93

Source: The online calculator at htpp://secure.itswebs.com/nsgc/niptcalculator/index.html which uses sensitivity and specificity from Gil et al. (2015).

with an invasive test. Any decision to terminate a pregnancy should not be based upon positive NIPT results alone.

While early trials focused on women from high-risk groups, more recent studies have demonstrated the clinical utility of NIPT in low-risk and average-risk women Although the use of NIPT in low-risk women is associated with a lower PPV than for higher-risk women, leading to more false-positive results, NIPT still outperforms conventional screening by a very considerable margin (Gregg et al. 2016).

NIPT for Other Trisomies. It is technically straightforward to expand NIPT to autosomes other than 13, 18, and 21, and in fact NIPT methods that use whole-genome sequencing already collect the necessary sequencing data. But the clinical utility of this information is not clear. Non-mosaic whole chromosome aneuploidy, other than the three common aneuploidies, typically results in fetal loss. In an ongoing pregnancy, the trisomic cells are often mosaic and confined to the placenta, and detection of these abnormalities may lead to parental anxiety and unnecessary diagnostic procedures. That is not to say that the detection of these "Rare Autosomal Trisomy" (RATs) might not be without clinical benefit. Finding a RAT at NIPT has been seen with more pregnancy complication (Lannoo et al. 2024) and, in rare instances, discovery of certain aneuploidies might have direct implication for the pregnancy—one example being the detection of trisomy 15 in cfDNA leading to the diagnosis of Prader-Willi syndrome due to uniparental disomy of chromosome 15 (Hong et al. 2023). Nevertheless, as of 2023, the American College of Medical Genetics and Genomics has recommended against screening for autosomal aneuploidies other than 13, 18, and 21 (Dungan et al 2023).

NIPT for Sex Chromosome Aneuploidies. NIPT for sex chromosome aneuploidies has a detection rate of >90% and a PPV of approximately 50%, similarly to the other common aneuploidies (Shear et al. 2023) (Table 21–3). But caution is needed Sex chromosome aneuploidies are more common than autosomal, in one series being detected in 1 in 272 amniocentesis samples (Forabosco et al. 2009). In consequence, inclusion of sex chromosome aneuploidies in an NIPT test will increase the overall number of invasive tests and the number of samples yielding a false-positive result. The phenotypes in the common sex chromosome abnormalities are typically much less severe than autosomal aneuploidies, and in some cases may not be clinically apparent (as discussed in the following Chapter 22). On the other hand, early identification of sex chromosome abnormalities might allow post-natal management to be optimized, with potential long-term benefit to the affected child (Martin et al. 2023). Careful pretest counseling should accompany NIPT for sex chromosome abnormalities, and some pregnant women may choose to restrict testing to autosomal trisomies.

Table 21–3. Sensitivity, Specificity and PPV of NIPT for Sex Chromosome Aneuploidies

ANEUPLOIDY	SENSITIVITY (%)	SPECIFICITY (%)	PPV (%)
Monosomy X	98.8	99.4	14.5%*
47,XXY	100	100	97.7
47,XXX	100	99.9	61.6
47,XYY	100	100	100

Note: These data are derived from pregnancies at high pretest risk for aneuploidy, and may not be generalizable to average-risk pregnancies. PPV = positive predictive value.
*The use of a paired-end cfDNA sequencing assay differentiates short (placental) from long (maternal) cfDNA fragments, and can improve the PPV for monosomy X to >60%, by removing false-positive calls associated with maternal monosomy X mosaicism (Scarff et al. 2023).
Source: The systematic review and meta-analysis of MA Shear et al., A systematic review and meta-analysis of cell-free DNA testing for detection of fetal sex chromosome aneuploidy, *Prenat Diagn* 43:133–143, 2023.

NIPT for Microdeletions, Microduplications, and Copy Number Variants. NIPT can be extended to detect microdeletions such as those of 1p36, 15q11q13, and 22q11.2. These microdeletions are associated with severe phenotypes, and on that basis they are appropriate for prenatal screening. NIPT can detect some microdel/dups with high sensitivity and low false-positive rate; but a concern is that, false-positive results will accumulate as greater proportions of the genome are analyzed, leading to unnecessary invasive tests (Gregg et al. 2016). Improved sequencing and analytical techniques may assuage this concern. Lefkowitz et al. (2016) retrospectively analyzed 1,166 NIPT samples, including 42 known to harbor CNVs: All but one of the 42 CNVs were detected and there was only one false-positive result, attesting to the feasibility of whole-genome CNV analysis using cfDNA. Zaninović et al. (2022) found rather wide ranges of reported sensitivity (from 20% to 100%), specificity (from 82% to 100%), and PPV (from 3% to 100%). Reflecting these uncertainties, the American College of Medical Genetics and Genomics recommended in 2023 offering NIPT for 22q11.2 deletion syndrome, but not for other CNVs (Dungan et al. 2023), whereas the American College of Obstetricians and Gynecologists (2020) does not support NIPT for any CNV.

False-Positive and False-Negative NIPT Results. Cell-free fetal DNA is, as noted above, placental in origin, and so NIPT by cfDNA shares the major pitfall of CVS, namely being susceptible to confined placental mosaicism (CPM; see Chapter 22). False-positive results due to CPM cannot be overcome by technical improvements (Brady et al. 2016). Accepting that NIPT results are, in principle, concordant with CVS findings, amniocentesis may be necessary to confirm that the aneuploidy is (if this is the case) confined to the placenta. In the event that NIPT shows trisomy for an imprintable chromosome, testing for uniparental disomy should be considered if amniocentesis is chosen.

Early and undetected co-twin demise ("vanished twin") may lead to a false-positive test result (Brady et al. 2016). Chromosome abnormalities are common in vanished twins, and the involuting placenta of an aneuploid vanished twin may continue to release aneuploid DNA into the maternal bloodstream for weeks after demise. Using an SNP-based technology to identify fetal haplotypes, Curnow et al. (2015) were able to identify haplotypes from a vanished twin in 0.18% of pregnancies tested, with fetal demise having occurred between two weeks and eight weeks prior to maternal blood sampling.

CNVs or mosaic aneuploidy in the mother may affect test interpretation. Unidentified maternal sex chromosome mosaicism (45,X/46,XX or 47,XXX/46,XX) is an important cause of false-positive NIPT results for sex chromosome abnormalities (Wang et al. 2014b). We have also found Y chromosome material in maternal DNA, which has led to a high-risk result for sex chromosome aneuploidy in the fetus. Less commonly, mosaicism in the mother for other chromosomes or chromosome segments can mislead (Brady et al. 2016). If NIPT is extended to CNVs, the possibility of unidentified CNVs being present in the mother and detected by NIPT will need to be considered, both in pretest counseling and in interpretation of results.

A particularly devastating cause of aneuploidy detectable in cfDNA is *maternal malignancy*. Ji et al. (2019) identified 41 cases of occult malignancy from a series of 1.93 million NIPT samples. Maternal malignancies were typically associated with a "tumor-like" aneuploidy profile, comprising copy number gains and losses across multiple chromosomes (a pattern that is unlikely to be mistaken for fetal aneuploidy). Heesterbeek et al. (2024) provide guidelines for the management of pregnant women who receive these challenging results.

Follow-Up Procedures Following Abnormal NIPT Results. Invasive testing is recommended to confirm a high-risk cfDNA finding, with CVS the preferred modality, in order to allow for a more timely return of results. In a minority of cases, the CVS result will be mosaic, and this will necessitate a second procedure (namely amniocentesis) in order to distinguish CPM from true fetal mosaicism. If mosaicism is likely, there is an argument for bypassing CVS and using amniocentesis as the first-line invasive test.

Grati et al. (2015) address this question by estimating the frequency with which a CVS, done after a high-risk cfDNA result, would need a follow-up amniocentesis due to suspected placental mosaicism. The authors did not actually do cfDNA testing, but rather modeled data based on results from more than 50,000 CVS karyotypes obtained from cytotrophoblast (direct preparation) and mesenchyme (long-term culture), and followed by confirmatory amniocentesis. Central to this modeling was the assumption that the fetal fraction of cfDNA originates mainly from the cytotrophoblast layer of the chorionic villus; and so, as noted above, the cfDNA test result should be concordant with direct rather than long-term cultures. The findings, along with the likelihood of mosaic CVS results being confirmed by amniocentesis, are shown in Table 21–4. Based on these interpretations, CVS is the recommended procedure following a high-risk cfDNA result for trisomy 21 or trisomy 18, but with the caveat of a 2%–4% risk of an inconclusive result, which would require a follow-up amniocentesis. For trisomy 13 and monosomy X, the benefit of an early diagnosis by CVS is to be balanced against the likelihood of an inconclusive result with an amniocentesis then needed (and ultrasonography may in any event have been clarifying).

NIPT for Twin Pregnancies. Judah et al. (2021) reviewed NIPT data for nearly 8,000 twin pregnancies for a meta-analysis. The performance of cfDNA testing for trisomy 21 in twin pregnancy was slightly less than that reported in singleton pregnancy (Table 21–5), but was nonetheless clearly superior to that of the first-trimester combined test or second-trimester biochemical testing. For trisomies 18 and 13, the detection rates were slightly lower than for singleton pregnancies, but confidence intervals were wide due to the smaller number of cases. The authors conclude that parents can be counseled

Table 21–4. Follow-Up Scenarios after a High-Risk cfDNA Result
Likelihood of Mosaicism at CVS Following High-Risk cfDNA Results for Common Aneuploidies, and Likelihood of Mosaicism at CVS Being Confirmed by Amniocentesis

ANEUPLOIDY	LIKELIHOOD THAT A HIGH-RISK cfDNA RESULT WILL BE FOLLOWED BY DETECTION OF MOSAICISM AT CVS (%)	LIKELIHOOD THAT A MOSAIC CVS RESULT WILL BE CONFIRMED BY AMNIOCENTESIS (%)
Trisomy 21	2	44
Trisomy 18	4	14
Trisomy 13	22	4
Monosomy X	59	26

CVS, chorion villus sampling.
Source: FR Grati et al., The type of feto-placental aneuploidy detected by cfDNA testing may influence the choice of confirmatory diagnostic procedure, *Prenat Diagn* 35:994–998, 2015.

that cfDNA testing in twin pregnancy is mainly useful in screening for trisomy 21, but that there is uncertainty concerning trisomies 18 and 13.

Experimental, Less Used, or Former Technologies

EARLY AMNIOCENTESIS

In the late 1980s, early (10–13 weeks) amniocentesis was proposed as an alternative to CVS. In a carefully controlled comparison, Nicolaides et al. (1994) found a 2%–3% additional fetal loss rate in early amniocentesis, and possibly a higher incidence of talipes among subsequently born children. Daniel et al. (1998), comparing 10–14 week procedures with 15 weeks and upward, observed that the early amniocentesis samples were not quite as satisfactory; multiple needle insertions were more often required; and the pregnancy loss rate was greater. On the whole, the differences were not great, other than the loss rate of 2.2% in the early group compared with 0.6% in the mid-trimester group. Similar figures were reported in Collins et al. (1998). In the Canadian Early and Midtrimester Amniocentesis Trial, the findings for 11wk 0d through to 13wk 6d were somewhat more disconcerting, with more complications and a higher culture failure rate (Delisle and Wilson 1999). The procedure is rarely undertaken now.

Table 21–5. Performance of cfDNA testing for Common Trisomies in Twin Pregnancies

	AFFECTED PREGNANCIES (N)	DETECTION RATE (%)	FALSE POSITIVE RATE (%)
Trisomy 21	137	99.0	0.02
Trisomy 18	50	92.8	0.01
Trisomy 13	11	94.7	0.10

Source: H Judah et al., Cell-free DNA testing of maternal blood in screening for trisomies in twin pregnancy: updated cohort study at 10–14 weeks and meta-analysis, *Ultrasound Obstet Gynecol* 58:178–189, 2021.

FETAL BLOOD SAMPLING

Fetal blood is aspirated by direct puncture of a blood vessel, usually in the umbilical cord (cordocentesis). The risk of fetal loss from the procedure is ~1% (Kosian et al. 2023). Before FISH analysis of uncultured cells (see above) came to be more widely used, cordocentesis was useful when speed of diagnosis was of the essence, in the setting of the detection of a fetal anomaly at ~18-week ultrasonography. The procedure once had a role in assisting resolution of mosaicism in amniotic fluid culture (Shalev et al. 1994), but this was largely replaced by the use of FISH.

PLACENTAL BIOPSY

In principle, this is the same as first-trimester CVS. The placenta is sampled by a transabdominal approach, and this is a straightforward procedure. The main application had been when a rapid result was needed, although newer methodologies have largely bypassed that imperative. An insufficient amount of amniotic fluid remains an indication.

FETAL CELL ISOLATION FROM MATERNAL BLOOD

In 1969, Walknowska et al. identified cells with a male karyotype during the cytogenetic analysis of lymphocyte cultures from pregnant women, and they recognized the potential to use these cells for prenatal diagnosis. The two important cell types that are released from the fetal tissue into the maternal circulation are the nucleated red blood cell and the trophoblast[2] (Dhallan et al. 2007; Maron and Bianchi 2007). Fetal cells circulating in maternal blood are an obvious target for noninvasive prenatal diagnosis, yet with a concentration of only one fetal cell in each 2–3 ml of maternal blood (Kølvraa et al. 2016), isolation is difficult. For this reason, cell-based NIPT approaches have fallen somewhat out of favor, particularly with the successful implementation of NIPT approaches that use cfDNA. Nonetheless, researchers continue to explore the potential of fetal cell–based techniques. A number of different techniques have been used to isolate fetal cells from maternal blood, after which various genetic methodologies can be applied, including FISH, PCR, whole-genome amplification, and short-read sequencing.

CELOCENTESIS

The extra-embryonic celom, which exists only during the first trimester, is a source for (non-dividing) cells originating from extra-embryonic mesoderm. Given its anatomical continuity with the cytotrophoblast, Makrydimas et al. (2006) comment that it could be thought of as "a liquid extension of the placenta." Celocentesis involves the transvaginal insertion of a needle into the celomic cavity and aspiration of 1mL fluid containing cells of fetal origin. The procedure has the attraction of an earlier timing (7–9 weeks) than CVS and NIPT, but so far its use has been limited by uncertainty about the safety of the technique, the low amount of DNA recovered, and by high levels of maternal cell contamination (Giambona et al. 2016). In practice, celocentesis has usually been applied for the early prenatal diagnosis of monogenic conditions, in particular hemoglobinopathies. Giambona et al. (2018) undertook celocentesis and isolated fetal cells from a large series of women whose pregnancies were at risk of thalassemia or sickle cell disease QF-PCR

[2] Fetal lymphocytes can also be isolated from the maternal circulation, but they can persist for many years, making them unsuitable for prenatal diagnosis.

for chromosomes 13, 18, 21, X, and Y was done primarily for the purpose of detecting maternal cell contamination, but also diagnosed pregnancies that were affected by trisomy 21, trisomy 13, and triploidy.

CYSTIC HYGROMA, PLEURAL EFFUSION, AND ASCITES

Cystic hygroma and fetal hydrops have a strong association with fetal aneuploidy, especially monosomy X. A concomitant oligohydramnios may make amniocentesis difficult. Fluid from cystic hygroma, ascites, and pleural effusion contains lymphocytes, and these cells can be analyzed using cytogenetic or molecular techniques within the time frame of a few days. In one small series of 14 pregnancies affected by hydrops, samples were collected from pleural fluid (n = 4), cystic hygroma (n = 5), and ascites (n = 6), and two cases of monosomy X were detected (Gole et al. 1997).

CERVICAL LAVAGE OR CYTOBRUSH

Trophoblast cells can migrate from the confines of the uterine cavity and enter the endocervical canal, and they can be collected for molecular analysis by endocervical irrigation and aspiration (lavage), or by insertion of a "cytobrush" (Bischoff and Simpson 2006). The attraction, in principle, is of diagnosis as early as five weeks, and a (relatively) noninvasive procedure. Cells of maternal origin outnumber fetal cells at a ratio of 2000:1 (Imudia et al. 2009), but fetal cells can be isolated by incubating with specifically binding antibodies attached to magnetic particles. Fetal cells are then separated with a magnet and subjected to molecular analysis (Fritz et al. 2015).

PROTEOMIC FINGERPRINTING

Proteomic fingerprinting of amniotic fluid assesses the expression profile of proteins coded from specific chromosomes, or otherwise expressed in the context of a specific aneuploidy, and this could be considered as a functional assay for trisomy (Vasani and Kumar 2019).

"PRIMUM NON NOCERE" AND PRACTICAL CONSIDERATIONS

"First, do no harm" is a cornerstone of medical practice. Yet, almost inevitably, having a prenatal diagnostic procedure causes anxiety. Rothman (1988), in her book *The Tentative Pregnancy*, is particularly critical of what she viewed as a medicalized distortion of the normal process of being pregnant. Hodge (1989) describes her personal experience of *Waiting for the Amniocentesis*, and we reproduce her letter in full:

> I drafted the following letter to the editor one week before I expected to hear the results of my amniocentesis:
>
> "I am 40 years old and 19 weeks pregnant with what will presumably be my third child. I am on the basic science faculty of a medical school. When I teach medical students about amniocentesis, I occasionally mention the difficulty for the woman of having to wait until well into the second trimester to receive her results.
>
> "I am in that situation myself now, awaiting my results. And before experiencing it, I was unprepared for two phenomena. One was just how difficult the wait is. Pregnancy is always a time of waiting, but now time has slowed down to an extent

I did not anticipate. The other, more disturbing phenomenon is how the waiting has affected my attitude toward the pregnancy. At many levels I deny that I really am pregnant "until after we get the results." I ignore the flutterings and kicks I feel; I talk of "if" rather than "when" the baby comes; I am reluctant to admit to others that I am pregnant. I dream frequently and grimly about second-trimester abortions. In some sense I am holding back on "bonding" with this child-to-be. This represents an unanticipated negative side effect of diagnostic amniocentesis. And all this, even though my risk of carrying a chromosomal abnormality is less than 2 percent.

"I presume I am not alone in these reactions, yet I have not seen this problem mentioned in the literature, nor did my physician or genetic counselor discuss it with me. I am writing now to bring it to the attention of clinicians with pregnant patients undergoing diagnostic amniocentesis. I suggest to both clinicians and their patients that, when weighing the relative risk and benefits of prenatal diagnosis performed later (amniocentesis) as compared with earlier (chorionic villus biopsy), they not underestimate the negative effects of a 4½ month wait before the woman knows if she is 'really' pregnant."

The next day, before I had mailed this letter, I received the results, and unfortunately they were the dreaded ones: trisomy 21. I have since then had the grim second-trimester abortion. From my current perspective of grief and shock, I encourage clinicians to help their patients avoid the denial described in my letter. My husband and I spared ourselves no pain by holding back emotionally. It has become a cultural expectation that one will keep one's pregnancy a secret until one has had the "all clear" from the amnio. One reasons, "If we get a bad result, we won't have to tell anyone." But I now believe that reasoning is wrong. After our bad result, my husband and I did tell everyone. Sympathy and support from our friends, family, and colleagues have helped us to survive the ordeal of aborting a wanted pregnancy. By keeping the loss a secret, we would have cut ourselves off from such support when the feared outcome did happen.

Not every couple will react this way, some preferring to keep their personal affairs private, but many will. The counselor needs to acknowledge these criticisms and to rise to the challenge of providing a sympathetic and skillful service to clients/patients according to their varying responses to deciding to have, undergoing, and waiting for the results of prenatal diagnosis, and then supporting those who do get an abnormal result.

Quite a few pregnant women are in any event against invasive prenatal testing. In a study of pregnant women (age 37 years or older) who had not undergone prenatal diagnosis in Victoria, Australia, 33% had actively declined, with the two main reasons being concern about the safety of the test and a conviction that they would not in any event have a termination (Halliday et al. 2001). Hill et al. (2016) studied preferences for prenatal tests for Down syndrome in nine countries, and found that pregnant women placed greatest emphasis on test safety and risk of miscarriage when choosing a prenatal test. In contrast, for health professionals, test accuracy was the most important factor in determining choice of prenatal test.

A practical question is pain: The thought of insertion of a needle or of a catheter sufficiently deeply to sample a pregnancy would naturally be cause for some apprehension. Csaba et al. (2006) surveyed a number of women having prenatal diagnosis in New York, asking them to quantify their anxiety ahead of the procedure (transabdominal CVS, transcervical CVS, or amniocentesis), and their perception of pain immediately afterward.

In each procedure, the pain was typically seen as "mild," and three-fourths of the women thought it was the same or less painful than they had been expecting. Those who were more anxious—mostly the younger and nulliparous—felt the pain more keenly, and thus special reassurance should be given to these women.

SCREENING FOR FETAL TRISOMY

In broad terms, "screening" describes testing a whole population, or a whole segment of population, for a condition that in fact only a (typically small) fraction will have. This criterion applies to pregnancy screening for Down syndrome (DS) or other trisomy. All, or at least many pregnant women in a population may be tested, but only a very few will turn out actually to have an affected pregnancy. A requirement of a screened condition is that the condition be well understood, and that an intervention be available. More precisely, screening in this context should meet three criteria: It should identify women who are at increased risk, prior to their having a definitive diagnostic test; it should be offered systematically to pregnant women who are considered to be at only baseline population risk; and it should be viewed as beneficial to those who receive it, in terms of either choosing termination or being prepared for the birth of a child with DS (Weisz and Rodeck 2006).

Until the implementation of NIPT, the screening tools used were the taking of a maternal blood sample and the performing of an ultrasonogram, and these methods remain in use. The methodology involves the analysis of data (maternal age, serum measurements, ultrasound findings) according to a sophisticated computed algorithm, in order to calculate a risk that the fetus is affected by DS. If the calculated risk is greater than that of a certain threshold risk figure (usually taken as 1 in 250), the pregnancy is regarded as being at "increased risk," and definitive testing is then offered. Since other aneuploidies can also influence the measured indices, the test procedure in practice becomes broader than just a trisomy 21 screen.

First-Trimester and Second-Trimester Biochemical Screening

Certain biochemical markers in the mother's serum may have altered concentrations, whether increased or decreased, if she is carrying a trisomic pregnancy; presumably, these differences reflect perturbation in the trisomic fetoplacental unit. An assessment is made of the degree to which each level differs from expectation, and these data are factored into an algorithm that takes into account the prior risk due to maternal age (Spencer 2007). Sophisticated computer packages are employed to calculate an overall risk figure.

The two first-trimester analytes most commonly measured are the β component of human chorionic gonadotropin (β-hCG) and pregnancy-associated plasma protein-A (PAPP-A), the former typically high and the latter low in a DS pregnancy. PAPP-A levels are influenced by mode of conception, being lower in pregnancies that are conceived using in vitro fertilization and leading to a higher rate of false-positive results in first-trimester screening for DS in these pregnancies (Amor et al. 2009). In the second trimester, the analytes measured in many jurisdictions comprise α-fetoprotein (AFP), estriol, β-hCG, and inhibin-A (four analytes; hence, the "quadruple test"[3]). In trisomy 21, the AFP is low, hCG high, uE3 low, and inhibin-A high.

With the increased uptake of noninvasive prenatal testing for DS, the question has arisen whether biochemical screening has a role in pregnancies that are also being screened by NIPT. Two arguments have been made in favor of retaining biochemical screening. The first is that although biochemical screening is aimed primarily at the detection of DS, in fact a range of other chromosome abnormalities may be seen, many of which would not be picked up on NIPT. The risk of a rare chromosome abnormality has been estimated to be 4% when PAPP-A levels are very low (<0.2 multiple of median [MoM]), and 7% when free β-hCG levels are very low (<0.2 MoM) (Petersen et al. 2014). Although it has also been argued, on the other hand, that the specific screening algorithms had not been set up for the purpose of finding rare chromosome abnormalities, and that using this screening to cast a wider net might have only a marginal benefit in terms of detection of other abnormalities but would yet imply a significant increase in the false-positive rate (Yaron et al. 2016).

The second argument in favor of retaining biochemical screening is that abnormal serum biochemistry, and particularly low levels of PAPP-A and free β-hCG, can give warning of third-trimester pregnancy complications such as pre-eclampsia, intrauterine growth restriction, and preterm birth (Sovio et al. 2024; Peris et al. 2024).

First-Trimester Ultrasonographic Screening

Ultrasonographic scanning is applied during the window of 11–14 weeks inclusive. This particular parameter is assessed: the degree to which the skin at the neck is separated from the underlying tissue by fluid (Figure 21–1). Since this fluid does not reflect the sound wave on the scan, it is referred to as "nuchal translucency"; "nuchal thickening" is another expression. Bekker et al. (2006) propose that the underlying cause is anomalous development of the lymphatic system in the region of the neck, and it appears that this development is susceptible to a chromosomal imbalance. An increased nuchal translucency is associated with DS, and combined with maternal age the detection rate is 69%–75%, for a false-positive rate of 5%–8% (Rink and Norton 2016). An increase in nuchal translucency is not specific to DS, being also observed in trisomy 13, trisomy 18, monosomy X, and triploidy. Bardi et al. (2020) have assessed various risks in the setting of the specific finding of an increased nuchal translucency, and these are summarized in Table 21–6. Other ultrasonographic markers of DS are absence of the fetal nasal bone, tricuspid regurgitation, and abnormal blood flow in the ductus venosus (Rao and Platt 2016).

A practical question is this: If, following the observation of an increased nuchal translucency a CVS or amniocentesis is done, and the chromosomes are normal, is there a residual risk for some other type of fetal abnormality? The main two risk categories are for single-gene disorders and fetal structural abnormalities. If the translucency resolves, and if no defects (with particular focus on the fetal heart) are seen at 14–16 weeks gestation, the prognosis is good, with a better than 95% chance of a baby with no major abnormalities. In fetuses with nuchal translucency ≥3.5 mm at 11–14 weeks gestation, normal microarray, and no other abnormalities on subsequent scans, the chance of a diagnostic variant on exome sequencing is only 2%, but is higher for nuchal translucencies ≥5 mm.

[3] The "double test" uses AFP and estriol; the "triple test" is AFP, estriol, and β-hCG.

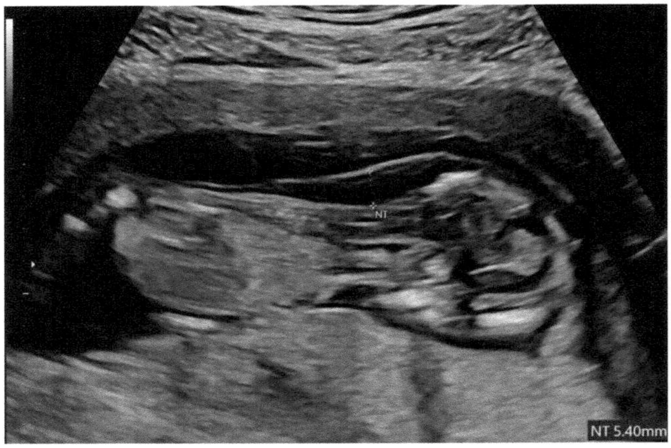

Figure 21-1. Nuchal Translucency.

Notes: Ultrasound image shows lateral view of the fetus. The two + markers delineate the degree of separation of the nuchal skin, in this case, 5.40 mm. Courtesy C Siles.

In the presence of additional ultrasound findings, the likelihood of a diagnostic variant increases to >20% (Mellis et al. 2022). Noonan syndrome or other "RASopathy" require consideration, accounting for about half of single-gene disorders in fetuses with a large nuchal translucency and normal karyotype (Bardi et al. 2020).

On the question of neurodevelopment, Hellmuth et al. (2017) followed up more than 220,000 euploid children who had been screened in the first trimester, and they found a sixfold increased risk of intellectual disability in children with a nuchal translucency above the 99th centile, although the absolute risk remained low (<1%). Buffin et al. (2021) followed up a cohort of 203 chromosomally normal infants with nuchal translucency >95th centile and 208 controls to age two years: They found that the developmental quotient (DQ) was slightly lower (108.6) in the increased nuchal translucency

Table 21-6. Implications of an Increased Nuchal Translucency

NUCHAL TRANSLUCENCY	TRISOMY 13/18/21 (%)	OTHER CHROMOSOMAL (%)	SINGLE GENE (%)*	STRUCTURAL ANOMALY (%)**	ALL ABNORMAL FETUSES (%)
95–99th centile	13	2.2	0.6	5.9	21
>99th centile	34	12	3.3	12	62
3.5–4.9 mm	25	6	1.2	11	43
5.0–6.4 mm	44	17	5.5	11	77
6.5-7.9 mm	51	12	2.6	17	83
≥8.0 mm	34	23	7.4	14	79

Notes: These data are based on 1901 pregnancies with NT ≥ 95th centile in the Netherlands, 2010–2016.
* 50% of single-gene disorders were Noonan syndrome, and the other 50% were various rare syndromes.
** The most common structural anomalies were cardiac (42%), multiple congenital anomalies (16%), urogenital (11%) and skeletal (7%).

Source: From F Bardi et al., Is there still a role for nuchal translucency measurement in the changing paradigm of first trimester screening? *Prenat Diagn* 40:197–205, 2020.

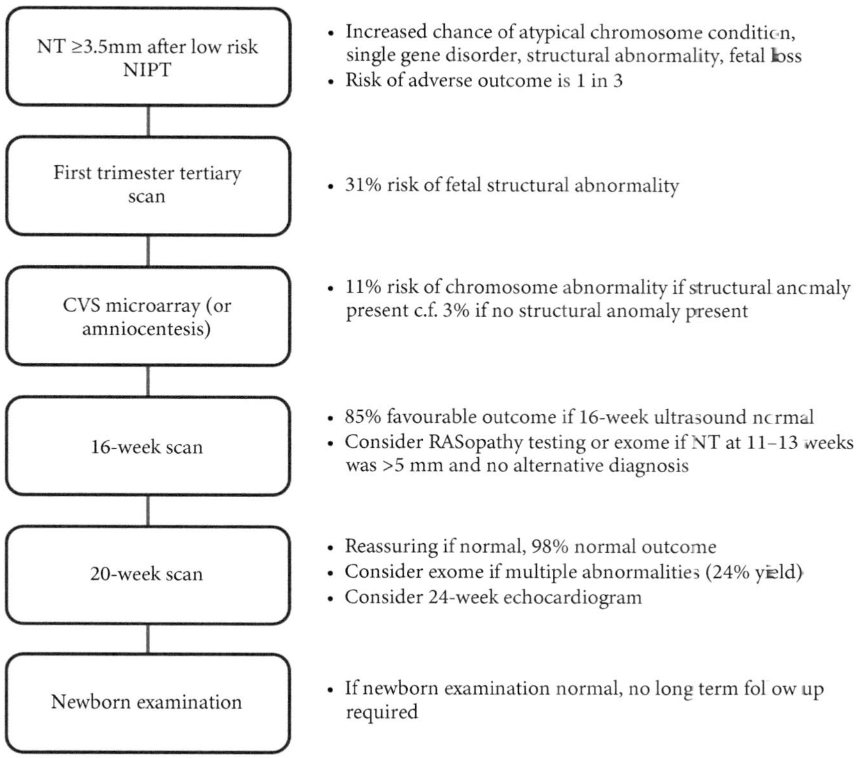

Figure 21–2. Interpreting an Increased Nuchal Translucency when NIPT has been Normal.

Notes: A flow diagram of diagnostic pathway for increased nuchal translucency and low-risk non-invasive prenatal testing

Source: Adapted from J Kelley et al., Increased nuchal translucency after low-risk noninvasive prenatal testing: What should we tell prospective parents? *Prenat Diagn* 41:1305–1315, 2021.

group compared to controls (112.8); however, both results were well within the expected range for age, and only one child in the increased nuchal translucency group had a DQ in the significantly impaired range of <70.

An increased nuchal translucency may also be detected after a low-risk NIPT result. Kelley et al. (2021) rehearse the key counseling points that apply here, noting that the chance of an adverse outcome increases with the nuchal translucency measurement size and the presence of other abnormalities on ultrasound. A summary of their approach is presented in Figure 21–2.

First-Trimester Combined Ultrasonography and Biochemical Screening

A better detection is achieved through a combination of first-trimester nuchal translucency assessment and the measurement of maternal serum-free β-hCG and PAPP-A. If the blood test is done first, these results can be held pending the ultrasound, and the combined figure can be available soon after the scan is done. Detection rates are typically >90%, for a false-positive rate of 5% or less (Santorum et al. 2017). The validity of this approach in more precisely targeting an increased-risk population is attested in the experience from Denmark, where a national program was put in place in 2004. The number of diagnostic procedures (amniocentesis or CVS) declined from 7,524 in 2000 to 3,510 in 2006; and yet, during the same period, the number of newborns with DS fell from approximately 50 to 30 per year (Ekelund et al. 2008).

While the prime focus of screening is on trisomy 21, a side benefit is the detection of other, and typically more severe, chromosomal disorders. Trisomy 13 and trisomy 18 both show reduced levels of β-hCG and PAPP-A at first-trimester screening, more so in trisomy 18, along with increased nuchal translucency or frank cystic hygroma. Few other trisomic pregnancies proceed through to the time of screening. Unsurprisingly, those that do so display abnormalities at screening. For example, in trisomy 22 at first-trimester screening, the β-hCG is very elevated, PAPP-A somewhat reduced, and fetal growth restriction is typical (Sifakis et al. 2008). In non-mosaic trisomy 9, the biochemistry is similar to that of trisomy 18 (Priola et al. 2007), and the same may apply in the mosaic case. In a triploid pregnancy, the biochemical indices at first-trimester screening are also quite abnormal, and very differently so according to the category of triploidy, digynic or diandric (p. 343). In the digynic form, β-hCG and PAPP-A are both much reduced, whereas in the diandric type, β-hCG is greatly elevated and PAPP-A marginally reduced. Likewise, ultrasonography is distinctly different, with severe growth restriction in the digynic type, and nearer normal growth but with an enlarged and partially molar placenta in diandric triploidy (Kagan et al. 2008).

Second-Trimester Ultrasonography

A fetal anatomic survey in the second trimester may lead to the diagnosis of DS through the detection of a major structural abnormality, such as a heart defect or duodenal atresia. In addition, a number of "soft signs" on second-trimester ultrasonographic fetal assessment point to an increased likelihood for DS. An advantage is that this procedure is often done routinely as part of normal obstetric management, and thus a de facto DS screen is added on, essentially at no additional cost. However, the observations do not lend themselves to a ready analysis in terms of adjusting the level of risk; furthermore, the frequency of these "soft signs" in normal fetuses leads to a high false-positive rate. A more rigorous approach is to adjust the patient's risk assessment using positive and negative likelihood ratios[4] which are available for each "soft sign" (Table 21–7).

Twin Pregnancies. In the case of biochemical screening, two fetoplacental units lead to the production of twice as much of the particular biochemical substance, which is then conveyed into the maternal bloodstream. Muller et al. (2003) examined the second-trimester analyte levels, and Spencer et al. (2008) the first-trimester analyte levels, in cohorts of twin pregnancies; and the MoM values were essentially double those of singleton pregnancies. The valid MoMs for risk evaluation can thus be derived by dividing the observed result by approximately 2. Intriguingly, monochorionic (and presumably monozygous) twins at first trimester have a somewhat lower PAPP-A mean (1.6 MoM)

[4] The Likelihood Ratio (LR) is the likelihood that a given test result would be expected in a patient with the target disorder (e.g., Down syndrome) compared to the likelihood that that same result would be expected in a patient without the target disorder.

Table 21–7. Positive and Negative Likelihood Ratios of Sonographic Markers for Trisomy 21

MARKER	POSITIVE LR	NEGATIVE LR	LR ISOLATED MARKER*
Intracardiac echogenic focus	5.8	0.80	0.95
Cerebral ventriculomegaly	27.5	0.94	3.81
Increased nuchal fold thickness	23.3	0.80	3.79
Echogenic bowel	11.4	0.90	1.65
Mild hydronephrosis	7.6	0.92	1.08
Short femur	4.8	0.74	0.78
Short humerus	3.7	0.80	0.61
Aberrant right subclavian artery	21.5	0.71	3.94
Absent/hypoplastic nasal bone	23.3	0.46	6.58

*Calculated by multiplying positive LR for given marker by negative LR for all other markers.
LR = likelihood ratio.

Source: Adapted from M Agathokleous et al., Meta-analysis of second-trimester markers for trisomy 21, *Ultrasound Obstet Gynecol* 41:247–261, 2013.

than do the dichorionic (2.1 MoM) (Madsen et al. 2011); if chorionicity is distinguishable at ultrasonography, adjustment can be made by applying the appropriate PAPP-A divisor. A theoretical complicating factor, in the case of one (dizygous) twin being trisomic 21, is that the normal co-twin might "dilute out" the abnormal serum biochemistry and thus invalidate the test result. However, in a large French study addressing a second-trimester population, such an effect, if present, was marginal (and not significant statistically), and screening in this setting was considered to be effective (Garchet-Beaudron et al. 2008).

Concerning the ultrasonography, nuchal translucency screening allows each twin to be assessed individually, and the detection rate for aneuploidy is similar to singleton pregnancies (Cleary-Goldman et al. 2005). For monochorionic twins, a single risk estimate can be calculated for the pregnancy using the average of the two nuchal translucency measurements, whereas for dichorionic twins, a specific risk is calculated for each twin. When first-trimester serum markers and nuchal translucency results are combined, a detection rate of 90% can be achieved, for a false-positive rate of 5.9% (Madsen et al. 2011).

Garchet-Beaudron et al. (2008) point out other issues relating to twin pregnancies. Logically, the age-related risk for DS might be expected to double in a dizygous twin pregnancy. But such logic appears not to apply; actual observation does not record such an increase. The technical procedures in the event of an increased-risk result are more demanding: double amniocentesis, with each sac sampled separately; and, if one twin is trisomic and selective termination is sought, the normal twin is placed at risk. Screening in twin pregnancies requires special expertise. In the case of a "vanishing twin" at the first trimester, as manifest by a second, empty sac, the PAPP-A level is artificially elevated and should be omitted from the risk calculation (Chaveeva et al. 2020).

As noted above, cfDNA testing is now the preferred screening methodology for twin pregnancies due to its superior performance (Judah et al. 2021), but first-trimester combined screening results can nonetheless be used to stratify twin pregnancies into low- and high-risk categories, with those at risk being offered follow-up cfDNA testing (Galeva et al. 2019).

Interpretation of Screening Results

What do these various figures—detection rate, false-positive rate, positive predictive value—mean? A little epidemiology is in order. Imagine a group of 10,000 pregnant women, of all ages. Assuming a birth prevalence for DS of 1.2 per 1,000, we can take it that 12 women would otherwise give birth to a baby with DS. If the particular screening approach has a detection rate of, for example, 85%, 10/12 of these DS pregnancies would be recognized as being at increased risk, and they could be identified at prenatal diagnosis. The remaining 15% who are carrying a DS fetus (2/12) would fail to be recognized. If the false-positive rate is, for example, 4%, 400 women would have an increased-risk report from screening, but they would go on to receive a normal result from the following amniocentesis or CVS. Putting these figures in the conventional format, we have (Table 21–8):

Table 21–8. Sensitivity, Positive Predictive Value, and Negative Predictive Value of DS Screening

TEST INTERPRETATION	FETUS WITH DS	FETUS NOT WITH DS	TOTAL
Test shows "increased risk"	10	400	410
Test shows "low risk"	2	9,588	9,590
Total	12	9,988	10,000

The *detection rate* (sensitivity) of the test is 10/12 (85%). Thus, 15% of women with a trisomic 21 fetus will be missed by the test. The *positive predictive value* of the test is only 10/410 (2.4%). Thus, 97.6% of women returning an "increased-risk" result will not have a baby with DS.[5] The *negative predictive value* is 9,588/9,590 (99.98%); in other words, a "low-risk" result means a 99.9% chance for an unaffected baby.

The false-positive rate is an important parameter. As noted earlier, this represents the fraction of women who will then go on to have an invasive definitive test that will return a normal chromosomal result. Clearly, the smaller this figure the better. The trade-off is this: the smaller the false-positive rate, the less the detection rate. To judge the effectiveness and acceptability of the screening, we can declare a false-positive rate that is desirable, and this would then determine what the detection rate will be; or, we can choose a preferred detection rate and accept the false-positive rate that this would incur. A typically desired false-positive rate is 5%; based upon this, the detection rate is noted as DR_5. Desired detection rates of 85% or 90% would come at a cost of false-positive rates noted as FPR_{85} and FPR_{90} (Weisz and Rodeck 2006).

THE UNDERSTANDING OF WOMEN WHO HAVE SCREENING

The interpretation of a DS screening test result to the patient is fraught with potential for confusion. The major pitfall is that an "increased-risk" test result may sometimes be understood by the woman and her medical advisor to mean that the pregnancy is likely to be affected. As we showed earlier, *many women who screen "positive" will go on to have a normal baby.* Counselors doing this work need a clear awareness of these issues so that they can enable their patients to understand, intuitively or explicitly, the concept

[5] Thus emphasizing the point that the expression to use is merely "increased risk," not "high risk."

and relevance of a low positive predictive value. The counselor is referred to Macintosh's (1994) essay "Perception of Risk" for a very readable and practical commentary upon these issues, and to Marteau and Dormandy (2001) for an overview of the complexity of the issues. The ideal is that those having a screening test for DS and other aneuploidies should have a basic awareness of the conditions and of the rationale of the screening procedure, and that their beliefs and perceptions and attitudes should be reasonably consonant with the aims and practice of the program.

The ideal has not necessarily been met. Jaques et al. (2004), in a paper provocatively titled "Do Women Know That Prenatal Testing Detects Fetuses with Down Syndrome?" surveyed responses from pregnant women 37 years old or older in Victoria, Australia, in 1998–1999; and the answer to their question was, disconcertingly, that "Down syndrome" was not mentioned as a reason for undergoing pregnancy testing in almost 40% of respondents. Not every woman will respond "rationally" to an increased-risk interpretation, according to the view of rationality as seen by the providers of the screening program. Those who enter into a screening program without being properly aware of the implications may find themselves "in an untenable situation—anxious about a positive result, but unwilling to incur the risks of diagnostic testing" (Kuppermann et al. 2006). Depressive symptoms, and thus a reduced capacity to make clear decisions, may be exacerbated in those with a predisposition, and Hippman et al. (2009) see a role for the counselor in recognizing this.

For those who are better informed, understanding is by no means a neutral matter, and Rapp (1999) refers to the role of women as "moral pioneers" in coming to terms with the ethical issues that readily available screening may, in these modern times, present. Susanne et al. (2006) assessed responses in women who had had what turned out to be a false-positive screening result, following them prospectively through the pregnancy and after the baby was born. Several declared that they had "withheld" their pregnancy and only returned to reacceptance after the normal chromosomal result from amniocentesis had been conveyed; nevertheless, most would have the same testing in a future pregnancy. Counselors need to be well attuned to these several complexities; and if a woman's family physician can share in the decision-making process, this is typically well received (Légaré et al. 2011).

NIPT differs from other prenatal tests by combining ease with high accuracy. Kristalijn et al. (2022) surveyed more than 4,500 women in the Netherlands and found that the vast majority of women who receive a low-risk result were positive about the experience and felt they had received sufficient information. However, those with increased-risk results were more likely to report negative feelings and anxiety, and to feel that they had not been sufficiently prepared for the result. This lack of preparedness is especially prominent for findings outside trisomies 21, 18, and 13. Lewit-Mendes (2023) report that people who received an increased chance of sex chromosome aneuploidy result at NIPT felt unprepared for the unanticipated complexity of the result, and were faced with making a time-sensitive decision for a condition they had not previously considered or even been aware of. Women who received increased-risk results for rare autosomal trisomies and structural chromosome abnormalities were similarly unprepared for these results (Bakkeren et al. 2024).

Kater-Kuipers et al. (2020) argue that the ease and routineness of NIPT challenges the notion of informed decision-making in prenatal testing, and propose a three-step counseling model in which three decision moments are distinguished and differently addressed: (1) professionals explore women's values concerning whether and why they wish to know whether their baby has a genetic disorder; (2) women receive layered medical-technical information and are asked to make a decision about screening; (3) during post-test counseling, women are supported in decision-making about the continuation or termination of their pregnancy.

Concerning the facts about DS itself in the context of pregnancy screening, the National Society of Genetic Counsellors (USA) has published a practice resource on communicating a prenatal or post-natal diagnosis of DS (Sheets et al. 2011). The authors recommend elements of a diagnosis conversation including genetic causes of DS and recurrence risks, recommendations for sensitively delivering a diagnosis of DS, essential information for the initial discussion of a diagnosis of DS, discussions of options of pregnancy management after a prenatal diagnosis, and DS resources; and they add that information about life outcomes is particularly valued by prospective parents.

Provision of a website or pamphlet is the simplest means of conveying information, and many clinics/jurisdictions produce their own material. It is a fine matter to judge what should be the level and tone of the information. Reviews of leaflets produced in the United Kingdom (Bryant et al. 2001) and Canada (Lawson et al. 2012) concluded that the viewpoints expressed were, in the main, weighted unduly negatively toward DS, and this is consistent with a broader criticism that genetic counseling primarily provides information consistent with the medical model of disabilities that focuses on problems to be fixed, as opposed to the social model, which prioritizes supports, services, and acceptance (Ijaz et al. 2025). It is true that information ought to be couched in such terms that it will be useful, in the fullest sense of that word, to the wide range of people for whom it is intended (and see p. 814). Equally, the comment can be made that attempting to neutralize negative aspects of DS may send a mixed message, since being given the option of abortion in order to avoid having a DS child rather plainly implies that having such a child may not be a desirable outcome. The view that is offered should be clear, accurate, and even-handed.[6]

Secular Trends in Prenatal Screening and Diagnosis of Aneuploidy

The population prevalence of Down syndrome has been influenced by three factors over the past half century: changes in maternal-age distribution (Chapter 13), improved survival, and advances in prenatal screening technologies and policies (Figure 21–3). Birth prevalence has fluctuated according to the changing maternal-age profile and to the take-up of prenatal diagnosis (Figures 21–4 and 21–5). In Europe, Australia, and New Zealand, the livebirth prevalence for DS has fallen, while in the USA there has been a modest increase (Figure 21–5). Another possible point to factor in to the overall picture may be a changing attitude toward pregnancy termination for an aneuploidy (Jacobs et al. 2016).

The increasing precision of screening has led to a reduction in the number of invasive procedures being done. Pynaker et al. (2024) analyzed data for the years 1976–2023 from Victoria, Australia, and noted that while the total number of invasive tests climbed

[6] These matters are dealt with in considerable detail in a document from the National Health Service of the United Kingdom, "Psychological Aspects of Genetic Screening of Pregnant Women and Newborns: A Systematic Review" (Green et al. 2004).

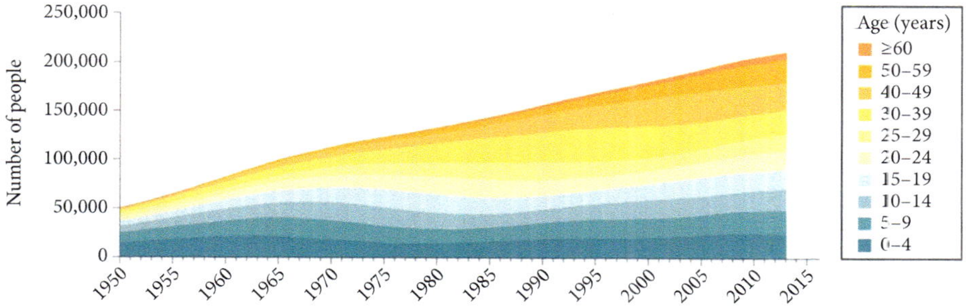

Figure 21–3. The Prevalence of Down Syndrome in the USA since the 1950s.

Notes: With increasing survival over the timeframe 1950s-2010s, the numbers of older DS individuals have been progressively increasing (yellow and orange bands, *above*), while the prevalence in children from the 1960s has been fairly constant. During this period, the US population doubled, from 150 million, to 310 million; and thus the fraction of DS among the whole population of children has been falling.

Source: From SE Antonarakis et al., Down syndrome, *Nat Rev Dis Primers* 6:9, 2020. Courtesy SE Antonarakis, and with the permission of Springer Nature.

steadily from 1976 to 2000, it then declined such that in 2023, fewer procedures were being done than at any time in the previous 35 years (Figure 21–6). At the same time, the number of prenatal diagnoses of DS was the highest recorded. This improved targeting reflected changes in the indications for invasive prenatal testing over the same period (Figure 21–7), and the number of invasive procedures performed per diagnosis of a major chromosome abnormality declined from 100 to two. Renshaw et al. (2013) have reported similar improvements in the United Kingdom, with the number of invasive procedures per syndrome diagnosis reducing from 46 to five between 1991 and 2010.

FETAL ULTRASONOGRAPHIC ANOMALIES

We have discussed above ultrasonography in the specific setting of targeted screening. Otherwise, a mid-trimester ultrasound examination is, of course, a routine part of

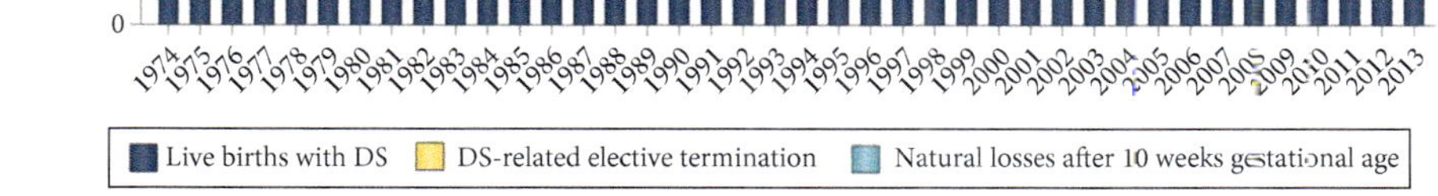

Figure 21–4. Down Syndrome Pregnancy Outcomes in the USA 1974–2013.

Notes: Livebirths and natural losses have increased fractionally over this timeframe, consonant with population growth. Prenatal diagnosis with termination expanded very substantially from the 1970s through to the turn of this century, but has remained fairly constant thereafter.

Source: From SE Antonarakis et al., Down syndrome, *Nat Rev Dis Primers* 6:9, 2020. Courtesy SE Antonarakis, and with the permission of Springer Nature.

22
CHROMOSOME ABNORMALITIES DETECTED AT PRENATAL DIAGNOSIS

THE MAIN FOCUS of chromosomal prenatal diagnosis had been upon trisomy 21, usually in the context of older childbearing age or of an increased-risk screening test. Trisomy 21 does remain, for most women and couples, the prime concern—the condition that most people are aware of—but with the sophistication of 21st century technology, the great majority of chromosomal imbalances are, in principle, diagnosable. Noninvasive prenatal testing—no more than a blood test for the woman—widens access and increases uptake very considerably. Routine fetal ultrasonography can detect quite subtle malformation, and genetic testing will often follow such a discovery. The counselor can expect to deal with a broad spectrum of chromosomal abnormality, presenting in the prenatal clinic.

DECISION-MAKING FOLLOWING PRENATAL DIAGNOSIS OF A CHROMOSOMAL ABNORMALITY

To some extent, the possibility of "other abnormalities besides Down syndrome" should have been raised at pretest counseling. But when a chromosomal abnormality is actually discovered, it is of course necessary to discuss in detail with prospective parents the implications of this particular abnormality, and to help them decide on a suitable course of action.

Outlines of the clinical consequences of these abnormalities follow, to serve as a basis for the decisions that these women and couples need to make. In transmitting the information, the counselor is obliged to be clear and accurate about the particular abnormality, and to take care that the couple's autonomy in the decision-making process is not compromised. A decision for or against termination is the immediate one to be made.

Hodgson et al. (2016) interviewed 102 women and men six weeks after diagnosis of fetal abnormality[1] and identified the following considerations in the decision about whether to terminate the pregnancy:

1. Uncertainty about the diagnosis or results
2. Uncertainty about the prognosis or severity
3. Expected survival
4. Worry about baby experiencing pain
5. Personal views on abortion and disability
6. Self-perceived ability to parent a disabled child
7. Potential for long-term care needs

[1] In this study the fetal abnormality was chromosomal in origin in 63% of affected pregnancies.

8. Societal treatment of people with disability
9. Impact on their other children
10. Impact on their career and finances
11. Potential maternal risks in pregnancy
12. Not the life they had imagined for their child
13. Fearing judgment of others
14. Societal views about abortion
15. Wondering what others would do in the same situation

Shaffer et al. (2006) undertook a large retrospective review (1983–2003), analyzing parental decisions in 816 prenatal diagnoses of a major aneuploidy, at a San Francisco clinic. Termination was chosen in 86% of autosomal trisomy and in 60% with a sex chromosome aneuploidy. Of the latter, the rates of termination increased progressively from XXX (40%) to XYY (57%), 45,X (65%), and XXY (70%), in parallel with a perceived severity of phenotype. The rates did not differ significantly during the 21-year period, to the slight surprise of these authors. Jacobs et al. (2016) assessed responses to the prenatal diagnosis of an aneuploidy in a Scottish population, observing a fall-off in the numbers choosing termination during the period 2000–2011. They suggested that this may have reflected "societal changes in accepting greater diversity" but acknowledged that "this interpretation is of course purely speculative." Finding a variant of uncertain clinical significance (VUS) is a more recent question, and while pregnancy termination is infrequently chosen, its discovery at prenatal diagnosis nonetheless imposes a considerable psychological burden on prospective parents (Lou et al. 2020; Libman et al. 2024). The simplicity of a blood test may have drawn many more into having a prenatal test, but this appears to have made little difference to the termination rates for DS, and indeed many parents have used NIPT for information, and have continued pregnancies in the context of a high risk of DS (Hill et al. 2016).

Trisomy 21

Skotko et al. (2009) emphasize the need for the person conveying the news of a Down syndrome (DS) result to be well informed, whether that be a counselor, obstetrician, or other health professional (and of course this qualification is scarcely confined to a diagnosis of DS). Ideally, the news should be given in person; but where that is not feasible, a phone call or telehealth appointment should be at a prearranged time. Parents who decide to continue a trisomy 21 pregnancy, versus those who have chosen termination, would presumably come from different points of view. Skotko and colleagues note that contact with a DS support group might be useful for some couples in deciding the fate of a DS pregnancy, although they do observe that few studies have assessed the views of those who have terminated a trisomic pregnancy, from whom the other face of the decision could be given a hearing.

A study of health professionals in Finland showed some inconsistency in comparing the points of view of midwives and public health nurses with the options available to their patients; and the acknowledgment was made that this difference could be viewed as a healthy sign, in recognizing that plurality of opinion is the way of the world (Jallinoja et al. 1999). Thus, most (79%) of these midwives and nurses agreed that all pregnant women should be offered a screening test, although only 44% personally accepted the

Table 22–1. Reasons for the Choice of DS Termination
The Five Most Acknowledged "Child-Related" Motivations of 71 Women Choosing Termination of a Trisomic 21 Pregnancy, from a Study Based in Eight Dutch Hospitals

MOTIVATION STATEMENT	PERCENTAGE OF WOMEN IN AGREEMENT WITH STATEMENT
I believed the child would never be able to function independently.	92
I considered the abnormality too severe.	90
I considered the burden for the child itself too heavy.	83
I worried about the care of the child after my/our death.	82
I considered the uncertainty about the consequences of the abnormality too high.	78

Source: From MJ Korenromp et al., Maternal decision to terminate pregnancy in case of Down syndrome, *Am J Obstet Gynecol* 196:149.e1–11, 2007.

concept of genetic abortion. An acceptance of abortion correlated with education and with a professional experience with DS patients. In the United States, Britt et al. (2000) studied 142 women who had had a prenatal diagnosis of trisomy 21, seen in Detroit over the period 1989–1998. Those who had already had children, and where the diagnosis of trisomy 21 was made earlier in the pregnancy, were more likely to choose termination. In the Netherlands, Korenromp et al. (2007) found that among women who had chosen termination following prenatal diagnosis of DS, "child-related" motivations (Table 22–1) were the most prevalent, but concerns about burden to the family were also important. Lou et al. (2020) discuss how some women detach themselves from the pregnancy, for example by using the term "fetus" and acting as if they were not pregnant, whereas others maintain attachment, such as by referring to the fetus as "our child." But these expressions of attachment and detachment sometimes coexist and may change over time.

Sex Chromosome Abnormality

NIPT has brought renewed focus on the prenatal diagnosis of sex chromosome aneuploidy (SCA). Prior to NIPT, very few SCAs were diagnosed prenatally, and these were mostly as incidental findings. Identifying SCA had not been an aim of prenatal screening; but sex chromosomes are now included in many NIPT tests (in part as a response to requests for fetal sex diagnosis). In Victoria, Australia, Loughry et al. (2023) reported a fivefold increase in the prenatal diagnosis of 47,XXY between 2005 and 2020, corresponding to the time of NIPT implementation. These matters now sharpen the question of what to tell prospective parents (White et al. 2023; Reimers et al. 2023) and of the associated ethical issues (Warton et al. 2023). Despite this, parents report being unprepared for the diagnosis of SCA when it actually happens (Lewit-Mendes et al. 2023).

Even prior to NIPT, views about SCA were evolving, generally in the direction of a more conservative response to the news of a chromosomal abnormality. In Denmark, Nielsen et al. (1986) reported that ~80% of prenatal diagnoses of sex chromosome aneuploidy at that time were followed by the choice of abortion. In an English/Finnish study from the same period, termination (in ~60% overall) was more likely to be chosen in the case of the XXY and 45,X karyotypes by younger parents with fewer previous children, and in all cases in which an ultrasonographic defect was identified (Holmes-Siedle et al. 1987). From a large survey of centers in five European countries covering the years 1986 to 1997, the rate of choice of termination with respect to XXY was 44% (Marteau et al. 2002). In a German study over a similar period, termination was chosen by a much smaller fraction, only 13%, among parents who had been given a prenatal diagnosis of 47,XXX, 47,XXY, or 47,XYY (in contrast, just 2% of parents at the same clinic decided to continue a pregnancy with trisomy 21) (Meschede et al. 1998). This may in part have reflected the practice of this clinic to emphasize the point that "the mean global IQ of around 90 falls well within the normal range and is compatible with a productive and socially well-adjusted life."

More recently, half of couples in a Chinese study elected to continue the pregnancy, but the choice to continue was very much dependent on the specific sex chromosome aneuploidy: 89% for 47,XYY, 85% for 47,XXX, 35% for 47,XXY, and just 7% for 45,X (Luo et al. 2024). In the specific case of Turner syndrome, from 19 registries in 10 countries across Europe from 1996 to 1998, 79% of parents chose termination if morphological abnormality (and in particular cystic hygroma) had been seen on ultrasonography, versus 42% in which the diagnosis had not been led into by an ultrasonographic defect (Baena et al. 2004). The poor post-natal survival associated with prenatally diagnosed cystic hygroma (Levy et al. 2021) is likely to have a major influence on decision-making.

The way in which information is given has an important impact, and counselors need to be well aware of the weight that parents, in some emotional turmoil at the news they have just received, may put upon the news given them. Consider the example of 47,XXY Klinefelter syndrome. In the European survey mentioned above, Marteau et al. (2002) assessed responses to the prenatal diagnosis of XXY when counseling had been given by obstetricians, pediatricians, midwives, health visitors, or genetics specialists. Women counseled solely by genetics specialists were more than twice as likely (a relative risk of 2.4) to continue the pregnancy versus those counseled either by other professionals or by other professionals along with a geneticist. It seems probable that these differences may reflect the style of counseling.

In a review of published reports, Jeon et al. (2012) noted the importance of these factors in influencing a decision: the specific type of sex chromosome abnormality, the gestational week at diagnosis, the parents' age, the providers' genetic expertise, and the number of children already had, or their desire for (more) children. They noted that among those parents choosing to continue a pregnancy, their socioeconomic status and ethnicity were particularly relevant. On the other hand, parents choosing termination were characterized by a fear or anxiety of having a child with a sex chromosome abnormality and also by having received directive counseling.

The desirability for a consistent approach, with access to accurate information, is to be emphasized, as is—of course—the requirement to enable women's choices to be well informed in the broadest sense, and for the counseling to be nondirective (Linden et al. 2002). Reimers et al. (2023) emphasize the importance of inclusive and non-stigmatizing language when discussing genetic diagnoses and of drawing upon the most up-to-date and unbiased SCA data. Beyond the clinic, there are support groups, public information resources, and communicating with other parents as means to become further informed about the implications of a SCA (in the short period of time during which a decision must be made), and Linden and colleagues note the pros and cons of taking these paths. As noted earlier with respect to trisomy 21, the views of those who had previously chosen to terminate a pregnancy are less readily accessible. The prime responsibility for putting couples in the best position to make an appropriate decision lies with the counselor.

As for subsequently informing the children from the pregnancies that are continued, Riggan et al. (2024) emphasize the importance of telling them of their sex chromosomal diagnosis and its implications in a timely, well informed, and sensitive manner.

"Microarray-Level" Rearrangement

Microarray analysis applied to prenatal samples can substantially increase the diagnostic pick-up (Figure 1–7). The other side of this two-edged sword is the fact that some micro-imbalances are not pathogenic, or may only be pathogenic in specific circumstances—for example when co-inherited with other variants from either parent. Indeed, one commentator wrote, somewhat provocatively, that prenatal array testing is likely "to produce a flood of information that is overwhelming, anxiety-producing, inconclusive, and misleading" (Shuster 2007); and Werner-Lin et al. (2016a) provide some testament, in documenting frustration and anxiety of couples receiving uncertain results, that this prediction may not have been entirely inaccurate.

A practical response is to limit reporting to those variants that reach a certain threshold in terms of evidence of pathogenicity, so that results of unclear clinical significance or with very low penetrance[2] are less often encountered (Armour et al. 2018; Maya et al. 2020). This approach is supported by data from McCoy et al. (2025), who followed up 46 children who had received VUS results in fetal life and found similar intellectual functioning and social functioning to those without a VUS. The counterpoint is that this approach will occasionally miss a clinically significant CNV.

Parental testing may shed further light, but will not necessarily resolve the question, particularly for CNVs of incomplete penetrance. Goh et al. (2025) pose the following: "Consider a family with an affected child who has a CNV with 20% penetrance that was inherited from a parent with a mild phenotype. In contrast, a different family may have the same CNV with no affected family members. Some may wonder if the likelihood of a relevant phenotype occurring in a newborn child identified prenatally with this CNV is 20% regardless of the scenario, while others might wonder if there are known mechanisms that could impact the chance of penetrance for this CNV."

Counselors need to be quite *au fait* with the interpretations and to maintain close liaison with expert scientists in the field (the science); they must also be aware of the particular subtleties that counseling in this circumstance will demand (the art) (Werner-Lin et al. 2016b). The uncertainty of a prenatal result, for those continuing the pregnancy, can flow over into the child's life: "They Can't Find Anything Wrong with Him, Yet," as Werner-Lin et al. (2017) title their paper apropos.

There are other ways in which the use of microarray is changing the face of prenatal chromosome analysis. The two notable categories are the identification of de novo balanced chromosome rearrangements, and very small marker chromosomes. Although typically benign, but not always so, these abnormalities have historically necessitated detailed counseling and cytogenetic follow-up, and they have been a cause of anxiety for patients. The fact that these abnormalities may be invisible on microarray is a feature of

[2] There is currently no consensus definition for low penetrance.

the methodology that is, perhaps, almost an advantage in the prenatal setting. The capacity for next-generation sequencing (NGS) methodologies—"post-microarray" testing, one could almost say—to clarify the nature of apparently balanced rearrangements, is mentioned on p. 24.

MOSAICISM: CONFINED, CONSTITUTIONAL, AND PSEUDO

Mosaicism is the bane of cytogenetic prenatal diagnosis. Most times, it turns out to have been a false alarm, and the mosaicism in villus tissue or amniocytes does not reflect a true constitutional mosaicism of the fetus. This is a problem for the laboratory to resolve, inasmuch as they are able. We may list these two major categories: confined placental mosaicism, and true constitutional fetal mosaicism. A third category, pseudomosaicism, refers to an abnormality that arose during tissue culture in vitro ("cultural artifact"), but with the embryonic and extra-embryonic tissues being chromosomally normal. Pseudomosaicism can be eliminated by analyzing uncultured cells, using DNA-based techniques.

A chromosomally abnormal cell line may exist only in the extra-embryonic tissues of the placenta (chorion, amnion), and the embryo is 46,N. This is confined placental mosaicism (CPM). CPM is encountered at CVS rather than at amniocentesis. It is uncommon that an observation of apparent CPM at CVS reflects a true constitutional mosaicism of the fetus. Grati (2014) offers an exhaustive treatment of the question of mosaicism at CVS, based upon an experience of more than 50,000 procedures, in which mosaicism was seen in 2.2%; of these, just 13% (0.3% of the total) proved to have a true fetal mosaicism (and see Table 22–2); she provides further authoritative review, with reference to the issues raised by noninvasive prenatal testing (Grati 2016).

Comparable fractions are seen on prenatal diagnosis by microarray: 1.8% of CVS, and 0.5% on amniocentesis, in the analysis of Carey et al. (2014). Mosaicism for copy number variants can also be detected by microarray: Gu et al. (2018) showed that 3.0%

Table 22–2. Different Types of Mosaicism Identified After Chorionic Villous Sampling*

TYPE	NATURE	TROPHOBLAST (DIRECT CVS, NIPT)	MESENCHYME (CULTURE CVS)	AMNIOCYTES	RELATIVE FREQUENCY
I	CPM	Abnormal	Normal	Normal	34.8% (308/886)
II	CPM	Normal	Abnormal	Normal	42.3% (375/886)
III	CPM	Abnormal	Abnormal	Normal	10.2% (90/886)
IV	TFM	Abnormal	Normal	Abnormal	1.6% (14/886)
V	TFM	Normal	Abnormal	Abnormal	5.8% (51/886)
VI	TFM	Abnormal	Abnormal	Abnormal	5.4% (48/886)

*Based upon a series of 52,673 CVS procedures, in which 1,136 (2.2%) showed mosaicism, and of which 886 had follow-up amniocentesis.

CPM = confined placental mosaicism; CVS = chorionic villous sampling; TFM = true fetal mosaicism.

Source: From Grati FR. Chromosomal mosaicism in human feto-placental development: Implications for prenatal diagnosis. *J Clin Med* 3:809–837, 2014.

of CVS[3] prenatal arrays samples were indicative of mosaicism, including submicroscopic CNVs. Likewise, the Danish study of Lund et al. (2020) identified mosaicism for a microscopic or submicroscopic CNV in 1.3% of uncultured CVS[3] samples as well as in 2.8% of samples having a mosaic autosomal or sex chromosome aneuploidy.[4] True fetal mosaicism was confirmed in 18% of mosaic whole chromosome aneuploidies, and in 25% of mosaic CNVs. A long-term follow-up study (Amor et al. 2006) is noted below.

Considerable discussion follows, but at the outset we emphasize that true mosaicism of the fetus is infrequently observed, and that *the majority of mosaicism identified at prenatal diagnosis, more especially at CVS, does not presage an abnormal baby.* It is important to keep this perspective in talking with parents (according to the particular attributes of the mosaicism, as we go on to discuss) and to avoid causing any more anxiety than that which an "abnormal" result inevitably brings.

Applied Embryology

Interpreting mosaicism obliges an understanding of the earliest events of development of the conceptus, as we now outline (Figure 22–1). The zygote undergoes successive mitoses to produce a ball of cells (the morula, at Day 4). The morula then cavitates to produce an inner cyst, and it becomes the blastocyst (Days 6 to 9 in Figure 22–1). The outermost layer of the blastocyst is composed of trophoblast, and this tissue becomes the outer investment of the chorionic villi. The inner cell mass protrudes into the blastocystic cavity, and this will give origin to the embryo. It comprises two different cellular layers, the epiblast and the hypoblast. In a 64-cell blastocyst, most cells are trophoblasts, the inner cell mass comprises about 16 cells, within which only about four (epiblast) cells will give rise to the embryo itself.

The hypoblast forms the spherical primary yolk sac (whose roof is, transiently, the ventral surface of the embryo). The primary yolk sac gives rise to the extra-embryonic mesoderm, sandwiched between itself and the outer cytotrophoblast and thus producing a three-layered sphere (Figure 22–1, Day 11). The mesodermal cells now invade the blastocystic cavity, and this mesodermal mass is in turn cavitated to produce the extra-embryonic celom such that there are outer and inner layers of extra-embryonic mesoderm (Figure 22–1, Day 13). The outer layer, underlying the trophoblast, gives rise to the mesenchymal core of the chorionic villus, and the inner layer becomes the outer (mesodermal) surface of the amniotic membrane. The amniotic cavity enlarges at the expense of the extra-embryonic celom (Figure 22–1, Week 4) and eventually obliterates it (by the end of the first trimester), with the mesodermal layer of the amnion fusing with the mesodermal layer of the chorion (Figure 22–1, Week 8).

> The epiblast gives rise to the amniotic cavity, the floor of which is the "dorsal" (ectodermal) surface of the embryo, and its roof is the amnion, these being continuous at their margins. Thus, the embryonic integument and the inner surface of the amniotic membrane—which are the source of the embryonic and amniotic epithelial cells present in amniotic fluid—have the same lineage. At the beginning of the third week,

[3] Both cytotrophoblastic and mesenchymal samples.

[4] The prevalence of CPM in this study was higher than most other studies, an observation that may be due at least in part to the indication for CVS being an increased-risk first trimester combined screen, a test which may itself enrich for CPM cases due to an association between low PAPP-A levels and CPM.

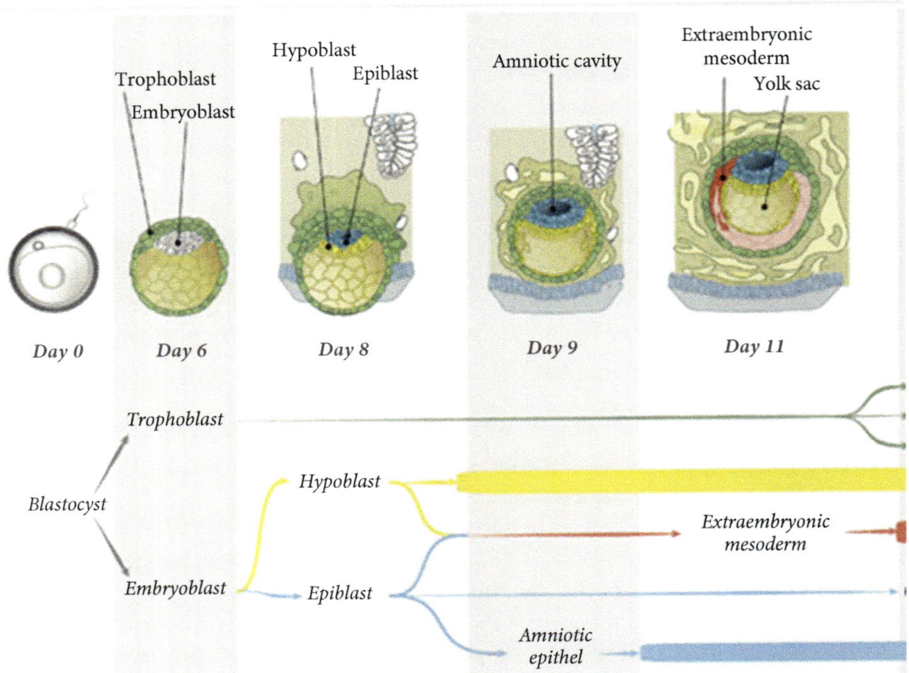

Figure 22–1. The timeline of embryogenesis, and the development of the different tissues.

Note: "Embryoblast" (day 6) is synonymous with Inner Cell Mass, and these cells include those which will give rise to the actual embryo. The unlabeled black and white cells shown at days 8 and 9 (upper right in each panel) represent decidua placentalis.

Source: From R Essers et al., Prevalence of chromosomal alterations in first-trimester spontaneous pregnancy loss, *Nat Med* 29:3233–3242, 2023. Courtesy A Salumets and MZ Esteki, and with the permission of Nature Medicine.

the primitive streak arises from the epiblast, and this in turn gives origin to both endoderm and intra-embryonic mesoderm. Endoderm gives origin, among other tissues, to urinary tract and lung epithelia–desquamated cells which contribute to the cellular population of amniotic fluid. Albeit that the extra- and intra-embryonic mesoderms have different origins, there may be migration of some intra-embryonic mesodermal cells into the (extra-embryonic) amniotic mesoderm. Cells from the latter add a minor fraction to the population of amniocytes, but have a proliferative advantage and may come to comprise most of the cells present following in vitro culture.

Amniocentesis is a procedure that samples cells having origin from the epiblast of the inner cell mass, and these cells rather closely reflect the true constitution of the embryo. *Chorionic villus sampling*, on the other hand, samples more distantly related cells: trophoblast cells (direct and short-term culture), which were the first lineage to differentiate from totipotent cells of the morula, and villus core cells (long-term culture), which reflect the more recently separated lineage of the extra-embryonic mesoderm. The differing origins of tissues sampled by different means are set out in Figure 22–3. *Noninvasive prenatal testing (NIPT)* samples cell-free DNA that originated from apoptotic trophoblast cells, and therefore is more closely related to CVS than to amniocentesis (indeed, it has been called a "liquid early CVS").

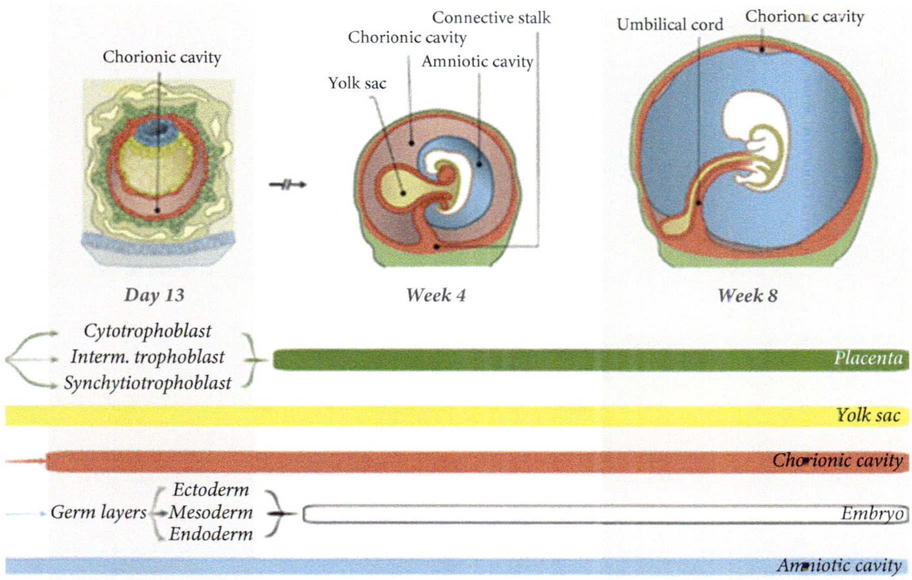

Figure 22–1. Continued.

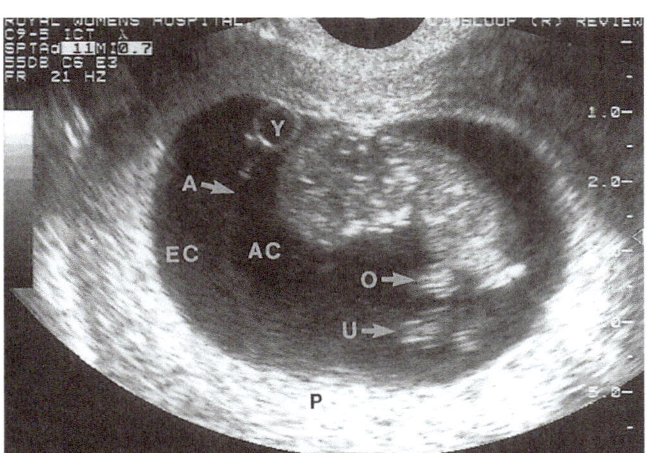

Figure 22–2. Ultrasound of the Embryo.

Notes: Ultrasound picture of embryo at 10–11 weeks gestational age, very close to actual size (note centimeter markers at right). Note amnion (A), amniotic cavity (AC), extra-embryonic celom (EC), umbilical cord (U), "physiological omphalocele" (O), yolk sac (Y), and placenta (P). The relative positions of embryo and other structures are similar to the depiction in Figure 22–1, Week 8.

Source: Courtesy HP Robinson.

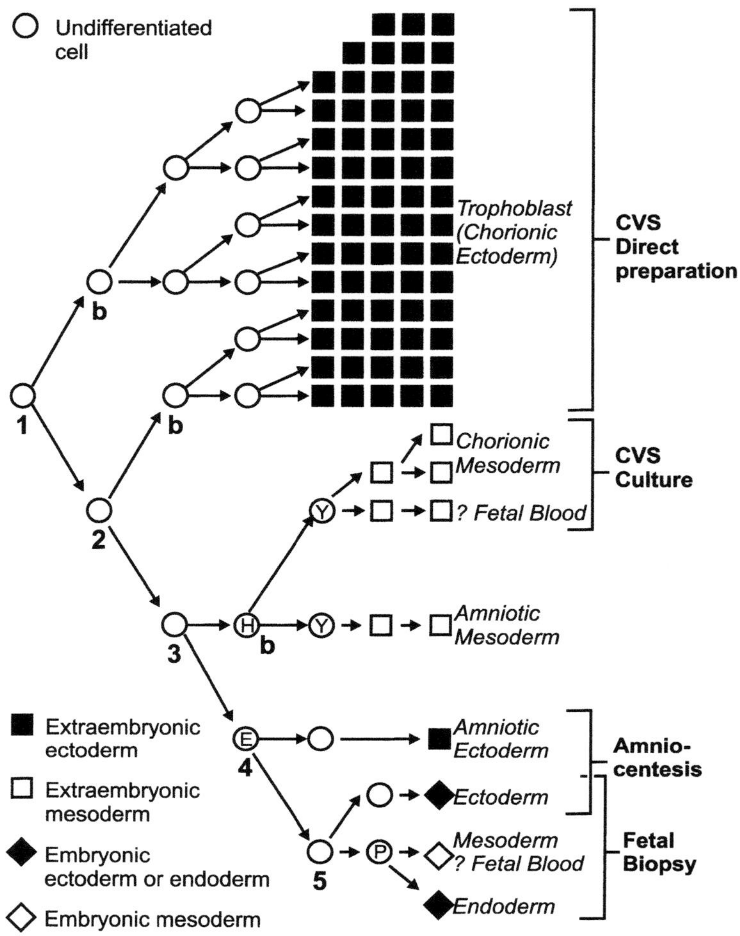

Figure 22–3. Cell Lineages vis a vis Prenatal Diagnostic Approaches.

Notes: The cell lineages arising from differentiation in the very early conceptus are shown, with respect to their relevance at prenatal diagnosis. The fertilized egg (1) produces a trophoblast precursor (1b) and a totipotent stem cell (2), which in turn forms another trophoblast precursor (2b) and a stem cell (3) that produces the inner cell mass. The inner cell mass divides into stem cells for hypoblast (3b) and epiblast (4). The epiblast cell(s) (5) produces embryonic ectoderm and primitive streak, and the latter is the source of embryonic mesoderm and endoderm. The cell lineages sampled at various prenatal diagnostic procedures are indicated at right. E, epiblast; H, hypoblast; P, primitive streak; Y, yolk sac.[a]

[a] This construction is to be compared with that of Kennerknecht et al. (1993b), in which three postzygotic mitoses occur, producing eight totipotent cells, before the cells begin to take on their tissue identities. Robinson et al. (2002) propose a further variation, with some cells of the embryonic mesoderm migrating into the (otherwise extra-embryonic) mesodermal layer of the amnion.

Source: From DW Bianchi et al., Origin of extra-embryonic mesoderm in experimental animals: Relevance to chorionic mosaicism in humans, *Am J Med Genet* 46: 542–550, 1993. Courtesy DW Bianchi, and with the permission of Wiley-Liss.

Mechanisms of Mosaicism

Mosaicism may involve aneuploidy for an intact chromosome or for an abnormal chromosome, along with a normal cell line. Two broad formats may apply, whereby the mosaicism arose: first, a mitotic error in an initially normal conceptus which gives rise to an abnormal cell line; or, second, an initially abnormal conceptus, typically due to a meiotic error, with a subsequent mitotic event generating a normal cell line (Figure 3–15). An "incomplete" trisomy rescue may generate a de novo sSMC (see below). The distribution of the normal and the abnormal cell lines in the fetus and the placenta depends upon the time and the place of the abnormal mitotic event. If, for example, a trisomic conceptus is "rescued" by the generation of a normal cell line, at a very early stage, in a cell that is going to give rise to the inner cell mass and to some of the extrafetal tissues, then the embryo may be 46,N, and the placenta will show mosaic trisomy. If rescue occurred at a later stage, the placenta might be entirely trisomic, with a mosaic trisomy of the fetus. These and other possible combinations are depicted in Figure 22–4. The eventual phenotype will be influenced by the tissue distribution of the cell

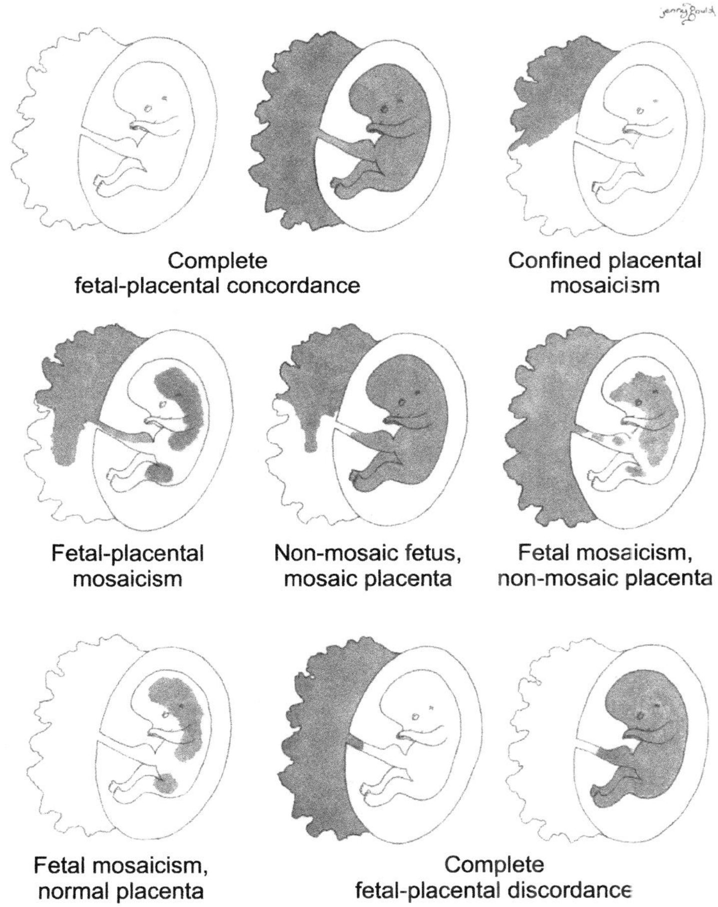

Figure 22–4. Types of Mosaicism of the Fetal-Placental Unit.

Notes: In each image, the fetus is depicted enclosed in its sac at right, with the chorionic villi comprising the placenta to left. Gray areas indicate an aneuploid cell line; white areas indicate karyotypic normality. In reality, the distributions of the two cell lines are unlikely to be as clear-cut as is shown here. In the examples showing placental mosaicism, the path taken by the sampling needle will determine whether the abnormality is detected or missed at chorionic villus sampling. The cartoon of the fetus, sac, and placenta is close to the form and about two-thirds of the size that actually exists at 10 weeks 0 days (gestational age as measured clinically, dated from the last menstrual period), when crown-rump length is approximately 30 mm.

Prediction of Phenotype in an Individual Mosaic Case

Elegant theorizing notwithstanding, the pragmatic observations from published cases in the literature provide the mainstay of the advice that the counselor may offer the parents in an individual case. (Large series are better than single case reports, which are better than anecdote.) Are mosaicisms for some particular chromosomes, or types of aberration, of more concern than others? What is a low enough level of mosaicism, if any such exists, to have a degree of confidence that the child will be physically and intellectually normal? We set out below summaries of the recorded examples from the literature, none of which necessarily provide a firm answer, but which may serve as the basis for discussion and counseling. The numbers in some are very small.

Another difficulty with these observational data is that, for the most part, the window of assessment of the child's phenotype was confined to the neonatal period. Of course, many children who are eventually diagnosed with significant disability may have been well grown and morphologically normal at birth, with normal functional neurology (inasmuch as this may be assessed in a baby). On the other hand, it is possible to overdiagnose problems in babyhood, as a child who subsequently develops normally may prove (Warburton 1991; Joyce et al. 2001). An important concern in mosaicism is that a cell line inaccessible to analysis—specifically, in the brain—might contain the abnormal chromosome, notwithstanding a normal karyotype in the post-natal tissues which are normally examined, namely blood or buccal mucosa, and possibly skin. If so, cognitive functioning could be compromised. Those few reports that include follow-up data for some years into childhood (Baty et al. 2001; Amor et al. 2006) are therefore most valuable. Nevertheless, no certainty can be offered, recognizing that every case of mosaicism will be unique, in terms of the extent and qualitative tissue distribution of the abnormal lineage.

CHORIONIC VILLUS CULTURE AND MOSAICISM, INCLUDING CONFINED PLACENTAL MOSAICISIM

CVS mosaicism is detected in about 2% of procedures at the 10- to 11-week mark. Mosaicism from an early mitotic error in a single cell can give rise to *confined* mosaicism (confined to placenta, or to fetus) or to *generalized* mosaicism (present in both fetus and placenta), according to the destined lineage of that cell; the broad range of possibilities is shown in Figure 22–4. Depending upon the timing and site of the event producing the mosaic state, the karyotypes observed at CVS will vary. The extreme form is complete discordance, with a non-mosaic 46,N karyotype in fetus and non-mosaic aneuploidy in CVS, or vice versa.[7]

Clearly, an important distinction to make, inasmuch as it is possible to do so, is between a mosaicism confined to the placenta (CPM) and causing little or no compromise of its function, and the presence of an aneuploid cell line extending into the fetus, plus or minus an important effect upon the ability of the placenta to support fetal development. Follow-up amniocentesis is certainly advisable: A normal result, which is very

[7] CPM is the main, but not the only, cause of discrepancy between the CVS and fetal/child karyotypes. One very rare explanation is that there was a resorbed co-twin with a different karyotype, with the sampling instrument having traversed its placental remnant (Tharapel et al. 1989).

often what eventuates, will substantially provide reassurance that the aneuploidy did not involve fetal tissue. In the large series of Grati (2014) as mentioned above, the great majority of mosaicism turned out to be CPM, with only a small fraction proving potentially to be true fetal mosaicism on follow-up amniocentesis. As shown in Table 22–2, Grati proposes the subclassification of CPM as follows: type I, aneuploidy confined to cytotrophoblast (recognized only at direct/short-term analysis); type II, aneuploidy confined to villous stroma; and type III, an aneuploid cell line in both cytotrophoblast and stroma. Since NIPT investigates the cytotrophoblast, it will detect only types I and III. A proviso is given in Daniel et al. (2004), who assess that on the order of 10% of CVS mosaicism for certain "rare chromosomes"[8] interpreted as CPM, may in fact reflect a cryptic fetal mosaicism that would not be detected at follow-up amniocentesis and which might or might not have important phenotypic consequence.

Origin of Trisomy in Confined Placental Mosaicism

Robinson et al. (1997) studied 101 cases in which CPM had been identified at CVS, seeking to establish correlates of the origin of the trisomy. Some CPM trisomies are usually of mitotic (somatic) origin, the zygote having been 46,N. Others typically arise meiotically, and the zygote was trisomic *ab initio*. They determined that the meiotic or mitotic origins of the trisomy are substantially chromosome-specific. For example, trisomy 8 CPM is characteristically the consequence of a mitotic event, while in contrast, almost all cases of CPM for trisomy 16 have arisen at maternal meiosis I. From a meiotic origin, "correction" may generate a 46,N karyotype in the fetus, but there is a risk for this to be associated with uniparental disomy. Thus, of the trisomy 16 CPM cases, about half displayed UPD(16) in the fetus. A meiotic origin of the CPM typically implies a more guarded prognosis than if the error had arisen somatically. Trisomy 2 at CVS (see below) is an example of a mosaicism that conveys quite different implications according the meiotic or mitotic mechanism of its generation.

Level III Mosaicism in CVS

Level III mosaicism in CVS raises an immediate concern. Management at this point (which will usually be around 12–13 weeks) is aimed at demonstrating, as much as possible, fetal normality—or, if it so transpires, confirming a true fetal mosaicism. Amniocentesis with rapid FISH analysis of a large number of cells, along with detailed ultrasonographic assessment of fetal morphology, is usually the next plan of action; or a microarray analysis might be performed on the uncultured amniocytes. In fact, the majority of cases will return normal results after this additional work-up, since the mosaicism is likely confined to the placenta.

A large body of data on level III mosaicism for autosomal trisomy was gathered by the European Collaborative Research Group on Mosaicism in CVS (EUCROMIC) (Hahnemann and Vejerslev 1997) comprising information on just over 92,000 CVS procedures, from 79 laboratories, during 1986–1994. Mosaicism (or non-mosaic feto-placental discrepancy) was seen in 650 (1.5%) cases. Of these, 192 were followed up

[8] In this study, chromosomes 5, 8, 9, 10, 11, 12, 14, 15, and 16.

in detail, with karyotyping of fetal fibroblasts, fetal blood, amniocytes, or neonatal tissues. Most (84% of the 192) represented CPM. The abnormal cell line was present in either trophoblast (type I CPM; in 50%), villus mesenchyme (type II CPM; in 30%), or both (type III CPM; in 20%). Comparable numbers are due to a single Italian laboratory based upon a total of 60,347 samples, of which 2.2% showed mosaicism (Malvestiti et al. 2015). Of the 1,001 of these going on to amniocentesis, in only 131 (13%; 0.2% of the whole) was a true fetal mosaicism actually demonstrated. A greater risk (18.6%) applied when the abnormality had been detected on villus culture. The likelihood of confirmation at amniocentesis varies considerably according to the specific chromosome abnormality, being greatest when the chromosome concerned was a sex chromosome, marker, or one of those involved in the common trisomies (Table 22–3). Malvestiti and colleagues emphasize the value and validity of follow-up amniocentesis.

Randomness of Sampling

The vagaries of sampling may influence the interpretation, as the following examples show. We followed to term a woman in whom first-trimester CVS had shown trisomy 7 mosaicism with 47,XY,+7 in three out of eight clones; and yet three out of four placental samples (one from each quadrant), and peripheral blood from the (normal) baby, karyotyped 46,XY. Just one placental sample, which was not histologically distinguishable from the others, was 47,+7 (Watt et al. 1991). Presumably, the CVS sampling catheter had traversed this unrepresentative region of the placenta, and most of the sample that was eventually analyzed came from here.

Table 22–3. Follow-Up Amniocentesis
Likelihood of Confirmation of a Mosaic Chorionic Villous Sampling Result at Follow-Up Amniocentesis, According to Type of Chromosome Aberration

ABERRATION	PHILLIPS ET AL. (1996)	HAHNEMANN AND VEJERSLEV (1997)	MALVESTITI ET AL. (2015)	COMBINED LIKELIHOOD OF CONFIRMATION
47,+mar	8/30		22/65	30/95 (31.6%)
Sex chromosome aneuploidies	17/109		51/153	68/262 (26.0%)
Common trisomies (13, 18, 21)	15/79	15/66	29/151	59/296 (20.0%)
Rearrangements	3/35		18/178	21/213 (9.9%)
Polyploidy	1/28		2/63	3/91 (3.3%)
Other autosomal trisomies	6/188	5/126	9/391	20/705 (2.8%)

Notes. These data include cases in which the abnormal cell line was detected only in trophoblast (type I CPM). A greater risk is expected when the abnormality has been detected on villus culture.
CPM = confined placental mosaicism.

Sources: Data of Phillips et al. (1996), Hahnemann and Vejerslev (1997), and Malvestiti et al. (2015).

Similarly, in a case of i(5p) diagnosis at CVS following the birth of the (normal) baby, we identified a region of placental mosaicism (Clement Wilson et al. 2002). De Pater et al. (1997) did a CVS in a pregnancy of 37 weeks gestation in which severe growth retardation and a heart defect had been identified, and this showed non-mosaic trisomy 22. However, from a simultaneous amniocentesis only two out of 10 clones were 47,XX,+22, the other eight being normal, and a cord blood from the (abnormal) baby gave a non-mosaic 46,XX karyotype. Skin fibroblasts demonstrated mosaicism, 47,XX,+22[7]/46,XX[25]. Of 14 placental biopsies studied by interphase FISH, only one showed trisomy 22 cells, and at a low (~20%) percentage. Again, it may be that a small focus of trisomic tissue happened to be in the path of the CVS sampling needle, and the sample was aspirated while the needle was at this very spot. (This case is an example of "fetal-placental mosaicism," as illustrated in Figure 22–4.) NIPT circumvents this question, in that effectively the whole placenta is sampled (Van Opstal et al. 2020) but with the counterpoint that low-level mosaicism detectable at CVS may be missed at NIPT (Lund et al. 2024).

Discordance between results of CVS and post-natal sampling of the placenta can extend to "micro-level" imbalances. Lund et al. (2021) followed up five cases of mosaicism for a copy number variant detected at CVS. Abnormalities were confirmed in post-natal placental biopsies in four of the five cases, but in two of these, the placental biopsy findings were more complex than in the original CVS. Thus, CVS mosaicism for CNVs may be unreliable in predicting fetal CNVs, and in this setting, counseling should focus on the option of amniocentesis, rather than the CNV region involved.

Different Trisomies

Certain CVS trisomies are more or less likely to reflect the same trisomy in the fetus, and the pattern and distribution of the cell lines are also indicative. Trisomy 21 mosaicism on CVS is the most likely to represent a true fetal trisomy 21, whether in the non-mosaic or mosaic state. A risk applies also with trisomies 8, 9, 12, 13, 15, 18, and 20. On the other hand, CPM or fetoplacental discrepancy for trisomies 2, 3, 5, 7, 10, 11, 14, 16, 17, and 22 was never, in the EUCROMIC series, confirmed at fetal or post-natal studies. In some trisomies, a true fetal mosaicism may exist, but at such a low level that there might be no discernible effect upon the phenotype. Klein et al. (1994) reported such a case, a child born of a pregnancy in which trisomy 8 was observed in 81% of CVS cultured cells, 0% of amniotic fluid cells, and in 60% of a placental biopsy at delivery: The child had 4% and 1% mosaicism in blood at 2 and 7 months of age and 0% on a skin fibroblast study, and was normal in appearance, growth, and developmental progress at age 30 months. Of course, any fetal morphologic defect shown on ultrasonography would indicate the very substantial probability of a major degree of true fetal mosaicism, and in that case the choice of termination is appropriately offered.

Prognosis

The child subsequently born provides the direct evidence of a harm, or not, due to CPM. Amor et al. (2006) undertook a detailed post-natal follow-up, from ages 4 to 11 years, of 36 children from a "CPM pregnancy" and compared their outcomes according to a

similar examples exist to disquiet the counselor (Terzoli et al. 1990; Vockley et al. 1991), but a sense of perspective is to be kept: For each autosome, only the tiniest number of level II mosaicisms (zero for most chromosomes) have turned out to reflect, in fact, a recognized true mosaicism of the fetus.

Level III Mosaicism at Amniocentesis

Hsu and Benn re-evaluated the issues in 1999, and they have set forth useful guidelines. These are presented in detail in Table 22–5. While every autosome has now had

Table 22–5. Amniocyte Pseudomosaicism/Mosaicism
Guidelines for Work-up for the Elucidation of Possible Amniocyte Pseudomosaicism/Mosaicism

FLASK METHOD	IN SITU METHOD
A. **Indications for Extensive Work-up**	
(1) Autosomal trisomy involving a chromosome 21, 18, 13; or 2, 5, 8, 9, 21, 18, 13; or 2, 5, 8, 9, 12, 14, 15, 16, 20, 22 (SC, MC)	(1) Autosomal trisomy involving a chromosome 12, 14, 15, 16, 20, 22 (SCo, MCo)
(2) Unbalanced structural rearrangement (MC)	(2) Unbalanced structural rearrangement (MCo)
(3) Marker chromosome (MC)	(3) Marker chromosome (MCo)
B. **Indications for Moderate Work-up**	
(4) Extra sex chromosome (SC, MC)	(4) Extra sex chromosome (SCo, MCo)
(5) Autosomal trisomy involving a chromosome 1, 3, 4, 6, 7, 10, 11, 17, 19 (SC, MC)	(5) Autosomal trisomy involving a chromosome 1, 3, 4, 6, 7, 10, 11, 17, 19 (SCo, MCo)
(6) 45,X (MC)	(6) 45,X (SCo, MCo)
(7) Monosomy (other than 45,X) (MC)	(7) Monosomy (other than 45,X) (SCo, MCo)
(8) Marker chromosome (SC)	(8) Marker chromosome (SCo)
(9) Balanced structural rea (MC)	(9) Balanced structural rea (MCo)
C. Standard, No Additional Work-up	
(10) 45,X (SC)	(10) Unbalanced structural rea (SCo)
(11) Unbalanced structural rea (SC)	(11) Balanced structural rea (SCo)
(12) Balanced structural rea (SC)	(12) Break at centromere with loss of one arm (SCo)
(13) Break at centromere with loss of one arm (SC)	(13) All single-cell abnormalities

Notes: Criteria for extensive (A), moderate (B), and standard (C) work-up: A. Forty cells (20 cells from each of two flasks, excluding those cells analyzed from the culture with the initial observation of abnormality), or 24 colonies (excluding those colonies analyzed from the vessel with the initial observation). B. Twenty cells (from the flask without the initial observation), or 12 colonies (from vessels without the initial observation). C. Twenty cells (10 from each of two independent cultures), or 15 colonies (from at least two independent vessels).
MC = multiple cells (single flask); MC_0 = multiple colonies (single dish); Rea = rearrangement; SC = single cell (single flask); SCo = single colony (single dish).
Source: From LY Hsu and PA Benn, Revised guidelines for the diagnosis of mosaicism in amniocytes, *Prenat Diagn* 19:1081–1082, 1999.

a mention as a mosaic trisomy at prenatal or post-natal diagnosis, some are very rare, and others are of questionable significance. Some reported associations may not necessarily have been causal. Hsu and Benn propose the stringent requirement that, before embarking upon an extensive work-up, there be in the literature, for the particular chromosome, "two, or more, well-documented independent reports of confirmed amniocyte mosaicism with abnormal pregnancy outcomes." The most extensive data treating the question are published in two reports from a collaboration of a number of American and Canadian laboratories: Hsu et al. (1997) with respect to the rare trisomies, and Wallerstein et al. (2000) on trisomies 13, 18, 20, and 21. We make much use of this material in the commentaries later, and every prenatal diagnosis laboratory will want to have a copy of these papers readily at hand. Ultrasonography provides useful adjunctive evidence, but apparent normality cannot be taken as a guarantee. Studies for uniparental disomy may need to be considered in the case of mosaicism for chromosomes known to be subject to imprinting. Further modifications to these guidelines can be anticipated, as new data come to hand.

It is wise to attempt confirmation of a diagnosis of mosaicism, either on multiple fetal samples following pregnancy termination, or on blood and placenta in an infant. A post-termination chromosome study that did not confirm the abnormality could cause parents great distress, particularly when no malformations are seen on fetal examination; and it needs deciding with them beforehand whether they wish to have the results. An unconfirmed abnormality could be misleading in a twin pregnancy in which the diagnostic sample had come from a vanishing abnormal twin, but the post-termination tissue had come from the normal co-twin (Griffiths et al. 1996). Fejgin et al. (1997) refer to the "hopeful possibility" of mosaicism as a comfort to parents, with the post-termination tissue having sampled only the normal cell line. It is true that even multiple tissue sampling cannot be taken as having ruled out mosaicism, and a diagnosis of "apparent phenotypic normality" in a fetus still leaves open that a functional brain defect could have come to pass.

Microarray Analysis of Uncultured Amniocytes

Microarray analysis of uncultured amniocentesis samples detects mosaicism about as often as does karyotyping; however, differences between the two methodologies mean that results are not always concordant. First, the detection of abnormal cell lines by microarray is limited to those present at fractions above 5%–10%, whereas karyotyping allows, at least in principle, the analysis of tens or even hundreds of cells. Second, selection pressure in culture may result in either an underestimate or overestimate of the true proportion of aneuploid cells. Third, karyotyping is superior to microarray for resolving some sex chromosome mosaics, particularly where there was a mixture of monosomic and trisomic cells (e.g. 45,X/47,XXX mosaics).

For most autosomal abnormalities, microarray on uncultured cells appears to be the optimal technique. Hao et al. (2020) compared microarray (on uncultured cells) and karyotype on 2,091 amniocentesis samples, and detected mosaicism in 13 cases (0.6%). Mosaic trisomy for an autosome was seen in seven samples, all of which were detected by microarray, but only four by karyotype. The percentage of autosomal aneuploid mosaicism on microarray was consistently higher than seen on karyotype, suggesting selection against the aneuploid cells in culture. In our experience, when the level of mosaicism in uncultured amniocytes exceeds 20%, the result is likely to be confirmed post-natally, at a similar percentage, in a saliva sample of the baby. In contrast, when the mosaicism in amniocytes is less than 20%, the result more likely represents CPM.

In the specific setting of follow-up of increased-risk NIPT results, Donze et al. (2024) analyzed concordance between microarray (uncultured cells) and karyotype in 204 amniocentesis samples, and found eight cases discordant for mosaicism. Five of these had mosaicism only in cultured cells, comprising low-level mosaicism for trisomies 8, 13, 16 and 22, and an isodicentric chromosome 9. By the authors' assessment, only two of these findings were clinically relevant (i.e., 1% of the 204 samples), and they argue that testing of amniocentesis samples after abnormal NIPT should be limited to SNP array on uncultured cells. Three cases had mosaicism detected only in uncultured cells, comprising mosaicism for trisomies 2, 9, and 22, of which at least one (trisomy 2) was clinically relevant. To conclude from these observations: following an abnormal NIPT result, SNP analysis based upon uncultured amniocytes, in order to confirm or exclude the finding, will almost always (96%) be concordant with the interpretation on cultured cells. Thus, SNP array may, of itself, suffice.

TWIN PREGNANCY, DISCORDANT KARYOTYPES

Discordant karyotypes may be observed in the setting of either dizygous (DZ) or monozygous (MZ) twinning (Figure 20–24). Selective termination of the abnormal twin is an option, although one that cannot ensure that the normal twin will be unharmed. Because twins may share circulations, the process of termination of the affected twin may lead to exsanguination of the normal one (Lewi et al. 2006). In MZ twins in which "trisomic rescue" has been the basis of one twin being karyotypically normal, a risk for UPD applies, and this would be a concern in the case of a "UPD-vulnerable" chromosome.

SPECIFIC ABNORMALITIES

In this section, we outline the risks for phenotypic abnormality of specific chromosomal abnormalities detected at prenatal diagnosis. Since the available data often derive from terminated pregnancies in which only major anomalies are recognized, many of these risk figures may be underestimates. For example, a trisomy 21 fetus may appear normal to the inexpert eye on external observation, but we naturally assume intellectual disability would have resulted; and the same may apply to several other chromosomal imbalances. New knowledge will continue to accumulate, and what appears here is printed on paper, not in stone.

The small number of aneuploidies that may exist in the true non-mosaic state are noted first. In the mosaic list, almost every chromosome is represented, although in the CVS section we do include also a few instances of non-mosaicism.

Autosomal Trisomy, Non-Mosaic

Trisomies 13 and 18 (and extremely rarely 8, 9, 14, and 22) are practically the only non-mosaic autosomal trisomies besides + 21 that are detected at amniocentesis. Others occur, but virtually all miscarry before the usual time of amniocentesis. CVS, on the other hand, is done at a gestational stage when a number of trisomies destined to abort have not yet done so.

Trisomies 13 and 18

There is a high likelihood of spontaneous abortion after amniocentesis, and it is somewhat higher if detection is at CVS. Won et al. (2005) determined a rate of fetal death in utero following amniocentesis-proven trisomy 18 of 32%, while Yamanaka et al. (2006) arrived at a figure of 27%; from a somewhat different viewpoint, Cavadino and Morris (2017) showed a 30% survival rate to term of prenatally diagnosed trisomy 18. Data for survival of a liveborn child are due to Vendola et al. (2010) and are set out in Table 22–6. Further data from Lakovschek et al. (2011), following prenatal diagnosis and a continued pregnancy, give live birth rates of 33% for trisomy 13 and 13% for trisomy 18, with deaths typically within days.

The outlook for a liveborn child is so bleak, with inevitable profound mental deficiency, barely a vestige of social response in those few who survive beyond early infancy (a capacity for communication limited to "body movement," vocalization, and facial expression; Liang et al. 2015), and typically a requirement for full nursing care, that termination is sought by the majority of couples. Nevertheless, views can vary, and some infants are having heart surgery or other intervention (Weaver et al. 2021; Kosiv et al. 2023; Song et al. 2023). Others may elect to continue the pregnancy but chose post-natal comfort care provided by trained palliative care teams (Bierer et al. 2024). Carey (2012) emphasizes the need to bring the parents fully into the making of any decisions, and Chung et al. (2017) describe a family's positive and rewarding experience of looking after their infant with trisomy 13, with the help of pediatric palliative care staff; a view to be acknowledged, in the spirit of recognizing the plurality of opinion that is seen in the world.

Trisomy 21

We expect most readers will have an expert appreciation of the predicted DS phenotype, but we do recommend Bull's (2020) review as a full and balanced account. Guidelines exist for the medical care of children and adolescents (Bull et al. 2022) and adults (Tsou et al. 2020). Marteau et al. (1994) appraised the views of obstetricians, geneticists, and genetic nurses to the prenatal diagnosis of DS, and recorded some remarkable differences.

Table 22–6. Trisomy Survival
Probabilities of Survival to 1 Week, 1 Month, and 1 Year, for Liveborn Infants with Trisomies 13, 18, and 21

	1 WEEK	1 MONTH	1 YEAR
Trisomy 13	0.42	0.20	0.03
Trisomy 18	0.52	0.30	0.03
Trisomy 21		0.98	0.95

Source: From C Vendola et al., Survival of Texas infants born with trisomies 21, 18, and 13, *Am J Med Genet* 152A:360–366, 2010.

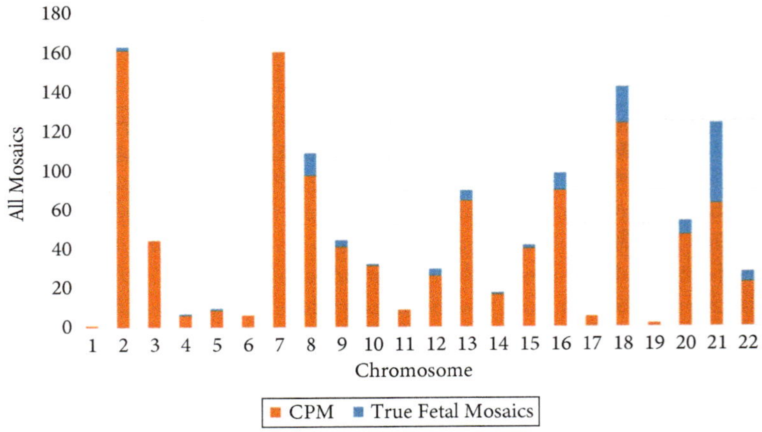

Figure 22–7. Mosaicism Outcomes at Prenatal Diagnosis.

Notes: This graph is derived from the data in Table 22-7. The increased risks associated with a prenatal diagnosis of mosaicism for trisomies 18 and 21, in particular, are evident.

or absence of a normal cell line is the key point: A fetal involvement is practically never seen if there is a normal cell line, and practically always seen if there is no normal cell line (MD Pertile, personal communication, 2002).

The general rule that Robinson et al. (1997) advance is this: CVS mosaicism due to a preconceptual (meiotic) error conveys a significant risk for fetal trisomy/UPD, whereas a postconceptual (somatic) error is usually innocuous. Mosaic trisomies 15, 16, and 22 are mostly in the former category, for example, whereas trisomies 3 and 7 are typically of mitotic origin, and mosaic trisomy 2 can be either.

The possibility remains for a residual effect due to (*1*) undetected (and presumably low-level) mosaic trisomy of the fetus, (*2*) uniparental disomy of the fetus, and (*3*) placental dysfunction as a consequence of a regional placental trisomy. The risks for these scenarios differ for different chromosomes, and we provide specific commentaries following.

Mosaic Trisomy 1 at Chorionic Villus Sampling. One case was recorded by Malvestiti et al. (2015), and it was not confirmed at amniocentesis.

Mosaic Trisomy 2 at Chorionic Villus Sampling and at NIPT. Two broad groups of trisomy 2 mosaicism are recognized (Robinson et al. 1997; Albrecht et al. 2001; Wolstenholme et al. 2001b). In the first, a majority (~90% of the total) are characterized by a small fraction of trisomic cells, and usually seen only in cultured mesenchymal cells. The pregnancy outcome is typically normal; in the series of Sago et al. (1997), 11/11 pregnancies had a normal outcome; and of the 77 cases reported by Malvestiti et al. (2015), none was confirmed at amniocentesis. It may be that these cases reflect a postzygotic generation of the trisomic lineage in a restricted region of chorionic tissue in an otherwise normal conceptus, and this small trisomic region has no discernible effect upon placental function. The second, minority group is presumed due to trisomy "correction" in a 47,+2 conceptus, from either a maternal or a paternal error. The level of trisomic cells in the CVS is typically high, up to 100%, with the involvement of both trophoblast and the mesenchymal core. In the series of Thomsen et al. (2024), 2/76 cases were confirmed at amniocentesis, and these had levels of mosaicism at CVS, as detected by microarray, of 80% and 69%. The placenta being substantially trisomic apparently compromises its function, and intrauterine growth retardation (IUGR) is a frequent observation, with a poor outcome (Roberts et al. 2003). One case is known of the very severe defect of "body stalk syndrome" associated with mosaic trisomy 2 at CVS (Smrcek et al. 2003). An atypical case in Chen et al. (2023c) attests to the variable levels of mosaicism between different tissues and the complexity of their interpretation. Following an initial trisomy 2 result at NIPT, the percentage of trisomic cells were, in chronological order:

11 week CVS, 100%;
20 week amniocentesis, 37% in cultured cells;
24 week amniocentesis, 28% FISH, 40% uncultured microarray, 0% cultured cells;
post-natal cord blood, 0%;
umbilical cord, 0%;
placenta, 23%; and
buccal swab at 6 weeks, 9%.

The child, who was born with growth retardation and also had maternal UPD(2), had normal development at one year.

Mosaic Trisomy 3 at Chorionic Villus Sampling. In the EUCROMIC study, of 10 cases with trisomy 3 at either short- or long-term culture, none proved to have fetal involvement, apart from one child with a normal karyotype at amniocentesis, and a very low 1/100 trisomy 3 count on blood as a newborn (Hahnemann and Vejerslev 1997). Similarly, none of the 27 cases reported by Malvestiti et al. (2015) or 14 cases of Thomsen et al. (2024) had fetal involvement. Zaslav et al. (2004) identified a case of trisomy 3, in which the initial amniocentesis showed 47,XX,+3[8]/46,XX[27], and a repeat procedure 47,XX,+3[1]/46,XX[18]. Fetal blood was normal in 100 cells. The baby was apparently normal at birth, except for IUGR. FISH of placenta demonstrated the trisomy 3; thus, it would likely have been found by CVS, had this been done.

Mosaic Trisomy 4 at Chorionic Villus Sampling. This is very rare: there were none in the EUCROMIC study and none of the four cases reported by Thomsen et al. (2024) were substantiated at amniocentesis. Malvestiti et al. (2015) did confirm one of their four cases by amniocentesis, and the pregnancy was terminated, the fetus having abnormalities of the heart, colon, and spleen. Two cases are noted in Kuchinka et al. (2001). In one case, subsequent amniocentesis gave a 46,XX karyotype, but fetal demise occurred at 30 weeks, associated with considerable growth retardation (although no externally observable malformations). UPD(4)mat was demonstrated. It remains open whether the unfortunate outcome was the consequence of the UPD or due to placental trisomy. The second case did not proceed to amniocentesis; biparental disomy 4 was demonstrated in the child. Follow-up at 1 year raised some reservation: Although development was judged to be normal, growth indices were low, including a head circumference at about the third centile (in other words, borderline microcephaly). To complicate the story, mother and child carried a balanced t(10;15).

The case in Marion et al. (1990), and followed up several years later (Brady et al. 2005), was actually an amniocentesis diagnosis, but since post-natal studies showed trisomy 4 mosaicism in the placenta, it is not unreasonable to consider this is a potential CVS example. The child, at age 14 years, had a low-normal intellect and some physical body asymmetries (of hand, ear, and breast). Blood was 46,XX; skin biopsy confirmed constitutional +4 mosaicism. In another case, Gentile et al. (2005)

identified mosaic trisomy 4 by amniocentesis (22% of cells). The pregnancy presented at 22 weeks gestation with micrognathia, abnormal brain development, and spinal and cardiac defects. At termination, trisomy 4 mosaicism was confirmed in placental and fetal skin cultured cells; the cord blood karyotype was normal. Molecular analysis excluded uniparental disomy of chromosome 4, but showed that the trisomy 4 was of maternal meiotic origin.

An extraordinary example of mosaic trisomy 4 at CVS with double mosaicism for trisomies 4 and 6 at amniocentesis, 47,XY +4/47,XY,+6/46,XY, is described in Wieczorek et al. (2003). The double trisomy mosaicism was confirmed on skin (but not blood) karyotyping in the child, whose phenotype, while certainly abnormal, was less so than might have been anticipated.

Mosaic Trisomy 5 at Chorionic Villus Sampling. Thomsen et al. (2024) recorded five cases, of which one was confirmed at amniocentesis. That pregnancy was investigated because of an increased-risk first-trimester screen, and trisomy 5 was identified in 2/25 cells at CVS and 2/100 cells at follow-up amniocentesis. The pregnancy continued to livebirth, but further follow-up was not provided. Only three cases are recorded in the EUCROMIC study; in none was a fetal trisomy subsequently shown (Hahnemann and Vejerslev 1997). Another three cases are listed in Malvestiti et al. (2015), again without fetal involvement. Chen et al. (2020a) report the diagnosis of CPM for trisomy 5 at CVS with follow-up amniocentesis showing maternal uniparental disomy for chromosome 5. The baby, born to a 45-year-old mother, also had Down syndrome, with no additional phenotypic features attributable to the CPM or UPD(5)mat.

Mosaic Trisomy 6 at Chorionic Villus Sampling. Very few examples are known. Malvestiti et al. (2015) record three cases, and Thomsen et al. (2024) four cases, none confirmed on amniocentesis. A detailed case report is given in Miller et al. (2001). A young mother had a 12-week CVS because of ultrasonographic anomalies (crown-rump length at 11-week size, nuchal translucency), with 60% of cells in short-term culture and 22% of long-term cells showing 47,XX,+6. Amniocentesis was declined. An abnormal heart rate at 25 weeks led to emergency delivery, and a growth-retarded infant with numerous anomalies was born. Her blood karyotype was normal, but trisomy 6 cells were found in placenta and umbilical cord samples. Growth indices remained below the third centile. On follow-up at age 2¾ years, neurodevelopmental progress was "near normal." Skin taken at the time of surgery showed 3% (hand) and 20% (inguinal area) mosaicism. The case in Kitamura et al. (2024) was ascertained via the detection of 47,XY,+6 in 20% of cells at amniocentesis, but post-natal analysis of the placenta showed trisomy 6 in 4% of cells. The baby was healthy at age 1 year, and the post-natal karyotype normal.

Mosaic Trisomy 7 at Chorionic Villus Sampling and at NIPT. This is typically a mitotically arising mosaicism. Kalousek et al. (1996) looked at 14 cases of trisomy 7 CVS mosaicism and feto-placental discordance, the fraction of trisomy ranging from 7% to 88% in 11, and with three showing 100%. Twelve infants were judged normal, and in the eight of these tested, all proved to have biparental inheritance. Two infants were of low birth weight, and the one of these tested was the only of the series with UPD and a meiotic origin; the cultured CVS in this case was 100% trisomic. In a case we studied, mentioned also above, three post-natal placental samples karyotyped normal, and one with trisomy 7; the baby was normal (Watt et al. 1991).

In the EUCROMIC study, of 32 cases with trisomy at either or both short- and long-term culture (including three with non-mosaic trisomy), none proved to have fetal involvement (Hahnemann and Vejerslev 1997). Similarly, of the 74 cases recorded by Malvestiti et al. (2015) and 55 cases by Thomsen et al. (2024), none were confirmed at amniocentesis. The conclusion is that the great majority of trisomy 7 mosaicism detected at CVS arises mitotically, does not imply a risk for UPD, is confined to the placenta, does not obviously compromise intrauterine growth, and is associated with the birth of a normal baby. Following detection of CPM for trisomy 7 at NIPT, however, an increased risk of low birth weight has been noted (Van Prooyen Schuurman et al. 2022).

Mosaic Trisomy 8 at Chorionic Villus Sampling and at NIPT. A well-recognized but highly variable post-natal phenotype (Warkany syndrome) accompanies trisomy 8 mosaicism, which may also include an increased risk for cancer (Altiner et al. 2016). Fetal defects are recorded on pathology examination (Jay et al. 1999). Typically, the mosaicism is the consequence of a post-zygotic nondisjunction in an initially 46,N conceptus (Danesino et al. 1998).[15] In the three-case series of Hahnemann and Vejerslev, Thomsen et al. and Malvestiti et al., there were a total of 102 cases, of which 13 were confirmed at amniocentesis. Thomsen et al. (2021) reviewed 60 cases of trisomy 8 mosaicism at CVS from the literature, and added 37 of their own. Fetal involvement was confirmed in 18 out of 97 pregnancies (19%), including eight pregnancies initially interpreted to be CPM following a normal amniocentesis, but subsequently seen as true fetal mosaicism. This circumstance calls to mind the scenario proposed by Wolstenholme (1996) True fetal mosaicism is typically associated with low levels of trisomy 8 in trophoblast cells (short-term CVS culture), high levels in extra-embryonic mesoderm (long-term CVS culture), and low levels in amniocytes and fetal blood cells.

Hu et al. (2022) report a case of trisomy 8 mosaicism initially detected at NIPT, and confirmed by the detection of 10% trisomy 8 cells at amniocentesis. Hydronephrosis and spinal irregularity were detected antenatally, and at three-year follow-up the child had language delay and facial asymmetry. A high risk NIPT result for trisomy 8 led to a diagnosis of paternal UPD(8) at amniocentesis in the case of Yu et al. (2022), with the child reported to be developing normally at age 3 years. In this case, the initial abnormality was likely a paternal meiotic error.

Mosaic Trisomy 9 at Chorionic Villus Sampling and at NIPT. Malvestiti et al. (2015) record 18 cases of mosaic trisomy 9 at CVS, none of which were confirmed at amniocentesis. In contrast, Thomsen et al. (2024) confirmed three of their 24 cases at amniocentesis. Saura et al. (1995) presented seven cases of trisomy 9, five of which gave a non-mosaic result, with the outcomes being abnormal in most. In the EUCROMIC study, of nine cases with trisomy 9 at either or both short- and long-term culture (including three with non-mosaic trisomy in one or both cultures), one proved to have fetal involvement (Hahnemann and Vejerslev 1997). This single case had non-mosaic trisomy at both short- and long-term culture. Slater et al. (2000) report a case of trisomy 9 non-mosaic at CVS, but with level II mosaicism found at amniocentesis, with only two cells 47,XX,+9. At fetal blood sampling, all 85 cells analyzed were 46,XX. Molecular studies revealed UPD(9)mat. A blood sample from the newborn infant had

[15] Trisomy 8 mosaicism of meiotic origin is sometimes found in miscarriage samples, but when detected post-natally, appears to cause a phenotype distinct from Warkany syndrome. Valind et al. (2014) detected trisomy 8 cells of meiotic origin in a Wilms tumor sample of an otherwise healthy 2 year old boy, and Baidas et al. (2014) made a similar finding in the bone marrow of an otherwise healthy 32 year old woman who presented with recurrent aphthous ulcers that were refractory to treatment.

Mosaic Trisomy 2 at Amniocentesis. In Hsu et al.'s (1997) survey, trisomy 2 conveyed the highest risk of any of the "rare trisomic" autosomes for an abnormal outcome, namely 90%, with a variable pattern of major defects. Wang et al. (2020b) provide a clear demonstration (Figure 22–8). It is probable that mosaic trisomy 2 detected at amniocentesis would be in the same group as the high-level mosaic CVS case (see above). Tuğ et al. (2017) report a case with severe fetal malformation initially identified on serum screening and ultrasonography, with amniocyte fractions 47,XX,+2[12]/46,XX[73].

A trisomic line in the fetus/child may take some diligence to find. Sago et al. (1997) reported a case in which there was level III mosaicism with trisomy 2 cells present in 27% of amniocytes (and biparental disomy). The child was severely abnormal, and while blood and skin karyotyped as 46,XY, 4% of liver cells were 47,+2. Similarly, Chen et al. (2013c) report a fetus with cardiac defect, polydactyly, and dysmorphism, and who had mosaic trisomy 2 at amniocentesis. Trisomy 2 cells had arisen due to maternal meiosis I error and comprised 100% of the placenta, 50% of the amniotic membrane, and 10% of the fetal liver, but fetal lung, skin, and blood showed a normal karyotype.

Mosaic Trisomy 3 at Amniocentesis. Only two cases were identified in Hsu et al.'s (1997) review, in one of which the child had multiple malformations, with the mosaicism confirmed on skin fibroblast culture. The child in the other case was normal. Marked intrauterine, and subsequently post-natal, growth restriction was the prominent feature in the cases in Zaslav et al. (2004) and Sheath et al. (2010); in both, development in early infancy was judged to be normal. Tang et al. (2017) provide further evidence that low-level mosaicism for trisomy 3 can be associated with a normal outcome. In their case, ascertained in the context of an increased-risk maternal serum screen and normal ultrasound, the prenatal detection of trisomy 3 in 10% of amniocytes and 3/200 cord blood lymphocytes was followed by the birth of a healthy baby girl, with a normal blood karyotype.

Mosaic Trisomy 4 at Amniocentesis. Hoyas et al. (2021) review ten cases, with normal and abnormal outcomes both, approximately proportional to the fraction of trisomic cells. Four cases had developed normally by age 1 year, with the percentage of + 4 cells between 8% and 31%; normal ultrasonography was a positive pointer. The case

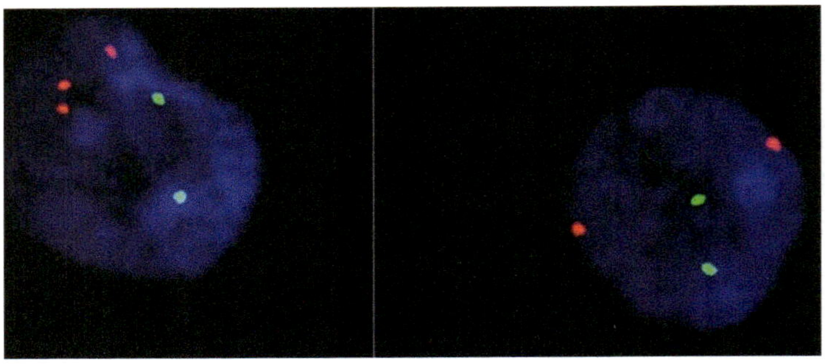

Figure 22–8. Trisomy 2 Mosaicism at Amniocentesis.

Notes: These images are of interphase FISH on uncultured amniocytes, two cells shown here. The red spots reflect a probe recognizing chromosome 2 centromere; the green is for chromosome 22, as a control. The cell at *left*, with three red spots, is trisomic; the cell at *right*, with two red spots, disomic. Second trimester NIPT results had indicated the chromosome 2 quantum to be increased. Follow-up amniocentesis showed mos 47,XY,+2[8]/46,XY[19]; ultrasonography at 24 weeks revealed fetal IUGR.

Source: From T Wang et al., Prenatal diagnosis of mosaic trisomy 2 and literature review, *Mol Cytogenet* 13:36, 2020. Courtesy L Guo, and with the permission of Springer Nature.

in Hoyas et al. is unique, of monozygous twins with discordant karyotypes: Twin A had multiple major structural anomalies and karyotyped non-mosaic trisomy 4 at amniocentesis, whereas the karyotype of Twin B was normal 46,XX. Trisomy 4 cells have never been detected in the peripheral blood of affected individuals.

Mosaic Trisomy 5 at Amniocentesis. Hsu et al. (1997) recorded five cases. In one, a high level of trisomic cells (80%) was associated nevertheless with a phenotypically and karyotypically normal infant. In two, the child was abnormal, both showing the mosaicism on post-natal study. Brown et al. (2009) and Bonasoni et al. (2022) describe cases in which a fetal heart defect had been the factor leading to an amniocentesis, with respective proportions of +5 cells of 50% and 19%. In both, autopsy analysis showed trisomy cells in several tissues, but not blood. A further case in Reittinger et al. (2017) may have reflected a "correction" of trisomy, as the severely malformed infant eventually born had, on peripheral blood analysis, uniparental disomy 5 (and no trisomy).

Mosaic Trisomy 6 at Amniocentesis. Hsu et al. (1997) recorded three cases, each with the same low-level (6%) trisomy in amniocytes, and each with a normal outcome. Reports are on record of the diagnosis following recognition of fetal defects at ultrasonography, the defects ranging from minor to severe (Wallerstein et al. 2002; Wegner et al. 2004; Destree et al. 2005). One case of fetal death in utero at 23 weeks was associated with 48% trisomy cells on fetal skin analysis (Cockwell et al. 2006). Chen et al. (2006b) report a case with low-level (3%–10%) mosaicism, with normal fetal blood karyotype, biparental inheritance, in which the parents chose termination, and the trisomy was absent on cultured fetal tissue. They suggest low-level trisomy 6 mosaicism may be a benign finding. A similar case, but with 20% mosaicism at amniocentesis, and where the parents chose to continue, is provided by Kitamura et al. (2024): the baby appeared healthy at birth, and post-natal cytogenetic investigations were normal.

Mosaic Trisomy 7 at Amniocentesis. Hsu et al. (1997) recorded eight cases, with fractions of trisomic cells ranging from 5% to 48%. Only one resulted in the birth of a phenotypically abnormal child, but low-level 47,XY,+7/46,XY mosaicism was confirmed in two phenotypically normal children on foreskin analysis. Warburton (2002) emphasized that this relatively low-risk assessment is the appropriate one to offer, and she notes also that UPD(7), while unlikely, may be worth testing for. A low-level mosaic case, taken to termination with pathology study and multiple fetal karyotyping, with entirely normal findings, led Chen et al. (2005a) to agree with the view that optimistic advice may usually be appropriate. A microarray-era example is that of Chen et al. (2024e) who identified 24% mosaicism for trisomy 7 in DNA from uncultured amniocytes, but a 46,XY karyotype in cultured amniocytes. At birth, the baby was assessed to be phenotypically normal, with no evidence of trisomy 7 in peripheral blood.

Other cases with a post-amniocentesis abnormal outcome (and in which ascertainment was necessarily biased) include the following: Mosaicism was verified post-natally on skin fibroblast analysis in the child reported in Kivirikko et al. (2002), in whom fetal blood sampling and mid-trimester ultrasonography had been normal; there was facial asymmetry and mild dysmorphism along with rather impressive hypomelanosis of Ito, while mental development was "considered to be within normal limits," although no detailed assessment had been done. The fraction of trisomic colonies in the 47,XX,+7/46,XX case of Bilimoria and Rothenberg (2003) was rather high, at 41%, and in addition uniparental heterodisomy was shown in the 46,XX line; the pregnancy had come to attention because of an increased-risk maternal serum screen. On a neonatal blood sample, all cells were 46,XX, while on the contrary, all placental cells analyzed were trisomic. The child was small for dates and had some minor anomalies. These authors mention an anecdote of a trisomy 7 mosaic woman "graduating from college and getting married." Petit et al. (2012) describe a case of IUGR leading to amniocentesis, which was interpreted at the time as normal. The child proved to be delayed in growth and development, and displayed hypomelanosis of Ito. Blood analysis showed 46,XY with maternal UPD(7). The skin fibroblast karyotype, however, was 47,XY,+7/46,XY; and restudy of stored amniocytes from long-term culture showed mosaic trisomy 7.

Mosaic Trisomy 8 at Amniocentesis. Counseling is difficult, and advice must be cautious. An observation of trisomy 8 in amniocytes predicts a distinct probability, but by no means a certainty, of the clinical syndrome, namely Warkany syndrome. It is not possible to put a good figure on the level of risk. Vice versa, a true fetal mosaicism may not necessarily be detected at amniocentesis. Lund et al. (2020) estimate that true fetal mosaicism is missed by amniocentesis in 11% of cases, and emphasize the importance of careful ultrasound, and the possible role of cordocentesis, as well as noting that microarray analysis of DNA from uncultured cells may inform the interpretation. A finding of apparently normal morphology at fetal examination following termination in some 47,+8/46,N pregnancies might be misleading, since the physical component of the clinical syndrome is relatively minor (Hsu et al. 1997). In the series of van Haelst et al. (2001), the two cases of trisomy 8 mosaicism detected at amniocentesis both turned out to be pseudomosaicism.

Mosaic Trisomy 9 at Amniocentesis. The risk is high (Chen et al. 2003a). Hsu et al. (1997) recorded data on 25 cases, with pregnancy termination being done in 21. Abnormality was identified in most of the 21, and mosaicism was confirmed in the seven having skin fibroblast studies. In the four pregnancies continuing, one abnormal child was born, with 47,+9/46,N mosaicism on blood karyotyping, the other three pregnancies resulting in apparently normal newborns. An overall figure of 56% applies for the risk that the fetus is abnormal. This high percentage figure is not surprising, and indeed it may well be an underestimate of the risk for functional abnormality in the child (intellect not being assessable in the newborn), considering the well-recorded phenotype of mosaic trisomy 9 in older individuals. A review of the outcomes in surviving individuals is given in Bruns and Campbell (2015).

Mosaic Trisomy 10 at Amniocentesis. In one case listed in Daniel et al. (2004), a 47,XX,+10[27]/46,XX[83] karyotype was associated with severe fetal defects, this observation being the basis of the referral for prenatal diagnosis. They were able to ascertain that the cause was a post-zygotic duplication of the maternal homolog.

Mosaic Trisomy 11 at Amniocentesis. Of the four reported examples, all have had a normal outcome. One child came from a pregnancy with a 26% fraction of trisomic cells, with 46,N findings on post-natal tissues, and followed through to 1 year of age. Basel-Vanagaite et al. (2006) raise the question that this mosaicism may typically be a benign finding.

Mosaic Trisomy 12 at Amniocentesis. This is one of the more frequently described mosaicisms, and often implies a high risk. Hsu et al. (1997) accumulated 23 cases, comprising 12 continuing pregnancies and 11 terminations. In most of those proceeding to fetal or neonatal fibroblast karyotyping, the mosaicism was subsequently confirmed, though most of the fetuses appeared to be normal. It is possible, however, that some subtle physical features, and possibly unsubtle neurological deficit, might have eventuated had these "normal" fetuses been born. The clinical range in the few recorded liveborn patients with true trisomy 12 mosaicism is quite variable, from lethality in the newborn period through to an otherwise normal man with Kartagener syndrome being investigated for infertility (DeLozier-Blanchet et al. 2000).

Of the 12 continuing pregnancies in Hsu et al. (1997) the outcomes were abnormal in five and grossly normal newborns in seven. Three of these normal infants followed for 5 months to 5 years were all judged to be continuing along normally, and Staals et al. (2003) add another 3-year-old to this list. The proportion of trisomic cells at amniocentesis apparently is not a very helpful guide in prognosis. In one case in Daniel et al. (2004), associated with fetal defect at 18-week termination, the trisomy had resulted from a post-zygotic duplication of one homolog.

Mosaic Trisomy 13 at Amniocentesis. The risk for abnormality is very high. A collaboration of 23 American and Canadian laboratories provided data on the outcomes of 25 prenatal diagnoses of 47,+13/46 mosaicism (Wallerstein et al. 2000). Care was taken to exclude cases in which ascertainment had been biased by abnormal ultrasonography. In 21, the pregnancies were terminated. Various abnormalities were identified in 10 of these; the range of percentages of abnormal amniocytes was very wide, 6%–94%, average 58%. No defect was detectable in the remaining 11 aborted fetuses, although the assessment was limited to simple inspection. Four pregnancies proceeded to apparently normal live birth; the percentages of abnormal amniocytes in these were lower, ranging from 5% to 13%. We mentioned above the very low-level mosaicism at a post-CVS follow-up amniocentesis in Delatycki et al. (1998), with a normal outcome.

Mosaic Trisomy 14 at Amniocentesis. Chen et al. (2013e) summarized 10 cases from the literature. In three of the 10 cases, the trisomy 14 resulted from an isochromosome 14. Four of the 10 pregnancies continued to term, from which three infants appeared normal, and one had multiple abnormalities resulting in neonatal death. Five pregnancies were terminated, in which four had multiple abnormalities, and one had micrognathia only. One pregnancy ended in intrauterine fetal death at 18 weeks gestation, in the absence of anatomical abnormality. A risk exists for UPD(14) over and above any defect due to the mosaic trisomy per se, and this should be checked.

Mosaic Trisomy 15 at Amniocentesis. Trisomy 15 is usually the consequence of a maternal meiosis I nondisjunction. Amniotic fluid mosaicism may well reflect a true mosaicism of the fetus. In Hsu et al. (1997), six of the 11 cases recorded had an abnormal outcome, the risk being greater when the trisomy level was higher (>40%). Zaslav et al. (1998) review seven cases of low-level mosaic trisomy 15 detected at prenatal diagnosis, in each the amniocentesis having been done for advanced maternal age. All seven chose to terminate, and a variety of defects were documented in most but not all. In their own case, the trisomic cell line in the initial amniocyte analysis was at a low level: 47,XX,+15[2]/46,XX[37]. Fetal tissues were also at low levels (lung 2%–5%, heart 8%–15%, skin 6%–10% on metaphase and interphase analysis, respectively), but the placenta showed 100% trisomy on metaphase analysis and 95% using FISH on interphase cells. These authors also document from the literature four cases of abnormal liveborns with trisomy 15 mosaicism. There is the additional question of UPD(15)mat, the considerable phenotypic consequence of which—that is, Prader-Willi syndrome—may be superadded upon that of a trisomy 15 mosaicism.

Chen et al. (2020c) identified discrepancy between a normal karyotype from cultured amniocytes, and a microarray result from uncultured amniocytes that detected 30% trisomy 15. The amniocentesis was repeated eight weeks later with a similar result, but with percentage of trisomy 15 reduced to 15%.[16] Biparental inheritance of chromosome 15 was confirmed, and the pregnancy proceeded to the delivery of a phenotypically normal but growth-retarded infant at 32 weeks of gestation. Trisomy 15 was absent from blood but detected in 2% of buccal mucosa cells, this confirming a low-level mosaicism in the child.

Mosaic Trisomy 16 at Amniocentesis. Neiswanger et al. (2006) reviewed the question of trisomy 16 mosaicism diagnosed prenatally, including 36 cases from amniocentesis; and they reported their own findings in three cases in which no prior CVS had been undertaken. Of these three, all had abnormal outcomes: IUGR but with normal cognitive development as judged at 14 months; IUGR and major malformations including cardiac dextroposition; and IUGR with hypoplastic left heart, leading to neonatal death. In their literature review, the figures for complication were as follows: infant death, 33%; prematurity, 64%; IUGR, 69%; physical anomalies, 75%; and just one assessed as a normal outcome, 3% (these figures being considerably worse than for CVS diagnosis). They note that level II mosaicism, in this context, may well reflect a true fetal mosaicism.

Thus, the earlier opinion of Hsu et al. (1998) is supported: "Mosaic trisomy 16 detected through amniocentesis is not a benign finding, but associated with a high risk of abnormal outcome, most commonly intrauterine growth retardation, congenital heart defect, developmental delay, and minor anomalies." Rieubland et al. (2009) diagnosed two cases post-natally, noting a considerable phenotypic difference between the two, one normally grown and developing at age 11 months, but with a severe hypospadias; the other with IUGR, body asymmetry, numerous physical anomalies, and dying at 7 months: yet further illustrating the challenge in offering advice at prenatal detection. Notwithstanding, we have seen an eventual apparently normal outcome, the child assessed at 2½ years of age, albeit that delivery by cesarean section at 36 weeks had been necessitated due to fetal distress with IUGR. Trisomy 16 had been detected at high level on CVS and at amniocentesis, and low-level (8%) post-natally on buccal mucosal cells (Coman et al. 2010a).

The question of an influence of UPD is open to argument. Scheuvens et al. (2017) proposed that UPD(16)mat is not of itself pathogenic, and that any associated phenotypic abnormality is actually the consequence of a cryptic trisomy 16 mosaicism; nevertheless, UPD was more frequent in those pregnancies in Neiswanger et al. (2006) with IUGR, and in the infants with anomalies. Yong et al. (2003) tested for UPD in a series of infants from mosaic trisomy 16 pregnancies, and the fraction with UPD(16) mat at 40% was close enough to the one-third expectation from random loss of one chromosome. These infants were more severely affected than those with biparental inheritance of 16. Mosaic trisomy 16 has a particular association with very low levels of pregnancy-associated plasma protein-A (PAPP-A) on first-trimester serum screening.

Mosaic Trisomy 17 at Amniocentesis. de Vries et al. (2013) summarized 28 cases from the literature, a proportion at least of which had arisen mitotically. The most common outcome (19 of the 28, 68%) was the birth of a healthy infant without evidence

[16] A reduction in trisomic cells over time is consistent with origin being primarily from the amnion, and with a progressive decline in the proportion of cells from the amnion compared to the proportion from the fetus.

of trisomy 17 in blood and/or fibroblasts. In nine cases the trisomy was confirmed on fibroblasts—six after birth, and three following termination of pregnancy. In seven of the nine cases of true mosaicism, trisomy was not detected in blood, suggesting selection against trisomic cells in this tissue and possibly explaining why so few post-natal cases are reported. In cases of true fetal mosaicism, the clinical phenotype includes cerebellar hypoplasia, ventricular septal defect, scoliosis, growth and intellectual retardation, and body asymmetry (Baltensperger et al. 2016). The longest follow-up is reported in Witters and Fryns (2008), a child at age 36 months who was significantly delayed, with a developmental age of 26 months.

And yet a number of normal outcomes are on record, as Abrams et al. (2005) document in their own case, with the child reportedly normal as a 2-year-old, and as they note similarly in a handful of other cases from the literature. They advise that an optimistic view is warranted, if the ultrasonography is normal. This view is supported in Chen et al. (2016b), whose patient had a prenatal diagnosis of 47,XX,+17[4]/46,XX[17], confirmed on repeat study with interphase FISH (5/105 cells); a normal child was in due course born, 46,XX on cord blood.[17] Chen et al. (2020b) report monozygous twins with discordant karyotypes at amniocentesis: Twin A had the mosaic karyotype 47,XX,+17[3]/46,XX[23], whereas Twin B was normal. At 2 year follow-up, the only discernable phenotype was preaxial polydactyly of the right hand in Twin A.

Mosaic Trisomy 18 at Amniocentesis. The risk is very high. In the collaboration of Wallerstein et al. (2000), 31 prenatal diagnoses of trisomy 18 mosaicism were available for review. In just over half of these, the abortuses (induced termination or natural abortion) were abnormal. In 11, no defects were discerned at fetal examination Just three pregnancies came to live birth, and these babies were apparently normal. The percentages of trisomic amniocytes in these three cases ranged from 2% to 20% (mean 9%), compared with 2%–95% (mean 37%) in those with abnormal outcome. A very rare abnormality is 45,X/47,XX,+18 mosaicism, in which the phenotype can vary from fairly mild to severe (Schluth-Bolard et al. 2009; Tyler et al. 2009).

Mosaic Trisomy 19 at Amniocentesis. A single case is recorded in Hsu et al. (1997), and in which there was a normal outcome at live birth.

Mosaic Trisomy 20 at Amniocentesis. This is one of the most commonly observed mosaic aneuploidies. Trisomy 20 may exist in three forms: as confined placental mosaicism, as placental-fetal mosaicism with an apparently normal phenotype in the child that is subsequently born, or as a fetal mosaicism with phenotypic consequence (Hsu et al. 1991). There may be no dysmorphic features, only some "soft" signs, or rarely an unambiguous facial dysmorphism; a characteristic if subtle syndrome is proposed (Willis et al. 2008). In certain fetal regions in which the trisomy may exist, in particular kidney and gut, the imbalance apparently has no discernible untoward effect, and in fact aneuploid cells may normally be cultured from urinary sediment. (Recognizing that amniotic fluid has a substantial contribution from fetal urine production, presumably some of the "amniotic fluid cells" from which the diagnosis of trisomy 20 had been made may have actually had origin from the fetal urinary tract.)

In the collaboration of Wallerstein et al. (2000) comprising 152 diagnoses, 10 (7%) were recorded with an abnormal outcome (six liveborns, four abortuses). There was

[17] The observation of 5/90 cells trisomic 17 on uncultured urinary cells from the child may well have reflected an occult constitutional mosaicism but not necessarily so, since a low level of trisomic cells can be a normal finding in this tissue.

correlation with the level of mosaicism: Abnormality was observed in 20% of infants where there had been >50% trisomic cells at amniocentesis, and in 5% of those with <50%. Baty et al. (2001) reviewed 17 cases in which follow-up of the children extended beyond 1 year, of whom 12 (71%) had developed normally. The remaining five had various degrees of speech and motor delay. A more optimistic interpretation comes from James et al. (2002), who tracked down all cases diagnosed at amniocentesis in New Zealand from 1991 to 2001, numbering 13, with follow-up well into childhood for nine of these (the longest to age 10 years). The range of the trisomic fraction of amniocytes was 8%–50%. All were essentially normal, except for one child who had minor anomalies at birth, resolving by 6 months of age, and deformation due to breech delivery may have been the cause, although weight was below the third centile; and in the only case in which termination was chosen, rather subtle (indeed borderline) external fetal anomalies were noted, and cultured tissue showed low-level (skin 2%, kidney 7%) trisomy mosaicism. Baty et al. (2001) followed up two cases with higher fractions of trisomic cells at amniocentesis, 83% and 57% in one, and of 90% in the other, and the children, at ages 9 and 8 years, respectively, were of normal intelligence and of essentially normal morphological appearance. Each did, however, display quite prominent hypomelanosis of Ito, presumably reflecting a fairly widespread distribution of a trisomic 20 lineage, at least in skin.

Nevertheless, reservation must remain. Reish et al. (1998) offer the sobering example of a 15-month-old child with considerably delayed gross and fine motor skills and poor language acquisition, who had 54% trisomic cells from a skin biopsy (a normal karyotype on peripheral blood). In the pregnancy, amniocentesis had shown a 45% mosaicism, fetal ultrasonography was normal, and the parents had been "cautiously counseled." Likewise, Wallerstein et al. (2005) report a child who had seemed normal at birth, and 46,XX on blood, but who went on to manifest a "pervasive developmental disorder." Trisomy 20 had been present in only 4/63 colonies at amniocentesis; trisomy was further documented in urinary sediment at age 4 years. They comment that "optimism regarding developmental outcome should be tempered with some caution."

Bianca et al. (2008) summarize the issues and advise along these lines: A second CVS or amniocentesis would add little value; fetal blood sampling is not useful, and neither is UPD analysis; the level of mosaicism does not predict outcome. This agrees with the views of some and contradicts others, as noted above; notwithstanding, Chen et al. (2023d) advise that low-level mosaic trisomy 20 at amniocentesis can be a transient and benign condition.

Mosaic Trisomy 21 at Amniocentesis. The risk for DS is very high. The collaborative study of Wallerstein et al. (2000) accumulated 96 cases for review. Half had an observably abnormal outcome, with confirmatory cytogenetic study performed in a minority. Most of these were fetuses post-termination with various abnormalities; six were liveborns, five of these with a clinical diagnosis of DS and one with an isolated heart defect. An apparently normal appearance (assessment limited to inspection in 39, autopsy in two) was recorded in 41 aborted fetuses. Among these, 20 were submitted to further cytogenetic analysis (repeat amniocentesis, fetal tissue, fetal blood, placenta), with eight showing 8%–90% trisomic cells, and 12 with 0%. Seven liveborns were normal, two being followed up beyond the newborn period; none had confirmatory karyotyping. The mean amniotic fluid proportion of trisomic cells was 17%, range 6%–31%, in these normal children. This compares with a mean of 35% in those with a demonstrably abnormal outcome. But even in the group with the lowest level of amniotic fluid trisomy (3%–10%) half had an abnormal outcome.

From the whole material, a risk for phenotypic abnormality of 50% should be seen as a minimum estimate, since subtler defects at fetal or neonatal assessment would have escaped notice, and a potential compromise of intellectual function was of course not assessable. However, the report in Chen et al. (2016c) illustrates that a confirmed true mosaicism in the child, if of low level (2/38 in this case, on post-natal cord blood), can be associated with phenotypic normality, at least as judged at age 7 months; two amniocenteses had returned trisomy 21 fractions of 5/53 and 6/26.

Mosaic Trisomy 22 at Amniocentesis. Chen et al. (2019) determined a very high risk for abnormality for 47,+22/46, with 14 out of 20 outcomes being abnormal. The mosaic trisomy 22 levels of the six normal cases ranged from 5% to 28%, which overlapped with the 3.6%–50% levels from the 14 abnormal cases. Growth retardation is the most common ultrasound finding, but a range of congenital anomalies are also seen. Berghella et al. (1998) described a normal fetal blood result following trisomy 22 mosaicism diagnosis at amniocentesis, but fetal skin biopsy showed 47,+22/46, and structural abnormalities were subsequently identified in the aborted fetus. Four cases are noted in the review of Wolstenholme et al. (2001a), these all having followed an initial detection at CVS. Three out of the four showed some degree of normal/trisomy mosaicism at fetal samplings post-termination. Leclercq et al. (2010) record a normal phenotypic outcome in a single case, followed up to age 4 years, albeit that the child showed the mosaicism on skin, in 6% of cells. Three other cases were abnormal at autopsy study (two following fetal death in utero, and one a medical termination).

Mosaic Partial Trisomy at Amniocentesis. It is not feasible to list here recorded cases, and each must be judged on its merits. One specific example is worth noting, in that it may represent simply cultural artifact associated with a fragile site. This is mosaicism for a del(10)(q23). Zaslav et al. (2002) document a case of 46,XY,del(10)(q23)[9]/46,XY[45] detected at amniocentesis. The phenotypically normal child had the del(10q) in only 3/100 blood cells, this culture having been stressed by growth in a low-folate medium. We are aware of a handful of essentially similar case, all involving 10q23, and none resulting in a documented abnormal child.

Polyploidy

TRIPLOIDY

Close to 100% of the time, triploidy aborts spontaneously, but in some cases not until the pregnancy is well advanced; those surviving through to the second or third trimester are usually digynic. In the prenatal diagnosis series of Lakovschek et al. (2011), in which no intervention was taken, no triploid infant was born alive. This being so, the offer of termination is appropriate when triploidy is diagnosed, particularly given the increased risk of maternal complications (Massalska et al. 2020). Cassidy et al. (1977) described the emotional turmoil suffered by the family when a triploid infant, predicted to die immediately, survived for the extraordinary period of 5 months.

The ultrasonographic observations are typically quite obvious, and include severe abnormalities of the brain, heart, and kidneys, limb defects, and oligohydramnios (Massalska et al. 2021). The ultrasonographic appearance of cystic placenta points to diandric triploidy, whereas digynic triploidy is characterized by asymmetric IUGR (p. 642). In general, cfDNA testing does not detect triploidy, but a very low fetal fraction may raise suspicion. Sarno et al. (1993) reported a unique case of complete placental/fetal discordance with triploidy on CVS and a normal diploid karyotype on amniocentesis and fetal blood sampling, with the birth of a normal baby; such a possibility warrants consideration where triploidy on CVS accompanies an ultrasonographically normal fetus.

True triploidy mosaicism is very rare (p. 345). Wegner et al. (2009) report a prenatal diagnosis, the pregnancy ending in fetal death in utero at 25 weeks, with the remarkable mixed-sex karyotype of 46,XX/69,XXY. Numerous abnormalities were revealed at anatomical pathological examination. They were able to demonstrate that the initial conception had been dispermic (one X- and one Y-bearing sperm) and that the 69,XXY lineage had arisen by the delayed incorporation of the Y-bearing male pronucleus into a cell with a 46,XX nucleus; they preferred the expression "mixoploidy" to describe this scenario. In the mosaic case of Mahon et al. (2022), amniocentesis showed 69,XXX[6]/46,XX[24], the procedure done on the basis of growth restriction. A growth-retarded and dysmorphic female infant was born at term; at age 15 months, she was clinically stable but developmentally delayed.

A very rare case is "hypotriploidy" with 68 chromosomes. One case of 68,XX hypotriploidy was diagnosed prenatally, following an ultrasound picture which was similar to that of classic digynic triploidy (Pasquini et al. 2010).

TETRAPLOIDY

Tetraploidy seen at prenatal diagnosis, in the context of normal ultrasonography, is usually an in vitro cultural artifact, or possibly a vestige from the blastocystic stage of normally occurring trophoblastic tetraploidy (Krieg et al. 2009). In their series of 76,104 CVSs, Grati et al. (2020) identified 72 cases (0.1%) of mosaic tetraploidy: All were confined to the placenta (32 CPM type I, 15 CPM type II, and 25 CPM type III), and there were no adverse perinatal outcomes. Balkan et al. (2012) tell a salutary story, concerning a pregnancy with an increased-risk screen, mild fetal pyelectasis and hyperechogenic bowel on ultrasound, and the amniocentesis showing non-mosaic 92,XXYY; but cordocentesis then demonstrating 46,XY, and a normal child subsequently born.

True tetraploidy is very rare, and Teyssier et al. (1997) recorded only 10 cases, two of which had been discovered at amniocentesis; further cases are listed in Stefanova et al. (2010), who describe their own case of a newborn who died at age 30 hours. Ultrasonographic demonstration of growth retardation and enlarged cerebral ventricles may be typical but rather non-specific signs.

While tetraploid/diploid mosaicism is almost always a cultural artifact, Edwards et al. (1994), having observed true normal/tetraploid mosaicism in two severely disabled individuals, nevertheless caution that a tetraploid cell line is not absolutely certain to be an innocuous finding. The 2½ year old child in Stefanova et al. (2010) with mosaic tetraploidy was quite abnormal. In a prenatal case, Meiner et al. (1998) showed 92,XXYY/46,XY mosaicism on fetal blood sampling following the diagnosis of non-mosaic 92,XXYY at amniocentesis, in the setting of growth retardation discovered at ultrasonography, and confirmed at subsequent fetal pathology study.

Structural Rearrangement

Structural rearrangements are seen in about 1 in 1,000 cytogenetic prenatal diagnoses (Warburton 1991). It is typically a matter of urgency to do parental chromosome studies, in order to distinguish between a familial or a de novo rearrangement in the fetus. If one parent is discovered to have the same apparently balanced autosomal rearrangement, and in the context of normal ultrasonographic anatomy, there is no firm evidence for an increased risk of fetal abnormality, and many would counsel to the effect of no discernibly increased risk. Sex chromosome rearrangements require separate attention.

De Novo Balanced Chromosome Rearrangement

A major difficulty posed by the de novo balanced chromosome rearrangement (BCR) seen at prenatal diagnosis is that, at the level of classical cytogenetic analysis, is "apparently balanced," and when the interpretation at ultrasonography is normal. But even with the highest resolution banding, a submicroscopic abnormality (deletion or duplication, or gene disruption) may still be present (Figure 5–25). However, now that microarray is often a first-line genetic test, the issue may be by-passed: De novo rearrangements with no copy number gain or loss will not be detected, and the test will be reported as normal.

When the prenatal diagnosis is made on classical methodology, the starting point is an acknowledgment that precedents are recorded for a de novo BCR having disrupted or compromised a locus, and therefore that the discovery of such a rearrangement at prenatal diagnosis could potentially herald an abnormal child. Of course, these translocations are to be taken seriously. Equally, the truly balanced translocation carrier state (every one of which in the world must have been de novo at some point in the near or distant past) is very familiar, as Chapter 5 attests at length. Very many translocations are indeed balanced, in terms of their functional genetic consequences. Thus, a normal child is very possible, and as the observations have shown, this is the more likely outcome.

Following a first-line test on classical cytogenetic analysis, microarray analysis should be offered as a second-tier test. In the study of De Gregori et al. (2007) of 14 prenatal diagnoses of de novo simple translocation, the ultrasonography being normal in 12, all proved to be balanced at the level of array-CGH. However, genomic sequencing around the breakpoints would be needed to detect a true disruption[13] of a gene (Ordulu et al. 2016).

Nevertheless, we should emphasize the pragmatic observation that most pregnancies with prenatal diagnosis of a de novo inversion or simple reciprocal translocation go on to produce a normal baby. Presumably, these normal cases reflect breakpoints in DNA that does not code for a gene or for a control element (or if a gene is disrupted, its haplostate is sufficient), and in which there is no concomitant microdeletion. Of course, abnormal ultrasonography dictates a different perspective. Thus, for example, when Price et al. (2005) identified growth and anatomical abnormalities suggestive of Cornelia de Lange syndrome (CdLS), the subsequent finding of a presumed de novo translocation (father not available for testing) 46,XX,t(3;5)(q21;p13) enabled a clear interpretation, the CdLS gene being located at 5p13, and presumably disrupted by the rearrangement.

[13] In the post-natal setting, Redin et al. (2017) performed whole genome sequencing on 273 patients with both a BCR and a congenital abnormality, and identified gene disruption in 35%, pathogenic genomic imbalances in 5% and disrupted topologically associated domains (TADs) in 7%.

On post-natal observation, one can be wise after the event. If a child with a particular phenotype has a rearrangement involving a breakpoint known to be in the region of a Mendelian locus, or of other recorded rearrangements producing the similar phenotype, the conclusion could reasonably be drawn that the cytogenetic abnormality was the cause of that abnormal phenotype. As just one example, a child with a de novo inv(7)(p22q21.3) having a particular split hand/foot malformation would invite the inference of a causal link, given the similarity of the limb defect with other 7q21.3q22 rearrangements (Cobben et al. 1995).

Empiric Risk Estimation. Warburton (1991) conducted a review of major laboratories in the United States and Canada over a 10-year period and collected data based on more than a third of a million procedures. We make frequent reference to this work. A de novo translocation was identified in about 1 in 2,000 amniocenteses, a Robertsonian translocation in about 1 in 9,000, and an inversion in 1 in 10,000 (all on classical methodology). In Warburton's study, serious malformations were identified in 6% of pregnancies with a de novo simple reciprocal translocation, either at elective termination or at live birth. This is some 3% above the background risk of approximately 3% for malformation and/or serious functional defect that applies to all pregnancies.

Thus, we may draw the inference that in approximately 3% of these de novo translocations, the chromosomal defect was causative. For a de novo inversion, peri- or paracentric, the risk from Warburton (1991) for phenotypic abnormality is 9.4%, which is 6%–7% over and above the background risk. The numerator is small, however, and the 95% confidence limits span 2%–25%. Since, in theory, a two-breakpoint inversion should not imply a greater risk than the two-break reciprocal translocation, the figure for this latter category as noted above, namely 3% (or a little above), might reasonably be seen as appropriate also for the inversion. Although if one breakpoint is in an acrocentric short arm, the risk might be that much less (Leach et al. 2005).

Warburton emphasized that the outcome data are imperfect, given the lack of long-term follow-up, and the questionable accuracy of phenotypic assessment in terminated pregnancies. Having made that point, she did then go on to say "there was no case in which a live birth originally reported as normal was later classified as abnormal after longer follow-up. In fact, the opposite tended to occur: Several cases described as having neonatal problems were later described as completely normal."

Follow-up Studies Small studies with follow-up into childhood have been undertaken (Gyejye et al. 2001), and these suggested that the figures presently offered are in the vicinity of the truth. We undertook detailed follow-up, to mean age 6 years, in 16 children with prenatally detected de novo balanced chromosome rearrangements (Sinnerbrink et al. 2013). One congenital anomaly (congenital hip dysplasia) was reported; but compared to population norms, no significant differences were observed with respect to health care needs, intelligence, or mental health.

A large collaborative exercise involving 29 Italian prenatal laboratories, covering the period 1983–2006, brought together the findings on a total of somewhat more than a quarter of a million diagnoses (amniocentesis, CVS, and fetal blood) (Giardino et al. 2009). From these, 246 de novo balanced rearrangements were identified: 177 reciprocal translocations, 45 Robertsonian translocations, 17 inversions, and seven complex chromosome rearrangements. But follow-up data, in the 80% of cases in which the pregnancy was continued, were insufficient to derive risk figures for clinical outcomes, due to logistic and legal considerations, albeit that the authors comment that "none of the newborns have been reported to display visible malformations."

Longer-term follow-up (mean 17 years) comes from a Danish registry study, based upon 41 individuals who had had a prenatal diagnosis of a de novo BCR in the absence of prenatal ultrasound anomalies (Halgren et al. 2018). Congenital malformations were neither more common nor more severe in BCR carriers than in matched controls, but the frequency of neurodevelopmental and/or neuropsychiatric disorder was significantly increased, 19.5% in BCR carriers compared with 8.3% in controls. This figure increased further, to 26.8% with longer clinical follow-up.

These disconcerting data, somewhat at odds with the foregoing, suggest that neurodevelopmental compromise, rather than congenital abnormalities, are the major morbidity associated with de novo BCRs, and that their impact may have been underestimated by previous studies, due to lack of follow-up. Microarray was normal in all 32 subjects of this series where it was performed, indicating a low prognostic value from this test. On the other hand, sequencing of breakpoints, performed retrospectively, was informative in 7/27 cases, detecting disrupted neurodevelopmental genes (*ARID1B, NPAS3, CELF4*), disruption of regulatory domains of known developmental genes (*ZEB2, HOXC*), and two complex BCRs with multiple breakpoints, all in fetuses with adverse outcomes. The authors recommend the sequencing of breakpoints in all pregnancies with de novo BCRs, but warn that this approach still has relatively low sensitivity (~50%) for the prediction of abnormal outcomes.

The "Carrier Fetus" Who Will Become a Carrier Adult. We discuss in Chapter 27 the issue of the genetic testing of children. In the case of prenatal diagnosis in which a de novo apparently balanced state is discovered, of course the child has already been tested, and "untesting" is not a practical matter. Consider the example of the mosaic test result mentioned below, the whole-arm translocation 46,XY,t(1;5)(p10;q10)/46,XY. Naturally, parents may want to know what reproductive implications this may have for their as-yet-unborn child. In this example, the genetic risk for the child will be, as the reader can readily determine, essentially that of a likely propensity to miscarriage, should the translocation cell line involve the gonad. It is the counselor's responsibility to communicate this sort of information in outline form to the parents, along with the advice that the child could, in the fullness of time, attend the clinic on his or her own behalf. The information must be clearly conveyed. It could be seen as a failure of the counselor's duty of care if in the next generation an affected child were born, the parents being unaware of the genetic risk (Burn et al. 1983; and p. 809).

DE NOVO BALANCED HETEROLOGOUS ROBERTSONIAN TRANSLOCATION

Heterologous Robertsonian translocations are present in 1 in 1000 persons, with similar proportions inherited and de novo (Shaffer et al. 1992). The great majority of de novo cases will be disomic, non-mosaic, and of biparental inheritance, and a normal phenotype is to be expected. The risk for phenotypic defect over and above the baseline is due to UPD and, theoretically, to occult mosaic trisomy.

For inherited balanced Robertsonian translocations, Moradkhani et al. (2019) surveyed 28 diagnostic laboratories, and arrived at a risk of UPD of 0.06% when a parent is a known carrier of a rob translocation involving chromosome 14 or 15, and the fetus carries the same translocation. Comparable data are not available for de novo robs, because they will seldom be ascertained, in the absence of a relevant family history. However, on post-natal observation, UPD is twice as common in de novo robs as in inherited robs (Moradkhani et al.). Given that ~half of Robertsonian translocations arise de novo, the risk of UPD, in the setting

De Novo Identifiable Supernumerary Chromosome of Substantial Size. An additional chromosome which is of sufficient size that it can be characterized on initial routine analysis as a deleted or rearranged form of a specific autosome will imply a very high risk of abnormality, approaching 100%, due to partial trisomy of that chromosome. Once a supernumerary chromosome has been identified, it is no longer referred to as an SMC; it is now described as a ring or derivative—for example, r(7), der(22), or neo(13q31), or whatever may be the precise description.

De Novo Small Supernumerary Marker Chromosome. De novo sSMCs have been described for most chromosomes (Liehr 2025b); two-thirds of sSMCs are acrocentric-derived (Dalprà et al. 2005). Huang et al. (2019) identified 40 de novo SMCs from 68,087 amniocentesis samples (1 in 1700), of which seven had a copy number gain detected on microarray, and could therefore be interpreted as pathogenic.

De Novo Minute Marker. The *very* small SMC (minSMC) may comprise only centromeric material and be harmless. We discuss a prenatal case on p. 626, a minSMC apparently comprising no more than chromosome 18 centromere; the child turned out to be normal. The tiny bisatellited microchromosome can be thought of as the reciprocal product of the Robertsonian rearrangement; these microchromosomes also are typically harmless (Liehr et al. 2021) (Figure 22–9).

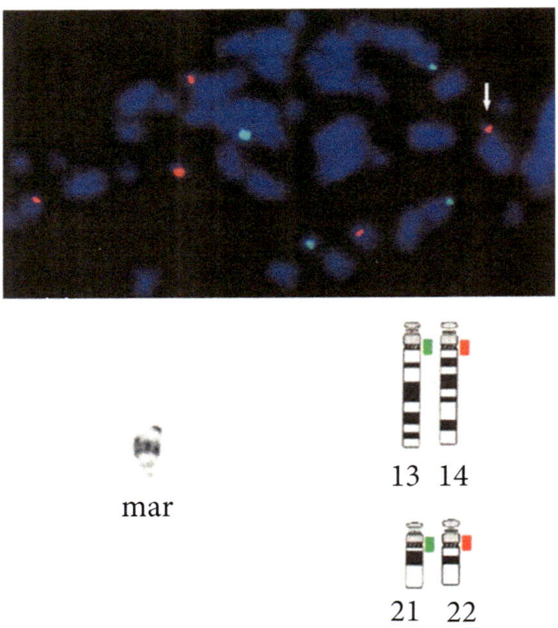

Figure 22–9. A De Novo Supernumerary Marker Chromosome at Amniocentesis.

Notes: Amniocentesis had been done on the basis of advanced maternal age. The very small marker chromosome (mar) was seen in all cells. FISH on cultured amniocytes with probes recognizing the centromeric region of acrocentric chromosomes 13 and 21 (green), and 14 and 22 (red), showed the marker (arrowed) to be derived from either 14 or 22. Having proven an acrocentric basis, the advice given could be optimistic. A healthy child was born.

Source: From CP Chen et al., Prenatal diagnosis and molecular cytogenetic characterization of a familial small supernumerary marker chromosome derived from the acrocentric chromosome 14/22, *Taiwan J Obstet Gynecol* 61:364–367, 2022. Courtesy CP Chen, and with the permission of Elsevier.

Supernumerary Marker Chromosome Outcomes. With precise cytogenetic characterization of an sSMC identified prenatally, using FISH and microarray (Jang et al. 2016), and with concomitant ultrasound examination, it should be possible precisely to categorize the genetic risk. Earlier published reports of liveborn children with various types of SMCs—a notably heterogeneous material—are mostly biased by ascertainment in favor of phenotypic abnormality. Series of prenatally diagnosed fetuses are deficient in that there is usually only a short-term follow-up of liveborn children, while pathological assessments following termination can only show major structural malformations (Warburton 1991). Brøndum-Nielsen and Mikkelsen (1995) report a 10-year experience in Glostrup, Denmark, during which nine de novo SMCs were identified. In seven cases, termination of pregnancy was chosen, with some of these showing defects at pathological examination; and in the two pregnancies continuing, one infant with a minute acrocentric-derived SMC was normal at birth, while one with a ring-like 17 was mildly delayed at age two years.

In the similar survey of Hastings et al. (1999a), data were presented on 31 prenatally diagnosed SMCs, of which 21 were de novo. In 10 of these 21 proceeding to FISH analysis, six being mosaic, five were shown to be 15-derived and three 14- or 22-derived; the remaining two included a r(8) and a der(16). Of the six in which the pregnancies continued, only the r(8) child was physically and developmentally abnormal. Repeating the point: With FISH and microarray, most sSMCs should admit of precise cytogenomic analysis, and the prenatal advice based upon knowledge of the specific involved segment.

Supernumerary Autosomal Ring Chromosomes. Autosomal ring chromosomes, as a supernumerary 47th chromosome, imply a high risk of phenotypic abnormality. They originate from a variety of chromosomes and contain euchromatin. Certain of these, in which only one arm of the chromosome is represented in the ring, are specifically recorded in association with phenotypic abnormality: r(1p), r(5p), r(7q), r(8q), r(9p), r(10p), r(20p), and r(20q) (Hastings et al. 1999a; Anderlid et al. 2001). Uniparental disomy may complicate the picture: James et al. (1995) and Anderlid et al. report supernumerary rings, from chromosomes 6 and 9, associated with UPD(6) and UPD(9), respectively. Very small rings, that might also have been categorized as sSMCs, might not necessarily cause an abnormal phenotype: For example, two infants in Kitsiou-Tzeli et al. (2009) born following prenatal diagnosis of 47,+r(20)/46,N mosaicism were judged normal in early infancy.

Autosomal Isochromosomes. Autosomal isochromosomes are typically seen in the mosaic state as a supernumerary isochromosome (or as isodicentric isochromosome), and thus the discovery of 47,+i/46,N (or 47,+idic/46,N) is always a concern, whether at a level II or even level I mosaicism.[21] Such a karyotype raises the prospect of an effective mosaic tetrasomy for the chromosomal arm concerned. A 46-chromosome karyotype in which one homolog is replaced by an isochromosome typically implies a trisomy for one arm of that chromosome, and monosomy for the other. These are certainly rare observations: In an amniocentesis-based survey from Italy, based on slightly less than 90,000 diagnoses, the most frequent were, in order, isochromosomes of 20q, 9p, 18p, and 12p, at approximately 1 in 30,000, 45,000, 45,000, and 90,000, respectively (Forabosco et al. 2009). Brief commentaries on these, and on certain other isochromosomes, follow.

[21] When microarray is used as the first-line test, a mosaic isochromosome may be mistaken for a duplication. For example, an isochromosome (4 copies), if present in 50% of cells, may be interpreted as a non-mosaic duplication (3 copies).

47,+i(5p). Blakey-Cheung et al. (2020) reviewed the literature and identified six cases where mosaic tetrasomy 5p had been diagnosed prenatally, but disconcertingly, an additional two cases where prenatal testing (one CVS and one amniocentesis) had been interpreted as normal, and a diagnosis of tetrasomy 5p was only made following the birth of a clinically affected child. Sijmons et al. (1993) assessed a dysmorphic and neurologically compromised child with a 5p isochromosome in 3/31 lymphocytes and 12/14 skin fibroblasts, and yet upon retrospective checking, only one of 217 cells from a stored short-term CVS culture was 47,XY,+i(5p).

We contrast this unfortunate experience with ours of seven cases of i(5p) mosaicism identified at CVS, six of which went on to follow-up amniocentesis (Clement Wilson et al. 2002). Three children were followed up to 2½, 3¼, and 4 years, and their normality was quite apparent. In one of these children, a circumscribed area of the placenta following delivery karyotyped 47,+i(5p), adjacent parts karyotyped 47,+i(5p)/46,N, and most of the placenta (and the child himself) had a normal karyotype. The CVS sampling had presumably needled this small region of confined placental i(5p) mosaicism. One pregnancy tested 100% i(5p) at CVS, and the parents chose termination; no i(5p) cells were detected from fetal skin culture. In another with a 65% load at CVS, a follow-up amniocentesis showed 45% of cells with the isochromosome, and post-termination tissues showed 15%–30%.

From the foregoing, we may conclude that a *CVS* diagnosis with a normal follow-up amniocentesis and with normal ultrasonography suggests, but cannot confirm, a normal child. As for the primary detection of i(5p) mosaicism at *amniocentesis*, only five cases are recorded, with all having an abnormal outcome (Blakey-Cheung et al. 2020). Grams et al. (2011) reported monozygotic twins who were discordant for i(5p) at CVS and amniocentesis; multiple abnormalities were seen on ultrasound in the affected twin, but the pregnancy ended in spontaneous loss of both twins at 18 weeks gestation.

47,+i(8p). López-Pajares et al. (2003) review the small number of reported cases. Two examples are given of discordance between amniocentesis (normal) and postnatal blood (tetrasomy 8p), an unusual pattern for isochromosomes (but cf. the i(9p) below). A disconcerting story is told in Nucaro et al. (2006): i(8p) mosaicism was seen at long-term cultured (but not short-term) CVS, with a normal result after amniocentesis, but resulting in a child severely disabled and epileptic, and with a 5% level of the i(8p) on blood.

47,+i(9p). The highly variable clinical picture and the subtleties of different breakpoints are discussed in Dhandha et al. (2002). Isochromosome mosaicism can be the basis of a false-negative test result at prenatal diagnosis. Thus, Eggermann et al. (1998) reported an abnormal baby born to a 39-year-old mother, in whom amniocentesis at 14 weeks gestation had returned a normal karyotype. On blood analysis, the child had an i(9p) in 32% of cells. From one skin biopsy, 50 cells had a normal karyotype, but on a second biopsy, five out of eight cells showed the i(9p) chromosome. Similarly, we have seen a girl with mosaicism for an isodicentric chromosome 9, in which microarray on DNA from uncultured amniocytes showed a copy number gain at 9p24.3q22.32, but karyotype on cultured cells was normal (Lee et al. 2025).

The particular attribute of the i(9p) is for blood, but not skin, to show the abnormality, and this is likely the explanation for its non-detection at amniocentesis. Pertile et al. (1996) support this interpretation, in their follow-up of a (non-mosaic) CVS diagnosis of idic(9)(q13). An extensive search at amniocentesis revealed a single abnormal colony, which might well otherwise have been missed. Finally, fetal blood sampling showed the idic(9) in 8% of cells. A more severe case is recorded in Tang et al. (2004), which showed the isochromosome in all amniocytes at 24 weeks, and in most blood and fibroblast cells from the very malformed infant (who died at 1 month of age).

47,+i(10p). A single case is on record, the diagnosis having been made following the recognition of fetal defects on ultrasonography (Wu et al. 2003).

47,+i(12p), Pallister-Killian Syndrome. The 12p isochromosome is the basis of the well-known Pallister-Killian syndrome. Salzano et al. (2018) review the prenatal profile. The fractions of abnormal cells detected at prenatal diagnosis can vary greatly. Bernert et al. (1992) showed in one example 100% of short-term CVS cells and 10% of amniotic fluid cells having the 47,+i(12p) karyotype, whereas in Kunz et al. (2009), at CVS the isochromosome was seen only in long-term culture; in both cases the pregnancies were terminated. Horn et al. (1995) reported a pregnancy in which CVS gave a 46,XY result on direct (17 cells) and cultured (eight cells) analysis (and 28 further cells on a retrospective study), and the abnormal newborn baby was 46,XY on a peripheral blood study (100 cells counted); at 18 months, a clinical diagnosis of Pallister-Killian syndrome was made, and the karyotype on skin fibroblast culture was 47,XY,+i(12p)/46,XY, with 85% of cells having the isochromosome. (Had it been an amniocentesis rather than CVS that had been done, abnormal cells would probably have been seen.) Classical karyotyping typically returns a normal result because the i(12p) is lost in stimulated lymphocyte cultures; thus, microarray on uncultured cells is the preferred prenatal test. Iso(12p) can also be detected by genome-wide cell-free DNA testing (Chau et al. 2020).

46,i(13q). A de novo "Robertsonian" translocation, leading to trisomy 13, is, in the majority of cases, actually an isochromosome, as discussed above.

Isodicentric 15. About half of all SMCs are an idic(15) (also referred to as pseudodicentric 15, or inverted duplication 15; and see p. 428). These are typically dicentric and bisatellited, although one of the centromeres may be suppressed. The smallest ones (smaller than chromosome 21q) appear to be harmless, but larger ones result in the "idic(15) syndrome," characterized by intellectual disability, epilepsy, and autistic features. The boundary between smaller and larger is in 15q12. The use of D15S10 or *SNRPN* FISH probes, which recognize sequences in 15q12q13, enables distinction of harmless and pathogenic chromosomes (Eggermann et al. 2002), a distinction that can also be made using microarray (Wang et al. 2004). Rare idic(15)s have been associated with UPD(15), and it may be warranted to check for this possibility (Hastings et al. 1999a).

47,+i(18p). Schinzel (2001) notes that more than 75 cases of 47,+i(18p) have been recorded. Multiple physical anomalies and a moderate to severe degree of intellectual disability characterize the clinical picture. Boyle et al. (2001) emphasize the plausibility of a premeiotic origin, and the caution therefore that gonadal mosaicism may exist in a parent, as they illustrate in their report of affected half-sisters. Iso(18p) has been diagnosed following a cfDNA result showing increased risk for trisomy 18 (Tamaki et al. 2020).

46,i(18q). The karyotype produces a combination of monosomy 18p and trisomy 18q. Chen et al. (1998) record that many 18q isochromosomes diagnosed prenatally are associated with very severe malformation, such as holoprosencephaly and cloacal dysgenesis. Levy-Mozziconacci et al. (1996) describe a case presenting at 22 weeks gestation with abnormal ultrasonography, and although the direct CVS was 46,XX in all cells, amniocentesis and fetal blood sampling showed the isochromosome (an isodicentric, in this instance) in all cells: an example of complete CVS-amniocentesis discordance.

aneuploidies influence brain function in such a way that the development of intellectual capacity, emotional maturity, and speech and language skills are affected to some extent; but none of these effects necessarily occurs, none is specific to sex chromosome aneuploidy, and some may be amenable to corrective intervention. There is considerable overlap with the XX and XY population. Hong et al. (2014) reviewed the cognitive and neurological aspects of sex chromosome aneuploidies and noted shared features across the sex chromosome aneuploidies, comprising impairments in executive functioning, motor skills, and higher-order social cognitive ability. In their comprehensive review, Tartaglia et al. (2020) note that although "the list of neurodevelopmental and psychological risks associated with SCT that can manifest from infancy into adulthood is long, marked variability in the presence and severity of these features is a consistent research finding."

Ratcliffe (1999) and Bender et al. (2001) provide long-term follow-up data, well into adulthood. Bender et al. followed eight 45,X, 10 47,XXX, and 11 47,XXY individuals through to an age range of 26–36 years, using siblings as controls, and noted the IQs of the aneuploid groups to be considerably less compared with the sibs. Nevertheless, the variation is wide, and these authors emphasize the point that "sex chromosome aneuploidy does not exert its influence in a vacuum, but rather interacts with the host of other genetic and environmental influences that collectively guide human development." As Le Gall et al. (2017) show, an independent, concomitant CNV can exacerbate the clinical, and especially the neurocognitive phenotype, and may indeed be the more significant factor. Children with sex chromosome aneuploidies seem more susceptible to either the good or the bad effects of a stable or of a dysfunctional family setting, than do their 46,XX and 46,XY siblings (Stewart et al. 1990; Bender et al. 1995). Children identified at prenatal diagnosis, a group biased toward higher socioeconomic status, may do better academically and socially than the cohorts followed from birth, although it was nevertheless true in the study of Linden and Bender (2002) that these children had "a strong risk for developmental problems, particularly for learning disabilities . . . [albeit that] these problems were not often severe." There may, however, be an increased risk for psychosis in childhood and adulthood (Kumra et al. 1998).

More prenatally ascertained cases are being found through noninvasive prenatal screenings, and this has provided both a need and an opportunity for follow-up of the children so diagnosed. A pioneering clinic in Colorado, the eXtraordinarY Kids Clinic, providing a multidisciplinary management for children and adolescents with a sex chromosome aneuploidy, has been well received by parents, and it may offer a useful model (Tartaglia et al. 2015). Figure 22–10 shows developmental data on the children in the eXtraordinarY Babies Study.

As well as the unbiased prenatally ascertained data, we now have (essentially) unbiased adult-derived information, with the genomic study of very large population-based cohorts giving insight into the long-term health and wellbeing of people with sex chromosome aneuploidy. Davis et al. (2025) utilized genomic and clinical data from the Million Veteran's Program in the USA to identify more than 1500 men with 47,XXY or 47,XYY. Of these, only 26% of XXY men and remarkable low of just 1% of XYY men had been diagnosed clinically. The study results showed that these men had successfully served in the military, with similar performance metrics to their XY peers, but were more likely to have a history of a broad range of medical and psychological conditions. Similar data come from 356 men with XXY or XYY identified from the UK Biobank, which

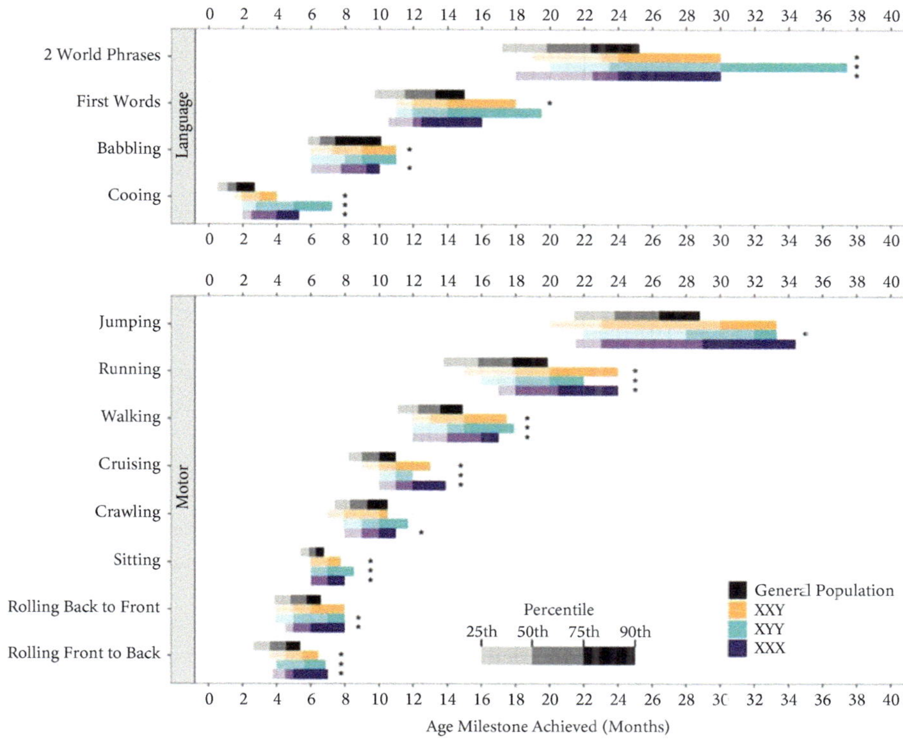

Figure 22–10. Developmental Progress in Children with a Sex Chromosome Trisomy.

Notes: Data were collected as part of the eXtraordinarY Babies Study, a prospective natural history of developmental and health trajectories in a prenatally identified sample of infants with sex chromosome trisomy (SCT). In all SCT conditions, compared with normative data, there was increased variability and a later median age of skill development across multiple gross motor and expressive language milestones. However, results also show significant overlap with the general pediatric population, suggesting that for many children with prenatally identified SCT, early milestones present within, or close to, the expected timeline.

Source: From T Thompson et al., Quantifying the spectrum of early motor and language milestones in sex chromosome trisomy, *MedRxiv in press* 2025. Courtesy N Tartaglia, and with the permission of the Cold Spring Harbor Laboratory.

identified surprisingly similar disease risks shared across XYY and XXY men, including increased risk of type 2 diabetes, atherosclerosis, and venous thrombosis (Zhao et al. 2022). Compared to XY men, men with sex chromosome trisomy were more likely to be taller, less likely to have a university or college degree, and more likely to live without a partner.

With the foregoing narrative in mind, what should parents say to others, if they decide to continue the pregnancy, after the prenatal diagnosis of an SCT? Should the family know, should they tell friends, and should school personnel be aware? And when should the child learn about his or her chromosomal condition? Linden et al. (2002) have considered these questions, and in general make a case for openness within the family, but see no need, indeed potential disadvantage, for those outside to be told.

We next outline the predicted outlook for the more commonly encountered sex chromosome aneuploidies. Attention is paid mostly to gonadal function and to intellectual and social development.

XXY (KLINEFELTER SYNDROME)

Almost certainly, the child becomes an infertile adult, although in recent times testicular sperm extraction with in vitro fertilization (IVF) has enabled a small number of men to become fathers (p. 475). Some have used gamete donation from a father or brother. Penile size is usually normal; the testes will be small. Androgen deficiency can be managed by replacement therapy with testosterone.[22] It may be that treatment induces a more masculine body habitus, improved self-esteem, vitality, ability to concentrate, and sexual interest (Nielsen 1990; Winter 1990). Gynecomastia may be present, transiently, in some 50%; if it persists, it can be treated surgically.

As an average statement, verbal IQ is reduced by some 18 points, and performance IQ by 11 points (Leggett et al. 2010). Learning difficulty at school is to be expected. Of 13 XXY boys studied by Walzer et al. (1990), 11 had persistent reading and spelling problems. Bender et al. (1993) note that a deficit in verbal fluency and reading is "the most homogeneous and consistent cognitive impairment found in any sex chromosome abnormality group," and this may reflect a specific dysfunction of the left cerebral hemisphere. Specific characteristics included a lowered level of motor activity, a pliant disposition, and a cautious approach to new situations; thus, in the classroom setting, they are perceived as "low-key children, well liked by their teachers, and presenting few behavioral management problems." Leggett et al. conclude that these boys "do not usually have major problems with social interaction and adaptation, although they may be timid and unassertive." Speculatively, the neural substrate of this passivity may reside in an underdevelopment of the amygdala, a brain nucleus that underpins aspects of social processing (Patwardhan et al. 2002).

Six Danish XXY boys were followed from birth to age 15–19 years by Nielsen and Wohlert (1991), and all but one needed remedial teaching. Their career plans were carpenter, draftsman, gardener, unskilled laborer, mechanic, and undecided. Stewart et al. (1990) comment that "XXY boys are unlikely to reach a level of personal and social development that is consistent with their family background." Ratcliffe (1999) commented upon a rate of psychiatric referral being above that of male controls (26% cf. 9%), with the neurotic score (not the antisocial score) being higher. (She also notes anecdotal mention of men from a Klinefelter clinic with professions including physician, engineer, minister, and accountant.) In a summary of psychosocial adaptation from several studies, recurring adjectives to describe the XXY personality were shy, immature, restrained, and reserved. In the Denver study, 11 young adults with XXY "appeared to have met the demands of early adulthood with fair success, although slightly less well than did their siblings"; they appeared to have a diminished insight into their own psychology (Bender et al. 1999). Their mean IQ of 91 compared with 109 in normal male sibling controls. We have noted above the ameliorative effect of growing up in a stable and supportive family. In a cohort of 934 Danish XXY males, the incidence of criminal convictions was 1.4 times that of controls, but this difference disappeared after adjusting for socioeconomic indices (Stochholm et al. 2012).

The origin of the extra X chromosome in XXY males may be maternal (60%) or paternal (40%), and Larsen et al. (2024) addressed the question of whether parent-of-origin influences might be a source of phenotypic variability within KS. In fact, deep

[22] A role for testosterone therapy in infancy to mimic the normal "mini-puberty" is controversial, and not routinely recommended (Aksglaede et al. 2020)

phenotyping in 58 XXY males, while identifying minor neuroanatomical differences, found no evidence of a substantial parent-of-origin effect on cognition, psychopathology or behavior.

White et al. (2023) addressed the question "What should we tell prospective parents?" and identified six key counseling points (Table 22–8).

Table 22–8. Key Counseling Points Following Prenatal Diagnosis of Klinefelter Syndrome

1. Genetic counseling by a clinician familiar with the issues and complexities of KS should be offered.
2. A review by a pediatric endocrinologist during the mini-puberty stage is recommended to assess the clinical +/− biochemical profile of each infant.
3. Testosterone replacement therapy during adolescence is the standard treatment for prevention of the sequalae of hypogonadatrophic hypogonadism in individuals with KS.
4. Discussions on fertility-preserving options should be introduced in late adolescence, depending on the individual maturity and wishes of the young person.
5. KS is associated with cognitive, language, and learning disabilities, attention and executive functioning difficulties, as well as internalizing and externalizing behavioral and psychological disorders; however, the rate of these neurodevelopmental outcomes may be over-reported due to ascertainment bias. Early diagnosis and intervention may improve outcomes.
6. The focus of antenatal counseling with parents emphasizes the role of appropriate screening and early management of evolving issues as the key to improved clinical outcomes.

Source: M White et al., Klinefelter Syndrome: What should we tell prospective parents? *Prenat Diagn* 43:240–249, 2023.

XXX

Physical development of the XXX female is generally unremarkable, although there is a tendency toward tallness. Gross and fine motor skills are likely to be somewhat impaired, and children are awkward and poorly coordinated. Pubertal development and fertility appear for the most part uncompromised. In a very few, genitourinary malformations (ovarian, uterine, renal, bladder) are recorded, of which the karyotype may or may not have been causal (Haverty et al. 2004; Linden and Bender 2002).

It is the neural substrate in which the important vulnerability applies (Otter et al. 2010). Thus, major concerns in childhood relate to intelligence and language development and poor self-confidence, and, in adulthood, psychosocial maladjustment and, occasionally, frank psychiatric disease. Full scale and verbal IQ is, on average, reduced by some 10–20 points. Language comprehension and use of speech are impaired in over half the cases. Learning difficulty is likely, and many will benefit from additional remedial teaching, but few require education outside the mainstream. In one small study of 11 girls, nine needed special education intervention, and one was placed in a class for disabled children (Bender et al. 1993). While girls who had been diagnosed prenatally do better than those ascertained post-natally (as naturally is to be expected), it remains true that their neurocognitive capacity is somewhat compromised (Wigby et al. 2016). They are likely to be more vulnerable if there is a concomitant CNV of reduced penetrance (González-Del Angel et al. 2023).

Harmon et al. (1998) and Bender et al. (1999) reported a longer follow-up in these young women, into adolescence and young adulthood, and documented difficult adaptation to the stresses of life. On a measure of social adjustment (in work, leisure, family, marital, parental), the XXX women scored significantly less well than their sisters. Their mean IQ was 82 (cf. sisters, 103). However, Ratcliffe (1999) described most XXX young women in the Edinburgh survey as "physically attractive, and displaying a common-sense attitude that counterbalanced their low educational achievements" (and relieved to be free of the pressure they had felt while at school). The observations in the similar study of Rovet et al. (1995) were more promising, although, as Harmon et al. point out, this was a group from a higher socioeconomic stratum, and presumably both genetic and environmental factors would have been more favorable. An XXX girl who might otherwise have had an IQ of 130 can yet do well despite a reduction to 110; to the contrary, a drop from 90 to 70 would be a considerable handicap. Many counselors will know from their own experience how variable can be the phenotype.

Davis et al. (2025) identified 61 XXX women enrolled in the Million Veterans Program, of whom 28% had been diagnosed clinically. The authors report a "more reassuring perspective to the trisomy X literature": Compared to their XX peers, women with XXX were 6 cm taller and had lower income and employment status, but there was little minimal difference in terms of health[23] and psychological concerns. In the UK Biobank, 110 women were identified with trisomy X (Tuke et al. 2019). They had had a normal menarche age, but went through menopause on average five years earlier than XX women; this did not seem to affect their fertility, as they had had a similar number of pregnancies and pregnancy losses as XX women. Nonetheless, 9% had experienced premature ovarian insufficiency (POI). They were found to have lower income, to be of below average cognitive ability, and more likely to live alone.

XYY

The multicenter prospective study documented in Evans et al. (1990) reviewed progress in 39 boys and young men. The particular physical attribute of the XYY male is increased stature. Sexual activity is normal, and fertility is apparently uncompromised. Motor proficiency may be impaired. While the IQ is in the normal range, it is usually lower than those of sibs or controls, and about half of XYY boys have a mild learning difficulty, and may display poor attentiveness and impulsivity in the classroom. There is an overlap in the cognitive profiles between individuals with Klinefelter syndrome and those with XYY syndrome, mainly characterized by deficits in executive function and language-related skills. The vignettes from the series of Ratcliffe et al. (1990) of 10 Scottish subjects who had left school give an idea of what XYY young men are capable of: One ran a market stall, two were chefs, and the others were a private in the army, a waiter, a supermarket assistant, a video shop assistant, a technician, a laborer, and one was training as a painter and decorator. In a cohort of children aged 8–16 years selected for the XYY karyotype having been diagnosed prenatally, and of higher socioeconomic status, a considerable range in academic ability was observed, with most coping satisfactorily, and IQs ranging from 100 to 147 (Linden and Bender 2002).

Perhaps the major concern is in psychosocial adaptation. These boys can have a low frustration tolerance, and some are prone to temper tantrums in childhood, progressing to aggressive behavior in teenage, and may need help to learn to cope with this. They may find it difficult to "read" social situations, and antisocial behavior is more common

[23] An increased risk was identified for kidney disease, congestive cardiac failure and glaucoma in women with 47,XXX.

(Ratcliffe 1999). The functioning of the family may be as much an ingredient as the karyotype in psychosocial development.

Fryns et al. (1995) identified 50 XYY males among 98,725 patients referred for chromosomal analysis, and they note that this fraction of 50/98,725, approximately 0.05%, is very close to the newborn incidence; they thus drew a conclusion that the XYY phenotype differs little from the norm. They do, however, acknowledge a high (86%) risk for psychosocial pathology in those XYY males with concomitant borderline intelligence. In Ratcliffe's follow-up report into adulthood, some disconcerting data are noted, not incongruent with the conclusions of Fryns et al. Psychiatric referrals were fivefold compared with male controls (47% cf. 9%), and the rate of criminal conviction was fourfold, the mean IQ of those convicted being lower than those who were not (although most offenses were minor and against property rather than persons). More reassuring data come from a cohort of 161 Danish XYY males, in which the incidence of criminal convictions was just 1.42 times that of controls, a difference which disappeared after adjusting for socioeconomic parameters (Stochholm et al. 2012).

In the data of the UK Biobank, only one of 143 men with XYY had been diagnosed clinically, emphasizing the bias in clinically ascertained cases (Zhao et al. 2022). Men with XYY were, on average, 7.9 cm taller than their XY counterparts, were less likely to have completed tertiary education, had below average cognitive abilities, and were more likely to live alone. As noted above, increased risk was observed for a range of common and potentially preventable diseases, including type 2 diabetes and cardiovascular diseases. In the Million Veteran's Study, Davis et al. (2024) also identified a surprisingly similar profile for common disease risk shared by XXY men and XYY men. The basis of these risks is unknown.

45,X (TURNER SYNDROME)

Unlike the foregoing three aneuploidies, monosomy X has a very high in utero lethality, peaking at around 12–15 weeks gestation. Spontaneous abortion follows amniocentesis-detected 45,X in three-fourths of cases (Hook 1983). But some survive pregnancy and are born as infants with Turner syndrome. Robinson et al. (1990) note that "variability among 45,X girls is considerable; and precise predictions about any child's prognosis are not possible." They also emphasized that "a supportive environment that provides stimulation and encouragement is of considerable importance." The traits following comprise the core phenotype:

- *Gonadal failure* with infertility is almost certain (Lippe 1991). In the survey of Sutton et al. (2006), infertility was seen, by the women with Turner syndrome themselves, as the most concerning component of the phenotype. Classically, a spontaneous onset of puberty, with breast development and onset of menses, has been regarded as being very infrequent, although Pasquino et al. (1997) propose that the fraction who enter a spontaneous puberty may be as high as 9%, and they suggest that earlier figures may have been biased downward by a policy, previously, of not karyotyping short girls who had had an onset of menstruation Most girls and women with Turner syndrome will require hormone replacement therapy for initiation of puberty, starting at 11-12 years old, continuing until the usual age of menopause (Gravholt et al. 2024). Spontaneous pregnancies are more likely in women who have a history of spontaneous menarche and a 45,X/46,XX karyotype.

Childbearing via ovum donation may be successful in some cases. The utility of oöcyte cryopreservation in girls and women with Turner syndrome is unknown.

- *Stature* will be short, and this is mostly due to haploinsufficiency of *SHOX*. In a study of adult Danish women with Turner syndrome, never having had growth hormone therapy, the average height (with standard deviation) was 147 cm ± 7 cm (4 feet 10 inches ± 2½ inches) (Gravholt and Weis Naeraa 1997), which may be slightly taller than in some other ethnic populations. Gravholt et al. report a deficit of about 20 cm compared with population mean. Growth hormone treatment results in a an approximately 1 cm gain in height for each year of treatment, such that most treated individuals will have a final height in the lower normal range.
- *Neuropsychological functioning* is impaired. The average IQ is reduced compared to siblings. At long-term follow-up in the Denver cohort (Bender et al. 1999), nine young women with 45,X had a mean lower IQ (85) compared with normal female sibling controls (104). Their educational achievements were, however, better than those of the XXX women from the same study: Eight were high school graduates, and five had college degrees. In one notable case, Reiss et al. (1993) report monozygous twins, one non-mosaic 45,X and the other 46,XX, the former's performance IQ being 18 points less than her sister, but the verbal IQs practically the same. In fact, girls with Turner syndrome appear possibly to have superior skills in some language domains compared to their 46,XX peers (Temple and Shephard 2012).

  Across the lifespan, development in the preschool years is largely normal, other than some delay in motor skills. At school age, a cognitive profile emerges characterized by relative strength in verbal abilities compared to non-verbal abilities. Vulnerabilities include handwriting, drawing, mathematics, attention, executive function (the ability to plan, organize, monitor, and execute multistep problem-solving processes), and visual-spatial appreciation with a lesser volume of the right parietal cerebral cortex (Gravholt et al. 2024). These cognitive differences continue into adolescence and adulthood. Difficulties initiating and maintaining social and intimate relationships are more common.
- *Certain physical differences* are associated, of which the major are neck webbing and cardiovascular malformation, of which coarctation (narrowing) of the aorta is the classic one (Birjiniuk et al. 2023). In the setting of prenatal diagnosis, fetal echocardiography should be performed, with post-natal follow-up within the first three days of life. Renal ultrasound should be performed at diagnosis to identify congenital anomalies of the kidney and urinary tract.
- *Morbidity* in adult life is increased and comprehensive management guidelines are available (Gravholt et al. 2024). Certain common diseases are more frequently seen: obesity, both insulin-dependent and insulin-resistant diabetes, hypothyroidism, heart disease, hypertension, stroke, and liver cirrhosis. Even in the absence of structural heart disease, lifelong cardiac surveillance is recommended due to the increased risk of aortic dissection. Weakness of the bones (osteoporosis) implies a risk for fracture.

The 45,X karyotype accounts for less than half of Turner syndrome diagnoses, and there is a range of variant forms (Table 15–2). The delineation of karyotype-phenotype correlations has been challenging due to small numbers, clinical heterogeneity, and the role of mosaicism, but some general karyotype-phenotype associations have been established, and these are listed in Table 15–3.

There is a possibility that Y-chromosome material may be present, even if the karyotype is apparently non-mosaic 45,X. Huang et al. (2002) reviewed 74 cases of 45,X diagnosed prenatally, most having been ascertained via, or discovered with, abnormal fetal ultrasonography. Of six with normal ultrasonography, three showed a male genital phenotype. The explanations, upon more detailed analysis, were as follows: In one, a segment of Yp was translocated to a chromosome 14, shown on FISH with an *SRY* probe; and in the other two, there was low-level mosaicism for an idic(Y) marker. Apparently normal male children were born. Some women with Turner syndrome who are 45,X on karyotyping may actually show Y sequences on molecular study, and these women do have a greater risk for gonadoblastoma (Mendes et al. 1999).

SEX CHROMOSOME POLYSOMY

The clinical pictures of the karyotypes 48,XXXX, 48,XXXY, 48,XXYY, 48,XYYY, 48,XXYY, 48,XXXY, 49,XXXXX, 49,XXXXY, 49,XXXYY, 49,XXYYY, and 49,XYYYY are outlined in Linden et al. (1995), Visootsak and Graham (2006), and Demily et al. (2017). The phenotypes may resemble commonly identified traits in the sex chromosome trisomies, such as impairment of language skills, executive function, and social adaptation, but with increased severity of these core phenotypic features, and with the addition of delayed developmental milestones and variable intellectual compromise (Hong and Reiss 2014). While the authors' comment is well taken that the current perception of the seriousness of phenotypic abnormality may have been overstated due to ascertainment bias, and indeed they describe normal (but low) IQs in some of the $2n = 48$ karyotypes, it remains true that most have intellectual impairment and abnormal behavior (Cammarata et al. 1999). Nuchal thickening is a frequent prenatal observation in 49,XXXXY (Peitsidis et al. 2009). Behavior in the 49,XXXXY male may modestly improve with testosterone therapy (Samango-Sprouse et al. 2023).

X AND Y CHROMOSOME MOSAICISM

True mosaicism involving the sex chromosomes seen at prenatal diagnosis presents a challenge in interpretation, and skilled ultrasonography, with respect to external genital anatomy, is central in determining the fetal gender. The problem is that the tissue analyzed at prenatal diagnosis may or may not reflect the distribution in the gonad. The presence of a Y chromosome in at least some gonadal tissue—or to be precise, the presence of the Y-borne *SRY* gene—will promote testicular development, which might or might not be complete, and which might or might not secrete male-inducing hormones. Thus, we may observe gender states from normal (although possibly infertile) female, through Turner-like female, genital ambiguity, mixed gonadal dysgenesis, even ovotesticular disorder of sex development (p. 763), to male with incomplete pubertal development, and to normal (although often infertile) male.

XX/XY Mosaicism. At prenatal karyotyping, this is usually pseudomosaicism resulting from the growth of maternal cells in a 46,XY pregnancy (Worton and Stern 1984). (Obviously, such pseudomosaicism would normally be undetected if the fetus is female.) Level III XX/XY mosaicism, curiously enough, is most likely to indicate a phenotypically normal female fetus in which the XY source is unknown, particularly when the XX cells predominate. A male "vanished twin" is a theoretical possibility (Worton and Stern), and indeed a quite plausible explanation given the frequency with which a twin pregnancy prior to seven weeks is followed some months later by the birth of a singleton baby (Sampson and de Crespigny 1992). Analysis of placental membranes after delivery in a pregnancy from which one twin has "vanished" can reveal a fetus papyraceous or a remnant empty sac (Nerlich et al. 1992). One can imagine tissue of the (male) twin remnant having been, by chance, in the path of the amniocentesis needle that sampled cells from the remaining (female) fetus.

A girl born following such a prenatal diagnosis (Hunter et al. 1982) was followed through to mid-adolescence, and her development was entirely normal (AGW Hunter, personal communication, 2002). A similar case was studied by I Hayes and A George (personal communication, 2009) with an XX:XY ratio of 90:10 on FISH of uncultured amniotic fluid, although non-mosaic 46,XX on cultured cells; ultrasonography indicated female external genital morphology. Following the birth of a normal girl, examination of seven sites from the placenta, and one site each from the cord and sac, all revealed a non-mosaic 46,XX complement, as did the cord blood sample.

A true fetal XX/XY karyotype is rare indeed, and it is more likely due to the fusion of two conceptuses—that is, XX//XY chimerism (but other mechanisms exist; see Chapter 24). Presumably depending upon the gonadal distribution of XX and XY cells, the genital anatomy will be male, female, or in between. Malan et al. (2007) report XX//XY chimerism at prenatal diagnosis, the child (subjected to pelvic ultrasonography) proving to be an apparently normal girl. Ovotesticular DSD, with imperfect or ambiguous genital anatomy, has been recorded from an XX/XY amniocentesis result with the same karyotype demonstrated in the child (Amor et al. 1999; Chen et al. 2005b, 2006e; Malan et al. 2007). Yaron et al. (1999) had a case presenting at amniocentesis with normal male morphology on ultrasound. The XX/XY mosaicism was confirmed on a second amniocentesis, and in due course on the normal male newborn infant (including on genital skin). Amor and colleagues note the point that intellectual compromise is not to be anticipated. Hughes et al. (2006) provide guidelines on management for children with intersex conditions. Infertility is predicted; but remarkably enough, one XX//XY man has fathered a child following IVF with retrieved sperm (Sugawara et al. 2005).

X/XY Mosaicism. Patients coming to medical attention with 45,X/46,XY mosaicism can be divided into three distinct groups based on their genitalia: typical female genitalia (variant of Turner syndrome), ambiguous genitalia (mixed gonadal dysgenesis), and normal male genitalia (Guzewicz et al. 2021). A risk for gonadal tumor applies (Müller et al. 1999). While post-natal cases often present with genital abnormality, at prenatal diagnosis a phenotypic male infant is the outcome in the considerable majority (90%–95%) of X/XY gestations—in other words, cases whose ascertainment was unbiased—and going through to birth (Hsu 1994; Huang et al. 2002). Fertility may be compromised, however, and other medical and neurodevelopmental manifestations of Turner syndrome such as short stature and cardiovascular defects may occasionally be present. We lack long-term follow-up data on prenatally ascertained cases (Alkhunaizi et al. 2024).

Of 14 pathology studies on fetuses post-termination in Chang et al. (1990), two had ovotestes and one a "precancerous" gonadal lesion. In a registry study that included mostly post-natally diagnosed cases, Stochholm et al. (2024) found that mortality rates were doubled in males and quadrupled in females with X/XY, and called for further research into the long-term health of these patients.

X/XX Mosaicism. Huang et al. (2002) reported their experience with 17 cases of X/XX mosaicism at amniocentesis. The ratios of X to XX cells ranged from 2:23 to 12:3. One case with IUGR (ratio 6:12) terminated in stillbirth, while the remaining 16 had normal ultrasonography. Of the eight cases continuing to term and for which information was available, two liveborn babies had the features of Turner syndrome (ratios 7:10 and 3:14), with the mosaicism confirmed post-natally in one of these. The remaining six (ratios ranging from 3:15 to 12:8) "reportedly had a normal female phenotype." To quote Huang et al., "The percentage of 45,X cells in amniocytes does not seem to be an indicator of pregnancy outcome, as there was considerable overlap between cases with normal and abnormal outcome." In a unique case of a monozygous twin pregnancy, one fetus showed nuchal swelling and the other appeared normal (Gilbert et al. 2002). Fetal blood sampling showed low-grade 45,X[2]/46,XX[23] mosaicism in the former and a normal 46,XX karyotype in the latter, in contrast to post-natal skin fibroblast karyotyping results of non-mosaic 45,X and 45,X[2]/46,XX[78], respectively.

Tokita and Sybert (2016) followed up 23 females with prenatally diagnosed 45,X/46,XX mosaicism, and noted the importance of accurate counseling in the context of increased detection of this karyotype by noninvasive prenatal testing. Follow-up was until mean age 11 years (range 0.1–27 years), and the mean percent aneuploidy was 42% at prenatal diagnosis and 23% in post-natal blood. Structural heart defects were documented in six females (26%), renal pathology in four (17%), and thyroid dysfunction in three (13%). No 45,X/46,XX female had formal IQ assessment, but persistent learning difficulties were reported in three (13%). Growth was comparable to population norms. Of the six patients older than 16 years, all had completed secondary school, and all had undergone spontaneous puberty. Results were compared with a cohort of 59 females with post-natally ascertained 45,X/46,XX mosaicism. Compared to the prenatally ascertained cohort, post-natally ascertained 45,X/46,XX females had shorter stature and a higher percentage aneuploidy in peripheral blood (40%); they also had a higher frequency of heart defects (39%), renal pathology (43%), and primary amenorrhea (50%). Combined data from both prenatally and post-natally ascertained cohorts suggest that the higher levels of percentage aneuploidy (on blood karyotype) were associated with an increased risk of congenital heart disease and a decreased chance of spontaneous menses, but not with the presence of other complications.

Insight into the long-term outlook well into adult age is gleaned from the UK Biobank data, and this offers some reassurance. 186 women with 45,X/46,XX mosaicism were included (Tuke et al. 2019). Most had not been diagnosed clinically, but presumably some would have been detected at prenatal diagnosis, had it been performed. This group of women had normal intelligence and household income, went through menarche and menopause at an average age, had an average number of children, were not at increased risk of pregnancy loss, and there was no evidence of increased risk of cardiac complications. The only difference noted compared to XX women was a 4 cm reduction in average height. Similarly, a number of healthy pregnant women have only been diagnosed themselves with X/XY mosaicism after receiving an abnormal cfDNA result (Steinfort et al. 2024).

X/XX/XXX, X/XXX, and XXX/XX Mosaicism. One reported case of X/XX/XXX mosaicism illustrates the difficulty in extrapolating the distribution of cell types from one tissue to another (Schwartz and Raffel 1992). Amniocentesis gave the proportions 16:64:20, respectively. Cord blood gave similar findings, although in placental tissue (chorion), the percentages were 2:57:41. The baby appeared normal. Huang et al. (2002) reported a case each of X/XXX and X/XX/XXX mosaicism diagnosed at amniocentesis, the former pregnancy producing a newborn with features of Turner syndrome, and the other a normal female.

As might be expected, the cardiovascular, renal and skeletal features of X/XXX are less severe than in non-mosaic monosomy X, and spontaneous puberty and pregnancy are more common (Tang et al. 2019). Sybert (2002) reviewed hers and others' data and concluded that ~60% of girls with X/XX/XXX and X/XXX could be predicted to have short stature and that "it is fair to suggest that residual ovarian function is possible, and to caution that premature ovarian failure is common." Klamut et al. (2024) noted that some features of Turner syndrome were more common in with X/XXX than with X/XX, and attributed this to the higher proportion of 45,X cells seen in the X/XXX girls.

XXY/XY Mosaicism. Up to 20% of Klinefelter syndrome are mosaic, and these men are, on average, more androgenized and have higher rates of fertility compared to their non-mosaic counterparts (Samplaski et al. 2014).

X/XYY and X/XY/XYY Mosaicism. The X/XYY and X/XY/XYY mosaic states are (necessarily) abnormal in post-natally ascertained cases, but prenatally diagnosed cases have consistently manifested an apparently normal male genital phenotype, albeit that the mosaicism may be confirmed in the child subsequently born (Pettenati et al. 1991; Hsu 1994). Presumably according to the distribution of X and XYY tissues, the gender in X/XYY mosaicism can be of either sex, or there can be ambiguity, these three states documented in one of the earliest reviews (Mulcahy et al. 1977). There is a tumor risk, and gonadoblastoma was identified at gonadectomy in a virilized female with mixed gonadal dysgenesis (Gibbons et al. 1999). Infertility is likely, but it may be treatable (Dale et al. 2002).

XXY/XX Mosaicism. XXY/XX is a rare karyotype that shows extreme clinical heterogeneity ranging from no abnormal phenotype to multiple physical and behavioral symptoms, and ambiguous genitalia with ovotestes (Guess et al. 2024). The phenotype presumably reflects the proportion and distribution of the XXY and XX cell lines.

STRUCTURALLY ABNORMAL SEX CHROMOSOME

X Chromosome Deletion. The possibility of an inherited X-autosome translocation should be checked by doing the mother's karyotype; it may transpire that she has the same karyotype.[24] Cytogenetically visible X chromosome deletions in the female, 46,X,del(Xp) or 46,X,del(Xq), predict the possibility, but not the certainty, of an incomplete form of Turner syndrome and/or premature ovarian failure (Chapter 15). Brown et al. (2001) describe a mother, of tall stature (5 feet 10 inches), having a prenatal diagnosis of del(X)(q22q26); she herself had the same karyotype, and "the parents took comfort in the observation that in the mother the deletion had no apparent phenotypic effect." A normal baby girl was born. Mother and daughter showed completely skewed X-inactivation, the abnormal X being consistently inactive.

In the male, the 46,Y,del(X) state would be nonviable for all but the very smallest cytogenetically visible deletions, and major abnormality would be probable for those pregnancies that might be viable.

X Chromosome Duplication. De novo X chromosome duplications in the female, 46,X,dup(X), may determine a nil, minor, or major phenotypic impairment accordingly, as the pattern of X-inactivation may or may not be protective and if a functional disomy is not prevented (Chapter 15). Zhang et al. (1997) provide detail according to the extent and site of the duplication in a review of post-natally diagnosed cases. Women with an

[24] X-autosome and Y-autosome rearrangements are discussed above, under De Novo Rearrangements, Apparently Balanced, and Unbalanced, respectively.

isodicentric X chromosome with Xq deletion are monosomic for genetic material distal to the Xq breakpoint and trisomic for the Xp arm. The phenotype typically includes primary or secondary amenorrhea, and other Turner syndrome features are lacking unless there is mosaicism for a 45,X cell line (Tsai et al. 2006). Normality has been reported with respect to an isodicentric X, idic(X)(q27) comprising practically a double copy of the X, identified prenatally with the abnormal chromosome being late replicating, and indeed one such child was "academically advanced and enrolled in a gifted and talented program." In contrast, isodicentric X chromosomes with Xp deletion are associated with a Turner syndrome phenotype. In the male, functional disomy for the duplicated segment would likely cause severe defects, often lethal in utero; this is likely the scenario in the case in the family described in Figure 22–11 with a concomitant del Xp and dup Xq.

X-Y Translocation. The most common form of the t(X;Y) has the X breakpoint in the distal short arm, at Xp22.3 or distal to Xp22, and the Y breakpoint at Yq11 or Yq12. The t(X;Y) arises during spermatogenesis by recombination due to highly similar sequences at these loci. The other, intact sex chromosome may be an X or a Y chromosome, and the two states differ as follows.

46,X,der(X)t(X;Y). A de novo X-Y translocation would be expected to herald a female child, who will likely have short stature due to *SHOX* haploinsufficiency but otherwise normal pubertal development and fertility, with a 50% risk to pass the t(X;Y) to male or female offspring (Daghsni et al. 2025). Intelligence is typically normal, but

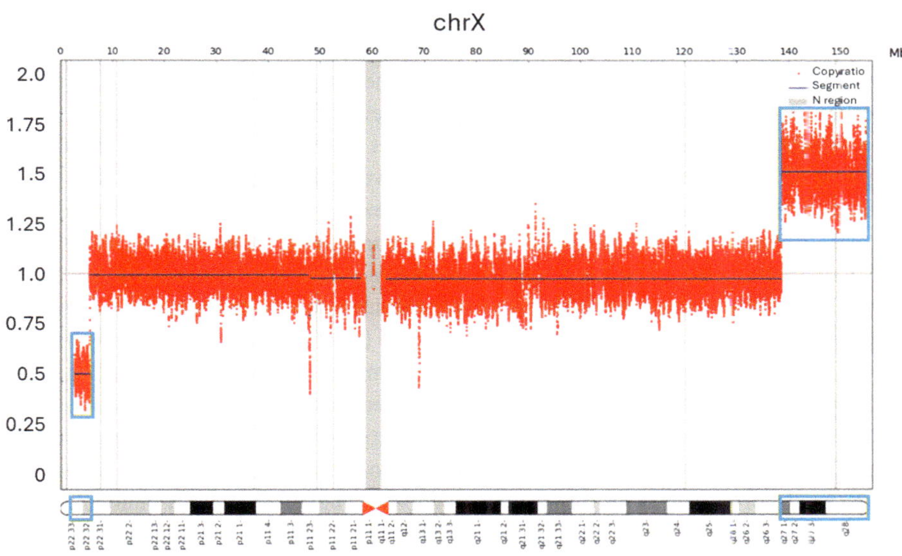

Figure 22–11. A Del/Dup X Chromosome in a Mother and her Fetus.

Notes: The mother was of short stature (150 cm), but otherwise normal. She had had four miscarriages, in one of which, a male, major fetal malformation (holoprosencephaly) had been identified. Ultrasonography in the current pregnancy had discovered multiple malformation. Amniocentesis gave a male result with an add(Xp22.2). Microarray of amniocyte DNA discovered 46,X,delXp22.33p22.32 and dupXp27.1q28. She herself had the same del/dup X chromosome. The fetal malformation likely reflected a functional distal Xq disomy including the *MECP2* locus, and a distal Xp monosomy, whereas the mother had been protected by favorable inactivation.

Source: From Q Lin et al., Prenatal detection and molecular cytogenetic characterization of Xp deletion and Xq duplication: a case report and literature review, *BMC Med Genomics* 17:57, 2024. Courtesy Q Lin, and with the permission of Springer Nature.

(rob) translocations, but chromosomal PGT-SR can likewise be applied to pericentric inversions and complex chromosome rearrangements.

Preimplantation Genetic Testing for Aneuploidy Screening (PGT-A)

PGT-A is the practice of evaluating embryos for chromosome aneuploidy in chromosomally normal parents. The rationale behind PGT-A is that a substantial number of human embryos are aneuploid, and certain patient populations, including couples of advanced maternal age or with histories of recurrent miscarriage and repeated implantation failure, may be predisposed to producing aneuploid embryos. Thus, aneuploidy is assumed to be an important reason that many IVF pregnancies fail. Logically, therefore, assessing the chromosome status of embryos, and discarding screened embryos that are aneuploid, should improve the proportion of transferred embryos that result in pregnancy.

PGT-A is also used in the setting of a couple who have had a previously chromosomally abnormal pregnancy, or a previous liveborn child with Down syndrome or other aneuploidy. Here, the risk of recurrence of the specific aneuploidy is usually low, and the benefit of PGT-A, at least in terms of risk reduction, is small. For couples who are naturally fertile, it is questionable whether such a small risk reduction justifies the use of IVF (with its associated small risks to both mother and baby); but for couples who are already using IVF because of infertility, the addition of PGT-A may be considered appropriate, and it may give the couple more confidence of a successful outcome.

Gender Selection

Gender diagnosis at PGT can be achieved via PGT-A, and may be appropriate in the context of a sex-related genetic risk, whether Mendelian or non-Mendelian—an example of the latter being autism (Amor and Cameron 2008). In practice, the use of sex-selection PGT has declined, as direct gene testing has become feasible for many sex-linked disorders. A notable exception is for males affected by an X-linked disease, who wish to avoid transmitting the faulty gene to their (female) offspring, a circumstance in which sex selection can substitute perfectly for a direct gene test.

EMBRYOLOGY PROCEDURES

Those who make the decision to embark upon chromosomal PGT will need to enroll (if not already) in an IVF program. In IVF, hormone treatment is given to stimulate the ovaries to produce a large number[2] of oöcytes in a single stimulated IVF cycle. Ovum "pick-up" is conducted by transvaginal endoscopy under ultrasound guidance. The ova are collected, and fertilization is achieved using either conventional IVF or intracytoplasmic sperm injection (ICSI).

[2] Preferably double figures; but if only a few, this does not per se betoken an increased risk for trisomy (Honorato et al. 2017).

On day 1, about 18 hours after exposure to sperm, the oöcytes are checked for the presence of two pronuclei and two polar bodies[3] as evidence that fertilization[4] has occurred. Shortly thereafter, syngamy will occur, and during the next 48 hours, the first few mitoses will have produced cleavage-stage embryos of six to eight cells. In the next 72 hours, these few cells give rise to 200–300 daughter cells, and this is the blastocyst stage (Figure 20–2).

> In the early days of IVF, embryos were transferred at the cleavage stage, on the assumption that the uterus would provide the best environment for the survival of the embryo, while also allowing assessment of embryo morphology, in order to select the best quality embryos for transfer. But during the 2010s, there was a shift in practice, with transfer now taking place on day 5 or 6, by which time the embryos have become blastocysts. This shift was facilitated by the improvement in embryo culture techniques, and supported by the observation that blastocysts appeared to have better implantation potential compared with cleavage-stage embryos; an observation subsequently confirmed in a Cochrane review, which showed that embryos transferred at the blastocyst stage were about 25% more likely to result in a live birth (Glujovsky et al. 2022). This picture likely reflects a "self-selection" whereby only the most viable embryos develop into blastocysts.

There are three types of PGT biopsy, done at three sequential stages of gametic and embryonic development: polar body biopsy, blastomere biopsy, and blastocyst (trophectoderm) biopsy. In practice, the great majority of PGT biopsies are done at the blastocyst stage.

Polar Body Analysis

Polar body (PB) genetic analysis (satisfyingly requiring recall of some elementary facts of biology) has been used for PGT (or "preconception diagnosis") in a few laboratories, and legal or logistic constraints against PGT in some jurisdictions have propelled interest (Verpoest et al. 2018; Oberle et al. 2024). The process of biopsy is illustrated in Figure 23–1, with the first and second polar bodies (PB1 and PB2) aspirated from beneath the "shell" of the zona pellucida. Both polar bodies are required for diagnosis, and they can be removed simultaneously or sequentially (Harper 2018). PB analysis allows a focus on the more vulnerable gamete—that is, the ovum—since the great majority of

[3] IVF laboratories use morphological assessment for the presence of two pronuclei as a "pseudo-genetic test" for ploidy. The rationale is that embryos with one pronucleus (2% of all embryos) are at high risk of haploidy, which is incompatible with embryo development; and embryos with three pronuclei (5% of all embryos) are at high risk of triploidy and its incumbent risk of miscarriage. However, Capalbo et al. (2024) argue that pronuclei number is a poor predictor of embryo ploidy, and that many livebirths have followed the transfer of embryos with 0, 1, or 3 pronuclei. They suggest that rather than discarding abnormally pronucleated embryos, PGT-A be applied to them as a more accurate ploidy assay, allowing those embryos that are euploid to be "rescued" for clinical use.

[4] Since fertilization in vitro can be observed as it actually happens, the fine detail of the process can be appreciated. The first act is penetration of the ovum by the sperm. To the embryologist, this is only the prelude to conception; the true moment of conception is the point at which the male and female pronuclei fuse, their chromosomes aligning on a common metaphase plate ("syngamy"). Once that event has taken place, the zygote has come into existence. At the first mitosis, it loses that name and becomes, in IVF parlance, a "cleavage-stage embryo," or simply an embryo.

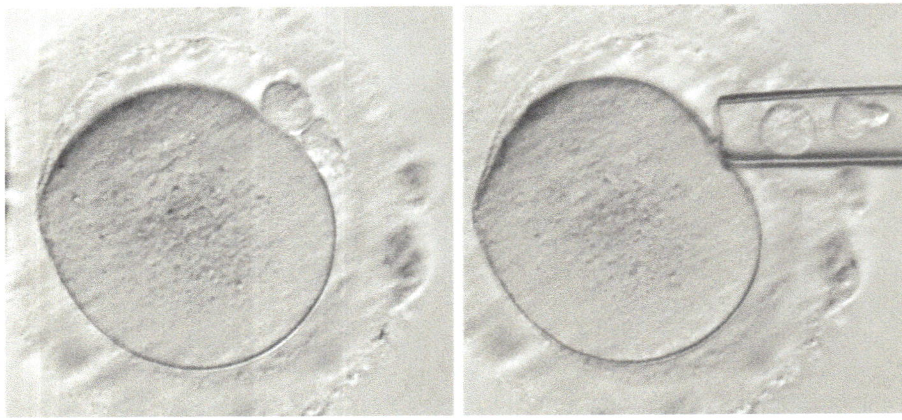

Figure 23–1. The process of polar body biopsy.

The egg (*left*) is held in place by a suction pipette, which is applied directly to the zona pellucida (the "shell" that invests the egg itself, seen in faint darker circular outline). The first and second polar bodies are located in the space between the zona pellucida and the egg's cell membrane. The egg is manipulated so that the polar bodies are at the 1 to 2 o'clock position. The pipette (*right*) has entered a laser-cut hole in the zona pellucida, and the two polar bodies have been aspirated into its lumen.

Source: From M Montag et al., Polar body biopsy: A viable alternative to preimplantation genetic testing and screening, *Reprod Biomed Online* 18 Suppl 1:6–11, 2009. Courtesy M Montag, and with the permission of Elsevier.

segregation errors leading to aneuploidy occur here, due either to nondisjunction, or to premature pre-division of sister chromatids. Disomic or nullisomic gametes could be identified and thus excluded from fertilization.

By way of example, imagine that the asterisked gametocyte at meiosis I in Figure 23–3 is PB1, and that the two chromosomes shown within it are chromosome 22s—that is, PB1 is disomic 22. The "empty" gamete to the right, therefore, would be a nullisomic 22 oöcyte, and thus of course to be discarded. Figure 23–2 shows an actual example, and while FISH is no longer used for this purpose, the colored probes provide an

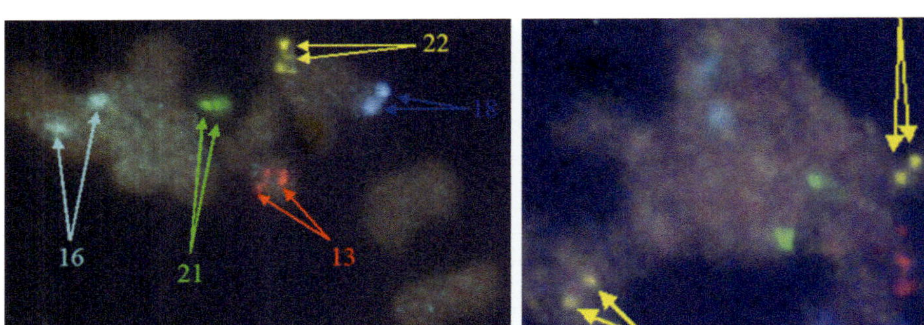

Figure 23–2. FISH Analysis of the First Polar Body. Normal Haploidy for Five Chromosomes (*left*), and Disomy 22 (*right*).

Notes: The 5-color FISH probes recognize chromosomes 13 (red), 16 (light blue), 18 (dark blue), 21 (green), and 22 (yellow). With each chromosome being two-chromatid, each has two colored spots. The arrows in the polar body at right indicate two no. 22 chromosomes, enabling an inference that the associated ovum is nullisomic 22.

Source: From F Vialard et al., Evidence of a high proportion of premature unbalanced separation of sister chromatids in the first polar bodies of women of advanced age, *Hum Reprod* 21:1172–1178, 2006. Courtesy F Vialard, and with the permission of Oxford University Press.

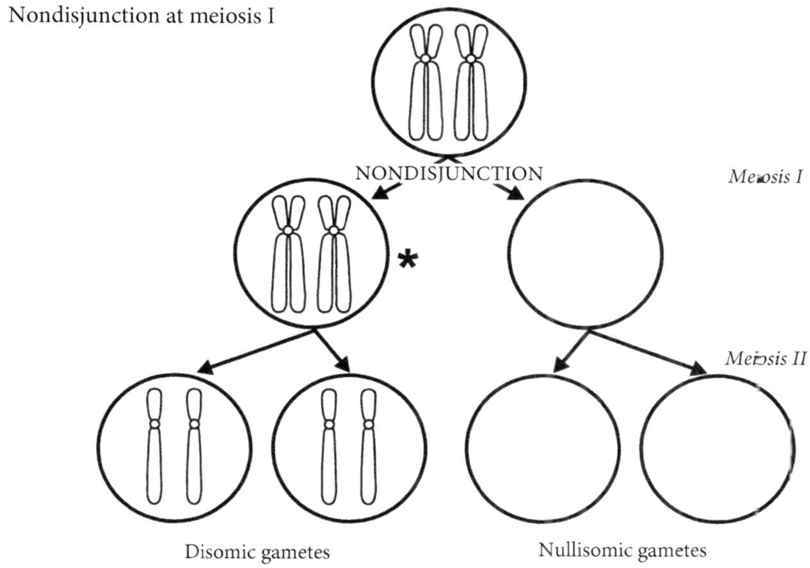

Figure 23–3. Nondisjunction Detected via Polar Body Analysis (Classical Scenario).

intuitive illustration. Preferably, the interpretation requires analysis of both PB1 and PB2 (Verpoest et al. 2018). The reader may determine, on study of Figure 23–4 with respect to pre-division of sister chromatids at meiosis, why analysis of just one PB could in some instances mislead. The asterisked cell at meiosis I could be, say, PB1, and tested as disomic, suggesting nullisomy of the egg; and yet the ovum alongside is actually monosomic normal. At meiosis II, the nullisomic PB2 (the fourth gamete of this row) allows the full picture to be interpreted: the opposite aneuploid results from PB1 and PB2, taken together, indicate a euploid egg.

Potential advantages of PB biopsy are that specimens are obtained earlier, and that the biopsy is less disruptive to the embryo. On the other hand, PB is expensive, given the need to test both polar bodies in every embryo, although new technologies may be more cost-effective (Oberle et al. 2024). It is time-consuming, and temporal constraints will stretch laboratory resources. The windows of opportunity for performing biopsy are narrow. Abnormalities arising in paternal meiosis, estimated to represent less than 10% of aneuploidies (Templado et al. 2013), will not be detected, nor will unbalanced structural rearrangements of paternal origin. PB biopsy will not detect mosaic post-zygotic aneuploidies. While PGT-A by microarray analysis of polar bodies may not increase live birth rate, there are less embryo transfers, with less requirement for cryopreservation and fewer miscarriages (Verpoest et al. 2018). The procedure may yet come to have a place (Madritsch et al. 2024).

Cleavage-Stage Biopsy (Day 3 Biopsy of a Blastomere)

In the early days of PGT, the usual approach was to remove one, or at most two,[5] cells (blastomeres) from each embryo on day 3. This required a hole to be made in the zona

[5] The live-birth rate is less when two cells are removed (De Vos et al. 2009).

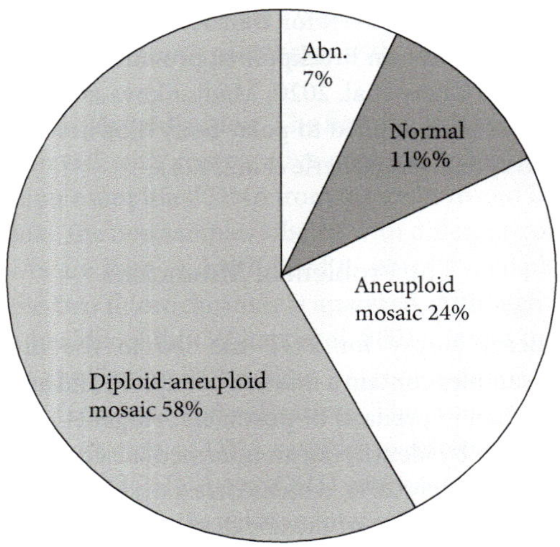

Figure 23–7. Chromosomal Status of Blastocysts.

Notes: Percentages of human blastocysts that have normal, abnormal and mosaic results, as detected by single cell sequencing in 55 embryos.

Source: Redrawn from EA Chavli et al., Single-cell DNA sequencing reveals a high incidence of chromosomal abnormalities in human blastocysts. *J Clin Invest* 2024:e174483, 2024. Courtesy EB Baart, and with the permission of the American Society for Clinical Investigation.

A landmark study in 2024 shed new light on the true extent of mosaicism, looking at every cell of blastocyst-stage embryos (Chavli et al. 2024). Remarkably, 82% of embryos contained at least some cells with numerical and/or structural abnormalities indicative of mosaic aneuploidy (Figure 23–7). Most of these embryos were euploid-aneuploid mosaic, with a range of numerical and structural abnormalities present. These findings represent a challenge of PGT-A, which relies on the genetics of the biopsied cell(s) being representative of the embryo as a whole (Figures 23–8); as such, the presence of mosaicism could mislead.

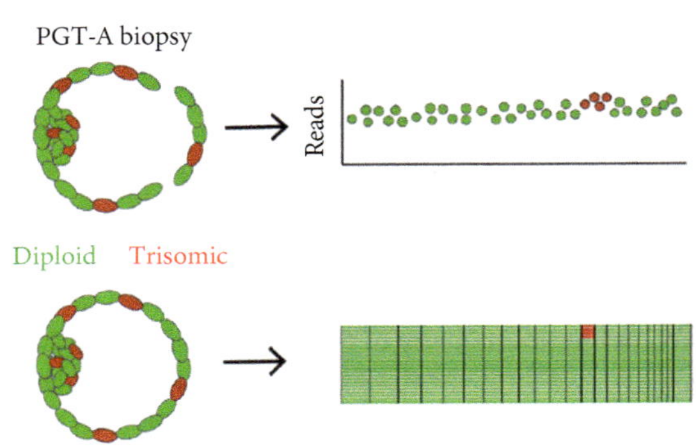

Figure 23–8. The Sensitivity of Blastocyst Biopsy, in the Detection of Mosaicism.

Notes: On trophectoderm biopsy at PGT-A (PGT for aneuploidy) using standard DNA methodology (*above*), mosaicism of less than 20% would likely be missed. Research using single-cell analyses of the whole embryo (*below*) could reveal otherwise undetectable mosaicism.

Source: From EA Chavli et al., Single-cell DNA sequencing reveals a high incidence of chromosomal abnormalities in human blastocysts. *J Clin Invest* 2024:e174483, 2024. Courtesy EB Baart, and with the permission of the American Society for Clinical Investigation.

PREIMPLANTATION GENETIC TESTING OUTCOMES

PGT for Aneuploidy

Every patient undergoing IVF has a risk to generate an aneuploid embryo. The risk varies according to individual factors, and these several factors may influence a decision in favor of PGT for Aneuploidy (PGT-A): advanced maternal age, recurrent implantation failure, recurrent pregnancy loss, unexplained infertility, and prior aneuploid conception. The aim of PGT-A is to improve the chance of a successful pregnancy by choosing only those embryos known to be euploid. Logically, it would seem that surely PGT-A would improve the odds. But the question is this: is PGT-A actually beneficial in practice?

The ability of NGS-based PGT-A accurately to predict a successful delivery was assessed in a large prospective, blinded, nonselection study in which 484 blastocysts were biopsied and transferred, but with PGT-A being performed only after clinical outcome was known (Figure 23–9). Out of 102 PGT-A aneuploid embryo transfers, 40% resulted in a biochemical pregnancy, but none ended in a live birth. On the other hand, from 312 PGT-A euploid transfers, 65% resulted in sustained implantation or delivery. The comparison is stark. While this study demonstrates the prognostic ability of NGS-based PGT-A, we yet await large randomized controlled trials to arrive at a definitive answer regarding the clinical benefit of PGT-A. Early research suggests an age-related difference. For older women, aged ≥35 years, PGT-A indeed appears to be effective in reducing the risk of miscarriage and results in a significantly higher birth rate. But no such benefit is observed in women younger than 35 (Simopoulou et al. 2021).

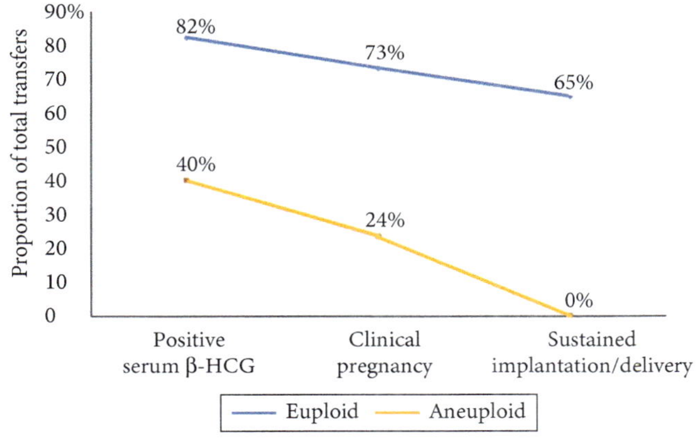

Figure 23–9. Outcomes Following Euploid and Aneuploid Embryo Transfer.

Notes: The two timelines reflect outcomes after the implantation at IVF of a euploid cf. an aneuploid embryo. The distinction in terms of outcome is very evident.

Source: From AW Tiegs et al., A multicenter, prospective, blinded, nonselection study evaluating the predictive value of an aneuploid diagnosis using a targeted next-generation sequencing-based preimplantation genetic testing for aneuploidy assay and impact of biopsy, *Fertil Steril* 115:627-637, 2021. Courtesy AW Tiegs, and with the permission of Elsevier.

> There are several reasons why PGT-A might not be as effective as logically expected. PGT-A remains a screening test, and as such is subject to a risk of false-positive and false-negative results. False-negative PGT-A would lead to embryos screened as euploid resulting in miscarriages, and to ongoing pregnancies in which aneuploidy is detected. Such observations, while rare (<1% of embryos transferred), are on record (Tiegs et al. 2016; Greco et al. 2023).

There are two main sources of false-positive and false-negative PGT-A results. First, PGT provides many opportunities for technical errors arising through the processes of embryo biopsy, whole genome amplification, and genetic analysis. Second, the phenomenon of mosaicism appears to be common, and potentially undermines the strategy of PGT-A by generating multiple pathways to misdiagnosis.

False-positive PGT-A results have been proven upon rebiopsy studies, but mostly are limited to mosaic and segmental aneuploidies. Non-mosaic full aneuploidies, which are typically of meiotic origin, are almost always confirmed at rebiopsy of the embryo. Similarly, if blastocysts testing non-mosaic aneuploid are transferred, only a very small fraction go through to successful normal live birth. At the request of parents, Barad et al. (2022) transferred 76 embryos that had been diagnosed at PGT-A with full chromosome aneuploidies. Five pregnancies resulted, but only one continued to live birth.[8] For fully euploid embryos, rebiopsy studies have found little evidence of false-negative results, with euploid PGT-A results confirmed in >99% of cases (Kim et al. 2022).

OUTCOMES FOLLOWING THE TRANSFER OF MOSAIC EMBRYOS

While a conservative approach, based on prenatal and pediatric experience with mosaicism, might have been to discard mosaic embryos, in fact the PGT-A literature allows otherwise, and two key facts are now understood. First, many healthy babies have been born following the transfer of mosaic aneuploid blastocysts; and second, pregnancies following transfer of mosaic embryos do not have an increased risk of untoward fetal or neonatal outcome. Indeed, if a mosaic embryo is transferred and a pregnancy results, in <1% is the mosaicism ever confirmed in the fetus or neonate (American Society for Reproductive Medicine 2023).

In the case of mosaic aneuploidies and non-mosaic segmental aneuploidies, between 40% and 80% are confirmed at rebiopsy (Victor et al. 2019; Girardi et al. 2020; Wu et al. 2021; Cascante et al. 2023). Aneuploidies that are *both* mosaic and segmental are particularly unlikely to be confirmed at rebiopsy, and in fact when these embryos are transferred, the livebirth rate is indistinguishable from that of euploid embryos (Grkovic et al. 2022).[9] Healthy livebirths have also been observed following the transfer of embryos diagnosed as non-mosaic segmental aneuploidy, but with a lower livebirth rate of about 25% (Besser et al. 2024), indicating that some of these embryos were actually mosaic.

Mosaicism does, however, have an impact upon the reproductive potential of the embryo: implantation rates are less, and miscarriage more so, compared to euploid embryos (Viotti et al. 2021). Risks vary with the type and extent of mosaicism (Figure 23–10). As noted above, embryos with low-level mosaicism of a single chromosome

[8] This embryo had been diagnosed at PGT-A with 46,XX,+14,-18.

[9] Yet, mosaic segmental aneuploidies at PGT-A are not always a benign finding. Barad et al. (2022) transferred an embryo diagnosed at PGT with mosaic dup(10)(q11.21-q21.1), and the outcome was the birth of a male infant non-mosaic for the dup(10), and with coarctation of the aorta.

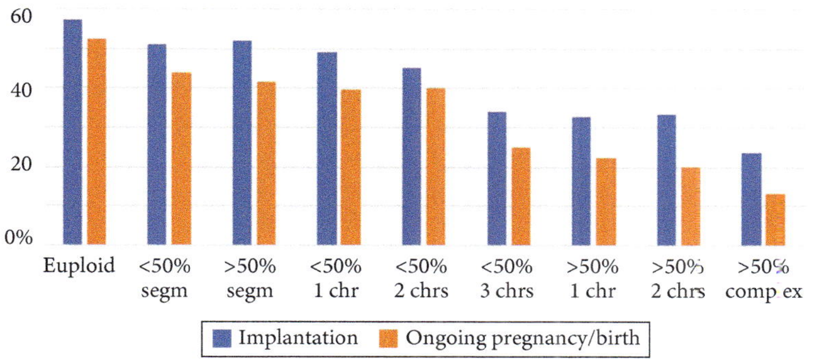

Figure 23–10. Outcomes after Transfer of Euploid and Mosaic Embryos.

Notes: Clinical outcomes of the euploid embryos are compared with mosaic groups, sorted according to mosaic level, and type (segmental cf. full aneuploidies). segm = segmental; chr = chromosome.

Source: Adapted from M Viotti et al., Using outcome data from one thousand mosaic embryo transfers to formulate an embryo ranking system for clinical use, *Fertil Steril* 115:1212–1224, 2021. Courtesy M Viotti, and with the permission of Elsevier

segment appear to have similar outcomes to euploid embryos. Conversely, these four factors are associated with worse clinical outcomes (Ma et al. 2022):

- Mosaicism level >50%
- Whole chromosomes involved
- Mosaicism for three or more chromosomes
- Mosaicism for both gain and loss

In light of this knowledge, couples can have the option of transferring mosaic embryos, but with an awareness of possible adverse outcomes including risks to the pregnancy and to the child to be born. The American Society for Reproductive Medicine (2023) provides guidance in this matter and has put forth these advisories that can guide decision-making:

- A lower percentage of mosaicism is associated with better rates of implantation and ongoing pregnancy.
- Higher-level mosaicism may predict a risk of adverse outcome, due to misdiagnosis of a true aneuploid embryo.
- Segmental mosaic aneuploidies have better ongoing pregnancy rates compared to whole chromosome mosaics.
- Although intuitively, mosaicism for one of the classic survivable aneuploidies (trisomies 13, 18, 21) might seem to pose a higher risk, in fact this appears not to be so.
- Monosomic and trisomic mosaicisms have similar pregnancy and miscarriage rates.
- Embryos with mosaic aneuploidies of three or more chromosomes do less well than those with one or two.
- Whether embryos with segmental mosaic aneuploidy versus those with whole chromosome mosaics differ in terms of risk, is not yet clarified.
- A theoretical risk of uniparental disomy (UPD) or confirmed placental mosaicism (CPM) in pregnancies from a mosaic embryo, in fact, seems not to apply.

In practice, mosaic embryos, as do the euploid, upon transfer follow a path to one of three outcomes: a failure of implantation, a miscarriage, or a live birth with no apparent abnormal phenotype. There does not seem to be an increased risk, vis-à-vis the euploid embryo, of pregnancy complications or abnormal prenatal or postnatal karyotypes. Viotti et al. (2023) collated data for more than 2,000 mosaic embryo transfers, including birth data for 488 infants, and results were largely reassuring. Birth outcomes showed no difference in birth weight or gestational age compared to euploid controls, and of the 488 livebirths, only one had a serious birth defect (a congenital heart defect). In three out of 250 cases (1.2%) where testing was performed in the pregnancy, there were fetal findings consistent with the previous PGT mosaic result (Viotti et al. 2023; Greco et al. 2023). The first was an embryo with low-level mosaicism for deletion of 1p36.33-p31.1, a finding that was confirmed at amniocentesis and in brain tissue from the products of conception after pregnancy termination. The second was an embryo with low-level mosaicism for trisomy 21 that was confirmed at CVS and amniocentesis, and the pregnancy terminated after the additional detection of ultrasound abnormalities. The third was an embryo with low-level mosaicism for duplication of 4q32.2q34.3 that was confirmed at CVS, with the pregnancy continuing to term, resulting in an infant with no birth defect. In addition to these three cases, Viotti et al. (2023) also identified two cases with prenatal mosaic results that were different from the original one detected with PGT-A, and assumed to be unrelated. Notably, this overall rate of 2% mosaic results at prenatal testing is not substantially different from the 1% to 2% mosaic results detected at CVS in the general population (Chapter 22).

Thus, in summary, the somewhat surprising conclusion is this: Mosaicism of the embryo, rather often, seems not to matter.

PGT for Structural Rearrangement (PGT-SR)

We have data from many thousands of reported PGT-SR cycles to call upon. Naturally, the risk that an embryo will be abnormal at PGT, not yet having been subject to survival pressure, is substantially—and often very substantially—higher than during the pregnancy or at birth.

Reciprocal Translocations. Xie et al. (2022) analyzed segregation fractions from the study of 10,846 blastocysts, from 2,253 couples, and tested by NGS as follows: normal (alternate) 46%, adjacent-1 31%, adjacent-2 12%, and 3:1, 4:0, and others all ~5%. Thus, slightly more than half were chromosomally imbalanced. These figures are averages derived from aggregated data, but of course each rcp translocation will have its own unique segregation pattern (as discussed at length in Chapter 5). Factors that reduce the proportion of alternate segregation are female sex of rcp carrier and involvement of an acrocentric chromosome (Figure 23–11). Alternate segregation is also favored if the translocated segment is of relatively large size, as a proportion of the chromosome arm (Xie et al. 2022).

Robertsonian Translocations. Segregation outcomes for rob translocations are more favorable than with rcp. Dang et al. (2023) tested 3,423 blastocysts with NGS, from 763 couples, and found the following: normal (alternate) 70%, adjacent 29%, and 3:0 in 0.7%. Alternate segregation was more frequent in male (82%) than in female (60%) carriers, the rates not varying with carrier age. Outcomes were similar across all rob translocations. One or more transferrable embryos were identified in 82% of cycles, and 57% of transferred embryos resulted in a live birth.

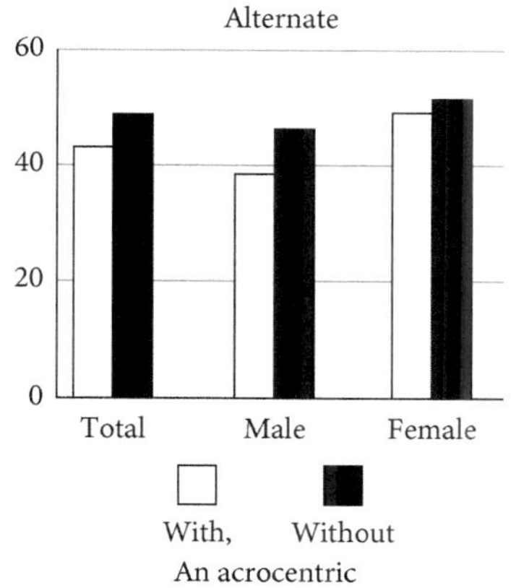

Figure 23–11. Alternate Segregation in Blastocysts.

Notes: These data show the impact of sex of reciprocal translocation carrier, and involvement of an acrocentric chromosome, on the proportion of embryos with alternate (balanced) segregation.

Source: From data in P Xie et al., Risk factors affecting alternate segregation in blastocysts from preimplantation genetic testing cycles of autosomal reciprocal translocations, *Front Genet* 13:880208, 2022.

Insertional Translocations. Zhang et al. (2023c) evaluated PGT-SR outcomes in 187 embryos from 23 couples, one of whom was an insertional translocation carrier, and found 30% of embryos were suitable for transfer (normal/balanced). Predictors of higher percentage of normal/balanced embryos were interchromosomal insertions (compared to intrachromosomal insertions) and male sex of carrier parent.

Pericentric Inversions. Xie et al. (2019) analyzed PGT-SR results for 379 embryos from couples, one of whom carried a pericentric inversion. Overall, 17% of blastocysts were unbalanced for the inversion, but unsurprisingly (Chapter 9), this varied with the size of the inversion segment. When the inverted segment was <57% of the chromosome length, only 8% were unbalanced, compared to 34% unbalanced when the inverted segment was >57% of the chromosome length. Overall, 51% of transferrable blastocysts resulted in a live birth.

Paracentric Inversions. As noted in Chapter 9, for paracentric inversions, unbalanced recombinant chromosomes are either acentric or dicentric, and typically do not lead to viable offspring. PGT-SR is rarely performed for paracentric inversions, but Xie et al. (2019) were able to study 197 blastocysts from couples, one of whom carried a paracentric inversion, and found unbalanced segregants in just 3.6%, representing a small fraction of the 30% of embryos that were aneuploid. After transfer, 63% of normal/balanced blastocysts resulted in a live birth.

Complex Balanced Chromosome Rearrangements (BCRs). When there is more than one balanced rearrangement, or a rearrangement involving more than two chromosomes, normal/balanced embryos are predicted to be scarce. Yet, there is still cause for some modest optimism that suitable embryos might be found. Li et al. (2020) collated PGT results for more than 200 embryos from couples with complex chromosome rearrangements, and found 12% were euploid (see also Chapter 10, Figure 10–13). Both partners of a couple carrying different balanced rearrangements is another challenging circumstance. Liu et al. (2021) report a couple where each partner carried a different reciprocal translocation: 46, XX,t(10;16)(q25.2;q12.1) and 46,XY,t(9;14)(p21.1;q12). They were advised of a low chance of success, but against the odds, two out of three blastocysts tested were found to be balanced/normal, and transfer of one of these embryos led to the birth of a healthy boy.

GENETIC COUNSELING

PGT is sufficiently complicated, not to mention expensive, that it will not usually be the first option for fertile couples wishing to avoid the birth of a child with a chromosomal disorder. High-risk scenarios, such as the person being a translocation carrier, might, however, warrant consideration sooner rather than later. Carriers of structural rearrangements may view access to the procedure as empowering, but equally may find the process stressful; discarding an embryo with an unbalanced rearrangement, having had a child with that condition, may raise uncomfortable ambiguities (Karatas et al. 2010). For infertile couples (whether or not there is a chromosomal basis of the infertility) who require an IVF procedure to conceive, advice about a place for PGT-A will need to be tempered by a continuing understanding of the biology of early human embryo development, and the fact that PGT is, as yet, an imperfect tool for predicting the health and viability of an embryo.

For couples presenting for PGT on the basis that one of them carries a chromosomal rearrangement, a number of points need to be raised.

The Reasons for Choosing PGT

Some couples may have had conventional prenatal diagnosis with successive terminations of pregnancies due to a high-risk translocation, and be unwilling to face this prospect again. It may be difficult to distinguish between two possibilities. Either, this may have been a run of bad luck, with an optimistic outlook for the next pregnancy as a realistic possibility and therefore allowing the counselor to suggest a further natural attempt; or, the series of abnormal pregnancies may reflect a strong predisposition of that translocation to generate unbalanced gametes. Avoiding the possibility of termination following conventional prenatal diagnosis is, for those who have had that experience, a strong motivation (Lavery et al. 2002).

The Limited Success Rate

As discussed above, many IVF/PGT procedures do not produce the desired end result of a "take-home baby," and the figures for PGT pregnancies are fairly similar to those applying to all IVF. For couples who require IVF in order to conceive (e.g., when a male translocation carrier also has oligospermia), the benefits of PGT—avoidance of transfer of nonviable embryos and reduced risk of miscarriage—are likely to outweigh the disadvantages, of which financial cost may be prominent. In contrast, couples who would otherwise have no difficulty conceiving may struggle weighing the pros and cons of IVF with PGT, compared to natural conception and conventional prenatal diagnosis (Kanavakis and Traeger-Synodinos 2002). In this comparison, the chances of ultimately having a healthy child may be similar between the two pathways, but the challenges of the two choices are very different. One study that compared livebirth rates in translocation couples who chose PGT-SR, against those choosing natural conception, found no difference in the livebirth rate, although the risk of miscarriage was less with PGT-SR (Ikuma et al. 2015). The counselor can help the couple in their decision-making by encouraging them to consider the relative merits and challenges of PGT versus natural conception. As noted below, the reality is, for those who face the dual challenge of advanced maternal age and a BCR, the chance of success may be low.

The Outlook at PGT-A

For PGT-A, a realistic consideration has to be that possibly not a single euploid embryo will be obtained from an IVF stimulation cycle. The risk for this unfortunate circumstance is at its lowest for women in the age range later 20s through early 30s, but rises steeply from the late 30s—and, as logically expected, this risk is mirrored by a fall, according to age, in the chance of retrieving at least one euploid embryo (Figure 23–12).

Maternal Age Considerations in PGT-SR

Given that PGT-SR typically also incorporates PGT-A, the additional impact of de novo aneuploidy will influence the proportion of embryos available for transfer. Whereas the proportion of embryos unbalanced for the parental rearrangement is constant, independent of parental age, the proportion of de novo aneuploid embryos will naturally increase with advancing maternal age.[10]

In a population with median maternal age of 30 years and de novo aneuploidy rate of 35%, Zhou et al. (2024) found that, after considering both unbalanced segregants of the balanced rearrangement and de novo aneuploidy, the proportion of embryos suitable for transfer was 30% for rcp translocations, 46% for rob translocations, and 57% for inversions (Table 23–1). By comparison, in a slightly older cohort with median maternal age 33 years, the de novo aneuploidy rate was 45%, and the proportion of embryos available for transfer was reduced to 19% for rcp translocations, 33% for rob translocations and 36% for inversions (Oğur et al. 2023). In the same study, the proportion of embryos with de novo aneuploidy was 59% in women ≥35 years, compared to 41% in women <35 years.

Hence, for women above age 35 years, the proportion of tested embryos that are suitable for transfer may be less than 20%, and a probable outcome of a PGT cycle may be that no embryo will be suitable for transfer. When suitable embryos are obtained, the outlook is considerably brighter regardless of maternal age, with around half of transferred euploid embryos leading to the birth of a healthy child (Oğur et al. 2023).

The Question of Mosaicism

The complexity and inherent imprecision of the interpretation of mosaic aneuploid findings are discussed above, and Moran et al. (2023) rehearse the challenges facing

[10] Embryos from translocation carriers appear to have a similar rate of de novo aneuploidy as the general population; that is, there is not a significant interchromosomal effect (ICE).

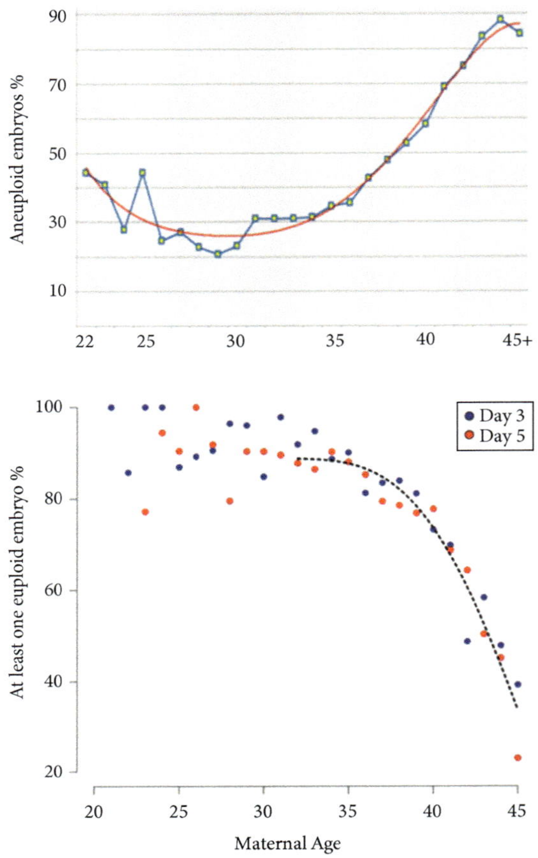

Figure 23–12. Maternal Age and Chance for Euploidy at PGT.

Notes: The relationship is shown between maternal age and the probability (*upper*) that *no* euploid blastocysts will be available from a single IVF cycle, or (*lower*) that at least one euploid embryo (day 3 or day 5) will be retrieved. These shapes of these two curves reflect each other, and show that the best chances lie between the maternal ages of the later twenties to the early thirties. The odds are a little less favorable in younger women, and a lot less in older.

Sources: From JM Franasiak et al., The nature of aneuploidy with increasing age of the female partner: a review of 15,169 consecutive trophectoderm biopsies evaluated with comprehensive chromosomal screening, *Fertil Steril* 101:656-663.e1, 2014, courtesy JM Franasiak, and with the permission of Elsevier; and from ZP Demko et al., Effects of maternal age on euploidy rates in a large cohort of embryos analyzed with 24-chromosome single-nucleotide polymorphism-based preimplantation genetic screening, *Fertil Steril* 105:1307–1313, 2016, courtesy ZP Demko, and with the permission of Elsevier.

counselors who have the task of conveying these uncertain findings to their patients. It is important that patients should be counseled prior to their IVF cycle about the possibility of mosaic results, including their frequency, difficulties in interpretation, and options regarding transfer. Considering this information, some couples might elect to decline PGT-A.

If one or more mosaic embryos are available for transfer, post-test counseling should discuss the question of lower implantation rates and higher miscarriage rates compared to euploid embryos, and the small (but poorly understood) risk of liveborn with aneuploidy (American Society for Reproductive Medicine 2023). In the event of an ongoing pregnancy, prenatal testing should be considered. Amniocentesis provides the

Table 23–1. Carriers of Balanced Rearrangements, and Blastocyst Results from PGT-SR

	RCP TRANSLOCATION (N=2943)	ROB TRANSLOCATION (N=927)	INVERSION (n=220)	COMPLEX BCR (n=39)	INSERT TRANSLOCATION (n=187)
Euploid	30%	46%	57%	46%	30%
Unbalanced BCR alone	36%	19%	7%	36%	44%
Unbalanced BCR and de novo aneuploid	16%	10%	6%	10%	9%
De novo aneuploid alone	18%	24%	30%	8%	16%
Total	100%	100%	100%	100%	100%
Total unbalanced BCR	52%	29%	13%	46%	53%
Total de novo aneuploid	34%	34%	36%	18%	25%

Notes: Biopsied trophectoderm cells were amplified using whole genome amplification and next-generation sequencing in order to detect numerical and segmental chromosome abnormalities. Complex BCR is defined as a BCR involving three or more chromosomes or with three or more breakpoints. Data on type of inversion was not provided. Mosaic embryos are included in the de novo aneuploid fraction.

Sources: Data of F. Zhou et al. Preimplantation genetic testing in couples with balanced chromosome rearrangement: a four-year period real-world retrospective cohort study. *BMC Pregnancy Childbirth* 24:86, 2024; and Z Zhang et al. Clinical outcomes in carriers of insertional translocation: a retrospective analysis of comprehensive chromosome screening results. *F S Rep* 5:55–62, 2023.

best representation of chromosome complement within fetal tissues, and therefore the best chance of detecting true fetal mosaicism, although being aware that even with amniocentesis, mosaicism may escape detection. CVS and NIPT may provide additional information, but it is possible that on very rare occasions confined trophoblast mosaicism might evolve into a confined placental mosaicism at CVS, and leave the question unanswered. UPD studies may be considered when the embryo mosaicism involves an imprintable chromosome.

Follow-up in the Pregnancy

Understandably, some couples will be unenthusiastic about an invasive procedure that could possibly put at risk the pregnancy in which there has been so much investment (Meschede et al. 1998). Nevertheless, couples need to be aware that chromosomal PGT cannot provide a "guarantee," although the misdiagnosis rate, for whatever reason, is very low when good-quality embryos are transferred. Prenatal testing should be offered. Ultrasonography may be an acceptable, if imperfect, compromise, only proceeding to CVS or amniocentesis if anomalies are detected. Noninvasive prenatal testing (NIPT) can target full aneuploidies, but consultation with the laboratory will be required to determine if unbalanced segregants of a translocation are detectable (Flowers et al. 2020).

Nature May Intervene

A natural pregnancy may be achieved while the couple waits for the IVF/PGT preparations to be made. For example, the adjacent-2 karyotype shown in Figure 5–15 came from culture of the products of conception of this couple's third miscarriage and no normal pregnancies, the woman being a t(13;16) carrier. The outlook did not seem very promising, and plans were being put in place for IVF; but the couple then reported a naturally conceived pregnancy in which amniocentesis showed a 46,XY karyotype.

The Children Resulting

Does PGT carry any risks to the embryo, pregnancy, or to the child? We may consider three categories of potential risk. First, there is a small risk of an embryo not surviving the biopsy process. With improvements in biopsy technique, this risk is now less than ½%; and although it is undoubtedly disappointing for a couple to lose an embryo in this way, the small risk is unlikely to deter couples from PGT. Second, might the biopsy procedure itself compromise the chance of success? In fact, this seems not to be so. In a review of nearly 500 PGT blastocyst transfers, Tiegs et al. (2021) found no difference in sustained implantation between the study group and an age-matched non-biopsied control group (48% vs. 46%).

The third and most important question relates to the child born from a PGT pregnancy. It is well recognized that there are differences, albeit small, in health between children conceived by IVF (without PGT) and naturally conceived children. IVF-conceived babies are more likely to be of low birth weight and to be born pre-term, and perinatal mortality and birth defects are more frequent (Halliday 2007; Halliday et al. 2010).

Nevertheless, it is reassuring that, in the longer term, the health of adult "IVFlings" appears to be similar to that of their in vivo–conceived counterparts (Halliday et al. 2019). For IVF in general, the usual counseling is for an absolute increase of approximately 1% in the risk of congenital abnormalities, compared to background risk.[11] The risk for Beckwith-Wiedemann syndrome in IVF babies generally is noted in Chapter 19, p. 551.

And, it is encouraging that IVF babies from PGT have no greater risk for pregnancy complication, neonatal outcomes, and birth defects, than IVFlings generally (Alteri et al. 2023; Van Heertum et al. 2024). Thus we may conclude that, in fact, there is likely no detrimental effect of embryo biopsy per se. Further, their health and development as children lie within a normal range (Ginström Ernstad et al. 2023). Perhaps unsurprisingly, for a child in whom so much has been invested, PGT infants score well on a scale of "warmth/affection" (measured by observing how infants may be cuddled and kissed, and how positively and kindly spoken to) (Banerjee et al. 2008).

[11] There is conflicting evidence regarding whether IVF conception increases the risk of chromosome abnormalities in offspring. If such a risk really exists, it is likely to be very low, and therefore IVF conception is not, in itself, an indication for chromosomal PGT.

Table 24–1. Major Genetic Categories of Differences of Sex Development (DSDs)

DSD GROUP	DISORDERS OF GONADAL DEVELOPMENT	DISORDERS OF HORMONE SYNTHESIS OR ACTION	UNCLASSIFIED DISORDERS
46,XY DSD	Complete or partial gonadal dysgenesis Ovotesticular DSD	Androgen biosynthesis defects Androgen insensitivity syndrome (AIS)	Complex syndromic DSD
46,XX DSD	Testicular DSD Ovotesticular DSD Primary ovarian insufficiency	Congenital adrenal hyperplasia (CAH)	Mayer-Rokitansky-Küster-Hauser syndrome Complex syndromic DSD
Sex chromosomal DSD	45,X 47,XXY 45,X/46,XY mixed gonadal dysgenesis 46,XX//46,XY chimerism		

Source: Adapted from M Cools et al., Caring for individuals with a difference of sex development (DSD): a Consensus Statement, *Nat Rev Endocrinol* 14:415–429, 2018.

(Müllerian and Wolffian) which enter a midline genital sinus, opening at the perineum. This opening is buttressed on each side by labioscrotal folds and capped above by a phallus. The basic plan of the genital ridge is laid down according to instruction from, in particular, the *WT1* and *NR5A1 (SF1)* genes. Failure of this process results in complete gonadal agenesis. Thereafter, the direction in which gonadal development proceeds is due to the activity of a number of genes on the sexual determination pathway, with *SRY* playing a central role. Finally, sex differentiation takes place through hormones produced by the gonads (Baetens et al. 2019).

The Key Role of the *SRY* and *SOX9* Genes

In the *absence* of *SRY*, but with input from *WNT4* and *RSPO1*, the gonad develops into an ovary, and the duct system develops into fallopian tubes and uterus. The genital sinus remains as an opening (the vagina), flanked and surmounted by labia and clitoris. The female state results. If a Y chromosome is *present*—or at least that part of the Y that contains *SRY*, the testis-determining gene—the male direction is taken. Transient expression of the *SRY* gene, beginning at embryonic day 41, calls into action *SOX9*, which in turn stimulates the *FGF9* gene; both *FGF9* and *SOX9* suppress *WNT4*, and the gonad becomes a testis. The testis, in turn, secretes hormones, of which androgen influences the genital tract to masculinize, and anti-Müllerian hormone causes regression of the female Müllerian ducts. A vas deferens forms from the duct system. The phallus enlarges. The labioscrotal folds fuse in the midline and accommodate the descending testes. The male state results.

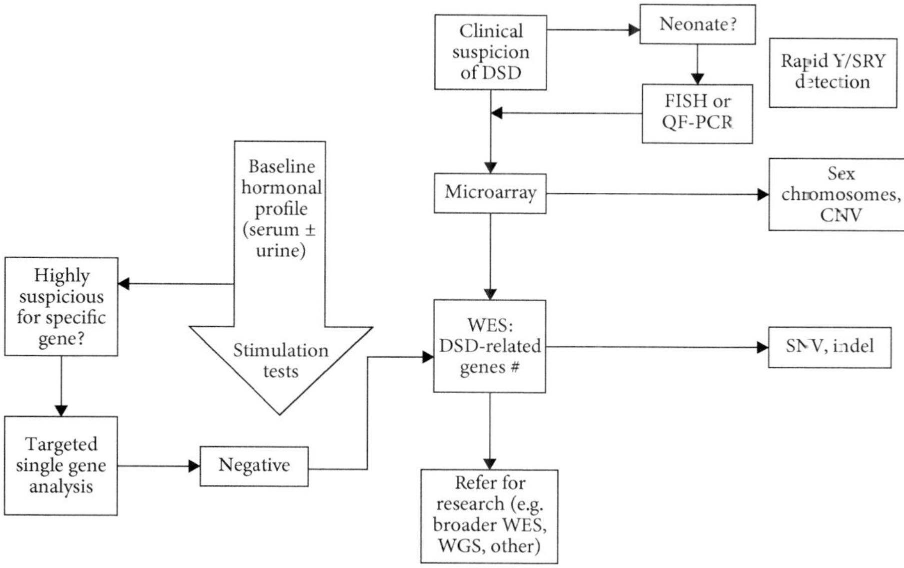

Figure 24–1. A recommended approach to genetic testing in a child with DSD.
Notes: #Targeted DSD-panel may be performed if WES is not available.
Source: Adapted from MA O'Connell et al., Establishing a molecular genetic diagnosis in children with differences of sex development: A clinical approach, *Horm Res Paediatr* 96:128-143, 2023. Courtesy A Sinclair.

Chromosome Testing in Differences of Sex Development

Classical cytogenetic testing[2] is often necessary to diagnose chromosomal DSDs accurately (Figure 24–1). The presence of *SRY* is routinely tested with FISH or QF-PCR, and chromosome microarray is used for initial chromosome assessment, allowing confirmation of chromosomal sex and detection of copy number changes affecting known or postulated DSD genes.[3] A standard microscope karyotype is undertaken to detect balanced translocations involving the sex chromosomes, and at least 30 cells should be examined in order to check for mosaicism. Molecular testing for *SRY* and *SOX9*, as well as many other specific DSD genes (e.g., *NR5A1*, *WNT4*, *SOX3*, *ARWT1*) per medium of a gene panel or exome sequencing approach, is a suitable adjunctive approach given the genotypic heterogeneity of the DSDs. Whole-genome sequencing enables the additional targeting of structural variants and regulatory elements of DSD genes in the non-coding genome, which may account for some undiagnosed DSDs (O'Connell et al. 2019; Délot and Vilain 2021). An example is a key regulatory element termed *RevSex* upstream of *SOX9*, which, when deleted, causes 46,XY DSD, and when duplicated causes 46,XX DSD (Benko et al. 2011).

[2] While our focus in this book is on the chromosomal state, necessarily here we must also refer, at least in outline, to molecular analysis: the two often go hand-in-hand in DSD diagnosis.

[3] Several genes in the pathways of sex development are known to have dose-dependent effects, including *SOX3*, *SOX9*, *WT1*, *DAX1*, and *WNT4*.

Chromosomal Differences of Sex Development in Girls and Women

XY OVARIAN DIFFERENCE OF SEXUAL DEVELOPMENT

The 46,XY karyotype in an otherwise normal girl with (apparently) completely normal female anatomy is a very rare observation. A single case is reported of a child who was a compound heterozygote for mutations in the *CBX2* gene, discovered only because of a discordant chromosome finding at prenatal diagnosis (Biason-Lauber et al. 2009). The internal genital tract was normal female, the gonads of normal ovarian appearance, and normal upon histology. *CBX2* may have a dual role in gonad development, promoting *SRY* and *SOX9* while repressing ovarian factors *WNT4* and *FOXL2* (Hart et al. 2022).

XY DIFFERENCE OF SEXUAL DEVELOPMENT, COMPLETE PURE GONADAL DYSGENESIS (SWYER SYNDROME)

Many cases of 46,XY gonadal dysgenesis are due to variants involving key transcription factors, along with their co-factors, that control the testicular developmental pathway (Elzaiat et al. 2022). When inherited, the rare *familial* forms provide a unique example of a Mendelian condition that can be inherited in an X-linked recessive, Y-linked, or sex-limited autosomal dominant or recessive mode. In the X-linked forms or autosomal forms, the XY female has a perfectly normal Y chromosome with a normal *SRY* testis-determining gene; the cause of the disorder is mutation in a gene (whether this be X-linked or autosomal) that affects a downstream event in testicular development.

Concerning the *X-linked* form, rearrangements at the Xp21.2 locus that either duplicate the *NR0B1* (*DAX1*) gene[4] or disrupt its regulatory elements account for some XY gonadal dysgenesis (Barbaro et al. 2012; Meinel et al. 2023). Larger duplications result in syndromic 46,XY gonadal dysgenesis and intellectual disability, whereas small duplications cause only gonadal dysgenesis (Ledig et al. 2012). Duplications of *NR0B1* have also been observed in several phenotypically normal males, indicating incomplete penetrance as observed in one male who transmitted a 1.1 Mb Xp21.2 duplication to his twin daughters (Veyt et al. 2024). He required IVF due to abnormal spermatogenesis, which may have reflected a mild manifestation of gonadal dysgenesis. Female 46,XX carriers of duplications involving *NR0B1* appear to have a normal female phenotype (Veyt et al. 2024).

As for the *Y-linked* form, there is a mutation in the *SRY* gene itself. In some Y-hemizygotes, the mutant gene has nevertheless been able to reach a threshold of operation that allows testis development, while in others with the same mutation it has not. Thus, for example, an XY male with a mutation in *SRY* may be a normal fertile man, while his XY child may be a daughter. The threshold is apparently all-or-nothing: Partial expression—that is, an intersex state—does not result (Jäger et al. 1992; Imai et al. 1999). A man may be a gonadal mosaic for an *SRY* deletion, as presumably was the father in Barbosa et al. (1995). Two daughters of his had XY DSD (one with gonadoblastoma) with a deletion of *SRY*, but he himself showed a normal *SRY* result; there were three other normal daughters and six normal sons. Similarly, Schmitt-Ney et al. (1995) describe two XY sisters and their XY half-sister with an *SRY* point mutation, whose father was shown to be mosaic for this mutation. These familial examples notwithstanding, sporadic occurrence is usual, and in ~15% of XY complete gonadal dysgenesis cases the *SRY* gene has a de novo mutation or rearrangement that abolishes its function of testis determination.

[4] Loss-of-function variants in *NR0B1* give rise to a different condition, X-linked congenital adrenal hypoplasia with hypogonadotropic hypogonadism.

The first *autosomal* gene for an XY DSD to be discovered was *DHH*, at 12q12. Homozygosity for this gene was identified in three of six apparently non-consanguineous Mexican-mestizo women with XY DSD, two of whom, not known to be related, had the same mutation (Canto et al. 2004). A number of autosomal dominant XY gonadal dysgenesis loci have since been identified, of which the major contributors are *NR5A1* (*SF1*), *MAP3K1*, and *DHX37* (Elzaiat et al. 2022).

The gonad in the autosomal form of XY DSD is dysgenetic and is seen as a "streak." The genital tract does not virilize. Familial "ovarian" malignancy was a notable observation in a sibship of three XY women (the karyotype presumed in two who had died at ages 19 and 20 years) described in Kempe et al. (2002).

XY DIFFERENCE OF SEXUAL DEVELOPMENT, COMPLETE ANDROGEN INSENSITIVITY SYNDROME

This is a Mendelian condition in which the locus happens to be on the X chromosome. In this condition, the defect lies further down the developmental path. The gonad becomes a testis and produces testosterone, but the genital tract, internal and external, is resistant to the effects of androgen. The inheritance is X-linked recessive, and the locus is the androgen receptor gene at Xq12. The individual appears externally very much as a female, but there is amenorrhea, and pubic and axillary hair is absent. Internally the vagina is short, and the uterus and tubes are represented only by remnants; the testes may be in the inguinal canal. Malignancy of the gonad, gonadoblastoma or dysgerminoma, is less of a concern than in Swyer syndrome, and is seen in only 1%–2% of patients with complete androgen insensitivity, although a greater risk, 15%, applies in partial insensitivity (Delli Paoli et al. 2023).

> One example is on record in which, in a sense, the X-linkage was directly visible to the cytogeneticist; that is, the X chromosome was abnormal, including the region containing the androgen receptor locus. An affected aunt and niece had the karyotype 46,Y,inv(X)(q11.2q27) and the connecting mother was 46,X,inv(X)(q11.2q27) (Xu et al. 2003). A unique case is that of androgen insensitivity due to uniparental disomy X in a woman with the XXY karyotype (Uehara et al. 1999a).

Chromosomal Differences of Sex Development in Boys and Men

XX TESTICULAR DIFFERENCE OF SEXUAL DEVELOPMENT

Most males with 46,XX testicular DSD ("XX males" in former parlance) arise from the presence of Yp material (rarely visible cytogenetically) on one of the X chromosomes, from occult XX/XXY mosaicism or from the inappropriate activity of a gene that is normally switched on only in response to a Y-originating genetic instruction. In approximately three-fourths of cases, the *SRY* gene is present, typically the consequence of an abnormal exchange between the X and Y during meiosis I in gametogenesis in the father and thus clearly a sporadic event. These cases are referred to as *SRY*$^+$ XX males, or *SRY*$^+$ XX testicular DSD. Délot and Vilain (2022) provide a full review.

The phenotype in males with *SRY*$^+$ XX testicular DSD shares with Klinefelter syndrome the phenotype of hypergonadotropic hypogonadism and near universal sterility, but differs in that height is normal and intelligence unimpaired (Ferguson-Smith et al. 1990). Margarit et al. (1998) describe six *SRY*$^+$ cases due to translocation of Yp material to Xp22.3, in whom different Y breakpoints could be identified but whose clinical phenotypes were very similar: normal intelligence, normal stature, and testicular atrophy with azoöspermia. In these *SRY*$^+$ cases, a more accurate cytogenetic designation would be 46,X,der(X)t(X;Y)—or more fully 46,X,der(X)t(X;Y)(p22.3;p11.2), though the exchange is not usually visible on standard cytogenetics—and so there is reference to this entity also in the section on the X;Y translocation (Chapter 6). Rare cases are known of a male with XX testicular DSD in whom the *SRY* gene had been translocated onto a terminal arm of an autosome (Dauwerse et al. 2006; Queralt et al. 2008).

Males with XX testicular DSD and having no *SRY* gene are denoted *SRY*$^-$ (Abalı and Guran 2024). The fact of male development being able to proceed (to some extent, at least) despite the lack of SRY product presumably reflects an inappropriate activation of the testis-determining cascade in an otherwise normal 46,XX embryo, either as a sporadic stochastic event or due to a particular genetic predisposition. Variants in at least a dozen genes encoding transcription factors and signaling molecules have been shown to cause 46,XX male DSD, their actions mediated either by decreased expression of genes involved in ovarian development (e.g., *WNT4, RSPO1, NR2F2*) or through overexpression of pro-testicular genes (e.g., *SOX9, SOX3, SOX10, DMRT1*). Overexpression of pro-testicular genes is frequently the result of gene duplication or of different copy number variants in the upstream promotor regions, and these may be detectable by microarray. A detailed review is provided by Ferrari et al. (2024).

Three cases are reported of males with 47,XXX chromosomes. In one well-studied example, the man was mildly intellectually disabled, with gynecomastia and hypogenitalism, and severe testicular atrophy on biopsy (Ogata et al. 2001). One X of the three was positive for *SRY*. In addition to an Xp-Yp interchange in paternal gametogenesis that produced the *SRY*-positive X chromosome, a coincidental maternal nondisjunction was responsible for a disomic X ovum. Thus, the combination at fertilization was XX(mat) + der(X)t(X;Y)(pat), giving 47,XX,der(X)t(X;Y) and appearing karyotypically as "47,XXX."

XX testicular DSD can be diagnosed prenatally, following the recognition that the chromosomal and ultrasonographic anatomical genders do not match, an observation that has become more frequent since the widespread adoption of noninvasive prenatal testing (Shen et al. 2023a).

45,X MALE

We refer to this rare condition on p. 178. Most (quite possibly all) "45,X males" have, in fact, a molecular translocation of the *SRY* gene to an autosome or to the X chromosome (and might therefore be thought of as a type of Y;autosome or X;Y translocation). In some, the underlying constitution might actually be an X/XY mosaicism.

Y ISOCHROMOSOMES

A Y isochromosome, idic(Y)(q11) in mosaic state with a 45,X line is a rare observation in individuals presenting with a disorder of sex development[5] (Manotas et al. 2020). The isochromosome presumably arises in paternal gametogenesis, with loss in an early mitosis of the embryo, to produce the 45,X line.

[5] The usual presentation with the idic(Yq) is infertility in an otherwise normal male (p. 481).

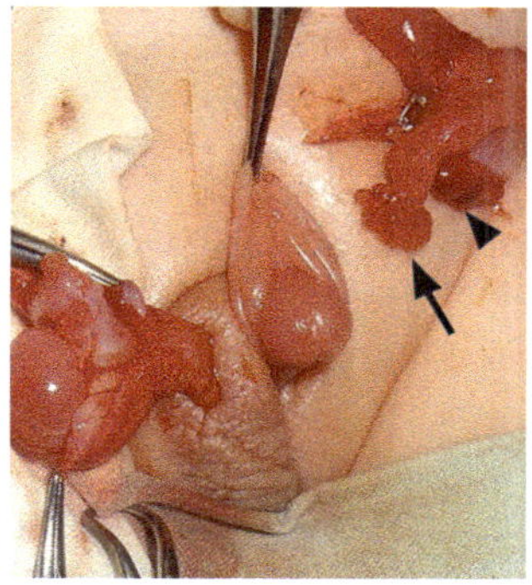

Figure 24–2. Ovotesticular DSD, surgical investigation in a newborn. At upper right, a fallopian tube has been delivered through the incision, its fimbriated opening (arrow) clearly evident, with an ovary (arrowhead) adjacent. At center, the forceps are retracting the prepuce of the phallus. At lower left, a testis has been delivered through the incision in the hemi-scrotum. The karyotype was mosaic XX/XY (or possibly chimeric XX//XY).

Ovotesticular Differences of Sex Development

The term *hermaphroditism*, of classical Greek derivation,[6] has lost favor among those so diagnosed; and the qualifiers "true" and "pseudo" were always somewhat arcane. These days, we speak of ovotesticular DSD. As that descriptor indicates, the defining feature is that the gonads comprise both ovarian and testicular elements. There may be a testis and an ovary (Figure 24–2), or one or both may be an ovotestis. The most common karyotype is 46,XX (thus XX ovotesticular DSD), seen in 60%; one-third have mosaicism with one cell line that includes Y chromosomal sequences, mostly 46,XX/46,XY; a few are 46,XY, and other more rare forms are known (Syryn et al. 2023). Ovotesticular DSD often presents with variation in genital appearance of the newborn such that sex cannot be determined from phenotype alone.

46,XX

Most 46,XX ovotesticular cases test negative on peripheral blood analysis for the *SRY* gene (Grinspon and Rey 2016). In some, there may be cryptic mosaicism within the gonad itself, with an island or islands of tissue containing the *SRY* gene or mosaic variants affecting other sex-determining genes (Ortenberg et al. 2002; Queipo et al. 2002). In terms of genetic causes, there is considerable overlap with 46,XX testicular DSD. In fact, it may be that 46,XX testicular DSD and 46,XX ovotesticular DSD are fundamentally the same genetic entity,[7] with ovotesticular DSD representing an intermediate or incomplete form of testicular DSD (Délot and Vilain 2022). A (relatively) common cause in these cases is duplication of the *RevSex* element that influences the activity of *SOX9* as noted above, this locus lying upstream of *SOX9* within 17q24.3 (Croft et al. 2018). Incomplete feminization has been described in several XX patients with duplications

[6] In Greek mythology, Hermaphroditus was the son of Aphrodite and Hermes. He was a handsome youth with whom the Naiad nymph Salmacis fell in love and prayed to be united with forever. The gods answered her prayer and merged their two bodies into one androgynous person.

[7] Délot and Vilain emphasize that despite shared genetic origins, the two conditions have very different complications and management.

of chromosome 22, a region now recognized to include the *SOX10* locus at 22q13.1 (Sreenivasan et al. 2022). A child with one gonad a testis and the other an ovary is described in Aleck et al. (1999); the karyotype in this child, who had presented with ambiguous genitalia, was 46,XX,rec(22)dup(22q) inv(22)(p13q13.1)mat.

Rare familial cases of 46,XX ovotesticular DSD may reflect a mutation, whether autosomal or X-linked (such as *RSPO1* or *NR5A1*) that induces the testis developmental cascade to proceed post-*SRY* stage (Domenice et al. 2016). Autosomal dominant variants might be transmitted through an unaffected 46,XY father, an example being duplication of *SOX9* enhancers (Cox et al. 2011). Intrafamilial phenotypic variability and incomplete penetrance expressivity is a feature in some affected families (Syryn et al. 2023). Slaney et al. (1998) describe the case of four 46,XX cousins with abnormal sexual differentiation. Three had 46,XX ovotesticular DSD, and one was a 46,XX male. The putative testis-development gene had been transmitted through two mothers. Affected distant relatives due to a familial X;Y translocation are noted on p. 180.

46,XY

XY ovotesticular DSD is rare indeed. The basis may be molecular rather than cytogenetic. For example, one non-mosaic 46,XY case had a post-zygotic mutation in *SRY* with SRY^+/SRY^- gonadal mosaicism (Braun et al. 1993). Presumably the SRY^+ line was responsible for the testicular elements in the gonad, and the SRY^- line for the ovarian elements.

XX/XY MOSAICISM

The mosaic XX/XY ovotesticular DSD state more usually results due to the fusion of twin XX and XY embryos (XX//XY chimerism).[8] Strain et al. (1998) reported a notable example of iatrogenic ovotesticular DSD which followed in vitro fertilization, presumably due to an XX and an XY embryo fusing; Malan et al. (2007) reached a similar conclusion in a case diagnosed prenatally and which could be referred to as "tetragametic chimerism." A further theoretical route is from the post-zygotic loss of the X and of the Y in separate cells of an initially 47,XXY conception (Niu et al. 2002). Hercent et al. (2019) reported the case of a 26-year-old infertile male who was initially diagnosed as a XX SRY^- male based on karyotype and absence of *SRY* in blood. Yet against expectation, a small number of sperm were obtained, and FISH studies showed equal numbers of X- and Y-bearing sperm, indicating that these gametes originated from normal XY cells.

X/XY, XXY/XX, AND OTHER MOSAICISMS

Other ovotesticular DSD mosaicisms include X/XY, XXY/XX, and X/X,idic(Yq). In the case in Röpke et al. (2007), a baby girl presenting with clitoral hypertrophy typed 46,XY on blood, but analysis of the removed dysgenetic gonads revealed X/XY mosaicism. On histological examination, the gonads contained testicular and ovarian elements. It was logically congruent that the XY state was observed more in the testicular component of the gonad, while cells with only an X chromosome predominated in the ovarian fraction. Kanaka-Gantenbein et al. (2007) report a boy, regarded as normal except for an undescended left testis, who presented as a 13-year-old with a left scrotal hemorrhage. In

[8] Fusion of zygotes with the same (XX/XX or XY/XY) chromosomal gender results in typical and fertile female or male individuals, and may only come to light if a SNP array is done for another reason.

fact, the undescended gonad was an ovary that had actually ovulated, and presumably this had been the cause of the bleed. There was a left hemi-uterus and fallopian tube; the testis, on the right, was dysgenetic. On both blood and testicular biopsy, the karyotype was 47,XXY/46,XX. As expected, given the presence of a male gonad albeit an imperfect one, *SRY* and *AZF* loci were present. Becker and Akhavan (2016) report an infant presenting with genital ambiguity in whom "the family made an initial gender assignment of female until patient preference could be elicited." The karyotype was 45,X[90]/46,X,idic(Yq)[10]; the isodicentric Y, with two copies of Yp, showed two copies of *SRY*. On laparoscopy, a normal-appearing uterus was seen; on the right, the gonad was an ovotestis and on the left, the gonad comprised only a "streak" (Figure 24–3). Prophylactic gonadectomy was done.

An extraordinary case is the family described in Haines et al. (2015), in which a phenotypically normal mother had a child with ovotesticular DSD, initially karyotyping as 46,XX, and mother and child were both subsequently shown to be heterozygous for an insertional translocation, 46,X,ins(X;1)(q27;q25.2q25.3). A 770 kb segment of chromosome 1 at q25.2q25.3 was translocated into the X chromosome, at Xq27, and this site is only 82 kb distant from the *SOX3* gene. *SOX3* may, in certain circumstances, have an *SRY*-like influence; and in this case, the inserted chromatin may have induced, or allowed, inappropriate *SOX3* activity, with its ectopic expression in one gonad (but not the other) producing a testis. Possibly, the mother's typical femaleness may have reflected a favorable X-inactivation. A somewhat similar circumstance is recorded in Ohnesorg et al. (2017), the case of a teenage male presenting with testicular pain, the gonad in fact proving to be an ovotestis. The karyotype was 46,XX, and *SRY*⁻, but upon multiplex ligation-dependent probe analysis (MLPA) he had a de novo ~300 kb duplication which included the upstream regulatory region for *SOX9*, at chr17:71.3-71.6 Mb.

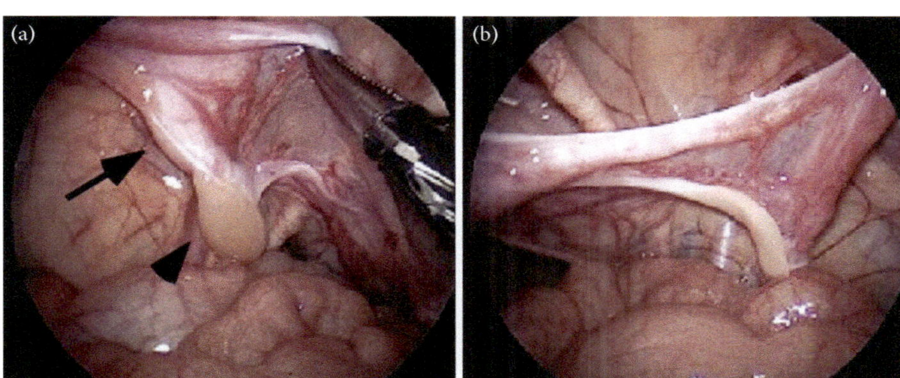

Figure 24–3. Gonadal observations at laparoscopy in an infant with an ovotesticular difference of sex development, having the karyotype 45,X/46,X,idic(Yq). The bilobar-appearing gonad on the child's right (*a*) is in part testicular (arrow) and in part ovarian (arrowhead). The gonad on the left (*b*) is a fibrotic "streak" (the curved structure in mid-field).

Source: From REN Becker and A Akhavan, Prophylactic bilateral gonadectomy for ovotesticular disorder of sex development in a patient with mosaic 45,X/46,X,idic(Y)q11.222 karyotype, *Urol Case Rep* 5:13–16, 2016. Courtesy REN Becker, and with the permission of Elsevier.

In most ovotesticular DSD, the molecular etiology remains unknown. In some, the basis of the defect may be a sporadic, inappropriate activation of the testicular developmental cascade in part of the gonadal tissue during its embryonic formation, as a stochastic event. Other genetic mechanisms postulated to play a role are non-coding variants, structural variants, epigenetic variation, and oligogenic inheritance (Délot and Vilain 2021). It is a curious and unexplained fact that ovotesticular DSD (mostly with a 46,XX karyotype) is far more common in the South African Black population than in Europeans (Wiersma 2004; Ganie et al. 2017).

A small number of pregnancies have been reported in women with ovotesticular DSD, both spontaneous and with assistance of IVF (Stancampiano et al. 2024). With regard to 46,XY ovotesticular DSD, Zayed et al. (2008) reported a man who had had surgery for removal of an intra-abdominal testicular seminoma which included ovarian elements. At the same operation, a uterus and tubes were identified and removed. A few years later he underwent testicular aspiration of the remaining gonad, which yielded sperm: These were used for intracytoplasmic sperm injection, and eventually a pregnancy resulted in the birth of a normal daughter. A similar case was reported by Sugawara et al. (2012).

Mixed Gonadal Dysgenesis

Mixed gonadal dysgenesis (MGD) is a phenotype that borders upon that of ovotesticular DSD. One gonad may be a streak (as the case in Figure 24–3b), and the other of apparently testicular form. The typical karyotype is 45,X/46,XY mosaicism; the body build and external genital phenotype can range very considerably from near-normal male, through ambiguity, to Turner-like female (Peng et al. 2024). Some with 46,XY on peripheral blood may show X/XY on analysis of the gonad, as Nishina-Uchida et al. (2015) show in an infant presenting as female with clitoromegaly and a gonad in the right labium majus. The removed gonad contained normal-appearing and abnormal testicular elements, undifferentiated gonadal tissue, Wolffian and Müllerian derivatives, and included nests of gonadoblastoma; 46,XY and 45,X cells could be demonstrated. The other gonad was a streak.

Rare Differences of Sex Development with Extragonadal Defects

A number of rare conditions exist in which sex reversal coexists with other physical differences, and in some, intellectual disability; the *SOX* loci have a notable role (Sreenivasan et al. 2022). One of the less rare of these conditions is campomelia (long bone bowing) with sex reversal. The usual cause is a mutation within the *SOX9* gene (at 17q24.3q25.1), this being one of the genes operating on the sexual differentiation pathway and which also influences limb bud mesenchymal development (Wagner et al. 1994). A cytogenetic form of this syndrome is seen in ~5% of affected individuals, who have an apparently balanced translocation disrupting the *SOX9* locus at 17q24.3q25.1 (Figure 3–18). Concerning *SOX10*, whose locus is at 22q13.1, Falah et al. (2017) describe a child presenting with Hirschsprung disease and Waardenburg syndrome type IV, and going on to develop a peripheral and central demyelination, who had male external

Table 24–2. Inheritance of Non-Syndromic 46,XY Gonadal Dysgenesis

MODE OF INHERITANCE	EXAMPLES
Sex-limited autosomal recessive	*DHH*
Sex-limited autosomal dominant	*DMRT1, DHX37, MAP3K1, NR5A1*
Y-linked	*SRY*
X-linked	Xp21.2 duplications involving *NR0B1* (*DAX1*)

Source: Adapted from L Mohnach et al., Nonsyndromic disorders of testicular development overview, *GeneReviews*, Seattle: University of Washington, 2022.

genitalia with intrascrotal gonads, the only genital abnormality being a first-degree hypospadias. He had a chromosome 22 duplication, 46,XX,dup(22)(q11.2q13), and was *SRY*-negative. Another syndrome is WT1 disorder, caused by heterozygous loss of *WT1* and characterized by 46,XY DSD, nephrotic syndrome, and high risk of Wilms tumor.[9] Otherwise, very many chromosomal conditions include a genital abnormality as part of an overall malformation syndrome.

GENETIC COUNSELING

XY Difference of Sexual Development, Complete Gonadal Dysgenesis (Swyer Syndrome)

FAMILIAL/INHERITED CASES

As noted above, the rare *familial* forms of XY gonadal dysgenesis provide an example of a Mendelian condition that can be inherited in a Y-linked, X-linked recessive, or sex-limited autosomal dominant or recessive mode (Table 24–2). Careful assessment of the pedigree may provide clues to the mode of inheritance, noting that phenotypic sex may not be concordant with chromosome sex and that expression of the DSD may be limited to the XY state. An individual with a sex-limited autosomal dominant difference of testicular development may have inherited the gene variant from their mother, or less commonly their mildly affected father. Autosomal recessive inheritance would be improbable in a multigenerational family tree, while on the other hand this mode would be strongly supported in a single affected sibship with more than one affected and in the setting of parental consanguinity. In the multigenerational scenario, a clear interpretation of autosomal versus X-linkage may not always be possible. The risk to the female carrier (as judged by position in the pedigree) to have an affected child would be a simple 25% if the X chromosome is implicated, but not readily calculable if a partially penetrant autosomal gene is the cause.

As noted above, more DSD genes are coming to be identified, with gene interrogation "panels" being developed (O'Connell et al. 2023), and genetic counseling will be better underpinned as this knowledge evolves. Although the XY female phenotype is close to that of a normal female (but of course associated with infertility) some couples may want to consider prenatal or preimplantation diagnosis. The use of cytogenetics or NIPT (XY chromosomes) and ultrasound morphology (female external genitalia)

[9] In WAGR syndrome, *WT1* is deleted in a contiguous gene deletion that also includes *PAX6* (p. 416).

25
PARTICULAR PHENOTYPES

Most chapters in this book start with the chromosome: an abnormality has been found, and we—the patient and counselor both—need to know more. Obviously enough, the discovery of a chromosomal abnormality then leads to a discussion about the phenotypic consequences, either as already seen in the person concerned, or in their family, or as a future possibility; and elsewhere in this book considerable detail attests apropos. In this chapter we take the opposite view and start with the phenotype: what particular phenotypes might be due to what particular chromosomal abnormality and which might therefore lead to a consideration for a chromosome analysis. We limit ourselves to a discussion of only a few conditions—the full range would require a new book!—namely, those in which a link to certain chromosomal scenarios has been well established and for which we consider some commentary might be useful. The reader may appreciate, in outline, the very broad extent of chromosomally caused disease with reference to the "malformation map" in Figure 3–20.

ALZHEIMER DISEASE

Familial autosomal dominant Alzheimer disease is due mostly to point mutation within *PSEN1*, with a minority due to mutation in *APP* (amyloid precursor protein) or *PSEN2*. A tiny fraction reflect a duplication of the *APP* locus. This may be as a CNV duplication (Figure 25–1) or as an insertion into another chromosome (Figures 14–79 and 14–80). The near-inevitable evolution of Alzheimer's in Down syndrome individuals as they enter middle age reflects this same *APP* dosage effect (Figure 13–2).

ATAXIA AND MOVEMENT DISORDERS

Much the most useful tool in identifying the genetic basis of an ataxia syndrome is mutation testing, either targeted according to the clinical picture presented or by way of a multiplex approach using a broad-band ataxia gene panel. But occasionally a microdeletion or a CNV might cause an intragenic deletion that could be missed on classical DNA methodology. An example is seen in spinocerebellar ataxia type 15 (SCA15) in which an intragenic deletion within *ITPR1* is a recognized cause of the disorder. Ghorbani et al. (2023) screened 338 cases of undiagnosed ataxia on SNP array and could establish a firm diagnosis in only two (who actually turned out to be related) with deletion-based SCA15. We mention on p. 422 the case of a woman diagnosed with autosomal recessive spastic ataxia of Charlevoix and Saguenay (ARSACS) due to a CNV on one chromosome removing the locus concerned and exposing a mutation on the other chromosome; or in other words, reducing a pathogenic variant on the other chromosome to hemizygosity.

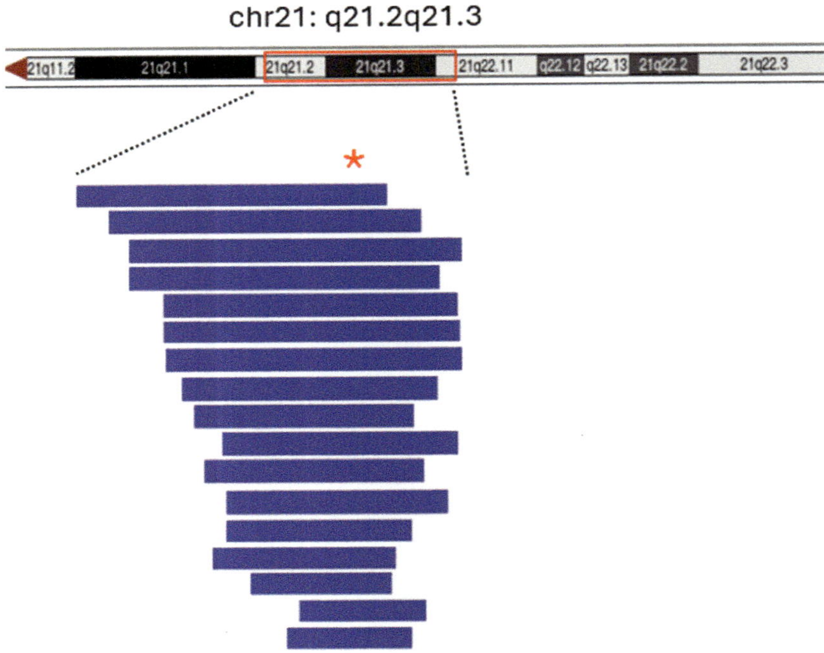

Figure 25–1. Duplications Encompassing *APP*.

Notes: These dup CNVs were identified in a series of cases of early-onset Alzheimer's disease. The asterisk shows the relative position of *APP*. Some have *APP* as the only contained gene, others are more extensive and include other loci. All but one were familial. The ages of onset were from 42 to 63 years, with ages at death from 42 to 68.

Source: From L Grangeon et al., Phenotype and imaging features associated with APP duplications, *Alzheimers Res Ther* 15:93, 2023. Courtesy L Grangeon, and with the permission of Springer Nature.

Parkinson disease, the classic movement disorder of adulthood, is somewhat more frequently seen in those with a sex chromosome aneuploidy and in those with the del 22q11.2, the latter chromosomal diagnosis not necessarily having been made before the onset of Parkinsonism (Carvalho et al. 2021). Movement disorders of *childhood* include ataxia, stereotypies, dystonia, chorea, tremor, myoclonus, paroxysmal dyskinesia, and spastic paraparesis. In the review of Soliani et al. (2023), the majority of such cases were seen in association with developmental delay/intellectual disability. Of the few with normal intellect, CNVs including these loci were ascertained: *NKX21, KMT2B,* and *HNRNPU* (which lies within 1q44, p. 381), *SGCE* (which lies within 7q21.3, p. 406), *PRRT2* (a locus within the proximal BP4-BP5 deletion 16p11.2, p. 433), and *NIPA1* (which is included within the Prader-Willi/Angelman segment, p. 426).

AUTISM

Autism is a frequent reason for a chromosome test to be requested (Ceylan et al. 2018; Jang et al. 2019). The term encompasses a wide range of symptomatology, acknowledged in the term "autism spectrum disorder." At one end of the spectrum there is Asperger syndrome, which may be seen with higher IQs and certain extraordinary intellectual abilities but with persistent difficulties with social interaction and communication; at the other, profound intellectual disability. More typically the autistic phenotype describes a person whose language development and educational ability may not be far below average but who cannot interact normally at a social level, who struggles with social reciprocity, and who lacks the psychological flexibility to accommodate to an unfamiliar environment. The formal definition also includes a communication deficit, restricted/repetitive behavior, and hyper- or hypo-reactivity to sensory input. A pre-eminent causative role of genetics is beyond argument (Khogeer et al. 2022). It is certainly common worldwide (Salari et al. 2022).

> If the term *autism spectrum disorder* may be seen as a somewhat "lumping" approach, chromosome testing might offer a "splitting" insight. That is to say, a chromosome abnormality, a del or a dup, is seen more particularly in children with more complex phenotypes where there is more likely to be intellectual disability, delay in motor milestones, and in whom there may also be a concomitant minor dysmorphology or growth disorder. This might be spoken of as "autism plus" (or "chromosomal autism") or on the other hand, perhaps from a standpoint of intellectual handicap with behavioral disorder, as the foregoing "plus autism." Another expression for this is "syndromic autism," which stands in contrast to "pure/idiopathic autism" (or "polygenic autism"). Subtle differences are seen in the autism of chromosomal syndromes versus pure autism (Bozhilova et al. 2023).

Certain chromosomal segments are particularly represented among the genomic imbalances observed in autism (Calle Sánchez et al. 2022; Raznahan et al. 2022; Fu et al. 2022; Wright et al. 2024), and Figures 25–2 and 25–3 draw attention accordingly. Chromosomes 15, 16, and 22 are obvious standouts, often occurring in the setting of a syndromic picture. In addition to the more commonly seen del/dups (Table 25–1), several other del/dups were recorded more than once in the large series of Wright and colleagues and include the following, seen in four or more cases: del 1q44, dup 2p25.3, del 2q37.3, del 5q34, del 6p21.33, dup 9q34.11, and dup 22q11.23. The 8p21.3 deletion is implicated in Cosemans et al. (2021). At the level of brain morphology, Modenato et al. (2021) analyzed brain MRI scans from patients with eight "neuropsychiatric" CNVs, documenting anatomical differences and thus confirming a direct physical effect due to the genomic imbalances (Figure 25–4). There is some genetic overlap with other neuropsychiatric conditions, including major depressive disorder, attention deficit hyperactivity disorder, and schizophrenia (Figure 18–6).

The male excess in autism has long been known. One contributor to this excess may be deletion at Xp22.11, a segment that includes the *DDX53* gene (Figure 25–5).

These several chromosomal culprit regions notwithstanding, the clinical return from a standard chromosome study is modest but important. In a study of 201 mostly (80%) self-referred cases in New Zealand (which excluded those with a previously identified causal CNV), 6% had a presumed or likely contributory del, dup, or translocation (Figure 25–6). From Iran, of 36 cases from 30 families, Ghasemi et al. (2022) found only two examples of a presumed contributory chromosome deletion or del/dup rearrangement. These fractions of about 5%–10%,[1] are typical. It remains the case that most

[1] This range is above the figure seen (3%) in the large study of Wright et al.; these latter authors suggest that their figure may be a more accurate reflection overall, due to a less stringent threshold of acceptance of the diagnosis.

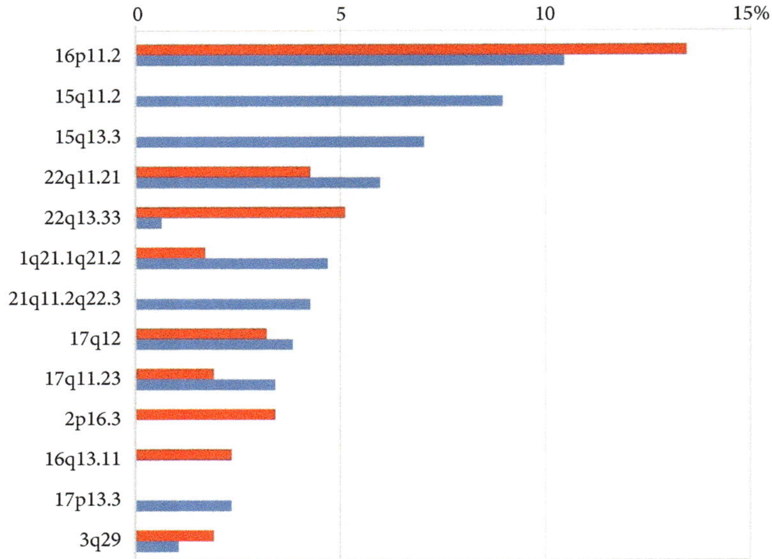

Figure 25–2. The Deletions and Duplications Most Commonly Associated with Autism.

Notes: Red = deletion, blue = duplication, for the 13 most commonly observed segments. The percentages shown here represent the fractions of all autism-associated del/dups. These data came from the study of 21,532 individuals, in a US-wide survey of autism: participants were recruited online and in-person at clinical sites across the country. The majority (83%) were minors at the time of enrolment, 8% were independent adults, and 9% were dependent adults enrolled by a parent. The ratio of males to females with autism was (as is quite typical) 3.3:1. Those with a CNV (as shown here) comprised only 3% of the whole cohort. The remarkable involvement of chromosomes 15, 16, and 22 is to be noted.

Source: Drawn from data in JR Wright et al., Return of genetic research results in 21,532 individuals with autism, *Genet Med* 26:101202, 2024.

autism will be categorized as polygenic (with many risk alleles identified; Mahjani et al. 2021; Wright et al. 2024) or idiopathic.

Genetic Counseling

Genetic testing in autism can be a fraught matter. What benefits might parents expect to see, and what reactions might they actually have (Lucas et al. 2022)? Having identified a putative autism-associated del/dup in a proband, a challenge for the counselor lies in conveying the interpretation. A particular sensitivity will apply if an invitation to proceed to parental sampling is accepted. If a del/dup has arisen de novo, a risk of recurrence (barring a gonadal mosaicism) is low indeed—assuming, that is, that the del/dup was truly causative (and a de novo CNV has a greater likelihood of having been causative than a familial CNV). This category will be seen not infrequently.

But if a parent proves to carry the same del/dup, there is a quandary to be faced. Might an astute and observant counselor see in that parent "microsigns" of autism? If so, how might such a delicate question be raised, if at all? And if there is a question of having further children, what sort of risk advice might be offered? The matters of nonpenetrance and variable expressivity, and the role of the familial background genome otherwise (Cirnigliaro et al. 2023), may become notions of considerable practical relevance.

The risk to transmit a del/dup will be a simple Mendelian 50%. But the question, then, of the modifying effect of the contribution of the other parent—why did the index child

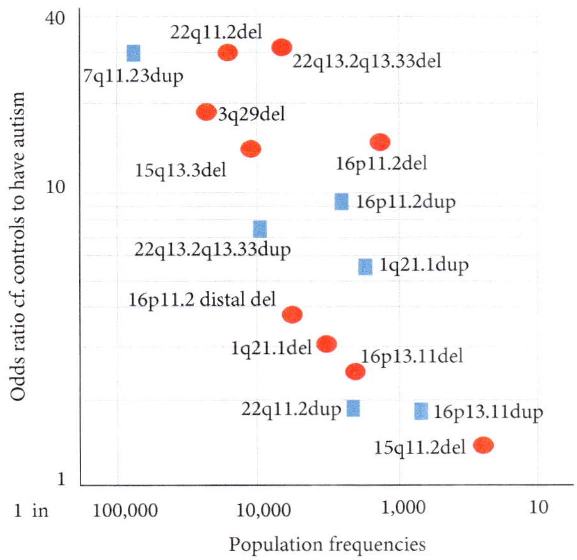

Figure 25–3. Frequencies of Certain Autism-Associated Deletions and Duplications.

Notes: The population frequencies are shown of certain cytogenetic abnormalities, and the likelihoods of their being associated with autism. Deletions are red circles, duplications blue squares. The imbalances range from a near-harmless effect due to the 15q11.2del, with an odds ratio barely over 1, and not uncommon in the general population (about 1 person in 300); and towards the other end of the scale, the "Williams duplication", 7q11.23dup, having a high risk to lead to autism (odds ratio about 30-fold), but also being a rare observation (near 1 in 100,000). In other words, the 15q11.2del is close to being non-penetrant, whereas the 7q11.23dup is fully penetrant.

Source: Redrawn as a composite figure from data of A Raznahan et al., Convergence and divergence of rare genetic disorders on brain phenotypes: A review, *JAMA Psychiatry*, 79:818-828, 2022; and JM Fu et al., Rare coding variation provides insight into the genetic architecture and phenotypic context of autism, *Nature Genet* 54, 1320–1331, 2022. Most estimates were very close between the two studies; where a difference was notable, an intermediate point was chosen.

have autism, but not the del/dup parent?—is certainly not simple. For the more commonly seen imbalances, the data displayed in Figure 25–3 and set out in Table C in the Appendix may give a sense of how potent is the functional impact (which is to say, the penetrance) in each, in terms of leading to an autism phenotype. The question may then arise of targeted testing in a future pregnancy.

- *Preimplantation Testing.* In the case of "pure" autism, the fact of a male predominance has led some to seek sex selection at PGT in order to choose a female embryo for a subsequent pregnancy[2] (Amor and Cameron 2008). With specific reference to "chromosomal autism" (in other words, CNV-associated) and in which a cognitive component is more likely to be a part of the phenotype, the clearest answer may come from PGT. Leahy et al. (2024) prove the point that PGT is feasible, and describe a 41-year-old mother from whom three of five embryos were dup15q11-13, and she herself then shown to be a carrier (but all five embryos being otherwise aneuploid). In principle, an embryo carrying this autism-associated duplication could be excluded from transfer; but in the awareness that the existence of autism is not necessarily predictable, were the

[2] In the extensive study of Fu et al. (2022) comprising a little over 20,000 autism cases, it is seen that this sex difference includes the particular category of CNV-associated autism.

Table 25–4. Translocations Associated with Various Cancer Risks

TRANSLOCATION	PROPOSED RELEVANT GENE	CANCER
t(1:13)(q21:q12)	*WAVE3*	Ganglioneuroblastoma
t(1;17)(p36.2;q11.2)	*NBPF1, ACCN1*	Neuroblastoma
t(1;18)(p36.1;q21.1)	*SMAD4*	Juvenile polyposis
t(5;7)(q22;p15)	*APC*	Polyposis coli
t(5;10)(q22;q25)	*APC*	Polyposis coli
t(5;18)(q35.1;q21.2)		Hodgkin lymphoma
t(5;22)(q14.1;q11.23)	*SMARCB1*	ATRT
t(5;22)(q35.1;q11.2)		NF2-associated medulloblastoma
t(7;22)(p21;q11.2)		Peripheral PNET
t(8;22)(q24.13;q11.21)	*TRC8*	Dysgerminoma
t(14;20)(q24;p12)	*RAD51L1, BMP2*	Thymoma
t(16;22)(p13.3;q11.2)	*SMARCB1*	ATRT
t(16;22)(p13.3;q11.2q12)		PNET

Notes: These translocations are apparently balanced, in the constitutional state and not otherwise causing a phenotype. ATRT = atypical teratoid/rhabdoid tumor; PNET = primitive neuroectodermal tumor; NF2 = neurofibromatosis type 2; RCC = renal cell cancer.

Sources: (Tables 25–2, 25–3, and 25–4) Aagaard et al. (2020), Betts et al. (2001), Blackburn et al. (2024), Bonne et al. (2007), Doyen et al. (2012), Gimelli et al. (2009), Hill et al. (2003), Järviaho et al. (2019), Kawamoto et al. (2017), Lovatel et al. (2023), Nicodème et al. (2005), Nunes et al. (2023), Panani et al. (2004), Panagopoulos et al. (2024), Poland et al. (2007), Ritter et al. (2015), Sahnane et al. (2016), Sawyer et al. (2003), Seo et al. (2015); Schoemaker et al. 2019; Smith et al. (2020), Sossey-Alaoui et al. (2002), Thibodeau et al. (2017), Vandepoele et al. (2008), Van der Luijt et al. (1995); Woodward et al. (2010).

pregnant women having had a blood test for cfDNA as part of prenatal screening for aneuploidy, in whom the result turned out to be non-reportable (Turriff et al. 2024).

CEREBRAL PALSY

Cerebral palsy is an "umbrella term" that describes a disorder of motor function resulting from maldevelopment or injury to the developing brain. A genetic etiology is found in a sizeable minority, with considerable heterogeneity that overlaps with genetic causes of intellectual disability and epilepsy (Lewis et al. 2021). CNVs account for ~10% of unselected cases (Oskoui et al. 2015).

DEVELOPMENTAL COORDINATION DISORDER

This condition is also called dyspraxia, or the "clumsy child syndrome." It is not uncommonly diagnosed in school-age children, quite often in coexistence with attention deficit disorder (Gibbs et al. 2007). In a relatively small Canadian cohort of such children the burden of CNV deletions or duplications in the 0.5 Mb–1.0 Mb range was significantly increased, and CNVs more often spanned brain-expressed genes compared with a control population (Mosca et al. 2016). Similarly, Cunningham et al. (2021) found that 91%

Table 25–5. Chromosomal Epilepsy Syndromes

EPILEPSY SYNDROME	CHROMOSOME
Del 1p36	1p36
Wolf-Hirschhorn syndrome	4p
Pallister Killian syndrome	12p
Trisomy 12p	12p
Ring 14 syndrome	14
Angelman syndrome	15q11q13
15q13.3 Microdeletion syndrome	15q13.3
InvDup (15)	15q11.2q13.1
Miller Dieker syndrome	17p13.3
18q− syndrome	18q22.1q23
Ring 20 syndrome	20
Down syndrome	21
Klinefelter syndrome	X

of children with neurodevelopmental CNVs screened positive for suspected developmental coordination disorder compared with 19% of controls.

EPILEPSY

Given the vulnerability of the brain to an incorrect genomic content, it is unsurprising that epilepsy is a frequent observation in many chromosomal disorders. Table 25–5 and Figure 25–7 show the classic chromosomal imbalances in which epilepsy is a particularly notable feature. A search for CNVs in children with epilepsy and neurodevelopmental delay may show a few with a pathogenic CNV, including del(16)p11.2 and del(1)p36 (Zhang et al. 2023b). A more detailed treatment of the particular case of epilepsy due to ring 20 appears in Chapter 11.

GUT

Malformations of the gastrointestinal system—notably duodenal atresia, jejunoileal atresia, and anorectal defects—have an association with certain chromosomal abnormalities. Meng and Jiang (2022) reviewed a series of prenatal diagnoses of a gut defect and showed a substantial increase in fetal chromosomal abnormality (34%) compared with the whole prenatally tested population (11%). Unsurprisingly, the rates were higher in those cases with concomitant other fetal malformation. Duodenal atresia is perhaps the classic example, being a well-recognized association with trisomy 21. Figure 25–8 shows a gut abnormality due to diaphragmatic hernia in trisomy 18, a defect reported in a number of different chromosomal abnormalities (Scott et al. 2022). As well as the classic trisomies, these segments were implicated in gastrointestinal defects in Meng and Jiang: 2p24, 3q, 4q24, and 10q26. A single case of a choledochal cyst in a child with dup 17q12 is reported in Kotalova et al. (2018); *HNF1B* is the likely relevant gene.

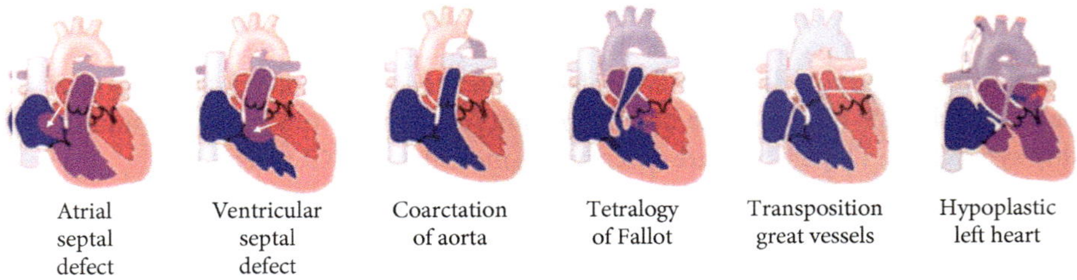

Figure 25–9. Heart Defects Associated with a Chromosomal Abnormality.

Notes: From left to right in the images in the diagram above, the severity of the defect increases. Blue represents venous blood returning to the heart; red is oxygenated blood; purple is mixed, due to a septal defect. Arrows show flow of blood across the atrial and ventricular septal defects, in a "left-to-right shunt".

Source: From S Zaidi and M Brueckner, Genetics and genomics of congenital heart disease, *Circ Res* 120:923–940, 2017, with the permission of Wolters Kluwer.

septal defect; the dup 1q21.1 syndrome (p. 380); and the 22q11 deletion syndrome, with a wide range and particularly involving outflow defects (Table 25–7). Tan et al. (2022) document CNVs associated with congenital heart defects.

KIDNEY

We have listed various abnormalities of the kidney and urinary system seen in the three classic trisomy syndromes (Amor et al. 2003). Deletion or duplication of 17q12 has a particular association with renal malformation, with *HNF1B* the likely gene of concern (Luo et al. 2024; Molina et al. 2023). Familial transmission of del17q12 is on record, with

Table 25–7. The Range of Cardiovascular Defects in the 22q11.2 Deletion Syndrome

		ASSOCIATED LESIONS						
DEFECT	FREQ	RAA	DAA	ASCA	BSVC	LSVC	MAPCA	VSD
Tetralogy of Fallot + pulmonary stenosis	19%	+	+	+	+			+
Tetralogy of Fallot + pulmonary atresia	22%	+				+	+	
Interrupted aortic arch	4%						+	
Ventricular septal defect	41%	+	+	+	+		+	+
Atrial septal defect	15%	+	+	+		+	+	+
Patent ductus arteriosus	11%							+
Aberrant subclavian artery	4%	+						
No cardiovascular defect	26%							

Notes: These observations were made from a series of 27 cases. ASCA = aberrant subclavian artery; B/LSVC = bilateral/left superior vena cava; MAPCAs = major aortopulmonary collateral arteries; RAA = right-sided aortic arch; VSD = ventricular septal defect. Tetralogy of Fallot = VSD, overriding aorta, pulmonary stenosis, and right ventricular hypertrophy

Source: CL Lee et al., 22q11.2 deletion syndrome in Taiwan: Clinical presentation and immune system status of patients, *Int J Med Sci* 20:1377–1385, 2023.

familial multicystic kidney disease (Aydın et al. 2022). Fetal hyperechogenic kidney is a sign that may be observed at prenatal ultrasonography; of the CNVs that may be identified in this setting, del17q12 is the most common (Huang et al. 2023b).

OLIGOSPERMIA, AZOÖSPERMIA

Oligospermia and azoöspermia (too few sperm, or none at all) is a frequent basis of male infertility. A chromosome abnormality is an occasional finding in the clinical work-up. A Robertsonian translocation is seen in 1½% to 3% of men presenting with oligospermia and a little under 1% of those with azoöspermia (Wiland et al. 2020). A reciprocal translocation is an infrequent finding (Chen and Zhou 2022). Klinefelter syndrome does not always present with the classic clinical picture, and it may take the recognition of infertility to arrive at that diagnosis. We refer elsewhere (p. 173) to the role of AZF deletions of the Y chromosome.

RARE UNDIAGNOSED DISEASES

To the practicing geneticist, rare diseases are common; one definition is a condition seen in fewer than 1 in 2,000 persons. A genomic study is often part of the investigative effort in such cases, and counselors will be familiar with the expression "diagnostic odyssey" (Kumar et al. 2023; Demidov et al. 2024). While Mendelian diagnoses are by far the most discovered in such broad-based genomic study, CNVs account for a notable minority (Figure 25–10). The categories of CNV thus identified are shown in Figure 25–11.

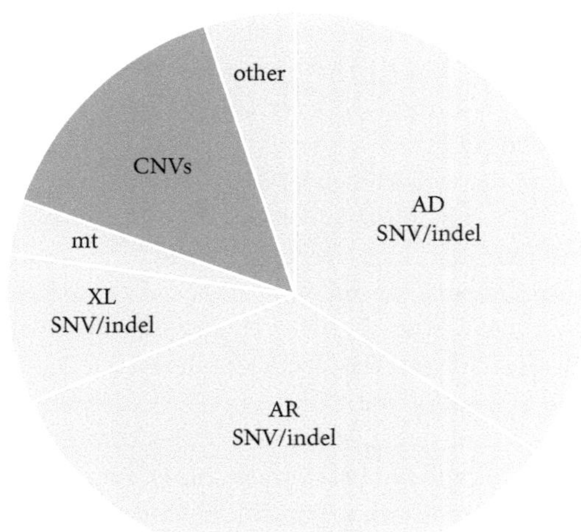

Figure 25–10. Discoveries at Genomic Diagnostic Odyssey.

Notes: These data are based upon findings at the retrospective analysis, on exome sequencing, of 2,100 consecutive index cases referred for genome sequencing, mostly (71%) pediatric, with 29% adults. There were no specific inclusion or exclusion criteria. A genomic diagnosis, as shown in the graph, was reached in close to one-half. The large majority were Mendelian, autosomal dominant (AD), recessive (AR), and X-linked (XL) single nucleotide variants (SNVs) or molecular-level insertions and deletions (indels). Mitochondrial diagnoses (mt) were made in 3%. Copy number variants (CNVs), the focus of our present interest, accounted for 15%.

Source: From F Guo et al., Evidence from 2100 index cases supports genome sequencing as a first-tier genetic test, *Genet Med* 26:100995, 2024. Courtesy M Hegde, and with the permission of Elsevier.

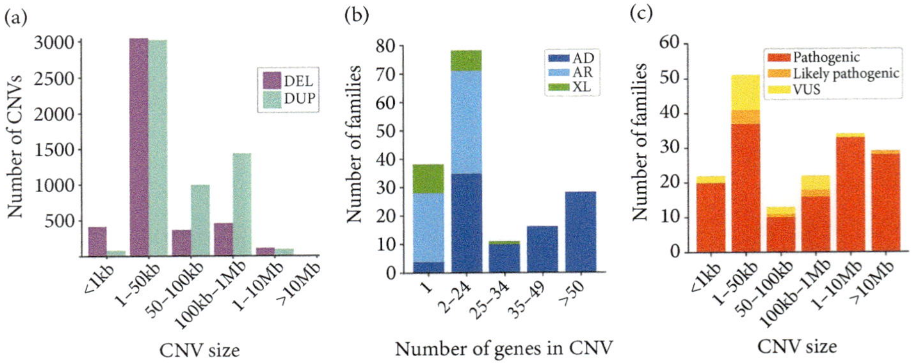

Figure 25–11. CNVs Discovered in Agnostic Testing.

Notes: These data reflect findings on 15,759 individuals from 6,633 families with undiagnosed rare disease. The CNV sizes vary (*a*) from <1 to >10 Mb, with most of 1-50 kb in size. The load of mendelian genes within CNVs is shown in (*b*), with most containing 2-24 genes. The considerable majority are assessed as being pathogenic (*c*).

Source: From G Lemire et al., Exome copy number variant detection, analysis, and classification in a large cohort of families with undiagnosed rare genetic disease, *Am J Hum Genet* 111:863–876, 2024. Courtesy G Lemire and A O'Donnell-Luria, and with the permission of the American Society of Human Genetics.

SCHIZOPHRENIA

Chromosomal copy-number variants are the basis of a minority of schizophrenia, which is otherwise a largely polygenically determined condition. The three CNVs in which a causative effect is well accepted are del(15)p13.3, dup(16)p11.2, and del(22)q11.2 (Sullivan et al. 2024). The case in a number of others is less secure, but nevertheless it is likely several of these will come to be seen as established genetic contributors to a schizophrenic phenotype (Figure 25–12). There are variants that are rare but with strong effects (highly penetrant), and those that are common but of weak effect (low penetrance) (Rees and Kirov 2021).

The most penetrant of the well-known CNVs is the del(22)q11.2 deletion, which is seen in 0.3% of those with schizophrenia versus 0.005% of control individuals: a sixty-fold difference. One in four del(22)q11 carriers develop the condition. Common polygenic risk factors may suffice to tip the genomic balance in these carriers such that schizophrenia evolves (Cleynen et al. 2021). A rare but apparently highly penetrant CNV is a 3.2 kb deletion at 10p15.2 (the locus of interest *PITRM1*) seen in a family in which schizophrenia is segregating practically as a dominant gene (Ormond et al. 2024).

The practice of genetic counseling in the case of this common (~1% of the population) psychiatric disorder is evolving (Besterman 2024). Psychiatric genetic counselors "are trained to use a holistic approach to explain the interplay between genetic and environmental factors contributing to psychiatric disorders, and to address the emotional concerns and questions of the patients" (Austin 2020). Such counseling may "improve the understanding of disease recurrence risk, increase objective and subjective genetics knowledge, and reduce internalized stigma, worry, and self-blame, in individuals with schizophrenia and their families" (Costain et al. 2014). Schizophrenia due to a CNV will comprise only a small fraction of all cases, and counseling in such cases will need to be specifically tailored apropos (Morris et al. 2022).

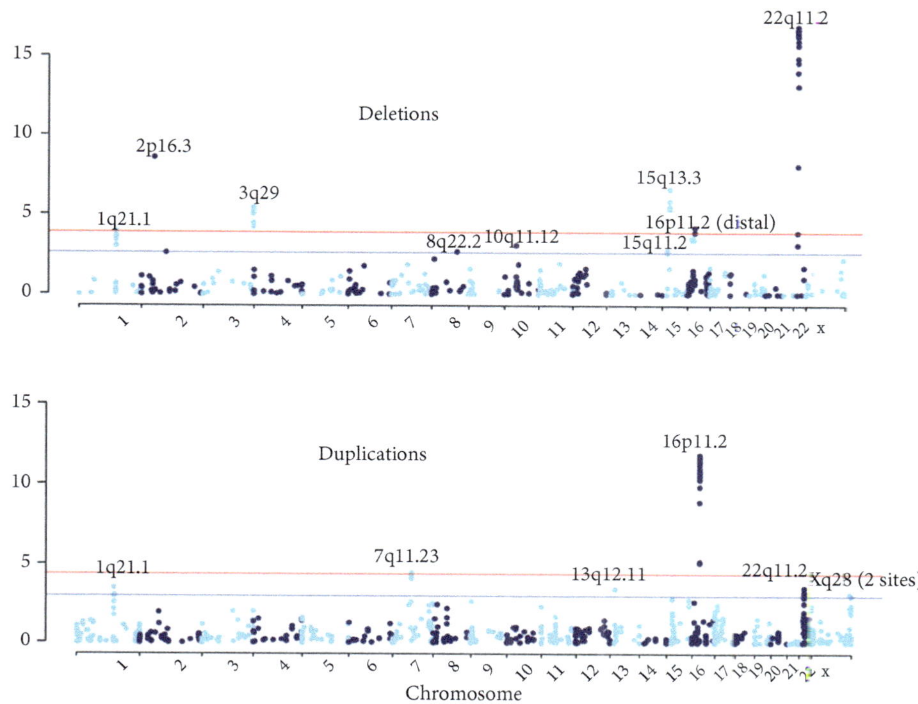

Figure 25–12. Deletions and Duplications Associated with Schizophrenia.

Notes: The Manhattan plot shows dels and dups that are observed in large cohorts of cases of schizophrenia. Those reaching levels of statistical significance are shown extending above the blue line (moderately significant) and above the orange line (highly significant) (the *y* axis calibrates a measure of significance). Del 22q11.2 and dup 16p11.2 are obvious stand-outs.

Source: From CR Marshall et al., Contribution of copy number variants to schizophrenia from a genome-wide study of 41,321 subjects, *Nat Genet* 49:27–35, 2016. Courtesy J Sebat, and with the permission of Springer Nature.

SKIN

Pigmentary mosaicism, which may exist as an isolated observation or along with other manifestations, has a strong correlation with a chromosome abnormality (e.g., Figures 3–22 and 11–9). In a literature review of 263 karyotyped cases, Kromann et al. (2018) found 42% to be cytogenetically abnormal. Figure 25–13 shows the different seven archetypical patterns of hyperpigmentation that may be observed. These authors recommend that a cytogenetic analysis should be a routine test in such patients. A separate type of pigmentary condition is the café-au-lait macule, well-known from its association with neurofibromatosis type 1 but also an occasional observation in individuals carrying an autosomal ring chromosome (Sodré et al. 2010).

SPEECH SOUND DISORDER

A speech sound disorder (SSD) affects articulation or phonetic structure (due to poor motor abilities associated with the production of speech-sounds) and phonology (an

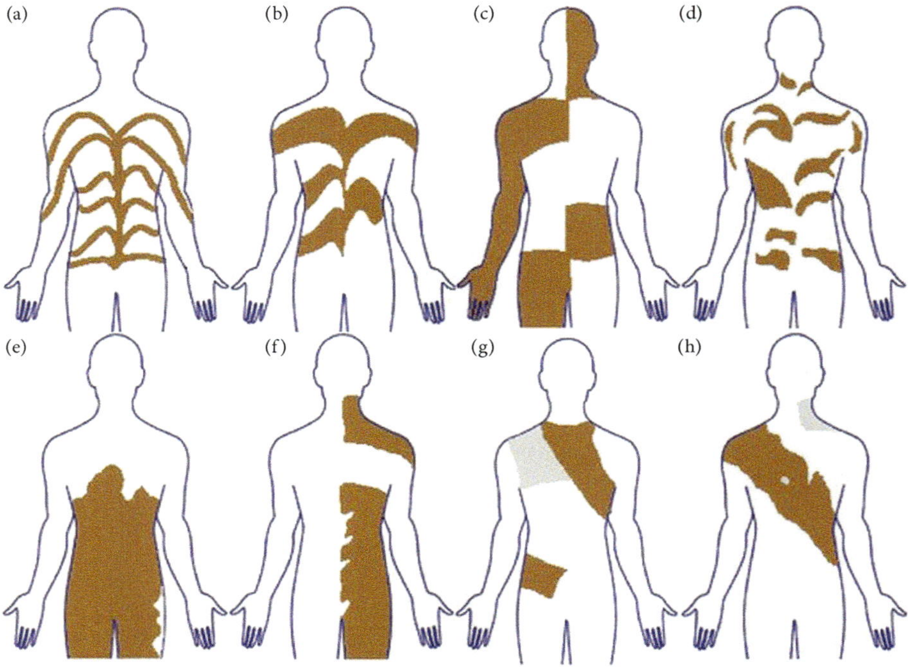

Figure 25–13. Patterns of Pigmentary Mosaicism.

Notes: Kromann et al. distinguish types *a* through *h*, as follows: (a) type 1a, (b) type 1b, (c) type 2, (d) type 3, (e) type 4, (f) type 5, (g) type 6 seen from the front, (h) type 6 seen from the back

Source: From AB Kromann et al., Pigmentary mosaicism: a review of original literature and recommendations for future handling, *Orphanet J Rare Dis* 13:39, 2018. Courtesy A Bygum, and with the permission of Springer Nature.

inability to apply linguistic rules to combine sounds to form words). In simple terms, it is an inability to put words together. It can be a component of autism, hearing impairment, or intellectual disability, but here we consider it as the predominant trait. In its more severe form, it is referred to as childhood apraxia of speech (CAS).

A genetic basis is common, and a number of loci are implicated (Morgan et al. 2024). We refer (Chapter 14) to deletions at 7q31, 12p13.33, and proximal 16p11.2 as being causative in cases with a broader neurofunctional phenotype. Chan et al. (2024) identify a number of other SSD-associated CNVs, including in particular deletions at 2q24.3, 6p12.3p12.2, and 11q23.2q23.3, in their study of families in which a proband had CAS, and other family members had a less severe SSD. Most cases were inherited; a few had arisen de novo.

SUDDEN INFANT DEATH

Brownstein et al. (2022) undertook CNV analysis in a large series of Sudden Unexplained Death in the Pediatric Age Group, ages at death from 1.5 months to 28 months; in five out of the 116 cases (4%) a presumed pathogenic deletion was identified (Table 25–8).

Table 25–8. Deletions and Duplications Seen in Sudden Unexplained Childhood Death.

SEGMENT	del/dup	SIZE
2p16.3*	del	108 kb
2p21	dup	2.8 kb
2p23.1	dup	174 kb
4q31.22 *	del	348 kb
5q13.2 *	del	1.8 Mb
7q36.3	dup	226 kb
8p23.2	del	223 kb
13q32.3	dup	117 kb
13q34	dup	140 kb
15q11.2 (×2)	del	245-246 kb
15q15.3 *	del	98 kb
22q11.21	dup	13.4 kb
22q13.33	dup	275 kb
Xp22.33 *	del	800 kb

Note: Sudden Unexplained Death in the Pediatric Age Group encompasses Sudden Infant Death Syndrome (under 1 year; "cot death") and Sudden Unexplained Death in Childhood (over 1 year). These cases came from a cohort of 116 Cases. In the five asterisked cases, the del was presumed to have been pathogenic; in the remainder, pathogenicity was considered likely. The dup2p21 and dup 22q11.21 were seen in the same child.

In an earlier such study, a del6p22, dup8q24.3, and del22q13.3 had been documented (Toruner et al. 2009).

Source: CA Brownstein et al., Copy number variation and structural genomic findings in 116 cases of sudden unexplained death between 1 and 28 months of age, *Adv Genet (Hoboken)* 4:2200012, 2022.

Additionally, a further nine cases had a deletion or a duplication that was assessed as being likely pathogenic, for a total 12% with a known or probably causative CNV. Brownstein and colleagues make the case for a chromosome study, along with exome sequencing, as a routine test in such cases.

BIOLOGY AND EPIDEMIOLOGY

Cancer Treatment

A majority of children and young adults who receive modern cancer treatment survive. Some treatments cause sterility, but in quite a number fertility is unscathed, or at any rate subsequently recovers (van Santen et al. 2020). For those who are potentially capable of having children, the question arises: Could there be an increased risk to have a child with a chromosomal abnormality? For most, in fact, the short answer may be apparently not. Longer answers follow.

The chemotherapeutic agents and radiation used to rid the body of cancer are essentially cellular toxins, some of which specifically target DNA or the mitotic apparatus. Thus, the starting hypothesis is that the chromosomes in exposed bystander tissues (and thinking specifically of the gonad) could be vulnerable. The fact that these treatments can damage chromosomes is well known, and this is actually the basis of one of the in vitro laboratory tests for ataxia-telangiectasia.[1] Rapidly dividing cells are the most vulnerable to anti-cancer treatments (this being, of course, the rationale for their use). This would suggest, in theory, a susceptibility for spermatogenesis in the postpubertal male (millions of cell divisions daily), along with a relative resistance in the prepubertal male child (male meiosis yet to commence) and in oögenesis from infancy through menopause in the female (cell division in suspension). In the male, the fact of a "blood-testis barrier" may offer a defense (Yauk et al. 2015); a selection against chromosomally imbalanced cells during gametogenesis may be another protective process.

The direct assessment of gametic chromosomes offers insight. A number of studies have used FISH to detect structural and numerical chromosome abnormalities in the sperm of men during and after chemotherapy treatment. From these, we may draw some broad generalizations regarding time course and sperm safety.

Tempest et al. (2008) studied men with testicular cancer treated with bleomycin-etoposide-cisplatin (BEP), and men with Hodgkin lymphoma treated with BEP: at six months after treatment, the frequencies of XY disomy and of nullisomy 13 and 21 were significantly increased. Aneuploidy frequencies declined at 18 months follow-up, though for some chromosomes remained elevated for up to 24 months. Rives et al. (2017) also studied sperm aneuploidy rate in a population of testicular cancer patients treated with either BEP chemotherapy or radiotherapy, and found a significant increase in sperm aneuploidy that mostly returned to baseline by 12 months (Figure 26–1).

Hodgkin lymphoma can be treated with radiotherapy and chemotherapy with Novantrone-Oncovin-Velban-Prednisone (NOVP). Frias et al. (2020) observed post-treatment increases in aneuploidies of chromosomes X, Y, 18, and 21, but which returned to baseline by six months. These authors extrapolated their findings genome-wide and estimated that the proportion of sperm with structural or numerical abnormalities would increase from a baseline of 1.6% to 16%, noting that most of these abnormalities would be lethal in early embryogenesis. They concluded there to be no excess risks for pregnancies conceived six months after the completion of therapy.

[1] Radiation and bleomycin, both having potent DNA-breaking properties, cause lymphocyte chromosome rearrangements in normal cells, and considerably more so in ataxia-telangiectasia cells.

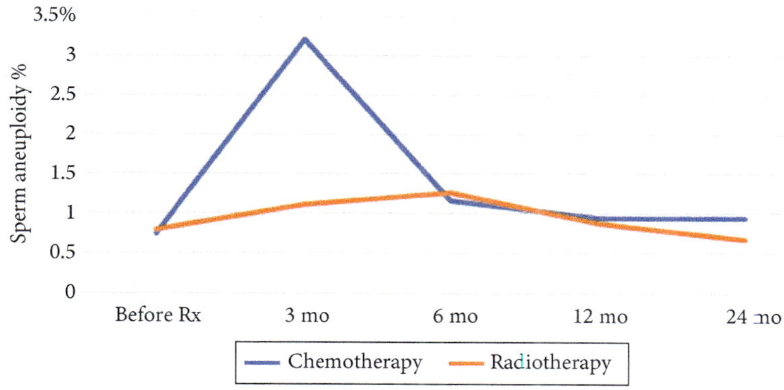

Figure 26–1. Sperm Chromosomes Pre and Post Cancer Treatments.

Notes: Longitudinal data on sperm aneuploidy rate in a population of testicular cancer patients treated with either bleomycin-etoposide-cisplatin chemotherapy or radiotherapy. Sperm aneuploidy was assessed using FISH for chromosomes X, Y and 18.

Source: Drawn from data in N Rives et al., Sperm aneuploidy after testicular cancer treatment: data from a prospective multicenter study performed within the French Centre d'Étude et de Conservation des Oeufs et du Sperme network, *Fertil Steril* 107:580–588.e1, 2017.

In practice, it is to the experience of the "therapeutic experiments" of oncological medicine that we mostly appeal: the in vivo observations of those who have survived their cancer, recovered from their treatment, and have gone on to have or to attempt to have children. Have the children shown any excess of cytogenetic abnormality? Outcomes from five large studies are summarized in Table 26–1. Collectively, these report on more than 50,000 children of cancer survivors and in fact, show no difference

Table 26–1. Outcomes from Six Large Studies of the Offspring of Childhood Cancer Survivors

SOURCES	COUNTRY	NO. OF OFFSPRING OF CANCER SURVIVORS	CHROMOSOME ABNORMALITIES		CLASS OF CONTROLS
			CASES (%)	CONTROLS (%)	
Byrne et al. (1998), Meistrich and Byrne (2002)	United States	2,198	0.20	0.10	Siblings
Ståhl et al. (2011)*	Denmark, Sweden	8,670	0.08	0.18	Population
Signorello et al. (2012)	United States	4,699	0.15		None
Seppänen et al. (2016)	Finland	6,862	0.06	0.07	Siblings
Nielsen et al. (2018)	Denmark	14,611	0.33	0.37	Siblings
Jin et al. (2024)**	South Korea	15,221	0.15	0.16	Population

*Included only offspring of male cancer survivors; ** included only offspring of female cancer survivors.

between the prevalence of chromosome abnormalities[2] in the offspring of cancer survivors when compared to the offspring of their cancer-free siblings or population controls. The prevalence of chromosome abnormalities is consistently ~1 in 600 regardless of the type of cancer, the age of cancer onset, the type and dosage of chemotherapy administered, and the use of radiotherapy. Data about miscarriage rates are in agreement: Green et al. (2009) followed up more than 4,000 pregnancies in which either the mother or the father was a cancer survivor, and they found no increase in the frequency of miscarriage in either group.

SPECIFIC THERAPIES

Chemotherapy. Lambertini et al. (2020) review the effects of various chemotherapy regimes on fertility, categorizing according to whether the risk of infertility is high, intermediate, low, or "unknown," the latter applying to most of the newer targeted and immunological therapies (Helgadottir et al. 2024). In both males and females, the risk of treatment-related infertility is highest for alkylating agents, radiotherapy that includes the gonads, and conditioning chemotherapy prior to bone marrow transplantation. Patients with an interest in future fertility should be referred for oncofertility assessment prior to commencing treatment.

Radiotherapy. Fertility is reduced in *females* who have had radiation therapy to the abdomen, and the risk of obstetric complication is increased. But their children appear to have no increased incidence of birth defects (Signorello et al. 2012; Seppänen et al. 2016). In the *male*, testicular radiotherapy causes a modest increase in sperm aneuploidy rate that returns to normal after 12 months (Figure 26–1). Ståhl et al. (2011) studied 2,488 children born one or more years after the diagnosis of testicular cancer in their father, most of whom would have been treated with radiotherapy, and there was no increase in congenital abnormalities in their children

Radioisotopes. Radioiodine is used in thyroid cancer and may cause transient oligospermia and amenorrhea in males and females, respectively, but its use appears to be of no risk for miscarriage or for congenital abnormality (Clement et al. 2015).

Infertility Associated with Cancer Therapy, and Prior Gamete Banking

Preservation of gametes prior to treatment for cancer is a logical management, and sperm banking as "fertility insurance" for boys and men with cancer is now considered routine (Menon et al. 2009). The American Society of Clinical Oncology recommends that the risk of infertility, and options for fertility preservation, be discussed with all patients of reproductive age (and with parents or guardians of children and adolescents) before starting treatment (Oktay et al. 2018). All patients who express an interest in fertility preservation should be referred to a reproductive specialist. For adult men, sperm cryopreservation is the only established fertility preservation method and should be done before starting chemotherapy. Cryopreservation of testicular tissue, which does not require sexual maturity, remains experimental. For adult women, both embryo and

[2] It is notable that these studies also detected no increase in the prevalence of non-chromosomal birth defects in the offspring of cancer survivors.

oöcyte cryopreservation are established methods or fertility preservation, while ovarian tissue cryopreservation remains experimental.

Diagnostic Radiology

Ionizing radiation is a well-known cause of cancer, and in theory could also cause gene mutations in the germ cells of exposed parents and lead to genetically mediated adverse outcomes in children inheriting the mutations. In practice, transgenerational effects of radiation have never been shown in human populations (Nakamura et al. 2023), and in general there is no convincing evidence for an increased risk of chromosome abnormalities in the offspring of parents who have been exposed to diagnostic radiology.

> A small effect may possibly exist for Down syndrome (DS) with respect to previous X-rays to the abdomen and pelvic area—that is, for X-rays in which the gonads may have been within or near the field of the film. In a study of 156 mothers and 149 fathers in whose DS children the "nondisjunctional parent" could be identified (using Q-banding polymorphisms), a history of X-ray exposure was more often recorded in older fathers and in younger mothers (Strigini et al. 1990). The odds ratio for the whole group was 1.85, although the lower limit of the 95% confidence interval was 1.0. If such an effect truly exists in younger mothers (and the statistics were borderline), it would seem that this slight influence becomes diluted as they get older and the age effect comes to be predominant.

Nonmedical Exposures

Radioactivity. The human germline may be relatively resistant to the damaging effects of radiation, compared with some animal models (Neel et al. 1990; Adriaens et al. 2009).[3] The atomic bomb blasts at Hiroshima and Nagasaki in 1945 were not followed by a statistically significant difference in the rate of chromosome abnormalities in children subsequently conceived, according to a study commenced in 1967 (Nakamura 2006). The study population comprised 8,322 individuals born 1946–1972, age range at the time of study 12–38 years, one or both of whose parents were within 2,000 meters of the hypocenter "ATB" (at the time of the bomb), alongside a contemporaneous local control group of 7,976 who were either more than 2,500 meters from the hypocenter or not present in the city. Sex chromosomal abnormalities were seen in 2.28 per 1,000 in the former group and in 3.01 per 1,000 of the latter. The only instance of autosomal trisomy was a 15-year-old with standard trisomy DS, whose father had been exposed at Hiroshima.

> Given the structure of this study, deceased younger children and infants with autosomal trisomy were not included, although it is also to be noted that in separate analyses in Neel and Schull (1991), no significant correlation existed between parental exposure ATB and the frequency of stillbirth or congenital malformations. More

[3] Of historic interest, a very early example of ill health due to radiation exposure is that of Marie Curie, who was awarded the Nobel Prize twice. One daughter of hers was a scientist, and she also won a Nobel Prize, and the other was a skilled pianist and gifted writer. A series of $n = 2$ is very small, but rather evidently there must have been normal chromosomal segregation in the meioses leading to these two daughters.

children of exposed parents had a small supernumerary abnormal chromosome than in controls (5 cf. 2, a difference not specifically commented upon in Awa et al. 1987). Of the balanced structural rearrangements, only two were confirmed as having arisen de novo (one each in the exposed and control groups). An earlier study with specific reference to clinically diagnosed DS in 9-month-old infants, undertaken during 1948–1954 before the chromosomal basis of DS was known, had shown no increase among offspring of 5,582 exposed cf. 9,452 unexposed mothers, and indeed the figures were in the other direction (0.54 cf. 1.27 per 1,000) and despite the exposed mothers being on average slightly older (Schull and Neel 1962).

The Chernobyl nuclear plant explosion occurred in April 1986, and a cloud of radioactivity was dispersed over Europe. With respect to DS, no subsequent rise in incidence was identified in a number of European countries apart from small clusters in Berlin and Belarus, the latter of interest in that the peak was confined to January 1987, nine months after the explosion (Little 1993; Zatsepin et al. 2007). In contrast, Bound et al. (1995) suggest a possible link between events in 1957 (a fire in a nuclear reactor) and the early 1960s (increased levels of fallout from nuclear testing) and peaks of DS prevalence in 1958 and 1963–1964 in the Fylde district of Lancashire, England. But by no means is a firm case made: *post hoc* does not necessarily mean *propter hoc*,[4] and some fluctuation is normal.

The same 1957 nuclear reactor accident had been proposed as the possible reason for a cluster of six cases of DS among the children of women who had attended the same high school in Dundalk, Ireland, during 1956–1957 when they would have been aged from 12 to 19 years. Of the 387 births to the former pupils from this period, the expectation would have been 0.69 children with DS. However, a stringent review of the evidence, including molecular analyses that showed one case to have arisen post-fertilization, led to the conclusion that in fact, chance alone was the probable basis for the "cluster" (Dean et al. 2000).

While the germline, at least from the evidence outlined earlier, is apparently resistant, the same cannot be said for the bone marrow. Numerous studies on radiation exposure have shown that stable chromosome rearrangements may be induced, as measured on peripheral blood samples. Indeed, it is proposed that these changes can be used as reliable biomarkers of exposure. Populations in whom this effect has been seen include Russian nuclear plant workers (comparing those exposed to plutonium and those to gamma rays) from 1949 to 1989; New Zealand navy personnel who had served on ships during nuclear bomb testing in the Pacific Ocean in the late 1950s; American radiation technologists who had begun practicing before 1950 (ages at the time of study 71–90 years); populations living near the Three Mile Island nuclear facility at the time of the 1979 accident; and even astronauts, unprotected by Earth's atmosphere from solar radiation (Durante et al. 2003; Hande et al. 2003; Sigurdson et al. 2008; Wahab et al. 2008; Little et al. 2021). We are unaware of any evidence that individuals exposed in these ways might have acquired any gonadal damage and that their children could have been at risk for a chromosomal disorder.

[4] *Post hoc, ergo propter hoc* (Latin) = Something happened after the event, and therefore it must have been due to the event.

Industrial Agents. The male gonad is protected by the blood-testis barrier (Li et al. 2016), but it is prudent to imagine that the protection may not necessarily be absolute. Paternal occupation provides a surrogate marker for a variety of potential industrial agents. Olshan et al. (1989) assessed the father's occupation for 1,000 DS children born in British Columbia from 1952 through 1973. Seven employment categories out of 59 showed odds ratios in the range 1.4–3.3, the lower confidence limit being not less than 0.9, in which exposure to various industrial agents could plausibly have occurred (including mechanics, janitors, metal workers, sawmill workers). But the increases in risk were small, and with 59 items under study there was of course the possibility of chance fluctuation. One category that might have seemed risky, namely "other chemical workers," in fact had the lowest odds ratio of all (0.2). Exposure to volatile oil (as studied following clean-up after an oil spill at sea) may damage the marrow, with chromosomal breakages observed in peripheral blood, but there is no indication of damage at the level of the gonad (Francés et al. 2016).

Given that most DS arises from maternal nondisjunction, maternal occupation may be more relevant. There may be an association between maternal socioeconomic status and meiosis II nondisjunction, suggesting that maternal occupational exposures might be relevant (Hunter et al. 2013). One study compared maternal occupation for 714 DS cases and 973 controls, and out of 19 occupational categories only one, "Life, Physical and Social Sciences" reached statistical significance, with an odds ratio of 1.57 (Keen et al. 2020). No specific occupational exposure could be discerned within this heterogeneous group, and the result may have arisen by chance.

Pesticides have biological activity, and it is reasonable to raise a case that distribution across the blood-testis barrier might follow inhalation, absorption, or ingestion, and that the local effect upon gonadal tissue might be toxic. Giulioni et al. (2022) reviewed 64 studies correlating pesticide-exposure male fertility and noted that many pesticides have been associated with altered sperm count, sperm motility, and sperm morphology. Regarding sperm chromosomal abnormality, data are more limited: some studies did and some did not show an increase in chromosomal defects. Of the numerous agents, the strongest case could be made for carbaryl and fenvalerate in particular as potentially causative of autosomal and gonosomal aneuploidy, with sex chromosome disomy the most frequent single abnormality.

The air we breathe, it is suggested, might convey mutagens in the form of industrial pollutants, and these might reach gonadal tissue (Somers and Cooper 2009). Farhi et al. (2014) found a borderline increased risk (odds ratio 1.14) for chromosome abnormalities in Israeli women exposed to high levels of air pollution in the first trimester, but these results were not confirmed by studies in China (Li et al. 2022b) and the United States (Ren et al. 2018), in which no association was seen between chromosome abnormalities and air pollution during the pre-conception period. In the male, Jurewicz et al. (2018) reviewed the impact of air pollution on a range of sperm parameters and found inconsistent results, with some studies suggesting an increase in sperm aneuploidy in men exposed to high air pollution and others finding no such difference.

Landfill sites contain toxic matter, which might in theory contaminate the air in nearby residential areas; but in an analysis based upon more than 6,000 such sites throughout the United Kingdom and comparing populations living within and beyond 2 kilometers of these sites, no differences in the prevalence of DS were observed (Jarup et al. 2007). However, older mothers living within one mile of industrial sites from which solvent and

27
ETHICAL ISSUES

Our focus in this book is largely on the biology of chromosomal defects and the reproductive implications that they may entail. Certain bioethical issues coming to be more formally defined in the late 20th and this century do, however, demand attention. Counselors must hold fast to these requirements: (1) that they act beneficently toward their patients,[1] and (2) that they strive to make their services accessible to those who may need them.

NONDIRECTIVE COUNSELING

In a Western ethos, the counselor is enjoined to respect the autonomy of the client, and this largely translates into the principle that counseling be nondirective. The principle may be more honored in the breach than in the observance, as Chańska and Grunt-Mejer (2022), in a Polish setting, discuss. In China, Dong et al. (2023) point to a need for education in this respect, as demand for genetic counseling "soars"; and South African counselors may struggle to adhere to the desideratum of nondirectiveness (Scott et al. 2024). Rentmeester (2001) comments that since it is "impossible for human language to convey facts purely, without any spoor of values," and since "risk cannot be appreciated without consideration of values," it is neither helpful nor indeed possible to try to be value-neutral.

There is a fine line between directive and detached counseling, a point well illustrated in Karp's (1983) deft essay, "The Terrible Question." Ingelfinger (1980) comments, admittedly in a somewhat different context: "A physician who merely spreads an array of vendibles in front of the patient and then says, 'Go ahead and choose, it's your life,' is guilty of shirking his duty, if not of malpractice." Rentmeester (2001) offers the refreshing advice that it is not necessarily unprofessional to answer a patient's question "What would you do?" It is the skill of the counselor that helps clients reach the decision that is, *for them*, the right one, and for the clients to feel satisfied that they have done so. How to balance nondirectiveness, while at the same time ensuring that patients do not lose an opportunity to achieve their best outcome, is outlined in Resnicow et al. (2022).

"GUILT" IN A CARRIER

Parental testing is often done in the case of a child having been diagnosed with a chromosomal abnormality, and occasionally one or other parent will be revealed as a balanced translocation carrier. Sometimes a chromosomal diagnosis may be made in an

[1] There seems no completely satisfactory word to use here, and we variably write of patients, clients, counselees, men and women, people, and "those whom we see."

older child or even an adult, where the parents will have held for years to the notion that obstetric misadventure, or a virus, or some other blameable event was the cause of the child's condition. Some people find it upsetting to have to readjust or to know that they may have been the source of the abnormality. They are likely to use words such as guilt, blame, and fault; others may approach the situation pragmatically (Kaneko et al. 2015). Helping these people to adjust to the new knowledge is a challenge for the counselor.

TESTING CHILDREN

To state the obvious, familial rearrangements are familial. It is very natural that parents would be concerned whether children they already have might be carriers, once an abnormality has been identified in one of them. Children, certainly, need to know their carrier status sooner or later. It is very unfortunate (and possibly creates an exposure to legal redress) if a failure to transmit information leads to another affected child unknowingly being born elsewhere in the family. Burn et al. (1983) reported a family with a translocation having been the cause of cri du chat syndrome in two generations, the genetic information not having flowed through to the people who really needed to know it. We have had a similar experience: a family with a t(4;12), concerning which we had gone to the lengths of deriving and publishing a recurrence-risk figure (Mortimer et al. 1980), and yet this information not traveling with a young man who had moved as a child from one country to another, and whose life was since changed by having had a daughter with partial 4p trisomy.

On the other hand, genetic counselors are attuned to the principle of not taking away a child's right to make, in the fullness of time, his or her own informed decision to learn about genetic risks he or she may face; thus, the principle is that the child's future autonomy is to be respected. The American Society of Human Genetics and the American College of Medical Genetics (1995) have determined that "timely medical benefit to the child should be the primary justification for genetic testing in children and adolescents." And, it is true that a balanced chromosomal rearrangement will have no influence upon a person's physical health other than, in due course, his or her reproductive health (and the issue is thus to be seen in a different light than testing for adult-onset disease). Questions are raised that testing could damage a child's self-esteem, distort the family's perceptions of the child, and have adverse effects upon the child's capacity to form future relationships (Clarke 1994). In France, testing a healthy child for the possibility of inheritance of a parental chromosome rearrangement may be unlawful (Hervé et al. 2015).

Parents' views are not without validity. Clayton (1995) commented that there is the possibility of conflict with parents as physicians come increasingly to act as advocates for the child's interests, but notes further that "children are generally ill-served if their parents feel they have not been listened to." She also draws the conclusion that this is a medico-ethical rather than a medico-legal issue. Vears et al. (2016) offer a similarly nuanced view. McConkie-Rosell et al. (1999) sought opinions from a group of 65 parents of fragile X children attending a national conference in Portland, Oregon, in 1996. They noted a "strong belief in a parental right to make the decision regarding carrier status in their children," with about half considering that they should have the right to decide when their child should be tested and informed of the result. The Genetic Interest Group in the United Kingdom gently chided the profession in commenting that "the vast majority of people are better able to understand the implications than they are often given credit for" and has enunciated the following principle: "After suitable counseling, parents have the right to make an informed choice about whether or not to have their children tested for carrier status. Ideally, children should only be tested when of an age to be involved in the decision" (Dalby 1995).

It may be that earlier concerns overstated the potential for harm. At least with respect to the Mendelian cancer-predisposing syndrome familial adenomatous polyposis, children having undergone predictive testing and receiving a positive gene test result experienced no increase in anxiety, depression, or loss of self-esteem (Michie et al. 2001). Indeed, Robertson and Savulescu (2001) see potential benefit to the child, and they support the view that as a general rule the parents' views should prevail and a request for predictive testing be respected. There is also the practical point that many parents will have had a prenatal karyotype from amniocentesis or chorionic villus sampling for one of their children-to-be; and it may not seem entirely logical to decline to test their other post-natal children. In an analogous Mendelian case, X-linked Duchenne muscular dystrophy, Helderman-van den Enden et al. (2013) go so far as to state "it is cruel to subject the parents to an ordeal, lasting years, with this dilemma [of their unborn or infant daughter possibly being a carrier]." Perhaps counselors' misattributed understanding of their clients' motivations may be hindering good communication (Vears et al. 2017).

From the foregoing, we conclude that a flexible stance is appropriate. Many parents will be satisfied (and possibly relieved) with the advice to leave testing until the child can decide. Equally, there will be occasions when acquiescence to a parental request is reasonable. Either the parent's mind is set at rest, or they know of the need to raise the issue with the child at a "suitable age," which should be with the assistance of the genetic counseling clinic. Bache et al. (2007) found that 9% of carriers in Denmark identified in childhood (or prenatally) had not been told as young adults; this observation led to a change in practice in that country, with a reminder letter being sent to the parents when their child reached the age of 18 years. The task for the counselor is to assist parents in deciding what age would be suitable for their child, and to convey the information in such a way that concern for the future is kept in perspective and the child's self-confidence is kept intact. And, the pragmatic imperative: the wish to avoid family distress due to avoidable births of abnormal children in the next generation, as outlined above.

FAMILY STUDIES

More widely, the parents' siblings and cousins could be carriers. Grandparental karyotypes may be useful in knowing which branch of a family to follow. The rights of individuals could potentially clash with the obligation that flows from belonging to a family: "No man is an island, entire unto himself," and some may see altruism as a duty. Austad (1996) proposes that the family's right to know about "sensitive genetic information" should take precedence over the individual's right *not* to know. He considers it "alarming to use the principle of autonomy to renounce the co-responsibility for others, in this case, relatives"; he goes on to state that "we cannot exclude ourselves from the genetic fellowship of fate into which we are born." Suslak et al. (1985) note that family members do not necessarily take on the responsibility of conveying information, and propose that counselors "may have a duty to transmit such information to at-risk relatives in light of the harm that may occur when information is withheld."

If counselors take pains to provide clear information and to do so sensitively, such studies should usually proceed without unfortunate consequence. A suitable approach in most families will be to ask the person coming to the clinic to take the responsibility of bringing the matter to the attention of relatives, with appropriate support from the counselor. A letter couched in terms that could be shown to other family members, and providing contact points for further information, is often useful. Forrest et al. (2007) reviewed many international sources and identified the following criteria seen as common obligations falling to the families and to the counselors who see them: (1) Individuals have a moral obligation to communicate genetic information to their family members; (2) genetic health professionals should encourage individuals to communicate this information to their family members; and (3) genetic health professionals should support individuals throughout the communication process. (We would add a caveat, now that microarray analysis has become the norm: The uncertainties of interpretation of many CNVs seen in routine clinical practice can complicate "cascade testing" to a degree that the exercise may become counterproductive and unhelpful.)

A more controversial question is whether genetic information can be disclosed by health professionals without patient consent, a circumstance that brings the duty of care of health professionals into conflict with privacy laws and professional regulations. The commonly held view is that such disclosure is appropriate when the genetic condition is severe and the information is actionable (Phillips et al. 2021a); however, whether actionability extends to reproductive implications (for example in the setting of a familial translocation) is less clear (Meggiolaro et al. 2020).

PREDICTIVE GENE TESTING: DELIBERATE AND INADVERTENT

Counselors are very familiar with the concept of predictive genetic testing—that is, offering genetic testing to people who are presently well but who are at risk for having inherited a particular genotype that may, at some stage in adult life, be the basis of the onset of disease. Its widest application is in the fields of cancer genetics and neurogenetics. With respect to rare translocations in the balanced state that may confer a predisposition to cancer, mention is made on pp. 781–2 and, over and above the reproductive implications of individuals being tested in such families, a cancer-associated risk will need to be assessed.

As for inadvertent testing, we may mention a 30-year-old woman we have seen, presenting with premature ovarian failure and having a karyotype to check for an X chromosome mosaicism but in whom trisomy 8 and a 14q;18q translocation were seen in 3/100 cells. She was otherwise in good health. This may well have been an "accidental" very early diagnosis of a lymphoma, and referral to a hematologist-oncologist—which was more than she had bargained for by having the test—was duly arranged. Nevertheless, although advice about a cancer risk may come as an "unwanted surprise," discovery of a chromosomal predisposition may in fact be lifesaving (Heald et al. 2007).

With the increasing application of microarray technology, the likelihood of discovering an incidental abnormality may now more frequently need to be taken into account when a chromosome test is ordered. We mention on pp. 446 and 454 the 17q21.31 and 21q21.3 duplications which may be the basis of a familial dementia. Schwarzbraun et al. (2009) report their experience in testing a 7-year-old girl with severe intellectual disability and mild dysmorphism, in whom microarray revealed a de novo microdeletion (774 kb; containing 47 genes) at 17p13.1, and this deletion was presumed to be the explanation for the clinical picture. One of the deleted 47 genes, however, happened to be *TP53*, and thus this deletion was considered effectively to represent a germline Li-Fraumeni[2] mutation. This was quite unanticipated information for the parents to deal with, and the issue was further complicated by the child's mental incapacity. Schluth-Bolard et al. (2010) consider this question, and they write:

> . . . the local Ethical Committee at the University Hospital of Lyon, France, suggested implementation of a plan to inform patients and their parents on the possibility of discovering pathology unrelated to mental retardation, and give them a month to carefully ponder on the possible consequences before signing the consent for study.

More pragmatically, they continue:

> If this period of reflection would be difficult to apply in clinical practice, the possibility of incidental findings should be discussed during pre-test counseling and information should be given during post-test counseling by a trained clinician, aware of the potential psychological impact of such findings.

Noninvasive prenatal testing (NIPT) may lead into unanticipated ethical minefields. An occasional inadvertent cancer diagnosis may be made (Dow et al. 2021). In a case reported in Sun et al. (2015), massive copy-number gains of chromosome 21 and some other chromosomes were observed, completely different from what would be seen in fetal trisomy; and in fact, the diagnosis was recurrence of a follicular lymphoma. Meschino et al. (2016) report the case of a woman who had had NIPT for trisomy 21 due to the ultrasound detection of two "soft markers" for Down syndrome and who also, as it happened, had a family history of early-onset Alzheimer disease. A dup(21) was identified, which included the Alzheimer-associated *APP* locus at 21q21.3 (but not the Down syndrome critical region). Thus, she and her unborn child had had an unwitting predictive genetic test for a dominantly inherited dementia (p. 454). Further to complicate the story, she had an identical twin sister. Meschino and colleagues debate the complicated issues that arose from this case, and they, along with Dow et al. (2021), rehearse lessons to be taken for those in the field.

THE STATUS OF EMBRYOS AT IN VITRO FERTILIZATION

Lejeune, the discoverer of trisomy 21, has commented and indeed provided extensive testimony on the ethical distinction between abortion and discarding an unwanted embryo. At a famous 1989 court case dealing with a dispute about IVF embryos in Blount County, Tennessee, he insisted on the point that human life commences at conception, and therefore that disposing of a zygote is in essence no different from the induced

[2] Li-Fraumeni syndrome is a dominantly inherited cancer-predisposition syndrome due to *TP53* germline mutation, with severe implications. The cancers include soft-tissue sarcoma in early childhood; in later childhood, osteosarcoma; and in young adulthood, breast, brain, and hematological malignancy. It is controversial whether medical surveillance should be offered in childhood.

abortion of an established pregnancy. A similar view has come from Alabama, and the concept of "extrauterine children" has been proposed, with one Justice referencing the "theologically based view of the sanctity of life adopted by the People of Alabama" from which it follows that "life cannot be wrongfully destroyed without incurring the wrath of a holy God" (Feinberg et al. 2024). Thus, providers of IVF in that state potentially could find themselves in the position of being charged under the Wrongful Death Act if stored embryos were allowed to succumb.

One Catholic thinker is of the opinion that "human personhood" of the embryo does not inhere until the stage at which embryonic cells have differentiated and the primitive streak has appeared (at about the end of the second week post-conception) (Ford 1988). Prior to that time when the "pro-embryo," as he prefers to call it, is only a *personne en devenir*, "we should resist the conceptual and linguistic temptation to attribute an unwarranted ontological unity to an actual multiplicity of developing human blastomeres." More liberally, Isaacs (2002) discusses the concept of a continuum in which the "moral status" of the fetus increases in value through pregnancy (and indeed after birth); and some couples seem intuitively to follow this line. Thus, the moral arguments of Lejeune and the Alabama legislature are not necessarily seen as convincing to those pragmatic couples who choose to have preimplantation diagnosis in order to avoid the predicament of having to decide upon a course of action following prenatal diagnosis of a chromosomal abnormality at chorionic villus sampling or amniocentesis.

Molecular methodologies, as we have already had cause to comment, bring with them ethical challenges. In a paper memorably titled "Embryos Without Secrets," Hens et al. (2013b) consider the new dimensions implied by the new methodologies. They conclude that microarray and potentially whole genome analysis may be a double-edged sword in the hands of those providing PGT, and they call for more discussion about "who should have the final say on which embryo to select." An embryo can be seen as a future person, and that being so, Hens et al. (2013a) point to an onerous responsibility upon the PGT clinician. These authors, while acknowledging the "principle of procreative beneficence" put forward by Savulescu and Kahane (2009), who consider that couples have a moral obligation (if reasonably feasible) to select the embryo whose life can be expected to be best, point out that the situation may not necessarily be straightforward. And in this 21st century, it may seem almost normal that artificial intelligence (AI) is being proposed as a means to select the best embryo (Afnan et al. 2021). The counselor working in an IVF clinic will need to keep abreast of these complex questions and to be aware of the vulnerabilities of the presenting couples.

PRENATAL DIAGNOSIS AND PREGNANCY TERMINATION FOR A CHROMOSOMAL ABNORMALITY

Prenatal diagnosis of a chromosome abnormality has been standard practice in many countries for half a century, initially via the methodology of amniocentesis and latterly based upon a maternal blood sample. Genetic counselors can have a key role in the implementation of such a service (Sánchez Marín and García González 2023). The level of acceptability of prenatal diagnosis, with termination in the case of a chromosomal abnormality having been identified, has largely plateaued in those jurisdictions in which the procedure is reasonably readily available. In Denmark, for example, over the period 2008–2021, the total numbers per year of terminations for an aneuploidy (mostly trisomies 13, 18, and 21, and sex chromosome aneuploidy) showed only the slightest increase. On the other hand, terminations for deletions and duplications rose substantially in the mid 2010s due to the introduction of methodologies capable of detecting these defects (Figure 27–1) (Raaby et al. 2024).

Legal barriers may arise in some jurisdictions. Abortion in Chile, formerly "allowed under no circumstances" (Casas and Vivaldi 2017), was the subject of legal review in 2017, with new legislation proposing decriminalization on the grounds of, inter alia, "an embryo or foetus suffering from a congenital structural anomaly or a genetic disorder incompatible with life outside the womb." The genetic branch of the Chilean Society of Pediatrics suggested changing the wording to "a congenital anomaly of poor prognosis," among which they would include trisomies 13 and 18 (Pardo Vargas et al. 2016).

In the United States, as Miller et al. (2000) commented, "there is perhaps no more divisive subject than abortion," as we now see in the 2010s–2020s. We have referred above to Alabama. A color-coded map illustrated on the website of the Center for Reproductive Rights shows state differences across the USA, on a scale from liberal through absolute prohibition. A review from 2023 comparing Down syndrome birth rates over the timeframe 2011–2018 in American states that did or did not impose a 20-week gestation abortion limit showed, unsurprisingly, a higher DS incidence in the restrictive states (Chaiken et al. 2023). Donley (2013) contends that such bans are in fact unconstitutional, and the interested reader possessed of a legal-oriented mindset is referred to her detailed and finely argued essay.

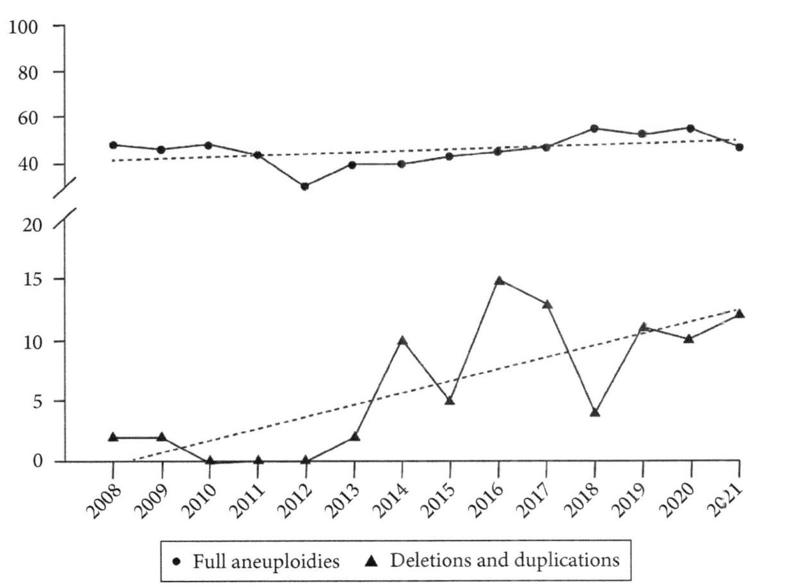

Figure 27–1. The numbers of terminations in central Denmark over the period 2002-2021, for the indications of an aneuploidy (*upper line*), and for a deletion or duplication (*lower line*).

Note: The baseline birth rate in this population is c. 14,000 per annum. Termination on the grounds of a fetal abnormality is available from 12 to 22 weeks gestation, but requires approval from a local Regional Abortion Council.

Source: From L Raaby et al., Has the introduction of increased genetic prenatal testing affected rates of termination of pregnancy due to fetal abnormality? *Prenat Diagn* 44:280–288, 2024. Courtesy L Raaby, and with the permission of John Wiley & Sons.

If prenatal testing is not made available, or if an abnormal result is reported but has not been passed on to the parents, the option of pregnancy termination is denied. Here, the legal concept of "wrongful birth" may be invoked. Frati et al. (2017) define this as referring ". . . to claims for alleged negligence where an opportunity has been lost to parents to terminate a pregnancy. These claims are often related to undetected fetal abnormalities, and involve a claim for damages by the parents of a child for, most importantly, the costs of bringing up the child." (This is to be distinguished from "wrongful life," or "the right not to be born"; Weber, 2001)[3] French courts made landmark decisions in 2000 and 2001 in which substantial financial compensation was granted to parents of children with Down syndrome. Whatever the legalities, the lesson for the counselor is that testing should be offered to those for whom it may be appropriate and legally available, and that they should be diligent and careful in ensuring that prenatal testing results are safely conveyed to the right person.

Intellectual Disability and Genetic Abortion

Intellectual disability is a condition for which many parents are unwilling to accept a significant recurrence risk—hardly remarkable, since intellectual function is such an obvious attribute of humanness. The great majority of those who chose to have prenatal diagnosis opt for pregnancy termination[4] if a chromosomal condition implying major cognitive impairment is identified. Some for whom abortion is not acceptable may nevertheless choose prenatal diagnosis for reassurance or for the preparedness that certain knowledge can allow. Community views on intellectual disability are changing, and the late 20th century saw something of an exodus from institutions and from special schools as the intellectually and psychologically disabled joined the "mainstream," some more successfully than others. Many syndromes, in this Internet age, have their own support groups, and these are often a source of advocacy. Counselors need to handle the tension inherent in these views and the views of parents who want to avoid having a disabled child; and the separate conflict that parents experience when a decision is taken to terminate an otherwise wanted pregnancy. As we discussed earlier, the doctrine of nondirective counseling is a central tenet of modern practice, and it is a test of counselors' professionalism that their own views not unduly influence the advice and counsel that they give. De Crespigny et al. (1998) document the experiences and comments of a number of couples in their book *Prenatal Testing: Making Choices in Pregnancy*, intended for the lay public. Walters (1995) and Tillisch (2001) offer personal perspectives. First, Walters:

[3] For example, a claim for wrongful life concerning cri du chat syndrome was brought on behalf of the child in a legal case in Australia, whose birth followed a failed vasectomy (Watson 2002). The claim failed, the judge finding it impossible to compare and to place values on impaired existence versus non-existence. The concept of wrongful life is fully explored in Botkin (1988), but he sidesteps the central issue thus: "Is not a glimpse of life better than no life at all? I would not presume to answer these questions—the truth is that we will never know." Differing views from different jurisdictions are outlined in Frati et al. (2017).

[4] A sensitivity in discussing the choice of abortion may be discerned in the following conversation with her genetic counselor that Urquhart (2016) had: She writes: "'What about cases where people want to change the management of their pregnancy?' I asked, using the euphemism for abortion I had learned during our counseling sessions, 'We would have to investigate other options,' she said."

> Defending the right of women who are carrying babies with Down's syndrome to have abortions is not pleasant. Anyone who does so is likely to sound heartless, especially if they have no first-hand experience. It is even harder for me. I am the father of a Down's syndrome baby. . . . It is the most painful thing I will ever say but my wife, Karen and I, wish she had had a test. If she had, we would have terminated the pregnancy. I must be a callous swine, mustn't I? . . . Her birth was a tragedy, but not so different to any tragedy that can strike out of the blue, such as a crippling accident. Just as we work to avoid other tragedies, I see nothing wrong in using Down's tests to avoid the tragedy of human handicap. . . . I know that I would rather not have existed at all than to be, like her, sentenced to a life of confusion, frustration, pain and possibly loneliness when Karen and I are gone. If I feel guilt, it is that I was responsible for her birth. To me that guilt is far worse than anything I would have felt had I prevented it.

Tillisch is the mother of a child with the del(1)(p36) syndrome (p. 376). Anomalies had been detected on ultrasonography during the pregnancy, but an amniocentesis returned a normal cytogenetic result. The child had a stormy neonatal course, and in due course the chromosomal defect was identified. Tillisch writes:

> I'm so thankful that the amniocentesis results were inaccurate. Since we didn't learn of Kasey's diagnosis until she was 9 months old, we were able to get to know, love, and admire Kasey as an individual, as our daughter. We didn't allow doctors to define her for us. . . . From a mother's perspective, Kasey's future is bright. She receives treatment and will soon go to a public school. We will allow Kasey to show us her potential, rather than labeling her "severely mentally retarded" and casting her off to be locked away from society. . . . My father once asked, if I could ever make Kasey "whole," would I? Without any hesitation, I answered: absolutely not. Adding the missing genes would make Kasey a different person, a stranger.

These differing, one could say polar views of parents find some parallels in the positions of those whom we could consider as the philosophers of our profession. Lejeune, in a provocative address to the American Society of Human Genetics in 1970, deplored the application of his original cytogenetic discovery to the prenatal diagnosis of Down syndrome. Epstein (2002) reflected some three decades later upon Lejeune's influence, and while not stepping back from the standpoint that prenatal diagnosis is a proper and valid medical procedure, he does acknowledge (as must we) that a plurality of views exists, and that the genetics community must be sensitive to and must respect the range of views in the community.

Brock (1995) discusses the philosophy of "wrongful handicap," addressing the question of whether not producing a child who would suffer has harmed that potential child, and he enunciates a principle that

> individuals are morally required not to let any possible child for whose welfare they are responsible experience serious suffering or limited opportunity if they can act so that, without imposing substantial burdens or costs on themselves or others, any alternative possible child for whose welfare they would be responsible will not experience serious suffering or limited opportunity.

This position (somewhat reflecting that of Savulescu and Kahane, 2009, above) could be seen as providing an ethically based framework for making a decision to terminate an abnormal pregnancy, and to conceive again.

There are some subtleties in the choice of language when fetal anomalies are uncovered by ultrasound, as De Crespigny et al. (1996, 1999) discuss. We speak of the pregnant woman as a mother, yet she is not; neither is her husband/partner as yet a father. Equally, the fetus is not a baby, not acquiring that status until ex utero existence is achieved. But of course many parents-to-be, not to mention professionals, use these words. Counselors should be sensitive to these subtleties. De Crespigny observes that if an ultrasonologist should discover a fetal defect, using the terms "baby" and "mother" may exert indirect pressure on the couple to continue the pregnancy: And yet, on the other hand, many women regard a fetus as a baby from the very beginning, others will be affronted if their doctor does not seem to recognize this difference between a fetus and a baby, which they may interpret as interfering with the pregnant woman's reproductive freedom. As always, counselors will need to know their patients and to judge the right words to use and the way to say them (Benkendorf et al. 2001).

In recent years there has been a move away from the traditional deficit-based approach in medicine toward having a focus that builds on a person's strengths. Parents may feel that medicalized, deficit-focused language used in relation to their children overlooks their inherent value, and implies deficiency compared with children without disabilities. This, in turn, has negative impacts on the emotional well-being of children and their families (Strnadová et al. 2023). The counselor will wish to be at pains to adhere to this evolving principle.

Uncertain Discoveries at Prenatal Microarray

Conveying uncertainty is more difficult than giving definite information. Much experience has been accumulated in the decade or so during which microarray has become the main means of chromosome diagnosis, but not every microdeletion or microduplication is well understood. There is the complicating factor that some of these abnormalities may be pathogenic only in certain circumstances—that is, they can be nonpenetrant. This becomes a particular issue in prenatal diagnosis: If a microdeletion/duplication is a "new" finding and not listed in any database, what does one say to the parents? Brady et al. (2014) consider this question and come down in favor of not mentioning such discoveries, and they argue that rather than undermining parental reproductive rights, in fact this policy prevents giving a false sense of autonomy. Stark et al. (2013) and de Jong et al. (2014) reach similar conclusions. An alternative viewpoint is proposed by McGillivray et al. (2012), who suggest nondisclosure may smack of paternalism, notwithstanding the distress that an uncertain interpretation may bring to bear. Counselors are well aware of these challenges and controversies, and in a survey of US and Canadian genetic counselors, just over half had reservations about giving "ambiguous results" and saw this as an ethical issue (Mikhaelian et al. 2013).

PREGNANCY AND THE INTELLECTUALLY DISABLED

One issue to test the caliber of the bioethicist (not to mention the counselor) is that of the rights of people with intellectual disability to have children (Elkins et al. 1986a). What of the person with Down syndrome, or some partial trisomy compatible with fertility, in whom a question of procreation arises? Zühlke et al. (1994) give an example in describing a man with Down syndrome who developed a relationship with a girl with intellectual disability living in the same house. She requested removal of an intrauterine contraceptive device, became pregnant, and the (chromosomally normal) baby was brought up by the maternal grandmother. A case in Queensland, Australia, of a couple both with Down syndrome wishing to marry and to have children, came to public attention in 2016 through a popular television program.

On the one hand, the right of the disabled person to experience parenthood is debated, and the American Academy of Pediatrics Committee on Bioethics (1990) expressed reservation about the sterilization of women with intellectual disability on the basis of anticipated hardship to others. On the other hand, Gillon (1987) notes that other people have the option of being sterilized, and those with intellectual disability should have the same right. The Law Lords in Great Britain concur that sterilization may be in the best interest of the disabled person herself (Brahams 1987). Parizot et al. (2019) rehearse the evolving landscape with respect to persons with Down syndrome wishing to have children and possibly needing access to fertility treatment, given the sub/infertility associated with the condition.

Many parents or guardians, not wishing to become "parental grandparents," favor contraception. Although some regard hysterectomy as having the double benefit of ensuring sterility and facilitating personal hygiene, Grover (2011) highlights the availability of effective and less invasive options that have additional benefits, such that hysterectomy is rarely necessary. The High Court of Australia decided in 1992 that the parents of a disabled child cannot themselves lawfully allow sterilization but that a court authorization is required, and noted that this requirement "ensures a hearing from those experienced in different ways in the care of those with intellectual disability and from those with experience of the long term social and psychological effects of sterilization" (Monahan 1992).

When a woman with severe intellectual disability due to a chromosomal defect is pregnant—or is pregnant by a man with disability, one or other of the couple having an unbalanced karyotype—and the pregnancy is recognized in time, the grounds for termination may be seen as substantial. The ethical issue arises over the difficulty (or impossibility) of securing the woman's informed consent versus the expressed wishes of her guardians. Martínez et al. (1993) report from Alabama a mother with cri du chat syndrome, who was severely disabled and had no speech, pregnant by an unknown male; and "although pregnancy termination had been desired by the patient's grandmother, social and legal limitations prevented access to this procedure."

Strnadová et al. (2022) review the wide range of reactions of people with intellectual disability to the question of whether they would like to have children, whether they would choose to have testing during a pregnancy, and how they might respond to the result, and note how this range of opinions mirrors that of the general population. Some less severely affected persons may not regard it as undesirable to have a child like themselves;

on the other hand, they may recognize their own disability and not wish to pass it on. We may perhaps read this into the brief report of Bobrow et al. (1992) of a man with Down syndrome fathering a child, the mother having had first-trimester prenatal diagnosis (the baby's karyotype was normal). There is the concept of imagining what a person with disability would want, were he or she intellectually competent to make a decision—a concept some would regard as paternalistic (and infringing personal autonomy) and that others might see as valid and common sense. The sociology rather than the biology will exercise the counselor's mettle in this uncommonly encountered situation.

> Two approaches to a modification of genetic counseling for those with intellectual disabilities have been described, and with respect to the particular example of Williams syndrome (Farwig et al. 2010). Watkins et al. (1989) teach basic facts to the counselee, using simplified language and repetition as needed. In discussion, they use yes/no rather than open-ended questions. In contrast, Finucane (1998) takes a psychosocial approach in which a more conversational style, focusing on feelings and attitudes, takes precedence over the provision of facts. She argues that most individuals with intellectual disability reason concretely (in Piagetian terms, are in the preoperational or concrete operational periods of development, rather than in the formal operational period), do not understand numbers or quantity reliably, and tend to act egocentrically. She advises that it is important for the goals set by the genetic counselor to be limited, specific, concrete, and related to the reason for referral.

The other party is the child. Is having good parenting a right? What of a child with normal karyotype born, for example, to a man carrying a dup(10)(p13p14) chromosome and a mother with idiopathic intellectual disability? How can the interests of the child and of the parents be resolved? This is an actual case that we have seen (Voullaire et al. 2000a): It was quite poignant as this man with mild disability, who had some insight into his own disability, struggled to understand how best he might be a father to his 46,XX baby and expressed sadness at the abnormal behavior displayed by his older 46,XY,dup(10) child. The capable and willing grandmother stepped into the breach; but when the daughter is older, and assuming she is of normal intelligence, how will the realization of her parents' abnormality affect her? Whether a child with normal intelligence in this sort of setting has a legal claim for "dissatisfied life" is an intriguing and as yet (to our knowledge) untested notion (Pelias and Shaw 1986).

PARTICIPATION IN RESEARCH

There is much yet to learn about clinical cytogenetics, and much of this cannot be done without patient participation (a rather obvious statement, and one that applies to medicine generally). It is, of course, well enshrined that patients who are potential recruitees should be fully informed of the implications for themselves of a study in which they might be invited to participate, and that they have the opportunity to decline without compromise of their own health care. Having made that point, one can see a reciprocity in providing a health care service: The patient who benefits (often at the expense of the state) could be seen as having a moral duty at least to consider an invitation to be involved in a bona fide research study. And having made that point, the reality is that rather often, patients are very willing to come forward, and they gain some satisfaction in feeling that they may be making a contribution toward the greater good. The altruism gene shines brightly in many people.

Rafii and Fortea (2023) propose that adults with Down syndrome would be willing to make themselves available for the study of anti-Alzheimer treatments, an approach that might prove of very wide benefit. Ramsay et al. (2009) examined the attitudes toward research participation of parents whose child had had an abnormality shown at prenatal ultrasound. To quote these authors:

> The balance falls between the possibility of causing upset to parents, particularly those with handicapped or ill children, and the possibility of gaining new knowledge that may prove important to parents deciding whether or not to continue their pregnancy after diagnosis of a fetal abnormality.

Their study in fact demonstrated that

> . . . the great majority of respondents indicated they would be happy to be contacted to provide information on their children's health and development. . . . Research ethics committees can be reassured that the risk of causing inappropriate and unnecessary parental distress by inviting them to take part in such studies is low.

THE COUNSELOR AS ETHICIST

From the foregoing, it is clear that the counselor must be well-attuned to the evolving landscape of what is regarded as proper ethical behavior. We do not, in this book, set ourselves up as moral arbiters; we can merely comment as we have above, that views change, practice matures, and counselors will, in simple terms, want to do their best by those they see in the clinic.

APPENDIXES

APPENDIX A

IDEOGRAMS OF HUMAN CHROMOSOMES

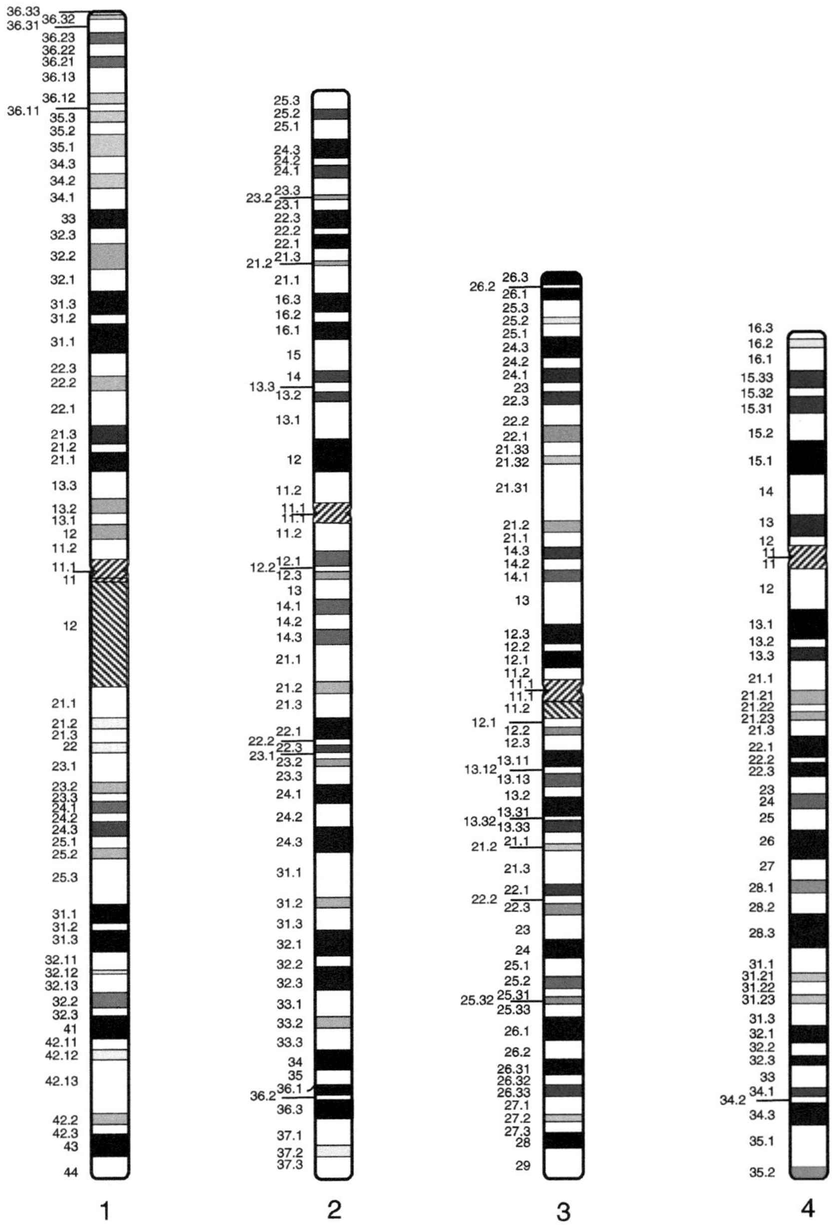

Figure A–1. These depictions represent the bands that can be distinguished at a very high level (850 band) of cytogenetic resolution. Different shadings and lengths of bands reflect actual intensities and lengths as observed by the cytogeneticist.

Source: From NL Chia, in ISCN 2024, An International System for Human Cytogenomic Nomenclature, *Cytogenet Genome Res* 164(Suppl 1):1–224, 2024. Courtesy NL Chia, and with the permission of Karger.

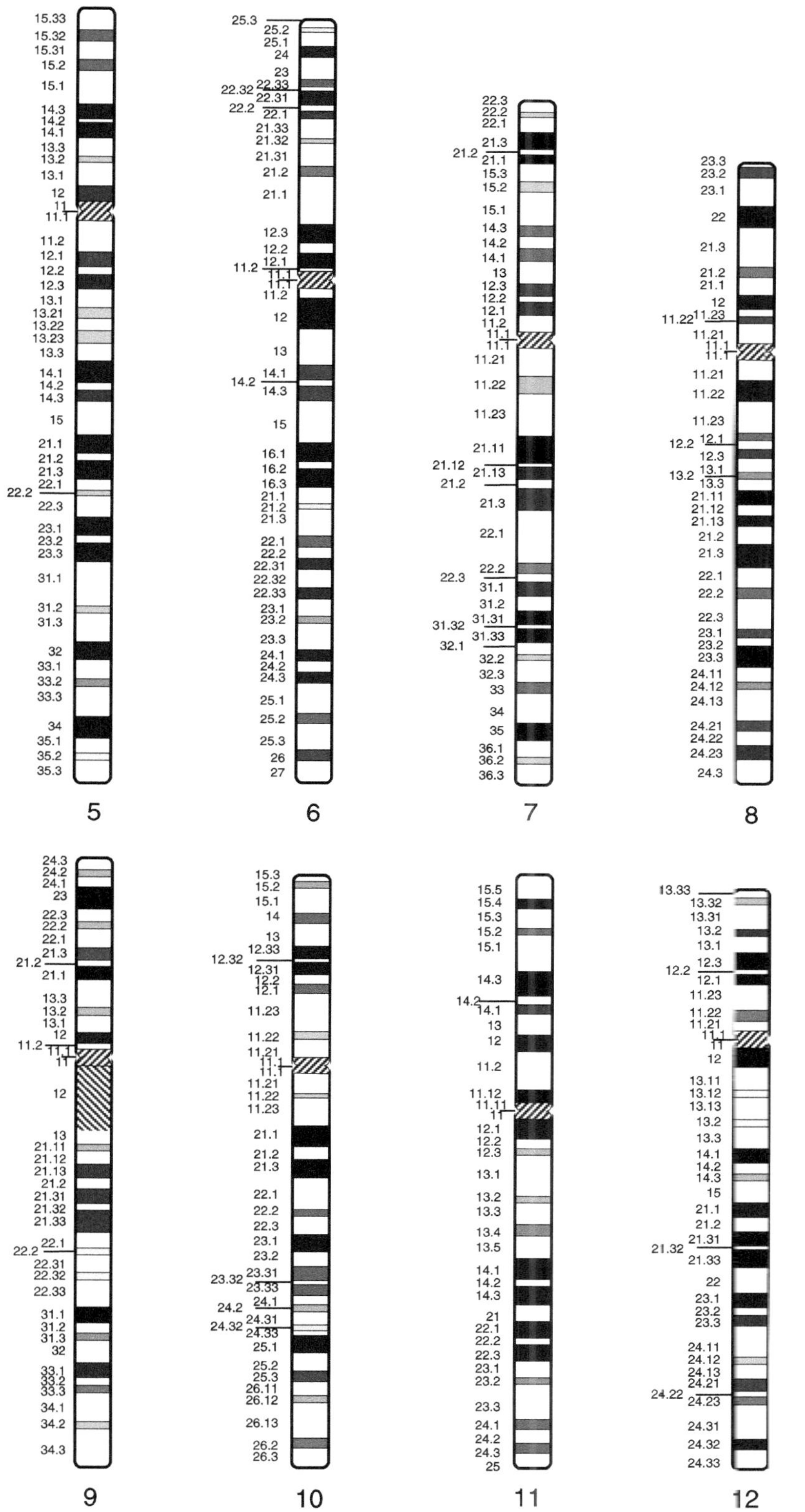

Figure A–1. Continued

Table A–1. The Nucleotide Content and Percentage of Haploid Autosomal Length (HAL) that Each Chromosome Constitutes

CHROMOSOME	Mb (hg38)	HAL % (hg38)	HAL % (DANIEL)
1	248.96	8.66	9.24
2	242.19	8.42	8.02
3	198.30	6.90	6.83
4	190.21	6.62	6.3
5	181.54	6.31	6.08
6	170.81	5.94	5.9
7	159.35	5.54	5.36
8	145.14	5.05	4.93
9	138.39	4.81	4.8
10	133.80	4.65	4.59
11	135.09	4.70	4.61
12	133.28	4.64	4.66
13	114.36	3.98	3.74
14	107.04	3.72	3.56
15	101.99	3.55	3.46
16	90.34	3.14	3.36
17	83.26	2.90	3.46
18	80.37	2.80	2.93
19	58.62	2.04	2.67
20	64.44	2.24	2.56
21	46.71	1.62	1.9
22	50.82	1.77	2.04
Autosomal length	2,875.00	100.00	
X	156.04		
Y	57.23		
Genome	3,088.27		

Source: From Daniel (1985), and UCSC Genome Browser.

APPENDIX B

ABBREVIATIONS AND CYTOGENETIC NOMENCLATURE

CYTOGENETICS HAS its own jargon and fondness for acronyms, and certain abbreviations are regularly used. The ICSN (itself an abbreviation for International System of Cytogenetic Nomenclature; ISCN, 2024) provides formally approved abbreviations, several of which are set out below (Table B–1) and, following this, we list another set of abbreviations (including a number of clinical expressions) that are used fairly frequently in this book and in many genetics journals and which should be familiar to the reader (Table B–2).

Table B–1. Some ISCN Abbreviations

add	Additional material of unknown origin
cht	Chromatid
del	Deletion
der	Derivative chromosome
dic	Dicentric chromosome
dn	De novo
dup	Duplication
fis	Fission (at the centromere)
fra	Fragile site
h	Heterochromatin
i	Isochromosome
idem	"The same" (to avoid repetition of complex description in a mosaic case)
ins	Insertion
dir ins	Direct insertion
inv ins	Inverted insertion
ish	In situ hybridization
inv	Inversion
mar	Marker chromosome
mat	Maternal origin
min	Minute chromosome
minus (–)	Loss of a whole chromosome
mos	Mosaic
neo	Neocentromere

(*continued*)

Table B–1. Continued

p	Short arm
pat	Paternal origin
plus (+)	Gain of a whole chromosome
q	Long arm
r	Ring
rcp	Reciprocal translocation
rea	Rearrangement
rec	Recombinant chromosome
rob	Robertsonian translocation
solidus (/)	Separates cell lines in describing mosaics. Two, as //, apply to chimerism
t	Translocation
tan	Tandem
tas	Telomeric association
ter	Terminal (end of chromosome arm)
upd	Uniparental disomy

Table B–2. Some Other Commonly Used Abbreviations

abn(X)	An abnormal X chromosome
aCGH	Array comparative genomic hybridization
AFP	Alpha-fetoprotein
arr	Array (microarray)
AS	Angelman syndrome
AT	Ataxia-telangiectasia
BAC	Bacterial artificial chromosome
CGH	Comparative genomic hybridization
CNV	Copy number variant
CpG	Cytosine-guanine DNA sequence
CPM	Confined placental mosaicism
CVS	Chorionic villus sampling
DGS	DiGeorge syndrome
DMR	Differentially methylated region
DS	Down syndrome
ECARUCA	European Cytogeneticists Association Register of Unbalanced Chromosome Aberrations
EEG	Electroencephalogram
ESAC	Extra structurally abnormal chromosome
ESHRE	European Society for Human Reproduction and Embryology
EUCROMIC	European Collaborative Research Group on Mosaicism in CVS
FA	Fanconi anemia

Table B–2. Continued

FISH	Fluorescence in situ hybridization
HAL	Haploid autosomal length
ICSI	Intracytoplasmic sperm injection
IUGR	Intrauterine growth retardation
IVF	In vitro fertilization
kb	Kilobases of DNA
LCRs	Low copy repeats
Mb	Megabases of DNA
MCA/MR	Multiple congenital anomalies/mental retardation
MLPA	Multiplex ligation-dependent probe analysis
MRI	Magnetic resonance imaging (an organ imaging modality)
mtDNA	Mitochondrial DNA
NAHR	Nonallelic homologous recombination
NGS	Next-generation sequencing
NHEJ	Nonhomologous end joining
NIPT	Noninvasive prenatal testing
NOR	Nucleolar organizing region
nt	Nucleotide
OMIM	Online Mendelian Inheritance in Man catalog
PAR (1 and 2)	Pseudoautosomal region (primary and secondary)
PB (1 and 2)	Polar body (first and second)
PCD	Premature centromere division
PCR	Polymerase chain reaction
PGD	Preimplantation diagnosis
PGD-A	Preimplantation diagnosis for aneuploidy screening
PND	Prenatal diagnosis
POF	Premature ovarian failure
PWACR	Prader-Willi/Angelman critical region
PWS	Prader-Willi syndrome
QF-PCR	Quantitative fluorescent polymerase chain reaction
RPL	Recurrent pregnancy loss
SCE	Sister chromatid exchange
SD	Standard deviation
SMC	Supernumerary marker chromosome
snoRNA	Small nucleolar RNA
SNP	Single nucleotide polymorphism
TS	Turner syndrome
UCSC	University of California at Santa Cruz (hosts a Genome Browser)
UPD	Uniparental disomy

The nomenclature has evolved to accommodate the growing complexity of cytogenetics, with the earlier nomenclatures issued since the first in 1960 often referred to by the name of the city in which the committee met (Denver, London, Chicago, Paris), and subsequently more anonymously as ISCN (year). Published papers from the earlier years will, of course, have used the nomenclature of their time. Many old papers remain a valuable resource, particularly case reports. The reader consulting these may therefore need to adjust and learn to handle earlier (generally simpler) versions of cytogenetic nomenclature.

APPENDIX C

PENETRANCE DATA FOR CERTAIN COPY NUMBER VARIANTS

Genomic coordinates of 82 copy number variants (CNVs) from nine studies and their pooled penetrance estimate from these nine studies compared against gnomAD controls, based on the systematic review of Goh et al. (2025). Penetrance is for a combination of intellectual disability, developmental delay, autism, congenital malformations, and miscellaneous other phenotypes depending on the studies involved in contributing data. It is to be noted that for many CNVs, the sample sizes are small and the confidence intervals of penetrance estimates are wide. Additional information about individual CNVs is presented in Chapters 14 and 18.

Copy number variant	Landmark Loci	Genomic coordinates (GRCh38) Mb (approximate)	Deletion/ Duplication	Penetrance (95% confidence interval) %
1p36 deletion and 1p36 duplication	*GABRD*	1:0.0–10.0	Del	100 (94–100)
			Dup	100 (85–100)
1q21.1 proximal deletion and 1q21.1 proximal duplication	*RBM8A*	1:144.0–144.5	Del	18 (9–27)
			Dup	9 (7–11)
1q21.1 distal deletion and 1q21.1 distal duplication	*GJA5*	1:147.1–147.9	Del	30 (23–38)
			Dup	19 (14–25)
2p16.3 deletion	*NRXN1*	2:49.9–51.0	Del	37 (21–51)
2q11.2 deletion	*TMEM127*	2:96.1–97.0	Del	10 (0–27)^{NS}
2q13 proximal deletion and 2q13 proximal duplication	*NPHP1*	2:110.1–110.2	Del	4 (3.6–5)^{NS}
			Dup	6 (4.8–7)^{NS}
2q23.1 deletion	*MBD5*	2:148.0–148.5	Del	100 (78–100)
2q37 deletion and 2q37 duplication	*HDAC4*	2:238.8–241.5	Del	100 (78–100)
			Dup	47 (0–100)^{NS}
3q29 deletion and 3q29 duplication	*DLG1*	3:196.0–197.6	Del	52 (33–80)
			Dup	67 (45–92)
4p16.3 deletion (Wolf-Hirschhorn Syndrome) and 4p16.3 duplication		4:1.9–2.0	Del	100 (74–100)
			Dup	37 (8–100)
5q35.3 deletion (Sotos Syndrome) and 5q35.3 duplication	*NSD1*	5:176.3–177.6	Del	100 (69–100)
			Dup	100 (31–100)
6p25 deletion and 6p25 duplication		6:0.2–6.1	Del	100 (80–100)
			Dup	100 (69–100)
6q16 deletion and 6q16 duplication	*SIM1*	6:100.37–100.50	Del	17 (0–100)^{NS}
			Dup	11 (0–48)^{NS}

(continued)

Copy number variant	Landmark Loci	Genomic coordinates (GRCh38) Mb (approximate)	Deletion/ Duplication	Penetrance (95% confidence interval) %
7q11.23 deletion (Williams-Beuren Syndrome) and 7q11.23 duplication		7:73.3–74.7	Del	93 (85–100)
			Dup	67 (50–87)
8p23.1 deletion and 8p23.1 duplication	*CLDN23, SOX7, GATA4*	8:8.2–12.0	Del	100 (77–100)
			Dup	100 (79–100)
9q34 deletion (Kleefstra syndrome) and duplication	*EHMT1*	9:134.9–138.29	Del	100 (76–100)
			Dup	100 (53–100)
10q23 deletion and 10q23 duplication	*NRG3, GRID1, BMPR1A*	10:80.2–87.0	Del	82 (62–100)
			Dup	27 (6–61)
13q12 deletion	*CRYL1*	13:20.2–20.4	Del	5 (3–8)^{NS}
15q11.2 deletion [BP1-BP2] and 15q11.2 duplication	*NIPA1, NIPA2*	15:22.8–23.1	Del	10 (9–12)
			Dup	5 (4–6)^{NS}
15q11.2 deletion [BP1-BP3] and 15q11.2 duplication (*NIPA1, NIPA2*, Prader-Willi Syndrome/Angelman Syndrome)		15:22.8–28.1	Del	100 (55–100)
			Dup	54 (40–73)
15q11q13 deletion [BP2-BP3] (Prader-Willi Syndrome/Angelman Syndrome) and 15q11q13 duplication		15:24.6–28.2	Del	100 (92–100)
			Dup	77 (65–88)
15q13.3 deletion [BP4-BP5] and 15q13.3 duplication	*CHRNA7*	15:30.8–32.2	Del	55 (45–66)
			Dup	8 (5–11)
15q13.3 smaller deletion and 15q13.3 smaller duplication	*CHRNA7* and *OTUD7A* only	15:31.7–32.2	Del	Insufficient data
			Dup	Insufficient data
15q24 deletion and 15q24 duplication	*BBS4, PML, SIN3A*	15:72.6–75.5	Del	100 (53–100)
			Dup	37 (7–100)
15q24.2q24.3 deletion and 15q24.2q24.3 duplication	*FBXO22, TSPAN3*	15:75.7–77.9	Del	69 (28–100)
			Dup	73 (31–100)
15q25.2 proximal deletion and 15q25.2 proximal duplication	*RPS17, HOMER2, BNC1*	15:82.5–84.1	Del	100 (0–100)^{NS}
			Dup	71 (24–100)
16p13.3 deletion (Rubinstein-Taybi Syndrome)	*CREBBP*	16:3.7–3.9	Del	82 (48–100)
16p13.11 deletion and 16p13.11 duplication	*MYH11*	16:15.4–16.2	Del	23 (18–29)
			Dup	10 (8–11)

Copy number variant	Landmark Loci	Genomic coordinates (GRCh38) Mb (approximate)	Deletion/ Duplication	Penetrance (95% confidence interval) %
16p12.2 deletion (previously 16p12.1 deletion) and 16p12.2 duplication (previously 16p12.1 duplication)	*CDR2*	16:21.9–22.5	Del	16 (12–20)
			Dup	5 (3–7)[NS]
16p11.2p12.2 deletion (previously 16p11.2p12.1) and 16p11.2p12.2 duplication (previously 16p11.2p12.1 duplication)		16:21.3–29.4	Del	100 (78–100)
			Dup	100 (69–100)
16p11.2 distal deletion and 16p11.2 distal duplication	*SH2B1*	16:28.8–29.1	Del	33 (24–44)
			Dup	16 (11–22)
16p11.2 proximal deletion and 16p11.2 proximal duplication	*TBX6*	16:29.6–30.2	Del	47 (40–55)
			Dup	33 (28–41)
17p13.3 deletion and 17p13.3 duplication	*YWHAE*	17:0.7–1.5	Del	100 (47–100)
			Dup	41 (15–65)
17p13.3 deletion and 17p13.3 duplication	*PAFAH1B1*	17:2.5–3.0	Del	100 (53–100)
			Dup	79 (34–100)
17p12 deletion (Hereditary Neuropathy with Liability to Pressure Palsies) and 17p12 duplication (Charcot Marie Tooth)*	*PMP22*	17:14.2–15.6	Del	2 (0–4)
			Dup	11 (6–17)
17p11.2 deletion (Smith-Magenis Syndrome) and 17p11.2 duplication (Potocki-Lupski Syndrome)	*RAI1*	17:16.8–20.6	Del	100 (82–100)
			Dup	92 (75–100)
17q11.2 deletion (Neurofibromatosis Type 1) and 17q11.2 duplication	*NF1*	17:30.8–31.9	Del	81 (61–100)
			Dup	74 (54–93)
17q12 deletion (Renal Cysts and Diabetes) and 17q12 duplication	*HNF1B*	17:36.5–37.9	Del	63 (45–85)
			Dup	20 (14–27)
17q21.31 deletion (Koolen-de Vries Syndrome) and 17q21.31 duplication	*MAPT, KANSL1*	17:45.6–46.1	Del	100 (88–100)
			Dup	69 (31–100)
17q23 deletion and 17q23 duplication	*TBX2, TBX4*	17:60.2–62.2	Del	100 (47–100)
			Dup	31 (0–100)[NS]
19p13.12 deletion		19:13.0–16.6	Del	100 (67–100)

(continued)

Copy number variant	Landmark Loci	Genomic coordinates (GRCh38) Mb (approximate)	Deletion/ Duplication	Penetrance (95% confidence interval) %
22q11.2 deletion Velocardiofacial Syndrome and 22q11.2 duplication	*TBX1*	22:18.3–21.2	Del Dup	86 (79–94) 19 (16–23)
22q11.2 distal deletion and 22q11.2 distal duplication	*BCR, MAPK1*	22:21.6–23.3	Del Dup	91 (74–100) 51 (32–77)
22q13.33 deletion Phelan-McDermid Syndrome and 22q13.33 duplication	*SHANK3*	22:50.7–50.7	Del Dup	93 (84–100) Insufficient data

Notes: Penetrance is for a combination of intellectual disability, developmental delay, autism, congenital malformations, and miscellaneous other phenotypes depending on the studies involved in contributing data. [NS]The prevalences of this CNV in control and affected cohorts are not significantly different (P > .05).

*The data for 17p12 exclude the fully penetrant nature of *PMP22* imbalance in causing a neuropathy. WHS = Wolf-Hirschhorn syndrome.

Source: From S Goh et al., A systematic review and pooled analysis of penetrance estimates of copy-number variants associated with neurodevelopment, *Genet Med* 27:101227, 2025. Courtesy S Goh, and with the permission of Elsevier.

REFERENCES

A

Aagaard KS, Brusgaard K, Miceikaite I, et al. Chromosomal translocation disrupting the SMAD4 gene resulting in the combined phenotype of Juvenile polyposis syndrome and Hereditary Hemorrhagic Telangiectasia. *Mol Genet Genomic Med* 8:e1498, 2020.

Aarabi M, Baumann J, Babcock M, et al. Chromosome 2q12.3-q13 copy number variants in patients with neurodevelopmental disorders: genotype-phenotype correlation and new hotspots. *Psychiatr Genet* 32:171–177, 2022.

Abalı ZY, Guran T. Diagnosis and management of non-CAH 46,XX disorders/differences in sex development. *Front Endocrinol (Lausanne)* 15:1354759, 2024.

Abarca-Barriga HH, Trubnykova M, Chavesta-Velásquez F, Barletta-Carrillo C, Ordoñez-Linares M, Rondón-Abuhadba A. Peruvian newborn male with 3p13 deletion syndrome encompassing the *FOXP1* gene: Review of the literature. *J Pediatr Genet* 9:270–278, 2020.

Abaied L, Trabelsi M, Chaabouni M, et al. A novel UBE3A truncating mutation in large Tunisian Angelman syndrome pedigree. *Am J Med Genet* 152A:141–146, 2010.

Abe KT, Rizzo IMPO, Coelho ALV, Sakai N Jr, Carvalho DR, Speck-Martins CE. 19q13.11 microdeletion: Clinical features overlapping ectrodactyly ectodermal dysplasia-clefting syndrome phenotype. *Clin Case Rep* 6:1300–1307, 2018.

Abeliovich D, Dagan J, Lerer I, Silberstein S, Katznelson MB, Frydman M. t(15;21)(q15;q22.1) pat resulting in partial trisomy and partial monosomy of chromosomes 15 and 21 in two offspring. *Am J Med Genet* 66:45–51, 1996.

Abeliovich D, Yagupsky P, Bashan N. 3:1 meiotic disjunction in a mother with a balanced translocation, 46,XX,t(5,14)(p15;q13) resulting in tertiary trisomy and tertiary monosomy offspring. *Am J Med Genet* 12:83–89, 1982.

Abrams DJ, Aronoff AR, Berend SA, Roa BB, Shaffer LG, Geier MR. Prenatal diagnosis of a homologous Robertsonian translocation involving chromosome 15. *Prenat Diagn* 21:676–679, 2001.

Abrams DJ, Augustyn AM, Geier MR. Prenatally diagnosed mosaic trisomy 17: A case report with two-year follow-up. *Prenat Diagn* 25:968–969, 2005.

Abrams L, Cotter PD. Prenatal diagnosis of de novo X;autosome translocations. *Clin Genet* 65:423–428, 2004.

Abreu LS, Brassesco MS, Moreira ML, Pina-Neto JM. Case report. Familial balanced translocation leading to an offspring with phenotypic manifestations of 9p syndrome. *Genet Mol Res* 13:4302–4310, 2014.

Abuelo DN, Barsel-Bowers G, Richardson A. Insertional translocations: Report of two new families and review of the literature. *Am J Med Genet* 31:319–329, 1988.

Abur U, Gunes S, Hekim N, Akar OS, Altundag E, Asci R. Clinical, cytogenomic, and molecular characterization of isodicentric Y-chromosome and prediction of testicular sperm retrieval outcomes in azoospermic and severe oligozoospermic infertile men. *J Assist Reprod Genet* 39:2799–2810, 2022.

Acreman ML, Bussolaro S, Raymond YC, Fantasia I, Rolnik DL, Da Silva Costa F. The predictive value of prenatal cell-free DNA testing for rare autosomal trisomies: A systematic review and meta-analysis. *Am J Obstet Gynecol* 228:292–305.e6, 2023.

Adachi M, Tachibana K, Asakura Y, Muroya K, Ogata T. Del(X)(p21.1) in a mother and two daughters: Genotype-phenotype correlation of Turner features. *Hum Genet* 106:306–310, 2000.

Adeyokunnu AA. The incidence of Down's syndrome in Nigeria. *J Med Genet* 19:277–279, 1982.

Adhvaryu SG, Peters-Brown T, Livingston E, Qumsiyeh MB. Familial supernumerary marker chromosome evolution through three generations. *Prenat Diagn* 18:178–181, 1998.

Adler A, Lee HL, McCulloh DH, et al. Blastocyst culture selects for euploid embryos: Comparison of blastomere and trophectoderm biopsies. *Reprod Biomed Online* 28:485–491, 2014.

Adriaens I, Smitz J, Jacquet P. The current knowledge on radiosensitivity of ovarian follicle development stages. *Hum Reprod Update* 15:359–377, 2009.

Amor DJ, Bentley K, Ryan J, et al. Human centromere repositioning "in progress." *Proc Natl Acad Sci USA* 101:6542–6547, 2004.

Amor DJ, Cameron C. PGD gender selection for non-Mendelian disorders with unequal sex incidence. *Hum Reprod* 23:729–734, 2008.

Amor DJ, Choo KHA. Neocentromeres: Role in human disease, evolution, and centromere study. *Am J Hum Genet* 71:695–714, 2002.

Amor DJ, De Crespigny L, Gardner RJM. Urinary tract defects and chromosomal disorders. In Flinter F (ed.), *The Genetics of Renal Disease*. Oxford, UK: Oxford University Press, 2003.

Amor D, Delatycki MB, Susman M, et al. 46,XX/46,XY at amniocentesis in a fetus with true hermaphroditism. *J Med Genet* 36:866–869, 1999.

Amor DJ, Halliday J. A review of known imprinting syndromes and their association with assisted reproduction technologies. *Hum Reprod* 23:2826–2834, 2008.

Amor DJ, Neo WT, Waters E, Heussler H, Pertile M, Halliday J. Health and developmental outcome of children following prenatal diagnosis of confined placental mosaicism. *Prenat Diagn* 26:443–448, 2006.

Amor DJ, Voullaire L, Bentley K, Savarirayan R, Choo KH. Mosaic monosomy of a neocentric ring chromosome maps brachyphalangy and growth hormone deficiency to 13q31.1–13q32.3. *Am J Med Genet* 133A:151–157, 2005.

Amor DJ, Xu JX, Halliday JL, et al. Pregnancies conceived using assisted reproductive technologies (ART) have low levels of pregnancy-associated plasma protein-A (PAPP-A) leading to a high rate of false-positive results in first trimester screening for Down syndrome. *Hum Reprod* 24:1330–1338, 2009.

Amyere M, Aerts V, Brouillard P, et al. Somatic uniparental isodisomy explains multifocality of glomuvenous malformations. *Am J Hum Genet* 92:188–196, 2013.

Anahory T, Hamamah S, Andreo B, et al. Sperm segregation analysis of a (13;22) Robertsonian translocation carrier by FISH: A comparison of locus-specific probe and whole chromosome painting. *Hum Reprod* 20:1850–1854, 2005.

Anastasiadou K, Silva M, Booth T, et al. Detection of chromosomal aneuploidy in ancient genomes. *Commun Biol* 7, 14, 2024.

Anderlid BM, Sahlén S, Schoumans J, et al. Detailed characterization of 12 supernumerary ring chromosomes using micro-FISH and search for uniparental disomy. *Am J Med Genet* 99:223–233, 2001.

Andó S, Koczok K, Bessenyei B, Balogh I, Ujfalusi A. Cytogenetic investigation of infertile patients in Hungary: A 10-year retrospective study. *Genes (Basel)* 13:2086, 2022.

Aneja K, Krishnan S. Prenatal ultrasound assisted diagnosis of de-novo terminal 7q deletion syndrome: A case report with literature review. *Radiol Case Rep* 20:756–760, 2024.

Angell R. First-meiotic-division nondisjunction in human oocytes. *Am J Hum Genet* 61:23–32, 1997.

Angell RR, Aitken RJ, van Look PF, Lumsden MA, Templeton AA. Chromosome abnormalities in human embryos after in vitro fertilization. *Nature* 303:336–338, 1983.

Anger GJ, Crocker S, McKenzie K, et al. X-linked deafness-2 (DFNX2) phenotype associated with a paracentric inversion upstream of POU3F4. *Am J Audiol* 23:1–6, 2014.

Anlaş Ö, Ölmez A, Karaman B, et al. Dicentric recombinant chromosome 18 due to maternal paracentric inversion analyzed by array CGH. *Mol Syndromol* 14:246–253, 2023.

Annable K, Donnenfeld AE, Fischer RL, Knops J. Prenatal diagnosis of a jumping translocation. *Prenat Diagn* 28:767–769, 2008.

Antoccia A, Kobayashi J, Tauchi H, Matsuura S, Komatsu K. Nijmegen breakage syndrome and functions of the responsible protein, NBS1. *Genome Dyn* 1:191–205, 2006.

Anton E, Blanco J, Egozcue J, Vidal F. Sperm studies in heterozygote inversion carriers: A review. *Cytogenet Genome Res* 111:297–304, 2005.

Anton E, Vidal F, Blanco J. Interchromosomal effect analyses by sperm FISH: Incidence and distribution among reorganization carriers. *Syst Biol Reprod Med* 57:268–278, 2011.

Antonarakis SE, Avramopoulos D, Blouin JL, Talbot CC, Schinzel AA. Mitotic errors in somatic cells cause trisomy 21 in about 4.5% of cases and are not associated with advanced maternal age. *Nat Genet* 3:146–150, 1993.

Antonarakis SE, Skotko BG, Rafii MS, et al. Down syndrome. *Nat Rev Dis Primers* 6:9, 2020.

Anzick S, Thurm A, Burkett S, et al. Chromoanasynthesis as a cause of Jacobsen syndrome. *Am J Med Genet* 182A:2533–2539, 2020.

Apacik C, Cohen M, Jakobeit M, et al. Two brothers with multiple congenital anomalies and mental retardation due to disomy (X)(q12→q13.3) inherited from the mother. *Clin Genet* 50:63–73, 1996.

Aradhya S, Smaoui N, Marble M, Lacassie Y. De novo duplication 11p13 involving the *PAX6* gene in a patient with neonatal seizures, hypotonia, microcephaly, developmental disability and minor ocular manifestations. *Am J Med Genet* 155A:442–444, 2011.

Archibald AD, Massie J, Smith MJ, Dalton DG, du Sart D, Amor DJ. Population-based genetic carrier screening for cystic fibrosis in Victoria. *Med J Aust* 200:205–206, 2014.

Ardalan A, Prieur M, Choiset A, Turleau C, Goutieres F, Girard-Orgeolet S. Intrachromosomal insertion mimicking a pericentric inversion: Molecular cytogenetic characterization of a three break rearrangement of chromosome 20. *Am J Med Genet* 138A:288–293, 2005.

Arens YHJM, Engelen JJM, Govaerts LCP, et al. Familial insertion (3;5)(q25.3;q22.1q31.3) with deletion or duplication of chromosome region 5q22.1–5q31.3 in ten unbalanced carriers. *Am J Med Genet* 130A:128–133, 2004.

Argiropoulos B, Carter M, Brierley K, et al. Discordant phenotypes in a mother and daughter with mosaic supernumerary ring chromosome 19 explained by a de novo 7q36.2 deletion and 7p22.1 duplication. *Am J Med Genet* 155A:885–991, 2011.

Aristidou C, Theodosiou A, Alexandrou A, et al. Exploring the genetic causality of discordant phenotypes in familial apparently balanced translocation cases using whole exome sequencing. *Genes (Basel)* 14:82, 2022.

Armour CM, Dougan SD, Brock JA, et al. Practice guideline: Joint CCMG-SOGC recommendations for the use of chromosomal microarray analysis for prenatal diagnosis and assessment of fetal loss in Canada. *J Med Genet* 55:215–221, 2018.

Armstrong L, McGowan-Jordan J, Brierley K, Allanson JE. De novo dup(X)(q22.3q26) in a girl with evidence that functional disomy of X material is the cause of her abnormal phenotype. *Am J Med Genet* 116A:71–76, 2003.

Arnedo N, Nogués C, Bosch M, Templado C. Mitotic and meiotic behaviour of a naturally transmitted ring Y chromosome: Reproductive risk evaluation. *Hum Reprod* 20:462–468, 2005.

Arora V, Aggarwal S, Bijarnia S, et al. Extending the phenotype and identification of a novel candidate gene for immunodeficiency in 5q11 microdeletion syndrome. *Mol Syndromol* 9:312–318, 2019.

Arsham MS, Barch MJ, Lawce HJ (eds.), *The AGT Cytogenetics Laboratory Manual*. John Wiley & Sons, Hoboken, 2017.

Ashley T, Gaeth AP, Inagaki H, et al. Meiotic recombination and spatial proximity in the etiology of the recurrent t(11;22). *Am J Hum Genet* 79:524–538, 2006.

Atli EI, Yalcintepe S, Atli E, Demir S, Mail C, Gurkan H. Clinical implications of chromosome 16 copy number variation. *Mol Syndromol* 13:184–192, 2022.

Attree O, Olivos IM, Okabe I, et al. The Lowe's oculocerebrorenal syndrome gene encodes a protein highly homologous to inositol polyphosphate-5-phosphatase. *Nature* 358:239–242, 1992.

Aughton DJ, AlSaadi AA, Canady AI, Lucas BM. Balanced reciprocal translocation mosaicism associated with an abnormal phenotype. *Am J Med Genet* 45:721–724, 1993.

Austad T. The right not to know—worthy of preservation any longer? An ethical perspective. *Clin Genet* 50:85–88, 1996.

Austin JC. Evidence-based genetic counseling for psychiatric disorders: A road map. *Cold Spring Harb Perspect Med* 10:a036608, 2020.

Auwerx C, Jõeloo M, Sadler MC, et al. Rare copy-number variants as modulators of common disease susceptibility. *Genome Med* 16:5, 2024a.

Auwerx C, Kutalik Z, Reymond A. The pleiotropic spectrum of proximal 16p11.2 CNVs. *Am J Hum Genet* 111:2309–2346, 2024b.

Avagliano L, Parenti I, Grazioli P, et al. Chromatinopathies: A focus on Cornelia de Lange syndrome. *Clin Genet* 97:3–11, 2020.

Avila M, Kirchhoff M, Marle N, et al. Delineation of a new chromosome 20q11.2 duplication syndrome including the *ASXL1* gene. *Am J Med Genet* 161A:1594–1598, 2013.

Awa AA, Honda T, Neriishi S, et al. Cytogenetic study of the offspring of atomic bomb survivors, Hiroshima and Nagasaki. In Obe G, Basler A (eds.), *Cytogenetics: Basic and Applied Aspects*. Berlin: Springer-Verlag, 1987.

Aydın C, Kıral E, Susam E, et al. A case of familial recurrent 17q12 microdeletion syndrome presenting with severe diabetic ketoacidosis. *Turk J Pediatr* 64:558–565, 2022.

Ayub S, Gadji M, Krabchi K, et al., Three new cases of terminal deletion of the long arm of chromosome 7 and literature review to correlate genotype and phenotype manifestations. *Am J Med Genet* 170A:896–907, 2016.

Ayukawa H, Tsukahara M, Fukuda M, Kondoh O. Recombinant chromosome 18 resulting from a maternal pericentric inversion. *Am J Med Genet* 50:323–325, 1994.

B

Baarends WM, van der Laan R, Grootegoed JA. DNA repair mechanisms and gametogenesis. *Reproduction* 121:31–39, 2001.

Babatz TD, Kumar RA, Sudi J, Dobyns WB, Christian SL. Copy number and sequence variants implicate APBA2 as an autism candidate gene. *Autism Res* 2:359–364, 2009.

Babbs C, Brown J, Horsley SW, et al. ATR-16 syndrome: Mechanisms linking monosomy to phenotype. *J Med Genet* 57:414–421, 2020.

Babu R, Shah U. Gender identity disorder (GID) in adolescents and adults with differences of sex development (DSD): A systematic review and meta-analysis. *J Pediatr Urol* 17:39–47, 2021.

Bache I, Brondum-Nielsen K, Tommerup N. Genetic counseling in adult carriers of a balanced chromosomal rearrangement ascertained in childhood: Experiences from a nationwide reexamination of translocation carriers. *Genet Med* 9:185–187, 2007.

Baena N, De Vigan C, Cariati E, et al. Prenatal detection of rare chromosomal autosomal abnormalities in Europe. *Am J Med Genet* 118A:319–327, 2003.

Baena N, De Vigan C, Cariati E, et al. Turner syndrome: Evaluation of prenatal diagnosis in 19 European registries. *Am J Med Genet* 129A:16–20, 2004.

Baetens D, Stoop H, Peelman F, et al. NR5A1 is a novel disease gene for 46,XX testicular and ovotesticular disorders of sex development. *Genet Med* 19:367–376, 2017.

Baetens D, Verdin H, De Baere E, Cools M. Update on the genetics of differences of sex development (DSD). *Best Pract Res Clin Endocrinol Metab* 33:101271, 2019.

Bagshawe KD, Lawler SD. Unmasking moles. *Br J Obstet Gynaecol* 89:255–257, 1982.

Bahçe M, Oõur G, Ýmirzalýoõlu N, et al. Repeated fetal loss in two related first cousin marriages with couples all carrying the same translocation t(13q;14q). *Eur J Hum Genet* 4:35–36, 1996.

Baidas S, Chen TJ, Kolev V, et al. Constitutional trisomy 8 mosaicism due to meiosis II non-disjunction in a phenotypically normal woman with hematologic abnormalities. *Am J Med Genet* 124A:383–387, 2004.

Baillie M. (1799) A series of engravings, accompanied with explanations, which are intended to illustrate the morbid anatomy of some of the most important parts of the human body. Ninth fasciculus. London, UK: W. Bulmer and Co. Facsimile edition prep. H Attwood, Melbourne University Press, 1985.

Baird ML, Heinig JA, Davis D, Sheets K, Kirkpatrick B, Starr DB. Chimeric germline tissue: Alleged father's genetic contribution to child found in semen sample but not in buccal sample. Paper presented at the International Symposium on Human Identification, Grapevine, TX, 2015.

Baker EK, Merton CF, Tan WH, Dudding-Byth T, Godler DE, Sadhwani A. Methylation analysis and developmental profile of two individuals with Angelman syndrome due to mosaic imprinting defects. *Eur J Med Genet* 65:104456, 2022.

Baker PR, Tsai AC, Springer M, et al. Male with mosaicism for supernumerary ring X chromosome: Analysis of phenotype and characterization of genotype using array comparative genome hybridization. *J Craniofac Surg* 21:1369–1375, 2010.

Bakhshi S, Joenje H, Schindler D, et al. A case report of a patient with microcephaly, facial dysmorphism, mitomycin-C-sensitive lymphocytes, and susceptibility to lymphoma. *Cancer Genet Cytogenet* 164:168–171, 2006.

Bakkeren IM, Henneman L, van Vliet-Lachotzki EH, et al. Psychological impact of additional findings detected by genome-wide Non-Invasive Prenatal Testing (NIPT): TRIDENT-2 study. *Eur J Hum Genet* 32:302–308, 2024.

Balakier H, Bouman D, Sojecki A, Librach C, Squire JA. Morphological and cytogenetic analysis of human giant oocytes and giant embryos. *Hum Reprod* 17:2394–2401, 2002.

Balasubramanian M, Barber JCK, Collinson MN, et al. Inverted duplication of 1q32.1 to 1q44 characterized by array CGH and review of distal 1q partial trisomy. *Am J Med Genet* 149A:793–797, 2009.

Balasubramanian M, Sithambaram S, Smith K. Inherited duplication of the short arm of chromosome 18p11.32-p11.31 associated with developmental delay/intellectual disability. *Clin Dysmorphol* 25:19–22, 2016.

Balci S, Unal A, Engiz O, et al. Bilateral periventricular nodular heterotopia, severe learning disability, and epilepsy in a male patient with 46,XY,der(19)t(X;19)(q11.1–11.2;p13.3). *Dev Med Child Neurol* 49:219–224, 2007.

Balci S, Zschocke J, Kotzot D, Ergün MA, Spreiz A. Formation of a familial ring chromosome 18 investigated by SNP-array analysis. *Am J Med Genet* 164A:1854–1856, 2014.

Baldwin EL, May LF, Justice AN, Martin CL, Ledbetter DH. Mechanisms and consequences of small supernumerary marker chromosomes: From Barbara McClintock to modern genetic-counseling issues. *Am J Hum Genet* 82:398–410, 2008.

Balkan M, Fidanboy M, Isi H, et al. A case of complete tetraploidy in amniocentesis with normal karyotype in subsequent cordocentesis. *J Pediatr Genet* 1:243–246, 2012.
Ballarati L, Rossi E, Bonati MT, et al. 13q Deletion and central nervous system anomalies: Further insights from karyotype-phenotype analyses of 14 patients. *J Med Genet* 44:e60, 2007.
Ballesta-Martínez MJ, López-González V, Dulcet LA, et al. Autosomal dominant oculoauriculovertebral spectrum and 14q23.1 microduplication. *Am J Med Genet* 161A:2030–2035, 2013.
Ballif BC, Rorem EA, Sundin K, et al. Detection of low-level mosaicism by array CGH in routine diagnostic specimens. *Am J Med Genet* 140:2757–2767, 2006.
Ballif BC, Rosenfeld JA, Traylor R, et al. High-resolution array CGH defines critical regions and candidate genes for microcephaly, abnormalities of the corpus callosum, and seizure phenotypes in patients with microdeletions of 1q43q44. *Hum Genet* 131:145–156, 2012.
Ballif BC, Theisen A, Rosenfeld JA, et al. Identification of a recurrent microdeletion at 17q23.1q23.2 flanked by segmental duplications associated with heart defects and limb abnormalities. *Am J Hum Genet* 86:454–461, 2010.
Ballout RA, El-Hattab AW, Schaaf CP, Cheung SW. Xq28 duplication syndrome, Int22h1/Int22h2 mediated. In: Adam MP, Feldman J, Mirzaa GM, Pagon RA, Wallace SE, Amemiya A (eds.), *GeneReviews*, Seattle: University of Washington, 1993–2024.
Balmer D, Baumer A, Röthlisberger B, Schinzel A. Severe intra-uterine growth retardation in a patient with maternal uniparental disomy 22 and a 22-trisomic placenta. *Prenat Diagn* 19:1061–1064, 1999.
Baltensperger A, Haischer G, Rohena L. Rare case of live born with confirmed mosaic trisomy 17 and review of the literature. *Clin Case Rep* 4:420–424, 2016.
Bandyopadhyay R, Heller A, Knox-DuBois C, et al. Parental origin and timing of de novo Robertsonian translocation formation. *Am J Hum Genet* 71:1456–1462, 2002.
Bandyopadhyay R, McCaskill C, Knox-Du Bois C, et al. Mosaicism in a patient with Down syndrome reveals post-fertilization formation of a Robertsonian translocation and isochromosome. *Am J Med Genet* 116A:159–163, 2003.
Banerjee I, Shevlin M, Taranissi M, et al. Health of children conceived after preimplantation genetic diagnosis: A preliminary outcome study. *Reprod Biomed Online* 16:376–381, 2008.
Bangun K, Kreshanti P, Tania V, Ariani Aswin Y, Menna C, Aurino L. Bilateral cleft lip and palate in ring chromosome 7 syndrome: A case report and review of clinical characteristics. *Cleft Palate Craniofac J* 61:527–533, 2024.
Baptista MJ, Fairbrother UL, Howard CM, et al. Heterotrisomy, a significant contributing factor to ventricular septal defect associated with Down syndrome? *Hum Genet* 107:476–482, 2000.
Barad DH, Albertini DF, Molinari E, Gleicher N. IVF outcomes of embryos with abnormal PGT-A biopsy previously refused transfer: A prospective cohort study. *Hum Reprod* 37:1194–1206, 2022.
Barbaro M, Cook J, Lagerstedt-Robinson K, Wedell A. Multigeneration inheritance through fertile XX carriers of an NR0B1 (DAX1) locus duplication in a kindred of females with isolated XY gonadal dysgenesis. *Int J Endocrinol* 2012:504904, 2012.
Barbaro M, Oscarson M, Schoumans J, Staaf J, Ivarsson SA, Wedell A. Isolated 46,XY gonadal dysgenesis in two sisters caused by a Xp21.2 interstitial duplication containing the *DAX1* gene. *J Clin Endocrinol Metab* 92:3305–3313, 2007.
Barber JC. Directly transmitted unbalanced chromosome abnormalities and euchromatic variants. *J Med Genet* 42:609–629, 2005.
Barber JCK, Ellis KH, Bowles LV, et al. Adenomatous polyposis coli and a cytogenetic deletion of chromosome 5 resulting from a maternal intrachromosomal insertion. *J Med Genet* 31:312–316, 1994.
Barber JCK, Rosenfeld JA, Graham JM, et al. Inside the 8p23.1 duplication syndrome; eight microduplications of likely or uncertain clinical significance. *Am J Med Genet* 167A:2052–2064, 2015.
Barber JCK, Sharp AJ, Hollox EJ, Tyson C. Copy number variation of the *REXO1L1* gene cluster; euchromatic deletion variant or susceptibility factor? *Eur J Hum Genet* 25:8–9, 2016.
Barbosa AS, Ferraz-Costa TE, Semer M, Liberman B, Moreira-Filho CA. XY gonadal dysgenesis and gonadoblastoma: A study in two sisters with a cryptic deletion of the Y chromosome involving the *SRY* gene. *Hum Genet* 95:63–66, 1995.
Bardi F, Bosschieter P, Verheij J, et al. Is there still a role for nuchal translucency measurement in the changing paradigm of first trimester screening? *Prenat Diagn* 40:197–205, 2020.
Barge-Schaapveld DQCM, Maas SM, Polstra A, Knegt LC, Hennekam RCM. The atypical 16p11.2 deletion: A not so atypical microdeletion syndrome? *Am J Med Genet* 155A:1066–1072, 2011.
Barinova IV, Voloshchuk IN, Chechneva MA, et al. [Twin gestation with regressive partial hydatidiform mole and coexisting live fetus]. *Arkh Patol* 84:44–50, 2022.

Benko S, Gordon CT, Mallet D, et al. Disruption of a long distance regulatory region upstream of SOX9 in isolated disorders of sex development. *J Med Genet* 48:825–830, 2011.

Benlian P, Foubert L, Gagne E, et al. Complete paternal isodisomy for chromosome 8 unmasked by lipoprotein lipase deficiency. *Am J Hum Genet* 59:431–436, 1996.

Benn P. Trisomy 16 and trisomy 16 mosaicism: A review. *Am J Med Genet* 79:121–133, 1998.

Benn PA, Hsu LYF. Evidence for preferential involvement of chromosome bands 6p21 and 13q14 in amniotic fluid cell balanced translocation pseudomosaicism. *Clin Genet* 29:116–121, 1986.

Benn P, Malvestiti F, Grimi B, Maggi F, Simoni G, Grati FR. Rare autosomal trisomies: Comparison of detection through cell-free DNA analysis and direct chromosome preparation of chorionic villus samples. *Ultrasound Obstet Gynecol* 54:458–467, 2019.

Benn P, Merrion K. Chromosome segregation of human nonhomologous Robertsonian translocations: Insights from preimplantation genetic testing. *Eur J Hum Genet* 33:711–717, 2025.

Bens S, Luedeke M, Richter T, et al. Mosaic genome-wide maternal isodiploidy: An extreme form of imprinting disorder presenting as prenatal diagnostic challenge. *Clin Epigenetics* 9:111, 2017.

Bensaid S, Bendahmane M, Loddo S, et al. Clinical and molecular cytogenetic studies of five new patients with 20q11q12 deletion and review of the literature: Proposition of two critical regions. *Am J Med Genet* 194A:e63580, 2024.

Berend SA, Feldman GL, McCaskill C, Czarnecki P, Van Dyke DL, Shaffer LG. Investigation of two cases of paternal disomy 13 suggests timing of isochromosome formation and mechanisms leading to uniparental disomy. *Am J Med Genet* 82:275–281, 1999.

Berend SA, Horwitz J, McCaskill C, Shaffer LG. Identification of uniparental disomy following prenatal detection of Robertsonian translocations and isochromosomes. *Am J Hum Genet* 66:1787–1793, 2000.

Berg JM, Korossy M. Down syndrome before Down: A retrospect. *Am J Med Genet* 102:205–211, 2001.

Bergemann E. Manifestation familiale du karyotype triplo-X. Communication préliminaire. *J Génét Hum* 10:370–371, 1962.

Bergère M, Wainer R, Nataf V, et al. Biopsied testis cells of four 47,XXY patients: Fluorescence in-situ hybridization and ICSI results. *Hum Reprod* 17:32–37, 2002.

Berghella V, Wapner RJ, Yang-Feng T, Mahoney MJ. Prenatal confirmation of true fetal trisomy 22 mosaicism by fetal skin biopsy following normal fetal blood sampling. *Prenat Diagn* 18:384–389, 1998.

Bernard V, Donadille B, Zenaty D, et al. Spontaneous fertility and pregnancy outcomes amongst 480 women with Turner syndrome. *Hum Reprod* 31:782–788, 2016.

Bernardini L, Capalbo A, D'Avanzo MG, et al. Five cases of supernumerary small ring chromosomes 1: Heterogeneity and genotype-phenotype correlation. *Eur J Med Genet* 50:94–102, 2007.

Bernasconi F, Karagüzel A, Celep F, et al. Normal phenotype with maternal isodisomy in a female with two isochromosomes: i(2p) and i(2q). *Am J Hum Genet* 59:1114–1118, 1996.

Berner AL, Bagci S, Wohlleber E, et al. Familial translocation t(6;20)(p21;p13) resulting in partial trisomy 6p and partial monosomy 20p: Report of a new case and review of the literature. *Cytogenet Genome Res* 136:308–313, 2012.

Bernert J, Bartels I, Gatz G, et al. Prenatal diagnosis of the Pallister-Killian mosaic aneuploidy syndrome by CVS. *Am J Med Genet* 42:747–750, 1992.

Bernicot I, Schneider A, Mace A, et al. Analysis using FISH of sperm and embryos from two carriers of rare rob(13;21) and rob(15;22) Robertsonian translocation undergoing PGD. *Eur J Med Genet* 55:245–251. 2012.

Bernier R, Steinman KJ, Reilly B, et al. Clinical phenotype of the recurrent 1q21.1 copy-number variant. *Genet Med* 18:341–349, 2016.

Bernkopf M, Abdullah UB, Bush SJ, et al. Personalized recurrence risk assessment following the birth of a child with a pathogenic de novo mutation. *Nat Commun* 14:853, 2023.

Berr C, Borghi E, Rethoré MO, Lejeune J, Alperovitch A. Risk of Down syndrome in relatives of trisomy 21 children: A case-control study. *Ann Génét* 33:137–140, 1990.

Bersu ET. Anatomical analysis of the developmental effects of aneuploidy in man: The Down syndrome. *Am J Med Genet* 5:399–420, 1980.

Bertelsen B, Nazaryan-Petersen L, Sun W, et al. A germline chromothripsis event stably segregating in 11 individuals through three generations. *Genet Med* 18:494–500, 2016.

Bertini V, Cambi F, Orsini A, et al. Phenotypic spectrum of *NFIA* haploinsufficiency: Two additional cases and review of the literature. *Genes (Basel)* 13:2249, 2022.

Bertini V, Valetto A, Uccelli A, et al. Molecular cytogenetic characterization of a de novo mosaic supernumerary ring chromosome 7: Report of a new patient. *Am J Med Genet* 146A:2955–2959, 2008a.

Bertini V, Valetto A, Uccelli A, Tarantino E, Simi P. Ring chromosome 21 and reproductive pattern: A familial case and review of the literature. *Fertil Steril* 90:2004, e1–5, 2008b.

Bertossi C, Cassina M, De Palma L, et al. 14q12 duplication including *FOXG1*: Is there a common age-dependent epileptic phenotype? *Brain Dev* 36:402–407, 2014.

Besser A, Weidenbaum E, Buldo-Licciardi J, McCaffrey C, Grifo J, Blakemore J. Healthy live births achieved from embryos diagnosed as non-mosaic segmental aneuploid. *J Assist Reprod Genet* 41:3379–3385, 2024.

Besterman AD. A genetics-guided approach to the clinical management of schizophrenia. *Schizophr Res* 267:462–469, 2024.

Bettio D, Baldwin EL, Carrozzo R, et al. Molecular cytogenetic and clinical findings in a patient with a small supernumerary r(8) mosaicism. *Am J Med Genet* 146A:247–250, 2008.

Bettio D, Levi Setti P, Bianchi P, Grazioli V. Trisomy 18 mosaicism in a woman with normal intelligence. *Am J Med Genet* 120A:303–304, 2003.

Betts DR, Greiner J, Feldges A, Caflisch U, Niggli FK. Constitutional balanced chromosomal rearrangements and neoplasm in children. *J Pediatr Hematol Oncol* 23:582–584, 2001.

Beverstock GC, Hansson K, Helderman-van den Enden AT, et al. A near false-negative finding of mosaic trisomy 21—A cautionary tale. *Prenat Diagn* 18:742–746, 1998.

Beygo J, Buiting K, Ramsden SC, Ellis R, Clayton-Smith J, Kanber D. Update of the EMQN/ACGS best practice guidelines for molecular analysis of Prader-Willi and Angelman syndromes. *Eur J Hum Genet* 27:1326–1340, 2019.

Bi X, Mulhern MS, Spiegel E, et al. 3' UTR Deletion of *FBXO28* in a patient with brain abnormalities and developmental delay. *Genes (Basel)* 14:1687, 2023.

Bianca S, Boemi G, Barrano B, et al. Mosaic trisomy 20: Considerations for genetic counseling. *Am J Med Genet* 146A:1897–1898, 2008.

Bianchi DW. Fetomaternal cell trafficking: A new cause of disease? *Am J Med Genet* 91:22–28, 2000.

Bianchi DW, Chudova D, Sehnert AJ, et al. Noninvasive prenatal testing and incidental detection of occult maternal malignancies. *JAMA* 314:162–169, 2015.

Bianchi DW, Wilkins-Haug LE, Enders AC, Hay ED. Origin of extraembryonic mesoderm in experimental animals: Relevance to chorionic mosaicism in humans. *Am J Med Genet* 46:542–550, 1993.

Biason-Lauber A, Konrad D, Meyer M, DeBeaufort C, Schoenle EJ. Ovaries and female phenotype in a girl with 46,XY karyotype and mutations in the *CBX2* gene. *Am J Hum Genet* 84:658–663, 2009.

Bidart M, El Atifi M, Miladi S, et al. Microduplication of the ARID1A gene causes intellectual disability with recognizable syndromic features. *Genet Med* 19:701–710, 2017.

Bielanska M, Tan SL, Ao A. Chromosomal mosaicism throughout human preimplantation development in vitro: Incidence, type, and relevance to embryo outcome. *Hum Reprod* 17:413–419, 2002.

Biesecker LG, Rosenberg M, Dziadzio L, et al. Detection of a subtle rearrangement of chromosome 22 using molecular techniques. *Am J Med Genet* 58:389–394, 1995.

Bierer R, Mladucky J, Anderson R, Carey JC. Parent narratives provide perspectives on the experience of care in trisomy 18. *Am J Med Genet* 196C:e32114, 2024.

Bildik G, Liang X, Sutton MN, Bast RC Jr, Lu Z. DIRAS3: An imprinted tumor suppressor gene that regulates RAS and PI3K-driven cancer growth, motility, autophagy, and tumor dormancy. *Mol Cancer Ther* 21:25–37, 2022.

Bilimoria KY, Rothenberg JM. Prenatal diagnosis of a trisomy 7/maternal uniparental heterodisomy 7 mosaic fetus. *Am J Med Genet* 118A:60–63, 2003.

Billes A, Pujalte M, Jedraszak G, et al. Possible incomplete penetrance of Xq28 int22h-1/int22h-2 duplication. *Clin Genet* 106:234–246, 2024.

Bint SM, Ogilvie CM, Flinter FA, Khalaf Y, Scriven PN. Meiotic segregation of Robertsonian translocations ascertained in cleavage-stage embryos—Implications for preimplantation genetic diagnosis. *Hum Reprod* 26:1575–1584, 2011.

Birca V, Myers KA. Genetic generalized epilepsy and intrafamilial phenotypic variability with distal 7q11.23 deletion. *Child Neurol Open* 9:2329048X221093173, 2022.

Birjiniuk A, Weisman AG, Laternser C, et al. Cardiovascular manifestations of Turner syndrome: Phenotypic differences between karyotype subtypes. *Pediatr Cardiol* 45:1407–1414, 2024.

Birkebaek NH, Cruger D, Hansen J, Nielsen J, Bruun-Petersen G. Fertility and pregnancy outcome in Danish women with Turner syndrome. *Clin Genet* 61:35–39, 2002.

Bisba M, Malamaki C, Constantoulakis P, Vittas S. Chromosome 15q11-q13 duplication syndrome: A review of the literature and 14 new cases. *Genes (Basel)* 15:1304, 2024.

Bischoff FZ, Simpson JL. Endocervical fetal trophoblast for prenatal genetic diagnosis. *Curr Opin Obstet Gynecol* 18:216–220, 2006.

Bisgaard AM, Kirchhoff M, Nielsen JE, et al. Chromosomal deletion unmasking a recessive disease: 22q13 deletion syndrome and metachromatic leukodystrophy. *Clin Genet* 75:175–179, 2009.

Bispo AV, Burégio-Frota P, Oliveira dos Santos L, et al. Y chromosome in Turner syndrome: Detection of hidden mosaicism and the report of a rare X;Y translocation case. *Reprod Fertil Dev* 26:1176–1182, 2014.

Bittel DC, Kibiryeva N, Butler MG. Expression of 4 genes between chromosome 15 breakpoints 1 and 2 and behavioral outcomes in Prader-Willi syndrome. *Pediatrics* 118:e1276–1283, 2006a.

Bittel DC, Kibiryeva N, Dasouki M, Knoll JH, Butler MG. A 9-year-old male with a duplication of chromosome 3p25.3p26.2: Clinical report and gene expression analysis. *Am J Med Genet* 140A:573–579, 2006b.

Bittel DC, Theodoro MF, Kibiryeva N, Fischer W, Talebizadeh Z, Butler MG. Comparison of X-chromosome inactivation patterns in multiple tissues from human females. *J Med Genet* 45:309–313, 2008.

Bittencourt MC, Morris MA, Chabod J, et al. Fortuitous detection of uniparental isodisomy of chromosome 6. *J Med Genet* 34:77–78, 1997.

Björck EJ, Anderlid BM, Blennow E. Maternal isodisomy of chromosome 9 with no impact on the phenotype in a woman with two isochromosomes: i(9p) and i(9q). *Am J Med Genet* 87:49–52, 1999.

Blagowidow N, Nowakowska B, Schindewolf E, et al. Prenatal screening and diagnostic considerations for 22q11.2 microdeletions. *Genes (Basel)* 14:160, 2023.

Blaicher W, Repa C, Schaller A. Acardiac twin pregnancy: Associated with trisomy 2: Case report. *Hum Reprod* 15:474–475, 2000.

Blackburn PR, McGee RB, Mostafavi R, et al. Constitutional balanced translocations involving SMARCB1: A rare cause of rhabdoid tumour predisposition syndrome. *Genes Chromosomes Cancer* 63:e23195, 2024.

Blakey-Cheung S, Parker P, Schlaff W, Monseur B, Keppler-Noreuil K, Al-Kouatly HB. Diagnosis and clinical delineation of mosaic tetrasomy 5p. *Eur J Med Genet* 63:103634, 2020.

Blair J, Tolmie J, Hollman AS, Donaldson MD. Phenotype, ovarian function, and growth in patients with 45,X/47,XXX Turner mosaicism: Implications for prenatal counseling and estrogen therapy at puberty. *J Pediatr* 139:724–728, 2001.

Blakey-Cheung S, Parker P, Schlaff W, Monseur B, Keppler-Noreuil K, Al-Kouatly HB. Diagnosis and clinical delineation of mosaic tetrasomy 5p. *Eur J Med Genet* 63:103634, 2020.

Blanco J, Farreras A, Egozcue J, Vidal F. Meiotic behavior of the sex chromosomes in a 45,X/46,X,r(Y)/46,X,dic r(Y) patient whose semen was assessed by fluorescence in situ hybridization. *Fertil Steril* 79:913–918, 2003.

Blanco J, Gabau E, Gomez D, et al. Chromosome 21 disomy in the spermatozoa of the fathers of children with trisomy 21, in a population with a high prevalence of Down syndrome: Increased incidence in cases of paternal origin. *Am J Hum Genet* 63:1067–1072, 1998.

Blazejewski SM, Bennison SA, Smith TH, Toyo-Oka K. Neurodevelopmental genetic diseases associated with microdeletions and microduplications of chromosome 17p13.3. *Front Genet* 9:80, 2018.

Blazina Š, Ihan A, Lovrecic L, Hovnik T. 11q terminal deletion and combined immunodeficiency (Jacobsen syndrome): Case report and literature review on immunodeficiency in Jacobsen syndrome. *Am J Med Genet* 170A:3237–3240, 2016.

Blennow E, Sahlén S, Inzunza J, Hovatta O, Nordenskjöld M, Malmgren H. Single cell CGH analysis of human preimplantation embryos from PGD patients with balanced structural chromosome aberrations. *Ann Génét* 44:s26, 2001.

Bliek J, Snijder S, Maas SM, et al. Phenotypic discordance upon paternal or maternal transmission of duplications of the 11p15 imprinted regions. *Eur J Med Genet* 52:404–408, 2009.

Blumenthal AL, Allanson JE. Turner syndrome in a mother and daughter: r(X) and fertility. *Clin Genet* 52:187–191, 1997.

Bobabilla-Morales L, Corona-Rivera A, Corona-Rivera JR, et al. Chromosome instability induced in vitro with mitomycin C in five Seckel syndrome patients. *Am J Med Genet* 123A:148–152, 2003.

Bobrow M, Barby T, Hajianpour A, Maxwell D, Yau SC. Fertility in a male with trisomy 21. *J Med Genet* 29:141, 1992.

Bocian E, Mazurczak T, Stanczak H. Paracentric inversion inv(18)(q21.1q23) in a woman with recurrent spontaneous abortions. *Am J Med Genet* 35:592–593, 1990.

Bodri D, Guillén JJ, Schwenn K, Casadesus S, Vidal R, Coll O. Poor outcome in oocyte donation after elective transfer of a single cleavage-stage embryo in Turner syndrome patients. *Fertil Steril* 91:1489–1492, 2009.

Boehmer ALM, Brinkmann O, Bruggenwirth H, et al. Genotype versus phenotype in families with androgen insensitivity syndrome. *J Clin Endocrinol Metab* 86:4151–4160, 2001.

Boente MDC, Bazan C, Montanari D. Cutis tricolor parvimaculata in two patients with ring chromosome 15 syndrome. *Pediatr Dermatol* 28:670–673, 2011.

Bofinger MK, Needham DF, Saldana LR, Sosnowski JP, Blough RI. 45,X/46,X,r(Y) karyotype transmitted by father to son after intracytoplasmic sperm injection for oligospermia: A case report. *J Reprod Med* 44:645–648, 1999.
Boghosian-Sell L, Mewar R, Harrison W, et al. Molecular mapping of the Edwards syndrome phenotype to two noncontiguous regions on chromosome 18. *Am J Hum Genet* 55:476–483, 1994.
Bohers E, Sarafan-Vasseur N, Drouet A, et al. Gradual reduction of BUBR1 protein levels results in premature sister-chromatid separation then in aneuploidy. *Hum Genet* 124:473–478, 2008
Boisseau P, Giraud M, Ternisien C, et al. An unexpected transmission of von Willebrand disease type 3: The first case of maternal uniparental disomy 12. *Haematologica* 96:1567–1568, 2011.
Boivin J, Appleton TC, Baetens P, et al. Guidelines for counselling in infertility: Outline version. *Hum Reprod* 16:1301–1304, 2001.
Bonaglia MC, Giorda R, Beri S, et al. Molecular mechanisms generating and stabilizing terminal 22q13 deletions in 44 subjects with Phelan/McDermid syndrome. *PLoS Genet* 7:e1002173, 2011.
Bonaglia MC, Zanotta N, Giorda R, D'Angelo G, Zucca C. Long-term follow-up of a patient with 5q31.3 microdeletion syndrome and the smallest de novo 5q31.2q31.3 deletion involving PURA. *Mol Cytogenet* 8:89, 2015.
Bonasoni MP, Comitini G, Tonni G, et al. Prenatal diagnosis of fetal trisomy 5 mosaicism with congenital pulmonary airway malformation type 3: A case report. *Fetal Pediatr Pathol* 41:516–522, 2022.
Bonati MT, Feresin A, Prontera P, et al. Contiguous gene syndromes and hearing loss: A clinical report of Xq21 deletion and comprehensive literature review. *Genes (Basel)* 15:677, 2024.
Bonduelle M, Van Assche E, Joris H, Keymolen K, Devroey P, Van Steirteghem A, Liebaers I. Prenatal testing in ICSI pregnancies: Incidence of chromosomal anomalies in 1586 karyotypes and relation to sperm parameters. *Hum Reprod* 17:2600–2614, 2002.
Bone KM, Chernos JE, Perrier R, et al. Mosaic trisomy 1q: A recurring chromosome anomaly that is a diagnostic challenge and is associated with a Fryns-like phenotype. *Prenat Diagn* 37:602–610, 2017.
Bonne A, Vreede L, Kuiper RP, et al. Mapping of constitutional translocation breakpoints in renal cell cancer patients: Identification of KCNIP4 as a candidate gene. *Cancer Genet Cytogenet* 179:11–18, 2007.
Bonnet C, Andrieux J, Béri-Dexheimer M, et al. Microdeletion at chromosome 4q21 defines a new emerging syndrome with marked growth restriction, mental retardation and absent or severely delayed speech. *J Med Genet* 47:377–384, 2010.
Bonnet C, Zix C, Grégoire MJ, et al. Characterization of mosaic supernumerary ring chromosomes by array-CGH: Segmental aneusomy for proximal 4q in a child with tall stature and obesity. *Am J Med Genet* 140:233–237, 2006.
Bonuccelli A, Valetto A, Orsini A, et al. Maternally derived 15q11.2-q13.1 duplication in a child with Lennox–Gastaut-type epilepsy and dysmorphic features: Clinical-genetic characterization of the family and review of the literature. *Am J Med Genet* 173A:556–560, 2017.
Bonus ML, McQueen DB, Ruderman R, et al. Relationship between paternal factors and embryonic aneuploidy of paternal origin. *Fertil Steril* 118:281–288, 2022.
Boonen SE, Hoffmann AL, Donnai D, Tümer Z, Ravn K. Diploid/triploid mosaicism: A rare event or an under-diagnosed syndrome? *Eur J Med Genet* 54:374–375, 2011.
Boonen SE, Mackay DJ, Hahnemann JM, et al. Transient neonatal diabetes, ZFP57, and hypomethylation of multiple imprinted loci: A detailed follow-up. *Diabetes Care* 36:505–512, 2013.
Boormans EM, Birnie E, Oepkes D, et al. Comparison of multiplex ligation-dependent probe amplification and karyotyping in prenatal diagnosis. *Obstet Gynecol* 115:297–303, 2010.
Børglum A, Nordentoft M, Hougaard DM, et al. Prevalence of rearrangements in the 22q11.2 region and population-based risk of neuropsychiatric and developmental disorders in a Danish population: A case-cohort study. *Lancet Psychiatry* 5:573–580, 2018.
Borgström B, Hreinsson J, Rasmussen C, et al. Fertility preservation in girls with Turner syndrome: Prognostic signs of the presence of ovarian follicles. *J Clin Endocrinol Metab* 94:74–80, 2009.
Borie C, Léger J, Dupuy O, et al. Translocation (Y;22) resulting in the loss of *SHOX* and isolated short stature. *Am J Med Genet* 125A:186–190, 2004.
Botkin JR. The legal concept of wrongful life. *JAMA* 259:1541–1545, 1988.
Bottani A, Robinson WP, DeLozier-Blanchet CD, et al. Angelman syndrome due to paternal uniparental disomy of chromosome 15: A milder phenotype? *Am J Med Genet* 51:35–40, 1994.
Bouassida M, Molina-Gomes D, Koraichi F, et al. The clinical value of optical genome mapping in the rapid characterization of RB1 duplication and 15q23q24.2 triplication, for more appropriate prenatal genetic counselling. *Mol Genet Genomic Med* 12:e2437, 2024.
Bouchlariotou S, Tsikouras P, Dimitraki M, et al. Turner's syndrome and pregnancy: Has the 45,X/47,XXX mosaicism a different prognosis? Own clinical experience and literature review. *J Matern Fetal Neonatal Med* 24:668–672, 2011.

Boué A, Gallano P. A collaborative study of the segregation of inherited chromosome structural rearrangements in 1356 prenatal diagnoses. *Prenat Diagn* 4 Spec No:45–67, 1984.

Bouhjar IB, Hannachi H, Zerelli SM, et al. Array-CGH study of partial trisomy 9p without mental retardation. *Am J Med Genet* 155A:1735–1739, 2011.

Bouman A, Schuitema A, Pfundt R, van de Zande G, Kleefstra T. Clinical delineation of a patient with trisomy 12q23q24. *Eur J Med Genet* 56:463–469, 2013.

Bouman A, van der Kevie-Kersemaekers AM, Huijsdens-van Amsterdam K, et al. Trisomy 4 mosaicism: Delineation of the phenotype. *Am J Med Genet* 170A:1040–1045, 2016.

Bound JP, Francis BJ, Harvey PW. Down's syndrome: Prevalence and ionising radiation in an area of north west England 1957–91. *J Epidemiol Community Health* 49:164–170, 1995.

Bourgois A, Bizaoui V, Colson C, et al. Phenotypic and genotypic characterization of 1q21.1 copy number variants: A report of 34 new individuals and literature review. *Am J Med Genet* 194A:e63457, 2024.

Bous SM, Solomon BD, Graul-Neumann L, Neitzel H, Hardisty EE, Muenke M. Holoprosencephaly-polydactyly/pseudotrisomy 13: A presentation of two new cases and a review of the literature. *Clin Dysmorphol* 21:183–190, 2012.

Bovie C, Holden ST, Schroer A, Smith E, Trump D, Raymond FL. Neurofibromatosis 2 in a patient with a de novo balanced reciprocal translocation 46,X,t(X;22)(p11.2;q11.2). *J Med Genet* 40:682–684, 2003.

Bowen P, Fitzgerald PH, Gardner RJM, Biederman B, Veale AM. Duplication 8q syndrome due to familial chromosome ins(10;8)(q21;q212q22). *Am J Med Genet* 14:635–646, 1983.

Bowser-Riley S, Buckton KE, Ratcliffe SG, Syme J. Inheritance of a ring 14 chromosome. *J Med Genet* 18:209–213, 1981.

Bowser-Riley SM, Griffiths MJ, Creasy MR, et al. Are double translocations double trouble? *J Med Genet* 25:326–331, 1988.

Boyd BM, Fang H, Allingham-Hawkins D, et al. Chromosomal translocation resolves a diagnostic odyssey for familial Ruvalcaba syndrome. *Am J Med Genet* 197A:e63847, 2025.

Boyd PA, Loane M, Garne E, Khoshnood B, Dolk H; EUROCAT working group. Sex chromosome trisomies in Europe: Prevalence, prenatal detection and outcome of pregnancy. *Eur J Hum Genet* 19:231–234, 2011.

Boyle J, Sangha K, Dill F, Robinson WP, Yong SL. Grandmaternal origin of an isochromosome 18p present in two maternal half-sisters. *Am J Med Genet* 101:65–69, 2001.

Bozhilova N, Welham A, Adams D, et al. Profiles of autism characteristics in thirteen genetic syndromes: A machine learning approach. *Mol Autism* 14:3, 2023.

Braddock SR, Henley KM, Potter KL, Nguyen HG, Huang TH. Tertiary trisomy due to a reciprocal translocation of chromosomes 5 and 21 in a four-generation family. *Am J Med Genet* 92:311–317, 2000.

Braddock SR, South ST, Schiffman JD, et al. Braddock–Carey syndrome: A 21q22 contiguous gene syndrome encompassing *RUNX1*. *Am J Med Genet* 170A:2580–2586, 2016.

Brady AN, May KM, Fernhoff PM. Mosaic trisomy 4: Long-term outcome on the first reported liveborn. *Am J Med Genet* 132:411–413, 2005.

Brady P, Brison N, Van Den Bogaert K, et al. Clinical implementation of NIPT—Technical and biological challenges. *Clin Genet* 89:523–530, 2016.

Brady PD, Delle Chiaie B, Christenhusz G, et al. A prospective study of the clinical utility of prenatal chromosomal microarray analysis in fetuses with ultrasound abnormalities and an exploration of a framework for reporting unclassified variants and risk factors. *Genet Med* 16:469–476, 2014.

Brahams D. House of Lords upholds decision to sterilise 17-year-old mentally handicapped girl. *Lancet* 1:1099–1100, 1987.

Brancati F, Mingarelli R, Dallapiccola B. Recurrent triploidy of maternal origin. *Eur J Hum Genet* 11:972–974, 2003.

Brand F, Vijayananth A, Hsieh TC, et al. Next-generation phenotyping contributing to the identification of a 4.7 kb deletion in KANSL1 causing Koolen-de Vries syndrome. *Hum Mutat* 43:1659–1665, 2022.

Braude P, Bolton V, Moore S. Human gene expression first occurs between the four- and eight-cell stages of preimplantation development. *Nature* 332:459–461, 1988.

Braun A, Kammerer S, Cleve H, Löhrs U, Schwarz HP, Kuhnle U. True hermaphroditism in a 46,XY individual, caused by a postzygotic somatic point mutation in the male gonadal sex-determining locus (*SRY*): Molecular genetics and histological findings in a sporadic case. *Am J Hum Genet* 52:578–585, 1993.

Braun-Falco M, Schempp W, Nevinny-Stickel-Hinzpeter C, Köhn FM. Azoospermia due to a unique de novo balanced reciprocal translocation (Y;1) (q12;q25). *J Androl* 28:647–651, 2007.
Brcic L, Underwood JF, Kendall KM, Caseras X, Kirov G, Davies W. Medical and neurobehavioural phenotypes in carriers of X-linked ichthyosis-associated genetic deletions in the UK Biobank. *J Med Genet* 57:692–698, 2020.
Breckpot J, Anderlid BM, Alanay Y, et al. Chromosome 22q12.1 microdeletions: Confirmation of the *MN1* gene as a candidate gene for cleft palate. *Eur J Hum Genet* 24:51–58, 2016.
Brender JD, Zhan FB, Langlois PH, Suarez L, Scheuerle A. Residential proximity to waste sites and industrial facilities and chromosomal anomalies in offspring. *Int J Hyg Environ Health* 211:50–58, 2008.
Brennan C, Smith ML, Baiduc RR, O'Connor L. Speech, language, hearing, and otopathology results from the international Smith-Magenis syndrome patient registry. *J Speech Lang Hear Res* 67:917–938, 2024.
Brewer C, Holloway S, Zawalnyski P, Schinzel A, FitzPatrick D. A chromosomal deletion map of human malformations. *Am J Hum Genet* 63:1153–1159, 1998.
Brewer C, Holloway S, Zawalnyski P, Schinzel A, FitzPatrick D. A chromosomal duplication map of malformations: Regions of suspected haplo- and triplolethality—and tolerance of segmental aneuploidy—in humans. *Am J Hum Genet* 64:1702–1708, 1999.
Brimble E, Reyes KG, Kuhathaas K, et al. Expanding genotype-phenotype correlations in FOXG1 syndrome: Results from a patient registry. *Orphanet J Rare Dis* 18:149, 2023.
Brioude F, Kalish JM, Mussa A, et al. Expert consensus document: Clinical and molecular diagnosis, screening and management of Beckwith-Wiedemann syndrome: An international consensus statement. *Nat Rev Endocrinol* 14:229–249, 2018.
Brisset S, Aboura A, Audibert F, et al. Discordant prenatal diagnosis of trisomy 21 due to mosaic structural rearrangements of chromosome 21. *Prenat Diagn* 23:461–469, 2003.
Brisset S, Capri Y, Briand-Suleau A, et al. Inherited 1q21.1q21.2 duplication and 16p11.2 deletion: A two-hit case with more severe clinical manifestations. *Eur J Med Genet* 58:497–501, 2015.
Brisset S, Izard V, Misrahi M, et al. Cytogenetic, molecular and testicular tissue studies in an infertile 45,X male carrying an unbalanced (Y;22) translocation: Case report. *Hum Reprod* 20:2168–2172, 2005.
Britt DW, Risinger ST, Miller V, Mans MK, Krivchenia EL, Evans MI. Determinants of parental decisions after the prenatal diagnosis of Down syndrome: Bringing in context. *Am J Med Genet* 93:410–416, 2000.
Brock DW. The non-identity problem and genetic harms—the case of wrongful handicaps. *Bioethics* 9:269–275, 1995.
Brøndum-Nielsen K, Mikkelsen M. A 10-year survey, 1980–1990, of prenatally diagnosed small supernumerary marker chromosomes, identified by FISH analysis: Outcome and follow-up of 14 cases diagnosed in a series of 12,699 prenatal samples. *Prenat Diagn* 15:615–619, 1995.
Brown LY, Alonso ML, Yu J, Warburton D, Brown S. Prenatal diagnosis of a familial Xq deletion in a female fetus: A case report. *Prenat Diagn* 21:27–30, 2001.
Brown N, Burgess T, Forbes R, et al. 5q31.3 Microdeletion syndrome: Clinical and molecular characterization of two further cases. *Am J Med Genet* 161A:2604–2608, 2013.
Brown S, Gersen S, Anyane-Yeboa K, Warburton D. Preliminary definition of a "critical region" of chromosome 13 in q32: Report of 14 cases with 13q deletions and review of the literature. *Am J Med Genet* 45:52–59, 1993.
Brown S, Higgins S, Hutchinson R, Bain S, Moore L, Haan E. A case of mosaicism for trisomy of chromosome 5 detected at amniocentesis. *Twin Res Hum Genet* 12:210, 2009.
Brownstein CA, Douard E, Haynes RL, et al. Copy number variation and structural genomic findings in 116 cases of sudden unexplained death between 1 and 28 months of age. *Adv Genet (Hoboken)* 4:2200012, 2022.
Brunet BCFK, Shen J, Cai L, et al. Preimplantation genetic testing for complex chromosomal rearrangement carriers by next-generation sequencing. *Reprod Biomed Online* 37:375–382, 2018.
Bruno DL, White SM, Ganesamoorthy D, et al. Pathogenic aberrations revealed exclusively by single nucleotide polymorphism (SNP) genotyping data in 5000 samples tested by molecular karyotyping. *J Med Genet* 48:831–839, 2011.
Bruns DA, Campbell E. Twenty-five additional cases of trisomy 9 mosaic: Birth information, medical conditions, and developmental status. *Am J Med Genet* 167A:997–1007, 2015.
Bruyère H, Rupps R, Kuchinka BD, Friedman JM, Robinson WP. Recurrent trisomy 21 in a couple with a child presenting trisomy 21 mosaicism and maternal uniparental disomy for chromosome 21 in the euploid cell line. *Am J Med Genet* 94:35–41, 2000.

Bruyère H, Speevak MD, Winsor EJ, et al. Isodicentric Yp: Prenatal diagnosis and outcome in 12 cases. *Prenat Diagn* 26:324–329, 2006.
Bryan J, Peters M, Pritchard G, Healey S, Payton D. A second case of intrauterine growth retardation and primary hypospadias associated with a trisomy 22 placenta but with biparental inheritance of chromosome 22 in the fetus. *Prenat Diagn* 22:137–140, 2002.
Bryant LD, Murray J, Green JM, Hewison J, Sehmi I, Ellis A. Descriptive information about Down syndrome: A content analysis of serum screening leaflets. *Prenat Diagn* 21:1057–1063, 2001.
Brzustowicz LM, Allitto BA, Matseoane D, et al. Paternal isodisomy for chromosome 5 in a child with spinal muscular atrophy. *Am J Hum Genet* 54:482–488, 1994.
Bu X, Li X, Zhou S, et al. Prenatal diagnosis of complete paternal uniparental isodisomy for chromosome 3: A case report. *Mol Cytogenet* 14:50, 2021.
Buckton KE, Newton MS, Collyer S, et al. Phenotypically normal individuals with an inversion (X) (p22q13) and the recombinant (X), dup q. *Ann Hum Genet* 45:159–168, 1981.
Budisteanu M, Papuc SM, Streata I, et al. The phenotypic spectrum of 15q13.3 region duplications: Report of 5 patients. *Genes (Basel)* 12:1025, 2021.
Budowle B, Capt C, Chakraborty R, Ge J. Paternity calculations in a di-spermy case. *Int J Legal Med* 131:339–343, 2017.
Buffin R, Fichez A, Decullier E, et al. Neurodevelopmental outcome at 2 years of corrected age in fetuses with increased nuchal translucency thickness and normal karyotype compared with matched controls. *Ultrasound Obstet Gynecol* 57:790–797, 2021.
Buffin-Meyer B, Richard J, Guigonis V, et al. Renal and extrarenal phenotypes in patients with *HNF1B* variants and chromosome 17q12 microdeletions. *Kidney Int Rep* 9:2514–2526, 2024.
Bugge M, Collins A, Hertz JM, et al. Non-disjunction of chromosome 13. *Hum Mol Genet* 16:2004–2010, 2007.
Bugge M, Collins A, Petersen MB, et al. Non-disjunction of chromosome 18. *Hum Mol Genet* 7:661–669, 1998.
Buiting K, Clayton-Smith J, Driscoll DJ, et al. Clinical utility gene card for: Angelman syndrome. *Eur J Hum Genet* 23:2015.
Buiting K, Dittrich B, Gross S, et al. Sporadic imprinting defects in Prader-Willi syndrome and Angelman syndrome: Implications for imprint-switch models, genetic counseling, and prenatal diagnosis. *Am J Hum Genet* 63:170–180, 1998.
Buiting K, Gross S, Lich C, Gillessen-Kaesbach G, el-Maarri O, Horsthemke B. Epimutations in Prader-Willi and Angelman syndromes: A molecular study of 136 patients with an imprinting defect. *Am J Hum Genet* 72:571–577, 2003.
Bukvic N, Cesarano C, Ceccarini C, et al. Characterization of the first adult de novo case of 46,X,der(Y)t(X;Y)(p22.3;q11.2). *Gene* 513:111–117, 2013.
Bull MJ. Down Syndrome. *N Engl J Med* 382:2344–2352, 2020.
Bullman H, Lever M, Robinson DO, Mackay DJ, Holder SE, Wakeling EL. Mosaic maternal uniparental disomy of chromosome 11 in a patient with Silver-Russell syndrome. *J Med Genet* 45:396–399, 2008.
Bunnell ME, Wilkins-Haug L, Reiss R. Should embryos with autosomal monosomy by preimplantation genetic testing for aneuploidy be transferred?: Implications for embryo selection from a systematic literature review of autosomal monosomy survivors. *Prenat Diagn* 37:1273–1280, 2017.
Burada F, Streata I, Ungureanu A, et al. Prenatal diagnosis of a pure 15q distal trisomy derived from a maternal pericentric inversion: A case report. *Exp Ther Med* 21:304, 2021.
Burgemeister AL, Daumiller E, Dietze-Armana I, et al. Continuing role for classical cytogenetics: Case report of a boy with ring syndrome caused by complete ring chromosome 4 and review of literature. *Am J Med Genet* 173A:727–732, 2017.
Burgess T, Brown NJ, Stark Z, et al. Characterization of core clinical phenotypes associated with recurrent proximal 15q25.2 microdeletions. *Am J Med Genet* 164A:2014a, 77–86.
Burgess T, Downie L, Pertile MD, et al. Monosomy 21 seen in live born is unlikely to represent true monosomy 21: A case report and review of the literature. *Case Rep Genet* 2014;2014:965401, 2014b.
Burgevin M, Lacroix A, Ollivier F, et al. Executive functioning in adolescents and adults with Silver-Russell syndrome. *PLoS One* 18:e0279745, 2023.
Burghel GJ, Khan U, Lin WY, Whittaker W, Banka S. Presence of pathogenic copy number variants (CNVs) is correlated with socioeconomic status. *J Med Genet* 57:70–72, 2020.
Burke LW, Wiley JE, Glenn CC, et al. Familial cryptic translocation resulting in Angelman syndrome: Implications for imprinting or location of the Angelman gene? *Am J Hum Genet* 58:777–784, 1996.

Burn J, Baraitser M, Butler LJ. An avoidable recurrence of cri du chat syndrome in the next generation. *Br Med J* 287:1287–1288, 1983.

Burns JP, Koduru PR, Alonso ML, Chaganti RS. Analysis of meiotic segregation in a man heterozygous for two reciprocal translocations using the hamster in vitro penetration system. *Am J Hum Genet* 38:954–964, 1986.

Burnside RD, Lose EJ, Dominguez MG, et al. Molecular cytogenetic characterization of two cases with constitutional distal 11q duplication/triplication. *Am J Med Genet* 149A:1516–1522, 2009.

Burnside RD, Pappas JG, Sacharow S, et al. Three cases of isolated terminal deletion of chromosome 8p without heart defects presenting with a mild phenotype. *Am J Med Genet* 161A:822–828, 2013.

Burssed B, Zamariolli M, Bellucco FT, Melaragno MI. Mechanisms of structural chromosomal rearrangement formation. *Mol Cytogenet* 15:23, 2022.

Butler MG. Prader-Willi syndrome and chromosome 15q11.2 BP1-BP2 region: A review. *Int J Mol Sci* 24:4271, 2023.

Butler MG, Hartin SN, Hossain WA, et al. Molecular genetic classification in Prader-Willi syndrome: A multisite cohort study. *J Med Genet* 56:149–153, 2019.

Byers HM, Adam MP, LaCroix A, et al. Description of a new oncogenic mechanism for atypical teratoid rhabdoid tumors in patients with ring chromosome 22. *Am J Med Genet* 173A:245–249, 2017.

Byrne J, Rasmussen SA, Steinhorn SC, et al. Genetic disease in offspring of long-term survivors of childhood and adolescent cancer. *Am J Hum Genet* 62:45–52, 1998.

C

Cafferkey M, Ahn JW, Flinter F, Ogilvie C. Phenotypic features in patients with 15q11.2(BP1-BP2) deletion: Further delineation of an emerging syndrome. *Am J Med Genet* 164A:1916–1922, 2014.

Calanchini M, Aye CYL, Orchard E, et al. Fertility issues and pregnancy outcomes in Turner syndrome. *Fertil Steril* 114:144–154, 2020.

Calle Sánchez X, Helenius D, Bybjerg-Grauholm J, et al. Comparing copy number variations in a Danish case cohort of individuals with psychiatric disorders. *JAMA Psychiatry* 79:59–69, 2022.

Callen DF, Eyre H, Fang YY, et al. Origins of accessory small ring marker chromosomes derived from chromosome 1. *J Med Genet* 36:847–853, 1999.

Callen DF, Eyre HJ, Ringenbergs ML, Freemantle CJ, Woodroffe P, Haan EA. Chromosomal origin of small ring marker chromosomes in man: Characterization by molecular genetics. *Am J Hum Genet* 48:769–782, 1991.

Callen DF, Sutherland GR. Normal female carrier and affected male half-sibs with t(X;5)(q13;p15): Location of a gene determining male genital development. *Clin Genet* 30:59–62, 1986.

Callen DF, Sutherland GR, Carter RF. A fertile man with tdic(Y;22): How a stable neo-X1X2Y sex-determining mechanism could evolve in man. *Am J Med Genet Suppl* 3:151–155, 1987.

Callen DF, Woollatt E, Sutherland GR. Paracentric inversions in man. *Clin Genet* 28:87–92, 1985.

Callier P, Faivre L, Pigeonnat S, et al. Contribution of array CGH in prognosis and genetic counselling of prenatally diagnosed supernumerary ring chromosome 20. *Prenat Diagn* 29:1002–1005, 2009.

Calounova G, Novotna D, Simandlova M, et al. Prader-Willi syndrome due to uniparental disomy in a patient with a balanced chromosomal translocation. *Neuro Endocrinol Lett* 27:579–585, 2006.

Cameron-Pimblett A, La Rosa C, King TFJ, Davies MC, Conway GS. The Turner syndrome life course project: Karyotype-phenotype analyses across the lifespan. *Clin Endocrinol (Oxf)* 87:532–538, 2017.

Cammarata M, Di Simone P, Graziano L, Giuffre M, Corsello G, Garofalo G. Rare sex chromosome aneuploidies in humans: Report of six patients with 48,XXYY, 49,XXXXY, and 48,XXXX karyotypes. *Am J Med Genet* 85:86–87, 1999.

Campbell LE, McCabe KL, Melville JL, Strutt PA, Schall U. Social cognition dysfunction in adolescents with 22q11.2 deletion syndrome (velo-cardio-facial syndrome): Relationship with executive functioning and social competence/functioning. *J Intellect Disabil Res* 59:845–859, 2015.

Campbell IM, Sheppard SE, Crowley TB, et al. What is new with 22q? An update from the 22q and You Center at the Children's Hospital of Philadelphia. *Am J Med Genet* 176A:2058–2069, 2018.

Campbell IM, Yuan B, Robberecht C, et al. Parental somatic mosaicism is underrecognized and influences recurrence risk of genomic disorders. *Am J Hum Genet* 95:173–182, 2014.

Campos AE, Rosenberg C, Krepischi A, et al. An apparently balanced complex chromosome rearrangement involving seven breaks and four chromosomes in a healthy female and segregation/recombination in her affected son. *Mol Syndromol* 12:312–320, 2021.

Campos G, Nel-Themaat L. Blastocoel fluid as an alternative source of DNA for minimally invasive PGT and biomarker of embryo competence. *Reprod Biomed Online* 49:104322, 2024.

Candelo E, Giraldo-Ocampo S, Nevado J, Lapunzina P, Pachajoa H. 2q31 microdeletion syndrome with the velocardiofacial phenotype and review of the literature: A case report. *BMC Pediatr* 24:641, 2024.

Canevini MP, Sgro V, Zuffardi O, et al. Chromosome 20 ring: A chromosomal disorder associated with a particular electroclinical pattern. *Epilepsia* 39:942–951, 1998.

Cannarella R, Mattina T, Condorelli RA, et al. Chromosome 15 structural abnormalities: Effect on *IGF1R* gene expression and function. *Endocr Connect* 6:528–539, 2017.

Cannon S, Clissold R, Sukcharoen K, et al. Recurrent 17q12 microduplications contribute to renal disease but not diabetes. *J Med Genet* 60:491–497, 2023.

Cans C, Cohen O, Lavergne C, Mermet MA, Demongeot J, Jalbert P. Logistic regression model to estimate the risk of unbalanced offspring in reciprocal translocations. *Hum Genet* 92:598–604, 1993.

Canto P, Söderlund D, Reyes E, Méndez JP. Mutations in the desert hedgehog (*DHH*) gene in patients with 46,XY complete pure gonadal dysgenesis. *J Clin Endocrinol Metab* 89:4480–4483, 2004.

Capalbo A, Cimadomo D, Coticchio G, Ottolini CS. An expert opinion on rescuing atypically pronucleated human zygotes by molecular genetic fertilization checks in IVF. *Hum Reprod* 39:1869–1878, 2024.

Carbone JF, Tuuli MG, Dicke JM, Macones GA, Odibo AO. Revisiting the risk for aneuploidy in fetuses with isolated pyelectasis. *Prenat Diagn* 31:566–570, 2011.

Cardoso C, Leventer RJ, Ward HL, et al. Refinement of a 400-kb critical region allows genotypic differentiation between isolated lissencephaly, Miller-Dieker syndrome, and other phenotypes secondary to deletions of 17p13.3. *Am J Hum Genet* 72:918–930, 2003.

Cardoso LCA, Moraes L, Camilo MJE, et al. Cytogenetic and molecular studies of an X;21 translocation previously diagnosed as complete monosomy 21. *Eur J Med Genet* 51:588–597, 2008.

Carella M, Spreafico F, Palumbo O, et al. Constitutional ring chromosome 11 mosaicism in a Wilms tumor patient: Cytogenetic, molecular and clinico-pathological studies. *Am J Med Genet* 152A:1756–1763, 2010.

Carey L, Scott F, Murphy K, et al. Prenatal diagnosis of chromosomal mosaicism in over 1600 cases using array comparative genomic hybridization as a first line test. *Prenat Diagn* 34:478–486, 2014.

Carey JC. Perspectives on the care and management of infants with trisomy 18 and trisomy 13: Striving for balance. *Curr Opin Pediatr* 24:672–678, 2012.

Carey JC, Lortz A, Mendel A, Battaglia A. Natural history study of adults with Wolf-Hirschhorn syndrome 2: Patient-reported outcomes study. *Am J Med Genet* 185A:2065–2069, 2021.

Carey JC, Viskochil DH. Status of the human malformation map: 2007. *Am J Med Genet* 143A:2868–2885, 2007.

Carrillo YD, Rueda-Gaitán P, Gualdrón O, et al. Diagnostic yield of chromosomal microarray in the largest Latino clinical cohort. *Am J Med Genet* 194A:218–225, 2024.

Carli D, Operti M, Russo S, et al. Clinical and molecular characterization of patients affected by Beckwith-Wiedemann spectrum conceived through assisted reproduction techniques. *Clin Genet* 102:314–323, 2022.

Carlson RJ, Quesnel A, Wells D, et al. Genetic heterogeneity and core clinical features of NOG-related-symphalangism spectrum disorder. *Otol Neurotol* 42:e1143–e1151, 2021.

Carmany EP, Bawle EV. Microduplication of 4p16.3 due to an unbalanced translocation resulting in a mild phenotype. *Am J Med Genet* 155A:819–824, 2011.

Carmichael H, Shen Y, Nguyen TT, Hirschhorn JN, Dauber A. Whole exome sequencing in a patient with uniparental disomy of chromosome 2 and a complex phenotype. *Clin Genet* 84:213–222, 2013.

Caroselli S, Figliuzzi M, Picchetta L, et al. Improved clinical utility of preimplantation genetic testing through the integration of ploidy and common pathogenic microdeletions analyses. *Hum Reprod* 38:762–775, 2023.

Carothers AD, Castilla EE, Dutra MG, Hook EB. Search for ethnic, geographic, and other factors in the epidemiology of Down syndrome in South America: Analysis of data from the ECLAMC project, 1967–1997. *Am J Med Genet* 103:149–156, 2001.

Carothers AD, Hecht CA, Hook EB. International variation in reported livebirth prevalence rates of Down syndrome, adjusted for maternal age. *J Med Genet* 36:386–393, 1999.

Carrera IA, de Zaldívar MS, Martín R, Begemann M, Soellner L, Eggermann T. Microdeletions of the 7q32.2 imprinted region are associated with Silver-Russell syndrome features. *Am J Med Genet* 170A:743–749, 2016.

Carter E, Heard P, Hasi M, et al. Ring 18 molecular assessment and clinical consequences. *Am J Med Genet* 167A:54–63, 2015.

Carter MT, Barrowman NJ, St Pierre SA, Emanuel BS, Boycott KM. Risk of breast cancer not increased in translocation 11;22 carriers: Analysis of 80 pedigrees. *Am J Med Genet* 152A:212–214, 2010.

Carter MT, St. Pierre SA, Zackai EH, Emanuel BS, Boycott KM. Phenotypic delineation of Emanuel syndrome (supernumerary derivative 22 syndrome): Clinical features of 63 individuals. *Am J Med Genet* 149A:1712–1721, 2009.

Carvalho V, Ferreira JJ, Correia Guedes L. Tremor and Parkinsonism in chromosomopathies—A systematic review. *Mov Disord* 36:2017–2025. 2021.

Carvalho CMB, Lupski JR. Mechanisms underlying structural variant formation in genomic disorders. *Nat Rev Genet* 17:224–238, 2016.

Carvalho CMB, Vasanth S, Shinawi M, et al. Dosage changes of a segment at 17p13.1 lead to intellectual disability and microcephaly as a result of complex genetic interaction of multiple genes. *Am J Hum Genet* 95:565–578, 2014.

Casas L, Vivaldi L. Pregnancies and fetal anomalies incompatible with life in Chile: Arguments and experiences in advocating for legal reform. *Health Hum Rights* 19:95–108, 2017.

Casas-Alba D, Nolasco GA, Díez-Juan M, Mezzatesta M, Balañá G, Fons C. Targeted therapy with galantamine in a pediatric patient with 15q13.3 deletion syndrome. *Am J Med Genet* 185A:3897–3899, 2021.

Cascante SD, Besser A, Lee HL, Wang F, McCaffrey C, Grifo JA. Blinded rebiopsy and analysis of noneuploid embryos with 2 distinct preimplantation genetic testing platforms for aneuploidy. *Fertil Steril* 120:1161–1169, 2023.

Casper AM, Durkin SG, Arlt MF, Glover TW. Chromosomal instability at common fragile sites in Seckel syndrome. *Am J Hum Genet* 75:654–660, 2004.

Cassidy and Allanson's Management of Genetic Syndrome, JC Carey, A Battaglia, D Viskochil, SB Cassidy (eds.), John Wiley & Sons, Hoboken, 2020.

Cassidy SB, Lai LW, Erickson RP, et al. Trisomy 15 with loss of the paternal 15 as a cause of Prader-Willi syndrome due to maternal disomy. *Am J Hum Genet* 51:701–708, 1992.

Cassidy SB, Whitworth T, Sanders D, Lorber CA, Engel E. Five month extrauterine survival in a female triploid (69,XXX) child. *Ann Génét* 20:277–279, 1977.

Castanet M, Mallya U, Agostini M, et al. Maternal isodisomy for chromosome 9 causing homozygosity for a novel *FOXE1* mutation in syndromic congenital hypothyroidism. *J Clin Endocrinol Metab* 95:4031–4036, 2010.

Castella M, Pujol R, Callén E, et al. Chromosome fragility in patients with Fanconi anaemia: Diagnostic implications and clinical impact. *J Med Genet* 48:242–250, 2011.

Castermans D, Thienpont B, Volders K, et al. Position effect leading to haploinsufficiency in a mosaic ring chromosome 14 in a boy with autism. *Eur J Hum Genet* 16:1187–1192, 2008.

Castiglia D, Castori M, Pisaneschi E, et al. Trisomic rescue causing reduction to homozygosity for a novel *ABCA12* mutation in harlequin ichthyosis. *Clin Genet* 76:392–397, 2009.

Castillo A, Kramer N, Schwartz CE, et al. 19q13.32 microdeletion syndrome: Three new cases. *Eur J Med Genet* 57:654–658, 2014.

Castori M, Bottillo I, Laino L, Morlino S, Grammatico B, Grammatico P. An additional patient with 3q27.3 microdeletion syndrome. *J Child Neurol* 30:500–504, 2015.

Castorina P, Selicorni A, Bedeschi F, Dalpra L, Larizza L. Genotype-phenotype correlation in two sets of monozygotic twins with Williams syndrome. *Am J Med Genet* 69:107–111, 1997.

Castronovo C, Rossetti R, Rusconi D, et al. Gene dosage as a relevant mechanism contributing to the determination of ovarian function in Turner syndrome. *Hum Reprod* 29:368–379, 2014.

Castronovo P, Gervasini C, Cereda A, et al. Premature chromatid separation is not a useful diagnostic marker for Cornelia de Lange syndrome. *Chromosome Res* 17:763–771, 2009.

Catelani ALPM, Krepischi ACV, Kim CA, et al. Chromosome imbalances in syndromic hearing loss. *Clin Genet* 76:458–464, 2009.

Caubit X, Gubellini P, Andrieux J, et al. TSHZ3 deletion causes an autism syndrome and defects in cortical projection neurons. *Nat Genet* 48:1359–1369, 2016.

Cavadino A, Morris JK. Revised estimates of the risk of fetal loss following a prenatal diagnosis of trisomy 13 or trisomy 18. *Am J Med Genet* 173A:953–958, 2017.

Ceccarini C, Sinibaldi L, Bernardini L, et al. Duplication 18q21.31-q22.2. *Am J Med Genet* 143A:343–348, 2007.

Cellini E, Disciglio V, Novara F, et al. Periventricular heterotopia with white matter abnormalities associated with 6p25 deletion. *Am J Med Genet* 158A:1793–1797, 2012.

Center for Reproductive Rights, https://reproductiverights.org/maps/abortion-laws-by-state/.

Cesaretti C, Spaccini L, Righini A, et al. Prenatal detection of 5q14.3 duplication including *MEF2C* and brain phenotype. *Am J Med Genet* 170A:1352–1357, 2016.

Cetin Z, Mihci E, Yakut S, Keser I, Karauzum SB, Luleci G. Pure and complete 12p trisomy due to a maternal centric fission of chromosome 12. *Am J Med Genet* 155A:349–352, 2011.

Ceylan AC, Citli S, Erdem HB, et al. Importance and usage of chromosomal microarray analysis in diagnosing intellectual disability, global developmental delay, and autism; and discovering new loci for these disorders. *Mol Cytogenet* 11:54, 2018.

Chai H, Ji W, Wen J, et al. Ring chromosome formation by intra-strand repairing of subtelomeric double stand breaks and clinico-cytogenomic correlations for ring chromosome 9. *Am J Med Genet* 182A:3023–3028, 2020.

Chaiken SR, Mandelbaum AD, Garg B, Doshi U, Packer CH, Caughey AB. Association between rates of Down syndrome diagnosis in states with vs without 20-week abortion bans from 2011 to 2018. *JAMA Netw Open* 6:e233684, 2023.

Chakravarti D, LaBella KA, DePinho RA. Telomeres: History, health, and hallmarks of aging. *Cell* 184:306–322, 2021.

Chalas C, Receveur A, Frydman N, et al. A case of germline mosaicism for a 7q32.1q33 deletion in a sperm donor: Consequences on pregnancy follow-up and recommendations. *Basic Clin Androl* 30:14, 2020.

Chamayou S, Sicali M, Lombardo D, Alecci C, Guglielmino A. The decision on the embryo to transfer after preimplantation genetic diagnosis for X-autosome reciprocal translocation in male carrier. *Mol Cytogenet* 11:63, 2018.

Chan CTJ, Clayton-Smith J, Cheng XJ, et al. Molecular mechanisms in Angelman syndrome: A survey of 93 patients. *J Med Genet* 30:895–902, 1993.

Chan CYZ, Baker EK, Francis D, Milner K, Amor DJ. Hexasomy of the 15q11q13 region: A detailed report and review of the literature. *Eur J Med Genet* 76:105023, 2025.

Chan ER, Benchek P, Miller G, et al. Importance of copy number variants in childhood apraxia of speech and other speech sound disorders. *Commun Biol* 7:1273, 2024.

Chance PF. Inherited focal, episodic neuropathies: Hereditary neuropathy with liability to pressure palsies and hereditary neuralgic amyotrophy. *Neuromolecular Med* 8:159–174, 2006.

Chandel D, Sanghavi P, Verma R. Clinical profile and cytogenetic correlations in females with primary amenorrhea. *Clin Exp Reprod Med* 50:192–199, 2023.

Chandrasekhar A, Mroczkowski HJ, Urraca N, et al. Genome sequencing detects a balanced pericentric inversion with breakpoints that impact the DMD and upstream region of POU3F4 genes. *Am J Med Genet* 194A:e63462, 2024.

Chanes B, Arriaza M, Lacassie Y. Lessons from a 30 year follow-up of monozygotic twins with discordant phenotype due to a ring 13 chromosomal mosaicism in one of them. *Am J Med Genet* 185A:1242–1246, 2021.

Chang HJ, Clark RD, Bachman H. The phenotype of 45,X/46,XY mosaicism: An analysis of 92 prenatally diagnosed cases. *Am J Hum Genet* 46:156–167, 1990.

Chang YS, Owen JP, Pojman NJ, et al. Reciprocal white matter alterations due to 16p11.2 chromosomal deletions versus duplications. *Hum Brain Mapp* 37:2833–2848, 2016.

Chańska W, Grunt-Mejer K. The directiveness that dare not speak its name. Views and attitudes of Polish clinical geneticists toward the nondirectiveness principle. *J Bioeth Inq* 19:557–569, 2022.

Chantot-Bastaraud S, Ravel C, Berthaut I, et al. Sperm-FISH analysis in a pericentric chromosome 1 inversion, 46,XY,inv(1)(p22q42), associated with infertility. *Mol Hum Reprod* 13:55–59, 2007.

Chantot-Bastaraud S, Stratmann S, Brioude F, et al. Formation of upd(7)mat by trisomic rescue: SNP array typing provides new insights in chromosomal nondisjunction. *Mol Cytogenet* 10:28, 2017.

Chapman CJ, Gardner RJM, Veale AMO. Segregation analysis of a large t(21q22q) family. *J Med Genet* 10:362–366, 1973.

Chau MHK, Lam DYM, Zhu X, et al. The utility of genome-wide cell-free DNA screening in the prenatal diagnosis of Pallister-Killian syndrome. *Prenat Diagn* 40:1005–1012, 2020.

Chaveeva P, Wright A, Syngelaki A, Konstantinidou L, Wright D, Nicolaides KH. First-trimester screening for trisomies in pregnancies with vanishing twin. *Ultrasound Obstet Gynecol* 55:326–331, 2020.

Chavli EA, Klaasen SJ, Van Opstal D, Laven JS, Kops GJ, Baart EB. Single-cell DNA sequencing reveals a high incidence of chromosomal abnormalities in human blastocysts. *J Clin Invest* 134:e174483, 2024.

Chawner SJ, Watson CJ, Owen MJ. Clinical evaluation of patients with a neuropsychiatric risk copy number variant. *Curr Opin Genet Dev* 68:26–34, 2021.

Check JH, Katsoff B, Summers-Chase D, Breitbart J. A case report supporting the concept that some women have a predisposition for maternal meiosis errors resulting in digyny. *Clin Exp Obstet Gynecol* 36:133–134, 2009.

Cheffins T, Chan A, Haan EA, et al. The impact of maternal serum screening on the birth prevalence of Down's syndrome and the use of amniocentesis and chorionic villus sampling in South Australia. *Br J Obstet Gynaecol* 107:1453–1459, 2000.

Chen CP. Mosaic isochromosome 20q at amniocentesis in a pregnancy associated with a favorable fetal outcome and cytogenetic discrepancy between cultured amniocytes and uncultured amniocytes. *Taiwan J Obstet Gynecol* 62:372–374, 2023a.

Chen CP. Genetic counseling of mosaicism for balanced or unbalanced translocation with a normal cell line at amniocentesis. *Taiwan J Obstet Gynecol* 63:618–623, 2024a.

Chen CP. Balanced Robertsonian translocation mosaicism of mosaic 45,XY,der(13;21) (q10;q10)/46,XY at amniocentesis in a pregnancy with a favorable outcome and no perinatal decrease of the cell line with the balanced Robertsonian translocation. *Taiwan J Obstet Gynecol* 63:572–574, 2024b.

Chen CP. Detection of mosaic ring chromosome 12 or 46,XY,r(12) (p13.3q24.33)/46, XY in a 37-year-old male associated with oligospermia but no other apparently phenotypic abnormalities. *Taiwan J Obstet Gynecol* 63:581–583, 2024c.

Chen CP, Chang TY, Guo WY, et al. Chromosome 17p13.3 deletion syndrome: aCGH characterization, prenatal findings and diagnosis, and literature review. *Gene* 532:152–159, 2013a.

Chen CP, Chen M, Chern SR, et al. Prenatal diagnosis and molecular cytogenetic characterization of mosaicism for a small supernumerary marker chromosome derived from ring chromosome 2. *Taiwan J Obstet Gynecol* 51:411–417, 2012.

Chen CP, Chen M, Su YN, et al. Mosaic small supernumerary marker chromosome 1 at amniocentesis: Prenatal diagnosis, molecular genetic analysis and literature review. *Gene* 529:169–175, 2013b.

Chen CP, Chen CY, Chern SR, et al. Molecular cytogenetic characterization of Xp22.32→pter deletion and Xq26.3→qter duplication in a male fetus associated with 46,Y,rec(X)dup(Xq) inv(X) (p22.3q26.3), a hypoplastic left heart, short stature, and maternal X chromosome pericentric inversion. *Taiwan J Obstet Gynecol* 55:705–711, 2016a.

Chen CP, Chen CY, Wu FT, et al. Prenatal diagnosis of a 14-Mb 11p11.2-p13 deletion by chromosome microarray analysis in a pregnancy with fetal recombinant chromosome 11 syndrome of rec(11) del(11)(p11.2p13)ins(11)(q21p11.2p13) and maternal intrachromosomal insertion of ins(11) (q21p11.2p13). *Taiwan J Obstet Gynecol* 63:913–917, 2024d.

Chen CP, Chen M, Ma GC, et al. Prenatal diagnosis and molecular cytogenetic characterization of a familial small supernumerary marker chromosome derived from the acrocentric chromosome 14/22. *Taiwan J Obstet Gynecol* 61:364–367, 2022.

Chen CP, Chen SW, Wu CY, et al. Molecular cytogenetic characterization of de novo concomitant proximal 21q deletion of 21q11.2q21.3 and distal Xp deletion of Xp22.33p22.2 due to an unbalanced X;21 translocation detected by amniocentesis. *Taiwan J Obstet Gynecol* 62:123–127, 2023b.

Chen CP, Chen YY, Chern SR, et al. Prenatal diagnosis of mosaic trisomy 2 associated with abnormal maternal serum screening, oligohydramnios, intrauterine growth restriction, ventricular septal defect, preaxial polydactyly, and facial dysmorphism. *Taiwan J Obstet Gynecol* 52:395–400, 2013c.

Chen CP, Chen CY, Chern SR, et al. Prenatal diagnosis of recurrent mosaic ring chromosome 13 of maternal origin. *Taiwan J Obstet Gynecol* 60:771–774, 2021a.

Chen CP, Chern SR, Chen LF, Chen WL, Wang W. Prenatal diagnosis of low-level mosaic trisomy 7 by amniocentesis. *Prenat Diagn* 25:1067–1069, 2005a.

Chen CP, Chern SR, Lee CC, Chen WL, Wang W. Prenatal diagnosis of interstitially satellited 6p. *Prenat Diagn* 24:430–433, 2004a.

Chen CP, Chern SR, Lee CC, et al. Prenatal diagnosis of de novo t(2;18;14)(q33.1;q12.2;q31.2), dup(5)(q34q34), del(7)(p21.1p21.1), and del(10)(q25.3q25.3) and a review of the prenatally ascertained de novo apparently balanced complex and multiple chromosomal rearrangements. *Prenat Diagn* 26:138–146, 2006a.

Chen CP, Chern SR, Lee CC, Town DD. Isochromosome 18q in a fetus with congenital megacystis, intra-uterine growth retardation and cloacal dysgenesis sequence. *Prenat Diagn* 18:1068–1074, 1998.

Chen CP, Chern SR, Lee PY, Town DD, Wang W. Prenatal diagnosis of low-level mosaic trisomy 6 by amniocentesis. *Prenat Diagn* 26:1093–1096, 2006b.

Chen CP, Chern SR, Sheu JC, et al. Prenatal diagnosis, sonographic findings and molecular genetic analysis of a 46,XX/46,XY true hermaphrodite chimera. *Prenat Diagn* 25:502–6, 2005b.

Chen CP, Chern SR, Town DD, Wang W, Liao YW. Fetoplacental and fetoamniotic chromosomal discrepancies in prenatally detected mosaic trisomy 9. *Prenat Diagn* 23:1019–1021, 2003a.

Chen CP, Chern SR, Wang LK, et al. Prenatal diagnosis of maternal uniparental disomy 5 by amniocentesis associated with confined placental mosaicism for trisomy 5 and fetal trisomy 21 in a pregnancy. *Taiwan J Obstet Gynecol* 59:938–940, 2020a.

Chen CP, Chern SR, Wu PS, et al. Monozygotic twins discordant for low-level mosaic trisomy 17 at amniocentesis in a pregnancy with a favorable outcome and a literature review of heterokaryotypic monozygotic twins at amniocentesis. *Taiwan J Obstet Gynecol* 59:306–313, 2020b.

Chen CP, Hsu TY, Ko TM, et al. Cytogenetic discrepancy between uncultured amniocytes and cultured amniocytes in mosaic trisomy 15 at amniocentesis. *Taiwan J Obstet Gynecol* 59:728–735, 2020c.

Chen CP, Huang MC, Chern SR, et al. Mosaic trisomy 22 at amniocentesis: Prenatal diagnosis and literature review. *Taiwan J Obstet Gynecol* 58:692–697, 2019.

Chen CP, Hwu YM, Yeh LF, Chern SR, Lee CC, Wang W. Successful triplet pregnancy and delivery after oocyte donation in an infertile female with chromosome mosaicism for monosomy X, partial trisomy X, and terminal Xp deletion. *Fertil Steril* 79:1231–1233, 2003b.

Chen CP, Lee CC, Chen WL, et al. Prenatal diagnosis of premature centromere division-related mosaic variegated aneuploidy. *Prenat Diagn* 24:19–25, 2004b.

Chen CP, Lee CC, Town DD, et al. Detection of euchromatic variants and unusual C band heterochromatin variants at genetic amniocentesis. *Genet Couns* 17:91–95, 2006c.

Chen CP, Lin SP, Lin CC, et al. Prenatal diagnosis of low-level mosaicism for a small XIST-negative supernumerary ring X chromosome in a nondysmorphic male fetus. *Prenat Diagn* 26:387–391, 2006d.

Chen CP, Lin SP, Sheu JC, Wang W, Tzen CY. Neonatal outcome of a prenatally detected 46,XX/46,XY true hermaphrodite. *Prenat Diagn* 26:185–186, 2006e.

Chen CP, Lin YH, Au HK, et al. Chromosome 15q overgrowth syndrome: Prenatal diagnosis, molecular cytogenetic characterization, and perinatal findings in a fetus with dup(15)(q26.2q26.3). *Taiwan J Obstet Gynecol* 50:359–365, 2011a.

Chen CP, Su YN, Chen YT, Chen WL, Hsu LJ, Wang W. Prenatal diagnosis of directly transmitted benign 4q12-q13.1 quadruplication associated with tandem segmental amplifications of the *LPHN3* gene. *Taiwan J Obstet Gynecol* 50:401–404, 2011b.

Chen CP, Su YN, Lin CC, et al. Genetic counseling of prenatally detected unbalanced t(Y;15)(q12;p13). *Genet Couns* 18:455–457, 2007.

Chen CP, Su YN, Lin SP, et al. Prenatal diagnosis and molecular cytogenetic characterization of a de novo interstitial duplication of 11q (11q22.3→q23.3) associated with abnormal maternal serum biochemistry. *Taiwan J Obstet Gynecol* 52:120–124, 2013d.

Chen CP, Wang KG, Ko TM, et al. Mosaic trisomy 14 at amniocentesis: Prenatal diagnosis and literature review. *Taiwan J Obstet Gynecol* 52:446–449, 2013e.

Chen CP, Wang LK, Chern SR, et al. Mosaic trisomy 17 at amniocentesis: Prenatal diagnosis, molecular genetic analysis, and literature review. *Taiwan J Obstet Gynecol* 55:712–717, 2016b.

Chen CP, Wang PT, Chern SR, et al. Prenatal diagnosis of a familial Y long-arm and chromosome 15 short-arm translocation inherited from a mother carrier. *Taiwan J Obstet Gynecol* 60:781–783, 2021b.

Chen CP, Wang YL, Chern SR, et al. Prenatal diagnosis and molecular cytogenetic characterization of low-level true mosaicism for trisomy 21 using uncultured amniocytes. *Taiwan J Obstet Gynecol* 55:285–287, 2016c.

Chen CP, Wu CY, Chern SR, et al. Prenatal diagnosis and molecular cytogenetic characterization of a de novo interchromosomal insertion of ins(1;8)(p22.1;q22q23). *Taiwan J Obstet Gynecol* 59:437–439, 2020d.

Chen CP, Wu FT, Chern SR, et al. Low-level mosaic trisomy 2 at amniocentesis in a pregnancy associated with positive NIPT and CVS results for trisomy 2, maternal uniparental disomy 2, perinatal progressive decrease of the aneuploid cell line, cytogenetic discrepancy between cultured amniocytes and uncultured amniocytes, intrauterine growth restriction and a favorable fetal outcome. *Taiwan J Obstet Gynecol.* 62:571–576, 2023c.

Chen CP, Wu FT, Pan YT, et al. Low-level mosaic trisomy 20 without uniparental disomy 20 at amniocentesis in a pregnancy associated with a favorable outcome, cytogenetic discrepancy between uncultured amniocytes and cultured amniocytes and perinatal progressive decrease of the aneuploid cell line. *Taiwan J Obstet Gynecol* 62:466–469, 2023d.

Chen CP, Wu FT, Pan YT, et al. Low-level mosaic trisomy 7 at amniocentesis in a pregnancy associated with cytogenetic discrepancy between cultured amniocytes and uncultured amniocytes, perinatal progressive decrease of the trisomy 7 cell line and a favorable fetal outcome. *Taiwan J Obstet Gynecol* 63:549–551, 2024e.

Chen CP, Wu FT, Pan YT, Wu PS, Lee MS, Wang W. Prenatal diagnosis of familial 3p26.3p25.3 deletion in a pregnancy associated with a favorable fetal outcome and asymptomatic carrier parent and family members in three generations. *Taiwan J Obstet Gynecol* 63:561–564, 2024f.

Chen E, Choe MA, Loughman WD, et al. Recurrent adjacent-2 segregation of a familial t(14;21)(q11.2;q11.2): Phenotypic comparison of two brothers and a paternal aunt inheriting the der(14). *Am J Med Genet A* 132A:164–70, 2005c.

Chen H, Young R, Mu X, et al. Uniparental isodisomy resulting from 46,XX,i(1p),i(1q) in a woman with short stature, ptosis, micro/retrognathia, myopathy, deafness, and sterility. *Am J Med Genet* 82:215–218, 1999.

Chen H, Yu CW, Wood MJ, Landry K. Mosaic trisomy 19 syndrome. *Ann Génét* 24:32–33, 1981.

Chen K, Chmait RH, Vanderbilt D, Wu S, Randolph L. Chimerism in monochorionic dizygotic twins: Case study and review. *Am J Med Genet* 161A:1817–1824, 2013f.

Chen M, Jiang H, Zhang C. Selected genetic factors associated with primary ovarian insufficiency. *Int J Mol Sci* 24:4423, 2023e.

Chen SH, Escudero T, Cekleniak NA, Sable DB, Garrisi MG, Munne S. Patterns of ovarian response to gonadotropin stimulation in female carriers of balanced translocation. *Fertil Steril* 83:1504–1509, 2005d.

Chen X, Zhou C. Reciprocal translocation and Robertsonian translocation in relation to semen parameters: A retrospective study and systematic review. *Andrologia* 54:e14262, 2022.

Chen Z, Chen H, Yuan K, et al. A 15q25.2 microdeletion phenotype for premature ovarian failure in a Chinese girl: A case report and review of literature. *BMC Med Genomics* 13:126, 2020e.

Cheng A, Dinulos MBP, Neufeld-Kaiser W, et al. 6q25.1 (*TAB2*) microdeletion syndrome Congenital heart defects and cardiomyopathy. *Am J Med Genet* 173A:1848–1857, 2017.

Cheng D, Yuan S, Yi D, et al. Analysis of molecular cytogenetic features and PGT-SR for two infertile patients with small supernumerary marker chromosomes. *J Assist Reprod Genet* 36:2533–2539, 2019.

Cheng EY, Chen YJ, Disteche CM, Gartler SM. Analysis of a paracentric inversion in human oocytes: Nonhomologous pairing in pachytene. *Hum Genet* 105:191–196, 1999.

Cheng SF, Rauen KA, Pinkel D, Albertson DG, Cotter PD. Xq chromosome duplication in males: Clinical, cytogenetic and array CGH characterization of a new case and review. *Am J Med Genet* 135A:308–313, 2005.

Chen-Shtoyerman R, Josefsberg Ben-Yehoshua S, Nissani R, Rosensaft J, Appelman Z. A prevalent Y;15 translocation in the Ethiopian Beta Israel community in Israel. *Cytogenet Genome Res* 136:171–174, 2012.

Cherian JD, Ta D, Smith J, Downs J, Leonard H. How families manage the complex medical needs of their children with *MECP2* duplication syndrome. *Children (Basel)* 10:1202, 2023.

Chernus JM, Allen EG, Zeng Z, et al. A candidate gene analysis and GWAS for genes associated with maternal nondisjunction of chromosome 21. *PLoS Genet* 15:e1008414, 2019.

Chetaille P, Preuss C, Burkhard S, et al. Mutations in *SGOL1* cause a novel cohesinopathy affecting heart and gut rhythm1. *Nat Genet* 46:1245–1249, 2014.

Chia N, Bousfield L, James S, Nelson J. Report of a severely retarded child with a duplication 18q derived from a paternal paracentric inversion (18q): A note of warning. *Bull Hum Genet Soc Australasia* 6:48, 1992.

Chiesa J, Hoffet M, Rousseau O, et al. Pallister-Killian syndrome [i(12p)]: First pre-natal diagnosis using cordocentesis in the second trimester confirmed by in situ hybridization. *Clin Genet* 54:294–302, 1998.

Chisholm CA, Bray MJ, Karns LB. Successful pregnancy in a woman with Bloom syndrome. *Am J Med Genet* 102:136–138, 2001.

Cho E, Yang TH, Shin ES, Byeon JH, Kim GH, Eun BL. Saethre-Chotzen syndrome with an atypical phenotype: Identification of *TWIST* microdeletion by array CGH. *Childs Nerv Syst* 29:2101–2104, 2013a.

Cho EH, Kim SY, Kim JK. A case of 9.7 Mb terminal Xp deletion including OA1 locus associated with contiguous gene syndrome. *J Korean Med Sci* 27:1273–1277, 2012a.

Cho SY, Goh DL, Lau KC, Ong HT, Lam CW. Microarray analysis unmasked paternal uniparental disomy of chromosome 12 in a patient with isolated sulfite oxidase deficiency. *Clin Chim Acta* 426:13–17, 2013b.

Cho SY, Ki CS, Jang JH, et al. Familial Xp22.33-Xp22.12 deletion delineated by chromosomal microarray analysis causes proportionate short stature. *Am J Med Genet* 158A:1462–1466 2012b.

Choi J, Lee H, Lee CG. Partial trisomy of 11q23.3-q25 inherited from a maternal low-level mosaic unbalanced translocation. *Am J Med Genet* 167A:1859–1864, 2015.

Chow JFC, Cheng HHY, Lau EYL, Yeung WSB, Ng EHY. Distinguishing between carrier and noncarrier embryos with the use of long-read sequencing in preimplantation genetic testing for reciprocal translocations. *Genomics* 112:494–500, 2020.

Chowdhury S, Bandholz AM, Parkash S, et al. Phenotypic and molecular characterization of 19q12q13.1 deletions: A report of five patients. *Am J Med Genet* 164A:62–69, 2014.

Christesen HT, Christensen LG, Löfgren ÅM, et al. Tissue variations of mosaic genome-wide paternal uniparental disomy and phenotype of multi-syndromal congenital hyperinsulinism. *Eur J Med Genet* 63:103632, 2020.

Chu C, Schwartz S, McPherson E. Paternal uniparental isodisomy for chromosome 14 in a patient with a normal 46,XY karyotype. *Am J Med Genet* 127A:167–171, 2004.

Chuang L, Wakui K, Sue WC, Su MH, Shaffer LG, Kuo PL. Interstitial deletion 11(p11.12p11.2) and analphoid marker formation results in inherited Potocki-Shaffer syndrome. *Am J Med Genet* 133A:180–183, 2005.

Chudley AE, Bauder F, Ray M, McAlpine PJ, Pena SD, Hamerton JL. Familial mental retardation in a family with an inherited chromosome rearrangement. *J Med Genet* 11:353–366, 1974.

Chung D, Haynes K, Haynes R. Surviving with trisomy 13: Provider and parent perspectives and the role of the pediatric palliative care program. *Am J Med Genet* 173A:813–815, 2017.

Ciaccio C, Redaelli S, Bentivegna A, et al. Unbalanced X;autosome translocations may lead to mild phenotypes and are associated with autoimmune diseases. *Cytogenet Genome Res* 160:80–84, 2020.

Cifuentes P, Navarro J, Míguez L, Egozcue J, Benet J. Sperm segregation analysis of a complex chromosome rearrangement, 2;22;11, by whole chromosome painting. *Cytogenet Cell Genet* 82:204–209, 1998.

Cignini P, Dinatale A, D'Emidio L, et al. Prenatal diagnosis of a fetus with de novo supernumerary ring chromosome 16 characterized by array comparative genomic hybridization. *AJP Rep* 1:29–32, 2011.

Cimadomo D, Capalbo A, Dovere L, et al. Leave the past behind: Women's reproductive history shows no association with blastocysts' euploidy and limited association with live birth rates after euploid embryo transfers. *Hum Reprod* 36:929–940, 2021.

Cinar C, Beyazyurek C, Ekmekci CG, Aslan C, Kahraman S. Sperm fluorescence in situ hybridization analysis reveals normal sperm cells for 14;14 homologous male Robertsonian translocation carrier. *Fertil Steril* 95:289.e5–9, 2011.

Cirigliano V, Voglino G, Ordoñez E, et al. Rapid prenatal diagnosis of common chromosome aneuploidies by QF-PCR: Results of 9 years of clinical experience. *Prenat Diagn* 29:40–49, 2009.

Cirillo E, Giardino G, Gallo V, et al. Intergenerational and intrafamilial phenotypic variability in 22q11.2 deletion syndrome subjects. *BMC Med Genet* 15:1, 2014.

Cirnigliaro M, Chang TS, Arteaga SA, et al. The contributions of rare inherited and polygenic risk to ASD in multiplex families. *Proc Natl Acad Sci USA* 120:e2215632120, 2023.

Città S, Buono S, Greco D, et al. 3q29 microdeletion syndrome: Cognitive and behavioral phenotype in four patients. *Am J Med Genet* 161A:3018–3022, 2013.

Ciuladaite Z, Preiksaitiene E, Utkus A, Kucinskas V. Relatives with opposite chromosome constitutions, rec(10)dup(10p)inv(10)(p15.1q26.12) and rec(10)dup(10q)inv(10)(p15.1q26.12), due to a familial pericentric inversion. *Cytogenet Genome Res* 144:109–113, 2014.

Clang DR, LaBaere RJ. Jacobsen syndrome: Chromosome deletion at llq23. *J Osteopath Med* 98:551–554, 2023.

Clarke A. The genetic testing of children: Working Party of the Clinical Genetics Society (UK). *J Med Genet* 31:785–797, 1994.

Clarke A. Harper's Practical Genetic Counselling, 8th edn. London: CRC Press, 2019.

Clayton EW. Removing the shadow of the law from the debate about genetic testing of children. *Am J Med Genet* 57:630–634, 1995.

Cleary-Goldman J, D'Alton ME, Berkowitz RL. Prenatal diagnosis and multiple pregnancy. *Semin Perinatol* 29:312–320, 2005.

Clement SC, Peeters RP, Ronckers CM, et al. Intermediate and long-term adverse effects of radioiodine therapy for differentiated thyroid carcinoma—A systematic review. *Cancer Treat Rev* 41:925–934, 2015.

Clement Wilson S, Susman M, Bain S, et al. Isochromosome 5p mosaicism at prenatal diagnosis: Observations and outcomes in six cases at chorionic villus sampling and one at amniocentesis. *Prenat Diagn* 22:681–685, 2002.

Cleynen I, Engchuan W, Hestand MS, et al. Genetic contributors to risk of schizophrenia in the presence of a 22q11.2 deletion. *Mol Psychiatry* 26:4496–4510, 2021.

Clouston HJ, Herbert M, Fenwick J, Murdoch AP, Wolstenholme J. Cytogenetic analysis of human blastocysts. *Prenat Diagn* 22:1143–1152, 2002.

Cobben JM, Verheij JBGM, Eisma WH, et al. Bilateral split hand/foot malformation and inv(7)(p22q21.3). *J Med Genet* 32:375–378, 1995.
Cockwell AE, Baker SJ, Connarty M, Moore IE, Crolla JA. Mosaic trisomy 6 and maternal uniparental disomy 6 in a 23-week gestation fetus with atrioventricular septal defect. *Am J Med Genet* 140:624–627, 2006.
Cockwell AE, James RS, Moore IE, Hatchwell E, Crolla JA. Clinical outcomes of adjacent segregation in a familial translocation t(8;18)(p21.3;p11.23). *J Med Genet* 33:515–517, 1996.
Coco R, Rahn MI, Estanga PG, Antonioli G, Solari AJ. A constitutional complex chromosome rearrangement involving meiotic arrest in an azoospermic male: Case report. *Hum Reprod* 19:2784–2790, 2004.
Codina-Pascual M, Oliver-Bonet M, Navarro J, et al. FISH characterization of a dicentric Yq (p11.32) isochromosome in an azoospermic male. *Am J Med Genet* 127A:302–306, 2004.
Cody JD, Hasi M, Soileau B, et al. Establishing a reference group for distal 18q-: Clinical description and molecular basis. *Hum Genet* 133:199–209, 2014.
Cody JD, Sebold C, Heard P, et al. Consequences of chromosome 18q deletions. *Am J Med Genet* 169C:265–280, 2015.
Coe BP, Witherspoon K, Rosenfeld JA, et al. Refining analyses of copy number variation identifies specific genes associated with developmental delay. *Nat Genet* 46:1063–1071, 2014.
Cohain JS, Buxbaum RE, Mankuta D. Spontaneous first trimester miscarriage rates per woman among parous women with 1 or more pregnancies of 24 weeks or more. *BMC Pregnancy Childbirth* 17:437, 2017.
Cohen MM. *The Child with Multiple Birth Defects* (2nd ed.). New York, NY: Oxford University Press, 1997.
Cohen O, Cans C, Mermet MA, Demongeot J, Jalbert P. Viability thresholds for partial trisomies and monosomies: A study of 1,159 viable unbalanced reciprocal translocations. *Hum Genet* 93:188–194, 1994.
Cohen O, Simonet M, Cans C, et al. Human reciprocal translocations: A new computer system for genetic counseling. *Ann Génét* 35:193–201, 1992.
Colijn MA. Phelan-McDermid syndrome-associated psychosis: A systematic review. *Acta Neuropsychiatr* 20:1–10, 2024.
Colijn MA, Smith CS, Thomas MA. Maternal 15q11.2-q13.1 duplication syndrome-associated psychosis and mania: A new case and review of the literature. *Psychiatr Genet* 34:1–7, 2024.
Collins BE, Neul JL. Rett syndrome and *MECP2* duplication syndrome: Disorders of MeCP2 dosage. *Neuropsychiatr Dis Treat* 18:2813–2835, 2022.
Collins RL, Glessner JT, Porcu E, et al. A cross-disorder dosage sensitivity map of the human genome. *Cell* 185:3041–3055.e25, 2022.
Collins VR, Webley C, Sheffield LJ, Halliday JL. Fetal outcome and maternal morbidity after early amniocentesis. *Prenat Diagn* 18:767–772, 1998.
Collinson MN, Fisher AM, Walker J, Currie J, Williams L, Roberts P. Inv(10)(p11.2q21.2), a variant chromosome. *Hum Genet* 101:175–180, 1997.
Collinson MN, Roberts SE, Crolla JA, Dennis NR. A familial balanced inverted insertion ins(15)(q15q13q11.2) producing Prader-Willi syndrome, Angelman syndrome and duplication of 15q11.2-q13 in a single family: Importance of differentiation from a paracentric inversion. *Am J Med Genet* 126A:27–32, 2004.
Colson C, Decamp M, Gruchy N, et al. High frequency of paternal iso or heterodisomy at chromosome 20 associated with sporadic pseudohypoparathyroidism 1B. *Bone* 123:145–152, 2019.
Coman DJ, Gardner RJM. Deletions that reveal recessive genes. *Eur J Hum Genet* 15:1103–1104, 2007.
Coman D, Gardner RJM, Pertile MD, Kannu P. Trisomy 16 mosaicism at chorionic villus sampling and amniocentesis with a normal physical and intellectual outcome. *Fetal Diagn Ther* 28:117–118, 2010a.
Coman D, Yaplito-Lee J, La P, et al. Three Mendelian disorders (chronic granulomatous disease, retinitis pigmentosa, ornithine transcarbamylase deficiency) in a young woman with an X chromosome deletion, del(X)(p11.4p21.1). *Mol Genet Metab* 99:329, 2010b.
Conlin LK, Kramer W, Hutchinson AL, et al. Molecular analysis of ring chromosome 20 syndrome reveals two distinct groups of patients. *J Med Genet* 48:1–9, 2011.
Conlin LK, Thiel BD, Bonnemann CG, et al. Mechanisms of mosaicism, chimerism and uniparental disomy identified by single nucleotide polymorphism array analysis. *Hum Mol Genet* 19:1263–1275, 2010.
Conn CM, Cozzi J, Harper JC, Winston RM, Delhanty JD. Preimplantation genetic diagnosis for couples at high risk of Down syndrome pregnancy owing to parental translocation or mosaicism. *J Med Genet* 36:45–50, 1999.

De Gregori M, Ciccone R, Magini P, et al. Cryptic deletions are a common finding in "balanced" reciprocal and complex chromosome rearrangements: A study of 59 patients. *J Med Genet* 44:750–762, 2007.

De John KO, De Quintal H, Mathibe MD, Albertus N, Opie JJ. A rare case of acute megakaryoblastic leukaemia with constitutional ring chromosome 21. *Br J Haematol* 202:912, 2023.

De Jong A, Dondorp WJ, Macville MVE, de Die-Smulders CEM, van Lith JMM, de Wert GMWR. Microarrays as a diagnostic tool in prenatal screening strategies: Ethical reflection. *Hum Genet* 133:163–172, 2014.

De la Paz-Gallardo MJ, García FS, de Haro-Muñoz T, et al. Quantitative-fluorescent-PCR versus full karyotyping in prenatal diagnosis of common chromosome aneuploidies in southern Spain. *Clin Chem Lab Med* 53:1333–1338, 2015.

De Lima LG, Guarracino A, Koren S, et al. The formation and propagation of human Robertsonian chromosomes. *BioRχiv, in press 2025.*

De Munck N, Bayram A, Elkhatib I, et al. Segmental duplications and monosomies are linked to in vitro developmental arrest. *J Assist Reprod Genet* 38:2183–2192, 2021.

De Pagter MS, van Roosmalen MJ, Baas AF, et al. Chromothripsis in healthy individuals affects multiple protein-coding genes and can result in severe congenital abnormalities in offspring. *Am J Hum Genet* 96:651–656, 2015.

De Pater JM, Schuring-Blom GH, van den Bogaard R, et al. Maternal uniparental disomy for chromosome 22 in a child with generalized mosaicism for trisomy 22. *Prenat Diagn* 17:81–86, 1997.

De Perdigo A, Gabriel-Robez O, Ratomponirina C, Rumpler Y. Synaptonemal complex analysis in a human male carrier of a 4;6 translocation: Heterosynapsis without previous homosynapsis. *Hum Genet* 86:279–282, 1991.

De Perdigo A, Gabriel-Robez O, Rumpler Y. Correlation between chromosomal breakpoint positions and synaptic behaviour in human males heterozygous for a pericentric inversion. *Hum Genet* 83:274–276, 1989.

De Ravel TJL, Keymolen K, van Assche E, et al. Post-zygotic origin of isochromosome 12p. *Prenat Diagn* 24:984–988, 2004.

De Ravel TJL, Legius E, Brems H, Van Hoestenberghe R, Gillis PH, Fryns JP. Hemifacial microsomia in two patients further supporting chromosomal mosaicism as a causative factor. *Clin Dysmorphol* 10:263–267, 2001.

De Rycke M, Liebaers I, Van Steirteghem A. Epigenetic risks related to assisted reproductive technologies: Risk analysis and epigenetic inheritance. *Hum Reprod* 17:2487–2494, 2002.

De Silva MG, Elliott K, Dahl HH, et al. Disruption of a novel member of a sodium/hydrogen exchanger family and *DOCK3* is associated with an attention deficit hyperactivity disorder-like phenotype. *J Med Genet* 40:733–740, 2003.

De Souza E, Halliday J, Chan A, Bower C, Morris JK. Recurrence risks for trisomies 13, 18, and 21. *Am J Med Genet* 149A:2716–2722, 2009.

De Souza LC, Sgardioli IC, Gil-da-Silva-Lopes VL, Vieira TP. A recognizable phenotype related to 19p13.12 microdeletion. *Am J Med Genet* 176A:1753–1759, 2018.

De Villena FPM, Sapienza C. Transmission ratio distortion in offspring of heterozygous female carriers of Robertsonian translocations. *Hum Genet* 108:31–36, 2001.

De Vos A, Staessen C, De Rycke M, et al. Impact of cleavage-stage embryo biopsy in view of PGD on human blastocyst implantation: A prospective cohort of single embryo transfers. *Hum Reprod* 24:2988–2996, 2009.

De Vries BBA, Eussen BHJ, van Diggelen OP, et al. Submicroscopic Xpter deletion in a boy with growth and mental retardation caused by a familial t(X;14). *Am J Med Genet* 87:189–194, 1999.

de Vries FA, Govaerts LC, Knijnenburg J, et al. Another rare prenatal case of post-zygotic mosaic trisomy 17. *Am J Med Genet A* 161A:1196–1199, 2013.

Del Gaudio D, Shinawi M, Astbury C, et al. Diagnostic testing for uniparental disomy: A points to consider statement from the American College of Medical Genetics and Genomics. *Genet Med* 22:1133–1141, 2020.

Del Llano E, Perrin A, Morel F, et al. Sperm meiotic segregation analysis of reciprocal translocations carriers: We have bigger FISH to fry. *Int J Mol Sci* 24:3664, 2023.

Dean G, Nevin NC, Mikkelsen M, et al. Investigation of a cluster of children with Down's syndrome born to mothers who had attended a school in Dundalk, Ireland. *Occup Environ Med* 57:793–804, 2000.

DeBault LE, Halmi KA. Familial trisomy 7 mosaicism. *J Med Genet* 12:200–203, 1975.

DeBose-Scarlett EM, Sullivan BA. Genomic and epigenetic foundations of neocentromere formation. *Annu Rev Genet* 55:331–348, 2021.

DeBrasi D, Genardi M, D'Agostino A, et al. Double autosomal/gonosomal mosaic aneuploidy: Study of nondisjunction in two cases with trisomy of chromosome 8. *Hum Genet* 95:519–525, 1995.
Del Gobbo GF, Yuan V, Robinson WP. Confined placental mosaicism involving multiple de novo copy number variants associated with fetal growth restriction: A case report. *Am J Med Genet* 185A:1908–1912, 2021.
Del Porto G, Di Fusco C, Baldi M, Grammatico P, D'Alessandro E. Familial centric fission of chromosome 4. *J Med Genet* 21:388–391, 1984.
Delahaye A, Khung-Savatovsky S, Aboura A, et al. Pre- and postnatal phenotype of 6p25 deletions involving the *FOXC1* gene. *Am J Med Genet* 158A:2430–2438, 2012.
Delatycki M, Gardner RJM. Three cases of trisomy 13 mosaicism and a review of the literature. *Clin Genet* 51:403–407, 1997.
Delatycki MB, Pertile MD, Gardner RJM. Trisomy 13 mosaicism at prenatal diagnosis: Dilemmas in interpretation. *Prenat Diagn* 18:45–50, 1998.
Delhanty JDA. Inherited aneuploidy: Germline mosaicism. *Cytogenet Genome Res* 133:136–140, 2011.
Delisle MF, Wilson RD. First trimester prenatal diagnosis: Amniocentesis. *Semin Perinatol* 23:414–423, 1999.
Delli Paoli E, Di Chiano S, Paoli D, Lenzi A, Lombardo F, Pallotti F. Androgen insensitivity syndrome: A review. *J Endocrinol Invest* 46:2237–2245, 2023.
Delobel B, Djlelati R, Gabriel-Robez O, et al. Y-autosome translocation and infertility: Usefulness of molecular, cytogenetic and meiotic studies. *Hum Genet* 102:98–102, 1998.
Délot EC, Vilain E. Towards improved genetic diagnosis of human differences of sex development. *Nat Rev Genet* 22:588–602, 2021.
Délot EC, Vilain EJ. Nonsyndromic 46,XX testicular disorders/differences of development. In: Adam MP, Feldman J, Mirzaa GM, et al. (eds.), *GeneReviews*, Seattle: University of Washington, 2022.
DeLozier-Blanchet CD, Roeder E, Denis-Arrue R, et al. Trisomy 12 mosaicism confirmed in multiple organs from a liveborn child. *Am J Med Genet* 95:444–449, 2000.
Demaerel W, Hosseinzadeh M, Nouri N, et al. Reciprocal 22q11.2 deletion and duplication in siblings with karyotypically normal parents. *Cytogenet Genome Res* 148:1–5, 2016.
Demarini DM. Declaring the existence of human germ-cell mutagens. *Environ Mol Mutagen* 53:166–172, 2012.
DeMarini DM. The mutagenesis moonshot: The propitious beginnings of the environmental mutagenesis and genomics society. *Environ Mol Mutagen* 61:8–24, 2020.
Demeer B, Andrieux J, Receveur A, et al. Duplication 16p13.3 and the *CREBBP* gene: Confirmation of the phenotype. *Eur J Med Genet* 56:26–31, 2013.
Demidov G, Yaldiz B, Garcia-Pelaez J, et al. Comprehensive reanalysis for CNVs in ES data from unsolved rare disease cases results in new diagnoses. *NPJ Genom Med* 9:49, 2024.
Demily C, Poisson A, Peyroux E, et al. Autism spectrum disorder associated with 49,XYYYY: Case report and review of the literature. *BMC Med Genet* 18:9, 2017.
Demko ZP, Simon AL, McCoy RC, Petrov DA, Rabinowitz M. Effects of maternal age on euploidy rates in a large cohort of embryos analyzed with 24-chromosome single-nucleotide polymorphism-based preimplantation genetic screening. *Fertil Steril* 105:1307–1313, 2016.
Deng C, Yi L, Mu Y, et al. Recent trends in the birth prevalence of Down syndrome in China: Impact of prenatal diagnosis and subsequent terminations. *Prenat Diagn* 35:311–318, 2015.
Deng HX, Abe K, Kondo I, et al. Parental origin and mechanism of formation of polysomy X: An XXXXX case and four XXXXY cases determined with RFLPs. *Hum Genet* 86:541–544, 1991.
Dentici ML, Bergonzini P, Scibelli F, et al. 7q11.23 microduplication syndrome: Clinical and neurobehavioral profiling. *Brain Sci* 10:839, 2020.
Depienne C, Nava C, Keren B, et al. Genetic and phenotypic dissection of 1q43q44 microdeletion syndrome and neurodevelopmental phenotypes associated with mutations in *ZBTB18* and *HNRNPU*. *Hum Genet* 136:463–479, 2017.
DeScipio C, Morrissette JD, Conlin LK, et al. Two siblings with alternate unbalanced recombinants derived from a large cryptic maternal pericentric inversion of chromosome 20. *Am J Med Genet* 152A:373–382, 2010a.
DeScipio C, Morrissette JD, Conlin LK, et al. Update on "Two Siblings with Alternate Unbalanced Recombinants Derived from a Large Cryptic Maternal Pericentric Inversion of Chromosome 20." *Am J Med Genet* 152A:1599, 2010b.

DesGroseilliers M, Beaulieu Bergeron M, Brochu P, Lemyre E, Lemieux N. Phenotypic variability in isodicentric Y patients: Study of nine cases. *Clin Genet* 70:145–150, 2006.

Destree A, Fourneau C, Dugauquier C, Rombout S, Sartenaer D, Gillerot Y. Prenatal diagnosis of trisomy 6 mosaicism. *Prenat Diagn* 25:354–357, 2005.

Deveault C, Qian JH, Chebaro W, et al. *NLRP7* mutations in women with diploid androgenetic and triploid moles: A proposed mechanism for mole formation. *Hum Mol Genet* 18:888–897, 2009.

Devi A, Benn PA. X-chromosome abnormalities in women with premature ovarian failure. *J Reprod Med* 44:321–324, 1999.

Devillard F, Guinchat V, Moreno-De-Luca D, et al. Paracentric inversion of chromosome 2 associated with cryptic duplication of 2q14 and deletion of 2q37 in a patient with autism. *Am J Med Genet* 152A:2346–2354, 2010.

Devine DH, Whitman-Elia G, Best RG, Edwards JG. Paternal paracentric inversion of chromosome 2: A possible association with recurrent pregnancy loss and infertility. *J Assist Reprod Genet* 17:293–296, 2000.

Devriendt K, Van Hoestenberghe R, Van Hole C, et al. Submicroscopic deletion in chromosome 22q11 in trizygous triplet siblings and their father: Clinical variability of 22q11 deletion. *Clin Genet* 51:246–249, 1997.

Dewhurst J. Fertility in 47,XXX and 45,X patients. *J Med Genet* 15:132–135, 1978.

Dhallan R, Guo X, Emche S, et al. A non-invasive test for prenatal diagnosis based on fetal DNA present in maternal blood: A preliminary study. *Lancet* 369:474–481, 2007.

Dhakar MB, Ilyas M, Jeong JW, Behen ME, Chugani HT. Frontal aslant tract abnormality on diffusion tensor imaging in an aphasic patient with 49,XXXXY syndrome. *Pediatr Neurol* 55:64–67, 2016.

Dhandha S, Hogge WA, Surti U, McPherson E. Three cases of tetrasomy 9p. *Am J Med Genet* 113:375–380, 2002.

Dharmadhikari AV, Kang SH, Szafranski P, et al. Small rare recurrent deletions and reciprocal duplications in 2q21.1, including brain-specific ARHGEF4 and GPR148. *Hum Mol Genet* 21:3345–3355, 2012.

Di Benedetto D, Musumeci SA, Avola E, et al. Definition of minimal duplicated region encompassing the *XIAP* and *STAG2* genes in the Xq25 microduplication syndrome. *Am J Med Genet* 164A:1923–1930, 2014.

Di Donato N, Klink B, Hahn G, Schrock E, Hackmann K. Interstitial deletion 1p36.32 in two brothers with a distinct phenotype—overgrowth, macrocephaly and nearly normal intellectual function. *Eur J Med Genet* 57:494–497, 2014.

Di Gregorio E, Riberi E, Belligni, EF, et al. Copy number variants analysis in a cohort of isolated and syndromic developmental delay/intellectual disability reveals novel genomic disorders, position effects and candidate disease genes. *Clin Genet* 92:415–422, 2017.

Di Mascio D, Khalil A, Rizzo G, et al. Risk of fetal loss following amniocentesis or chorionic villus sampling in twin pregnancy: Systematic review and meta-analysis. *Ultrasound Obstet Gynecol* 56:647–655, 2020.

Di-Battista A, Favilla BP, Zamariolli M, et al. Premature ovarian insufficiency is associated with global alterations in the regulatory landscape and gene expression in balanced X-autosome translocations. *Epigenetics Chromatin* 16:19, 2023.

Di-Battista A, Meloni VA, da Silva MD, Moysés-Oliveira M, Melaragno MI. Unusual X-chromosome inactivation pattern in patients with Xp11.23-p11.22 duplication: Report and review. *Am J Med Genet* 170A:3271–3275, 2016.

Di Benedetto D, Musumeci SA, Avola E, et al. Definition of minimal duplicated region encompassing the XIAP and STAG2 genes in the Xq25 microduplication syndrome. *Am J Med Genet* 164A:1923–1930, 2014

Digilio MC, Bernardini L, Consoli F, et al. Congenital heart defects in recurrent reciprocal 1q21.1 deletion and duplication syndromes: Rare association with pulmonary valve stenosis. *Eur J Med Genet* 56:144–149, 2013.

Dimitrov B, Balikova I, de Ravel T, et al. 2q31.1 microdeletion syndrome: Redefining the associated clinical phenotype. *J Med Genet* 48:98–104, 2011.

Dimitrov BI, de Ravel T, Van Driessche J, et al. Distal limb deficiencies, micrognathia syndrome, and syndromic forms of split hand foot malformation (SHFM) are caused by chromosome 10q genomic rearrangements. *J Med Genet* 47:103–111, 2010.

Dimitrov BI, Ogilvie C, Wieczorek D, et al. 3p14 deletion is a rare contiguous gene syndrome: Report of 2 new patients and an overview of 14 patients. *Am J Med Genet* 167:1223–1230, 2015.

Ding Q, Ouyang Q, Xi X, Wang X, Shen Y, Wang H. Maternal chromosome 4 heterodisomy/isodisomy and Bβ chain Trp323X mutation resulting in severe hypodysfibrinogenaemia. *Thromb Haemost* 108:654–661, 2012.

DiPietro JA, Cristofalo EA, Voegtline KM, Crino J. Isolated prenatal choroid plexus cysts do not affect child development. *Prenat Diagn* 31:745–749, 2011.

Dittner-Moormann S, Reschke M, Biewald E, et al. 13q deletion syndrome resulting from balanced chromosomal rearrangement in father: The significance of parental karyotyping. *Mol Cytogenet* 23;13:31, 2020.

Drmic IE, MacKinnon Modi B, McConnell B, et al. Neurodevelopmental functioning in probands and non-proband carriers of 22q11.2 microduplication. *Am J Med Genet* 188A:2999–3008, 2022.

Dobek WA, Kim HG, Walls CA, et al. Long-term follow-up of females with unbalanced X;Y translocations-reproductive and nonreproductive consequences. *Mol Cytogenet* 8:13, 2015.

Dobyns WB, Mirzaa G, Christian SL, et al. Consistent chromosome abnormalities identify novel polymicrogyria loci in 1p36.3, 2p16.1-p23.1, 4q21.21-q22.1, 6q26-q27, and 21q2. *Am J Med Genet* 146A:1637–1654, 2008.

Docherty LE, Kabwama S, Lehmann A, et al. Clinical presentation of 6q24 transient neonatal diabetes mellitus (6q24 TNDM) and genotype-phenotype correlation in an international cohort of patients. *Diabetologia* 56:758–762, 2013.

Doelken SC, Seeger K, Hundsdoerfer P, Weber-Ferro W, Klopocki E, Graul-Neumann L. Proximal and distal 15q25.2 microdeletions—genotype-phenotype delineation of two neurodevelopmental susceptibility loci. *Am J Med Genet* 161A:218–224, 2012.

Doğer E, Çakiroglu Y, Ceylan Y, Ulak E, Özdamar Ö, Çaliskan E. Reproductive and obstetric outcomes in mosaic Turner's syndrome: A cross-sectional study and review of the literature. *Reprod Biol Endocrinol* 13:59, 2015.

Doheny KF, Rasmussen SA, Rutberg J, et al. Segregation of a familial balanced (12;10) insertion resulting in Dup(10)(q21.2q22.1) and Del(10)(q21.2q22.1) in first cousins. *Am J Med Genet* 69:188–193, 1997.

Dolan M, Berry SA, Rubin KR, Hirsch B. Deletion and duplication of 11p13–11p14: Reciprocal aberrations derived from a paternal insertion. *Am J Med Genet* 155A:2775–2783, 2011.

Dolcetti A, Silversides CK, Marshall CR, et al. 1q21.1 microduplication expression in adults. *Genet Med* 15:282–289, 2013.

Dolk H, Loane M, Garne E, et al. Trends and geographic inequalities in the prevalence of Down syndrome in Europe, 1980–1999. *Rev Epidemiol Sante Publique* 53:2S87–2S95, 2005.

Domaradzka J, Deperas M, Obersztyn E, et al. A placental trisomy 2 detected by NIPT evolved in a fetal small Supernumerary Marker Chromosome (sSMC). *Mol Cytogenet* 14:18, 2021.

Domenice S, Zamboni Machado A, Moraes Ferreira F, et al. Wide spectrum of NR5A1-related phenotypes in 46,XY and 46,XX individuals. *Birth Defects Res C Embryo Today* 108:309–320, 2016.

Domínguez MG, Rivera H, Aguilar-Lemarroy A, et al. Two familial intrachromosomal insertions with maternal dup(6)(p22.3p25.3) or dup(2)(q24.2q32.1) in recombinant offspring. *Clin Dysmorphol* 26:209–216, 2017.

Domínguez MG, Rivera H, Dávalos-Pulido RM, Dávalos-Rodríguez IP. A paternal t(6;22)(q25.3;p12) leading to a deleted and satellited der(6) in a short-lived infant. *J Clin Lab Anal* 34:e23355, 2020.

Dominguez MG, Rivera H, Vasquez AI, Hernandez-Zaragoza G, Rivas F. Interchange trisomy 21 by t(1;21)(p22;q22)mat. *Genet Couns* 12:363–367, 2001.

Donaghue C, Mann K, Docherty Z, Mackie Ogilvie C. Detection of mosaicism for primary trisomies in prenatal samples by QF-PCR and karyotype analysis. *Prenat Diagn* 25:65–72, 2005.

Donate A, Estop AM, Giraldo J, Templado C. Paternal age and numerical chromosome abnormalities in human spermatozoa. *Cytogenet Genome Res* 148:241–248, 2016.

Dong D, Xiong S, Nichini E, et al. Applying and assessing the PEERS model on genetic counseling training in China: A mixed-method approach. *Front Med (Lausanne)* 9:986851, 2023.

Dong Z, Chau MHK, Zhang Y, et al. Low-pass genome sequencing-based detection of absence of heterozygosity: Validation in clinical cytogenetics. *Genet Med* 23:1225–1233, 2021.

Dong Z, Jiang L, Yang C, et al. A robust approach for blind detection of balanced chromosomal rearrangements with whole-genome low-coverage sequencing. *Hum Mutat* 35:625–636, 2014.

Dong Y, Li J, Zeng Z, et al. Growth retardation and congenital heart disease in a boy with a ring chromosome 6 of maternal origin. *Mol Cytogenet* 15:9, 2022.

Dong Z, Wang H, Chen H, et al. Identification of balanced chromosomal rearrangements previously unknown among participants in the 1000 Genomes Project: Implications for interpretation of structural variation in genomes and the future of clinical cytogenetics. *Genet Med* 20:697–707, 2018.

Dong Z, Zhang J, Hu P, et al. Low-pass whole-genome sequencing in clinical cytogenetics: A validated approach. *Genet Med* 18:940–948, 2016.

Donley G. Does the constitution protect abortions based on fetal anomaly? Examining the potential for disability-selective abortion bans in the age of prenatal whole genome sequencing. *Michigan J Gender Law* 20:291–328, 2013.

Faivre L, Morichon-Delvallez N, Viot G, et al. Prenatal diagnosis of a satellited non-acrocentric chromosome derived from a maternal translocation (10;13)(p13;p12) and review of literature. *Prenat Diagn* 19:282–286, 1999.

Faivre L, Portnoï MF, Pals G, et al. Should chromosome breakage studies be performed in patients with VACTERL association? *Am J Med Genet* 137:55–58, 2005.

Faivre L, Radford I, Viot G, et al. Cerebellar ataxia and mental retardation in a child with an inherited satellited chromosome 4q. *Ann Génét* 43:35–38, 2000.

Falah N, Posey JE, Thorson W, et al. 22q11.2q13 duplication including SOX10 causes sex-reversal and peripheral demyelinating neuropathy, central dysmyelinating leukodystrophy, Waardenburg syndrome, and Hirschsprung disease. *Am J Med Genet* 173A:1066–1070, 2017.

Falek A, Schmidt R, Jervis GA. Familial de Lange syndrome with chromosome abnormalities. *Pediatrics* 37:92–101, 1966.

Falik-Borenstein TC, Korenberg JR, Schreck RR. Confined placental chimerism: Prenatal and postnatal cytogenetic and molecular analysis, and pregnancy outcome. *Am J Med Genet* 50:51–56, 1994.

Falik-Borenstein TC, Pribyl TM, Pulst SM, et al. Stable ring chromosome 21: Molecular and clinical definition of the lesion. *Am J Med Genet* 42:22–28, 1992.

Fan H, Zhou Z, Zheng W, et al. Homozygous variants in CDC23 cause female infertility characterized by oocyte maturation defects. *Hum Genet* 142:1621–1631, 2023a.

Fan J, Senaratne TN, Liu JY, et al. Outcomes of two different unbalanced segregations from a maternal t(4;10)(q33;p15.1) translocation. *BMC Med Genomics* 16:65, 2023b.

Fan YS, Siu VM, Jung JH, Farrell SA, Côté GB. Direct duplication of 8p21.3→p23.1: A cytogenetic anomaly associated with developmental delay without consistent clinical features. *Am J Med Genet* 103:231–234, 2001.

Fanciulli M, Pasini E, Malacrida S, et al. Copy number variations and susceptibility to lateral temporal epilepsy: A study of 21 pedigrees. *Epilepsia* 55:1651–1658, 2014.

Fang HH, Liu SY, Wang YF, Chiang CM, Liu CC, Lin CM. Phenotypic features of a microdeletion in chromosome band 20p13: A case report and review of the literature. *Mol Genet Genomic Med* 7:e00739, 2019.

Fannemel M, Barøy T, Holmgren A, et al. Haploinsufficiency of XPO1 and USP34 by a de novo 230 kb deletion in 2p15, in a patient with mild intellectual disability and cranio-facial dysmorphisms. *Eur J Med Genet* 57:513–519, 2014.

Farag TI, Krishna Murthy DS, Al-Awadi SA, et al. Robertsonian translocation t dic (14p;22p) with regular trisomy 21: A possible interchromosomal effect? *Ann Génét* 30:189–192, 1987.

Farah LMS, Nazareth HRdeS, Dolnikoff M, Delascio D. Balanced homologous translocation t(22q22q) in a phenotypically normal woman with repeated spontaneous abortions. *Humangenetik* 28:357–360, 1975.

Faraut T, Mermet MA, Demongeot J, Cohen O. Cooperation of selection and meiotic mechanisms in the production of imbalances in reciprocal translocations. *Cytogenet Cell Genet* 88:15–21, 2000.

Faravelli F, Murdolo M, Marangi G, Bricarelli FD, Di Rocco M, Zollino M. Mother to son amplification of a small subtelomeric deletion: A new mechanism of familial recurrence in microdeletion syndromes. *Am J Med Genet* 143A:1169–1173, 2007.

Farhi A, Boyko V, Almagor J, et al. The possible association between exposure to air pollution and the risk for congenital malformations. *Environ Res* 135:173–80, 2014.

Farrell SA, Chow G. Intrachromosomal insertion of chromosome 7. *Clin Genet* 41:299–302, 1992.

Farrell SA, Fan YS. Balanced nonacrocentric whole-arm reciprocal translocations: A de novo case and literature review. *Am J Med Genet* 55:423–426, 1995.

Farwig K, Harmon AG, Fontana KM, Mervis CB, Morris CA. Genetic counseling of adults with Williams syndrome: A first study. *Am J Med Genet* 154C:307–315, 2010.

Fassihi H, Lu L, Wessagowit V, et al. Complete maternal isodisomy of chromosome 3 in a child with recessive dystrophic epidermolysis bullosa but no other phenotypic abnormalities. *J Invest Dermatol* 126:2039–2043, 2006.

Fatemi N, Salehi N, Pignata L, et al. Biallelic variant in cyclin B3 is associated with failure of maternal meiosis II and recurrent digynic triploidy. *J Med Genet* 58:783–788, 2021.

Favier R, Akshoomoff N, Mattson S, Grossfeld P. Jacobsen syndrome: Advances in our knowledge of phenotype and genotype. *Am J Med Genet C Semin Med Genet* 169:239–250, 2015.

Federman DD. Mapping the X-chromosome: Mapping its p's and q's. *N Engl J Med* 317:161–162, 1987.

Feenstra I, Hanemaaijer N, Sikkema-Raddatz B, et al. Balanced into array: Genome-wide array analysis in 54 patients with an apparently balanced de novo chromosome rearrangement and a meta-analysis. *Eur J Hum Genet* 19:1152–1160, 2011.

Feinberg RS, Sinha MS, Cohen IG. The Alabama embryo decision—The politics and reality of recognizing "extrauterine children". *JAMA* 331:1083–1084, 2024.

Fejgin MD, Arbel-DeRowe Y, Shul N, Amiel A. A false-positive diagnosis of Turner syndrome by amniocentesis. *Prenat Diagn* 17:88–89, 1997.

Feldman B, Ebrahim SAD, Hazan SL, et al. Routine prenatal diagnosis of aneuploidy by FISH studies in high-risk pregnancies. *Am J Med Genet* 90:233–238, 2000.

Feldman B, Kramer RL, Ebrahim SAD, Wolff DJ, Evans MI. Prenatal evaluation of a de novo X;9 translocation. *Am J Med Genet* 85:476–478, 1999.

Fénichel P, Letur H. Procréation et syndrome de Turner: Quelles recommandations avant, pendant et après la grossesse? *Gynécol Obstét Fertil* 36:891–897, 2008.

Ferfouri F, Bernicot I, Schneider A, Haquet E, Hédon B, Anahory T. Is the resulting phenotype of an embryo with balanced X-autosome translocation, obtained by means of preimplantation genetic diagnosis, linked to the X inactivation pattern? *Fertil Steril* 105:1035–1046, 2016.

Ferfouri F, Clement P, Molina Gomes D, et al. Is classic pericentric inversion of chromosome 2 inv(2)(p11q13) associated with an increased risk of unbalanced chromosomes? *Fertil Steril* 92:1497, e1–4, 2009.

Ferguson-Smith MA. Prenatal chromosome analysis and its impact on the birth incidence of chromosome disorders. *Br Med Bull* 39:355–364, 1983.

Ferguson-Smith MA. Human cytogenetics at Johns Hopkins Hospital, 1959-1962. *Am J Med Genet* 185A:3236–3241, 2021.

Ferguson-Smith MA, Cooke A, Affara NA, Boyd E, Tolmie JL. Genotype-phenotype correlations in XX males and their bearing on current theories of sex determination. *Hum Genet* 84:198–202, 1990.

Fernández RM, Sánchez J, García-Díaz L, et al. Interstitial 10p deletion derived from a maternal ins(16;10)(q22;p13p15.2): Report of the first familial case of 10p monosomy affecting two familial members of different generations. *Am J Med Genet* 170A:1268–1273, 2016.

Fernández Hernández L, Alcántara Ortigoza MA, Ramos Angeles SE, González-Del Angel A. Cleft lip palate in a patient with 5q14.3 deletion syndrome: A possible unreported feature? *Cytogenet Genome Res* 161:556–563, 2021.

Fernández-Rebollo E, Lecumberri B, Garin I, et al. New mechanisms involved in paternal 20q disomy associated with pseudohypoparathyroidism. *Eur J Endocrinol* 163:953–962, 2010.

Ferrari MTM, Silva ESDN, Nishi MY, Batista RL, Mendonca BB, Domenice S. Testicular differentiation in 46,XX DSD: An overview of genetic causes. *Front Endocrinol (Lausanne)* 15:1385901, 2024.

Ferrario A, Aliu N, Rieubland C, Vuilleumier S, Grabe HM, Escher P. Expanding genotype/phenotype correlation in 2p11.2-p12 microdeletion syndrome. *Genes (Basel)* 14:2222, 2023.

Ferraris A, Bernardini L, Sabolic Avramovska V, et al. Dandy-Walker malformation and Wisconsin syndrome: Novel cases add further insight into the genotype-phenotype correlations of 3q23q25 deletions. *Orphanet J Rare Dis* 8:75, 2013.

Ferrier RA, Lowry RB, Lemire EG, Stoeber GP, Howard J, Parboosingh JS. Father-to-son transmission of an X-linked gene: A case of paternal sex chromosome heterodisomy. *Am J Med Genet* 149A:2871–2873, 2009.

Fickelscher I, Liehr T, Watts K, et alThe variant inv(2)(p11.2q13) is a genuinely recurrent rearrangement but displays some breakpoint heterogeneity. *Am J Hum Genet* 81:847–856, 2007.

Field LL, Tobias R, Robinson WP, Paisey R, Bain S. Maternal uniparental disomy of chromosome 1 with no apparent phenotypic effects. *Am J Hum Genet* 63:1216–1220, 1998.

Fieremans N, Bauters M, Belet S, et al. De novo MECP2 duplications in two females with intellectual disability and unfavorable complete skewed X-inactivation. *Hum Genet* 133:1359–1367, 2014.

Filges I, Manokhina I, Peñaherrera MS, et al. Recurrent triploidy due to a failure to complete maternal meiosis II: Whole-exome sequencing reveals candidate variants. *Mol Hum Reprod* 21:339–346, 2015.

Filges I, Röthlisberger B, Wenzel F, Heinimann K, Huber AR, Miny P. Mosaic ring chromosome 8: Clinical and array-CGH findings in partial trisomy 8. *Am J Med Genet* 146A:2837–2841, 2008.

Filho AB, Souza J, Faucz FR, et al. Somatic/gonadal mosaicism in a syndromic form of ectrodactyly, including eye abnormalities, documented through array-based comparative genomic hybridization. *Am J Med Genet* 155A:1152–1156, 2011.

Finley J, Hay S, Oldzej J, et al. The genomic basis of sporadic and recurrent pregnancy loss: A comprehensive in-depth analysis of 24,900 miscarriages. *Reprod Biomed Online* 45:125–134, 2022.

Finucane B. Acculturation in women with mental retardation and its impact on genetic counseling. *J Genet Couns* 7:31–47, 1998.

Firth H. Chorion villus sampling and limb deficiency—Cause or coincidence? *Prenat Diagn* 17:1313–1330, 1997.

Fitzgerald PH, Archer SA, Morris CM. Evidence for the repeated primary non-disjunction of chromosome 21 as a result of premature centromere division (PCD). *Hum Genet* 72:58–62, 1986.

Flejter WL, Finlinson D, Root S, Nguyen W, Brothman AR, Viskochil D. Familial ring (19) chromosome mosaicism: Case report and review. *Am J Med Genet* 66:276–280, 1996.

Flipsen-ten Berg K, van Hasselt PM, Eleveld MJ, et al. Unmasking of a hemizygous WFS1 gene mutation by a chromosome 4p deletion of 8.3 Mb in a patient with Wolf-Hirschhorn syndrome. *Eur J Hum Genet* 15:1132–1138, 2007.

Florea A, Caba L, Grigore AM, et al. Hydatidiform mole — Between chromosomal abnormality, uniparental disomy and monogenic variants: A narrative review. *Life (Basel)* 13:2314, 2023.

Flori E, Doray B, Rudolf G, et al. Failure of prenatal diagnosis of diploid-triploid mosaicism after amniocentesis. *Clin Genet* 63:328–331, 2003.

Flowers NJ, Burgess T, Giouzeppos O, et al. Genome-wide noninvasive prenatal screening for carriers of balanced reciprocal translocations. *Genet Med* 22:1944–1955, 2020.

Fonseca AC, Bonaldi A, Bertola DR, Kim CA, Otto PA, Vianna-Morgante AM. The clinical impact of chromosomal rearrangements with breakpoints upstream of the SOX9 gene: Two novel de novo balanced translocations associated with acampomelic campomelic dysplasia. *BMC Med Genet* 14:50, 2013.

Fonseca-Pedrero E, Debbané M, Schneider M, Badoud D, Eliez S. Schizotypal traits in adolescents with 22q11.2 deletion syndrome: Validity, reliability and risk for psychosis. *Psychol Med* 46:1005–1013, 2016.

Forabosco A, Percesepe A, Santucci S. Incidence of non-age-dependent chromosomal abnormalities: A population-based study on 88965 amniocenteses. *Eur J Hum Genet* 17:897–903, 2009.

Ford CE, Jones KW, Miller OJ, et al. The chromosomes in a patient showing both mongolism and the Klinefelter syndrome. *Lancet* 1:709–710, 1959.

Ford NM. When Did I Begin? Cambridge, UK: Cambridge University Press, 1988.

Foresta C, Moro E, Ferlin A. Y chromosome microdeletions and alterations of spermatogenesis. *Endocr Rev* 22:226–239, 2001.

Forman EJ. Morphology matters: Are all euploid blastocyst created equal? *Fertil Steril* 107:573–574, 2017.

Forrest LE, Delatycki MB, Skene L, Aitken M. Communicating genetic information in families—A review of guidelines and position papers. *Eur J Hum Genet* 15:612–618, 2007.

Forrester MB, Merz RD. Epidemiology of triploidy in a population-based birth defects registry, Hawaii, 1986–1999. *Am J Med Genet* 119A:319–323, 2003a.

Forrester MB, Merz RD. Maternal age-specific Down syndrome rates by maternal race/ethnicity, Hawaii, 1986–2000. *Birth Defects Res* 67:625–629, 2003b.

Forsberg LA. Loss of chromosome Y (LOY) in blood cells is associated with increased risk for disease and mortality in aging men. *Hum Genet* 136:657–663, 2017.

Foudila T, Söderström-Anttila V, Hovatta O. Turner's syndrome and pregnancies after oocyte donation. *Hum Reprod* 14:532–535, 1999.

Fowler DM, Rehm HL. Will variants of uncertain significance still exist in 2030? *Am J Hum Genet* 111:5–10, 2024.

Fragouli E, Alfarawati S, Spath K, et al. The origin and impact of embryonic aneuploidy. *Hum Genet* 132:1001–1013, 2013.

Fragouli E, Wells D, Doshi A, Gotts S, Harper JC, Delhanty JD. Complete cytogenetic investigation of oocytes from a young cancer patient with the use of comparative genomic hybridisation reveals meiotic errors. *Prenat Diagn* 26:71–76, 2006.

Franasiak JM, Forman EJ, Hong KH, et al. The nature of aneuploidy with increasing age of the female partner: A review of 15,169 consecutive trophectoderm biopsies evaluated with comprehensive chromosomal screening. *Fertil Steril* 101:656–663.e1, 2014.

Franasiak JM, Olcha M, Shastri S, et al. Embryonic aneuploidy does not differ among genetic ancestry according to continental origin as determined by ancestry informative markers. *Hum Reprod* 31:2391–2395, 2016.

França MM, Mendonca BB. Genetics of ovarian insufficiency and defects of folliculogenesis. *Best Pract Res Clin Endocrinol Metab* 36:101594, 2022.

Francés A, Hildur K, Barberà JA, et al. Persistence of breakage in specific chromosome bands 6 years after acute exposure to oil. *PLoS One* 11:e0159404, 2016.

Francis DI, Stark Z, Scheffer IE, et al. Comparing saliva and blood for the detection of mosaic genomic abnormalities that cause syndromic intellectual disability. *Eur J Hum Genet* 31:521–525, 2023.

Franz EA, Chiaroni-Clarke R, Woodrow S, et al. Congenital mirror movements: Phenotypes associated with DCC and RAD51 mutations. *J Neurol Sci*, 351:140–145, 2015.

Fraser FC. Does paternal exposure to Agent Orange cause birth defects? *Am J Med Genet* 149A:835–836, 2009.

Frati P, Fineschi V, Di Sanzo M, et al. Preimplantation and prenatal diagnosis, wrongful birth and wrongful life: A global view of bioethical and legal controversies. *Hum Reprod Update* 23:338–357, 2017.

Freitas ÉL, Gribble SM, Simioni M, et al. A familial case with interstitial 2q36 deletion: Variable phenotypic expression in full and mosaic state. *Eur J Med Genet* 55:660–665, 2012.

Frias S, Van Hummelen P, Meistrich ML, Wyrobek AJ. Meiotic susceptibility for induction of sperm with chromosomal aberrations in patients receiving combination chemotherapy for Hodgkin lymphoma. *PLoS One* 15:e0242218, 2020.

Fritz B, Greber-Platzer S, Frischer T, et al. Familial cryptic translocation with del 4q34→qter and dup 12pter→p13 in sibs with tracheal stenosis: Clinical, classical and molecular cytogenetic studies and CGH analyses from archival placental tissues evidencing tertiary trisomy 4 in one abortion specimen. *Am J Med Genet* 94:271–280, 2000.

Fritz R, Kohan-Ghadr HR, Sacher A, et al. Trophoblast retrieval and isolation from the cervix (TRIC) is unaffected by early gestational age or maternal obesity. *Prenat Diagn* 35:1218–1222, 2015.

Frumkin T, Peleg S, Gold V, et al. Complex chromosomal rearrangement—a lesson learned from PGS. *J Assist Reprod Genet* 34:1095–1100, 2017.

Fryburg JS, Dimaio MS, Yang-Feng TL, Mahoney MJ. Follow-up of pregnancies complicated by placental mosaicism diagnosed by chorionic villus sampling. *Prenat Diagn* 13:481–494, 1993.

Fryns JP, Bulcke J, Hens L, Van den Berghe H. Balanced transmission of centromeric fission products in man. *Hum Genet* 54:127–128, 1980.

Fryns JP, Kleczkowska A, Kubień E, Van den Berghe H. On the excess of mental retardation and/or congenital malformations in apparently balanced reciprocal translocations: A critical review of the Leuven data 1966–1991. *Genet Counsel* 2:185–194, 1992.

Fryns JP, Kleczkowska A, Kubien E, Van den Berghe H. XYY syndrome and other Y chromosome polysomies: Mental status and psychosocial functioning. *Genet Couns* 6:197–206, 1995.

Fryns JP, Van den Berghe H, Schrander-Stumpel C. Kabuki (Niikawa-Kuroki) syndrome and paracentric inversion of the short arm of chromosome 4. *Am J Med Genet* 53:204–205, 1994.

Fu J, Wang T, Fu Z, et al. Case Report: A case report and literature review of 3p deletion syndrome. *Front Pediatr* 10;9:618059, 2021.

Fu JM, Satterstrom FK, Peng M, et al. Rare coding variation provides insight into the genetic architecture and phenotypic context of autism. *Nat Genet* 54:1320–1331, 2022.

Fu M, Chen M, Guo N, et al. Molecular genetic analysis of 1,980 cases of male infertility. *Exp Ther Med* 26:345, 2023.

Fujimoto M, Nakamura Y, Iwaki T, et al. Angelman syndrome with mosaic paternal uniparental disomy suggestive of mitotic nondisjunction. *J Hum Genet* 68:87–90, 2023.

Fukunaga M. Immunohistochemical characterization of p57Kip2 expression in tetraploid hydropic placentas. *Arch Pathol Lab Med* 128:897–900, 2004.

Fung WL, Butcher NJ, Costain G, et al. Practical guidelines for managing adults with 22q11.2 deletion syndrome. *Genet Med* 17:599–609, 2015.

Furuya K, Sasaki Y, Takeuchi T, Urita Y. Characteristics of 22q 11.2 deletion syndrome undiagnosed until adulthood: An example suggesting the importance of psychiatric manifestations. *BMJ Case Rep* bcr2014:208903, 2015.

Fuster C, Miguez L, Miró R, Rigola MA, Perez A, Egozcue J. Familial complex chromosome rearrangement ascertained by in situ hybridisation. *J Med Genet* 34:164–166, 1997.

Futaki M, Liu JM. Chromosomal breakage syndromes and the BRCA1 genome surveillance complex. *Trends Mol Med* 7:560–565, 2001.

G

Gabbett MT, Peters GB, Carmichael JM, Darmanian AP, Collins FA. Prader-Willi syndrome phenocopy due to duplication of Xq21.1-q21.31, with array CGH of the critical region. *Clin Genet* 73:353–359, 2008.

Gabriel AS, Thornhill AR, Ottolini CS, et al. Array comparative genomic hybridisation on first polar bodies suggests that non-disjunction is not the predominant mechanism leading to aneuploidy in humans. *J Med Genet* 48:433–437, 2011.

Gabriel-Robez O, Rumpler Y. The meiotic pairing behaviour in human spermatocytes carrier of chromosome anomalies and their repercussions on reproductive fitness. I: Inversions and insertions. *A European collaborative study. Ann Génét* 37:3–10, 1994.

Ghosh S, Feingold E, Dey SK. Etiology of Down syndrome: Evidence for consistent association among altered meiotic recombination, nondisjunction, and maternal age across populations. *Am J Med Genet* 149A:1415–1420, 2009.

Giambona A, Leto F, Passarello C, et al. Fetal aneuploidy diagnosed at celocentesis for early prenatal diagnosis of congenital hemoglobinopathies. *Acta Obstet Gynecol Scand* 97:312–321, 2018.

Giambona A, Leto F, Damiani G, et al. Identification of embryo-fetal cells in celomic fluid using morphological and short-tandem repeats analysis. *Prenat Diagn* 36:973–978, 2016.

Giardino D, Corti C, Ballarati L, et al. Prenatal diagnosis of a de novo complex chromosome rearrangement (CCR) mediated by six breakpoints, and a review of 20 prenatally ascertained CCRs. *Prenat Diagn* 26:565–570, 2006.

Giardino D, Corti C, Ballarati L, et al. De novo balanced chromosome rearrangements in prenatal diagnosis. *Prenat Diagn* 29:257–265, 2009.

Giardino D, Finelli P, Russo S, et al. Small familial supernumerary ring chromosome 2: FISH characterization and genotype-phenotype correlation. *Am J Med Genet* 111:319–323, 2002.

Giaroli G, Bass N, Strydom A, Rantell K, McQuillin A. Does rare matter? Copy number variants at 16p11.2 and the risk of psychosis: A systematic review of literature and meta-analysis. *Schizophr Res* 159:340–346, 2014.

Gibbons B, Tan SY, Yu CC, Cheah E, Tan HL. Risk of gonadoblastoma in female patients with Y chromosome abnormalities and dysgenetic gonads. *J Paediatr Child Health* 35:210–213, 1999.

Gibbons RJ. α-Thalassemia, mental retardation, and myelodysplastic syndrome. *Cold Spring Harb Perspect Med* 2:a011759, 2012.

Gibbs J, Appleton J, Appleton R. Dyspraxia or developmental coordination disorder? Unravelling the enigma. *Arch Dis Child* 92:534–539, 2007.

Gidoni YS, Takefman J, Holzer HE, et al. Cryopreservation of a mother's oocytes for possible future use by her daughter with Turner syndrome: Case report. *Fertil Steril* 90:e9–12, 2008.

Giglio S, Broman KW, Matsumoto N, et al. Olfactory receptor-gene clusters, genomic-inversion polymorphisms, and common chromosome rearrangements. *Am J Hum Genet* 68:874–883, 2001.

Giglio S, Calvari V, Gregato G, et al. Heterozygous submicroscopic inversions involving olfactory receptor-gene clusters mediate the recurrent t(4;8)(p16;p23) translocation. *Am J Hum Genet* 71:276–285, 2002.

Giglio S, Pirola B, Arrigo G, et al. Opposite deletions/duplications of the X chromosome: Two novel reciprocal rearrangements. *Eur J Hum Genet* 8:63–70, 2000.

Giguet-Valard AG, Thevenin C, Dreux S, et al. Antenatal description of large 4q13.2q21.23 deletion and outcomes. *Mol Genet Genomic Med* 12:e2397, 2024.

Gil MM, Quezada MS, Revello R, Akolekar R, Nicolaides KH. Analysis of cell-free DNA in maternal blood in screening for fetal aneuploidies: Updated meta-analysis. *Ultrasound Obstet Gynecol* 45:249–66, 2015.

Gilardi JL, Perrotin F, Paillet C, et al. Prenatal diagnosis of trisomy 21 by i(21q): A rare case of fetoplacental chromosomal discrepancy. *Prenat Diagn* 22:856–858, 2002.

Gilbert B, Yardin C, Briault S, et al. Prenatal diagnosis of female monozygotic twins discordant for Turner syndrome: Implications for prenatal genetic counselling. *Prenat Diagn* 22:697–702, 2002.

Gilling M, Dullinger JS, Gesk S, et al. Breakpoint cloning and haplotype analysis indicate a single origin of the common Inv(10)(p11.2q21.2) mutation among northern Europeans. *Am J Hum Genet* 78:878–883, 2006.

Gillon R. On sterilising severely mentally handicapped people. *J Med Ethics* 13:59–61, 1987.

Giltay JC, Kastrop PM, Tiemessen CH, van Inzen WG, Scheres JM, Pearson PL. Sperm analysis in a subfertile male with a Y;16 translocation, using four-color FISH. *Cytogenet Cell Genet* 84:67–72, 1999.

Gimelbrant A, Hutchinson JN, Thompson BR, Chess A. Widespread monoallelic expression on human autosomes. *Science* 318:1136–1140, 2007.

Gimelli S, Beri S, Drabkin HA, et al. The tumor suppressor gene TRC8/RNF139 is disrupted by a constitutional balanced translocation t(8;22)(q24.13;q11.21) in a young girl with dysgerminoma. *Mol Cancer* 8:52, 2009.

Gimelli S, Stathaki E, Béna F, et al. Recurrent microdeletion 2q21.1: Report on a new patient with neurological disorders. *Am J Med Genet* 164A:801–805, 2014.

Ginsberg NA, Cadkin A, Strom C, Bauer-Marsh E, Verlinsky Y. Prenatal diagnosis of 46,XX male fetuses. *Am J Obstet Gynecol* 180:1006–1007, 1999.

Ginsburg C, Fokstuen S, Schinzel A. The contribution of uniparental disomy to congenital development defects in children born to mothers at advanced childbearing age. *Am J Med Genet* 95:454–460, 2000.

Ginström Ernstad E, Hanson C, Wånggren K, et al. Preimplantation genetic testing and child health: A national register-based study. *Hum Reprod* 38:739–750, 2023.

Giorda R, Bonaglia MC, Milani G, et al. Molecular and cytogenetic analysis of the spreading of X inactivation in a girl with microcephaly, mild dysmorphic features and t(X;5)(q22.1;q31.1). *Eur J Hum Genet* 16:897–905, 2008.

Giordano JL, Wapner RJ. Genomics of stillbirth. *Semin Perinatol* 48:151866, 2024.

Girardi L, Serdarogullari M, Patassini C, et al. Incidence, origin, and predictive model for the detection and clinical management of segmental aneuploidies in human embryos. *Am J Hum Genet* 106:525–534, 2020.

Girirajan S, Rosenfeld JA, Coe BP, et al. Phenotypic heterogeneity of genomic disorders and rare copy-number variants. *N Engl J Med* 367:1321–1331, 2012.

Girirajan S, Rosenfeld JA, Cooper GM, et al. A recurrent 16p12.1 microdeletion supports a two-hit model for severe developmental delay. *Nat Genet* 42:203–209, 2010.

Girisha KM, Rajasekhar M, Gopinath PM, Satyamoorthy K. Balanced translocation in mother leading to interchange trisomy 21? *Genet Couns* 21:183–185, 2010.

Giulioni C, Maurizi V, Castellani D, et al. The environmental and occupational influence of pesticides on male fertility: A systematic review of human studies. *Andrology* 10:1250–1271, 2022

Glass IA, Rauen KA, Chen E, et al. Ring chromosome 15: Characterization by array CGH *Hum Genet* 118:611–617, 2006.

Glassford MR, Rosenfeld JA, Freedman AA, Zwick ME, Mulle JG; Unique Rare Chromosome Disorder Support Group. Novel features of 3q29 deletion syndrome: Results from the 3q29 registry. *Am J Med Genet* 170A:999–1006, 2016.

Glasson EJ, Sullivan SG, Hussain R, Petterson BA, Montgomery PD, Bittles AH. The changing survival profile of people with Down's syndrome: Implications for genetic counselling. *Clin Genet* 62:390–393, 2002.

Glujovsky D, Quinteiro Retamar AM, Alvarez Sedo CR, Ciapponi A, Cornelisse S, Blake D. Cleavage-stage versus blastocyst-stage embryo transfer in assisted reproductive technology. *Cochrane Database Syst Rev* 5:CD002118, 2022.

Godfrey M, Udhnani M, Lee NR. A case report of the neurocognitive and behavioral phenotype of mosaic trisomy 14. *Neurocase* 24:250–254, 2018.

Goetzinger L, Starks RD, Dillahunt K, Major H, Nagy JM, Sidhu A. Interstitial duplication of 20q11.22q13.11: A case report and review of literature. *Mol Genet Genomic Med* 9:e1755, 2021.

Goh S, Thiyagarajan L, Dudding-Byth T, Pinese M, Kirk EP. A systematic review and pooled analysis of penetrance estimates of copy-number variants associated with neurodevelopment. *Genet Med* 27:101227, 2025.

Goitia V, Oquendo M, Stratton R. Case of 7p22.1 microduplication detected by whole genome microarray (REVEAL) in workup of child diagnosed with autism. *Case Rep Genet* 2015:212436, 2015.

Golden WL, Sudduth KW, Burnett SH, Kelly TE. Mosaicism in Prader-Willi syndrome: Detection using fluorescent in situ hybridization. *Am J Med Genet* 85:424–425, 1999.

Goldman ASH, Hultén MA. Chromosome in situ suppression hybridisation in human male meiosis. *J Med Genet* 29:98–102, 1992.

Goldman ASH, Martin RH, Johannisson R, et al. Meiotic and sperm chromosome analysis in a male carrier of an inverted insertion (3;10)(q13.2;p14p13). *J Med Genet* 29:460–464, 1992.

Gole L, Crolla JA, Thomas SN, Jacobs PA, Dennis NR. Characterization of breakpoints in the GABRG3 and TSPY genes in a family with a t(Y;15)(p11.2;q12). *Am J Med Genet* 125A:177–180, 2004.

Gole LA, Anandakumar C, Bongso A, Chua TM, Wong YC, Ratnam SS. Analysis of cystic hygroma, ascitic, and pleural fluids by conventional lymphocyte culture and fluorescent in situ hybridization. *Prenat Diagn* 17:1151–1157, 1997.

Golzio C, Guirchoun J, Ozilou C, et al. Cytogenetic and histological features of a human embryo with homogeneous chromosome 8 trisomy. *Prenat Diagn* 26:1201–1205, 2006.

Gómez-Laguna L, Martínez-Herrera A, Reyes-de la Rosa ADP, et al. Nance-Horan syndrome in females due to a balanced X;1 translocation that disrupts the NHS gene: Familial case report and review of the literature. *Ophthalmic Genet* 39:56–62, 2018.

Gonzalez XV, Mora F, Arshad F, et al. Detection of germline mosaicism for Robertsonian translocation 14;14: A case report. *J Reprod Infertil* 25:66–71, 2024.

González-Del Angel A, Alcántara-Ortigoza MA, Ramos S, Algara-Ramírez C, Hernández-Hernández MA, Saenger-Rivas L. Unusual trisomy X phenotype associated with a concurrent heterozygous 16p11.2 deletion: Importance of an integral approach for proper diagnosis. *Int J Mol Sci* 24:14643, 2023.

Goodall J. Helping a child to understand her own testicular feminisation. *Lancet* 337:33–35, 1991.

Gordon CT, Attanasio C, Bhatia S, et al. Identification of novel craniofacial regulatory domains located far upstream of SOX9 and disrupted in Pierre Robin sequence. *Hum Mutat* 35:1011–1020, 2014.

Gorski JL, Kistenmacher ML, Punnett HH, Zackai EH, Emanuel BS. Reproductive risks for carriers of complex chromosome rearrangements: Analysis of 25 families. *Am J Med Genet* 29:247–261, 1988.

Goumy C, Beaufrère AM, Francannet C, et al. Prenatal detection of mosaic isochromosome 20q: A fourth report with abnormal phenotype. *Prenat Diagn* 25:653–655, 2005.

Gouveia MP, Coutinho I, Teixeira V, d'Oliveira R, Venâncio M, Moreno A. Do you know this syndrome? Dyspigmentation along the Blaschko lines caused by trisomy 7 mosaicism. *An Bras Dermatol* 91:837–839, 2016.

Gradek GA, Kvistad PH, Houge G. Monosomy 8 rescue gave cells with a normal karyotype in a mildly affected man with 46,XY,r(8) mosaicism. *Eur J Med Genet* 49:292–297, 2006.

Graham EJ, Vermeulen M, Vardarajan B, et al. Somatic mosaicism of sex chromosomes in the blood and brain. *Brain Res* 1721:146345, 2019.

Graham JH, Schlachetzki JCM, Yang X, Breuss MW. Genomic mosaicism of the brain: Origin, impact, and utility. *Neurosci Bull* 40:759–776, 2024.

Grams SE, Argiropoulos B, Lines M, et al. Genotype-phenotype characterization in 13 individuals with chromosome Xp11.22 duplications. *Am J Med Genet* 170A:967–977, 2016.

Grams SE, Rand L, Norton ME. Complete isochromosome 5p in one fetus of a monochorionic twin pair. *Prenat Diagn* 31:605–607, 2011.

Grande M, Stergiotou I, Borobio V, Sabrià J, Soler A, Borrell A. Heterotrisomy recurrence risk: A practical maternal age-dependent approach for excess trisomy 21 risk calculation after a previous autosomal trisomy. *J Matern Fetal Neonatal Med* 30:1613–1615, 2017.

Grange DK, Garcia-Heras J, Kilani RA, Lamp S. Trisomy 20q13→20qter in a girl with multiple congenital malformations and a recombinant chromosome 20 inherited from a paternal inversion (20)(p13q13.1): Clinical report and review of the trisomy 20q phenotype. *Am J Med Genet* 137A:308–312, 2005.

Grangeon L, Charbonnier C, Zarea A, et al. Phenotype and imaging features associated with APP duplications. *Alzheimers Res Ther* 15:93, 2023.

Granocchio E, Pollina E, De Salvatore M, et al. 22q13.33 duplication involving SHANK3 gene: A boy and his mother with "persistent" language and speech sound disorder. *Psychiatr Genet* 34:19–23, 2024.

Grati FR. Chromosomal mosaicism in human feto-placental development: Implications for prenatal diagnosis. *J Clin Med* 3:809–837, 2014.

Grati FR. Implications of fetoplacental mosaicism on cell-free DNA testing: A review of a common biological phenomenon. *Ultrasound Obstet Gynecol* 48:415–423, 2016.

Grati FR, Bajaj K, Malvestiti F, et al. The type of feto-placental aneuploidy detected by cfDNA testing may influence the choice of confirmatory diagnostic procedure. *Prenat Diagn* 35:994–998, 2015.

Grati FR, Ferreira J, Benn P, et al. Outcomes in pregnancies with a confined placental mosaicism and implications for prenatal screening using cell-free DNA. *Genet Med* 22:309–316, 2020.

Grau Madsen S, Uldbjerg N, Sunde L, Becher N; Danish Fetal Medicine Study Group; Danish Clinical Genetics Study Group. Prognosis for pregnancies with trisomy 16 confined to the placenta: A Danish cohort study. *Prenat Diagn* 38:1103–1110, 2018.

Gravholt CH, Andersen NH, Christin-Maitre S, et al. Clinical practice guidelines for the care of girls and women with Turner syndrome. *Eur J Endocrinol* 190:G53–G151, 2024.

Gravholt CH, Weis Naeraa R. Reference values for body proportions and body composition in adult women with Ullrich-Turner syndrome. *Am J Med Genet* 72:403–408, 1997.

Graw SL, Sample T, Bleskan J, Sujansky E, Patterson D. Cloning, sequencing, and analysis of inv8 chromosome breakpoints associated with recombinant 8 syndrome. *Am J Hum Genet* 66:1138–4411, 2000.

Grayton HM, Fernandes C, Rujescu D, Collier DA. Copy number variations in neurodevelopmental disorders. *Prog Neurobiol* 99:81–91, 2012.

Greally JM, Neiswanger K, Cummins JH, et al. A molecular anatomical analysis of mosaic trisomy 16. *Hum Genet* 98:86–90, 1996.

Greco E, Minasi MG, Fiorentino F. Healthy babies after intrauterine transfer of mosaic aneuploid blastocysts. *N Engl J Med* 373:2089–2090, 2015.

Greco E, Yakovlev P, Kornilov N, et al. Two clinical case reports of embryonic mosaicism identified with PGT-A persisting during pregnancy as true fetal mosaicism. *Hum Reprod* 38:315–323. 2023.

Green DM, Sklar CA, Boice JD Jr, et al. Ovarian failure and reproductive outcomes after childhood cancer treatment: Results from the Childhood Cancer Survivor Study. *J Clin Oncol* 27:2374–2381, 2009.

Green JM, Hewison J, Bekker HL, Bryant LD, Cuckle HS. Psychosocial aspects of genetic screening of pregnant women and newborns: A systematic review. *Health Technol Assess (UK)* 8:No. 33, 2004.

Greer PL, Hanayama R, Bloodgood BL, et al. The Angelman Syndrome protein Ube3A regulates synapse development by ubiquitinating arc. *Cell* 140:704–16, 2010.

Greger V, Knoll JHM, Wagstaff J, et al. Angelman syndrome associated with an inversion of chromosome 15q11.2q24.3. *Am J Hum Genet* 60:574–580, 1997.

Gregg AR, Skotko BG, Benkendorf JL, et al. Noninvasive prenatal screening for fetal aneuploidy, 2016 update: A position statement of the American College of Medical Genetics and Genomics. *Genet Med* 18:1056–1065, 2016.

Gregor A, Krumbiegel M, Kraus C, Reis A, Zweier C. De novo triplication of the MAPT gene from the recurrent 17q21.31 microdeletion region in a patient with moderate intellectual disability and various minor anomalies. *Am J Med Genet* 158A:1765–1770, 2012.

Griffin DK, Brezina PR, Tobler K, et al. The human embryonic genome is karyotypically complex, with chromosomally abnormal cells preferentially located away from the developing fetus. *Hum Reprod* 38:180–188, 2023.

Griffiths MJ, Miller PR, Stibbe HM. A false-positive diagnosis of Turner syndrome by amniocentesis. *Prenat Diagn* 16:463–466, 1996.

Grinspon RP, Rey RA. Disorders of sex development with testicular differentiation in SRY-negative 46,XX individuals: Clinical and genetic aspects. *Sex Dev* 10:1–11, 2016.

Grkovic S, Traversa MV, Livingstone M, McArthur SJ. Clinical re-biopsy of segmental gains-the primary source of preimplantation genetic testing false positives. *J Assist Reprod Genet* 39:1313–1322, 2022.

Gross M, Hanenberg H, Lobitz S, et al. Reverse mosaicism in Fanconi anemia: Natural gene therapy via molecular self-correction. *Cytogenet Genome Res* 98:126–135, 2002.

Grossmann V, Höckner M, Karmous-Benailly H, et al. Parental origin of apparently balanced de novo complex chromosomal rearrangements investigated by microdissection, whole genome amplification, and microsatellite-mediated haplotype analysis. *Clin Genet* 78:548–553, 2010.

Groupe de Cytogénéticiens Français. Pericentric inversions in man: A French collaborative study. *Ann Génét* 29:129–168, 1986a.

Groupe de Cytogénéticiens Français. Paracentric inversions in man: A French collaborative study Ann Génét 29:169–176, 1986b.

Grover SR. Gynaecological issues in adolescents with disability. *J Paediatr Child Health* 47:610–613, 2011.

Gruchy N, Barreau M, Kessler K, Gourdier D, Leporrier N. A paternally transmitted complex chromosomal rearrangement (CCR) involving chromosomes 2, 6, and 18 includes eight breakpoints and five insertional translocations (ITs) through three generations. *Am J Med Genet* 152A:185–190, 2010.

Gruchy N, Blondeel E, Le Meur N, et al. Pregnancy outcomes in prenatally diagnosed 47,XXX and 47,XYY syndromes: A 30-year French, retrospective, multicentre study. *Prenat Diagn* 36:523–529, 2016.

Gruhn JR, Hoffmann ER. Errors of the egg: The establishment and progression of human aneuploidy research in the maternal germline. *Annu Rev Genet* 56:369–390, 2022.

Gruhn JR, Zielinska AP, Shukla V, et al. Chromosome errors in human eggs shape natural fertility over reproductive life span. *Science* 365:1466–1469, 2019.

Gu C, Li K, Li R, et al. Chromosomal aneuploidy associated with clinical characteristics of pregnancy loss. *Front Genet* 12:667697, 2021.

Gu S, Jernegan M, Van den Veyver IB, Peacock S, Smith J, Breman A. Chromosomal microarray analysis on uncultured chorionic villus sampling can be complicated by confined placental mosaicism for aneuploidy and microdeletions. *Prenat Diagn* 38:858–865, 2018.

Gu S, Yuan B, Campbell IM, et al. Alu-mediated diverse and complex pathogenic copy-number variants within human chromosome 17 at p13.3. *Hum Mol Genet* 24:4061–4077, 2015.

Guadagnolo D, Mastromoro G, Torres B, et al. Duplication at 19q13.32q13.33 segregating with neuropsychiatric phenotype in a three-generation family: Towards the definition of a critical region. *Genes (Basel)* 14:2157, 2023.

Guarracino A, Buonaiuto S, de Lima LG, et al. Recombination between heterologous human acrocentric chromosomes. Nature 617:335–343, 2023.

Gubb SJA, Brcic L, Underwood JFG, et al. Medical and neurobehavioural phenotypes in male and female carriers of Xp22.31 duplications in the UK Biobank. *Hum Mol Genet* 29:2872–2881, 2020.

Guediche N, Brisset S, Benichou JJ, et al. Chromosomal breakpoints characterization of two supernumerary ring chromosomes 20. *Am J Med Genet* 152A:464–471, 2010.

Gueiderikh A, Maczkowiak-Chartois F, Rosselli F. A new frontier in Fanconi anemia: From DNA repair to ribosome biogenesis. *Blood Rev* 52:100904, 2022.

Guess T, Wheeler FC, Yenamandra A, et al. A multicenter analysis of individuals with a 47,XXY/46,XX karyotype. *Genet Med* 26:101212, 2024.

Guha S, Rees E, Darvasi A, et al. Implication of a rare deletion at distal 16p11.2 in schizophrenia. *JAMA Psychiatry* 70:253–260, 2013.

Gül S, Vloeberghs V, Gies I, Goossens E. Testicular mosaicism in non-mosaic postpubertal Klinefelter patients with focal spermatogenesis and in non-mosaic prepubertal Klinefelter boys. *Hum Reprod* 39:2210–2220, 2024.

Guo F, Liu R, Pan Y, et al. Evidence from 2100 index cases supports genome sequencing as a first-tier genetic test. *Genet Med* 26:100995, 2024.

Gur RC, Bearden CE, Jacquemont S, et al. Neurocognitive profiles of 22q11.2 and 16p11.2 deletions and duplications. *Mol Psychiatry* 30:379–387, 2025.

Giudice-Nairn P, Downs J, Wong K, et al. The incidence, prevalence and clinical features of MECP2 duplication syndrome in Australian children. *J Paediatr Child Health* 55:1315–1322, 2019.

Guha Sarkar P, Dalmia S, Khatri P. A case report on recurrent partial moles in three consecutive pregnancies. *J Obstet Gynaecol* 2022 42:1591–1592, 2022.

Guilherme RS, Klein E, Hamid A, et al. Human ring chromosomes—New insights for their clinical significance. *Balkan J Med Genet* 16:13–20, 2013.

Guilherme RS, Meloni VF, Kim CA, et al. Mechanisms of ring chromosome formation, ring instability and clinical consequences. *BMC Med Genet* 12:171, 2011.

Guilherme RS, Meloni VF, Kim CA, et al. Mechanisms of ring chromosome formation, ring instability and clinical consequences. *BMC Med Genet* 12:171, 2011.

Guilherme RS, Meloni VA, Perez AB, et al. Duplication 9p and their implication to phenotype. *BMC Med Genet* 15:142, 2014.

Guilherme RS, Meloni VA, Takeno SS, et al. Twenty-year cytogenetic and molecular follow-up of a patient with ring chromosome 15: A case report. *J Med Case Rep* 6:283, 2012.

Guilherme RS, Moysés-Oliveira M, Dantas AG, et al. Position effect modifying gene expression in a patient with ring chromosome 14. *J Appl Genet* 57:183–187, 2016.

Guimiot F, Dupont C, Fuentes-Duarte A, et al. Maternal transmission of interstitial 8p23.1 deletion detected during prenatal diagnosis. *Am J Med Genet* 161A:208–213, 2013.

Guioli S, Incerti B, Zanaria E, et al. Kallmann syndrome due to a translocation resulting in an X/Y fusion gene. *Nat Genet* 1:337–340, 1992.

Guo J, He WB, Dai L, et al. Mosaic variegated aneuploidy syndrome with tetraploid, and predisposition to male infertility triggered by mutant CEP192. *HGG Adv* 5:100256, 2024.

Gupta K, Czerminski JT, Lawrence JB. Trisomy silencing by XIST: Translational prospects and challenges. *Hum Genet* 143:843–855, 2024.

Gupta N, Dalvi R, Koppaka N, Mandava S. Balanced reciprocal translocation: Multiple chromosome rearrangements in an infertile female. *J Hum Reprod Sci* 12:72–74, 2019.

Gurunath S, Pandian Z, Anderson RA, Bhattacharya S. Defining infertility—a systematic review of prevalence studies. *Hum Reprod Update* 17:575–588, 2011.

Guttenbach M, Kohn FM, Engel W, Schmid M. Meiotic nondisjunction of chromosomes 1, 17, 18, X, and Y in men more than 80 years of age. *Biol Reprod* 63:1727–1729, 2000.

Guvendag Guven ES, Dilbaz S, Ceylaner S, et al. An uncommon complementary isochromosome of 46,XY, i(9)(p10),i(9)(q10) in an infertile oligoasthenoteratozoospermic man. *Fertil Steril* 95:290, e5–8, 2011.

Guzé C, Qin N, Kelly J, et al. Isochromosome 22 in trisomy 22 mosaic with five cell lines. *Am J Med Genet* 124A:79–84, 2004.

Guzewicz L, Howell S, Crerand CE, et al. Clinical phenotype and management of individuals with mosaic monosomy X with Y chromosome material stratified by genital phenotype. *Am J Med Genet* 185A:1437–1447, 2021.

Gyejye A, Anyane-Yeboa K, Warburton D. Follow-up of 30 children with de novo balanced rearrangements and supernumerary marker chromosomes diagnosed at amniocentesis. *Am J Hum Genet* 69:208, 2001.

H

Haapaniemi Kouru K, Malmgren H, White I, Rodriguez Sanchez A, Syk Lundberg E. Meiotic segregation analyses of reciprocal translocations in spermatozoa and embryos: No support for predictive value regarding PGD outcome. *Reprod Biomed Online* 34:645–652, 2017.

Habecker-Green J, Naeem R, Goh W, Pflueger S, Murray M, Cohn G. Reproduction in a patient with trisomy 8 mosaicism: Case report and literature review. *Am J Med Genet* 75:382–385, 1998.

Habhab W, Mau-Holzmann U, Singer S, et al. Pre- and postnatal findings in a patient with a recombinant chromosome rec(8)(qter→q21.11::p23.3→qter) due to a paternal pericentric inversion inv(8)(p23.3q21.11) and review of the literature. *Am J Med Genet* 182A:2680–2684, 2020.
Hadjiathanasiou CG, Brauner R, Lortat-Jacob S, et al. True hermaphroditism: Genetic variants and clinical management. *J Pediatr* 125:738–744, 1994.
Hadzsiev K, Dávid D, Szabó G, Czakó M, Melegh B, Kosztolányi G. Partial trisomy of the pericentromeric region of chromosome 5 in a girl with Binder phenotype. *Cytogenet Genome Res* 144:190–195, 2014.
Hagleitner MM, Lankester A, Maraschio P, et al. Clinical spectrum of immunodeficiency, centromeric instability and facial dysmorphism (ICF syndrome). *J Med Genet* 45:93–99, 2008.
Hahnemann JM, Nir M, Friberg M, Engel U, Bugge M. Trisomy 10 mosaicism and maternal uniparental disomy 10 in a liveborn infant with severe congenital malformations. *Am J Med Genet* 138A:150–154, 2005.
Hahnemann JM, Vejerslev LO. European Collaborative Research on Mosaicism in CVS (EUCROMIC)—Fetal and extrafetal cell lineages in 192 gestations with CVS mosaicism involving single autosomal trisomy. *Am J Med Genet* 70:179–187, 1997.
Haines B, Hughes J, Corbett M, et al. Interchromosomal insertional translocation at Xq26.3 alters SOX3 expression in an individual with XX male sex reversal. *J Clin Endocrinol Metab* 100:E815–820, 2015.
Hajianpour A, Murer-Orlando M, Docherty Z. Germ line mosaicism for chromosome 5 "cri-du-chat" deletion? *Am J Hum Genet* 49:217, 1991.
Halgren C, Nielsen NM, Nazaryan-Petersen L, et al. Risks and recommendations in prenatally detected de novo balanced chromosomal rearrangements from assessment of long-term outcomes. *Am J Hum Genet* 102:1090–1103, 2018.
Hall BD. Recurrence risk in de novo 21q21q translocation Down syndrome. *Am J Med Genet* 22:417–418, 1985.
Hallast P, Ebert P, Loftus M, et al. Assembly of 43 human Y chromosomes reveals extensive complexity and variation. *Nature* 621:355–364, 2023.
Hallast P, Kibena L, Punab M, et al. A common 1.6 mb Y-chromosomal inversion predisposes to subsequent deletions and severe spermatogenic failure in humans. *Elife* 10:e65420, 2021.
Halliday J. Outcomes of IVF conceptions: Are they different? *Best Pract Res Clin Obstet Gynaecol* 21:67–81, 2007.
Halliday J, Lewis S, Kennedy J, et al. Health of adults aged 22 to 35 years conceived by assisted reproductive technology. *Fertil Steril* 112:130–139, 2019.
Halliday JL, Ukoumunne OC, Baker HWG, et al. Increased risk of blastogenesis birth defects, arising in the first 4 weeks of pregnancy, after assisted reproductive technologies. *Hum Reprod* 25 59–65, 2010.
Halliday JL, Warren R, McDonald G, Rice PL, Bell RJ, Watson LF. Prenatal diagnosis for women aged 37 years and over: To have or not to have. *Prenat Diagn* 21:842–847, 2001.
Halliday JL, Watson LF, Lumley J, Danks DM, Sheffield LJ. New estimates of Down syndrome risks at chorionic villus sampling, amniocentesis, and livebirth in women of advanced maternal age from a uniquely defined population. *Prenat Diagn* 15:455–465, 1995.
Hamilton MJ, Newbury-Ecob R, Holder-Espinasse M, et al. Rubinstein-Taybi syndrome type 2: Report of nine new cases that extend the phenotypic and genotypic spectrum. *Clin Dysmorphol* 25:135–145, 2016.
Hammoud I, Molina Gomes D, Bergere M, Wainer R, Selva J, Vialard F. Sperm chromosome analysis of an infertile patient with a 95% mosaic r(21) karyotype and normal phenotype. *Fertil Steril* 91:930, e13–15, 2009.
Hamvas A, Nogee LM, Wegner DJ, et al. Inherited surfactant deficiency caused by uniparental disomy of rare mutations in the surfactant protein-B and ATP binding cassette, subfamily a, member 3 genes. *J Pediatr* 155:854–859.e1, 2009.
Han JC, Thurm A, Golden Williams C, et al. Association of brain-derived neurotrophic factor (BDNF) haploinsufficiency with lower adaptive behaviour and reduced cognitive functioning in WAGR/11p13 deletion syndrome. *Cortex* 49:2700–2710, 2013.
Han JY, Lee HJ, Lee YM, Park J. Complete penetrance but different phenotypes in a Korean family with maternal interstitial duplication at 15q11.2-q13.1: A case report. *Children (Basel)* 8:313, 2021.
Han JY, Shin JH, Han MS, Je GH, Shaffer LG. Microarray detection of a de novo der(X)t(X;11)(q28;p13) in a girl with premature ovarian failure and features of Beckwith-Wiedemann syndrome. *J Hum Genet* 51:641–643, 2006.
Hande MP, Azizova TV, Geard CR, et al. Past exposure to densely ionizing radiation leaves a unique permanent signature in the genome. *Am J Hum Genet* 72:1162–1170, 2003.

Hornak M, Vozdova M, Musilova P, et al. Comprehensive meiotic segregation analysis of a 4-breakpoint t(1;3;6) complex chromosome rearrangement using single sperm array comparative genomic hybridization and FISH. *Reprod Biomed Online* 29:499–508, 2014.

Horsthemke B, Buiting K. Imprinting defects on human chromosome 15. *Cytogenet Genome Res* 113:292–299, 2006.

Hoshi N, Fujita M, Mikuni M, et al. Seminoma in a postmenopausal woman with a Y;15 translocation in peripheral blood lymphocytes and a t(Y;15)/45,X Turner mosaic pattern in skin fibroblasts. *J Med Genet* 35:852–856, 1998.

Hosoki K, Takano K, Sudo A, Tanaka S, Saitoh S. Germline mosaicism of a novel UBE3A mutation in Angelman syndrome. *Am J Med Genet* 138A:187–189, 2005.

Hosseinirad H, Yadegari P, Mohanazadeh Falahieh F, et al. Disorders of sex development and female reproductive capacity: A literature review. *Syst Biol Reprod Med* 67:323–336, 2021.

Houcinat N, Llanas B, Moutton S, et al. Homozygous 16p13.11 duplication associated with mild intellectual disability and urinary tract malformations in two siblings born from consanguineous parents. *Am J Med Genet* 167A:2714–2719, 2015.

Hovatta O. Ovarian function and in vitro fertilization (IVF) in Turner syndrome. *Pediatr Endocrinol Rev* 9 (Suppl 2):713–717, 2012.

Hovhannisyan G, Harutyunyan T, Aroutiounian R, Liehr T. DNA copy number variations as markers of mutagenic impact. *Int J Mol Sci* 20:4723, 2019.

Hoyas PC, Tárrega ER, Vázquez Rodríguez S, Quiroga de la Cruz R, Diago Almela V, Perales Marín A. Monozygotic twins discordant for trisomy 4: A case report and a literature review. *J Obstet Gynaecol* 41:147–149, 2021.

Hsieh JC, Van Den Berg D, Kang H, Hsieh CL, Lieber MR. Large chromosome deletions, duplications, and gene conversion events accumulate with age in normal human colon crypts. *Aging Cell* 12:269–279, 2013.

Hsu CC, Lee IW, Su MT, et al. Triple genetic identities for the complete hydatidiform mole, placenta and co-existing fetus after transfer of a single in vitro fertilized oocyte: Case report and possible mechanisms. *Hum Reprod* 23:2686–2691, 2008.

Hsu CF. Contextual effects on the figurative processing of nouns and verbs in people with Williams syndrome. *Res Dev Disabil* 134:104429, 2023.

Hsu LYF. Phenotype/karyotype correlations of Y chromosome aneuploidy with emphasis on structural aberrations in postnatally diagnosed cases. *Am J Med Genet* 53:108–140, 1994.

Hsu LYF, Benn PA. Revised guidelines for the diagnosis of mosaicism in amniocytes. *Prenat Diagn* 19:1081–1082, 1999.

Hsu LYF, Kaffe S, Jenkins EC, et al. Proposed guidelines for diagnosis of chromosome mosaicism in amniocytes based on data derived from chromosome mosaicism and pseudomosaicism studies. *Prenat Diagn* 12:555–573, 1992.

Hsu LYF, Kaffe S, Perlis TE. A revisit of trisomy 20 mosaicism in prenatal diagnosis—An overview of 103 cases. *Prenat Diagn* 11:7–15, 1991.

Hsu LYF, Yu MT, Neu RL, et al. Rare trisomy mosaicism diagnosed in amniocytes, involving an autosome other than chromosomes 13, 18, 20, and 21: Karyotype/phenotype correlations. *Prenat Diagn* 17:201–242, 1997.

Hsu LYF, Yu MT, Richkind KE, et al. Incidence and significance of chromosome mosaicism involving an autosomal structural abnormality diagnosed prenatally through amniocentesis: A collaborative study. *Prenat Diagn* 16:1–28, 1996.

Hu H, Yao H, Dong Y, et al. Distinct karyotypes in two offspring of a man with jumping translocation karyotype 45,XY,der(16)t(16;22)(q24;q11.2), -22 [59]/45,XY,der(1)t(1;22)(p36;q11.2), -22 [11]/45,XY,der(22)t(22;22)(p13;q11.2), -22 [10]. *Am J Med Genet* 164A:2048–2053, 2014.

Hu J, Ou Z, Infante E, Kochmar SJ, et al. Chromosome 12q13.13q13.13 microduplication and microdeletion: A case report and literature review. *Mol Cytogenet* 10:24, 2017.

Hu J, Yan K, Jin P, Yang Y, Sun Y, Dong M. Prenatal diagnosis of trisomy 8 mosaicism, initially identified by cffDNA screening. *Mol Cytogenet* 15:39, 2022.

Hu L, Wei Y, Luo K, et al. Clinical outcomes in carriers of complex chromosomal rearrangements: A retrospective analysis of comprehensive chromosome screening results in seven cases. *Fertil Steril* 109:486–492, 2018.

Hu X, Ayala SS, Dyer L, Guan Q, Pena L. A rare case of postnatal mosaic trisomy 12 with severe congenital heart disease and literature review. *Am J Med Genet* 185A:1864–1869, 2021.

Huang B, Prensky L, Thangavelu M, Main D, Wang S. Three consecutive triploidy pregnancies in a woman: Genetic predisposition? *Eur J Hum Genet* 12:985–986, 2004.

Huang B, Thangavelu M, Bhatt S, Sandlin CJ, Wang S. Prenatal diagnosis of 45,X and 45,X mosaicism: The need for thorough cytogenetic and clinical evaluations. *Prenat Diagn* 22:105–110, 2002.

Huang MH, Lee C, Chang JS, et al. Retrospectively investigating the 12-year experience of prenatal diagnosis of small supernumerary marker chromosomes through array comparative genomic hybridization. *Taiwan J Obstet Gynecol* 58:139–144, 2019.

Huang N, Zhou J, Lu W, et al. Characteristics and clinical evaluation of X chromosome translocations. *Mol Cytogenet* 16:36, 2023a.

Huang R, Fu F, Zhou H, et al. Prenatal diagnosis in the fetal hyperechogenic kidneys: Assessment using chromosomal microarray analysis and exome sequencing. *Hum Genet* 142:835–847, 2023b.

Hudson DF, Amor DJ, Boys A, et al. Loss of RMI2 increases genome instability and causes a Bloom-like syndrome. *PLoS Genet* 12:e1006483, 2016.

Hughes IA, Houk C, Ahmed SF, Lee PA. Consensus statement on management of intersex disorders. *Arch Dis Child* 91:554–563, 2006.

Huang B, Prensky L, Thangavelu M, Main D, Wang S. Three consecutive triploidy pregnancies in a woman: Genetic predisposition? *Eur J Hum Genet* 12:985–986, 2004.

Huang B, Thangavelu M, Bhatt S, J Sandlin C, Wang S. Prenatal diagnosis of 45,X and 45,X mosaicism: The need for thorough cytogenetic and clinical evaluations. *Prenat Diagn* 22:105–110, 2002.

Huang MH, Lee C, Chang JS, et al. Retrospectively investigating the 12-year experience of prenatal diagnosis of small supernumerary marker chromosomes through array comparative genomic hybridization. *Taiwan J Obstet Gynecol* 58:139–144, 2019.

Huguet G, Schramm C, Douard E, et al. Genome-wide analysis of gene dosage in 24,092 individuals estimates that 10,000 genes modulate cognitive ability. *Mol Psychiatry* 26:2663–2676, 2021.

Huijsdens-van Amsterdam K, Page-Christiaens L, Flowers N, et al. Isochromosome 21q is overrepresented among false-negative cell-free DNA prenatal screening results involving Down syndrome. *Eur J Hum Genet* 26:1490–1496, 2018.

Huisman EJ, Brooimans AR, Mayer S, et al. Patients with chromosome 11q deletions are characterized by inborn errors of immunity involving both B and T lymphocytes. *J Clin Immunol* 42:1521–1534, 2022.

Hujoel MLA, Sherman MA, Barton AR, et al. Influences of rare copy-number variation on human complex traits. *Cell* 185:4233–4248.e27, 2022.

Hultén M, Armstrong S, Challinor P, et al. Genomic imprinting in an Angelman and Prader-Willi translocation family. *Lancet* 338:638–639, 1991.

Hultén MA, Jonasson J, Iwarsson E, et al. Trisomy 21 mosaicism: We may all have a touch of Down syndrome. *Cytogenet Genome Res* 139:189–192, 2013.

Hung PH, Froenicke L, Lin CY, et al. Effects of environmental tobacco smoke in vivo on rhesus monkey semen quality, sperm function, and sperm metabolism. *Reprod Toxicol* 27:140–148, 2009.

Hunt PA, Hassold TJ. Sex matters in meiosis. *Science* 296:2181–2183, 2002.

Hunter A, Brierley K, Tomkins D. 46,XX/46XY chromosome complement in amniotic fluid cell culture followed by the birth of a normal female child. *Prenat Diagn* 2:127–131, 1982.

Hunter AGW, Allanson JE. Follow-up study of patients with Wiedemann-Beckwith syndrome with emphasis on the change in facial appearance over time. *Am J Med Genet* 51:102–107, 1994.

Hunter JE, Allen EG, Shin M, et al. The association of low socioeconomic status and the risk of having a child with Down syndrome: A report from the National Down Syndrome Project. *Genet Med* 15:698–705, 2013.

Hurd LM, Thacker MM, Okenfuss E, et al. Aneurysmal bone cysts and pathologic fracture associated with supernumerary ring chromosome 6 in two unrelated patients. *Am J Med Genet* 173A:3205–3210, 2017.

Hussain SZ, Evans AL, Ahmed OA, et al. Non-syndromic mental retardation segregating with an apparently balanced t(1;17) reciprocal translocation through three generations. *Am J Med Genet* 95:99–104, 2000.

Huynh MT, Gérard M, Ranguin K, et al. Novel interstitial 2q12.3q13 microdeletion predisposes to developmental delay and behavioral problems. Neurogenetics 22:195–206, 2021a.

Huynh MT, Riteau AS, Moradkhani K, et al. Structural abnormalities of chromosome 8 and fetoplacental discrepancy: A second case report and review of fetal phenotype of 8p inverted duplication deletion syndrome. *Eur J Med Genet* 64:104118, 2021b.

Hwang SH, Lee SM, Seo EJ, et al. A case of male infertility with a reciprocal translocation t(X;14)(p11.4;p12). *Korean J Lab Med* 27:139–142, 2007.

Hyon C, Mansour-Hendili L, Chantot-Bastaraud S, et al. Deletion of CPEB1 gene: A rare but recurrent cause of premature ovarian insufficiency. *J Clin Endocrinol Metab* 101:2099–2104, 2016.

Hysert M, Bruyère H, Côté GB, et al. Prenatal cytogenetic assessment and inv(2)(p11.2q13). *Prenat Diagn* 26:810–813, 2006.

I

Ideraabdullah FY, Vigneau S, Bartolomei MS. Genomic imprinting mechanisms in mammals. *Mutat Res* 647:77–85, 2008.

Ijaz MR, Trepanier AM, Kleinert HL, Weiss SM, Meredith SH. Parent-reported genetic counselor adherence to the NSGC practice resource for communicating a potential prenatal diagnosis: Impact on the Down syndrome diagnosis experience. *J Genet Couns*, 34:e1948,2025.

Ikuma S, Sato T, Sugiura-Ogasawara M, Nagayoshi M, Tanaka A, Takeda S. Preimplantation genetic diagnosis and natural conception: A comparison of live birth rates in patients with recurrent pregnancy loss associated with translocation. *PLoS One* 10:e0129958, 2015.

Imai A, Takagi A, Tamaya T. A novel sex-determining region on Y (SRY) missense mutation identified in a 46,XY female and also in the father. *Endocr J* 46:735–739, 1999.

Imudia AN, Suzuki Y, Kilburn BA, et al. Retrieval of trophoblast cells from the cervical canal for prediction of abnormal pregnancy: A pilot study. *Hum Reprod* 24:2086–2092, 2009.

Inbar-Feigenberg M, Choufani S, Cytrynbaum C, et al. Mosaicism for genome-wide paternal uniparental disomy with features of multiple imprinting disorders: Diagnostic and management issues. *Am J Med Genet* 161A:13–20, 2013.

Indrieri A, van Rahden VA, Tiranti V, et al. Mutations in COX7B cause microphthalmia with linear skin lesions, an unconventional mitochondrial disease. *Am J Hum Genet* 91:942–949, 2012.

Ingelfinger FJ. Arrogance. *N Engl J Med* 303:1507–1511, 1980.

Inoue T, Yagasaki H, Nishioka J, et al. Molecular and clinical analyses of two patients with UPD(16)mat detected by screening 94 patients with Silver-Russell syndrome phenotype of unknown aetiology. *J Med Genet* 56:413–418, 2019.

Ioannides Y, Lokulo-Sodipe K, Mackay DJ, Davies JH, Temple IK. Temple syndrome: Improving the recognition of an underdiagnosed chromosome 14 imprinting disorder—An analysis of 51 published cases. *J Med Genet* 51:495–501, 2014.

Ioannou D, Fortun J, Tempest HG. Meiotic nondisjunction and sperm aneuploidy in humans. *Reproduction* 157:R15–R31, 2019.

Iourov IY, Zelenova MA, Vorsanova SG, Voinova VV, Yurov YB. 4q21.2q21.3 duplication: Molecular and nneuropsychological aspects. *Curr Genomics* 19:173–178, 2018.

Irani M, Reichman D, Robles A, et al. Morphologic grading of euploid blastocysts influences implantation and ongoing pregnancy rates. *Fertil Steril* 107:664–670, 2017.

Isaacs D. What is the value of a human baby? *J Paediatr Child Health* 38:608–609, 2002.

ISCN 2024—An International System for Human Cytogenomic Nomenclature. *Cytogenet Genome Res* 164(Suppl 1):1–224, 2024.

Iselius L, Lindsten J, Aurias A, et al. The 11q;22q translocation: A collaborative study of 20 new cases and analysis of 110 families. *Hum Genet* 64:343–355, 1983.

Ishii F, Fujita H, Nagai A, et al. Case report of rec(7)dup(7q)inv(7)(p22q22) and a review of the recombinants resulting from parental pericentric inversions on any chromosomes. *Am J Med Genet* 73:290–295, 1997.

Ishikawa S, Ishikawa M, Tokuda T, et al. Japanese family with an autosomal dominant chromosome instability syndrome: A new neurodegenerative disease? *Am J Med Genet* 94:265–270, 2000.

Ishikiriyama S, Tonoki H, Shibuya Y, Chin S, Harada N, Abe K, Niikawa N. Waardenburg syndrome type I in a child with de novo inversion (2)(q35q37.3). *Am J Med Genet* 33:505–507, 1989.

Isles AR, Ingason A, Lowther C, et al. Parental origin of interstitial duplications at 15q11.2-q13.3 in schizophrenia and neurodevelopmental disorders. *PLoS Genet* 12:e1005993, 2016.

Ismail A, Ahid F, Thong MK, Zakaria Z. Terminal microdeletion of chromosome 18 in a Malaysian boy characterized with few features of typical 18q- deletion syndrome: A case report. *J Med Case Rep* 17:250, 2023.

Itoh N, Becroft DMO, Reeve AE, Morison IM. Proportion of cells with paternal 11p15 uniparental disomy correlates with organ enlargement in Wiedemann-Beckwith syndrome. *Am J Med Genet* 92:111–116, 2000.

Itsara A, Wu H, Smith JD, et al. De novo rates and selection of large copy number variation. *Genome Res* 20:1469–1481, 2010.

Ivanova AD, Semenova ML. Chromosomal aberrations as a biological phenomenon in human embryonic development. *Acta Naturae* 15:27–36, 2023.

Iwarsson E, Kvist U, Hultén MA. Disomy 21 in spermatozoa and the paternal origin of trisomy 21 Down syndrome. *Mol Cytogenet* 8:67, 2015.

Iwata-Otsubo A, Darr KR, Torres-Martinez W, Hodge JC. Genotype-phenotype correlation of distal 2q37 deletions. *Cytogenet Genome Res* 162:237–243, 2022.

Iype T, Alakbarzade V, Iype M, et al. A large Indian family with rearrangement of chromosome 4p16 and 3p26.3 and divergent clinical presentations. *BMC Med Genet* 16:104, 2015.

Izumi K, Culler D, Solomon B, Muenke M, Parikh A. Submicroscopic familial chromosomal translocation between 7q and 12p mimicking an autosomal dominant holoprosencephaly syndrome. *Clin Genet* 78:402–404, 2010.

J

Jackson KE, Tsien F, Marble M. Phenotypic features in a boy with monosomy 18 mosaicism. *Am J Med Genet* 95:229–32, 2000.

Jacobs M, Cooper SA, McGowan R, Nelson SM, Pell JP. Pregnancy outcome following prenatal diagnosis of chromosomal anomaly: A record linkage study of 26,261 pregnancies. *PLoS One* 11:e0166909, 2016.

Jacobs P, Dalton P, James R, et al. Turner syndrome: A cytogenetic and molecular study. *Ann Hum Genet* 61:471–483, 1997.

Jacobs PA. Mutation rates of structural chromosome rearrangements in man. *Am J Hum Genet* 33:44–54, 1981.

Jacobs PA, Strong JA. A case of human intersexuality having a possible XXY sex-determining mechanism. *Nature* 183:302–303, 1959.

Jacobsen P, Hauge M, Henningsen K, Hobolth N, Mikkelsen M, Philip J. An (11;21) translocation in four generations with chromosome 11 abnormalities in the offspring: A clinical, cytogenetical, and gene marker study. *Hum Hered* 23:568–585, 1973.

Jacquemont S, Reymond A, Zufferey F, et al. Mirror extreme BMI phenotypes associated with gene dosage at the chromosome 16p11.2 locus. *Nature* 478:97–102, 2011.

Jacquin C, Landais E, Poirsier C, et al. 1p36 deletion syndrome: Review and mapping with further characterization of the phenotype, a new cohort of 86 patients. *Am J Med Genet* 191A:445–458, 2023.

Jafari-Ghahfarokhi H, Moradi-Chaleshtori M, Liehr T, Hashemzadeh-Chaleshtori M Teimori H, Ghasemi-Dehkordi P. Small supernumerary marker chromosomes and their correlation with specific syndromes. *Adv Biomed Res* 4:140, 2015.

Jäger RJ, Harley VR, Pfeiffer RA, Goodfellow PN, Scherer G. A familial mutation in the testis-determining gene SRY shared by both sexes. *Hum Genet* 90:350–355, 1992.

Jalbert P, Jalbert H, Sele B. Types of imbalances in human reciprocal translocations: Risks at birth. In Daniel A (ed.), *The Cytogenetics of Mammalian Autosomal Rearrangements*. New York, NY: Liss, 1988.

Jalbert P, Jalbert H, Sele B, et al. Partial trisomy for the long arms of chromosome no. 5 due to insertion and further "aneusomie de recombinaison." *J Med Genet* 12:418–423, 1975.

Jalbert P, Sele B, Jalbert H. Reciprocal translocations: A way to predict the mode of imbalanced segregation by pachytene-diagram drawing. *Hum Genet* 55:209–222, 1980.

Jallinoja P, Santalahti P, Toiviainen H, Hemminki E. Acceptance of screening and abortion for Down syndrome among Finnish midwives and public health nurses. *Prenat Diagn* 19:1015–1022, 1999.

James PA, Gibson K, McGaughran J. Prenatal diagnosis of mosaic trisomy 20 in New Zealand. *Aust NZ J Obstet Gynaecol* 42:486–489, 2002.

James RS, Ellis K, Pettay D, Jacobs PA. Cytogenetic and molecular study of four couples with multiple trisomy 21 pregnancies. *Eur J Hum Genet* 6:207–212, 1998.

James RS, Temple IK, Dennis NR, Crolla JA. A search for uniparental disomy in carriers of supernumerary marker chromosomes. *Eur J Hum Genet* 3:21–26, 1995.

James WD, Roth R, Fitzgerald M. Ring 20 syndrome: A call to action. *Epilepsia* 65:1147–1148, 2024.

Jamsheer A, Sowinska A, Simon D, Jamsheer-Bratkowska M, Trzeciak T, Latos-Bielenska A. Bilateral radial agenesis with absent thumbs, complex heart defect, short stature, and facial dysmorphism in a patient with pure distal microduplication of 5q35.2–5q35.3. *BMC Med Genet* 14:13, 2013.

Jang W, Chae H, Kim J, et al. Identification of small marker chromosomes using microarray comparative genomic hybridization and multicolor fluorescent in situ hybridization. *Mol Cytogenet* 9:61, 2016.

Jang W, Kim Y, Han E, et al. Chromosomal microarray analysis as a first-tier clinical diagnostic test in patients with developmental delay/intellectual disability, autism spectrum disorders, and multiple congenital anomalies: A prospective multicenter study in Korea. *Ann Lab Med* 39:299–310, 2019.

Janke D. Centric fission of chromosome no. 7 in three generations. *Hum Genet* 60:200–201, 1982.

Khalifa Y, Hassan HY, Weise A, Liehr T, Alkhayyat H. Molecular cytogenetic and phenotypic characterization of Phelan McDermid and 22q13 duplication syndrome: A case report. *Mol Cytogenet* 15:52, 2022.

Khan SA, Theunissen TW. Modeling X-chromosome inactivation and reactivation during human development. *Curr Opin Genet Dev* 82:102096, 2023.

Khan WA, Cohen N, Scott SA, Pereira EM. Familial inheritance of the 3q29 microdeletion syndrome: Case report and review. *BMC Med Genomics* 12:51, 2019.

Khawajkie Y, Buckett W, Nguyen NMP, et al. Recurrent triploid digynic conceptions and mature ovarian teratomas: Are they different manifestations of the same genetic defect? *Genes Chromosomes Cancer* 56:832–840, 2017.

Khogeer AA, AboMansour IS, Mohammed DA. The role of genetics, epigenetics, and the environment in ASD: A mini review. *Epigenomes* 6:15, 2022.

Kher AS, Chattopadhyay A, Datta S, Kanade S, Sreenivasan VK, Bharucha BA. Familial mosaic Turner syndrome. *Clin Genet* 46:382–383, 1994.

Kim ED, Bischoff FZ, Lipshultz LI, Lamb DJ. Genetic concerns for the subfertile male in the era of ICSI. *Prenat Diagn* 18:1349–1365, 1998.

Kim EY, Kim YK, Kim MK, et al. A case of de novo duplication of 15q24-q26.3. *Korean J Pediatr* 54:267–271, 2011.

Kim H, Lee KS, Kim AK, et al. A chemical with proven clinical safety rescues Down-syndrome-related phenotypes in through DYRK1A inhibition. *Dis Model Mech* 9:839–848, 2016.

Kim HJ, Cho E, Park JB, Im WY, Kim HJ. A Korean family with KBG syndrome identified by ANKRD11 mutation, and phenotypic comparison of ANKRD11 mutation and 16q24.3 microdeletion. *Eur J Med Genet* 58:86–94, 2015.

Kim IW, Khadilkar AC, Ko EY, Sabanegh ES. 47,XYY syndrome and male infertility. *Rev Urol* 15:188–196, 2013.

Kim J, Tao X, Cheng M, et al. The concordance rates of an initial trophectoderm biopsy with the rest of the embryo using PGTseq, a targeted next-generation sequencing platform for preimplantation genetic testing-aneuploidy. *Fertil Steril* 117:315–323, 2022.

Kim JK, Jeong JE, Choi JM, Kim GH, Yoo HW. A female with typical fragile-X phenotype caused by maternal isodisomy of the entire X chromosome. *J Hum Genet* 65:551–555, 2020.

Kim JW, Lee SY, Hur CY, Lim JH, Park CK. Clinical outcomes of preimplantation genetic testing for aneuploidy in high-risk patients: A retrospective cohort study. *Clin Exp Reprod Med* 51:75–84, 2024.

Kim JW, Park SY, Ryu HM, et al. Molecular and clinical characteristics of 26 cases with structural Y chromosome aberrations. *Cytogenet Genome Res* 136:270–277, 2012.

Kim MK, Seok HH, Kim YS, et al. Molecular genetic and cytogenetic characterization of a partial Xp duplication and Xq deletion in a patient with premature ovarian failure. *Gene* 534:54–59, 2014.

Kim SH, Park MJ, Cho EH, Kim S, Yoo SJ. Different parental origins of supernumerary X chromosomes in brothers with Klinefelter syndrome: A case report. *Medicine (Baltimore)* 98:e17838, 2019.

Kim SR, Choi EJ, Kim TY, et al. Midtrimester amniocentesis for prenatal diagnosis. *J Genet Med* 5:125–130, 2008.

Kim SY, Wohler E, Gutierrez MJ, Sadreameli C, Kossoff E, Sobreira NL. Ring chromosome 17 syndrome—A case report and discussion of diagnostic methods. *Am J Med Gen* 197:e63925, 2025.

Kimura R, Kamino K, Yamamoto M, et al. The DYRK1A gene, encoded in chromosome 21 Down syndrome critical region, bridges between beta-amyloid production and tau phosphorylation in Alzheimer disease. *Hum Mol Genet* 16:15–23, 2007.

King DA, Fitzgerald TW, Miller R, et al. A novel method for detecting uniparental disomy from trio genotypes identifies a significant excess in children with developmental disorders. *Genome Res* 24:673–687, 2014.

King PH, Waldrop R, Lupski JR, Shaffer LG. Charcot-Marie-Tooth phenotype produced by a duplicated PMP22 gene as part of a 17p trisomy-translocation to the X chromosome. *Clin Genet* 54:413–416, 1998.

Kircheisen R, Schroeder-Kurth T. Familiäres blasenmolen-syndrom und genetische aspekte dieser gestörten trophoblastentwicklung. *Geburtshilfe Frauenheilkd* 51:569–571, 1991.

Kirkpatrick G, Chow V, Ma S. Meiotic recombination, synapsis, meiotic inactivation and sperm aneuploidy in a chromosome 1 inversion carrier. *Reprod Biomed Online* 24:91–100, 2012.

Kirkpatrick G, Ferguson KA, Gao H, et al. A comparison of sperm aneuploidy rates between infertile men with normal and abnormal karyotypes. *Hum Reprod* 23:1679–1683, 2008.

Kitamura N, Ito Y, Kawai T, et al. Clinical course and genetic analysis of a case of the amniocentesis showing chromosome 6 trisomy mosaicism. *Taiwan J Obstet Gynecol* 63:418–421, 2024.

Kitsiou-Tzeli S, Manolakos E, Lagou M, et al. Characterization of a prenatally assessed de novo supernumerary minute ring chromosome 20 in a phenotypically normal male. *Mol Cytogenet* 2:8, 2009.

Kivirikko S, Salonen R, Salo A, von Koskull H. Prenatally detected trisomy 7 mosaicism in a dysmorphic child. *Prenat Diagn* 22:541–544, 2002.
Kızıltan K, Özbezen Kızıltan E, Yerlikaya Oral E, Akgün Doğan Ö, Ersoy M, Karaçetin G. Very early-onset schizophrenia with accompanying obsessive-compulsive symptoms: A case report of a female with 16p13.11 duplication. *Psychiatry Clin Psychopharmacol* 34:356–360, 2024.
Klaassen P, Duijff S, Swanenburg de Veye H, et al. Explaining the variable penetrance of CNVs: Parental intelligence modulates expression of intellectual impairment caused by the 22q11.2 deletion. *Am J Med Genet* 171B:790–796, 2016.
Klamut N, Bothwell S, Carl AE, et al. Prevalence, diagnostic features, and medical outcomes of females with Turner syndrome with a trisomy X cell line (45,X/47,XXX): Results from the InsighTS Registry. *Am J Med Genet* 194A:e63819, 2024.
Kleczkowska A, Fryns JP, Van den Berghe H. Pericentric inversions in man: Personal experience and review of the literature. *Hum Genet* 75:333–338, 1987.
Kleczkowska A, Fryns JP, Vinken L, van den Berghe H. Effect of balanced X/autosome translocations on sexual and physical development: A personal experience in 4 patients. *Clin Genet* 27:147–152, 1985.
Kleffmann W, Zink AM, Lee JA, et al. 5q31 microdeletions: Definition of a critical region and analysis of LRRTM2, a candidate gene for intellectual disability. *Mol Syndromol* 3:68–75, 2012.
Klein J, Graham JM, Platt LD, Schreck R. Trisomy 8 mosaicism in chorionic villus sampling: Case report and counselling issues. *Prenat Diagn* 14:451–454, 1994.
Klein OD, Backstrand K, Cotter PD, Marco E, Sherr E, Slavotinek A. Case report: Y;6 translocation with deletion of 6p. *Clin Dysmorphol* 14:93–96, 2005.
Kleinendorst L, van Haelst MM. Mirror hand movements caused by a deletion of the DCC gene. *JAMA Neurol* 81:187, 2024.
Klimczak AM, Patel DP, Hotaling JM, Scott RT Jr. Role of the sperm, oocyte, and embryo in recurrent pregnancy loss. *Fertil Steril* 115:533–537 2021.
Klitzman R, Bezborodko E, Chung WK, Appelbaum PS. Receiving de novo genetic diagnoses for autism with intellectual disability: Parents' views of impacts on families' reproductive decisions. *J Community Genet* 15:85–96, 2024
Knebel S, Pasantes JJ, Thi DA, Schaller F, Schempp W. Heterogeneity of pericentric inversions of the human Y chromosome. *Cytogenet Genome Res* 132:219–226, 2011.
Knegt AC, Li S, Engelen JJM, Bijlsma EK, Warburton PE. Prenatal diagnosis of a karyotypically normal pregnancy in a mother with a supernumerary neocentric 13q21→13q22 chromosome and balancing reciprocal deletion. *Prenat Diagn* 23:215–220, 2003.
Knight MA, Hernandez D, Diede SJ, et al. A duplication at chromosome 11q12.2–11q12.3 is associated with spinocerebellar ataxia type 20. *Hum Mol Genet* 17:3847–3853, 2008.
Knijnenburg J, van Haeringen A, Hansson KB, et al. Ring chromosome formation as a novel escape mechanism in patients with inverted duplication and terminal deletion. *Eur J Hum Genet* 15:548–555, 2007.
Knudson AG, Jr. Mutation and cancer: Statistical study of retinoblastoma. *Proc Natl Acad Sci USA* 68:820–823, 1971.
Kofoed AWS, Kristiansen SS, Miranda MJ, Rubboli G, Johannesen KM. Differences in manifestations of epilepsy and developmental delay in PURA syndrome and 5q31 microdeletions. *Clin Genet* 106:386–393, 2024.
Kojis TL, Gatti RA, Sparkes RS. The cytogenetics of ataxia telangiectasia. *Cancer Genet Cytogenet* 56:143–156, 1991.
Kokkonen H, Leisti J. An unexpected recurrence of Angelman syndrome suggestive of maternal germline mosaicism of del(15)(q11q13) in a Finnish family. *Hum Genet* 107:83–85, 2000.
Kolbasin LN, Dubrovskaya TA, Salnikova GB, et al. Family case of Potocki-Lupski syndrome. *Mol Cytogenet* 17:6, 2024.
Kolgeci S, Azemi M, Ahmeti H, Dervishi Z, Sopjani M, Kolgeci J. Recurrent abortions and Down syndrome resulting from Robertsonian translocation 21q;21q. *Med Arch* 66:350–352, 2012.
Kølvraa S, Singh R, Normand EA, et al. Genome-wide copy number analysis on DNA from fetal cells isolated from the blood of pregnant women. *Prenat Diagn* 36:1127–1134, 2016.
Kompanje EJO. The earliest description of an autopsy on a case of Roberts syndrome reported in 1672: Some additions. *Am J Med Genet* 149A:1610–1611, 2009.
Kondo Y, Mizuno S, Ohara K, et al. Two cases of partial trisomy 21 (pter-q22.1) without the major features of Down syndrome. *Am J Med Genet* 140:227–232, 2006.
Kong GW, Cao Y, Huang J, et al. Prenatal detection of 10q22q23 duplications: Dilemmas in phenotype prediction. *Prenat Diagn* 36:1211–1216, 2016.

Konialis C, Hagnefelt B, Sevastidou S, et al. Uncovering recurrent microdeletion syndromes and subtelomeric deletions/duplications through non-selective application of a MLPA-based extended prenatal panel in routine prenatal diagnosis. *Prenat Diagn* 31:571–577, 2011.

Koochek M, Harvard C, Hildebrand MJ, et al. 15q duplication associated with autism in a multiplex family with a familial cryptic translocation t(14;15)(q11.2;q13.3) detected using array-CGH. *Clin Genet* 69:124–134, 2006.

Koolen DA, Dupont J, de Leeuw N, et al. Two families with sibling recurrence of the 17q21.31 microdeletion syndrome due to low-grade mosaicism. *Eur J Hum Genet* 20:729–733, 2012.

Koolen DA, Pfundt R, Linda K, et al. The Koolen-de Vries syndrome: A phenotypic comparison of patients with a 17q21.31 microdeletion versus a KANSL1 sequence variant. *Eur J Hum Genet* 24:652–659, 2016.

Korenberg JR, Chen XN, Schipper R, et al. Down syndrome phenotypes: The consequences of chromosomal imbalance. *Proc Natl Acad Sci USA* 91:4997–5001, 1994.

Korenromp MJ, Page-Christiaens GCML, van den Bout J, Mulder EJH, Visser GHA. Maternal decision to terminate pregnancy in case of Down syndrome. *Am J Obstet Gynecol* 196:149.e1–11, 2007.

Kornfield MS, Parker P, Rubin E, et al. Patients with recurrent pregnancy loss have similar embryonic preimplantation genetic testing aneuploidy rates and in vitro fertilization outcomes to infertility patients. *F S Rep* 3:342–348, 2022.

Kort JD, McCoy RC, Demko Z, Lathi RB. Are blastocyst aneuploidy rates different between fertile and infertile populations? *J Assist Reprod Genet* 35:403–408, 2018.

Kosaki R, Migita O, Takahashi T, Kosaki K. Two distinctive classic genetic syndromes, 22q11.2 deletion syndrome and Angelman syndrome, occurring within the same family. *Am J Med Genet* 149A:702–705, 2009.

Kosian P, Gloning KP, Germer U, et al. Maternal risk factors and their effect on outcome and procedure-related complications in cordocentesis: A multicenter retrospective study. *J Clin Med* 12:6841, 2023.

Kosiv KA, Mercurio MR, Carey JC. The common trisomy syndromes, their cardiac implications, and ethical considerations in care. *Curr Opin Pediatr* 35:531–537, 2023.

Koskinen S, Onnelainen T, de la Chapelle A, Kere J. A rare reciprocal translocation (12;21) segregating for nine generations. *Hum Genet* 92:509–512, 1993.

Kosztolányi G. Does "ring syndrome" exist? An analysis of 207 case reports on patients with a ring autosome. *Hum Genet* 75:174–179, 1987.

Kosztolányi G, Brecevic L, Bajnòczky K, Schinzel A, Riegel M. Mosaic supernumerary ring chromosome 1 in a three-generational family: 10-year follow-up report. *Eur J Med Genet* 54:152–156, 2011.

Kosztolányi G, Méhes K, Hook EB. Inherited ring chromosomes: An analysis of published cases. *Hum Genet* 87:320–324, 1991.

Kotalova R, Dusatkova P, Drabova J, et al. Choledochal cyst with 17q12 chromosomal duplication. *Ann Hum Genet* 82:48–51, 2018.

Kotani T, Tsuda H, Ito Y, et al. Prenatal diagnosis of distal 13q deletion syndrome in a fetus with esophageal atresia: A case report and review of the literature. *J Med Case Rep* 16:481, 2022.

Kotzot D. Abnormal phenotypes in uniparental disomy (UPD): Fundamental aspects and a critical review with bibliography of UPD other than 15. *Am J Med Genet* 82:265–274, 1999.

Kotzot D. Complex and segmental uniparental disomy (UPD): Review and lessons from rare chromosomal complements. *J Med Genet* 38:497–507, 2001.

Kotzot D. Review and meta-analysis of systematic searches for uniparental disomy (UPD) other than UPD 15. *Am J Med Genet* 111:366–375, 2002.

Kotzot D. Complex and segmental uniparental disomy updated. *J Med Genet* 45:545–556, 2008a.

Kotzot D. Prenatal testing for uniparental disomy: Indications and clinical relevance. *Ultrasound Obstet Gynecol* 31:100–105, 2008b.

Kousoulidou L, Tanteles G, Moutafi M, Sismani C, Patsalis PC, Anastasiadou V. 263.4 kb deletion within the TCF4 gene consistent with Pitt-Hopkins syndrome, inherited from a mosaic parent with normal phenotype. *Eur J Med Genet* 56:314–318, 2013.

Kouvidi E, Zachaki S, Tsarouha H, et al. Female reproductive ageing and chromosomal abnormalities in a large series of women undergoing IVF. *Cytogenet Genome Res* 161:551–555, 2021.

Kowalczyk M, Tomaszewska A, Podbiol-Palenta A, et al. A familial deletion of 16q21 characterized by an SNP array and associated with a normal phenotype. *Am J Med Genet* 161A:1501–1504, 2013.

Kovaleva NV. Germ-line transmission of trisomy 21: Data from 80 families suggest an implication of grandmaternal age and a high frequency of female-specific trisomy rescue. *Mol Cytogenet* 3:7, 2010.

Kovaleva NV. Increased risk of tisomy 21 in offspring of carriers of balanced non-contributing autosomal rearrangements is not explained by interchromosomal effect. *Genetika* 49:259–268, 2013.

Kovaleva NV. Resolving paradoxes of Robertsonian translocations. In Larramendy M, Soloneski S (eds.), *Cytogenetics—Past, Present and Further Perspectives*. IntechOpen, 2019.

Kovaleva NV, Cotter PD. Somatic/gonadal mosaicism for structural autosomal rearrangements: Female predominance among carriers of gonadal mosaicism for unbalanced rearrangements. *Mol Cytogenet* 9:8, 2016.

Kovaleva NV, Shaffer LG. Under-ascertainment of mosaic carriers of balanced homologous acrocentric translocations and isochromosomes. *Am J Med Genet* 121A:180–187, 2003.

Koza SA, Tabet AC, Bonaglia MC, et al. Consensus recommendations on counselling in Phelan-McDermid syndrome, with special attention to recurrence risk and to ring chromosome 22. *Eur J Med Genet* 66:104773, 2023.

Kozel BA, Barak B, Kim CA, et al. Williams syndrome. *Nat Rev Dis Primers* 7:42, 2021.

Kozma C, Slavotinek AM, Meck JM. Segregation of a t(1;3) translocation in multiple affected family members with both types of adjacent-1 segregants. *Am J Med Genet* 124A:118–128, 2004.

Kozma K, Bembea M, Jurca CM, et al. Greig cephalopolysyndactyly contiguous gene syndrome: Case report and literature review. *Genes (Basel)* 12:1674, 2021.

Kramer RL, Jarve RK, Yaron Y, et al. Determinants of parental decisions after the prenatal diagnosis of Down syndrome. *Am J Med Genet* 79:172–174, 1998.

Krausz C, Casamonti E. Spermatogenic failure and the Y chromosome. *Hum Genet* 136:637–655, 2017.

Krieg SA, Lathi RB, Behr B, Westphal LM. Normal pregnancy after tetraploid karyotype on trophectoderm biopsy. *Fertil Steril* 92:1169, e10, 2009.

Kristalijn SA, White K, Eerbeek D, Kostenko E, Grati FR, Bilardo CM. Patient experience with non-invasive prenatal testing (NIPT) as a primary screen for aneuploidy in the Netherlands. *BMC Pregnancy Childbirth* 22:782. 2022.

Kromann AB, Ousager LB, Ali IKM, Aydemir N, Bygum A. Pigmentary mosaicism: A review of original literature and recommendations for future handling. *Orphanet J Rare Dis* 13:39, 2018.

Kruszka P, Addissie YA, McGinn DE, et al. 22q11.2 deletion syndrome in diverse populations. *Am J Med Genet* 173A:879–888, 2017.

Krzeminska D, Steinfeld C, Cloez JL, et al. Prenatal diagnosis of Williams syndrome based on ultrasound signs. *Prenat Diagn* 29:710–712, 2009.

Kubicek D, Hornak M, Horak J, et al. Incidence and origin of meiotic whole and segmental chromosomal aneuploidies detected by karyomapping. *Reprod Biomed Online* 38:330–339, 2019.

Kubota T, Nonoyama S, Tonoki H, et al. A new assay for the analysis of X-chromosome inactivation based on methylation-specific PCR. *Hum Genet* 104:49–55, 1999.

Kuchinka BD, Barrett IJ, Moya G, et al. Two cases of confined placental mosaicism for chromosome 4, including one with maternal uniparental disomy. *Prenat Diagn* 21:36–39, 2001.

Kuechler A, Hauffa BP, Köninger A, et al. An unbalanced translocation unmasks a recessive mutation in the follicle-stimulating hormone receptor (FSHR) gene and causes FSH resistance. *Eur J Hum Genet* 18:656–661, 2010.

Kühl H, Röttger S, Heilbronner H, Enders H, Schempp W. Loss of the Y chromosomal PAR2-region in four familial cases of satellited Y chromosomes (Yqs). *Chromosome Res* 9:215–222, 2001.

Kulharya AS, Mills Lovell C, Flannery DB. Unusual mosaic karyotype resulting from adjacent 1 segregation of t(11;22): Importance of performing skin fibroblast karyotype in patients with unexplained multiple congenital anomalies. *Am J Med Genet* 113:367–370, 2002.

Kumar A, Cassidy SB, Romero L, Schwartz S. Molecular cytogenetics of a de novo interstitial deletion of chromosome arm 6q in a developmentally normal girl. *Am J Med Genet* 86:227–231, 1999.

Kumar RD, Saba LF, Streff H, et al. Clinical genome sequencing: Three years' experience at a tertiary children's hospital. *Genet Med* 25:100916, 2023.

Kumra S, Wiggs E, Krasnewich D, et al. Brief report: Association of sex chromosome anomalies with childhood-onset psychotic disorders. *J Am Acad Child Adolesc Psychiatry* 37:292–296, 1998.

Kung A, Munné S, Bankowski B, Coates A, Wells D. Validation of next-generation sequencing for comprehensive chromosome screening of embryos. *Reprod Biomed Online* 31:760–769, 2015.

Kunz J, Schoner K, Stein W, Rehder H, Fritz B. Tetrasomy 12p (Pallister-Killian syndrome): Difficulties in prenatal diagnosis. *Arch Gynecol Obstet* 280:1049–1053, 2009.

Kuo PL. Maternal trisomy 21 mosaicism and recurrent spontaneous abortion. *Fertil Steril* 78:432–433, 2002.

Kupchik GS, Barrett SK, Babu A, Charria-Ortiz G, Velinov M, Macera MJ. Atypical 18p- syndrome associated with partial trisomy 16p in a chromosomally unbalanced child of consanguineous parents with an identical balanced translocation. *Eur J Med Genet* 48:57–65, 2005.

Kuppermann M, Learman LA, Gates E, et al. Beyond race or ethnicity and socioeconomic status: Predictors of prenatal testing for Down syndrome. *Obstet Gynecol* 107:1087–1097, 2006.

Kurahashi H, Emanuel BS. Unexpectedly high rate of de novo constitutional t(11;22) translocations in sperm from normal males. *Nat Genet* 29:139–140, 2001.

Kurahashi H, Sakamoto M, Ono J, Honda A, Okada S, Nakamura Y. Molecular cloning of the chromosomal breakpoint in the LIS1 gene of a patient with isolated lissencephaly and balanced t(8;17). *Hum Genet* 103:189–192, 1998.

Kurnit DM, Aldridge JF, Matsuoka R, Matthysse S. Increased adhesiveness of trisomy 21 cells and atrioventricular canal malformations in Down syndrome: A stochastic model. *Am J Med Genet* 20:385–399, 1985.

Kuroda K. A review of the optimization of thyroid function, thrombophilia, immunity and uterine milieu treatment strategy for recurrent implantation failure and recurrent pregnancy loss. *Reprod Med Biol* 23:e12561, 2024.

Kuroda S, Usui K, Sanjo H, et al. Genetic disorders and male infertility. *Reprod Med Biol* 19:314–322, 2020.

Kuroda Y, Ohashi I, Saito T, et al. Deletion of UBE3A in brothers with Angelman syndrome at the breakpoint with an inversion at 15q11.2. *Am J Med Genet* 164A:2873–2878, 2014.

Kuroda Y, Saito T, Nagai J, et al. Microdeletion of 19p13.3 in a girl with Peutz-Jeghers syndrome, intellectual disability, hypotonia, and distinctive features. *Am J Med Genet* 167A:389–393, 2015.

Kurtas NE, Xumerle L, Leonardelli L, et al. Small supernumerary marker chromosomes: A legacy of trisomy rescue? *Hum Mutat* 40:193–200, 2019.

Kurtulgan HK, Özer L, Yildirim ME, et al. Recombinant chromosome with partial 14 q trisomy due to maternal pericentric inversion. *Mol Cytogenet* 8:92, 2015.

Kushwaha S, Stinnett V, Zou YS, Murry JB. (2024). Live-born autosomal ring chromosomes at the Johns Hopkins Hospital cytogenomics laboratory: Case series—Spanning 52 years of experience in a single center. *Am J Med Genet* 194A:253–267, 2024.

Kutteh WH, Papas RS, Maisenbacher MK, Dahdouh EM. Role of genetic analysis of products of conception and PGT in managing early pregnancy loss. *Reprod Biomed Online* 49:103738, 2024.

Kuznetsova IL, Uralsky LI, Tyazhelova TV, Andreeva TV, Rogaev EI. Mosaic loss of the Y chromosome in human neurodegenerative and oncological diseases. *Vavilovskii Zhurnal Genet Selektsii* 27:502–511, 2023.

Kvarnung M, Lindstrand A, Malmgren H, et al. Inherited mosaicism for the supernumerary marker chromosome in cat eye syndrome: Inter- and intra-individual variation and correlation to the phenotype. *Am J Med Genet* 158A:1111–1117, 2012.

L

La Cour Sibbesen E, Jespersgaard C, Alosi D, Bisgaard AM, Tümer Z. Ring chromosome 9 in a girl with developmental delay and dysmorphic features: Case report and review of the literature. *Am J Med Genet* 161A:1447–1452, 2013.

La Marca A, Capuzzo M, Longo M, et al. The number and rate of euploid blastocysts in women undergoing IVF/ICSI cycles are strongly dependent on ovarian reserve and female age. *Hum Reprod* 37:2392–2401, 2022.

Labade AS, Chiang ZD, Comenho C, et al. Expansion *in situ* genome sequencing links nuclear abnormalities to hotspots of aberrant euchromatin repression. BioRχiv, *in press, 2025.* doi:10.1101/2024.09.24.614614.

Labonne JDJ, Shen Y, Kong IK, Diamond MP, Layman LC, Kim HG. Comparative deletion mapping at 1p31.3-p32.2 implies NFIA responsible for intellectual disability coupled with macrocephaly and the presence of several other genes for syndromic intellectual disability. *Mol Cytogenet* 9:24, 2016.

Labonne JDJ, Vogt J, Reali L, Kong IK, Layman LC, Kim HG. A microdeletion encompassing PHF21A in an individual with global developmental delay and craniofacial anomalies. *Am J Med Genet* 167A:3011–3018, 2015.

Lacaria M, Srour M, Michaud JL, et al. Expansion of the clinical phenotype of the distal 10q26.3 deletion syndrome to include ataxia and hyperemia of the hands and feet. *Am J Med Genet* 173:1611–1619, 2017.

Lacassie Y, Arriaza MI, Vargas A, La Motta I. Ring 2 chromosome: Ten-year follow-up report. *Am J Med Genet* 85:117–122, 1999.

Lacbawan FL, White BJ, Anguiano A, et al. Rare interstitial deletion (2)(p11.2p13) in a child with pericentric inversion (2)(p11.2q13) of paternal origin. *Am J Med Genet* 87:139–142, 1999.

Lachlan KL, Youings S, Costa T, Jacobs PA, Thomas NS. A clinical and molecular study of 26 females with Xp deletions with special emphasis on inherited deletions. *Hum Genet* 118:640–651, 2006.

Lagier-Tourenne C, Ginglinger E, Alembik Y, et al. Two cousins with partial trisomy 12q and monosomy 12p recombinants of a familial pericentric inversion of the chromosome 12. *Am J Med Genet* 125A:77–85, 2004.

Lagirand-Cantaloube J, Ciabrini C, Charrasse S, et al. Loss of centromere cohesion in aneuploid human oocytes correlates with decreased kinetochore localization of the Sac proteins Bub1 and Bubr1. *Sci Rep* 7:44001, 2017.

Lakovschek IC, Streubel B, Ulm B. Natural outcome of trisomy 13, trisomy 18, and triploidy after prenatal diagnosis. *Am J Med Genet* 155A:2626–33, 2011.

Lambertini M, Peccatori FA, Demeestere I, et al. Fertility preservation and post-treatment pregnancies in post-pubertal cancer patients: ESMO Clinical Practice Guidelines. *Ann Oncol* 31:1664–1678, 2020.

Lammert DB, Miedema D, Ochotorena J, et al. Central and peripheral dysmyelination in a 3-year-old girl with ring chromosome 18. *Clin Case Rep* 7:2087–2091, 2019.

Lamotte A, Martinez G, Devillard F, et al. Is sperm FISH analysis still useful for Robertsonian translocations? Meiotic analysis for 23 patients and review of the literature. *Basic Clin Androl* 28:5, 2018.

Lanasa MC, Hogge WA. X chromosome defects as an etiology of recurrent spontaneous abortion. *Semin Reprod Med* 18:97–103, 2000.

Langlois S, Yong PJ, Yong SL, et al. Postnatal follow-up of prenatally diagnosed trisomy 16 mosaicism. *Prenat Diagn* 26:548–558, 2006.

Lannoo L, Van Den Bogaert K, Brison N, et al. Rare autosomal trisomies and adverse perinatal outcomes. N Engl J Med 391:184–185, 2024.

Lannoo L, van Straaten K, Breckpot J, et al. Rare autosomal trisomies detected by non-invasive prenatal testing: An overview of current knowledge. *Eur J Hum Genet* 30:1323–1330, 2022.

Larsen IG, Moses RG, Seifert BA, et al. Deep screening for X chromosome parent-of-origin effects on neurobehavioral and neuroanatomical phenotypes in 47,XXY Klinefelter syndrome. *Biol Psychiatry Glob Open Sci* 4:100391, 2024.

LaSalle JM. Epigenomic signatures reveal mechanistic clues and predictive markers for autism spectrum disorder. *Mol Psychiatry* 28:1890–1901, 2023.

Lathi RB, Liebert CA, Brookfield KF, et al. Conjugated bisphenol A in maternal serum in relation to miscarriage risk. *Fertil Steril* 102:123–128, 2014.

Lau NM, Huang JY, MacDonald S, et al. Feasibility of fertility preservation in young females with Turner syndrome. *Reprod Biomed Online* 18:290–295, 2009.

Lau TK, Fung HYM, Rogers MS, Cheung KL. Racial variation in incidence of trisomy 21: Survey of 57,742 Chinese deliveries. *Am J Med Genet* 75:386–388, 1998.

Laufer-Cahana A, Krantz ID, Bason LD, Lu FM, Piccoli DA, Spinner NB. Alagille syndrome inherited from a phenotypically normal mother with a mosaic 20p microdeletion. *Am J Med Genet* 112:190–193, 2002.

Laursen RJ, Tüttelmann F, Humaidan P, Elbæk HO, Alsbjerg B, Röpke A. Azoospermia and ring chromosome 9—A case report. *J Assist Reprod Genet* 32:293–296, 2015.

Laver TW, Wakeling MN, Caswell RC, et al. Chromosome 20p11.2 deletions cause congenital hyperinsulinism via the loss of FOXA2 or its regulatory elements. *Eur J Hum Genet* 32:813–818, 2024.

Lavery SA, Aurell R, Turner C, et al. Preimplantation genetic diagnosis: Patients' experiences and attitudes. *Hum Reprod* 17:2464–2467, 2002.

Lawson KL, Carlson K, Shynkaruk JM. The portrayal of Down syndrome in prenatal screening information pamphlets. *J Obstet Gynaecol Can* 34:760–768, 2012.

Layman LC, Tho SPT, Clark AD, Kulharya A, McDonough PG. Phenotypic spectrum of 45,X/46,XY males with a ring Y chromosome and bilaterally descended testes. *Fertil Steril* 91:791–797, 2009.

Lazzaro SJ, Speevak MD, Farrell SA. Recombinant Down syndrome: A case report and literature review. *Clin Genet* 59:128–130, 2001.

Le H, Jin E, Jewell A, Jackson-Cook C, Haskell GT, Couser N. Chromosome 6p25 deletion syndrome: A case report and review of ophthalmic features. *Am J Med Genet* 191A:1639–1645, 2023.

Le Caignec C, Boceno M, Jacquemont S, Nguyen The Tich S, Rival JM, David A. Inherited ring chromosome 8 without loss of subtelomeric sequences. *Ann Genet* 47:289–296, 2004.

Le Caignec C, Boceno M, Saugier-Veber P, et al. Detection of genomic imbalances by array based comparative genomic hybridisation in fetuses with multiple malformations. *J Med Genet* 42:121–128, 2005.

Le Fevre A, Beygo J, Silveira C, et al. Atypical Angelman syndrome due to a mosaic imprinting defect: Case reports and review of the literature. *Am J Med Genet* 173A:753–757, 2017.

Le Gall J, Nizon M, Pichon O, et al. Sex chromosome aneuploidies and copy-number variants: A further explanation for neurodevelopmental prognosis variability? *Eur J Hum Genet* 25:930–934, 2017.

Leach NT, Cole SM, Sandstrom DJ, Weremowicz S. A novel pericentric inversion of chromosome 14 involving the rRNA gene cluster. *Prenat Diagn* 25:620–621, 2005.

Leach NT, Cole SM, Sandstrom DJ, Weremowicz S. A novel pericentric inversion of chromosome 14 involving the rRNA gene cluster. *Prenat Diagn* 25:620–621, 2005.

Leahy D, Marin D, Xu J, Eccles J, Treff NR. High-resolution PGT-A results in incidental identification of patients with small pathogenic copy number variants. *J Assist Reprod Genet* 41:121–126, 2024.

Lebedev IN, Karamysheva TV, Elisaphenko EA, et al. Prenatal diagnosis of small supernumerary marker chromosome 10 by array-based comparative genomic hybridization and microdissected chromosome sequencing. *Biomedicines* 9:1030, 2021.

Lebo RV, Milunsky J, Higgins AW, Loose B, Huang XL, Wyandt HE. Symmetric replication of an unstable isodicentric Xq chromosome derived from isolocal maternal sister chromatid recombination. *Am J Med Genet* 85:429–437, 1999.

Lebre AS, Morinière V, Dunand O, Bensman A, Morichon-Delvallez N, Antignac C. Maternal uniparental heterodisomy of chromosome 17 in a patient with nephropathic cystinosis. *Eur J Hum Genet* 17:1019–1023, 2009.

Leclercq S, Baron X, Jacquemont ML, Cuillier F, Cartault F. Mosaic trisomy 22—Five new cases with variable outcomes: Implications for genetic counselling and clinical management. *Prenat Diagn* 30:168–172, 2010.

Lecoquierre F, Cassinari K, Chambon P, et al. Patients with 10q22.3q23.1 recurrent deletion syndrome are at risk for juvenile polyposis. *Eur J Med Genet* 63:103773, 2020.

Ledbetter DH, Zachary JM, Simpson JL, et al. Cytogenetic results from the U.S. Collaborative Study on CVS. *Prenat Diagn* 12:317–345, 1992.

Ledig S, Hiort O, Scherer G, et al. Array-CGH analysis in patients with syndromic and non-syndromic XY gonadal dysgenesis: Evaluation of array CGH as diagnostic tool and search for new candidate loci. *Hum Reprod* 25:2637–2646, 2010.

Ledig S, Hiort O, Wünsch L, Wieacker P. Partial deletion of DMRT1 causes 46,XY ovotesticular disorder of sexual development. *Eur J Endocrinol* 167:119–124, 2012.

Lee et al. *2025 TBA*

Lee AJ, Nam DE, Choi YJ, et al. Paternal gender specificity and mild phenotypes in Charcot-Marie-Tooth type 1A patients with de novo 17p12 rearrangements. *Mol Genet Genomic Med* 8:e1380, 2020.

Lee BH, Kasparis C, Chen B, et al. Setleis syndrome due to inheritance of the 1p36.22p36.21 duplication: Evidence for lack of penetrance. *J Hum Genet* 60:717–722, 2015.

Lee CG, Cho E, Ahn YM. Maternally inherited autosomal dominant intellectual disability caused by 16p13.3 microduplication. *Eur J Med Genet* 59:210–214, 2016.

Lee CL, Lin SM, Chen MR, et al. 22q11.2 deletion syndrome in Taiwan: Clinical presentation and immune system status of patients. *Int J Med Sci* 20:1377–1385, 2023.

Lee J, Stanley JR, Vaz SA, et al. Down syndrome with pure partial trisomy 21q22 due to a paternal insertion (4;21) uncovered by uncultured amniotic fluid interphase FISH. *Am J Med Genet* 132A:206–208, 2005.

Leegte B, Sikkema-Raddatz B, Hordijk R, et al. Three cases of mosaicism for balanced reciprocal translocations. *Am J Med Genet* 79:362–365, 1998.

Leffler M, Christie L, Hackett A, et al. Further delineation of dosage-sensitive K/L mediated Xq28 duplication syndrome includes incomplete penetrance. *Clin Genet* 103:681–687, 2023.

Lefkowitz RB, Tynan JA, Liu T, et al. Clinical validation of a noninvasive prenatal test for genomewide detection of fetal copy number variants. *Am J Obstet Gynecol* 215:227.e1–16, 2016.

Lefort G, Blanchet P, Belgrade N, et al. Stable dicentric duplication-deficiency chromosome 14 resulting from crossing-over within a maternal paracentric inversion. *Am J Med Genet* 113:333–338, 2002.

Lefort G, Blanchet P, Chaze AM, et al. Cytogenetic and molecular study of a jumping translocation in a baby with Dandy-Walker malformation. *J Med Genet* 38:67–73, 2001.

Légaré F, St-Jacques S, Gagnon S, et al. Prenatal screening for Down syndrome: A survey of willingness in women and family physicians to engage in shared decision-making. *Prenat Diagn* 31 319–326, 2011.

Leggett V, Jacobs P, Nation K, Scerif G, Bishop DV. Neurocognitive outcomes of individuals with a sex chromosome trisomy: XXX, XYY, or XXY: A systematic review. *Dev Med Child Neurol* 52:119–129, 2010.

Lehmann KJ, Kovac JR, Xu J, Fischer MA. Isodicentric Yq mosaicism presenting as infertility and maturation arrest without altered SRY and AZF regions. *J Assist Reprod Genet* 29:939–942, 2012.

Lei M, Mitsuhashi S, Miyake N, et al. Translocation breakpoint disrupting the host SNHG14 gene but not coding genes or snoRNAs in typical Prader-Willi syndrome. *J Hum Genet* 64:647–652, 2019.

Leichtman DA, Schmickel RD, Gelehrter TD, Judd WJ, Woodbury MC, Meilinger KL. Familial Turner syndrome. *Ann Intern Med* 89:473–476, 1978.

Leisti JT, Kaback MM, Rimoin DL. Human X-autosome translocations: Differential inactivation of the X chromosome in a kindred with an X-9 translocation. *Am J Hum Genet* 27:441–453, 1975.

Lejeune H, Brosse A, Groupe Fertipreserve, Plotton I. Fertilité dans le syndrome de Klinefelter. *Presse Méd* 43:162–170, 2014.

Lejeune J. Types et contretypes. *J Génét Hum* 15 (Suppl):20–32, 1966.

Lejeune J. The William Allan Memorial Award Lecture: On the nature of men. *Am J Hum Genet* 22:121–128, 1970.

Lejeune J, Gautier M, Turpin R. Étude des chromosomes somatiques de neuf enfants mongoliens. *Comp Rend Hebd Séances Acad Sci* 248:1721–1722, 1959.

Lejeune J, Lafourcade J, Berger R, et al. Trois cas de délétion partielle du bras court d'un chromosome 5. *Comp Rend Hebd Séances Acad Sci* 257:3098–3102, 1963.

Lek M, Karczewski KJ, Minikel EV, et al. Analysis of protein-coding genetic variation in 60,706 humans. *Nature* 536:285–291, 2016.

Leka-Emiri S, Petrou V, Manolakos E, et al. 17p13.1 microduplication syndrome in a child, familial short stature, and growth hormone deficiency: A case report and review of the literature. *Mol Syndromol* 9:300–305, 2019.

Lekszas C, Nanda I, Vona B, et al. Unbalanced segregation of a paternal t(9;11)(p24.3;p15.4) translocation causing familial Beckwith-Wiedemann syndrome: A case report. *BMC Med Genomics* 12:83, 2019.

Lemire G, Sanchis-Juan A, Russell K, et al. Exome copy number variant detection, analysis, and classification in a large cohort of families with undiagnosed rare genetic disease. *Am J Hum Genet* 111:863–876, 2024.

Lemyre E, der Kaloustian VM, Duncan AMV. Stable non-Robertsonian dicentric chromosomes: Four new cases and a review. *J Med Genet* 38:76–79, 2001.

Leng M, Li G, Zhong L, Hou H, Yu D, Shi Q. Abnormal synapses and recombination in an azoospermic male carrier of a reciprocal translocation t(1;21). *Fertil Steril* 91:1293.e17–22, 2009.

Leonard NJ, Tomkins DJ. Diploid/tetraploid/t(1;6) mosaicism in a 17-year-old female with hypomelanosis of Ito, multiple congenital anomalies, and body asymmetry. *Am J Med Genet* 112:86–90, 2002.

Leonard S, Bower C, Petterson B, Leonard H. Survival of infants born with Down's syndrome: 1980–96. *Paediatr Perinat Epidemiol* 14:163–171, 2000.

Lespinasse J, Gicquel C, Robert M, Le Bouc Y. Phenotypic and genotypic variability in monozygotic triplets with Turner syndrome. *Clin Genet* 54:56–59, 1998.

Lespinasse J, Hoffmann P, Lauge A, et al. Chromosomal instability in two siblings with gonad deficiency: Case report. *Hum Reprod* 20:158–162, 2005.

Lessel D, Vaz B, Halder S, et al. Mutations in *SPRTN* cause early onset hepatocellular carcinoma, genomic instability and progeroid features. *Nat Genet* 46:1239–1244, 2014.

Lestou VS, Desilets V, Lomax BL, et al. Comparative genomic hybridization: A new approach to screening for intrauterine complete or mosaic aneuploidy. *Am J Med Genet* 92:281–284, 2000.

Levitas AS, Reid CS. An angel with Down syndrome in a sixteenth century Flemish Nativity painting. *Am J Med Genet* 116A:399–405, 2003.

Levy AT, Berghella V, Al-Kouatly HB. Outcome of 45,X fetuses with cystic hygroma: A systematic review. *Am J Med Genet* 185A:26–32, 2021.

Levy B, Dunn TM, Hirschhorn K, Kardon N. Jumping translocations in spontaneous abortions. *Cytogenet Cell Genet* 88:25–29, 2000.

Levy B, Sigurjonsson S, Pettersen B, et al. Genomic imbalance in products of conception: Single-nucleotide polymorphism chromosomal microarray analysis. *Obstet Gynecol* 124:202–209, 2014.

Levy M, Shohat M, Kahana S, et al. Proximal 1q21 duplication: A syndrome or a susceptibility locus? *Am J Med Genet* 191A:2551–2557, 2023.

Levy T, Holder JL Jr, Horrigan JP, et al. An open-label study evaluating the safety and efficacy of AMO-01 for the treatment of seizures in Phelan-McDermid syndrome. *HGG Adv*, 6:100393, 2025.

Levy-Mozziconacci A, Piquet C, Scheiner C, et al. i(18q) in amniotic and fetal cells with a normal karyotype in direct chorionic villus sampling: Cytogenetics and pathology. *Prenat Diagn* 16:1156–1159, 1996.

Lewi L, Blickstein I, Van Schoubroeck D, et al. Diagnosis and management of heterokaryotypic monochorionic twins. *Am J Med Genet* 140:272–275, 2006.

Lewin B. *Genes V*. New York, NY: Oxford University Press, 1994.

Lewis AH, Chugh A, Sobotka SA. Behavioral outbursts in a child with a deletion syndrome, generalized epilepsy, global developmental delay, and failure to thrive. *Pediatr Ann* 47:e130–e134, 2018.

Lewis SA, Shetty S, Wilson BA, et al. Insights from genetic studies of cerebral palsy. *Front Neurol* 11:625428, 2021.

Lewit-Mendes MF, Robson H, Kelley J, et al. Experiences of receiving an increased chance of sex chromosome aneuploidy result from non-invasive prenatal testing in Australia: "A more complicated scenario than what I had ever realized". *J Genet Couns* 32:213–223, 2023.

Li C. A prenatally recognizable malformation syndrome associated with a recurrent post-zygotic chromosome rearrangement der(Y)t(Y;1)(q12:q21). *Am J Med Genet* 152A:2339–2341, 2010.

Li G, Iqbal F, Wang L, et al. Meiotic defects and decreased expression of genes located around the chromosomal breakpoint in the testis of a patient with a novel 46,X,t(Y;1)(p11.3;p31) translocation. *Int J Mol Med* 40:367–377, 2017.

Li G, Shi W, Niu W, et al. The influence of balanced complex chromosomal rearrangements on preimplantation embryonic development potential and molecular karyotype. *BMC Genomics* 21:326, 2020.

Li H, Lu L, Yao Y, et al. Perinatal outcomes of prenatal cases testing positive for trisomy 9 by noninvasive prenatal testing. *Taiwan J Obstet Gynecol* 61:965–970, 2022a.

Li JW, Qian YJ, Mao SJ, et al. Clinical features associated with maternal uniparental disomy for chromosome 6. *Mol Cytogenet* 17:18, 2024a.

Li L, Zhang N, Wu X, et al. Exposure to air pollution is associated with congenital anomalies in the population born by in vitro fertilization. *Environ Res* 207:112161, 2022b.

Li LL, Dong Y, Wang RX, An N, Yun X, Liu RZ. Sperm aneuploidy and implications for genetic counseling in a pedigree of three t(1;3) balanced translocation carriers. *Genet Mol Res* 14:5003–5009, 2015.

Li M, Glass J, Du X, et al. Trisomy 9 mosaic syndrome: Sixteen additional patients with new and/or less commonly reported features, literature review, and suggested clinical guidelines. *Am J Med Genet* 185A:2374–2383, 2021a.

Li M, Squire JA, Weksberg R. Molecular genetics of Wiedemann-Beckwith syndrome. *Am J Med Genet* 79:253–259, 1998.

Li N, Tang EI, Cheng CY. Regulation of blood-testis barrier by actin binding proteins and protein kinases. *Reproduction* 151:R29–41, 2016.

Li P, Dupont B, Hu Q, et al. The past, present, and future for constitutional ring chromosomes: A report of the international consortium for human ring chromosomes. *HGG Adv* 3:100139, 2022c.

Li S, Chen M, Zheng PS. Analysis of parental abnormal chromosomal karyotype and subsequent live births in Chinese couples with recurrent pregnancy loss. *Sci Rep* 11:20298, 2021b.

Li S, Hassed S, Mulvihill JJ, Nair AK, Hopcus DJ. Double trisomy. *Am J Med Genet* 124A:96–98, 2004.

Li S, Li H, Gao Y, et al. Identification of cryptic balanced translocations in couples with unexplained recurrent pregnancy loss based upon embryonic PGT-A results. *J Assist Reprod Genet* 41:171–184, 2024b.

Li Y, Zhou R, Xia Z, et al. Reproductive outcomes in couples with recurrent pregnancy loss after embryonic chromosomal microarray analysis. *J Assist Reprod Genet* 41:161–170, 2024c.

Li Z, Liu J, Li H, et al. Phenotypic expansion of the interstitial 16p13.3 duplication: A case report and review of the literature. *Gene* 531:502–505, 2013.

Liang B, Yu D, Zhao W, et al. Clinical findings and genetic analysis of patients with copy number variants involving 17p13.3 using a single nucleotide polymorphism array: A single-center experience. *BMC Med Genomics* 15:268, 2022a

Liang CA, Braddock BA, Heithaus JL, Christensen KM, Braddock SR, Carey JC. Reported communication ability of persons with trisomy 18 and trisomy 13. *Dev Neurorehabil* 18:322–329, 2015.

Liang M, Suresh B, Bareke E, et al. A homozygous stop codon in HORMAD2 in a patient with recurrent digynic triploid miscarriage. *Mol Genet Genomic Med* 12:e2402, 2024.

Liang Y, Xie Y, Kong S, et al. Complex chromosomal rearrangement causes male azoospermia: A case report and literature review. *Front Genet* 13:792539, 2022b.

Liang Z, Wen Q, Li J, Zeng D, Huang P. A systematic review and meta-analysis: Clinical outcomes of recurrent pregnancy failure resulting from preimplantation genetic testing for aneuploidy. *Front Endocrinol (Lausanne)* 14:1178294, 2023.

Liao C, Li DZ. Should sex chromosomes be excluded from use in QF-PCR in prenatal samples with a molecular referral? *Am J Med Genet* 164A:2404–2406, 2014.

Liao YP, Wang CJ, Liang M, Hu XM, Wu Q. Analysis of genetic characteristics and reproductive risks of balanced complex chromosome rearrangement carriers in China. *Yi Chuan* 39:396–412, 2017.

Libman V, Macarov M, Friedlander Y, et al. Women's attitudes towards disclosure of genetic information in pregnancy with varying levels of penetrance. *Prenat Diagn* 44:270–279, 2024.

Lichtenbelt KD, Hochstenbach R, van Dam WM, Eleveld MJ, Poot M, Beemer FA. Supernumerary ring chromosome 7 mosaicism: Case report, investigation of the gene content, and delineation of the phenotype. *Am J Med Genet* 132A:93–100, 2005.

Liehr T. Cases with uniparental disomy. https://cs-tl.de/DB/CA/UPD/0-Start.html, 2025a.

Liehr T. Small supernumerary marker chromosomes. https://cs-tl.de/DB/CA/sSMC/0-Start.html, 2025b.

Liehr T. Uniparental disomy is a chromosomic disorder in the first place. *Mol Cytogenet* 15:5, 2022.

Liehr T, Starke H, Weise A, Lehrer H, Claussen U. Multicolor FISH probe sets and their applications. *Histol Histopathol* 19:229–237, 2004.

Liehr T, Stumm M, Wegner RD, et al. 10p11.2 to 10q11.2 is a yet unreported region leading to unbalanced chromosomal abnormalities without phenotypic consequences. *Cytogenet Genome Res* 124:102–105, 2009.

Liehr T, Utine GE, Trautmann U, et al. Neocentric small supernumerary marker chromosomes (sSMC)—Three more cases and review of the literature. *Cytogenet Genome Res* 118:31–37, 2007.

Liehr T, Weise A, Mrasek K, et al. Recombinant chromosomes resulting from parental pericentric inversions—Two new cases and a review of the literature. *Front Genet* 10:1165, 2019.

Liehr T, Williams HE, Ziegler M, Kankel S, Padutsch N, Al-Rikabi A. Small supernumerary marker chromosomes derived from chromosome 14 and/or 22. *Mol Cytogenet* 14:13, 2021.

Lim AST, Lim TH, Kee SK, Chieng R, Tay SK. Sperm segregation patterns by fluorescence in situ hybridization studies of a 46,XY,t(2;6) heterozygote giving rise to a rare triploid product of conception with a 69,XXY,t(2;6)(p12;q24)der(6)t(2;6)(p12;q24)pat karyotype. *Am J Med Genet* 117A:172–176, 2003.

Lim AST, Su LC. Mosaic trisomy 18 male with normal intelligence who fathered a normal baby girl. *Am J Med Genet* 76:365–366, 1998.

Lim BC, Min BJ, Park WY, et al. A unique phenotype of 2q24.3–2q32.1 duplication: Early infantile epileptic encephalopathy without mesomelic dysplasia. *J Child Neurol* 29:260–264, 2014.

Lim CK, Cho JW, Song IO, Kang IS, Yoon YD, Jun JH. Estimation of chromosomal imbalances in preimplantation embryos from preimplantation genetic diagnosis cycles of reciprocal translocations with or without acrocentric chromosomes. *Fertil Steril* 90:2144–2151, 2008.

Lim ECP, Ng ISL, Yong MH, Yon HY, Brett MSY, Tan EC. De novo trisomy 12p in twin girls with different levels of mosaicism. *Am J Med Genet* 161A:1702–1705, 2013.

Lim HH, Kil HR, Koo SH. Incidence, puberty, and fertility in 45,X/47,XXX mosaicism: Report of a patient and a literature review. *Am J Med Genet* 173A:1961–1964, 2017a.

Lim Z, Downs J, Wong K, Ellaway C, Leonard H. Expanding the clinical picture of the *MECP2* duplication syndrome. *Clin Genet* 91:557–563, 2017b.

Lin A, Clasen L, Lee NR, et al. Mapping the stability of human brain asymmetry across five sex-chromosome aneuploidies. *J Neurosci* 35:140–145, 2015.

Lin A, Vajdi A, Kushan-Wells L, et al. Reciprocal copy number variations at 22q11.2 produce distinct and convergent neurobehavioral impairments relevant for schizophrenia and autism spectrum disorder. *Biol Psychiatry* 88:260–272, 2020.

Lin CC, Hsieh YY, Wang CH, et al. Prenatal detection and characterization of a small supernumerary marker chromosome (sSMC) derived from chromosome 22 with apparently normal phenotype. *Prenat Diagn* 26:898–902, 2006.

Lin HY, Lee CL, Fran S, et al. Epigenotype, genotype, and phenotype analysis of Taiwanese patients with Silver-Russell syndrome. *J Pers Med* 11:1197, 2021a.

Lin I, Afshar Y, Goldstein J, et al. Central 22q11.2 deletion (LCR22 B-D) in a fetus with severe fetal growth restriction and a mother with severe systemic lupus erythematosus: Further evidence of CRKL haploinsufficiency in the pathogenesis of 22q11.2 deletion syndrome. *Am J Med Genet* 185A:3042–3047, 2021b.

Lin Q, Liang C, Du B, et al. Prenatal detection and molecular cytogenetic characterization of Xp deletion and Xq duplication: A case report and literature review. *BMC Med Genomics* 17:57, 2024.

Lin SP, Huang SY, Tu ME, et al. Netherton syndrome: Mutation analysis of two Taiwanese families. *Arch Dermatol Res* 299:145–150, 2007.

Lin Y, Wei Z, Zhang L, et al. Homozygous missense variations of APC12 cause meiotic metaphase I arrest in oocytes and female infertility. *Am J Obstet Gynecol* 232:547.e1–547.e17, 2025.

Liñán A, Lawrenz B, El Khatib I, et al. Clinical reassessment of human embryo ploidy status between cleavage and blastocyst stage by next generation sequencing. *PLoS One* 13:e0201652, 2018.

Linden MG, Bender BG. Fifty-one prenatally diagnosed children and adolescents with sex chromosome abnormalities. *Am J Med Genet* 110:11–18, 2002.

Linden MG, Bender BG, Robinson A. Sex chromosome tetrasomy and pentasomy. *Pediatrics* 96:672–682, 1995.

Linden MG, Bender BG, Robinson A. Genetic counseling for sex chromosome abnormalities. *Am J Med Genet* 110:3–10, 2002.

Lindenbaum RH, Clarke G, Patel C, Moncrieff M, Hughes JT. Muscular dystrophy in an X;1 translocation female suggests that Duchenne locus is on X chromosome short arm. *J Med Genet* 16:389–392, 1979.

Lindenbaum RH, Hultén M, McDermott A, Seabright M. The prevalence of translocations in parents of children with regular trisomy 21: A possible interchromosomal effect? *J Med Genet* 22:24–28, 1985.

Liou JD, Chen CP, Breg WR, Hobbins JC, Mahoney MJ, Yang-Feng TL. Fetal blood sampling and cytogenetic abnormalities. *Prenat Diagn* 13:1–8, 1993.

Liou JD, Ma YY, Gibson LH, et al. Cytogenetic and molecular studies of a familial paracentric inversion of Y chromosome present in a patient with ambiguous genitalia. *Am J Med Genet* 70:134–137, 1997.

Lippe B. Turner syndrome. *Endocrinol Metab Clin North Am* 20:121–152, 1991.

Little J. The Chernobyl accident, congenital anomalies and other reproductive outcomes. *Paediatr Perinat Epidemiol* 7:121–151, 1993.

Little MP, Wakeford R, Hatch M, Ainsbury EA, Tawn EJ. Chromosome aberrations in a group of people exposed to radioactive releases from the Three Mile Island nuclear accident and inferences for radiation effects. *Radiat Res* 195:584–589, 2021.

Liu A, Genovese G, Zhao Y, et al. Genetic drivers and cellular selection of female mosaic X chromosome loss. *Nature* 631:134–141, 2024a.

Liu D, Chen C, Huang Q, et al. Preimplantation genetic testing for complex chromosomal rearrangements: Clinical outcomes and potential risk factors. *Front Genet* 15:1401549, 2024b.

Liu D, Chen C, Zhang X, et al. Successful birth after preimplantation genetic testing for a couple with two different reciprocal translocations and review of the literature. *Reprod Biol Endocrinol* 19:58. 2021.

Liu L, Li XB, Zi XH, et al. A novel hemizygous SACS mutation identified by whole exome sequencing and SNP array analysis in a Chinese ARSACS patient. *J Neurol Sci* 362:111–114, 2016.

Liu P, Yuan B, Carvalho CMB, et al. An organismal CNV mutator phenotype restricted to early human development. *Cell* 168:830–842.e7, 2017.

Liu Q, Zhou WJ, Huang ZH, et al. Exploring the impact of pericentric inversion of chromosome 9 on fertility in sperm donors. *Asian J Androl* 26:302–307, 2024c.

Liu S, Wang Z, Wei S, et al. Gray matter heterotopia, mental retardation, developmental delay, microcephaly, and facial dysmorphisms in a boy with ring chromosome 6: A 10-year follow-up and literature review. *Cytogenet Genome Res* 154:201–208, 2018.

Liu S, Zheng J, Liu X, et al. Comprehensive analysis of three female patients with different types of X/Y translocations and literature review. *Mol Cytogenet* 16:7, 2023.

Liu W, Zhang H, Wang J, et al. Prenatal diagnosis of complete maternal uniparental isodisomy of chromosome 4 in a fetus without congenital abnormality or inherited disease-associated variations. *Mol Cytogenet* 8:85, 2015.

Liu XY, Fan Q, Wang J, et al. Higher chromosomal abnormality rate in blastocysts from young patients with idiopathic recurrent pregnancy loss. *Fertil Steril* 113:853–864, 2020.

Liu Y, Lan X, Lu J, et al. Preimplantation genetic testing for aneuploidy could not improve cumulative live birth rate among 705 couples with unexplained recurrent implantation failure. *Appl Clin Genet* 17:1–13, 2024d.

Ljubicic ML, Jørgensen A, Aksglaede L, et al. Serum concentrations and gonadal expression of INSL3 in eighteen males with 45,X/46,XY mosaicism. *Front Endocrinol (Lausanne)* 12:709954, 2021.

Lledó B, Ortiz JA, Morales R, et al. The paternal effect of chromosome translocation carriers observed from meiotic segregation in embryos. *Hum Reprod* 25:1843–1848, 2010.

Lloveras E, Canellas A, Cirigliano V, Català V, Cerdan C, Plaja A. Supernumerary ring chromosome: An etiology for Pallister-Killian syndrome? *Fetal Diagn Ther* 34:172–175, 2013.

Loeffler J, Soelder E, Erdel M, et al. Muellerian aplasia associated with ring chromosome 8p12q12 mosaicism. *Am J Med Genet* 116A:290–294, 2003.

Lonardo F, Di Natale P, Lualdi S, et al. Mucopolysaccharidosis type II in a female patient with a reciprocal X;9 translocation and skewed X chromosome inactivation. *Am J Med Genet* 164A:2627–2632, 2014.

Looijenga LH, Hersmus R, Oosterhuis JW, Cools M, Drop SL, Wolffenbuttel KP. Tumor risk in disorders of sex development (DSD). *Best Pract Res Clin Endocrinol Metab* 21:480–495, 2007.

Lopes F, Torres F, Soares G, van Karnebeek CD, et al. The role of *AKT3* copy number changes in brain abnormalities and neurodevelopmental disorders: Four new cases and literature review. *Front Genet* 10:58, 2019.

López-Expósito I, Bafalliu JA, Santos M, Fuster C, Puche-Mira A, Guillén-Navarro E. Intrachromosomal partial triplication of chromosome 13 secondary to a paternal duplication with mild phenotypic effect. *Am J Med Genet* 146A:1190–1194, 2008.

López-Garrido MP, Carrascosa-Romero MC, Montero-Hernández M, Serrano-Martínez CM, Sánchez-Sánchez F. Case Report: Precision genetic diagnosis in a case of Dyggve-Melchior-Clausen syndrome reveals paternal isodisomy and heterodisomy of chromosome 18 with imprinting clinical implications. *Front Genet* 13:1005573, 2022.

López-Pajares I, Delicado A, Lapunzina P, et al. Tetrasomy 8p: Discordance of amniotic fluid and blood karyotypes. *Am J Med Genet* 118A:353–357, 2003.

López Pajares I, Villa O, Salido M, et al. Euchromatic variant 16p+: Implications in prenatal diagnosis. *Prenat Diagn* 26:535–538, 2006.

Lorda-Sánchez I, Diego-Alvarez D, Ayuso C, de Alba MR, Trujillo MJ, Ramos C. Trisomy 2 due to a 3:1 segregation in an abortion studied by QF-PCR and CGH. *Prenat Diagn* 25:934–938, 2005.

Lostchuck E, Poulton A, Halliday J, Hui L. Population-based trends in invasive prenatal diagnosis for ultrasound-based indications: Two decades of change from 1994 to 2015. *Ultrasound Obstet Gynecol* 53:503–511, 2019.Lou S, Lomborg K, Lewis C, Riedijk S, Petersen OB, Vogel I. "It's probably nothing, but . . . " Couples' experiences of pregnancy following an uncertain prenatal genetic result. *Acta Obstet Gynecol Scand* 99:791–801, 2020.

Loughry L, Pynaker C, White M, Halliday J, Hui L. State-wide increase in prenatal diagnosis of klinefelter syndrome on amniocentesis and chorionic villus sampling: Impact of non-invasive prenatal testing for sex chromosome conditions. *Prenat Diagn* 43:156–161, 2023.

Loup V, Bernicot I, Janssens P, et al. Combined FISH and PRINS sperm analysis of complex chromosome rearrangement t(1;19;13): An approach facilitating PGD. *Mol Hum Reprod* 16:111–116, 2010.

Louvrier C, Egea G, Labalme A, et al. Characterization of a de novo supernumerary neocentric ring chromosome derived from chromosome 7. *Cytogenet Genome Res* 147:111–117, 2015.

Lovatel VL, Bueno AP, Kós EAA, et al. A novel constitutional t(3;8)(p26;q21) and *ANKRD26* and *SRP72* variants in a child with myelodysplastic neoplasm: Clinical implications. *J Clin Med* 12:3171, 2023.

Loviglio MN, Leleu M, Männik K, et al., 2p15 Consortium; 16p11.2 Consortium. Chromosomal contacts connect loci associated with autism, BMI and head circumference phenotypes. *Mol Psychiatry* 22:836–849, 2017.

Lowther C, Mehrjouy MM, Collins RL, et al. Balanced chromosomal rearrangements offer insights into coding and noncoding genomic features associated with developmental disorders. *MedRχiv*. in press 2022.

Lowry RB, Chernos JE, Connelly MS, Wyse JP. Interstitial deletions at 6q14.1q15 associated with developmental delay and a marfanoid phenotype. *Mol Syndromol* 4:280–284, 2013.

Lowry RB, Sibbald B, Bedard T. *Alberta Congenital Anomalies Surveillance System: Eighth Report 1980–2007*. Edmonton, Alberta, Canada: Alberta Health and Wellness, 2009.

Lowther C, Costain G, Stavropoulos DJ, et al. Delineating the 15q13.3 microdeletion phenotype: A case series and comprehensive review of the literature. *Genet Med* 17:149–157, 2015.

Lu Y, Qin M, He Q, et al. How the extra X chromosome impairs the development of male fetal germ cells. *Nature* 635:960–968, 2024.

Lubinsky MS. Kouska's fallacy: The error of the divided denominator. *Lancet* 2:1449–1450, 1986.

Lubs HA. A marker X chromosome. *Am J Hum Genet* 21:231–244, 1969.

Lucas HM, Lewis AM, Lupo PJ, Schaaf CP. Parental perceptions of genetic testing for children with autism spectrum disorders. *Am J Med Genet* 188A:178–186, 2022.

Lugli L, Malacarne M, Cavani S, Pierluigi M, Ferrari F, Percesepe A. A 12.4 Mb direct duplication in 19q12-q13 in a boy with cardiac and CNS malformations and developmental delay. *J Appl Genet* 52:335–339, 2011.

Lühmann JL, Schmidt G, Auber B, et al. Parallel deletion and duplication at 7q11.23 in a silent carrier for two reciprocal syndromic disorders. *Am J Med Genet* 191A:1849–1857, 2023.

Luijsterburg AJM, van der Zee DC, Gaillard JLJ, et al. Chorionic villus sampling and end-artery disruption of the fetus. *Prenat Diagn* 17:71–76, 1997.

Luk HM, Ivan Lo FM, Sano S, et al. Silver-Russell syndrome in a patient with somatic mosaicism for upd(11)mat identified by buccal cell analysis. *Am J Med Genet* 170A:1938–1941, 2016.

Lund ICB, Becher N, Christensen R, et al. Prevalence of mosaicism in uncultured chorionic villus samples after chromosomal microarray and clinical outcome in pregnancies affected by confined placental mosaicism. *Prenat Diagn* 40:244–259, 2020.

Lund ICB, Becher N, Graakjaer J, et al. Mosaicism for copy number variations in the placenta is even more difficult to interpret than mosaicism for whole chromosome aneuploidy. *Prenat Diagn* 41:668–680, 2021.

Lund ICB, Becher N, Lildballe D, et al. Use of cell-free non-invasive prenatal testing in pregnancies affected by placental mosaicism. *Prenat Diagn* 44:562–571, 2024.

Luo K, Lan Y, Xie P, et al. Next-generation sequencing analysis of embryos from mosaic patients undergoing in vitro fertilization and preimplantation genetic testing. *Fertil Steril* 112:291–297.e3, 2019.

Luo X, Liu W, Hu L, et al. Prenatal diagnosis, pregnancy determination and follow up of sex chromosome aneuploidy screened by non-invasive prenatal testing from 122 453 unselected singleton pregnancies: A retrospective analysis of 7-year experience. *Congenit Anom (Kyoto)* 64:99–106, 2024.

Luo Y, Xu C, Sun Y, Wang L, Chen S, Jin F. Different segregation patterns in five carriers due to a pericentric inversion of chromosome 1. *Syst Biol Reprod Med* 60:367–372, 2014.

Lupski JR. Cognitive phenotypes and genomic copy number variations. *JAMA* 313:2029–2030, 2015.

Lurie IW. A critical region for ulnar defects in patients with 4q deletions may be narrowed. *Clin Dysmorphol* 25:133, 2016.

Lustosa-Mendes E, dos Santos AP, Viguetti-Campos NL, Vieira TP, Gil-da-Silva-Lopes VL. A boy with partial dup(18q)/del(18p) due to a maternal pericentric inversion: Genotype-phenotype correlation and risk of recombinant chromosomes based on systematic review of the literature. *Am J Med Genet* 173A:143–150, 2017.

Luukkonen TM, Mehrjouy MM, Pöyhönen M, et al. Breakpoint mapping and haplotype analysis of translocation t(1;12)(q43;q21.1) in two apparently independent families with vascular phenotypes. *Mol Genet Genomic Med* 6:56–68, 2018.

Lybaek H, Ørstavik KH, Prescott T, et al. An 8.9 Mb 19p13 duplication associated with precocious puberty and a sporadic 3.9 Mb 2q23.3q24.1 deletion containing *NR4A2* in mentally retarded members of a family with an intrachromosomal 19p-into-19q between-arm insertion. *Eur J Hum Genet* 17:904–910, 2009.

M

Ma S, Yuen BH, Penaherrera M, Koehn D, Ness L, Robinson W. ICSI and the transmission of X-autosomal translocation: A three-generation evaluation of X;20 translocation: Case report. *Hum Reprod* 18:1377–1382, 2003.

Ma Y, Liu LW, Liu Y, et al. Which type of chromosomal mosaicism is compatible for embryo transfer: A systematical review and meta-analysis. *Arch Gynecol Obstet* 306:1901–1911, 2022.

Maan AA, Eales J, Akbarov A, et al. The Y chromosome: A blueprint for men's health? *Eur J Hum Genet* 25:1181–1188, 2017.

Maas NMC, Van Vooren S, Hannes F, et al. The t(4;8) is mediated by homologous recombination between olfactory receptor gene clusters, but other 4p16 translocations occur at random. *Genet Couns*18:357–365, 2007.

Maas SM, Shaw AC, Bikker H, et al. Phenotype and genotype in 103 patients with tricho-rhino-phalangeal syndrome. *Eur J Med Genet* 58:279–92, 2015.

MacDermot KD, Jack E, Cooke A, et al. Investigation of three patients with the "ring syndrome," including familial transmission of ring 5, and estimation of reproductive risks. *Hum Genet* 85:516–520, 1990.

MacDonald JR, Ziman R, Yuen RK, Feuk L, Scherer SW. The Database of Genomic Variants: A curated collection of structural variation in the human genome. *Nucleic Acids Res* 42:D986–992, 2014.

MacDonald M, Hassold T, Harvey J, Wang LH, Morton NE, Jacobs P. The origin of 47,XXY and 47,XXX aneuploidy: Heterogeneous mechanisms and role of aberrant recombination. *Hum Mol Genet* 3:1365–1371, 1994.

Machlitt A, Kuepferling P, Bommer C, Koerner H, Chaoui R. Prenatal diagnosis of trisomy 1q21-qter: Case report and review of literature. *Am J Med Genet* 134A:207–211, 2005.

Macintosh MCM. Perception of risk. In Grudzinskas JG, Chard T, Chapman M, Cuckle H (eds.), *Screening for Down's syndrome*. Cambridge, UK: Cambridge University Press, 1994.

Mackay D, Bliek J, Kagami M, et al. First step towards a consensus strategy for multi-locus diagnostic testing of imprinting disorders. *Clin Epigenetics* 14:143, 2022.

Mackie A. Using cell-free fetal DNA as a diagnostic and screening test: Current understanding and uncertainties. *BJOG* 124:47, 2017.

Mackie Ogilvie C, Scriven PN. Meiotic outcomes in reciprocal translocation carriers ascertained in 3-day human embryos. *Eur J Hum Genet* 10:801–806, 2002.

Mackie Ogilvie C, Watson S, Braude P, Pickering S, Scriven PN. Preimplantation genetic diagnosis for a carrier of a Y;autosome translocation resulting in a healthy male offspring. *Fertil Steril* 94:1529, e11–14, 2010.

Madan K. Paracentric inversions: A review. *Hum Genet* 96:503–515, 1995.

Madan K. Balanced complex chromosome rearrangements—Reproductive aspects. A review. *Am J Med Genet* 158A:947–963, 2012.

Madan K. Natural human chimeras: A review. *Eur J Med Genet* 63:103971, 2020.

Madan K, Hompes PGA, Schoemaker J, Ford CE. X-autosome translocation with a breakpoint in Xq22 in a fertile woman and her 47,XXX infertile daughter. *Hum Genet* 59:290–296, 1981.

Madan K, Kleinhout J. First trimester abortions associated with a translocation t(1;20)(p36;p11). *Hum Genet* 76:109, 1987.

Madan K, Lundberg ES. Low grade mosaicism for X aneuploidy in women referred for recurrent abortions. *Eur Cytogeneticists Assoc Newslett* 35:9–12, 2015.

Madan K, Menko FH. Intrachromosomal insertions: A case report and a review. *Hum Genet* 89:1–9, 1992.

Madan K, Nieuwint AWM. Reproductive risks for paracentric inversion heterozygotes: Inversion or insertion? That is the question. *Am J Med Genet* 107:340–343, 2002.

Madan K, Nieuwint AWM, van Bever Y. Recombination in a balanced complex translocation of a mother leading to a balanced reciprocal translocation in the child: Review of 60 cases of balanced complex translocations. *Hum Genet* 99:806–815, 1997.

Madariaga ML, Rivera H. Familial inv(X)(p22q22): Ovarian dysgenesis in two sisters with del Xq and fertility in one male carrier. *Clin Genet* 52:180–183, 1997.

Maddirevula S, Coskun S, Awartani K, Alsaif H, Abdulwahab FM, Alkuraya FS. The human knockout phenotype of *PADI6* is female sterility caused by cleavage failure of their fertilized eggs. *Clin Genet* 91:344–345, 2017.

Mademont-Soler I, Morales C, Madrigal I, et al. Prenatal diagnosis of two different unbalanced forms of an inherited (Y;12) translocation. *Am J Med Genet* 149A:2820–2823, 2009.

Madian A, Eid MM, Shahin AAB, Mazen I, El-Bassyouni HT, Eid OM. Detection of low-grade mosaicism and its correlation with hormonal profile, testicular volume, and semen quality in a cohort of Egyptian Klinefelter and Klinefelter-like patients. *Reprod Biol* 20:259–263, 2020.

Madjunkova S, Sundaravadanam Y, Antes R, et al. Detection of structural rearrangements in embryos. *N Engl J Med* 382:2472–2474, 2020.

Madritsch S, Arnold V, Haider M, et al. Aneuploidy detection in pooled polar bodies using rapid nanopore sequencing. *J Assist Reprod Genet* 41:1261–1271, 2024.

Madsen HN, Ball S, Wright D, et al. A reassessment of biochemical marker distributions in trisomy 21-affected and unaffected twin pregnancies in the first trimester. *Ultrasound Obstet Gynecol* 37:38–47, 2011.

Maeda K, Imoto I, Kaji T, Yoshida Y, Nakayama S, Irahara M. Case of non-mosaic trisomy 20 in amniotic fluid cultures without anomalies in the fetus: Cytogenetic discrepancy between amniocytes and fetal blood. *J Obstet Gynaecol Res* 41:141–144, 2015.

Magee AC, Humphreys MW, McKee S, Stewart M, Nevin NC. De novo direct duplication 2 (p12→p21) with paternally inherited pericentric inversion 2p11.2 2q12.2. *Clin Genet* 54:65–69, 1998a.

Magee AC, Nevin NC, Armstrong MJ, McGibbon D, Nevin J. Ullrich-Turner syndrome: Seven pregnancies in an apparent 45,X woman. *Am J Med Genet* 75:1–3, 1998b.

Magenis E, Webb MJ, Spears B, Opitz JM. Blaschkolinear malformation syndrome in complex trisomy-7 mosaicism. *Am J Med Genet* 87:375–383, 1999.

Magini P, Poscente M, Ferrari S, et al. Cytogenetic and molecular characterization of a recombinant X chromosome in a family with a severe neurologic phenotype and macular degeneration. *Mol Cytogenet* 8:58, 2015.

Mahjani B, De Rubeis S, Gustavsson Mahjani C. et al. Prevalence and phenotypic impact of rare potentially damaging variants in autism spectrum disorder. Molecular Autism 12:65, 2021.

Mahmood R, Brierley CH, Faed MJW, Mills JA, Delhanty JDA. Mechanisms of maternal aneuploidy: FISH analysis of oocytes and polar bodies in patients undergoing assisted conception. *Hum Genet* 106:620–626, 2000.

Mahmoud R, Leonenko A, Butler MG, et al. Influence of molecular classes and growth hormone treatment on growth and dysmorphology in Prader-Willi syndrome: A multicenter study. *Clin Genet* 100:29–39, 2021.

Mahon O, Fox Á, Lynch SA, Cunningham K. Use of tissue samples in diagnosing diploid triploid mosaicism. *BMJ Case Rep* 15:e252779, 2022.

Martínez-Jacobo L, Ortíz-López R, Rizo-Méndez A, et al. Clinical and molecular delineation of duplication 9p24.3q21.11 in a patient with psychotic behavior. *Gene* 560:124–127, 2015.

Martínez-Juárez A, Uribe-Figueroa L, Quintana-Palma M, Razo-Aguilera G, Sevilla-Montoya R. Pure trisomy 2p syndrome in two siblings with an unbalanced translocation and minimal terminal 12q monosomy characterized by high-density microarray. *Cytogenet Genome Res* 142:249–254, 2014.

Martínez-Pasarell O, Templado C, Vicens-Calvet E, Egozcue J, Nogués C. Paternal sex chromosome aneuploidy as a possible origin of Turner syndrome in monozygotic twins: Case report. *Hum Reprod* 14:2735–2738, 1999.

Martinez-Portilla RJ, Pauta M, Hawkins-Villarreal A, et al. Added value of chromosomal microarray analysis over conventional karyotyping in stillbirth work-up: Systematic review and meta-analysis. *Ultrasound Obstet Gynecol* 53:590–597, 2019.

Martorell MR, Martínez-Pasarell O, Lopez O, et al. Chromosome 16 abnormalities in embryos and in sperm from a male with a fragile site at 16q22.1. *Cytogenet Genome Res* 142:134–139, 2014.

Mas J, Sabouni R, Bocca S. A novel male 2;4;14 complex chromosomal translocation with normal semen parameters but 100% embryonic aneuploidy. *J Assist Reprod Genet* 35:907–912, 2018.

Massalska D, Bijok J, Kucińska-Chahwan A, et al. Maternal complications in molecularly confirmed diandric and digynic triploid pregnancies: Single institution experience and literature review. *Arch Gynecol Obstet* 301:1139–1145, 2020.

Massalska D, Bijok J, Kucińska-Chahwan A, et al. Triploid pregnancy—Clinical implications. *Clin Genet* 100:368–375, 2021.

Mastenbroek S, Twisk M, van der Veen F, Repping S. Preimplantation genetic screening: A systematic review and meta-analysis of RCTs. *Hum Reprod Update* 17:454–466, 2011.

Mastromoro G, Guadagnolo D, Khaleghi, et al. Molecular approaches in fetal malformations, dynamic anomalies and soft markers: Diagnostic rates and challenges—systematic review of the literature and meta-analysis. *Diagnostics (Basel)* 12:575, 2022.

Mastrorosa FK, Rozanski AN, Harvey WT, et al. Complete chromosome 21 centromere sequences from a Down syndrome family reveal size asymmetry and differences in kinetochore attachment. *BioRχiv*, in press 2025.

Masuno M, Imaizumi K, Ishii T, Kimura J, Kuroki Y. Supernumerary ring chromosome 5 identified by FISH. *Am J Med Genet* 84:381, 1999.

Matalon R, Supple P, Wyandt H, Rosenthal IM. Transmission of ring 14 chromosome from mother to two sons. *Am J Med Genet* 36:381–385, 1990.

Mateu-Brull E, Rodrigo L, Peinado V, et al. Interchromosomal effect in carriers of translocations and inversions assessed by preimplantation genetic testing for structural rearrangements (PGT-SR). *J Assist Reprod Genet* 36:2547–2555, 2019.

Matorras R, Pérez-Fernández S, Mercader A, et al. Lessons learned from 64,071 embryos subjected to PGT for aneuploidies: Results, recurrence pattern and indications analysis. *Reprod Biomed Online* 49:103979, 2024.

Matsukura H, Nagamori M, Miya K, Yorifuji T. MODY3, renal cysts, and Dandy-Walker variants with a microdeletion spanning the HNF1A gene. *Clin Nephrol* 88:162–166, 2017.

Matsuo M, Muroya K, Nanao K, et al. Mother and daughter with 45,X/46,X,r(X)(p22.3q28) and mental retardation: Analysis of the X-inactivation patterns. *Am J Med Genet* 91:267–272, 2000.

Mattina T, Palumbo O, Stallone R, et al. Interstitial 16p13.3 microduplication: Case report and critical review of genotype-phenotype correlation. *Eur J Med Genet* 55:747–752, 2012.

Maurin ML, Arfeuille C, Sonigo P, et al. Large duplications can be benign copy number variants: A case of a 3.6-Mb Xq21.33 duplication. *Cytogenet Genome Res* 151:115–118, 2017.

Maurin ML, Labrune P, Brisset S, et al. Molecular cytogenetic characterization of a 4p15.1-pter duplication and a 4q35.1-qter deletion in a recombinant of chromosome 4 pericentric inversion. *Am J Med Genet* 149A:226–231, 2009.

Maya I, Kahana S, Agmon-Fishman I, et alL. The phenotype of 15 cases with rare 8q24.13-q24.3 deletions-A new syndrome or still an enigma? *Am J Med Genet* 185A:1461–1467, 2021.

Maya I, Perlman S, Shohat M, et al. Should we report 15q11.2 BP1-BP2 deletions and duplications in the prenatal setting? *J Clin Med* 9:2602, 2020.

Maya I, Vinkler C, Konen O, et al. Abnormal brain magnetic resonance imaging in two patients with Smith-Magenis syndrome. *Am J Med Genet* 164A:1940–1946, 2014.

Mazen IM, Kamel AK, Mohamed AM, et al. Unique karyotype: mos 46,X,dic(X;Y)(p22.33;p11.32)/45,X/45,dic(X;Y)(p22.33;p11.32) in an Egyptian patient with ovotesticular disorder of sexual development. *Sex Dev* 7:235–243, 2013.

Mazzaschi RL, Love DR, Hayes I, George A. Inheritance of a ring chromosome 21 in a couple undergoing in vitro fertilization (IVF): A case report. *Case Rep Genet* 2011:158086, 2011.

McClarren J, Donnenfeld AE, Ravnan JB. Prenatal diagnosis of an unexpected interstitial 22q11.2 deletion causing truncus arteriosus and thymic hypoplasia in a ring 22 chromosome derived from a maternally inherited paracentric inversion. *Prenat Diagn* 26:1212–1215, 2006.

McConkie-Rosell A, Spiridigliozzi GA, Rounds K, et al. Parental attitudes regarding carrier testing in children at risk for fragile X syndrome. *Am J Med Genet* 82:206–211, 1999.

McConnell V, Derham R, McManus D, Morrison PJ. Mosaic monosomy 14: Clinical features and recognizable facies. *Clin Dysmorphol* 13:155–160, 2004.

McCool C, Spinks-Franklin A, Noroski LM, Potocki L. 2017. Potocki-Shaffer syndrome in a child without intellectual disability—The role of *PHF21A* in cognitive function. *Am J Med Genet* 173A:716–720, 2017.

McCormack A, Claxton K, Ashton F, et al. Microarray testing in clinical diagnosis: An analysis of 5,300 New Zealand patients. *Mol Cytogenet* 9:29, 2016.

McCoy J, Pynaker C, Lewis S, et al. Childhood outcomes of fetal genomic copy number variants: the prenatal microarray cohort study, 24 June 2025, PREPRINT (Version 1) available at Research Square [https://doi.org/10.21203/rs.3.rs-6952328/v1].

McCoy RC. Mosaicism in preimplantation human embryos: When chromosomal abnormalities are the norm. *Trend* Blackburn *s Genet* 33:448–463, 2017.

McCoy RC, Demko ZP, Ryan A, et al. Evidence of selection against complex mitotic-origin aneuploidy during preimplantation development. *PLoS Genet* 11:e1005601, 2015.

McCoy RC, Summers MC, McCollin A, Ottolini CS, Ahuja K, Handyside AH. Meiotic and mitotic aneuploidies drive arrest of in vitro fertilized human preimplantation embryos. *Genome Med* 15:77, 2023.

McDermott H, Johnson JL. Is the prevalence of Down syndrome births in Hawai'i increasing? *Hawaii Med J* 70:72–76, 2011.

McDonald-McGinn DM, Emanuel BS, Zackai EH. 22q11.2 deletion syndrome. In Pagon RA, Adam MP, Ardinger HH, et al. (eds.), *GeneReviews*. Seattle, WA: University of Washington, 2013.

McElyea SD, Starbuck JM, Tumbleson-Brink DM, et al. Influence of prenatal EGCG treatment and Dyrk1a dosage reduction on craniofacial features associated with Down syndrome. *Hum Mol Genet* 25:4856–4869, 2016.

McFadden DE, Jiang R, Langlois S, Robinson WP. Dispermy—Origin of diandric triploidy: Brief communication. *Hum Reprod* 17:3037–3038, 2002.

McFadden DE, Langlois S. Parental and meiotic origin of triploidy in the embryonic and fetal periods. *Clin Genet* 58:192–200, 2000.

McFadden DE, Friedman JM. Chromosome abnormalities in human beings. *Mutat Res* 396:129–140, 1997.

McFadden DE, Robinson WP. Phenotype of triploid embryos. *J Med Genet* 43:609–612, 2006.

McGillivray G, Begg L, Billson VR, et al. Trisomy 3: The supported "natural" history. Poster presented at Annual Scientific Meeting of the Human Genetics Society Australasia, 2004.

McGillivray G, Rosenfeld JA, Gardner RJM, Gillam LH. Genetic counselling and ethical issues with chromosome microarray analysis in prenatal testing. *Prenat Diagn* 32:389–395, 2012.

McGowan KD, Weiser JJ, Horwitz J, et al. The importance of investigating for uniparental disomy in prenatally identified balanced acrocentric rearrangements. *Prenat Diagn* 22:141–143, 2002.

McKenzie LJ, Cisneros PL, Torsky S, et al. Preimplantation genetic diagnosis for a known cryptic translocation: Follow-up clinical report and implication of segregation products. *Am J Med Genet* 121A:56–59, 2003.

McPadden J, Helm BM, Spangler BB, Ross LP, Boles DB, Schrier Vergano SA. Mosaic trisomy 15 in a liveborn infant. *Am J Med Genet* 167A:821–825, 2015.

McRae AM, Duncan J, Drackley A, et al. Further delineation of the proximal 15p11.2 microdeletion syndrome: Novel findings among 22 new individuals. *Am J Med Genet* 197A:e63873, 2025.

McStay B. The p-arms of human acrocentric chromosomes play by a different set of rules. *Annu Rev Genomics Hum Genet* 24:63–832023.

Mears AJ, el-Shanti H, Murray JC, McDermid HE, Patil SR. Minute supernumerary ring chromosome 22 associated with cat eye syndrome: Further delineation of the critical region. *Am J Hum Genet* 57:667–673, 1995.

Mefford HC, Cook J, Gospe SM. Epilepsy due to 20q13.33 subtelomere deletion masquerading as pyridoxine-dependent epilepsy. *Am J Med Genet* 158A:3190–3195, 2012.

Meggiolaro N, Barlow-Stewart K, Dunlop K, Newson AJ, Fleming J. Disclosure to genetic relatives without consent—Australian genetic professionals' awareness of the health privacy law. *BMC Med Ethics* 21:13, 2020.

Mehra S, Christ L, Jeng L, Zinn AB, Schwartz S. Characterization of a familial balanced rec(13) in a child with mild MR and his half-sibling with two structurally rearranged chromosomes 13. *Am J Med Genet* 137:217–221, 2005.

Mei C, Fedorenko E, Amor DJ, et al. Deep phenotyping of speech and language skills in individuals with 16p11.2 deletion. *Eur J Hum Genet* 26:676–686, 2018.

Mei Y, Lin Y, Chen Y, et al. Preimplantation genetic testing for aneuploidy optimizes reproductive outcomes in recurrent reproductive failure: A systematic review. *Front Med (Lausanne)* 11:1233962, 2024.

Meinel JA, Yumiceba V, Künstner A, et al. Disruption of the topologically associated domain at Xp21.2 is related to 46,XY gonadal dysgenesis. *J Med Genet* 60:469–476, 2023.

Meiner A, Holland H, Reichenbach H, Horn LC, Faber R, Froster UG. Tetraploidy in a growth-retarded fetus with a thick placenta. *Prenat Diagn* 18:864–865, 1998.

Meistrich ML, Byrne J. Genetic disease in offspring of long-term survivors of childhood and adolescent cancer treated with potentially mutagenic therapies. *Am J Hum Genet* 70:1069–1071, 2002.

Mekkawy M, Kamel A, El-Ruby M, et al. Isodicentric Y chromosomes in Egyptian patients with disorders of sex development (DSD). *Am J Med Genet* 158A:1594–1603, 2012.

Mekkawy MK, Kamel AK, Thomas MM, et al. Clinical and genetic characterization of ten Egyptian patients with Wolf-Hirschhorn syndrome and review of literature. *Mol Genet Genomic Med* 9:e1546, 2021.

Melichar VO, Guth S, Hellebrand H, et al. A male infant with a 9.6 Mb terminal Xp deletion including the OA1 locus: Limit of viability of Xp deletions in males. *Am J Med Genet* 143:135–141, 2007.

Melis D, Genesio R, Boemio P, et al. Clinical description of a patient carrying the smallest reported deletion involving 10p14 region. *Am J Med Genet* 158A:832–835, 2012.

Mellis R, Eberhardt RY, Hamilton SJ, et al. Fetal exome sequencing for isolated increased nuchal translucency: Should we be doing it? *BJOG* 129:52–61, 2022.

Melnyk AR, Ahmed I, Taylor JC. Prenatal diagnosis of familial ring 21 chromosome. *Prenat Diagn* 15:269–273, 1995.

Melo JB, Estevinho A, Saraiva J, Ramos L, Carreira IM. Cutis aplasia as a clinical hallmark for the syndrome associated with 19q13.11 deletion: The possible role for *UBA2* gene. *Mol Cytogenet* 8:21, 2015.

Mendes JRT, Strufaldi MWL, Delcelo R, et al. Y-chromosome identification by PCR and gonadal histopathology in Turner's syndrome without overt Y-mosaicism. *Clin Endocrinol* 50:19–26, 1999.

Mendes M, Chen DZ, Engchuan W, et al. Chromosome X-wide common variant association study in autism spectrum disorder. *Am J Hum Genet* 112:135–153, 2025.

Meng X, Jiang L. Prenatal detection of chromosomal abnormalities and copy number variants in fetuses with congenital gastrointestinal obstruction. *BMC Pregnancy Childbirth* 22:50, 2022.

Meng Y, Yang J, Tian C, Qiao J. Identification of a 6-month-old baby with a combination of WAGR and Potocki-Shaffer contiguous deletion syndromes by SNP array testing. *Hereditas* 157:23, 2020.

Menon S, Rives N, Mousset-Siméon N, et al. Fertility preservation in adolescent males: Experience over 22 years at Rouen University Hospital. *Hum Reprod* 24:37–44, 2009.

Meossi C, Carrer A, Ciaccio C, et al. Clinical features and magnesium levels: Novel insights in 15q11.2 BP1-BP2 copy number variants. *J Intellect Disabil Res* 67:679–689, 2023.

Mercer CL, Lachlan K, Karcanias A, et al. Detailed clinical and molecular study of 20 females with Xq deletions with special reference to menstruation and fertility. *Eur J Med Genet* 56:1–6, 2013.

Mercier S, Bresson JL. Analysis of chromosomal equipment in spermatozoa of a 46,XY/47,XY/+8 male by means of multicolour fluorescent in situ hybridization: Confirmation of a mosaicism and evaluation of risk for offspring. *Hum Genet* 99:42–46, 1997.

Meredith MM, Crabb B, Vargas M, Hirsch BA. Chimerism for 20q11.2 microdeletion of *GDF5* explains discordant phenotypes in monochorionic-diamniotic twins. *Am J Med Genet* 73A:3182–3188, 2017.

Merrill A, Rosenblum-Vos L, Driscoll DA, Daley K, Treat K. Prenatal diagnosis of Fanconi anemia (Group C) subsequent to abnormal sonographic findings. *Prenat Diagn* 25:20–22, 2005.

Merrion K, Maisenbacher M. Pericentric inversion (inv) 9 variant-reproductive risk factor or benign finding? *J Assist Reprod Genet* 36:2557–2561, 2019.

Mertzanidou A, Spits C, Nguyen HT, Van de Velde H, Sermon K. Evolution of aneuploidy up to day 4 of human preimplantation development. *Hum Reprod* 28:1716–1724, 2013.

Meschede D, Froster UG, Bergmann M, Nieschlag E. Familial pericentric inversion of chromosome 1 (p34q23) and male infertility with stage specific spermatogenic arrest. *J Med Genet* 31:573–575, 1994.

Meschede D, Louwen F, Nippert I, Holzgreve W, Miny P, Horst J. Low rates of pregnancy termination for prenatally diagnosed Klinefelter syndrome and other sex chromosome polysomies. *Am J Med Genet* 80:330–334, 1998.

Meschino WS, Miller K, Bedford HM. Incidental detection of familial APP duplication An unusual reason for a false positive NIPT result of trisomy 21. *Prenat Diagn* 36:382–384, 2016.

Meyer E, Lim D, Pasha S, et al. Germline mutation in *NLRP2* (*NALP2*) in a familial imprinting disorder (Beckwith-Wiedemann Syndrome). *PLoS Genet* 5:e1000423, 2009.

Meza-Espinoza JP, González-García JR, Nieto-Marín N, et al. Chromosomal instability in a patient with ring chromosome 14 syndrome: A case report. *Mol Cytogenet* 17:17, 2024.

Mi L, Yao R, Guo W, Wang J, Zhang G, Ye X. Concurrent de novo MACF1 mutation and inherited 16p13.11 microduplication in a preterm newborn with hypotonia, joint hyperlaxity and multiple congenital malformations: A case report. *BMC Pediatr* 24:528, 2024.

Micale M, Insko J, Ebrahim SAD, Adeyinka A, Runke C, Van Dyke DL. Double trisomy revisited—A multicenter experience. *Prenat Diagn* 30:173–176, 2010.

Miceli M, Failla P, Saccuzzo L, et al. Trait-driven analysis of the 2p15p16.1 microdeletion syndrome suggests a complex pattern of interactions between candidate genes. *Genes Genomics* 45:491–505, 2023.

Michaelis RC, Velagaleti GVN, Jones C, et al. Most Jacobsen syndrome deletion breakpoints occur distal to *FRA11B*. *Am J Med Genet* 76:222–228, 1998.

Michelson RJ, Weinert T. Closing the gaps among a web of DNA repair disorders. *Bioessays* 22:966–969, 2000.

Michie S, Bobrow M, Marteau TM. Predictive genetic testing in children and adults: A study of emotional impact. *J Med Genet* 38:519–526, 2001.

Middleton FA, Trauzzi MG, Shrimpton AE, et al. Complete maternal uniparental isodisomy of chromosome 4 in a subject with major depressive disorder detected by high density SNP genotyping arrays. *Am J Med Genet* 141B:28–32, 2006.

Midro AT, Panasiuk B, Stasiewicz-Jarocka B, et al. Risk estimates for carriers of chromosome reciprocal translocation t(4;9)(p15.2;p13). *Clin Genet* 58:153–155, 2000.

Midro AT, Panasiuk B, Stasiewicz-Jarocka B, et al. Recurrence risks for different pregnancy outcomes and meiotic segregation analysis of spermatozoa in carriers of t(1;11)(p36.22;q12.2). *J Hum Genet* 59:667–674, 2014.

Midro AT, Stengel-Rutkowski S, Stene J. Experiences with risk estimates for carriers of chromosomal reciprocal translocations. *Clin Genet* 41:113–122, 1992.

Midro AT, Wiland E, Panasiuk B, Lesniewicz R, Kurpisz M. Risk evaluation of carriers with chromosome reciprocal translocation t(7;13)(q34;q13) and concomitant meiotic segregation analyzed by FISH on ejaculated spermatozoa. *Am J Med Genet* 140:245–256, 2006.

Midro AT, Zollino M, Wiland E, et al. Meiotic and pedigree segregation analyses in carriers of t(4;8)(p16;p23.1) differing in localization of breakpoint positions at 4p subband 4p16.3 and 4p16.1. *J Assist Reprod Genet* 33:189–197, 2016.

Miga KH, Eichler EE. Envisioning a new era: Complete genetic information from routine telomere-to-telomere genomes. *Am J Hum Genet* 110:1832–1840, 2023.

Migeon B. *Females Are Mosaics: X Inactivation and Sex Differences in Disease*. New York, NY: Oxford University Press, 2007.

Mighton C, Noor A, Watkins N, et al. Validation of low-pass genome sequencing for prenatal diagnosis. *Prenat Diagn* 44:443–453, 2024.

Mihajlović AI, Byers C, Reinholdt L, FitzHarris G. Spindle assembly checkpoint insensitivity allows meiosis-II despite chromosomal defects in aged eggs. *EMBO Rep* 24:e57227, 2023.

Mihci E, Velagaleti GV, Ensenauer R, Babovic-Vuksanovic D. The phenotypic spectrum of trisomy 2: Report of two new cases. *Clin Dysmorphol* 18:201–204, 2009.

Mikhaelian M, Veach PM, MacFarlane I, LeRoy BS, Bower M. Prenatal chromosomal microarray analysis: A survey of prenatal genetic counselors' experiences and attitudes. *Prenat Diagn* 33:371–377, 2013.

Mikwar M, MacFarlane AJ, Marchetti F. Mechanisms of oocyte aneuploidy associated with advanced maternal age. *Mutat Res Rev Mutat Res* 785:108320, 2020.

Milazzo JP, Rives N, Mousset-Siméon N, Macé B. Chromosome constitution and apoptosis of immature germ cells present in sperm of two 47,XYY infertile males. *Hum Reprod* 21:1749–1758, 2006.

Morales C, Madrigal I, Esqué T, et al. Duplication/deletion mosaicism of the 7q(21.1→31.3) region. *Am J Med Genet* 143:179–183, 2007a.

Morales C, Soler A, Bruguera J, et al. Pseudodicentric 22;Y translocation transmitted through four generations of a large family without phenotypic repercussion. *Cytogenet Genome Res* 116:319–323, 2007b.

Moran OM, Flamenbaum K, Myles Reid D, et al. Challenges experienced by genetic counselors while they provided counseling about mosaic embryos. *F S Rep* 4:353–360, 2023.

Morandi A, Bonnefond A, Lobbens S, et al. A girl with incomplete Prader-Willi syndrome and negative MS-PCR, found to have mosaic maternal UPD-15 at SNP array. *Am J Med Genet* 167A:2720–2726, 2015.

Morel F, Duguépéroux I, McElreavey K, et al. Transmission of an unbalanced (Y;1) translocation in Brittany, France. *J Med Genet* 39:e52, 2002.

Morel F, Fellmann F, Roux C, Bresson JL. Meiotic segregation analysis by FISH investigation of spermatozoa of a 46,Y,der(X),t(X;Y)(qter→p22::q11→qter) carrier. *Cytogenet Cell Genet* 92:63–68, 2001.

Morel F, Laudier B, Guérif F, et al. Meiotic segregation analysis in spermatozoa of pericentric inversion carriers using fluorescence in-situ hybridization. *Hum Reprod* 22:136–141, 2007.

Morel Y, Mebarki F, Forest MG. What are the indications for prenatal diagnosis in the androgen insensitivity syndrome? Facing clinical heterogeneity of phenotypes for the same genotype. *Eur J Endocrinol* 130:325–326, 1994.

Morgan A, Lenarduzzi S, Cappellani S, et al. Genomic studies in a large cohort of hearing impaired Italian patients revealed several new alleles, a rare case of uniparental disomy (UPD) and the importance to search for copy number variations. *Front Genet* 9:681, 2018.

Morgan AT, Amor DJ, St John MD, Scheffer IE, Hildebrand MS. Genetic architecture of childhood speech disorder: A review. *Mol Psychiatry* 29:1281–1292, 2024.

Mori MA, Huertas H, Pinel I, Giralt P, Martínez-Frías ML. Trisomy 13 in the child of two carriers of a 13/15 translocation. *Am J Med Genet* 20:17–20, 1985.

Morison LD, Kennis MGP, Rots D, et al. Expanding the phenotype of Kleefstra syndrome: Speech, language and cognition in 103 individuals. *J Med Genet* 61:578–585, 2024.

Morleo M, Franco B. Microphthalmia with Linear Skin Defects Syndrome. In: Adam MP, Feldman J, Mirzaa GM, et al. (eds.), *GeneReviews*. University of Washington, Seattle; 1993–2024.

Morleo M, Iaconis D, Chitayat D, et al. Disruption of the IQSEC2 transcript in a female with X;autosome translocation t(X;20)(p11.2;q11.2) and a phenotype resembling X-linked infantile spasms (ISSX) syndrome. *Mol Med Rep* 1:33–39, 2008.

Morleo M, Pramparo T, Perone L, et al. Microphthalmia with linear skin defects (MLS) syndrome: Clinical, cytogenetic, and molecular characterization of 11 cases. *Am J Med Genet* 137A:190–198, 2005.

Morokawa H, Kamiya M, Wakui K, et al. Myelodysplastic syndrome in an infant with constitutional pure duplication 1q41-qter. *Hum Genome Var* 5:6, 2018.

Morris A, Boyd E, Dhanjal S, et al. Two years' prospective experience using fluorescence in situ hybridization on uncultured amniotic fluid cells for rapid prenatal diagnosis of common chromosomal aneuploidies. *Prenat Diagn* 19:546–551, 1999.

Morris CA, Mervis CB, Paciorkowski AP, et al. 7q11.23 duplication syndrome: Physical characteristics and natural history. *Am J Med Genet* 167A:2916–2935; 2015.

Morris E, Inglis A, Austin J. Psychiatric genetic counseling for people with copy number variants associated with psychiatric conditions. *Clin Genet* 102:369–378, 2022.

Morris JK, Alberman E. Trends in Down's syndrome live births and antenatal diagnoses in England and Wales from 1989 to 2008: Analysis of data from the National Down Syndrome Cytogenetic Register. *BMJ* 339:b3794, 2009.

Morris JK, Alberman E, Scott C, Jacobs P. Is the prevalence of Klinefelter syndrome increasing? *Eur J Hum Genet* 16:163–170, 2008.

Morris JK, Mutton DE, Alberman E. Revised estimates of the maternal age specific live birth prevalence of Down's syndrome. *J Med Screen* 9:2–6, 2002.

Morris JK, Mutton DE, Alberman E. Recurrences of free trisomy 21: Analysis of data from the National Down Syndrome Cytogenetic Register. *Prenat Diagn* 25:1120–1128, 2005.

Morris JK, Wald NJ, Mutton DE, Alberman E. Comparison of models of maternal age-specific risk for Down syndrome live births. *Prenat Diagn* 23:252–258, 2003.

Mortimer JG, Chewings WE, Gardner RJM. A further report on a kindred with cases of 4p trisomy and monosomy. *Hum Hered* 30:58–61, 1980.

Mosca SJ, Langevin LM, Dewey D, et al. Copy-number variations are enriched for neurodevelopmental genes in children with developmental coordination disorder. *J Med Genet* 53:812–819, 2016.

Mottola F, Santonastaso M, Ronga V, Finelli R, Rocco L. Polymorphic rearrangements of human chromosome 9 and male infertility: New evidence and impact on spermatogenesis. *Biomolecules* 13:729, 2023.

Moustakli E, Zikopoulos A, Skentou C, Bouba I, Dafopoulos K, Georgiou I. Evolution of minimally invasive and non-invasive preimplantation genetic testing: An overview. *J Clin Med* 13:2160, 2024.

Moysés-Oliveira M, Giannuzzi G, Fish RJ, et al. Inactivation of AMMECR1 is associated with growth, bone, and heart alterations. *Hum Mutat* 39:281–291, 2018.

Moysés-Oliveira M, Guilherme RS, Meloni VA, et al. X-linked intellectual disability related genes disrupted by balanced X-autosome translocations. *Am J Med Genet Neuropsychiatr Genet* 168B:669–677, 2015.

Mroczkowski HJ, Arnold G, Schneck FX, Rajkovic A, Yatsenko SA. Interstitial 10p11.23-p12.1 microdeletions associated with developmental delay, craniofacial abnormalities, and cryptorchidism. *Am J Med Genet* 164A:2623–2626, 2014.

Mu W, Tochen L, Bertsch C, Singer HS, Barañano KW. Intracranial calcifications and dystonia associated with a novel deletion of chromosome 8p11.2 encompassing *SLC20A2* and *THAP1*. *BMJ Case Rep* 12:e228782, 2019.

Muhlhauser A, Susiarjo M, Rubio C, et al. Bisphenol A effects on the growing mouse oocyte are influenced by diet. *Biol Reprod* 80:1066–1071, 2009.

Mulcahy MT, Jenkyn J, Mackellar A. 45,X/47,XYY mosaicism. *J Med Genet* 14:218–221, 1977.

Mulchandani S, Bhoj EJ, Luo M, et al. Maternal uniparental disomy of chromosome 20: A novel imprinting disorder of growth failure. *Genet Med* 18:309–315, 2016.

Mules EH, Stamberg J. Reproductive outcomes of paracentric inversion carriers: Report of a liveborn dicentric recombinant and literature review. *Hum Genet* 67:126–131, 1984.

Mulle JG. The 3q29 deletion confers >40-fold increase in risk for schizophrenia. *Mol Psychiatry* 20:1028–1029, 2015.

Mulle JG, Pulver AE, McGrath JA, et al. Reciprocal duplication of the Williams-Beuren syndrome deletion on chromosome 7q11.23 is associated with schizophrenia. *Biol Psychiatry* 75:371–377, 2014.

Mullegama SV, Elsea SH. Clinical and molecular aspects of MBD5-associated neurodevelopmental disorder (MAND). *Eur J Hum Genet* 24:1235–1243, 2016.

Mullegama SV, Rosenfeld JA, Orellana C, et al. Reciprocal deletion and duplication at 2q23.1 indicates a role for MBD5 in autism spectrum disorder. *Eur J Hum Genet* 22:57–63, 2014.

Mullen SA, Carvill GL, Bellows S, et al. Copy number variants are frequent in genetic generalized epilepsy with intellectual disability. *Neurology* 81:1507–1514, 2013.

Muller EA, Aradhya S, Atkin JF, et al. Microdeletion 9q22.3 syndrome includes metopic craniosynostosis, hydrocephalus, macrosomia, and developmental delay. *Am J Med Genet* 158A:391–399, 2012.

Muller F, Dreux S, Dupoizat H, et al. Second-trimester Down syndrome maternal serum screening in twin pregnancies: Impact of chorionicity. *Prenat Diagn* 23:331–335, 2003.

Muller F, Rebiffé M, Taillandier A, Oury JF, Mornet E. Parental origin of the extra chromosome in prenatally diagnosed fetal trisomy 21. *Hum Genet* 106:340–344, 2000.

Müller J, Ritzén EM, Ivarsson SA, Rajpert-De Meyts E, Norjavaara E, Skakkebæk NE. Management of males with 45,X/46,XY gonadal dysgenesis. *Horm Res* 52:11–14, 1999.

Müller J, Skakkebæk NE. Gonadal malignancy in individuals with sex chromosome anomalies. *Birth Defects Orig Artic Ser* 26:247–255, 1990.

Mumusoglu S, Telek SB, Ata B. Preimplantation genetic testing for aneuploidy in unexplained recurrent pregnancy loss: A systematic review and meta-analysis. *Fertil Steril* 123:121–136, 2025.

Mundhofir FE, Smeets D, Nillesen W, et al. Monosomy 9pter and trisomy 9q34.11qter in two sisters due to a maternal pericentric inversion. *Gene* 511:451–454, 2012.

Munné S. Analysis of chromosome segregation during preimplantation genetic diagnosis in both male and female translocation heterozygotes. *Cytogenet Genome Res* 111:305–309, 2005.

Munné S, Bahçe M, Schimmel T, Sadowy S, Cohen J. Case report: Chromatid exchange and predivision of chromatids as other sources of abnormal oocytes detected by preimplantation genetic diagnosis of translocations. *Prenat Diagn* 18:1450–1458, 1998a.

Munné S, Escudero T, Sandalinas M, Sable D, Cohen J. Gamete segregation in female carriers of Robertsonian translocations. *Cytogenet Cell Genet* 90:303–308, 2000.

Munné S, Scott R, Sable D, Cohen J. First pregnancies after preconception diagnosis of translocations of maternal origin. *Fertil Steril* 69:675–681, 1998b.

Murakami H, Enomoto Y, Kumaki T, Aida N, Kurosawa K. Nanopore long-read sequencing analysis reveals ZIC1 dysregulation caused by a de novo 3q inversion with a breakpoint located 7 kb downstream of ZIC1. *J Hum Genet* 69:47–52, 2024.

Muroya K, Yamamoto K, Fukushima Y, Ogata T. Ring chromosome 21 in a boy and a derivative chromosome 21 in the mother: Implication for ring chromosome formation. *Am J Med Genet* 110:332–337, 2002.

Murphy AJ, Cheng C, Williams J, et al. Genetic and epigenetic features of bilateral Wilms tumor predisposition in patients from the Children's Oncology Group AREN18B5-Q. *Nat Commun* 14:8006, 2023.

Murphy EA, Chase GA. *Principles of Genetic Counseling*. Chicago, IL: Year Book, 1975.

Musgrave SM, Taylor J, Whitford W, et al., Genetic diagnostic outcomes from a 10-year research programme in autism in Aotearoa New Zealand. *J Roy Soc New Zealand* 55:2464–2480, 2024.

Mussa A, Russo S, De Crescenzo A, et al. (Epi)genotype-phenotype correlations in Beckwith-Wiedemann syndrome. *Eur J Hum Genet* 24:183–190, 2016.

Mutter M, Binkert F, Schinzel A. Down syndrome livebirth rate in the eastern part of Switzerland between 1980 and 1996 stays constant in spite of growing numbers of prenatally diagnosed and subsequently terminated cases. *Prenat Diagn* 22:835–836, 2002.

Myers KA, Bennett MF, Hildebrand MS, et al. Transcriptome analysis of a ring chromosome 20 patient cohort. *Epilepsia* 62:e22–e28, 2021a.

Myers KA, Marini C, Carvill GL, et al. Phenotypic spectrum of seizure disorders in MBD5-associated neurodevelopmental disorder. *Neurol Genet* 7:e579, 2021b.

Myers KA, Wallis MJ, Fitt GJ, Sarnat HB, Newton MR. Blake's pouch cyst in 13q deletion syndrome: Posterior fossa malformations may occur due to disruption of multiple genes. *Am J Med Genet* 173A:2442–2445, 2017.

N

Nadal M, Moreno S, Pritchard M, Preciado MA, Estivill X, Ramos-Arroyo MA. Down syndrome: Characterisation of a case with partial trisomy of chromosome 21 owing to a paternal balanced translocation (15;21)(q26;q22.1) by FISH. *J Med Genet* 34:50–54, 1997.

Nadal M, Valiente A, Domènech A, Pritchard M, Estivill X, Ramos-Arroyo MA. Hereditary neuropathy with liability to pressure palsies: Two cases with a reciprocal translocation t(16;17)(q12;11.2) interrupting the *PMP22* gene. *J Med Genet* 37:396–398, 2000.

Nagai T, Shimokawa O, Harada N, et al. Postnatal overgrowth by 15q-trisomy and intrauterine growth retardation by 15q-monosomy due to familial translocation t(13;15): Dosage effect of *IGF1R*? *Am J Med Genet* 113:173–177, 2002.

Nagarsheth NP, Mootabar H. Prenatal diagnosis of mosaic tetrasomy 21q confirmed by fluorescence in situ hybridization. *Clin Genet* 51:260–263, 1997.

Nagle C, Hodges R, Wolfe R, Wallace EM. Reporting Down syndrome screening results: Women's understanding of risk. *Prenat Diagn* 29:234–239, 2009.

Nagy O, Kárteszi J, Elmont B, Ujfalusi A. Case report: Expressive speech disorder in a family as a hallmark of 7q31 deletion involving the *FOXP2* gene. *Front Pediatr* 9:664548, 2021.

Nakamura N. Genetic effects of radiation in atomic-bomb survivors and their children: Past, present and future. *J Radiat Res* 47 (Suppl B):B67–73, 2006.

Nakamura N, Yoshida N, Suwa T. Three major reasons why transgenerational effects of radiation are difficult to detect in humans. *Int J Radiat Biol* 15:1–15, 2023.

Nakano T, Ammae M, Satoh M, Mizuno S, Nakaoka Y, Morimoto Y. Analysis of clinical outcomes and meiotic segregation modes following preimplantation genetic testing for structural rearrangements using aCGH/NGS in couples with balanced chromosome rearrangement. *Reprod Med Biol* 21:e12476, 2022.

Nakka P, Pattillo Smith S, O'Donnell-Luria AH, et al. Characterization of prevalence and Health consequences of uniparental disomy in four million individuals from the general population. *Am J Hum Genet* 105:921–932, 2019.

Nap AW, Van Golde RJ, Tuerlings JH, et al. Reproductive decisions of men with microdeletions of the Y chromosome: The role of genetic counselling. *Hum Reprod* 14:2166–2169, 1999.

Nardelli A, Laskoski LV, Luiz AF, Silveira MAD, d'Arce LPG. Occurrence of mosaic trisomy 22 and pericentric inversion of chromosome 9 in a patient with a good prognosis. *BMC Med Genomics* 16:286, 2023.

Nardmann J, Tranebjærg L, Horsthemke B, Lüdecke HJ. The tricho-rhino-phalangeal syndromes: Frequency and parental origin of 8q deletions. *Hum Genet* 99:638–643, 1997.

Nascimento CG, Prota JRM, Sgardioli IC, et al. Rare 15q21.1q22.31 duplication due to a familial chromosomal insertion and diagnostic investigation in a carrier of balanced chromosomal rearrangement and intellectual disability. *Genes (Basel)* 14:885, 2023.

Natera de Benito D, García-Pérez MA, Martínez-Granero MÁ, Izquierdo-López L. A patient with a duplication of chromosome 3p (p24.1p26.2): A comparison with other partial 3p trisomies. *Am J Med Genet* 164A:548–550, 2014.

Natesan SA, Bladon AJ, Coskun S, et al. Genome-wide karyomapping accurately identifies the inheritance of single-gene defects in human preimplantation embryos in vitro. *Genet Med* 16:838–845, 2014.

Natsuga K, Nishie W, Arita K, et al. Complete paternal isodisomy of chromosome 17 in junctional epidermolysis bullosa with pyloric atresia. *J Invest Dermatol* 130:2671–2674, 2010.

Navarro-Cobos MJ, Balaton BP, Brown CJ. Genes that escape from X-chromosome inactivation: Potential contributors to Klinefelter syndrome. *Am J Med Genet* 184C:225–238, 2020.

Neas KR, Yip MY, James C, Kirk EPE. Patient with a non-mosaic isodicentric Yp and mild developmental delay. *Am J Med Genet* 137:223–224, 2005.

Neel JV, Schull WJ. *The Children of Atomic Bomb Survivors: A Genetic Study.* Washington, DC: National Academy Press, 1991.

Neel JV, Schull WJ, Awa AA, et al. The children of parents exposed to atomic bombs: Estimates of the genetic doubling dose of radiation for humans. *Am J Hum Genet* 46:1053–1072, 1990.

Neeman B, Sudhakar S, Biswas A, et al. Sotos syndrome: Deep neuroimaging phenotyping reveals a high prevalence of malformations of cortical development. *Am J Neuroradiol* 45:1570–1577, 2024.

Neira-Fresneda J, Potocki L. Neurodevelopmental disorders associated with abnormal gene dosage: Smith-Magenis and Potocki-Lupski syndromes. *J Pediatr Genet* 4:159–167, 2015.

Neiswanger K, Hohler PM, Hively-Thomas LB, McPherson EW, Hogge WA, Surti U. Variable outcomes in mosaic trisomy 16: Five case reports and literature analysis. *Prenat Diagn* 26:454–461, 2006.

Neitzel H, Neumann LM, Schindler D, et al. Premature chromosome condensation in humans associated with microcephaly and mental retardation: A novel autosomal recessive condition. *Am J Hum Genet* 70:1015–1022, 2002.

Németh AH, Gallen IW, Crocker M, Levy E, Maher E. Klinefelter-like phenotype and primary infertility in a male with a paracentric Xq inversion. *J Med Genet* 39:E28, 2002.

Neri G. A possible explanation for the low incidence of gonosomal aneuploidy among the offspring of triplo-X individuals. *Am J Med Genet* 18:357–364, 1984.

Neri G, Opitz JM. Down syndrome: Comments and reflections on the 50th anniversary of Lejeune's discovery. *Am J Med Genet* 149A:2647–2654, 2009.

Neri G, Romana Di Raimo F. Long time no see: The type and contre-type concept. *Eur J Hum Genet* 18:135–136, 2010.

Nerlich A, Wisser J, Krone S. Placental findings in "vanishing twins." *Geburtshilfe Frauenheilkd* 52:230–234, 1992.

Neu RL, Brar HS, Koos BJ. Prenatal diagnosis of inv(X)(q12q28) in a male fetus. *J Med Genet* 25:52–53, 1988a.

Neu RL, Kousseff BG, Hardy DE, et al. Trisomy 3p23→pter and monosomy 11q23→qter in an infant with two translocation carrier parents. *J Med Genet* 25:631–633, 1988b.

Neu RL, Valentine FA, Gardner LI. Segregation of a t(14q22q) chromosome in a large kindred. *Clin Genet* 8:30–36, 1975.

Neumann AA, Robson LG, Smith A. A 15p+ variant shown to be a t(Y;15) with fluorescence in situ hybridisation. *Ann Génét* 35:227–230, 1992.

Nevado J, de Torres ML, Fernández L, et al. Unusual four-generation chromosome-22 rearrangement: When "normality" masks abnormality. *Am J Med Genet* 149A:1561–1564, 2009.

Nevado J, Rosenfeld JA, Mena R, et al. PIAS4 is associated with macro/microcephaly in the novel interstitial 19p13.3 microdeletion/microduplication syndrome. *Eur J Hum Genet* 23:1615–1626, 2015.

Newberg MT, Francisco RG, Pang MG, et al. Cytogenetics of somatic cells and sperm from a 46,XY/45,X mosaic male with moderate oligoasthenoteratozoospermia. *Fertil Steril* 69:146–148, 1998.

Newbury DF, Mari F, Sadighi Akha E, et al. Dual copy number variants involving 16p11 and 6q22 in a case of childhood apraxia of speech and pervasive developmental disorder. *Eur J Hum Genet* 21:361–365, 2013.

Ngo AD, Taylor R, Roberts CL, Nguyen TV. Association between Agent Orange and birth defects: Systematic review and meta-analysis. *Int J Epidemiol* 35:1220–1230, 2006.

Nguyen HH, Umapathi KK, Bokowski JW, Hogan K, Hart A, Li MH. Mosaic trisomy 16 associated with left lung agenesis, abnormal left arm, and right pulmonary artery stenosis: Expanding the phenotype and review of the literature. *J Pediatr Genet* 11:324–332, 2020.

Pérez-Palma E, Saarentaus E, Ravoet M, et al. Duplications at 19q13.33 in patients with neurodevelopmental disorders. *Neurol Genet* 4:e210, 2018.

Pergament E, Confino E, Zhang JX, Roscetti L, Xien Chen P, Wellman D. Recurrent triploidy of maternal origin. *Prenat Diagn* 20:561–563, 2000.

Periquito I, Carrusca C, Morgado J, Robalo B, Pereira C, de Lurdes Sampaio M. Familial Turner syndrome: The importance of information. *J Pediatr Endocrinol Metab* 29:617–620, 2016.

Peris M, Crompton K, Shepherd DA, Amor DJ. The association between human chorionic gonadotropin and adverse pregnancy outcomes: A systematic review and meta-analysis. *Am J Obstet Gynecol* 230:118–184, 2024.

Peron A, Catusi I, Recalcati MP, et al. Ring chromosome 20 syndrome: Genetics, clinical characteristics, and overlapping phenotypes. *Front Neurol* 11:613035, 2020.

Perrin A, Douet-Guilbert N, Le Bris MJ, et al. Segregation of chromosomes in sperm of a t(X;18)(q11;p11.1) carrier inherited from his mother: Case report. *Hum Reprod* 23:227–230, 2008.

Perrin A, Douet-Guilbert N, Le Bris MJ, et al. Increased aneuploidy rates in spermatozoa of a male carrier of a trisomy 18 mosaicism. *Int J Androl* 32:231–234, 2009a.

Perrin A, Vialard F, Douet-Guilbert N, et al. Meiotic segregation of X-autosome translocation in two carriers and implications for assisted reproduction. *Reprod Biomed Online* 18:850–855, 2009b.

Perry J, Slater HR, Choo KHA. Centric fission—Simple and complex mechanisms. *Chromosome Res* 12:627–640, 2004.

Perry J, White SM, Nouri S, et al. Unstable Robertsonian translocations der(13;15)(q10;q10): Heritable chromosome fission without phenotypic effect in two kindreds. *Am J Med Genet* 136:25–30, 2005.

Pertile MD, Halks-Miller M, Flowers N, et al. Rare autosomal trisomies, revealed by maternal plasma DNA sequencing, suggest increased risk of feto-placental disease. *Sci Transl Med* 9:1240, 2017.

Pertile MD, Ryan JT, Kelley JL, Webber LM. Prenatal diagnosis of tetrasomy 9p. *Bull Hum Genet Soc Australasia* 9:43, 1996.

Peter B, Scherer N, Liang WS, Pophal S, Nielsen C, Grebe TA. A phenotypically diverse family with an atypical 22q11.2 deletion due to an unbalanced 18q23;22q11.2 translocation. *Am J Med Genet A* 185:1532–1537, 2021.

Peters SU, Fu C, Suter B, et al. Characterizing the phenotypic effect of Xq28 duplication size in MECP2 duplication syndrome. *Clin Genet* 95:575–581, 2019.

Petersen MB, Adelsberger PA, Schinzel AA, Binkert F, Hinkel GK, Antonarakis SE. Down syndrome due to de novo Robertsonian translocation t(14q;21q): DNA polymorphism analysis suggests that the origin of the extra 21q is maternal. *Am J Hum Genet* 49:529–536, 1991.

Petersen OB, Vogel I, Ekelund C, et al. Potential diagnostic consequences of applying non-invasive prenatal testing: Population-based study from a country with existing first-trimester screening. *Ultrasound Obstet Gynecol* 43:265–271. 2014.

Petit F, Holder-Espinasse M, Duban-Bedu B, et al. Trisomy 7 mosaicism prenatally misdiagnosed and maternal uniparental disomy in a child with pigmentary mosaicism and Russell- Silver syndrome. *Clin Genet* 81:265–271, 2012.

Petrova E, Neuner C, Haaf T, et al. A boy with an LCR3/4-flanked 10q22.3q23.2 microdeletion and uncommon phenotypic features. *Mol Syndromol* 5:19–24, 2014.

PetrykA, Kanakatti Shankar R, Giri N, et al. Endocrine disorders in Fanconi anemia: Recommendations for screening and treatment. *J Clin Endocrinol Metab* 100:803–811, 2015.

Pettenati MJ, Rao PN, Phelan MC, et al. Paracentric inversions in humans: A review of 446 paracentric inversions with presentation of 120 new cases. *Am J Med Genet* 55:171–187, 1995.

Pettenati MJ, Rao PN, Weaver RG, Thomas IT, McMahan MR. Inversion (X)(p11.4q22) associated with Norrie disease in a four generation family. *Am J Med Genet* 45:577–580, 1993.

Pettenati MJ, Von Kap-Herr C, Jackle B, et al. Rapid interphase analysis for prenatal diagnosis of translocation carriers using subtelomeric probes. *Prenat Diagn* 22:193–197, 2002.

Pettenati MJ, Wheeler M, Bartlett DJ, et al. 45,X/47,XYY mosaicism: Clinical discrepancy between prenatally and postnatally diagnosed cases. *Am J Med Genet* 39:42–47, 1991.

Petter C, Moreira LMA, Riegel M. Towards new approaches to evaluate dynamic mosaicism in ring chromosome 13 syndrome. *Case Rep Genet* 2019:7250838, 2019.

Pettersson M, Grochowski CM, Wincent J, et al. Cytogenetically visible inversions are formed by multiple molecular mechanisms. *Hum Mutat* 41:1979–1998, 2020.

Peycheva V, Kamenarova K, Ivanova N, et al. Chromosomal microarray analysis of Bulgarian patients with epilepsy and intellectual disability. *Gene* 667:45–55, 2018.

Pfeiffer RA, Loidl J. Mirror image duplications of chromosome 21. Three new cases and discussion of the mechanisms of origin. *Hum Genet* 62:361–363, 1982.

Pflueger S, Golden J, Troiano R, Gasparini R, Marini T. Fission of familial (13;22) Robertsonian translocation resulting in fetal mosaicism. *Am J Hum Genet* 49:283, 1991.

Pham J, Shaw C, Pursley A, et al. Somatic mosaicism detected by exon-targeted, high-resolution aCGH in 10,362 consecutive cases. *Eur J Hum Genet* 22:969–978, 2014.

Phelan MC, Crawford EC, Bealer DM. Mental retardation in South Carolina III: Chromosome aberrations. *Proc Greenwood Genet Center* 15:45–60, 1996.

Phelan MC, Rogers RC, Stevenson RE. Multiple, compound, and complex chromosome rearrangements. *Proc Greenwood Genet Center* 9:19–37, 1990.

Phelan MC, Stevenson RE, Anderson EV, Jr. Recombinant chromosome 9 possibly derived from breakage and reunion of sister chromatids within a paracentric inversion loop. *Am J Med Genet* 46:304–308, 1993.

Philipp T, Feichtinger W, Van Allen MI, Separovic E, Reiner A, Kalousek DK. Abnormal embryonic development diagnosed embryoscopically in early intrauterine deaths after in vitro fertilization: A preliminary report of 23 cases. *Fertil Steril* 82:1337–1342, 2004.

Philipp T, Philipp K, Reiner A, Beer F, Kalousek DK. Embryoscopic and cytogenetic analysis of 233 missed abortions: Factors involved in the pathogenesis of developmental defects of early failed pregnancies. *Hum Reprod* 18:1724–1732, 2003.

Phillips A, Borry P, Van Hoyweghen I, Vears DF. Disclosure of genetic information to family members: A systematic review of normative documents. *Genet Med* 23:2038–2046, 2021a.

Phillips EA, Caluseriu O, Schlade-Bartusiak K, Chernos J, McLeod DR, Thomas MA. Clinical and molecular characterization of an almost complete ring chromosome 4 in two sisters, with recurrence due to gonadal mosaicism. *Clin Dysmorphol* 30:173–176, 2021b.

Phillips OP, Tharapel AT, Lerner JL, Park VM, Wachtel SS, Shulman LP. Risk of fetal mosaicism when placental mosaicism is diagnosed by chorionic villus sampling. *Am J Obstet Gynecol* 174:850–855, 1996.

Phung V, Singh KE, Danon S, Tan CA, Dabagh S. Non-mosaic trisomy 22 and congenital heart surgery using the shared decision making model: A case report. *BMC Pediatr* 23:122, 2023.

Piard J, Mignot B, Arbez-Gindre F, et al. Severe sex differentiation disorder in a boy with a 3.8 Mb 10q25.3-q26.12 microdeletion encompassing *EMX2*. *Am J Med Genet* 164A:2618–2622, 2014.

Pignata L, Sparago A, Palumbo O, et al. Mosaic segmental and whole-chromosome upd(11)mat in Silver-Russell syndrome. *Genes (Basel)* 12:581, 2021.

Pinchefsky E, Laneuville L, Srour M. Distal 22q11.2 Microduplication: Case report and review of the literature. *Child Neurol Open* 4:2329048X17737651, 2017.

Pinho MJ, Neves R, Costa P, et al. Unique t(Y;1)(q12;q12) reciprocal translocation with loss of the heterochromatic region of chromosome 1 in a male with azoospermia due to meiotic arrest: A case report. *Hum Reprod* 20:689–696, 2005.

Pinto MR, Fonseca e Silva ML, Aguiar J, Quelhas I, Lima MR. Supernumerary ring chromosome 20 in a mother and her child. *Am J Med Genet* 133A:193–196, 2005.

Pinto-Escalante D, Ceballos-Quintal JM, Castillo-Zapata I, Canto-Herrera J. Full mosaic monosomy 22 in a child with DiGeorge syndrome facial appearance. *Am J Med Genet* 76:150–153, 1998.

Pinto Leite R, Pinto M. Prenatal detection of an inverted X chromosome in a male fetus. *Prenat Diagn* 21:233, 2001.

Pipiras E, Dupont C, Chantot-Bastaraud S, et al. Structural chromosomal mosaicism and prenatal diagnosis. *Prenat Diagn* 24:101–103, 2004.

Pires de Oliveira-Sobrinho R, Bispo LM, Heleno JL, Rojas Ayala FR, Reis F, Vieira TP, Steiner CE. Microdeletion 1p32p31 Presenting with Moyamoya Disease and Incomplete Hippocampal Inversion. *Mol Syndromol* 15:225–231, 2024.

Pirollo LM, Salehi LB, Sarta S, et al. A new case of prenatally diagnosed pentasomy X: Review of the literature. *Case Rep Obstet Gynecol* 2015:935202, 2015.

Pivnick EK, Wilroy RS, Summitt JB, Tucker B, Herrod HG, Tharapel AT. Adjacent-2 disjunction of a maternal t(9;22) leading to duplication 9pter→q22 and deficiency of 22pter→q11.2. *Am J Med Genet* 37:92–96, 1990.

Pizzo L, Andrieux J, Amor DJ, Girirajan S. Clinical utility gene card for: 16p12.2 microdeletion. *Eur J Hum Genet* 25, 2017.

Pizzo L, Jensen M, Polyak A, et al. Rare variants in the genetic background modulate cognitive and developmental phenotypes in individuals carrying disease-associated variants. *Genet Med* 21:816–825, 2019.

Plaisancié J, Bouneau L, Cances C, et al. Distal 10q monosomy: New evidence for a neurobehavioral condition? *Eur J Med Genet* 57:47–53, 2014.

Plaja A, Mediano C, Cano L, et al. Prenatal diagnosis of a rare chromosomal instability syndrome: Variegated aneuploidy related to premature centromere division (PCD). *Am J Med Genet* 117A:85–86, 2003.

Plesser Duvdevani M, Pettersson M, et al. Whole-genome sequencing reveals complex chromosome rearrangement disrupting NIPBL in infant with Cornelia de Lange syndrome. *Am J Med Genet* 182A:1143–1151, 2020.

Pober BR. Williams-Beuren syndrome. *N Engl J Med* 362:239–252, 2010.

Poirsier C, Landais E, Bednarek N, et al. Report on 3 patients with 12p duplication including *GRIN2B*. *Eur J Med Genet* 57:185–194, 2014.

Poland KS, Azim M, Folsom M, et al. A constitutional balanced t(3;8)(p14;q24.1) translocation results in disruption of the TRC8 gene and predisposition to clear cell renal cell carcinoma. *Genes Chromosomes Cancer* 46:805–812, 2007.

Politi C, Grillone K, Nocera D, et al. Non-invasive prenatal test analysis opens a Pandora's box: Identification of very rare cases of SRY-positive healthy females, segregating for three generations thanks to preferential inactivation of the XqYp translocated chromosome. *Genes (Basel)* 15:103, 2024.

Pollin TI, Dobyns WB, Crowe CA, Ledbetter DH, Bailey-Wilson JE, Smith AC. Risk of abnormal pregnancy outcome in carriers of balanced reciprocal translocations involving the Miller-Dieker syndrome (MDS) critical region in chromosome 17p13.3. *Am J Med Genet* 85:369–375, 1999.

Poluha A, Bernaciak J, Jaszczuk I, Kędzior M, Nowakowska BA. Molecular and clinical characterization of new patient with 1,08 Mb deletion in 10p15.3 region. *Mol Cytogenet* 10:34, 2017.

Poot M. Beware of hemizygous deletions that may unmask deleterious variants. *Mol Syndromol* 3:45–46, 2012.

Poot M, Haaf T. Mechanisms of origin, phenotypic effects and diagnostic Implications of complex chromosome rearrangements. *Mol Syndromol* 6:110–134, 2015.

Poot M, Hochstenbach R. Prevalence and phenotypic impact of Robertsonian translocations. *Mol Syndromol* 12:1–11, 2021.

Portoian-Shuhaiber S, Al-Awadi S, Farag TI, Sundareshan TS, Jindal HR, Al-Rashied AA. Clinical findings in an Arab boy with ring (14)(mos 46,XY,r(14)/45,XY,-14). *Ann Genet* 29:122–124, 1986.

Poszewiecka B, Gogolewski K, Karolak JA, Stankiewicz P, Gambin A. PhaseDancer: A novel targeted assembler of segmental duplications unravels the complexity of the human chromosome 2 fusion going from 48 to 46 chromosomes in hominin evolution. *Genome Biol* 24:205, 2023.

Potocki L, Chen KS, Park SS, et al. Molecular mechanism for duplication 17p11.2—The homologous recombination reciprocal of the Smith-Magenis microdeletion. *Nat Genet* 24:84–87, 2000.

Potok O, Schlade-Bartusiak K, Perrier R, et al. Paternal uniparental isodisomy for chromosome 14 in a child with normal karyotype, resulting from malsegregation of maternal Robertsonian translocation. *Eur J Hum Genet* 17 (Supp 2):P03.147, 2009.

Power S, Meaney S, O'Donoghue K. The incidence of fatal fetal anomalies associated with perinatal mortality in Ireland. *Prenat Diagn* 40:549–556, 2020.

Practice Committee of the American Society for Reproductive Medicine. Evaluation and treatment of recurrent pregnancy loss: A committee opinion. *Fertil Steril* 98:1103–1111, 2012.

Practice Committees of the American Society for Reproductive Medicine and the Genetic Counseling Professional Group. Clinical management of mosaic results from preimplantation genetic testing for aneuploidy of blastocysts: A committee opinion. *Fertil Steril* 120:973–982, 2023.

Pradhan M, Dalal A, Khan F, Agrawal S. Fertility in men with Down syndrome: A case report. *Fertil Steril* 86:1765, e1–3, 2006.

Prasad C, Wagstaff J. Genotype and phenotype in Angelman syndrome caused by paternal UPD 15. *Am J Med Genet* 70:328–329, 1997.

Prasasya R, Grotheer KV, Siracusa LD, Bartolomei MS. Temple syndrome and Kagami-Ogata syndrome: Clinical presentations, genotypes, models and mechanisms. *Hum Mol Genet* 29(R1):R107–R116, 2020.

Preis S, Majewski F. Monozygotic twins concordant for Rubinstein-Taybi syndrome: Changing phenotype during infancy. *Clin Genet* 48:72–75, 1995.

Presunto M, Mariana M, Lorigo M, Cairrao E. The effects of Bisphenol A on human male infertility: A review of current epidemiological studies. *Int J Mol Sci* 24:12417, 2023.

Price HA, Roberts SH, Laurence KM. Homozygous paracentric inversion 12 in a mentally retarded boy: A case report and review of the literature. *Hum Genet* 75:101–108, 1987.

Price N, Bahra M, Griffin D, Hanna G, Stock A. Cornelia de Lange Syndrome in association with a balanced reciprocal translocation involving chromosomes 3 and 5. *Prenat Diagn* 25:602–603, 2005.

Prieto F, Badia L, Asensi F, Roques V. Two reciprocal translocations t(9p+;13q-) and t(13q-;21q+): A study of the families. *Hum Genet* 54:7–11, 1980.

Priola V, De Vivo A, Imbesi G, Azzerboni A, Triolo O. Trisomy 9 associated with maternal serum screening results positive for trisomy 18: Case report and review of the literature. *Prenat Diagn* 27:1167–1169, 2007.

Priolo M, Schanze D, Tatton-Brown K, et al. Further delineation of Malan syndrome. *Hum Mutat* 39:1226–1237, 2018.

Pritchard MA, Kola I. The "gene dosage effect" hypothesis versus the "amplified developmental instability" hypothesis in Down syndrome. *J Neural Transm Suppl* 57:293–303, 1999.

Prontera P, Buldrini B, Aiello V, et al. Trisomy 15 mosaicism owing to familial reciprocal translocation t(1;15): Implication for prenatal diagnosis. *Prenat Diagn* 26:571–576, 2006.

Prontera P, Ottaviani V, Isidori I, Stangoni G, Donti E. Xq12-q13.3 duplication: Evidence of a recurrent syndrome. *Ann Neurol* 72:821–822, 2012.

Pruccoli J, Graziano C, Locatelli C, Maltoni L, Sheikh Maye HA, Cordelli DM. Expanding the neurological phenotype of ring chromosome 10 syndrome: A case report and review of the literature. *Genes (Basel)* 12:1513, 2021.

Puck MH. Some considerations bearing on the doctrine of self-fulfilling prophecy in sex chromosome aneuploidy. *Am J Med Genet* 9:129–137, 1981.

Punnett A, Teshima I, Heon E, et al. Unique insertional translocation in a childhood Wilms' tumor survivor detected when his daughter developed bilateral retinoblastoma. *Am J Med Genet* 120A:105–109, 2003.

Purandare SM, Lee J, Hassed S, et al. Ring chromosome 9 [r(9)(p24q34)]: A report of two cases. *Am J Med Genet* 138A:229–235, 2005.

Purvis-Smith SG, Saville T, Manass S, et al. Uniparental disomy 15 resulting from "correction" of an initial trisomy 15. *Am J Hum Genet* 50:1348–1350, 1992.

Putoux A, Labalme A, André JM, et al. Jacobsen and Beckwith-Wiedemann syndromes in a child with mosaicism for partial 11pter trisomy and partial 11qter monosomy. *Am J Med Genet* 161A:331–337, 2013.

Puvabanditsin S, Garrow E, Razi S, et al. A Y/15 translocation in a 45,X male with Prader-Willi syndrome. *Genet Couns* 18:417–421, 2007.

Pylyp L, Zukin V, Mykytenko D, Spinenko L. A rare non-Robertsonian translocation with chromosome fusion der(5;15)(q35.3;q10): Segregation analysis in male meiosis and preimplantation embryos. *Cytogenet Genome Res* 142:161–166, 2014.

Pynaker C, Hui L, Halliday J. *Annual report on Prenatal Diagnosis in Victoria 2023*, The Victorian Prenatal Diagnosis Database, Murdoch Children's Research Institute, 2024

Q

Qi Z, Jeng LJ, Slavotinek A, Yu J. Haploinsufficiency and triploinsensitivity of the same 6p25.1p24.3 region in a family. *BMC Med Genomics* 8:38, 2015.

Qian Y, Liu J, Yang Y, et al. Paternal low-level mosaicism caused *SATB2*-associated syndrome. *Front Genet* 10:630. 2019.

Qiao Y, Badduke C, Tang F, et al. Whole exome sequencing of families with 1q21.1 microdeletion or microduplication. *Am J Med Genet* 173A:1782–1791, 2017.

Qin S, Wang X, Wang J, et al. Verification of a cryptic t(Y;15) translocation in a male with an apparent 45,X karyotype. *Mol Cytogenet* 15:3, 2022.

Quack B, Speed RM, Luciani JM, Noel B, Guichaoua M, Chandley AC. Meiotic analysis of two human reciprocal X-autosome translocations. *Cytogenet Cell Genet* 48:43–47, 1988.

Quan F, Janas J, Toth-Fejel S, Johnson DB, Wolford JK, Popovich BW. Uniparental disomy of the entire X chromosome in a female with Duchenne muscular dystrophy. *Am J Hum Genet* 60:160–165, 1997.

Queipo G, Zenteno JC, Peña R, et al. Molecular analysis in true hermaphroditism: Demonstration of low-level hidden mosaicism for Y-derived sequences in 46,XX cases. *Hum Genet* 111:278–283, 2002.

Quenby S, Gallos ID, Dhillon-Smith RK, et al. Miscarriage matters: The epidemiological, physical, psychological, and economic costs of early pregnancy loss. *Lancet* 397:1658–1667, 2021.

Quentin S, Cuccuini W, Ceccaldi R, et al. Myelodysplasia and leukemia of Fanconi anemia are associated with a specific pattern of genomic abnormalities that includes cryptic RUNX1/AML1 lesions. *Blood* 117:e161–70, 2011.

Queralt R, Madrigal I, Vallecillos MA, et al. Atypical XX male with the *SRY* gene located at the long arm of chromosome 1 and a 1qter microdeletion. *Am J Med Genet* 146A:1335–1340, 2008.

Quigley DI, McDonald MT, Krishnamuthy V, et al. Triploid mosaicism in a 45,X/69,XXY infant. *Am J Med Genet* 138A:171–174, 2005.

Quinonez SC, Gelehrter TD, Uhlmann WR. A Marfan syndrome-like phenotype caused by a neocentromeric supernumerary ring chromosome 15. *Am J Med Genet* 173A:268–273, 2017a.

Quinonez SC, Hedera P, Barr M, et al. Maternal intrachromosomal insertional translocation leads to recurrent 1q21.3q23.3 deletion in two siblings. *Am J Med Genet* 158A:2591–2601, 2012.

Quinonez SC, Park JM, Rabah R, et al. 9p partial monosomy and disorders of sex development: Review and postulation of a pathogenetic mechanism. *Am J Med Genet* 161A:1882–1896, 2013.

Quinonez SC, Seeley AH, Lam C, Glover TW, Barshop BA, Keegan CE. Paracentric inversion of chromosome 21 leading to disruption of the *HLCS* gene in a family with holocarboxylase synthetase deficiency. *JIMD Rep* 34:55–61, 2017b.

Quiñones-Pérez B, VanNoy GE, Towne MC, et al. Three-generation family with novel contiguous gene deletion on chromosome 2p22 associated with thoracic aortic aneurysm syndrome. *Am J Med Genet* 176A:560–569, 2018.

Quintela I, Fernandez-Prieto M, Gomez-Guerrero L, et al. A 6q14.1-q15 microdeletion in a male patient with severe autistic disorder, lack of oral language, and dysmorphic features with concomitant presence of a maternally inherited Xp22.31 copy number gain. *Clin Case Rep* 3:415–423, 2015.

R

Raaby L, Lou S, Ivarsen RRL, Sørensen J, Larsen OH, Vogel I. Has the introduction of increased genetic prenatal testing affected rates of termination of pregnancy due to fetal abnormality? *Prenat Diagn* 44:280–288, 2024.

Raca G, Astbury C, Behlmann A, et al. Points to consider in the detection of germline structural variants using next-generation sequencing: A statement of the American College of Medical Genetics and Genomics. *Genet Med* 25:100316, 2023.

Radwan M, Wielgomas B, Dziewirska E, et al. Urinary bisphenol A levels and male fertility. *Am J Mens Health* 12:2144–2151, 2018.

Rafalko JM, Caldwell S, Tynan J, Almasri E, Weinblatt V, McCullough R. Impact of mosaicism ratio on positive predictive value of cfDNA screening. *Prenat Diagn* 41:28–34, 2021.

Rafii MS, Fortea J. Down Syndrome in a new era for Alzheimer disease. *JAMA* 330:2157–2158, 2023.

Rajangam S, Michaelis RC, Velagaleti GVN, et al. Down syndrome with biparental inheritance of der(14q21q) and maternally derived trisomy 21: Confirmation by fluorescent in situ hybridization and microsatellite polymorphism analysis. *Am J Med Genet* 70:43–47, 1997.

Rajcan-Separovic E, Robinson WP, Stephenson M, et al. Recurrent trisomy 15 in a female carrier of der(15)t(Y;15)(q12;p13). *Am J Med Genet* 99:320–324, 2001.

Rajesh H, Freckmann ML, Chapman M. Azoospermia and paternal autosomal ring chromosomes: Case report and literature review. *Reprod Biomed Online* 23:466–470, 2011.

Raleigh D, Nguyen M, Chen W, Zakimi N, Mirchia K, Lucas CH. Pan-cancer copy number variant analysis identifies optimized size thresholds and co-occurrence models for individualized risk-stratification. *Nat Commun* 16:6024, 2025.

Ralph A, Scott F, Tiernan C, et al. Maternal uniparental isodisomy for chromosome 14 detected prenatally. *Prenat Diagn* 19:681–684, 1999.

Ramalingam A, Zhou XG, Fiedler SD, et al. 16p13.11 duplication is a risk factor for a wide spectrum of neuropsychiatric disorders. *J Hum Genet* 56:541–544, 2011.

Ramírez-Velasco A, Rivera H. A further rec(X)dup p and compilation of 23 cases. Comment on "Molecular Genetic and Cytogenetic Characterization of a Partial Xp Duplication and Xq Deletion in a Patient with Premature Ovarian Failure" by Kim et al. *Gene* 548:155–157, 2014.

Ramsay L, Howe DT, Wellesley D. Parental attitude to participating in long-term follow-up studies of their children's health after in utero diagnosis of abnormalities. *Prenat Diagn* 29:207–212, 2009.

Rana B, Lambrese K, Mendola R, et al. Identifying parental and cell-division origins of aneuploidy in the human blastocyst. *Am J Hum Genet* 110:565–574, 2023.

Ranganath P, Agarwal M, Phadke SR. Angelman syndrome and prenatally diagnosed Prader-Willi syndrome in first cousins. *Am J Med Genet* 155A:2788–2790, 2011.

Rao R, Platt LD. Ultrasound screening: Status of markers and efficacy of screening for structural abnormalities. *Semin Perinatol* 40:67–78, 2016.

Rapp R. *Testing Women, Testing the Fetus: The Social Impact of Amniocentesis in America.* New York, NY: Routledge, 1999.

Ratcliffe S. Long-term outcome in children of sex chromosome abnormalities. *Arch Dis Child* 80:192–195, 1999.

Ratcliffe SG, Butler GE, Jones M. Edinburgh study of growth and development of children with sex chromosome abnormalities: IV. *Birth Defects Orig Artic Ser* 26:1–44, 1990.

Rath A, Sethi P, Jena SK, Mitra S. Familial recurrent molar pregnancy: Positive for KHDC3L gene mutation. *BMJ Case Rep* 16:e254435, 2023.

Rauen KA, Bitts SM, Li L, Golabi M, Cotter PD. Tandem duplication mosaicism: Characterization of a mosaic dup(5q) and review. *Clin Genet* 60:366–370, 2001.

Rauen KA, Golabi M, Cotter PD. Fertility in a female with mosaic trisomy 8. *Fertil Steril* 79:206–208, 2003.

Raun N, Mailo J, Spinelli E, et al. Quantitative phenotypic and network analysis of 1q44 microdeletion for microcephaly. *Am J Med Genet* 173A:972–977, 2017.

Ravaei A, Emanuele M, Nazzaro G, Fadiga L, Rubini M. Placental DNA methylation profile as predicting marker for autism spectrum disorder (ASD). *Mol Med* 29:8, 2023.

Ravel C, Berthaut I, Bresson JL, Siffroi JP. Prevalence of chromosomal abnormalities in phenotypically normal and fertile adult males: Large-scale survey of over 10,000 sperm donor karyotypes. *Hum Reprod* 21:1484–1489, 2006a.

Ravel C, Chantot-Bastaraud S, Siffroi JP, Escalier D, Antoine JM, Mandelbaum J. Tail stump syndrome associated with chromosomal translocation in two brothers attempting intracytoplasmic sperm injection. *Fertil Steril* 86:719, e1–7, 2006b.

Raziel A, Friedler S, Schachter M, Kasterstein E, Strassburger D, Ron-El R. Increased frequency of female partner chromosomal abnormalities in patients with high-order implantation failure after in vitro fertilization. *Fertil Steril* 78:515–519, 2002.

Raznahan A, Won H, Glahn DC, Jacquemont S. Convergence and divergence of rare genetic disorders on brain phenotypes: A review. *JAMA Psychiatry*, 79:818–828, 2022.

Redaelli S, Maitz S, Crosti F, et al. Refining the phenotype of recurrent rearrangements of chromosome 16. *Int J Mol Sci* 20:1095, 2019.

Redaelli S, Sala E, Roncaglia N, et al. Severe intrauterine growth restriction and trisomy 15 confined placental mosaicism: A case report and review of literature. *Prenat Diagn* 25:140–147, 2005.

Reddy KS. Double trisomy in spontaneous abortions. *Hum Genet* 101:339–345, 1997.

Reddy KS. The conundrum of a jumping translocation (JT) in CVS from twins and review of JTs. *Am J Med Genet* 152A:2924–2936, 2010.

Reddy KS, Sulcova V. Pathogenetics of 45,X/46,XY gonadal mosaicism. *Cytogenet Cell Genet* 82:52–57, 1998.

Reddy KS, Sulcova V, Siassi B. Two sibs with Wolf-Hirschhorn and DiGeorge deletions resulting from an unbalanced chromosome rearrangement, 45,XX/XY, der(4)t(4;22) (p16.3;q11.2) mat,-22. *J Med Genet* 33:852–855, 1996.

Reddy UM, Page GP, Saade GR, et al. Karyotype versus microarray testing for genetic abnormalities after stillbirth. *N Engl J Med* 367:2185–2193, 2012.

Redin C, Brand H, Collins RL, et al. The genomic landscape of balanced cytogenetic abnormalities associated with human congenital anomalies. *Nat Genet*, 49:36–45, 2017.

Rees E, Kirov G. Copy number variation and neuropsychiatric illness. *Curr Opin Genet Dev* 68:57–63, 2021.

Rees E, Walters JT, Chambert KD, et al. CNV analysis in a large schizophrenia sample implicates deletions at 16p12.1 and SLC1A1 and duplications at 1p36.33 and *CGNL1*. *Hum Mol Genet* 23:1669–1676, 2014.

Regal JA, Festerling TA, Buis JM, Ferguson DO. Disease-associated MRE11 mutants impact ATM/ATR DNA damage signaling by distinct mechanisms. *Hum Mol Genet* 22:5146–5159, 2013.

Regan L, Rai R, Saravelos S, Li TC; Royal College of Obstetricians and Gynaecologists. Recurrent miscarriage green-top guideline No. 17. *BJOG* 130:e9–e39, 2023.

Reid R, Sepulveda W, Kyle PM, Davies G. Amniotic fluid culture failure: Clinical significance and association with aneuploidy. *Obstet Gynecol* 87:588–592, 1996.

Reimers R, High F, Kremen J, Wilkins-Haug L. Prenatal diagnosis of sex chromosome aneuploidy-What do we tell the prospective parents? *Prenat Diagn* 43:250–260, 2023.

Reinehr T, Jauch A, Zoll B, Engel U, Bartels I, Andler W. Short stature in a mother and daughter caused by familial der(X)t(X;X)(p22.1–3;q26). *Am J Med Genet* 102:81–85, 2001.

Reish O, Wolach B, Amiel A, Kedar I, Dolfin T, Fejgin M. Dilemma of trisomy 20 mosaicism detected prenatally: Is it an innocent finding? *Am J Med Genet* 77:72–75, 1998.

Reiss AL, Freund L, Plotnick L, et al. The effects of X monosomy on brain development: Monozygotic twins discordant for Turner's syndrome. *Ann Neurol* 34:95–107, 1993.

Reittinger AM, Helm BM, Boles DJ, Gadi IK, Schrier Vergano SA. A prenatal diagnosis of mosaic trisomy 5 reveals a postnatal complete uniparental disomy of chromosome 5 with multiple congenital anomalies. *Am J Med Genet* 173A:2528–2533, 2017.

Ren H, Chow V, Ma S. Meiotic behaviour and sperm aneuploidy in an infertile man with a mosaic 45,X/46,XY karyotype. *Reprod Biomed Online* 31:783–789, 2015.

Ren S, Haynes E, Hall E, et al. Periconception exposure to air pollution and risk of congenital malformations. *J Pediatr* 193:76–84.e6, 2018.

Rendeiro P, Gonçalves R, Freixo JP, et al. A case of parental transmission of Koolen-de Vries syndrome. Poster presented at the American College of Medical Genetics meeting, Tampa, 2016.

Rendtorff ND, Karstensen HG, Lodahl M, et al. Identification and analysis of deletion breakpoints in four Mohr-Tranebjærg syndrome (MTS) patients. *Sci Rep* 12:14959, 2022.

Renshaw R, Ellis K, Jacobs P, Morris J. Antenatal screening for Down syndrome: A quantitative demonstration of the improvements over the past 20 years. *J Health Serv Res Policy* 18:195–201, 2013.

Rentmeester CA. Value neutrality in genetic counseling: An unattained ideal. *Med Health Care Philos* 4:47–51, 2001.

Repnikova EA, Astbury C, Reshmi SC, et al. Microarray comparative genomic hybridization and cytogenetic characterization of tissue-specific mosaicism in three patients. *Am J Med Genet* 158A:1924–1933, 2012.

Resnicow K, Delacroix E, Chen G, et al. Motivational interviewing for genetic counseling: A unified framework for persuasive and equipoise conversations. *J Genet Couns* 31:1020–1031, 2022.

Rethoré MO, Blois MC, Peeters M, Popowski P, Pangalos C, Lejeune J. Pure partial trisomy of the short arm of chromosome 5. *Hum Genet* 82:296–298, 1989.

Revah-Politi A, Ganapathi M, Bier L, et al. Loss-of-function variants in *NFIA* provide further support that *NFIA* is a critical gene in 1p32-p31 deletion syndrome: A four patient series. *Am J Med Genet* 173A:3158–3164, 2017.

Ribeiro Dias Barroso C, Silveira Gomes L, Abrantes Silvestre V, Yamada Utagawa C. Cutis tricolor parvimaculata in ring chromosome 15 syndrome: A case report. *Pediatr Dermatol* 35:e204–e205, 2018.

Riccaboni A, Lalatta F, Caliari I, Bonetti S, Somigliana E, Ragni G. Genetic screening in 2,710 infertile candidate couples for assisted reproductive techniques: Results of application of Italian guidelines for the appropriate use of genetic tests. *Fertil Steril* 89:800–808, 2008.

Ricciardello A, Tomaiuolo P, Persico AM. Genotype-phenotype correlation in Phelan-McDermid syndrome: A comprehensive review of chromosome 22q13 deleted genes. *Am J Med Genet* 185A:2211–2233, 2021.

Rice AM, McLysaght A. Dosage sensitivity is a major determinant of human copy number variant pathogenicity. *Nat Commun* 8:14366, 2017.

Richards S, Aziz N, Bale S, et al. Standards and guidelines for the interpretation of sequence variants: A joint consensus recommendation of the American College of Medical Genetics and Genomics and the Association for Molecular Pathology. *Genet Med* 17:405–424, 2015.

Rickman L, Fiegler H, Shaw-Smith C, et al. Prenatal detection of unbalanced chromosomal rearrangements by array CGH. *J Med Genet* 43:353–361, 2006.

Ried T, Schröck E, Ning Y, Wienberg J. Chromosome painting: A useful art. *Hum Mol Genet* 7:1619–1626, 1998.

Riegel M, Wisser J, Baumer A, Schinzel A. Postzygotic isochromosome formation as a cause for false-negative results from chorionic villus chromosome examinations. *Prenat Diagn* 26:221–225, 2006.

Rieger M, Krumbiegel M, Reuter MS, Schützenberger A, Reis A, Zweier C. 7q31.2q31.31 deletion downstream of FOXP2 segregating in a family with speech and language disorder. *Am J Med Genet* 182A:2737–2741, 2020.

Riehmer V, Erger F, Herkenrath P, et al. A heritable microduplication encompassing *TBL1XR1* causes a genomic sister-disorder for the 3q26.32 microdeletion syndrome. *Am J Med Genet* 173A:2132–2138, 2017.

Rieubland C, Francis D, Houben L, Corrie S, Bankier A, White SM. Two cases of trisomy 16 mosaicism ascertained postnatally. *Am J Med Genet* 149A:1523–1528, 2009.

Riggan KA, Gross B, Close S, Weinberg A, Allyse MA. Prenatal genetic diagnosis of a sex chromosome aneuploidy: Parent experiences. *J Genet Couns* 30:1407–1417, 2021.

Riggan KA, Ormond KE, Allyse MA, Close S. Evidence-based recommendations for delivering the diagnosis of X & Y chromosome multisomies in children, adolescents, and young adults: An integrative review. *BMC Pediatr* 24:263, 2024.

Riggs ER, Andersen EF, Cherry AM, et al. Technical standards for the interpretation and reporting of constitutional copy-number variants: A joint consensus recommendation of the American College of Medical Genetics and Genomics (ACMG) and the Clinical Genome Resource (ClinGen). *Genet Med* 22:245–257, 2020.

Rigola MA, Baena N, Català V, et al. A 11.7-Mb paracentric Inversion in chromosome 1q detected in prenatal diagnosis associated with familial intellectual disability. *Cytogenet Genome Res* 146:109–114, 2015.

Riley KN, Catalano LM, Bernat JA, et al. Recurrent deletions and duplications of chromosome 2q11.2 and 2q13 are associated with variable outcomes. *Am J Med Genet* 167A:2664–2673, 2015.

Rim JH, Kim JA, Yoo J. A novel 1.13 Mb interstitial duplication at 19q13.32 causing developmental delay and microcephaly in a pediatric patient: The first Asian case reports. *Yonsei Med J* 58:1241–1244, 2017.

Rink BD, Norton ME. Screening for fetal aneuploidy. *Semin Perinatol* 40:35–43, 2016.

Ritter DI, Haines K, Cheung H, et al. Identifying gene disruptions in novel balanced de novo constitutional translocations in childhood cancer patients by whole-genome sequencing. *Genet Med* 17:831–835, 2015.

Rittinger O, Krabichler B, Kronberger G, Kotzot D. Clinical, cytogenetic, and molecular findings in a patient with a 46,XX,del(18)(q22)/46,XX,idic(18)(q22) karyotype. *Eur J Med Genet* 58:603–607, 2015.

Rivas F, García-Esquivel L, Rivera H, Jimenez ME, Gonzalez RM, Cantú JM. Inv(4)(p16q21): A five-generation pedigree with 24 carriers and no recombinants. *Clin Genet* 31:97–101, 1987.

Rivera H, Cantú JM. Centric fission consequences in man. *Ann Génét* 29:223–225, 1986.

Rivera H, Domínguez MG, Vásquez-Velásquez AI, Lurie IW. De novo dup p/del q or dup q/del p rearranged chromosomes: Review of 104 cases of a distinct chromosomal mutation. *Cytogenet Genome Res* 141:58–63, 2013.

Rives N, Walschaerts M, Setif V, et al. Sperm aneuploidy after testicular cancer treatment: Data from a prospective multicenter study performed within the French Centre d'Étude et de Conservation des Oeufs et du Sperme network. *Fertil Steril* 107:580–588.e1, 2017.

Rives N, Siméon N, Milazzo JP, Barthélémy C, Macé B. Meiotic segregation of sex chromosomes in mosaic and non-mosaic XYY males: Case reports and review of the literature. *Int J Androl* 26:242–249, 2003.

Robbins WA, Vine MF, Truong KY, Everson RB. Use of fluorescence in situ hybridization (FISH) to assess effects of smoking, caffeine, and alcohol on aneuploidy load in sperm of healthy men. *Environ Mol Mutagen* 30:175–183, 1997.

Roberts E, Dunlop J, Davis GS, Churchill D, Davison EV. A further case of confined placental mosaicism for trisomy 2 associated with adverse pregnancy outcome. *Prenat Diagn* 23:564–565, 2003.

Roberts JL, Buckley RH, Luo B, et al. CD45-deficient severe combined immunodeficiency caused by uniparental disomy. *Proc Natl Acad Sci USA* 109:10456–10461, 2012.

Roberts P, Williams J, Sills MA. A case of two inversion (10) recombinants in a family. *J Med Genet* 26:461–464, 1989.

Robertson S, Savulescu J. Is there a case in favour of predictive genetic testing in young children? *Bioethics* 15:26–49, 2001.

Robilliard R, Caylan M. Infantile presentation of 3q26.33–3q27.2 deletion syndrome. *BMJ Case Rep* 13:e233215, 2020.

Robinson A, Bender BG, Borelli JB, Puck MH, Salbenblatt JA, Winter JSD. Sex chromosomal aneuploidy: Prospective and longitudinal studies. *Birth Defects Orig Artic Ser* 22:23–71, 1986.

Robinson A, Bender BG, Linden MG, Salbenblatt JA. Sex chromosome aneuploidy: The Denver Prospective Study. *Birth Defects Orig Artic Ser* 26:59–115, 1990.

Robinson WP, Barrett IJ, Bernard L, et al. Meiotic origin of trisomy in confined placental mosaicism is correlated with presence of fetal uniparental disomy, high levels of trisomy in trophoblast, and increased risk of fetal intrauterine growth restriction. *Am J Hum Genet* 60:917–927, 1997.

Robinson WP, Bernasconi F, Basaran S, et al. A somatic origin of homologous Robertsonian translocations and isochromosomes. *Am J Hum Genet* 54:290–302, 1994.

Robinson WP, Bernasconi F, Lau A, McFadden DE. Frequency of meiotic trisomy depends on involved chromosome and mode of ascertainment. *Am J Med Genet* 84:34–42, 1999.

Robinson WP, Binkert F, Bernasconi F, Lorda-Sánchez I, Werder EA, Schinzel AA. Molecular studies of chromosomal mosaicism: Relative frequency of chromosome gain or loss and possible role of cell selection. *Am J Hum Genet* 56:444–451, 1995.

Robinson WP, Binkert F, Gine R, et al. Clinical and molecular analysis of five inv dup(15) patients. *Eur J Hum Genet* 1:37–50, 1993.

Robinson WP, Christian SL, Kuchinka BD, et al. Somatic segregation errors predominantly contribute to the gain or loss of a paternal chromosome leading to uniparental disomy for chromosome 15. *Clin Genet* 57:349–358, 2000.

Robinson WP, Kuchinka BD, Bernasconi F, et al. Maternal meiosis I non-disjunction of chromosome 15: Dependence of the maternal age effect on level of recombination. *Hum Mol Genet* 7:1011–1019, 1998.
Robinson WP, McFadden DE, Barrett IJ, et al. Origin of amnion and implications for evaluation of the fetal genotype in cases of mosaicism. *Prenat Diagn* 22:1076–1085, 2002.
Robinson WP, McFadden DE, Stephenson MD. The origin of abnormalities in recurrent aneuploidy/polyploidy. *Am J Hum Genet* 69:1245–1254, 2001.
Robinson WP, McGillivray B, Friedman JM. Pregnancy and postnatal outcome of mosaic isochromosome 20q. *Prenat Diagn* 27:143–145, 2007.
Robinson WP, McGillivray B, Lewis ME, Arbour L, Barrett I, Kalousek DK. Prenatally detected trisomy 20 mosaicism. *Prenat Diagn* 25:239–244, 2005.
Rodrigo L, Peinado V, Mateu E, et al. Impact of different patterns of sperm chromosomal abnormalities on the chromosomal constitution of preimplantation embryos. *Fertil Steril* 94:1380–1386, 2010.
Rodriguez JD, Bhat SS, Meloni I, et al. Intellectual disability, midface hypoplasia, facial hypotonia, and Alport syndrome are associated with a deletion in Xq22.3. *Am J Med Genet* 152A:713–717, 2010.
Rodríguez L, Diego-Alvarez D, Lorda-Sánchez I, et al. A small and active ring X chromosome in a female with features of Kabuki syndrome. *Am J Med Genet* 146A:2816–2821, 2008.
Rodrigues Alves Barbosa V, Maroilley T, Diao C, Colvin-James L, Perrier R, Tarailo-Graovac M. Single variant, yet "double trouble": TSC and KBG syndrome because of a large de novo inversion. *Life Sci Alliance* 22:e202302115, 2024.
Rodriguez-Purata J, Lee J, Whitehouse M, et al. Embryo selection versus natural selection: How do outcomes of comprehensive chromosome screening of blastocysts compare with the analysis of products of conception from early pregnancy loss (dilation and curettage) among an assisted reproductive technology population? *Fertil Steril* 104:1460–1466.e1–12, 2015.
Rodriguez-Revenga L, Badenas C, Madrigal I, et al. 46,XY,18q+/46,XY,18q- mosaicism in a fragile X prenatal diagnosis. *Prenat Diagn* 25:448–450, 2005.
Rogers JC, Harris DJ, Pasztor LM. Reciprocal translocation 4;11 with both adjacent-1 segregants viable within a family. *Clin Genet* 51:250–256, 1997.
Rogers JF. Clinical delineation of proximal and distal partial 13q trisomy. *Clin Genet* 25:221–229, 1984.
Rogers JG, Voullaire L, Gold H. Monozygotic twins discordant for trisomy 21. *Am J Med Genet* 11:143–146, 1982.
Rogers R, Mardy A. Chorionic villous testing versus amniocentesis after abnormal noninvasive prenatal testing. *Clin Obstet Gynecol* 66:595–606, 2023.
Rohrback S, Siddoway B, Liu CS, Chun J. Genomic mosaicism in the developing and adult brain. *Dev Neurobiol* 78:1026–1048, 2018.
Romain DR, Columbano-Green LM, Whyte S, et al. Familial paracentric inversion of 1p. *Am J Med Genet* 14:629–634, 1983.
Romanelli V, Meneses HN, Fernández L, et al. Beckwith-Wiedemann syndrome and uniparental disomy 11p: Fine mapping of the recombination breakpoints and evaluation of several techniques. *Eur J Hum Genet* 19:416–421, 2011.
Romano C, Ferranti S, Mencarelli MA, Longo I, Renieri A, Grosso S. 17p13.3 microdeletion including YWHAE and CRK genes: Towards a clinical characterization. *Neurol Sci* 41:2259–2262, 2020.
Ronzoni L, Grassi FS, Pezzani L, et al. 7p22.1 microduplication syndrome: Refinement of the critical region. *Eur J Med Genet* 60:114–117, 2017.
Rooney DE (Ed.) *Human Cytogenetics: Constitutional Analysis*, 3rd Edn. Oxford University Press, 2023.
Röpke A, Kalinski T, Mohnike K, et al. Distribution of sex chromosomes in dysgenetic gonads of mixed type. *Cytogenet Genome Res* 116:146–151, 2007.
Rose CSP, Patel P, Reardon W, Malcolm S, Winter RM. The *TWIST* gene, although not disrupted in Saethre-Chotzen patients with apparently balanced translocations of 7p21, is mutated in familial and sporadic cases. *Hum Mol Genet* 6:1369–1373, 1997.
Rosenberg AGW, Wellink CM, Tellez Garcia JM, et al. Health problems in adults with Prader-Willi syndrome of different genetic subtypes: Cohort study, meta-analysis and review of the literature. *J Clin Med* 11:4033, 2022.
Rosenbusch B, Schneider M, Gläser B, Brucker C. Cytogenetic analysis of giant oocytes and zygotes to assess their relevance for the development of digynic triploidy. *Hum Reprod* 17:2388–2393, 2002.
Rosenfeld JA, Coe BP, Eichler EE, Cuckle H, Shaffer LG. Estimates of penetrance for recurrent pathogenic copy-number variations, *Genet Med* 15:478–481, 2013.
Rosenkrantz JL, Carbone L. Investigating somatic aneuploidy in the brain: Why we need a new model. *Chromosoma* 126:337–350, 2017.

Rossi E, Messa J, Zuffardi O. Ring syndrome: Still true? *J Med Genet* 45:766–768, 2008.
Rossi C, Siffroi JP, Ruosso L, et al. Chromosomal segregation analysis and HOST-based sperm selection in a complex reciprocal translocation carrier. *J Assist Reprod Genet* 40:33–40, 2023.
Rothenmund H, Chudley AE, Dawson AJ. Familial transmission of a small supernumerary marker chromosome 8 identified by FISH: An update. *Am J Med Genet* 72:339–342, 1997.
Röthlisberger B, Kotzot D. Recurrence risk in de novo structural chromosomal rearrangements. *Am J Med Genet* 143A:1708–1714, 2007.
Röthlisberger B, Kotzot D, Brecevic L, et al. Recombinant balanced and unbalanced translocations as a consequence of a balanced complex chromosomal rearrangement involving eight breakpoints in four chromosomes. *Eur J Hum Genet* 7:873–883, 1999.
Rothman BK. *The Tentative Pregnancy: Prenatal Diagnosis and the Future of Motherhood*. London, UK: Pandora Press, 1988.
Rots D, Rooney K, Relator R, et al. Refining the 9q34.3 microduplication syndrome reveals mild neurodevelopmental features associated with a distinct global DNA methylation profile. *Clin Genet* 105:655–660, 2024.
Rougeulle C, Lalande M. Angelman syndrome: How many genes to remain silent? *Neurogenet* 1:229–237, 1998.
Rovet J, Netley C, Bailey J, Keenan M, Stewart D. Intelligence and achievement in children with extra X aneuploidy: A longitudinal perspective. *Am J Med Genet* 60:356–363, 1995.
Rowland RE, Edwards LA, Podd JV. Elevated sister chromatid exchange frequencies in New Zealand Vietnam War veterans. *Cytogenet Genome Res* 116:248–251, 2007.
Roy SF, Bastian BC, Maguiness S, et al. Multiple desmoplastic Spitz nevi with BRAF fusions in a patient with ring chromosome 7 syndrome. *Pigment Cell Melanoma Res* 34:987–993, 2012.
Rubio C, Simón C, Vidal F, et al. Chromosomal abnormalities and embryo development in recurrent miscarriage couples. *Hum Reprod* 18:182–188, 2003.
Rudnicka AR, Wald NJ, Huttly W, Hackshaw AK. Influence of maternal smoking on the birth prevalence of Down syndrome and on second trimester screening performance. *Prenat Diagn* 22:893–897, 2002.
Ruggeri A, Dulcetti F, Miozzo M, et al. Prenatal search for UPD 14 and UPD 15 in 83 cases of familial and de novo heterologous Robertsonian translocations. *Prenat Diagn* 24:997–1000, 2004.
Rumpler Y. Meiotic studies in animal models. *Ann Génét* 44:s18, 2001.
Rusconi D, Negri G, Colapietro P, et al. Characterization of 14 novel deletions underlying Rubinstein-Taybi syndrome: An update of the *CREBBP* deletion repertoire. *Hum Genet* 134:613–626, 2015.
Russell LM, Strike P, Browne CE, Jacobs PA. X chromosome loss and ageing. *Cytogenet Genome Res* 116:181–185, 2007.
Russo S, Finelli P, Recalcati MP, et al. Molecular and genomic characterisation of cryptic chromosomal alterations leading to paternal duplication of the 11p15.5 Beckwith-Wiedemann region. *J Med Genet* 43:e39, 2006.
Ryu SW, Yoon JH, Kim DW, et al. Identification of a complex intrachromosomal inverted insertion in the long arm of chromosome 9 as a cause of tuberous sclerosis complex in a Korean family. *Mol Genet Genomic Med* 12:e2330, 2024.

S

Sá R, Ferraz L, Barros A, Sousa M. The Klinefelter syndrome and testicular sperm retrieval outcomes. *Genes (Basel)* 14:647, 2023.
Saal HM, Harbison MD, Netchine I. Silver-Russell Syndrome. In: Adam MP, Feldman J, Mirzaa GM, et al. (eds.), *GeneReviews*. University of Washington, Seattle; 1993–2024.
Saadallah N, Hultén M. A complex three breakpoint translocation involving chromosomes 2, 4, and 9 identified by meiotic investigations of a human male ascertained for subfertility. *Hum Genet* 71:312–320, 1985.
Sabatini PJB, Ejaz R, Stavropoulos DJ, Mendoza-Londono R, Joseph-George AM. Stable transmission of an unbalanced chromosome 21 derived from chromoanasynthesis in a patient with a *SYNGAP1* likely pathogenic variant. *Mol Cytogenet* 11:50, 2018.
Sabbaghian M, Meybodi AM, Rahimian M, Sadighi Gilani MA. Occurrence of 47,X,-(X)(q10),Y Klinefelter variant with hypogonadotropic hypogonadism. *Fertil Steril* 96:e115–117, 2011.
Sacharow S, Li D, Fan YS, Tekin M. Familial 16q24.3 microdeletion involving *ANKRD11* causes a KBG-like syndrome. *Am J Med Genet* 158A:547–552, 2012.
Sachs ES, Jahoda MGJ, Los FJ, Pijpers L, Wladimiroff JW. Trisomy 21 mosaicism in gonads with unexpectedly high recurrence risks. *Am J Med Genet Suppl* 7:186–188, 1990.
Sagi-Dain L, Goldberg Y, Peleg A, et al. The rare 13q33-q34 microdeletions: Eight new patients and review of the literature. *Hum Genet* 138:1145–1153, 2019.

Sago H, Chen E, Conte WJ, et al. True trisomy 2 mosaicism in amniocytes and newborn liver associated with multiple system abnormalities. *Am J Med Genet* 72:343–346, 1997.

Sahinturk S, Ozemri Sag S, Ture M, et al. A fertile patient with 45X/47XXX mosaicism. *Genet Couns* 26:29–34, 2015.

Sahnane N, Bernasconi B, Carnevali I, et al. Disruption of the *APC* gene by t(5;7) translocation in a Turcot family. *Cancer Genet* 209:107–111,2016.

Sahoo T, Bacino CA, German JR, et al. Identification of novel deletions of 15q11q13 in Angelman syndrome by array-CGH: Molecular characterization and genotype-phenotype correlations. *Eur J Hum Genet* 15:943–949, 2007.

Sahoo T, Theisen A, Sanchez-Lara PA, et al. Microdeletion 20p12.3 involving *BMP2* contributes to syndromic forms of cleft palate. *Am J Med Genet* 155A:1646–1653, 2011.

Sahraeean S, Jebelli A, Shahbazi Z, Piryaei F. Homozygosity for Robertsonian translocation (14q;15q) in a newborn with a familial history of recurrent Abortion and newborns affected by hepatosplenomegaly: A case report. *J Reprod Infertil* 24:301–305, 2023.

Saitoh S, Buiting K, Cassidy SB, et al. Clinical spectrum and molecular diagnosis of Angelman and Prader-Willi syndrome patients with an imprinting mutation. *Am J Med Genet* 68:195–206, 1997.

Saitta SC, Harris SE, McDonald-McGinn DM, et al. Independent de novo 22q11.2 deletions in first cousins with DiGeorge/velocardiofacial syndrome. *Am J Med Genet* 124A:313–317, 2004.

Sakakibara Y, Hashimoto S, Nakaoka Y, Kouznetsova A, Höög C, Kitajima TS. Bivalent separation into univalents precedes age-related meiosis I errors in oocytes. *Nat Commun* 6:7550, 2015.

Sakazume S, Kido Y, Murakami N, Matsubara T, Numabe H. Additional patients with 4q deletion: Severe growth delay and polycystic kidney disease associated with 4q21q22 loss. *Pediatr Int* 57:880–883, 2015.

Salari N, Rasoulpoor S, Rasoulpoor S, et al. The global prevalence of autism spectrum disorder: A comprehensive systematic review and meta-analysis. *Ital J Pediatr* 48:112, 2022.

Salima S, Wibowo MH, Dewayani BM, Nisa AS, Alkaff FF. Recurrent partial hydatidiform mole: A case report of seven consecutive molar pregnancies. *Int J Womens Health* 15:1239–1244, 2023.

Salo P, Ignatius J, Simola KOJ, Tahvanainen E, Kaariainen H. Clinical features of nine males with molecularly defined deletions of the Y chromosome long arm. *J Med Genet* 32:711–715, 1995.

Salomon LJ, Bernard JP, Nizard J, Ville Y. First-trimester screening for fetal triploidy at 11 to 14 weeks: A role for fetal biometry. *Prenat Diagn* 25:479–483, 2005.

Salpietro V, Manole A, Efthymiou S, Houlden H. A review of copy number variants in inherited neuropathies. *Curr Genomics* 19:412–419, 2018.

Salpietro V, Ruggieri M, Mankad K, et al. A de novo 0.63 Mb 6q25.1 deletion associated with growth failure, congenital heart defect, underdeveloped cerebellar vermis, abnormal cutaneous elasticity and joint laxity. *Am J Med Genet* 167A:2042–2051, 2015.

Salzano E, Raible SE, Kaur M, et al. Prenatal profile of Pallister-Killian syndrome: Retrospective analysis of 114 pregnancies, literature review and approach to prenatal diagnosis. *Am J Med Genet* 176A:2575–2586, 2018.

Samango-Sprouse CA, Hamzik MP, Gropman E, et al. The behavioral profile of 49,XXXXY and the potential impact of testosterone replacement therapy. *Genet Med* 25:100847, 2023.

Samango-Sprouse C, Kirkizlar E, Hall MP, et al. Incidence of X and Y chromosomal aneuploidy in a large child bearing population. *PLoS One* 11:e0161045, 2016.

Samarasekera T, Willats E, Green MP, Hardy T, Rombauts L, Zander-Fox D. Impact of male age on paternal aneuploidy: Single-nucleotide polymorphism microarray outcomes following blastocyst biopsy. *Reprod Biomed Online* 47:103245, 2023.

Samplaski MK, Lo KC, Grober ED, Millar A, Dimitromanolakis A, Jarvi KA. Phenotypic differences in mosaic Klinefelter patients as compared with non-mosaic Klinefelter patients. *Fertil Steril* 101:950–955, 2014.

Sampson A, de Crespigny LC. Vanishing twins: The frequency of spontaneous fetal reduction of a twin pregnancy. *Ultrasound Obstet Gynecol* 2:107–109, 1992.

Sams EI, Ng JK, Tate V, et al. From karyotypes to precision genomics in 9p deletion and duplication syndromes. *HGG Adv* 3:100081, 2021.

Samura O, Nakaoka Y, Miharu N. Sperm and oocyte chromosomal abnormalities. *Biomolecules* 13:1010, 2023.

Sánchez J, Fernández R, Madruga M, Bernabeu-Wittel J, Antiñolo G, Borrego S. Somatic and germ-line mosaicism of deletion 15q11.2-q13 in a mother of dyzigotic twins with Angelman syndrome. *Am J Med Genet* 164A:370–376, 2014.

Sánchez-Herrero Á, Carmona-Talavera D, García-Verdevio ME, Hernando-Espinilla A, Estañ-Capell N. Mosaic trisomy 5: Prenatal genetic diagnosis and outcomes of a new case. *J Pediatr Genet* 12:64–68, 2020.

Sánchez Marín JP, García González E. Dilemas bioéticos en diagnóstico prenatal: Test prenatal no invasivo y nuevas tecnologías. *Cuad Bioet* 34:219–232, 2023.
Sanderson B, Leach C, Zein M, et al. Bilateral severe microphthalmia in a neonate with trisomy 8 mosaicism: A new finding. *Am J Med Genet* 185A:534–538, 2021.
Sandrin-Garcia P, Macedo C, Martelli LR, et al. Recurrent 22q11.2 deletion in a sibship suggestive of parental germline mosaicism in velocardiofacial syndrome. *Clin Genet* 61:380–383, 2002.
Sang Q, Zhou Z, Mu J, Wang L. Genetic factors as potential molecular markers of human oocyte and embryo quality. *J Assist Reprod Genet* 38:993–1002, 2021.
Sanlaville D, Prieur M, de Blois MC, et al. Functional disomy of the Xq28 chromosome region. *Eur J Hum Genet* 13:579–585, 2005.
Sano S, Thel MC, Walsh K. Mosaic loss of Y chromosome in white blood cells: Its impact on men's health. *Physiology (Bethesda)* 38:0, 2023.
Santorum M, Wright D, Syngelaki A, Karagioti N, Nicolaides KH. Accuracy of first-trimester combined test in screening for trisomies 21, 18 and 13. *Ultrasound Obstet Gynecol* 49:714–720, 2017.
Sarno AP, Moorman AJ, Kalousek DK. Partial molar pregnancy with fetal survival: An unusual example of confined placental mosaicism. *Obstet Gynecol* 82:716–719, 1993.
Sarri C, Douzgou S, Kontos H, et al. 35-year follow-up of a case of ring chromosome 2: Array-CGH analysis and literature review of the ring syndrome. *Cytogenet Genome Res* 145:6–13, 2015.
Sasaki T, Tonoki H, Soejima H, Niikawa N. A 4 Mb cryptic deletion associated with inv(8)(q13.1q24.11) in a patient with trichorhinophalangeal syndrome type I. *J Med Genet* 34:335–339, 1997.
Sasi R, Senft J, Spruill M, Rej S, Perrotta PL. Double Robertsonian translocations in an infertile patient with macrocytic anemia: A case report. *Mol Cytogenet* 13:14, 2020.
Sato K, Iwakoshi M, Shimokawa O, et al. Angelman syndrome caused by an identical familial 1,487-kb deletion. *Am J Med Genet* 143:98–101, 2007.
Saura R, Longy M, Serville F, Chokairi O, Froute MF. Abnormal phenotype in a child with a "balanced" translocation 8/12 in mosaic state. *Am J Med Genet* 28:1021–1023, 1987.
Saura R, Traore W, Taine L, et al. Prenatal diagnosis of trisomy 9. Six cases and a review of the literature. *Prenat Diagn* 15:609–614, 1995.
Savage AR, Petersen MB, Pettay D, et al. Elucidating the mechanisms of paternal non-disjunction of chromosome 21 in humans. *Hum Mol Genet* 7:1221–1227, 1998.
Savarese M, Grandone A, Perone L, et al. Familial trisomy 6p in mother and daughter. *Am J Med Genet* 161A:1675–1681, 2013.
Savarirayan R, Bankier A. Acampomelic campomelic dysplasia with de novo 5q;17q reciprocal translocation and severe phenotype. *J Med Genet* 35:597–599, 1998.
Savulescu J, Kahane G. The moral obligation to create children with the best chance of the best life. *Bioethics* 23:274–290, 2009.
Savva GM, Morris JK, Mutton DE, Alberman E. Maternal age-specific fetal loss rates in Down syndrome pregnancies. *Prenat Diagn* 26:499–504, 2006.
Savva GM, Walker K, Morris JK. The maternal age-specific live birth prevalence of trisomies 13 and 18 compared to trisomy 21 (Down syndrome). *Prenat Diagn* 30:57–64, 2010.
Sawyer JR, Sammartino G, Husain M, Linskey ME. Constitutional t(16;22)(p13.3;q11.2 approximately 12) in a primitive neuroectodermal tumor of the pineal region. *Cancer Genet Cytogenet* 142:73–76, 2003.
Sawyer JR, Swanson CM, Wheeler G, Cunniff C. Chromosome instability in ICF syndrome: Formation of micronuclei from multibranched chromosomes 1 demonstrated by fluorescence in situ hybridization. *Am J Med Genet* 56:203–209, 1995.
Saxov KR, Strandberg-Larsen K, Pristed SG, Bruun NH, Kesmodel US. Maternal alcohol consumption and the risk of miscarriage in the first and second trimesters: A systematic review and dose-response meta-analysis. *Acta Obstet Gynecol Scand* 102:821–832, 2023.
Scala M, Bradley CA, Howe JL, et al. Genetic variants in DDX53 contribute to autism spectrum disorder associated with the Xp22.11 locus. *Am J Hum Genet* 112:154–167, 2025.
Scarff KL, Flowers N, Love CJ, et al. Performance of a cell-free DNA prenatal screening test, choice of prenatal procedure, and chromosome conditions identified during pregnancy after low-risk cell-free DNA screening. *Prenat Diagn* 43:213–225. 2023.
Schaaf CP, Wiszniewska J, Beaudet AL. Copy number and SNP arrays in clinical diagnostics. *Annu Rev Genomics Hum Genet* 12:25–51, 2011.
Schaap AHP, van der Pol HG, Boer K, Leschot NJ, Wolf H. Long-term follow-up of infants after transcervical chorionic villus sampling and after amniocentesis to compare congenital abnormalities and health status. *Prenat Diagn* 22:598–604, 2002.

Schecter A, Constable JD. Commentary: Agent Orange and birth defects in Vietnam. *Int J Epidemiol* 35:1230–1232, 2006.
Scherer S, *Guide to the Human Genome*, Cold Spring Harbor Laboratory Press, Woodbury: New York, 2010.
Scherer SW, Gripp KW, Lucena J, et al. Observation of a parental inversion variant in a rare Williams-Beuren syndrome family with two affected children. *Hum Genet* 117:383–388, 2005.
Scheuvens R, Begemann M, Soellner L, et al. Maternal uniparental disomy of chromosome 16 (upd(16)mat): Clinical features are rather caused by (hidden) trisomy 16 mosaicism than by upd(16)mat itself. *Clin Genet* 92:45–51, 2017.
Schinzel A. *Catalogue of Unbalanced Chromosome Aberrations in Man.* New York, NY: de Gruyter, 2001.
Schinzel AA, Adelsberger PA, Binkert F, Basaran S, Antonarakis SE. No evidence for a paternal interchromosomal effect from analysis of the origin of nondisjunction in Down syndrome patients with concomitant familial chromosome rearrangements. *Am J Hum Genet* 50:288–293, 1992.
Schinzel AA, Riegel M, Baumer A, et al. Long-term follow-up of four patients with Langer-Giedion syndrome: Clinical course and complications. *Am J Med Genet* 161A:2216–2225, 2013.
Schinzel AA, Robinson WP, Binkert F, Torresani T, Werder EA. Exclusively paternal X chromosomes in a girl with short stature. *Hum Genet* 92:175–178, 1993.
Schlessel JS, Brown WT, Lysikiewicz A, Schiff R, Zaslav AL. Monozygotic twins with trisomy 18: A report of discordant phenotype. *J Med Genet* 27:640–642, 1990.
Schluth-Bolard C, Sanlaville D, Labalme A, et al. Unexpected diagnosis of 45,X/47,XX,+18 mosaicism in a girl with mild phenotype. *Am J Med Genet* 149A:2584–2587, 2009.
Schluth-Bolard C, Sanlaville D, Labalme A, et al. 17p13.1 microdeletion involving the *TP53* gene in a boy presenting with mental retardation but no tumor. *Am J Med Genet* 152A:1278–1282, 2010.
Schluth-Bolard C, Till M, Rafat A, et al. Monosomy 19pter and trisomy 19q13-qter in two siblings arising from a maternal pericentric inversion: Clinical data and molecular characterization. *Eur J Med Genet* 51:622–630, 2008.
Schmickel RD. Contiguous gene syndromes: A component of recognizable syndromes. *J Pediatr* 109:231–241, 1986.
Schmidt L, Münster K. Infertility, involuntary infecundity, and the seeking of medical advice in industrialized countries 1970–1992: A review of concepts, measurements and results. *Hum Reprod* 10:1407–1418, 1995.
Schmidt M, Du Sart D. Functional disomies of the X chromosome influence the cell selection and hence the X inactivation pattern in females with balanced X-autosome translocations: A review of 122 cases. *Am J Med Genet* 42:161–169, 1992.
Schmidt T, Bartels I, Liehr T, Burfeind P, Zoll B, Shoukier M. A family with an inverted tandem duplication 5q22.1q23.2. *Cytogenet Genome Res* 139:65–70, 2013
Schmitt-Ney M, Thiele H, Kaltwasser P, Bardoni B, Cisternino M, Scherer G. Two novel *SRY* missense mutations reducing DNA binding identified in XY females and their mosaic fathers. *Am J Hum Genet* 56:862–869, 1995.
Schmutz SM, Pinno E. Morphology alone does not make an isochromosome. *Hum Genet* 72:253–255, 1986.
Schnabel F, Smogavec M, Funke R, Pauli S, Burfeind P, Bartels I. Down syndrome phenotype in a boy with a mosaic microduplication of chromosome 21q22. *Mol Cytogenet* 11:62, 2018.
Schneider M, Forrester S, Crain V, Kimonis V. A further case of coincidental Prader-Willi and Klinefelter syndromes. *Am J Med Genet* 126A:213–214, 2004.
Schoemaker MJ, Jones ME, Higgins CD, Wright AF; United Kingdom Clinical Cytogenetics Group; Swerdlow AJ. Mortality and cancer incidence in carriers of balanced Robertsonian translocations: A national cohort study. *Am J Epidemiol* 188:500–508, 2019.
Scholz NB, Bolund L, Nyegaard M, et al. Triploidy—Observations in 154 diandric cases. *PLoS One* 10:e0142545, 2015.
Schönewolf-Greulich B, Ravn K, Hamborg-Petersen B, Brøndum-Nielsen K, Tümer Z. Segregation of a 4p16.3 duplication with a characteristic appearance, macrocephaly, speech delay and mild intellectual disability in a 3-generation family. *Am J Med Genet* 161A:2358–2362, 2013.
Schönherr N, Meyer E, Roos A, Schmidt A, Wollmann HA, Eggermann T. The centromeric 11p15 imprinting centre is also involved in Silver-Russell syndrome. *J Med Genet* 44:59–63, 2007.
Schoolcraft WB, Keller JL, Schlenker T. Excellent embryo quality obtained from vitrified oocytes. *Reprod Biomed Online* 19:820–823, 2009.
Schorderet DF, Friedman C, Disteche CM. Pericentric inversion of the X chromosome: Presentation of a case and review of the literature. *Ann Génét* 34:98–103, 1991.

Schouten JP, McElgunn CJ, Waaijer R, Zwijnenburg D, Diepvens F, Pals G. Relative quantification of 40 nucleic acid sequences by multiplex ligation-dependent probe amplification. *Nucleic Acids Res* 30:e57, 2002.

Schubert T, Schaaf CP. MAGEL2 (patho-)physiology and Schaaf-Yang syndrome. *Dev Med Child Neurol* 67:35–48, 2025.

Schüle B, Albalwi M, Northrop E, et al. Molecular breakpoint cloning and gene expression studies of a novel translocation t(4;15)(q27;q11.2) associated with Prader-Willi syndrome. *BMC Med Genet* 6:18, 2005.

Schull WJ, Neel JV. Maternal radiation and mongolism. *Lancet* 279:537–538, 1962.

Schultz LM, Knighton A, Huguet G, et al. Copy-number variants differ in frequency across genetic ancestry groups. *HGG Adv* 5:100340, 2024.

Schwartz S, Raffel LJ. Prenatal detection of 45,X/46,XX/47,XXX mosaicism through amniocentesis: Mosaicism confirmed in cord blood, amnion, and chorion. *Prenat Diagn* 12:1043–1046, 1992.

Schwarzbraun T, Obenauf AC, Langmann A, et al. Predictive diagnosis of the cancer prone Li-Fraumeni syndrome by accident: New challenges through whole genome array testing. *J Med Genet* 46:341–344, 2009.

Schwendemann WD, Contag SA, Wax JR, et al. Sonographic findings in trisomy 9. *J Ultrasound Med* 28:39–42, 2009.

Schwinger E, Mikkelsen M, Niesen M. Familial balanced (7;11;21) translocation and Down's syndrome in two siblings. *Clin Genet* 7:304–307, 1975.

Sciurano RB, Rahn IM, González Arias B, et al. Selective advantage of euploid spermatocytes I in an azoospermic 47,XYY man with gonadal mosaicism. *Hum Reprod* 34:568–573, 2019.

Scott DA, Gofin Y, Berry AM, Adams AD. Underlying genetic etiologies of congenital diaphragmatic hernia. *Prenat Diagn* 42:373–386, 2022.

Scott JA, Wenger SL, Steele MW, Chakravarti A. Down syndrome consequent to a cryptic maternal 12p;21q chromosome translocation. *Am J Med Genet* 56:67–71, 1995.

Scott M, Watermeyer J, Wessels TM. "We are just not sure what that means or if it's relevant": Uncertainty when gathering family history information in South African prenatal genetic counselling consultations. *Soc Sci Med* 342:116555, 2024.

Scott RH, Douglas J, Baskcomb L, et al. Constitutional 11p15 abnormalities, including heritable imprinting center mutations, cause nonsyndromic Wilms tumor. *Nat Genet* 40:1329–1334, 2008a.

Scott RH, Douglas J, Baskcomb L, et al. Methylation-specific MLPA (MS-MLPA) robustly detects and distinguishes 11p15 abnormalities associated with overgrowth and growth retardation. *J Med Genet* 45:106–113, 2008b.

Scott Schwoerer J, Laffin J, Haun J, Raca G, Friez MJ, Giampietro PF. MECP2 duplication: Possible cause of severe phenotype in females. *Am J Med Genet* 164A:1029–1034, 2014.

Scriven PN. X;autosome translocations do not follow the normal rules and more caution is advised for PGD. *Hum Reprod Online* November 2013, in response to Van Echten-Arends et al., Preimplantation genetic diagnosis for X; autosome translocations: Lessons from a case of misdiagnosis. *Hum Reprod* 28:3141–3145, 2013.

Scriven PN, Bint SM, Davies AF, Ogilvie CM. Meiotic outcomes of three-way translocations ascertained in cleavage-stage embryos: Refinement of reproductive risks and implications for PGD. *Eur J Hum Genet* 22:748–753, 2014.

Scriven PN, Flinter FA, Braude PR, Ogilvie CM. Robertsonian translocations--reproductive risks and indications for preimplantation genetic diagnosis. *Hum Reprod* 16:2267–2273, 2001.

Scriven PN, Handyside AH, Mackie Ogilvie C. Chromosome translocations: Segregation modes and strategies for preimplantation genetic diagnosis. *Prenat Diagn* 18:1437–1449, 1998.

Scuffins J, Keller-Ramey J, Dyer L, et al. Uniparental disomy in a population of 32,067 clinical exome trios. *Genet Med* 23:1101–1107, 2021.

Sebold C, Soileau B, Heard P, et al. Whole arm deletions of 18p: Medical and developmental effects. *Am J Med Genet* 167A:313–323, 2015.

Sedat J, McDonald A, Cang H, et al. A proposed unified interphase nucleus chromosome structure: Preliminary preponderance of evidence. *Proc Natl Acad Sci USA* 119:e2119101119, 2022.

Seemanová E, Sperling K, Neitzel H, et al. Nijmegen breakage syndrome (NBS) with neurological abnormalities and without chromosomal instability. *J Med Genet* 43:218–224, 2006.

Sefik E, Duan K, Li Y, Sholar B, et al. Structural deviations of the posterior fossa and the cerebellum and their cognitive links in a neurodevelopmental deletion syndrome. *Mol Psychiatry* 29:3395–3411, 2024.

Segarra-Casas A, Yépez VA, Demidov G, et al. An integrated transcriptomics and genomics approach detects an X/autosome translocation in a female with Duchenne muscular dystrophy. *Int J Mol Sci* 25:7793, 2024.

Shohat M, Legum C, Romem Y, Borochowitz Z, Bach G, Goldman B. Down syndrome prevention program in a population with an older maternal age. *Obstet Gynecol* 85:368–373, 1995.
Shuib S, McMullan D, Rattenberry E, et al. Microarray based analysis of 3p25-p26 deletions (3p- syndrome). *Am J Med Genet* 149A:2099–2105, 2009.
Shuman C, Kalish JM, Weksberg R. Beckwith-Wiedemann Syndrome. In: Adam MP, Feldman J, Mirzaa GM, et al. (eds.), *GeneReviews*. University of Washington, Seattle, 1993–2024.
Shuster E. Microarray genetic screening: A prenatal roadblock for life? *Lancet* 369:526–529, 2007.
Shuttleworth GE. Mongolian imbecility. *Br Med J* 2:661–665, 1909.
Sifakis S, Eleftheriades M, Kappou D, et al. Prenatal diagnosis of proximal partial trisomy 1q confirmed by comparative genomic hybridization array: Molecular cytogenetic analysis, fetal pathology and review of the literature. *Birth Defects Res A Clin Mol Teratol* 100:284–293, 2014.
Sifakis S, Karkaletsi M, Christopoulou S, et al. Distinctive pattern of first trimester maternal serum biochemical markers in trisomy 22 pregnancies. *Prenat Diagn* 28:1174–1176, 2008.
Siggberg L, Ala-Mello S, Jaakkola E, et al. Array CGH in molecular diagnosis of mental retardation—A study of 150 Finnish patients. *Am J Med Genet* 152A:1398–1410, 2010.
Signorello LB, Mulvihill JJ, Green DM, et al. Congenital anomalies in the children of cancer survivors: A report from the childhood cancer survivor study. *J Clin Oncol* 30:239–245, 2012.
Sigurdardottir S, Goodman BK, Rutberg J, Thomas GH, Jabs EW, Geraghty MT. Clinical, cytogenetic, and fluorescence in situ hybridization findings in two cases of "complete ring" syndrome. *Am J Med Genet* 87:384–390, 1999.
Sigurdson AJ, Bhatti P, Preston DL, et al. Routine diagnostic X-ray examinations and increased frequency of chromosome translocations among U.S. radiologic technologists. *Cancer Res* 68:8825–8831, 2008.
Sijmons RH, Leegte B, van Lingen RA, et al. Tetrasomy 5p mosaicism in a boy with delayed growth, hypotonia, minor anomalies, and an additional isochromosome 5p [46,XY/47,XY, + i(5p)]. *Am J Med Genet* 47:559–562, 1993.
Sikkema-Raddatz B, Bouman K, Verschuuren-Bemelmans CC, de Jong B. Trisomy 12 mosaicism in CVS culture confirmed in the fetus. *Prenat Diagn* 19:1176–1177, 1999.
Sikkema-Raddatz B, Castedo S, Te Meerman GJ. Probability tables for exclusion of mosaicism in prenatal diagnosis. *Prenat Diagn* 17:115–118, 1997a.
Sikkema-Raddatz B, Verschuuren-Bemelmans CC, Kloosterman M, de Jong B. A 46,XX,der(13;14)(q10;q10),+21 child born after a 45,XX,der(13;14)(q10;q10) chromosomal finding in CVS. *Prenat Diagn* 17:1086–1088, 1997b.
Silipigni R, Milani D, Tolva G, et al. Complex genomic alterations and intellectual disability: An interpretative challenge. *J Intellect Disabil Res* 65:113–124, 2021.
Silipigni R, Monfrini E, Baccarin M, et al. Familial duplication/deletion of 1q42.13q43 as meiotic consequence of an intrachromosomal insertion in chromosome 1. *Cytogenet Genome Res* 153:73–80, 2017.
Silverstein S, Lerer I, Sagi M, Frumkin A, Ben-Neriah Z, Abeliovich D. Uniparental disomy in fetuses diagnosed with balanced Robertsonian translocations: Risk estimate. *Prenat Diagn* 22:649–651, 2002.
Simón C, Rubio C, Vidal F, et al. Increased chromosome abnormalities in human preimplantation embryos after in-vitro fertilization in patients with recurrent miscarriage. *Reprod Fertil Dev* 10:87–92, 1998.
Simonstein F, Mashiach-Eizenberg M. Attitudes toward autism spectrum disorders among students of allied health professions. *J Genet Couns* 25:1276–1285, 2016.
Simopoulou M, Sfakianoudis K, Maziotis E, et al. PGT-A: Who and when? A systematic review and network meta-analysis of RCTs. *J Assist Reprod Genet* 38:1939–1957, 2021.
Simsek L, Zamani AG, Taskapu HH, Yildirim MS. A rare case in literature: Isochromosome Xq in Klinefelter syndrome. *Andrologia* 51:e13253, 2019.
Singer S, Gazou A, Sturm M, et al. New euchromatic variant dup(11)(p15.3p15.1) transmitted through two generations defined by low coverage whole genome sequencing. *Am J Med Genet* 185A:3053–3056, 2021.
Singh P, Fragoza R, Blengini CS, et al. Human MLH1/3 variants causing aneuploidy, pregnancy loss, and premature reproductive aging. *Nat Commun* 12:5005, 2021.
Singh R, Gardner RJM, Crossland KM, Scheffer IE, Berkovic SF. Chromosomal abnormalities and epilepsy: A review for clinicians and gene hunters. *Epilepsia* 43:127–140, 2002a.
Singh SM, Murphy B, O'Reilly R. Monozygotic twins with chromosome 22q11 deletion and discordant phenotypes: Updates with an epigenetic hypothesis. *J Med Genet* 39:e71, 2002b.

Sinnerbrink IB, Sherwen A, Meiser B, et al. Long-term health and development of children diagnosed prenatally with a de novo apparently balanced chromosomal rearrangement. *Prenat Diagn* 33:831–838, 2013.

Šípek A, Panczak A, Mihalová R, et al. Pericentric inversion of human chromosome 9 epidemiology study in Czech males and females. *Folia Biol (Praha)* 61:140–146, 2015.

Sirchia SM, Garagiola I, Colucci G, et al. Trisomic zygote rescue revealed by DNA polymorphism analysis in confined placental mosaicism. *Prenat Diagn* 18:201–206, 1998.

Sirera Sirera P, García-Payá E, Olivas García J, Jadraque Rodríguez R, Hernández Romero SD. Maternally inherited deletion encompassing the RTL1as and MEG8 genes of the human 14q32 imprinted region in a patient with a mild Kagami-Ogata syndrome phenotype. *Am J Med Genet* 191A:2225–2231, 2023.

Sismani C, Anastasiadou V, Kousoulidou L, et al. 9 Mb familial duplication in chromosome band Xp22.2–22.13 associated with mental retardation, hypotonia and developmental delay, scoliosis, cardiovascular problems and mild dysmorphic facial features. *Eur J Med Genet* 54:e510–515, 2011.

Sismani C, Rapti SM, Iliopoulou P, et al. Novel pericentric inversion inv(9)(p23q22.3) in unrelated individuals with fertility problems in the Southeast European population. *J Hum Genet* 65:783–795, 2020.

Sivasankaran A, Murthy K, Oruganti VP, Deenadayalu A, R, Samuel C, Kandukuri LR. De-novo 'pure' partial trisomy (6)(p22.3→pter): A case report and review of the literature. *Clin Dysmorphol* 26:26–32, 2017.

Sklower Brooks SS, Genovese M, Gu H, Duncan CJ, Shanske A, Jenkins EC. Normal adaptive function with learning disability in duplication 8p including band p22. *Am J Med Genet* 78:114–117, 1998.

Skotko BG, Kishnani PS, Capone GT. Prenatal diagnosis of Down syndrome: How best to deliver the news. *Am J Med Genet* 149A:2361–2367, 2009.

Skraban CM, Wells CF, Markose P, et al. *WDR26* haploinsufficiency causes a recognizable syndrome of intellectual disability, seizures, abnormal gait, and distinctive facial features. *Am J Hum Genet* 101:139–148, 2017.

Skuse DH, James RS, Bishop DVM, et al. Evidence from Turner's syndrome of an imprinted X-linked locus affecting cognitive function. *Nature* 387:705–708, 1997.

Slaney SF, Chalmers IJ, Affara NA, Chitty LS. An autosomal or X linked mutation results in true hermaphrodites and 46,XX males in the same family. *J Med Genet* 35:17–22, 1998.

Slater H, Bruno D, Ren H, et al. Improved testing for CMT1A and HNPP using multiplex ligation-dependent probe amplification (MLPA) with rapid DNA preparations: Comparison with the interphase FISH method. *Hum Mutat* 24:164–171, 2004.

Slater H, Shaw JH, Bankier A, Forrest SM, Dawson G. UPD 13: No indication of maternal or paternal imprinting of genes on chromosome 13. *J Med Genet* 32:493, 1995.

Slater H, Shaw JH, Dawson G, Bankier A, Forrest SM. Maternal uniparental disomy of chromosome 13 in a phenotypically normal child. *J Med Genet* 31:644–646, 1994.

Slater HR, Nouri S, Earle E, Lo AW, Hale LG, Choo KHA. Neocentromere formation in a stable ring 1p32-p36.1 chromosome. *J Med Genet* 36:914–918, 1999.

Slater HR, Ralph A, Daniel A, Worthington S, Roberts C. A case of maternal uniparental disomy of chromosome 9 diagnosed prenatally and the related problem of residual trisomy. *Prenat Diagn* 20:930–932, 2000.

Slavotinek A, Gaunt L, Donnai D. Paternally inherited duplications of 11p15.5 and Beckwith-Wiedemann syndrome. *J Med Genet* 34:819–826, 1997.

Slavotinek A, Misceo D, Htun S, et al. Biallelic variants in the RNA exosome gene EXOSC5 are associated with developmental delays, short stature, cerebellar hypoplasia and motor weakness. *Hum Mol Genet* 29:2218–2239, 2020.

Slim R, Fisher R, Milhavet F, et al. Biallelic NLRP7 variants in patients with recurrent hydatidiform mole: A review and expert consensus. *Hum Mutat* 43:1732–1744, 2022.

Slimani W, Jelloul A, Al-Rikabi A, et al. Small supernumerary marker chromosomes (sSMC) and male infertility: Characterization of five new cases, review of the literature, and perspectives. *J Assist Reprod Genet* 37:1729–1736, 2020.

Sloboda N, Sorlin A, Valduga M, et al. Deletion of chr7p22 and chr15q11: Two familial cases of immune deficiency: Extending the phenotype toward dysimmunity. *Front Immunol* 10:1871, 2019.

Sloter E, Nath J, Eskenazi B, Wyrobek AJ. Effects of male age on the frequencies of germinal and heritable chromosomal abnormalities in humans and rodents. *Fertil Steril* 81:925–943, 2004.

Smajlagić D, Lavrichenko K, Berland S, et al. Population prevalence and inheritance pattern of recurrent CNVs associated with neurodevelopmental disorders in 12,252 newborns and their parents. *Eur J Hum Genet* 29:205–215, 2021.

Smeets DFCM, Hamel BCJ, Nelen MR, et al. Prader-Willi syndrome and Angelman syndrome in cousins from a family with a translocation between chromosomes 6 and 15. *N Engl J Med* 326:807–811, 1992.

Smith A, Deng ZM, Beran R, Woodage T, Trent RJ. Familial unbalanced translocation t(8;15)(p23.3;q11) with uniparental disomy in Angelman syndrome. *Hum Genet* 93:471–473, 1994.

Smith A, Robson L. Low frequency of inherited deletions of 22q11. *Am J Med Genet* 85:513–514, 1999.

Smith A, Watt AJ, Cummins M, Gardner RJM, Wilson M. A small one-band paracentric inversion inv (4) (p15.3p16.3). *Ann Génét* 35:161–163, 1992.

Smith ACM, Spuhler K, Williams TM, McConnell T, Sujansky E, Robinson A. Genetic risk for recombinant 8 syndrome and the transmission rate of balanced inversion 8 in the Hispanic population of the southwestern United States. *Am J Hum Genet* 41:1083–1103, 1987.

Smith CS, Riddell M, Badalato L, Au PYB. Adults with paternal UPD14 causing Kagami-Ogata syndrome: Case report and review of the literature. *Am J Med Genet* 194A:e63625, 2024.

Smith K, Lowther G, Maher E, Hourihan T, Wilkinson T, Wolstenholme J. The predictive value of findings of the common aneuploidies, trisomies 13, 18 and 21, and numerical sex chromosome abnormalities at CVS: Experience from the ACC U.K. collaborative study. *Prenat Diagn* 19:817–826, 1999.

Smith PS, Whitworth J, West H, et al. Characterization of renal cell carcinoma-associated constitutional chromosome abnormalities by genome sequencing. *Genes Chromosomes Cancer* 59:333–347, 2020.

Smolen C, Jensen M, Dyer L, et al. Assortative mating and parental genetic relatedness contribute to the pathogenicity of variably expressive variants. *Am J Hum Genet* 110:2015–2028, 2023.

Smrcek JM, Germer U, Krokowski M, et al. Prenatal ultrasound diagnosis and management of body stalk anomaly: Analysis of nine singleton and two multiple pregnancies. *Ultrasound Obstet Gynecol* 21:322–328, 2003.

Snijders AM, Nowak N, Segraves R, et al. Assembly of microarrays for genome-wide measurement of DNA copy number. *Nat Genet* 29:263–264, 2001.

Snijders RJM, Sebire NJ, Nicolaides KH. Maternal age and gestational age-specific risk for chromosomal defects. *Fetal Diagn Ther* 10:356–367, 1995.

Sobotka V, Vozdova M, Heracek J, Rubes J. A rare Robertsonian translocation rob(14;22) carrier with azoospermia, meiotic defects, and testicular sperm aneuploidy. *Syst Biol Reprod Med* 61:245–250, 2015.

Söderström-Anttila V, Pinborg A, Karnis MF, Reindollar RH, Paulson RJ. Should women with Turner syndrome be allowed to carry their own pregnancies? *Fertil Steril* 112:220–225, 2019.

Sodré CP, Guilherme RS, Meloni VF, et al. Ring chromosome instability evaluation in six patients with autosomal rings. *Genet Mol Res* 9:134–143, 2010.

Soemedi R, Topf A, Wilson IJ, et al. Phenotype-specific effect of chromosome 1q21.1 rearrangements and GJA5 duplications in 2436 congenital heart disease patients and 6760 controls. *Hum Mol Genet* 21:1513–1520, 2012.

Sohn YB, Lee CG, Ko JM, et al. Clinical and genetic spectrum of 18 unrelated Korean patients with Sotos syndrome: Frequent 5q35 microdeletion and identification of four novel *NSD1* mutations. *J Hum Genet* 58:73–77, 2013.

Soileau B, Hasi M, Sebold C, et al. Adults with chromosome 18 abnormalities. *J Genet Couns* 24:663–674, 2015.

Solé M, Blanco J, Valero O, Vergés L, Vidal F, Sarrate Z. Altered bivalent positioning in metaphase I human spermatocytes from Robertsonian translocation carriers. *J Assist Reprod Genet* 34:131–138, 2017.

Soler A, Badenas C, Margarit E, Madrigal I, Muñoz M, Borobio V, Sánchez A. A 92,XXXY miscarriage consecutive to a digynic triploid pregnancy. *Cytogenet Genome Res* 149:258–261, 2016.

Soler A, Margarit E, Queralt R, et al. Paternal isodisomy 13 in a normal newborn infant after trisomy rescue evidenced by prenatal diagnosis. *Am J Med Genet* 90:291–293, 2000.

Soler A, Salami C, Balmes I, et al. Pericentric X chromosome in a family. *Clin Genet* 20:234–235, 1981.

Soler A, Sánchez A, Carrió A, et al. Recombination in a male carrier of two reciprocal translocations involving chromosomes 14, 14', 15, and 21 leading to balanced and unbalanced rearrangements in offspring. *Am J Med Genet* 134A:309–314, 2005.

Soler-Alfonso C, Carvalho CM, Ge J, et al. CHRNA7 triplication associated with cognitive impairment and neuropsychiatric phenotypes in a three-generation pedigree. *Eur J Hum Genet* 22:1071–1076, 2014.

Soliani L, Alcalá San Martín A, Balsells S, Hernando-Davalillo C, Ortigoza-Escobar JD. Chromosome microarray analysis for the investigation of deletions in pediatric movement disorders: A systematic review of the literature. *Mov Disord Clin Pract* 10:547–557, 2023.

Somers CM, Cooper DN. Air pollution and mutations in the germline: Are humans at risk? *Hum Genet* 125:119–130, 2009.

Somprasit C, Aguinaga M, Cisneros PL, et al. Paternal gonadal mosaicism detected in a couple with recurrent abortions undergoing PGD: FISH analysis of sperm nuclei proves valuable. *Reprod Biomed Online* 9:225–230, 2004.

Sønderby IE, van der Meer D, Moreau C, et al. 1q21.1 distal copy number variants are associated with cerebral and cognitive alterations in humans. *Transl Psychiatry* 11:182, 2021.

Song IG, Shin SH, Cho YM, Lim Y. Survival of children with trisomy 18 associated with the presence of congenital heart disease and intervention in the Republic of Korea. *BMC Pediatr* 23:252, 2023.

Song J, Li X, Sun L, et al. A family with Robertsonian translocation: A potential mechanism of speciation in humans. *Mol Cytogenet* 9:48, 2016.

Sossey-Alaoui K, Su G, Malaj E, Roe B, Cowell JK. WAVE3, an actin-polymerization gene, is truncated and inactivated as a result of a constitutional t(1;13)(q21;q12) chromosome translocation in a patient with ganglioneuroblastoma. *Oncogene* 21:5967–74, 2002.

South ST, Rope AF, Lamb AN, et al. Expansion in size of a terminal deletion: A paradigm shift for parental follow-up studies. *J Med Genet* 45:391–395, 2008a.

South ST, Swensen JJ, Maxwell T, Rope A, Brothman AR, Chen Z. A new genomic mechanism leading to cri-du-chat syndrome. *Am J Med Genet* 140:2714–2720, 2006.

South ST, Whitby H, Battaglia A, Carey JC, Brothman AR. Comprehensive analysis of Wolf-Hirschhorn syndrome using array CGH indicates a high prevalence of translocations. *Eur J Hum Genet* 16:45–52, 2008.

South ST, Whitby H, Maxwell T, Aston E, Brothman AR, Carey JC. Co-occurrence of 4p16.3 deletions with both paternal and maternal duplications of 11p15: Modification of the Wolf-Hirschhorn syndrome phenotype by genetic alterations predicted to result in either a Beckwith-Wiedemann or Russell-Silver phenotype. *Am J Med Genet* 146A:2691–2697, 2008b.

Sovio U, Gaccioli F, Cook E, et al. Association between adverse pregnancy outcome and placental biomarkers in the first trimester: A prospective cohort study. *BJOG* 131:823–831, 2024.

Sowińska-Seidler A, Socha M, Jamsheer A. Split-hand/foot malformation—Molecular cause and implications in genetic counseling. *J Appl Genet* 55:105–115, 2014.

Sparago A, Cerrato F, Vernucci M, Ferrero GB, Silengo MC, Riccio A. Microdeletions in the human *H19* DMR result in loss of *IGF2* imprinting and Beckwith-Wiedemann syndrome. *Nat Genet* 36:958–960, 2004.

Sparkes RL, Shetty S, Chernos JE, Mefford HC, Micheil Innes A. Interstitial deletion of 11q in a mother and fetus: Implications of directly transmitted chromosomal imbalances for prenatal genetic counseling. *Prenat Diagn* 29:283–286, 2009.

Speed RM. Meiotic configurations in female trisomy 21 foetuses. *Hum Genet* 66:176–180, 1984.

Speevak MD, Farrell SA. Charcot-Marie-Tooth 1B caused by expansion of a familial myelin protein zero (MPZ) gene duplication. *Eur J Med Genet* 56:566–569, 2013.

Speevak MD, Smart C, Unwin L, Bell M, Farrell SA. Molecular characterization of an inherited ring (19) demonstrating ring opening. *Am J Med Genet* 121A:141–145, 2003.

Spena S, Duga S, Asselta R, et al. Congenital afibrinogenaemia caused by uniparental isodisomy of chromosome 4 containing a novel 15-kb deletion involving fibrinogen Aalpha-chain gene. *Eur J Hum Genet* 12:891–898, 2004.

Spencer K. Aneuploidy screening in the first trimester. *Am J Med Genet* 145C:18–32, 2007.

Spencer K, Kagan KO, Nicolaides KH. Screening for trisomy 21 in twin pregnancies in the first trimester: An update of the impact of chorionicity on maternal serum markers. *Prenat Diagn* 28:49–52, 2008.

Spinner NB, Saitta SC, Delaney DP, et al. Intracytoplasmic sperm injection (ICSI) with transmission of a ring(Y) chromosome and ovotesticular disorder of sex development in offspring. *Am J Med Genet* 146A:1828–1831, 2008.

Spittel H, Kubek F, Kreskowski K, et al. Mitotic stability of small supernumerary marker chromosomes: A study based on 93 immortalized cell lines. *Cytogenet Genome Res* 142:151–160, 2014.

Srebniak MI, Diderich KE, Noomen P, Dijkman A, de Vries FA, van Opstal D. Abnormal non-invasive prenatal test results concordant with karyotype of cytotrophoblast but not reflecting abnormal fetal karyotype. *Ultrasound Obstet Gynecol* 44:109–111, 2014.

Srebniak MI, Jehee FS, Joosten M, et al. Non-invasive prenatal diagnosis for translocation carriers—YES please or NO go? *Acta Obstet Gynecol Scand* 100:2036–2043, 2021.

Srebniak MI, van Zutven LJ, Petit F, et al. Interstitial 6q21q23 duplication—variant of variable phenotype and incomplete penetrance or benign duplication? *Mol Cytogenet* 9:43, 2016.

Sreenivasan R, Gonen N, Sinclair A. SOX genes and their role in disorders of sex development. *Sex Dev* 16:80–91, 2022.

Staals JE, Schrander-Stumpel CT, Hamers G, Fryns JP. Prenatal diagnosis of trisomy 12 mosaicism: Normal development of a 3 years old female child. *Genet Couns* 14:233–237, 2003.

Stabile M, Angelino T, Caiazzo F, et al. Fertility in a i(Xq) Klinefelter patient: Importance of XIST expression level determined by qRT-PCR in ruling out Klinefelter cryptic mosaicism as cause of oligozoospermia. *Mol Hum Reprod* 14:635–640, 2008.

Staebler M, Donner C, Van Regemorter N, et al. Should determination of the karyotype be systematic for all malformations detected by obstetrical ultrasound? *Prenat Diagn* 25:567–573, 2005.

Stagi S, Lapi E, Pantaleo M, et al. A *SOX3* (Xq26.3–27.3) duplication in a boy with growth hormone deficiency, ocular dyspraxia, and intellectual disability: A long-term follow-up and literature review. *Hormones (Athens)* 13:552–560, 2014.

Stagi S, Lapi E, Pantaleo M, et al. A new case of de novo 6q24.2-q25.2 deletion on paternal chromosome 6 with growth hormone deficiency: A twelve-year follow-up and literature review. *BMC Med Genet* 16:69, 2015.

Stahl BC, Patil SR, Syrop CH, Sparks AE, Wald M. Supernumerary minute ring chromosome 14 in a man with primary infertility and left varicocele. *Fertil Steril* 87:1213, e1–3, 2007.

Ståhl O, Boyd HA, Giwercman A, et al. Risk of birth abnormalities in the offspring of men with a history of cancer: A cohort study using Danish and Swedish national registries. *J Natl Cancer Inst* 103:398–406, 2011.

Stalker HJ, Williams CA. Genetic counseling in Angelman syndrome: The challenges of multiple causes. *Am J Med Genet* 77:54–59, 1998.

Stallard R, Krueger S, James RS, Schwartz S. Uniparental isodisomy 13 in a normal female due to transmission of a maternal t(13q13q). *Am J Med Genet* 57:14–18, 1995.

Stamberg J, Thomas GH. Unusual supernumerary chromosomes: Types encountered in a referred population, and high incidence of associated maternal chromosome abnormalities. *Hum Genet* 72:140–144, 1986.

Stancampiano MR, Meroni SLC, Bucolo C, Russo G. 46,XX differences of sex development outside congenital adrenal hyperplasia: Pathogenesis, clinical aspects, puberty, sex hormone replacement therapy and fertility outcomes. *Front Endocrinol (Lausanne)* 15:1402579, 2024.

Stankiewicz P. One pedigree we all may have come from—did Adam and Eve have the chromosome 2 fusion? *Mol Cytogenet* 9:72, 2016.

Stankiewicz P, Sen P, Bhatt SS, et al. Genomic and genic deletions of the *FOX* gene cluster on 16q24.1 and inactivating mutations of *FOXF1* cause alveolar capillary dysplasia and other malformations. *Am J Hum Genet* 84:780–791, 2009.

Stankiewicz P, Thiele H, Baldermann C, et al. Phenotypic findings due to trisomy 7p15.3-pter including the TWIST locus. *Am J Med Genet* 103:56–62, 2001.

Stankiewicz P, Thiele H, Schlicker M, et al. Duplication of Xq26.2-q27.1, including *SOX3*, in a mother and daughter with short stature and dyslalia. *Am J Med Genet* 138:11–17, 2005.

Stanley KE, Giordano J, Thorsten V, et al. Causal genetic variants in stillbirth. *N Engl J Med* 383:1107–1116, 2020.

Staples AJ, Sutherland GR, Haan EA, Clisby S. Epidemiology of Down syndrome in South Australia, 1960–89. *Am J Hum Genet* 49:1014–1024, 1991.

Starbuck JM, Cole TM, Reeves RH, Richtsmeier JT. The Influence of trisomy 21 on facial form and variability. *Am J Med Genet* 173A:2861–2872, 2017.

Stark Z, Gillam L, Walker SP, McGillivray G. Ethical controversies in prenatal microarray. *Curr Opin Obstet Gynecol* 25:133–137, 2013.

Starosta RT, Jensen N, Couteranis S, et al. Using a new analytic approach for genotyping and phenotyping chromosome 9p deletion syndrome. *Eur J Hum Genet* 32:1095–1105, 2024.

Starr LJ, Truemper EJ, Pickering DL, Sanger WG, Olney AH. Duplication of 20qter and deletion of 20pter due to paternal pericentric inversion: Patient report and review of 20qter duplications. *Am J Med Genet* 164A:2020–2024, 2014.

Stasiewicz-Jarocka B, Haus O, Van Assche E, et al. Genetic counseling in carriers of reciprocal chromosomal translocations involving long arm of chromosome 16. *Clin Genet* 66:189–207, 2004.

Stasiewicz-Jarocka B, Raczkiewicz B, Kowalczyk D, Zawada M, Midro AT. Genetic risk of families with t(1;2)(q42;q33) GTG, RHG, QFQ, FISH. *Ginekol Pol* 71:1262–1272, 2000.

Stefanou EG, Crocker M, Boon A, Stewart H. Cryptic mosaicism for monosomy 20 identified in renal tract cells. *Clin Genet* 70:228–232, 2006.

Stefanova I, Jenderny J, Kaminsky E, et al. Mosaic and complete tetraploidy in live-born infants: Two new patients and review of the literature. *Clin Dysmorphol* 19:123–127, 2010.

Stefansson H, Meyer-Lindenberg A, Steinberg S, et al. CNVs conferring risk of autism or schizophrenia affect cognition in controls. *Nature* 505:361–366, 2014.

Steffensen EH, Skakkebaek A, Gadsbøll K, et al. Inclusion of sex chromosomes in noninvasive prenatal testing in Asia, Australia, Europe and the USA: A survey study. *Prenat Diagn* 43:144–155, 2023.

Stein QP, Boyle JG, Crotwell PL, et al. Prenatally diagnosed trisomy 20 mosaicism associated with arachnoid cyst of basal cistern. *Prenat Diagn* 28:1169–1170, 2008.

Steinbach P. Excess of mental retardation and/or congenital malformation in reciprocal translocations in man. *Hum Genet* 73:379, 1986.

Steinberg C, Zackai EH, Eunpu DL, Mennuti MT, Emanuel BS. Recurrence rate for de novo 21q21q translocation Down syndrome: A study of 112 families. *Am J Med Genet* 17:523–530, 1984.

Steinberg Warren N, Soukup S, King JL, St JDP. Prenatal diagnosis of trisomy 20 by chorionic villus sampling (CVS): A case report with long-term outcome. *Prenat Diagn* 21:1111–1113, 2001.

Steinbusch CVM, van Roozendaal KEP, Tserpelis D, et al. Somatic mosaicism in a mother of two children with Pitt-Hopkins syndrome. *Clin Genet* 83:73–77, 2013.

Steiner B, Masood R, Rufibach K, et al. An unexpected finding: Younger fathers have a higher risk for offspring with chromosomal aneuploidies. *Eur J Hum Genet* 23:466–472, 2015.

Steinfort K, Fransen E, Blaumeiser B, Janssens K. Monocentric study on the performance of noninvasive prenatal testing on cell-free DNA for the detection of monosomy X. *Prenat Diagn* 44:1210–1217, 2024.

Steinman KJ, Spence SJ, Ramocki MB, et al. 16p11.2 deletion and duplication: Characterizing neurologic phenotypes in a large clinically ascertained cohort. *Am J Med Genet* 170A:2943–2955, 2016.

Stelzer Y, Sagi I, Yanuka O, Eiges R, Benvenisty N. The noncoding RNA IPW regulates the imprinted *DLK1-DIO3* locus in an induced pluripotent stem cell model of Prader-Willi syndrome. *Nat Genet* 46:551–557, 2014.

Stemkens D, Broekmans FJ, Kastrop PM, Hochstenbach R, Smith BG, Giltay JC. Variant Klinefelter syndrome 47,X,i(X)(q10),Y and normal 46,XY karyotype in monozygotic adult twins. *Am J Med Genet* 143A:1906–1911, 2007.

Stene J. Detection of higher recurrence risk for age-dependent chromosome abnormalities with an application to trisomy G1 (Down's syndrome). *Hum Hered* 20:112–122, 1970.

Stene J. Comments on methods and results in: Sherman et al., "Segregation Analysis of Balanced Pericentric Inversions in Pedigree Data." *Clin Genet* 30:95–107, 1986.

Stene J, Stengel-Rutkowski S. Genetic risks of familial reciprocal and Robertsonian translocation carriers. In Daniel A (ed.), *The Cytogenetics of Mammalian Autosomal Rearrangements*. New York, NY: Liss, 1988.

Stengel-Rutkowski S, Stene J, Gallano P. Risk estimates in balanced parental reciprocal translocations. *Monogr Ann Génétique* 1–147, 1988.

Stephenson MD, Awartani KA, Robinson WP. Cytogenetic analysis of miscarriages from couples with recurrent miscarriage: A case-control study. *Hum Reprod* 17:446–451, 2002.

Stern C, Pertile M, Norris H, Hale L, Baker HGW. Chromosome translocations in couples with in-vitro fertilization implantation failure. *Hum Reprod* 14:2097–2101, 1999.

Stern S, Biron D, Moses E. Transmission of trisomy decreases with maternal age in mouse models of Down syndrome, mirroring a phenomenon in human Down syndrome mothers. *BMC Genet* 17:105, 2016.

Stetten G, Escallon CS, South ST, McMichael JL, Saul DO, Blakemore KJ. Reevaluating confined placental mosaicism. *Am J Med Genet* 131:232–239, 2004.

Stevens SJC, Smeets EEJGL, Blom E, et al. Identical cryptic partial monosomy 20pter and trisomy 20qter in three adult siblings due to a large maternal pericentric inversion: Detection by MLPA and breakpoint mapping by SNP array analysis. *Am J Med Genet* 149A:2226–2230, 2009.

Stewart DA, Bailey JD, Netley CT, Park E. Growth, development, and behavioral outcome from mid-adolescence to adulthood in subjects with chromosome aneuploidy: The Toronto Study. *Birth Defects Orig Artic Ser* 26:131–188, 1990.

Stipoljev F, Stanojevic M, Kurjak A. Familial pericentric inversion of chromosome 4: inv(4)(p16.1q12). *Clin Genet* 61:386–388, 2002.

Stochholm K, Bojesen A, Jensen AS, Juul S, Gravholt CH. Criminality in men with Klinefelter's syndrome and XYY syndrome: A cohort study. *BMJ Open* 2:e000650, 2012.

Stochholm K, Holmgård C, Davis SM, Gravholt CH, Berglund A. Incidence, prevalence, age at diagnosis, and mortality in individuals with 45,X/46,XY mosaicism: A population-based registry study. *Genet Med* 26:100987, 2024.

Stoklasova J, Kaprova J, Trkova M, et al. A rare variant of Turner syndrome in four sequential generations: Effect of the interplay of growth hormone treatment and estrogens on body proportion. *Horm Res Paediatr* 86:349–356, 2016

Stokman MF, Oud MM, van Binsbergen E, et al. De novo 14q24.2q24.3 microdeletion including *IFT43* is associated with intellectual disability, skeletal anomalies, cardiac anomalies, and myopia. *Am J Med Genet* 170:1566–1569, 2016.

Stokowski R, Wang E, White K, et al. Clinical performance of non-invasive prenatal testing (NIPT) using targeted cell-free DNA analysis in maternal plasma with microarrays or next generation sequencing (NGS) is consistent across multiple controlled clinical studies. *Prenat Diagn* 35:1243–1246, 2015.

Strain L, Dean JCS, Hamilton MPR, Bonthron DT. A true hermaphrodite chimera resulting from embryo amalgamation after in vitro fertilization. *N Engl J Med* 338:166–169, 1998.

Strain L, Warner JP, Johnston T, Bonthron DT. A human parthenogenetic chimaera. *Nat Genet* 11:164–169, 1995.

Strauss G, Mott K, Klopocki E, Schulze H. Thrombocytopenia Absent Radius (TAR)-Syndrome: From current genetics to patient self-empowerment. *Hamostaseologie* 43:252–260, 2023.

Strazisar M, Cammaerts S, van der Ven K, et al. *MIR137* variants identified in psychiatric patients affect synaptogenesis and neuronal transmission gene sets. *Mol Psychiatry* 20:472–481, 2015.

Strehle EM, Yu L, Rosenfeld JA, et al. Genotype-phenotype analysis of 4q deletion syndrome: Proposal of a critical region. *Am J Med Genet* 158A:2139–2151, 2012.

Strigini P, Pierluigi M, Forni GL, et al. Effect of X-rays on chromosome 21 nondisjunction. *Am J Med Genet Suppl* 7:155–159, 1990.

Strnadová I, Loblinzk J, Scully JL, et al. "I am not a number!" Opinions and preferences of people with intellectual disability about genetic healthcare. *Eur J Hum Genet* 31:1057–1065, 2023.

Strnadová I, Nevin SM, Scully JL, Palmer EE. The opinions and experiences of people with intellectual disability regarding genetic testing and genetic medicine: A systematic review. *Genet Med* 24:535–548, 2022.

Stumm M, Müsebeck J, Tönnies H, et al. Partial trisomy 9p12p21.3 with a normal phenotype. *J Med Genet* 39:141–144, 2002.

Stylianou CE, Wiggins GAR, Lau VL, et al. Germline copy number variants and endometrial cancer risk. *Hum Genet* 143:1481–1498, 2024.

Su MT, Liang YL, Chen JC, Sun HS, Chang FM, Kuo PL. Non-mosaic uniparental trisomy 16 presenting with asplenia syndrome and placental abruption: A case report and literature review. *Eur J Med Genet* 56:197–201, 2013.

Su P, Ding H, Huang D, et al. A 4.6 kb genomic duplication on 20p12.2–12.3 is associated with brachydactyly type A2 in a Chinese family. *J Med Genet* 48:312–316, 2011.

Sudha T, Gopinath PM. Homologous Robertsonian translocation (21q21q) and abortions. *Hum Genet* 85:253–255, 1990.

Sudik R, Jakubiczka S, Nawroth F, Gilberg E, Wieacker PF. Chimerism in a fertile woman with 46,XY karyotype and female phenotype. *Hum Reprod* 16:56–58, 2001.

Sugawara N, Kimura Y, Araki Y. Successful second delivery outcome using refrozen thawed testicular sperm from an infertile male true hermaphrodite with a 46,XX/46,XY karyotype: Case report. *Hum Cell* 25:96–99, 2012.

Sugawara N, Kimura Y, Araki Y. Case report: A successful pregnancy outcome in a patient with non-mosaic Turner syndrome (45, X) via in vitro fertilization. *Hum Cell* 26:41–43, 2013.

Sugawara N, Tokunaga Y, Maeda M, Komaba R, Araki Y. A successful pregnancy outcome using frozen testicular sperm from a chimeric infertile male with a 46,XX/46,XY karyotype: Case report. *Hum Reprod* 20:147–148, 2005.

Sukenik-Halevy R, Sukenik S, Koifman A, et al. Clinical aspects of prenatally detected congenital heart malformations and the yield of chromosomal microarray analysis. *Prenat Diagn* 36:1185–1191, 2016.

Süleyman M, Oğuz S, Kaykı G, et al. A very rare case of a newborn with tetrasomy 9p and literature review. *Turk J Pediatr* 64:171–178, 2022.

Sullivan PF, Yao S, Hjerling-Leffler J. Schizophrenia genomics: Genetic complexity and functional insights. *Nat Rev Neurosci* 25:611–624, 2024.

Šumanovic-Glamuzina D, Lozic B, Iwanowski PS, et al. Limited survivability of unbalanced progeny of carriers of a unique t(4;19)(p15.32;p13.3): A study in multiple generations. *Mol Cytogenet* 10:29, 2017.

Sun F, Oliver-Bonet M, Turek PJ, Ko E, Martin RH. Meiotic studies in an azoospermic human translocation (Y;1) carrier. *Mol Hum Reprod* 11:361–364, 2005.

Sun K, Jiang P, Chan KC, et al. Plasma DNA tissue mapping by genome-wide methylation sequencing for noninvasive prenatal, cancer, and transplantation assessments. *Proc Natl Acad Sci USA* 112:E5503–5512, 2015.

Sun L, Wen J, Chu G, Lai G, He R. [Prenatal genetic diagnosis of a case with ring chromosome 13]. *Zhonghua Yi Xue Yi Chuan Xue Za Zhi* 40:1455–1460, 2023.

Sund KL, Khattar D, Boomer T, et al. Confirmatory testing illustrates additional risks for structural sex chromosome abnormalities in fetuses with a non-invasive prenatal screen positive for monosomy X. *Am J Med Genet* 184C:294–301, 2020.

Sundvall L, Lund H, Niemann I, Jensen UB, Bolund L, Sunde L. Tetraploidy in hydatidiform moles. *Hum Reprod* 28:2010–2020, 2013.

Sung PL, Chang SP, Wen KC, et al. Small supernumerary marker chromosome originating from chromosome 10 associated with an apparently normal phenotype. *Am J Med Genet* 149A:2768–2774, 2009.

Suntharesan J, Apperley L, Senniappan S. 45,X male—Rare case of unbalanced translocation of Y chromosome to chromosome 2 presenting with developmental delay, learning difficulty and obesity. *Endocrinol Diabetes Metab Case Rep* 2022:22–0320, 2022.

Surace C, Berardinelli F, Masotti A, et al. Telomere shortening and telomere position effect in mild ring 17 syndrome. *Epigenetics Chromatin* 7:1, 2014.

Susanne GO, Sissel S, Ulla W, Charlotta G, Sonja OL. Pregnant women's responses to information about an increased risk of carrying a baby with Down syndrome. *Birth* 33:64–73, 2006.

Susiarjo M, Hassold TJ, Freeman E, Hunt PA. Bisphenol A exposure in utero disrupts early oogenesis in the mouse. *PLoS Genet* 3:e5, 2007.

Suslak L, Price DM, Desposito F. Transmitting balanced translocation carrier information within families: A follow-up study. *Am J Med Genet* 20:227–232, 1985.

Sutherland GR. Rare fragile sites. *Cytogenet Genome Res* 100:77–84, 2003.

Sutherland GR, Callen DF, Gardner RJM. Paracentric inversions do not normally generate monocentric recombinant chromosomes. *Am J Med Genet* 59:390–392, 1995.

Sutherland GR, Gardiner AJ, Carter RF. Familial pericentric inversion of chromosome 19, inv(19)(p13q13) with a note on genetic counseling of pericentric inversion carriers. *Clin Genet* 10:54–59, 1976.

Sutton VR, McAlister WH, Bertin TK, et al. Skeletal defects in paternal uniparental disomy for chromosome 14 are re-capitulated in the mouse model (paternal uniparental disomy 12). *Hum Genet* 113:447–451, 2003.

Swillen A, Devriendt K, Vantrappen G, et al. Familial deletions of chromosome 22q11: The Leuven experience. *Am J Med Genet* 80:531–532, 1998.

Sybert VP. Phenotypic effects of mosaicism for a 47,XXX cell line in Turner syndrome. *J Med Genet* 39:217–220, 2002.

Sybert VP. Turner Syndrome. In Cassidy SB, Allanson JE (eds.), *Management of Genetic Syndromes* (2nd edn.). Hoboken, NJ: John Wiley & Sons, 2005.

Syryn H, Van De Vijver K, Cools M. Ovotesticular difference of sex development: Genetic background, histological features, and clinical management. *Horm Res Paediatr* 96:180–189, 2023.

Szafranski P, Gambin T, Dharmadhikari AV, et al. Pathogenetics of alveolar capillary dysplasia with misalignment of pulmonary veins. *Hum Genet* 135:569–586, 2016.

Szafranski P, Von Allmen GK, Graham BH, et al. 6q22.1 microdeletion and susceptibility to pediatric epilepsy. *Eur J Hum Genet* 23:173–179, 2015.

T

Tabet AC, Aboura A, Gérard M, et al. Molecular characterization of a de novo 6q24.2q25.3 duplication interrupting *UTRN* in a patient with arthrogryposis. *Am J Med Genet* 152A:1781–1788, 2010.

Tabet AC, Pilorge M, Delorme R, et al. Autism multiplex family with 16p11.2p12.2 microduplication syndrome in monozygotic twins and distal 16p11.2 deletion in their brother. *Eur J Hum Genet* 20:540–546, 2012.

Tabet AC, Verloes A, Pilorge M, et al. Complex nature of apparently balanced chromosomal rearrangements in patients with autism spectrum disorder. *Mol Autism* 6:19, 2015.

Tabolacci E, Zollino M, Lecce R, et al. Two brothers with 22q13 deletion syndrome and features suggestive of the Clark-Baraitser syndrome. *Clin Dysmorphol* 14:127–132, 2005.

Tachdjian G, Aboura A, Benkhalifa M, et al. De novo interstitial direct duplication of Xq21.1q25 associated with skewed X-inactivation pattern. *Am J Med Genet* 131:273–280, 2004.

Tadros S, Wang R, Waters JJ, et al. Inherited 2q23.1 microdeletions involving the *MBD5* locus. *Mol Genet Genomic Med* 5:608–613, 2017.

Tagaya M, Mizuno S, Hayakawa M, Yokotsuka T, Shimizu S, Fujimaki H. Recombination of a maternal pericentric inversion results in 22q13 deletion syndrome. *Clin Dysmorphol* 17:19–21, 2008.

Takagi M, Hoshino A, Bousset K, et al. Bone marrow failure and immunodeficiency associated with human RAD50 variants. *J Clin Immunol* 2023 43:2136–2145, 2023.

Takahashi S, Kyogoku H, Hayakawa T, et al. Embryonic genome instability upon DNA replication timing program emergence. *Nature* 633:686–694, 2024.

Takeuchi A, Ehara H, Ohtani K, et al. Live birth prevalence of Down syndrome in Tottori, Japan, 1980–1999. *Am J Med Genet* 146A:1381–1386, 2008.

Talantova OE, Koltsova AS, Tikhonov AV, et al. Prenatal detection of trisomy 2: Considerations for genetic counseling and testing. *Genes (Basel)* 14:913, 2023.

Talaulikar VS, Conway GS, Pimblett A, Davies MC. Outcome of ovarian stimulation for oocyte cryopreservation in women with Turner syndrome. *Fertil Steril* 111:505–509, 2019.

Talkowski ME, Mullegama SV, Rosenfeld JA, et al. Assessment of 2q23.1 microdeletion syndrome implicates *MBD5* as a single causal locus of intellectual disability, epilepsy, and autism spectrum disorder. *Am J Hum Genet* 89:551–563, 2011.

Tamaki Y, Katagiri Y, Umemura N, Takeshita N, Morita M. Noninvasive prenatal testing aids identification of tetrasomy 18p: A case report. *Case Rep Womens Health* 27:e00236, 2020.

Tamura M, Isojima T, Kawashima M, et al. Detection of hereditary 1,25-hydroxyvitamin d-resistant rickets caused by uniparental disomy of chromosome 12 using genome-wide single nucleotide polymorphism array. *PLoS One* 10:e0131157, 2015.

Tan H, Huang Q, Liu D, et al. Effects of carrier's sex on the outcome of embryos and pregnancies in 412 couples undergoing preimplantation genetic testing for structural rearrangements. *Gene* 933:148989, 2025.

Tan M, Wang X, Liu H, et al. Genetic diagnostic yield and novel causal genes of congenital heart disease. *Front Genet* 13:941364, 2022.

Tan Q, Potter KJ, Burnett LC, et al. Prader-Willi-like phenotype caused by an atypical 15q11.2 microdeletion. *Genes (Basel)* 11:128, 2020.

Tan TY, Aftimos S, Worgan L, et al. Phenotypic expansion and further characterisation of the 17q21.31 microdeletion syndrome. *J Med Genet* 46:480–489, 2009.

Tan TY, Collins A, James PA, et al. Phenotypic variability of distal 22q11.2 copy number abnormalities. *Am J Med Genet* 155A:1623–1633, 2011.

Tan VJ, Liu T, Arifin Z, et al. Third-generation single-molecule sequencing for preimplantation genetic testing of aneuploidy and segmental imbalances. *Clin Chem* 69:881–889, 2023.

Tan YQ, Tan YQ, Cheng DH. Whole-genome mate-pair sequencing of apparently balanced chromosome rearrangements reveals complex structural variations: Two case studies. *Mol Cytogenet* 13:15, 2020.

Tanabe H, Ijiri M, Takahashi K, et al. Genomic insights into familial adenomatous polyposis: Unraveling a rare case with whole APC gene deletion and intellectual disability. *Hum Genome Var* 11:13, 2024.

Tang R, Lin L, Guo Z, Hou H, Yu Q. Ovarian reserve evaluation in a woman with 45,X/47,XXX mosaicism: A case report and a review of literature. *Mol Genet Genomic Med* 7:e00732, 2019.

Tang W, Boyd BK, Hummel M, Wenger SL. Prenatal diagnosis of tetrasomy 9p. *Am J Med Genet* 126A:328, 2004.

Tang W, Wu Y, Liu J, Ren W. Prenatal diagnosis of low-level trisomy 3 mosaicism. *Taiwan J Obstet Gynecol* 56:114–115, 2017.

Tang X, Du Y, Chen M, et al. Relationships among maternal monosomy X mosaicism, maternal trisomy, and discordant sex chromosome aneuploidies. *Clin Chim Acta* 554:117770, 2024.

Tan-Sindhunata G, Castedo S, Leegte B, et al. Molecular cytogenetic characterization of a small, familial supernumerary ring chromosome 7 associated with mental retardation and an abnormal phenotype. *Am J Med Genet* 92:147–152, 2000.

Tartaglia NR, Howell S, Sutherland A, Wilson R, Wilson L. A review of trisomy X (47,XXX). *Orphanet J Rare Dis* 5:8, 2010.

Tartaglia N, Howell S, Davis S, et al. Early neurodevelopmental and medical profile in children with sex chromosome trisomies: Background for the prospective eXtraordinarY babies study to identify early risk factors and targets for intervention. *Am J Med Genet* 184C:428–443, 2020.

Tartaglia NR, Howell S, Wilson R, et al. The eXtraordinarY Kids Clinic: An interdisciplinary model of care for children and adolescents with sex chromosome aneuploidy. *J Multidiscip Health* 8:323–334, 2015.

Tassano E, Biancheri R, Denegri L, et al. Heterozygous deletion of *CHL1* gene: Detailed array-CGH and clinical characterization of a new case and review of the literature. *Eur J Med Genet* 57:626–629, 2014.

Tassano E, Giacomini T, Severino M, et al. Characterization of the phenotype associated with microduplication reciprocal to NF1 microdeletion syndrome. *Cytogenet Genome Res* 152:22–28, 2017.

Tassano E, Ronchetto P, Calcagno A, et al. 'Distal 16p12.2 microdeletion' in a patient with autosomal recessive deafness-22. *J Genet* 98:56, 2019.

Tatton-Brown K, Douglas J, Coleman K, et al. Multiple mechanisms are implicated in the generation of 5q35 microdeletions in Sotos syndrome. *J Med Genet* 42:307–313, 2005.

Tatton-Brown K, Pilz DT, Örstavik KH, et al. 15q overgrowth syndrome: A newly recognized phenotype associated with overgrowth, learning difficulties, characteristic facial appearance, renal anomalies and increased dosage of distal chromosome 15q. *Am J Med Genet* 149A:147–154, 2009.

Tayebi N, Khodaei H. Secondary amenorrhea associated with 46,X,der(X)t(X;X)(p22;p22). *Taiwan J Obstet Gynecol* 50:223–224, 2011.

Taylor AMR, Rothblum-Oviatt C, Ellis NA, et al. Chromosome instability syndromes. *Nat Rev Dis Primers* 5:64, 2019.

Taylor H, Yerlioglu D, Phen C, et al. mTOR inhibitors reduce enteropathy, intestinal bleeding and colectomy rate in patients with juvenile polyposis of infancy with PTEN-BMPR1A deletion. *Hum Mol Genet* 30:1273–1282, 2021.

Tekin M, Jackson-Cook C, Buller A, et al. Fluorescence in situ hybridization detectable mosaicism for Angelman syndrome with biparental methylation. *Am J Med Genet* 95:145–149, 2000.

Tello C, Darling A, Lupo V, Ortez CI, Pérez-Dueñas B, Espinós C. Twin-sisters with *PLA2G6*-associated neurodegeneration due to paternal isodisomy of the chromosome 22 following in vitro fertilization. *Clin Genet* 92:117–118, 2017.

Tempest HG, Ko E, Chan P, Robaire B, Rademaker A, Martin RH. Sperm aneuploidy frequencies analysed before and after chemotherapy in testicular cancer and Hodgkin's lymphoma patients. *Hum Reprod* 23:251–258, 2008.

Tempest HG, Simpson JL. Why are we still talking about chromosomal heteromorphisms? *Reprod Biomed Online* 35:1–2, 2017.

Templado C, Donate A, Giraldo J, Bosch M, Estop A. Advanced age increases chromosome structural abnormalities in human spermatozoa. *Eur J Hum Genet* 19:145–151, 2011.

Templado C, Uroz L, Estop A. New insights on the origin and relevance of aneuploidy in human spermatozoa. *Mol Hum Reprod* 19:634–643, 2013.

Temple CM, Shephard EE. Exceptional lexical skills but executive language deficits in school starters and young adults with Turners syndrome: Implications for X chromosome effects on brain function. *Brain Lang* 120:345–359, 2012.

Temple IK, Cockwell A, Hassold T, Pettay D, Jacobs P. Maternal uniparental disomy for chromosome 14. *J Med Genet* 28:511–514, 1991.

Temple IK, Gardner RJ, Robinson DO, et al. Further evidence for an imprinted gene for neonatal diabetes localised to chromosome 6q22-q23. *Hum Mol Genet* 5:1117–21, 1996.

Tempone Cardoso Penna G, de Rezende Lelot G, de Rezende Lelot AL, et al. Effect of recombinant human growth hormone treatment in a patient with short stature associated with the ring chromosome 17 syndrome. *Case Rep Pediatr* 2023:6686511, 2023.

Ten SK, Chin YM, Noor PJ, Hassan K. Cytogenetic studies in women with primary amenorrhea. *Singapore Med J* 31:355–359, 1990.

Tennakoon J, Kandasamy Y, Alcock G, Koh TH. Edwards syndrome with double trisomy. *Singapore Med J* 49:e190–191, 2008.

Tenorio J, Nevado J, González-Meneses A, et al. Further definition of the proximal 19p13.3 microdeletion/microduplication syndrome and implication of PIAS4 as the major contributor. *Clin Genet* 97:467–476, 2020.

Termsarasab P, Yang AC, Reiner J, Mei H, Scott SA, Frucht SJ. Paroxysmal kinesigenic dyskinesia caused by 16p11.2 microdeletion. *Tremor Other Hyperkinet Mov* 4:274, 2014.

Terzoli G, Lalatta F, Lobbiani A, Simoni G, Colucci G. Fertility in a 47,XXY patient: Assessment of biological paternity by deoxyribonucleic acid fingerprinting. *Fertil Steril* 58:821–822, 1992.

Terzoli G, Rossella F, Biscaglia M, Simoni G. True fetal mosaicism revealed by a single abnormal colony in amniocyte culture. *Prenat Diagn* 10:273–274, 1990.

Teshima IE, Winsor EJT, Van Allen MI. Trisomy 18 and a constitutional maternal translocation (2;18). *Am J Med Genet* 43:759–761, 1992.
Teyssier M, Gaucherand P, Buenerd A. Prenatal diagnosis of a tetraploid fetus. *Prenat Diagn* 17:474–478, 1997.
Teyssier M, Moreau N. Transmission familiale d'un chromosome 22 remanié [r(22) ou 22p0?] chez deux femmes normales. *Ann Génét* 28:116–118, 1985.
Teyssier M, Rafat A, Pugeat M. Case of (Y;1) familial translocation. *Am J Med Genet* 46:339340, 1993.
Thapa M, Asamoah A, Gowans GC, et al. Molecular characterization of distal 4q duplication in two patients using oligonucleotide array-based comparative genomic hybridization (oaCGH) analysis. *Am J Med Genet* 164A:1069–1074, 2014.
Tharapel AT, Elias S, Shulman LP, Seely L, Emerson DS, Simpson JL. Resorbed co-twin as an explanation for discrepant chorionic villus results: Non-mosaic 47,XX,+16 in villi (direct and culture) with normal (46,XX) amniotic fluid and neonatal blood. *Prenat Diagn* 9:467–472, 1989.
Tharapel AT, Michaelis RC, Velagaleti GVN, et al. Chromosome duplications and deletions and their mechanisms of origin. *Cytogenet Cell Genet* 85:285–290, 1999.
Tharapel SA, Lewandowski RC, Tharapel AT, Wilroy RS, Jr. Phenotype-karyotype correlation in patients trisomic for various segments of chromosome 13. *J Med Genet* 23:310–315, 1986.
Therman E, Laxova R, Susman B. The critical region on the human Xq. *Hum Genet* 85:455–461, 1990.
Therman E, Susman B, Denniston C. The nonrandom participation of human acrocentric chromosomes in Robertsonian translocations. *Ann Hum Genet* 53:49–65, 1989.
Thevenon J, Callier P, Andrieux J, et al. 12p13.33 microdeletion including *ELKS/ERC1*, a new locus associated with childhood apraxia of speech. *Eur J Hum Genet* 21:82–88, 2013.
Thevenon J, Callier P, Poquet H, et al. 3q27.3 microdeletional syndrome: A recognisable clinical entity associating dysmorphic features, marfanoid habitus, intellectual disability and psychosis with mood disorder. *J Med Genet* 51:21–27, 2014.
Thibodeau ML, Steinraths M, Brown L, et al. Genomic and cytogenetic characterization of a balanced translocation disrupting NUP98. *Cytogenet Genome Res* 152:117–121, 2017.
Thienpont B, Béna F, Breckpot J, et al. Duplications of the critical Rubinstein-Taybi deletion region on chromosome 16p13.3 cause a novel recognisable syndrome. *J Med Genet* 47:155–161, 2010.
Thierry G, Bénéteau C, Pichon O, et al. Molecular characterization of 1q44 microdeletion in 11 patients reveals three candidate genes for intellectual disability and seizures. *Am J Med Genet* 158A:1633–1640, 2012.
Thomas NS, Morris JK, Baptista J, Ng BL, Crolla JA, Jacobs PA. De novo apparently balanced translocations in man are predominantly paternal in origin and associated with a significant increase in paternal age. *J Med Genet* 47:112–115, 2010.
Thompson DJ, Genovese G, Halvardson J, et al. Genetic predisposition to mosaic Y chromosome loss in blood. *Nature* 575:652–657, 2019.
Thompson T, Bothwell S, Janusz J, et al. Quantifying the spectrum of early motor and language milestones in sex chromosome trisomy. *MedRχiv* in print 2025.
Thomsen SH, Lund ICB, Bache I, Becher N, Vogel I. Placental mosaicism for autosomal trisomies: Comprehensive follow-up of 528 Danish cases (1983–2021). *Am J Obstet Gynecol MFM* 6:101497, 2024.
Thomsen SH, Lund ICB, Fagerberg C, Bache I, Becher N, Vogel I. Trisomy 8 mosaicism in the placenta: A Danish cohort study of 37 cases and a literature review. *Prenat Diagn* 41:409–421, 2021.
Thorsson T, Russell WW, El-Kashlan N, et al. Chromosomal imbalances in patients with congenital cardiac defects: A meta-analysis reveals novel potential critical regions involved in heart development. *Congenit Heart Dis* 10:193–208, 2015.
Tian Q, Xu LL, Li DZ. Parental germline mosaic transmission of 5p13.2 microduplication in two siblings of a Chinese family. *J Obstet Gynaecol* 42:701–703, 2022.
Tiegs AW, Hodes-Wertz B, McCulloh DH, Munné S, Grifo JA. Discrepant diagnosis rate of array comparative genomic hybridization in thawed euploid blastocysts. *J Assist Reprod Genet* 33:893–897, 2016.
Tiegs AW, Tao X, Zhan Y, et al. A multicenter, prospective, blinded, nonselection study evaluating the predictive value of an aneuploid diagnosis using a targeted next-generation sequencing-based preimplantation genetic testing for aneuploidy assay and impact of biopsy. *Fertil Steril* 115:627–637, 2021.
Tiepolo L, Zuffardi O. Localization of factors controlling spermatogenesis in the nonfluorescent portion of the human Y chromosome long arm. *Hum Genet* 34:119–124, 1976.
Tillisch DL. Chromosome deletions. Looking beyond disability. *Lancet* 358 (Suppl):S10, 2001.
Tim-Aroon T, Jinawath N, Thammachote W, et al. 1q21.3 deletion involving GATAD2B: An emerging recurrent microdeletion syndrome. *Am J Med Genet* 173A:766–770, 2017.

Ting NS, Chen YH, Chen SF, Chen PC. Successful live twin birth through IVF/ICSI from a couple with an infertile father with pericentric inversion of chromosome 9 (p12q13): A case with a high aneuploidy rate. *Medicina (Kaunas)* 58:1646, 2022.

Tiranti V, Lamantea E, Uziel G, et al. Leigh syndrome transmitted by uniparental disomy of chromosome 9. *J Med Genet* 36:927–928, 1999.

Tobler KJ, Zhao Y, Ross R, et al. Blastocoel fluid from differentiated blastocysts harbors embryonic genomic material capable of a whole-genome deoxyribonucleic acid amplification and comprehensive chromosome microarray analysis. *Fertil Steril* 104:418–425, 2015.

Tokita MJ, Chow PM, Mirzaa G, et al. Five children with deletions of 1p34.3 encompassing *AGO1* and *AGO3*. *Eur J Hum Genet* 23:761–765, 2015.

Tokita MJ, Sybert VP. Postnatal outcomes of prenatally diagnosed 45,X/46,XX. *Am J Med Genet* 170A:1196–1201, 2016.

Tomkins DJ. Unstable familial translocations: A t(11;22)mat inherited as a t(11;15). *Am J Hum Genet* 33:745–751, 1981.

Tommerup N. Mendelian cytogenetics: Chromosome rearrangements associated with Mendelian disorders. *J Med Genet* 30:713–727, 1993.

Tommerup N, Fonseca AC, Mehrjouy MM, et al. Interpretation of NGS-mapped chromosomal breakpoints: The importance of healthy controls. Poster presented at the European Human Genetics conference, Copenhagen, 2017.

Tong J, Jiang J, Niu Y, Zhang T. Do chromosomal inversion carriers really need preimplantation genetic testing? *J Assist Reprod Genet* 39:2573–2579, 2022a.

Tong J, Niu Y, Wan A, Zhang T. Effect of parental origin and predictors for obtaining a euploid embryo in balanced translocation carriers. *Reprod Biomed Online* 44:72–79, 2022b.

Tong J, Zhao XM, Wan AR, Zhang T. PGT or ICSI? The impression of NGS-based PGT outcomes in nonmosaic Klinefelter syndrome. *Asian J Androl* 23:621–626, 2021.

Tonk V, Schultz RA, Christian SL, Kubota T, Ledbetter DH, Wilson GN. Robertsonian (15q;15q) translocation in a child with Angelman syndrome: Evidence of uniparental disomy. *Am J Med Genet* 66:426–428, 1996.

Tonk VS, Jesurun CA, Morgan DL, Lockhart LH, Velagaleti GV. Molecular cytogenetic characterization of a recombinant chromosome rec(22)dup(22q)inv(22)(p13q12.2). *Am J Med Genet* 124A:92–95, 2004.

Tonyan ZN, Puppo IL, Saifitdinova AF, Vavilova TV, Glotov AS. Assessment of quadrivalent characteristics influencing chromosome segregation by analyzing human preimplantation embryos from reciprocal translocation carriers. *Comp Cytogenet* 18:1–13, 2024.

Torfs CP, Christianson RE. Anomalies in Down syndrome individuals in a large population-based registry. *Am J Med Genet* 77:431–438, 1998.

Torfs CP, Christianson RE. Effect of maternal smoking and coffee consumption on the risk of having a recognized Down syndrome pregnancy. *Am J Epidemiol* 152:1185–1191, 2000.

Torisu H, Yamamoto T, Fujiwaki T, et al. Girl with monosomy 1p36 and Angelman syndrome due to unbalanced der(1) transmission of a maternal translocation t(1;15)(p36.3;q13.1). *Am J Med Genet* 131:94–98, 2004.

Torres EM. Consequences of gaining an extra chromosome. *Chromosome Res* 31:24, 2023.

Torres F, Barbosa M, Maciel P. Recurrent copy number variations as risk factors for neurodevelopmental disorders: Critical overview and analysis of clinical implications. *J Med Genet* 53:73–90, 2016.

Toruner GA, Kurvathi R, Sugalski R, et al. Copy number variations in three children with sudden infant death. *Clin Genet* 76:63–68, 2009.

Tosca L, Brisset S, Petit FM, et al. Recurrent 70.8 Mb 4q22.2q32.3 duplication due to ovarian germinal mosaicism. *Eur J Hum Genet* 18:882–888, 2010.

Tóth A, Gaál M, László J. Familial pericentric inversion of the Y chromosome. *Ann Génét* 27:60–61, 1984.

Towner DR, Shaffer LG, Yang SP, Walgenbach DD. Confined placental mosaicism for trisomy 14 and maternal uniparental disomy in association with elevated second trimester maternal serum human chorionic gonadotrophin and third trimester fetal growth restriction. *Prenat Diagn* 21:395–398, 2001.

Tranebjaerg L, Petersen A, Hove K, Rehder H, Mikkelsen M. Clinical and cytogenetic studies in a large (4;8) translocation family with pre- and postnatal Wolf syndrome. *Ann Génét* 27:224–229, 1984.

Trask BJ. Human cytogenetics: 46 chromosomes, 46 years and counting. *Nat Rev Genet* 3:769–778, 2002.

Treff NR, Thompson K, Rafizadeh M, et al. SNP array-based analyses of unbalanced embryos as a reference to distinguish between balanced translocation carrier and normal blastocysts. *J Assist Reprod Genet* 33:1115–1119, 2016.

Trimborn M, Grueters A, Neitzel H, Tönnies H. First small supernumerary ring chromosome carrying 10q euchromatin in a patient with mild phenotype characterized by molecular cytogenetic techniques and review of the literature. *Cytogenet Genome Res* 108:278–282, 2005.

Tritto V, Bettinaglio P, Mangano E, et al. Genetic/epigenetic effects in NF1 microdeletion syndrome: Beyond the haploinsufficiency, looking at the contribution of not deleted genes. *Hum Genet* 143:775–795, 2024.

Tropeano M, Ahn JW, Dobson RJ, et al. Male-biased autosomal effect of 16p13.11 copy number variation in neurodevelopmental disorders. *PLoS One* 8:e61365, 2013.

Trpchevska N, Dimova I, Arabadji T, et al. A family study of complex chromosome rearrangement involving chromosomes 1, 8, and 11 and its reproductive consequences. *J Assist Reprod Genet* 34:659–669, 2017.

Tsai AC, Fine CA, Yang M, Walton CS, Beischel L, Johnson JP. De novo isodicentric X chromosome: 46,X,idic(X)(q24), and summary of literature. *Am J Med Genet* 140:923–930, 2006.

Tsai AC, Gibby T, Beischel L, McGavran L, Johnson JP. A child with Angelman syndrome and trisomy 13 findings due to associated paternal UPD 15 and segmental UPD 13. *Am J Med Genet* 126A:208–212, 2004.

Tsai LP, Liao HM, Chen YJ, Fang JS, Chen CH. A novel microdeletion at chromosome 2q31.1–31.2 in a three-generation family presenting duplication of great toes with clinodactyly. *Clin Genet* 75:449–456, 2009.

Tschare L, Ennemoser A, Carli L, Vaccari E, Feichtinger M. Impact of maternally derived meiotic aneuploidies on early embryonic development in vitro. *J Assist Reprod Genet* 40:2715–2723, 2023.

Tseng LH, Chuang SM, Lee TY, Ko TM. Recurrent Down's syndrome due to maternal ovarian trisomy 21 mosaicism. *Arch Gynecol Obstet* 255:213–216, 1994.

Tsezou A, Hadjiathanasiou C, Gourgiotis D, et al. Molecular genetics of Turner syndrome: Correlation with clinical phenotype and response to growth hormone therapy. *Clin Genet* 56:441–446, 1999.

Tsou AY, Bulova P, Capone G, et al. Medical care of adults with Down syndrome: A clinical guideline. *JAMA* 324:1543–1556, 2020.

Tsuboyama M, Iqbal MA. CHL1 deletion is associated with cognitive and language disabilities—Case report and review of literature. *Mol Genet Genomic Med* 9:e1725, 2021.

Tucci A, Ciaccio C, Scuvera G, Esposito S, Milani D. *MIR137* is the key gene mediator of the syndromic obesity phenotype of patients with 1p21.3 microdeletions. *Mol Cytogenet* 9:80, 2016.

Tucker ME, Garringer HJ, Weaver DD. Phenotypic spectrum of mosaic trisomy 18: Two new patients, a literature review, and counseling issues. *Am J Med Genet* 143:505–517, 2007.

Tuck-Muller CM, Chen H, Martínez JE, et al. Isodicentric Y chromosome: Cytogenetic, molecular and clinical studies and review of the literature. *Hum Genet* 96:119–129, 1995.

Tuğ E, Karacaaltincaba D, Yirmibeş Karaoğuz M, Saat H, Özek A. Confirmation of the prenatal mosaic trisomy 2 via fetal USG and cytogenetic analyses. *J Matern Fetal Neonatal Med* 18:1–12, 2017.

Tug E, Karaoguz MY, Bakir A. An interchange trisomy resulted in Down syndrome. *Genet Couns* 27:429–431, 2016.

Tuke MA, Ruth KS, Wood AR, et al. Mosaic Turner syndrome shows reduced penetrance in an adult population study. *Genet Med* 21:877–886, 2019.

Tümer Z, López-Hernández JA, Netchine I, et al. Structural and sequence variants in patients with Silver-Russell syndrome or similar features—Curation of a disease database. *Hum Mutat* 39:345–364, 2018.

Tunç E, Ilgaz S. Robertsonian translocation (13;14) and its clinical manifestations: A literature review. *Reprod Biomed Online* 45:563–573, 2022.

Turchi G, Bernardo P, Consales A, Bilo L, Coppola A. Xq25 microduplication syndrome: A further contribution to its definition. A case report and review of the literature. *Clin Dysmorphol* 29:90–96, 2020.

Turgut NE, Boynukalin FK, Gultomruk M, Yarkiner Z, Abali R, Bahceci M. The number of prior pregnancy losses does not impact euploidy rates in young patients with idiopathic recurrent pregnancy loss. *Arch Gynecol Obstet* 308:1567–1575, 2023.

Türkyılmaz A, Cimbek EA, Çebi AH, Acar Arslan E, Karagüzel G. De novo pure partial trisomy 6p associated with facial dysmorphism, developmental delay, brain anomalies, and primary congenital hypothyroidism. *Mol Syndromol* 14:35–43, 2023.

Turner C, Dennis NR, Skuse DH, Jacobs PA. Seven ring (X) chromosomes lacking the *XIST* locus, six with an unexpectedly mild phenotype. *Hum Genet* 106:93–100, 2000.

Turner JMA. Meiotic sex chromosome inactivation. *Development* 134:1823–1831, 2007.

Turner TN, Yi Q, Krumm N, et al. denovo-db: A compendium of human de novo variants. *Nucleic Acids Res* 45:D804–811, 2017.

Turnpenny PD, Pigott RW. Deletion 22q11 syndrome: Acknowledging a lost eponym as we say farewell to an acronym. *J Med Genet* 38:271–273, 2001.

Turriff AE, Annunziata CM, Malayeri AA, et al. Prenatal cfDNA sequencing and incidental detection of maternal cancer. *N Engl J Med* 391:2123–2132, 2024.

Tüysüz B, Collin A, Arapoglu M, Suyugül N. Clinical variability of Waardenburg-Shah syndrome in patients with proximal 13q deletion syndrome including the endothelin-B receptor locus. *Am J Med Genet* 149A:2290–2295, 2009.

Tyler CT, Rice GM, Grady M, Raca G. Mild clinical presentation in a child with prenatally diagnosed 45,X/47,XX,+18 mosaicism. *Am J Med Genet* 149A:2588–2592, 2009.

Tyshchenko N, Lurie I, Schinzel A. Chromosomal map of human brain malformations. *Hum Genet* 124:73–80, 2009.

Tyson C, Dawson AJ, Bal S, et al. Molecular cytogenetic investigation of two patients with Y chromosome rearrangements and intellectual disability. *Am J Med Genet* 149A:490–495, 2009.

Tyson C, Sharp AJ, Hrynchak M, et al. Expansion of a 12-kb VNTR containing the *REXO1L1* gene cluster underlies the microscopically visible euchromatic variant of 8q21.2. *Eur J Hum Genet* 22:458–463, 2014.

Tzancheva M, Kaneva R, Kumanov P, Williams G, Tyler-Smith C. Two male patients with ring Y: Definition of an interval in Yq contributing to Turner syndrome. *J Med Genet* 36:549–553, 1999.

U

Uchida IA, Freeman VCP. Trisomy 21 Down syndrome: II. Structural chromosome rearrangements in the parents. *Hum Genet* 72:118–122, 1986.

Uehara S, Tamura M, Nata M, et al. Complete androgen insensitivity in a 47,XXY patient with uniparental disomy for the X chromosome. *Am J Med Genet* 86:107–111, 1999a.

Uehara S, Yaegashi N, Maeda T, et al. Risk of recurrence of fetal chromosomal aberrations: Analysis of trisomy 21, trisomy 18, trisomy 13, and 45,X in 1,076 Japanese mothers. *J Obstet Gynaecol Res* 25:373–379, 1999b.

Uematsu A, Yorifuji T, Muroi J, et al. Parental origin of normal X chromosomes in Turner syndrome patients with various karyotypes: Implications for the mechanism leading to generation of a 45,X karyotype. *Am J Med Genet* 111:134–139, 2002.

Uhlmann F. SMC complexes: From DNA to chromosomes. *Nat Rev Mol Cell Biol* 17:399–412, 2016.

Ujfalusi A, Nagy O, Bessenyei B, et al. 22q13 microduplication syndrome in siblings with mild clinical phenotype: Broadening the clinical and behavioral spectrum. *Mol Syndromol* 11:146–152, 2020.

Unda BK, Chalil L, Yoon S, et al. Impaired OTUD7A-dependent Ankyrin regulation mediates neuronal dysfunction in mouse and human models of the 15q13.3 microdeletion syndrome. *Mol Psychiatry* 28:1747–1769. 2023.

Unterberger I, Dobesberger J, Schober H, et al. A further case of familial ring chromosome 20 mosaicism - molecular characterization of the ring and review of the literature. *Eur J Med Genet* 62:103564, 2019.

Urban M, Bommer C, Tennstedt C, et al. Ring chromosome 6 in three fetuses: Case reports, literature review, and implications for prenatal diagnosis. *Am J Med Genet* 108:97–104, 2002.

Urioste M, Martínez-Frías ML, Bermejo E, et al. Short rib-polydactyly syndrome and pericentric inversion of chromosome 4. *Am J Med Genet* 49:94–97, 1994.

Uroz L, Templado C. Meiotic non-disjunction mechanisms in human fertile males. *Hum Reprod* 27:1518–1524, 2012.

Urquhart E. Clairvoyance. *Am J Med Genet* 170A:1242–1244, 2016.

Urquhart JE, Williams SG, Bhaskar SS, Bowers N, Clayton-Smith J, Newman WG. Deletion of 19q13 reveals clinical overlap with Dubowitz syndrome. *J Hum Genet* 60:781–785, 2015.

Usui D, Shimada S, Shimojima K, et al. Interstitial duplication of 2q32.1-q33.3 in a patient with epilepsy, developmental delay, and autistic behavior. *Am J Med Genet* 161A:1078–1084, 2013.

V

Valetto A, Bertini V, Toschi B, Simi P. A 47,XX,+der(21)t(8;21)(q24.2;q21.1) karyotype in a patient with mild intellectual disability, cleft lip, Hashimoto thyroiditis and hirsutism. *Am J Med Genet* 161A:2389–2392, 2013.

Valind A, Pal N, Asmundsson J, Gisselsson D, Holmquist Mengelbier L. Confined trisomy 8 mosaicism of meiotic origin: A rare cause of aneuploidy in childhood cancer. *Genes Chromosomes Cancer* 53:634–638, 2014.

Vals MA, Kahre T, Mee P, et al. Familial 1.3-Mb 11p15.5p15.4 duplication in three generations causing Silver-Russell and Beckwith-Wiedemann syndromes. *Mol Syndromol* 6:147–151, 2015.

Van L, Heung T, Reyes NGD, et al. Real-world treatment of schizophrenia in adults with a 22q11.2 microdeletion: Traitement dans le monde réel de la schizophrénie chez des adultes atteints du syndrome de microdélétion 22q11.2. *Can J Psychiatry*, 70:160–170, 2025.

Van Bon BWM, Balciuniene J, Fruhman G, et al. The phenotype of recurrent 10q22q23 deletions and duplications. *Eur J Hum Genet* 19:400–408, 2011.

Van Bon BWM, Coe BP, Bernier R, et al. Disruptive de novo mutations of *DYRK1A* lead to a syndromic form of autism and ID. *Mol Psychiatry* 21:126–132, 2016.

Van Bon BWM, Koolen DA, Brueton L, et al. The 2q23.1 microdeletion syndrome: Clinical and behavioural phenotype. *Eur J Hum Genet* 18:163–170, 2010.

Van Bon BWM, Mefford HC, Menten B, et al. Further delineation of the 15q13 microdeletion and duplication syndromes: A clinical spectrum varying from non-pathogenic to a severe outcome. *J Med Genet* 46:511–523, 2009.

Van Buggenhout GJ, Pijkels E, Holvoet M, Schaap C, Hamel BC, Fryns JP. Cri du chat syndrome: Changing phenotype in older patients. *Am J Med Genet* 90:203–215, 2000.

Van Cauwenberghe J, Beckers S, Coremans P. Nonmosaic isodicentric Y chromosome: A rare cause of azoospermia—From genetics to clinical practice. *Case Rep Endocrinol* 25;2020:8828740, 2020.

Van de Laar I, Rabelink G, Hochstenbach R, Tuerlings J, Hoogeboom J, Giltay J. Diploid/triploid mosaicism in dysmorphic patients. *Clin Genet* 62:376–382, 2002.

Van den Berg C, Van Opstal D, Polak-Knook J, Galjaard RJ. (Potential) false-negative diagnoses in chorionic villi and a review of the literature. *Prenat Diagn* 26:401–408, 2006.

Van den Berg DJ, Francke U. Roberts syndrome: A review of 100 cases and a new rating system for severity. *Am J Med Genet* 47:1104–1123, 1993.

Van den Berg MM, van Maarle MC, van Wely M, Goddijn M. Genetics of early miscarriage. *Biochim Biophys Acta* 1822:1951–1959, 2012.

van den Boogaard ML, Thijssen PE, Aytekin C, et al. Expanding the mutation spectrum in ICF syndrome: Evidence for a gender bias in ICF2. *Clin Genet* 92:380–387, 2017.

Van der Burgt CJAM, Merkx GFM, Janssen AH, Mulder JC, Suijkerbuijk RF, Smeets DFCM: Partial trisomy for 5q and monosomy for 12p in a liveborn child as a result of a complex five breakpoint chromosome rearrangement in a parent. *J Med Genet* 29:739–741, 1992.

Van der Crabben SN, Hennus MP, McGregor GA, et al. Destabilized *SMC5/6* complex leads to chromosome breakage syndrome with severe lung disease. *J Clin Invest* 126:2881–2892, 2016.

Van der Lelij P, Chrzanowska KH, Godthelp BC, et al. Warsaw breakage syndrome, a cohesinopathy associated with mutations in the XPD helicase family member *DDX11/ChlR1*. *Am J Hum Genet* 86:262–266, 2010.

Van der Lugt NM, Weerts MJA, Veenma DCM, et al. 5q35 duplication syndrome: Narrowing the critical region on the distal side and further evidence of intrafamilial variability and expression. *Am J Med Genet* 191A:835–841, 2023.

Van der Luijt RB, Tops CM, Khan PM, et al. Molecular, cytogenetic, and phenotypic studies of a constitutional reciprocal translocation t(5;10)(q22;q25) responsible for familial adenomatous polyposis in a Dutch pedigree. *Genes Chromosomes Cancer* 13:192–202, 1995.

Van der Steen SL, Riedijk SR, Verhagen-Visser J, et al. The psychological impact of prenatal diagnosis and disclosure of susceptibility loci: First impressions of parents' experiences. *J Genet Couns* 25:1227–1234, 2016.

Van der Veken LT, Dieleman MMJ, Douben H, et al. Low grade mosaic for a complex supernumerary ring chromosome 18 in an adult patient with multiple congenital anomalies. *Mol Cytogenet* 3:13, 2010.

Van der Werf IM, Buiting K, Czeschik C, et al. Novel microdeletions on chromosome 14q32.2 suggest a potential role for non-coding RNAs in Kagami-Ogata syndrome. *Eur J Hum Genet* 24:1724–1729, 2016.

VanDerwerken D. Bayesian assessment of genetic risk in families with a balanced translocation. *J Genet Couns* 24:541–547, 2015.

Van Dijck A, van der Werf IM, Reyniers E, et al. Five patients with a chromosome 1q21.1 triplication show macrocephaly, increased weight and facial similarities. *Eur J Med Genet* 58:503–508, 2015.

Van Dyke DL, Weiss L, Roberson JR, Babu VR. The frequency and mutation rate of balanced autosomal rearrangements in man estimated from prenatal genetic studies for advanced maternal age. *Am J Hum Genet* 35:301–308, 1983.

Van Echten-Arends J, Coonen E, Reuters B, et al. Preimplantation genetic diagnosis for X;autosome translocations: Lessons from a case of misdiagnosis. *Hum Reprod* 28:3141–3145, 2013.

Van Haelst MM, Van Opstal D, Lindhout D, Los FJ. Management of prenatally detected trisomy 8 mosaicism. *Prenat Diagn* 21:1075–1078, 2001.

Van Heertum K, DeVilbiss EA, Goldfarb J, Mumford SL, Weinerman R. Does embryo biopsy, independent of vitrification, impact perinatal outcomes? An analysis of perinatal outcomes following preimplantation genetic testing biopsy in fresh and frozen embryo transfer cycles. *F S Rep* 5:47–54, 2024.

Van Hemel JO, Eussen HJ. Interchromosomal insertions: Identification of five cases and a review. *Hum Genet* 107:415–432, 2000.

Van Hummelen P, Manchester D, Lowe X, Wyrobek AJ. Meiotic segregation, recombination, and gamete aneuploidy assessed in a t(1;10)(p22.1;q22.3) reciprocal translocation carrier by three- and four-probe multicolor FISH in sperm. *Am J Hum Genet* 61:651–659, 1997.

Van Karnebeek CDM, Hennekam RCM. Associations between chromosomal anomalies and congenital heart defects: A database search. *Am J Med Genet* 84:158–166, 1999.

Van Kogelenberg M, Ghedia S, McGillivray G, et al. Periventricular heterotopia in common microdeletion syndromes. *Mol Syndromol* 1:35–41, 2010.

Van Opstal D, Eggenhuizen GM, Joosten M, et al. Noninvasive prenatal testing as compared to chorionic villus sampling is more sensitive for the detection of confined placental mosaicism involving the cytotrophoblast. *Prenat Diagn* 40:1338–1342, 2020.

Van Opstal D, van den Berg C, Galjaard RJH, Los FJ. Follow-up investigations in uncultured amniotic fluid cells after uncertain cytogenetic results. *Prenat Diagn* 21:75–80, 2001.

Van Prooyen Schuurman L, Sistermans EA, Van Opstal D, et al. Clinical impact of additional findings detected by genome-wide non-invasive prenatal testing: Follow-up results of the TRIDENT-2 study. *Am J Hum Genet* 109:1344, 2022.

Van Rahden VA, Fernandez-Vizarra E, Alawi M, et al. Mutations in *NDUFB11*, encoding a complex I component of the mitochondrial respiratory chain, cause microphthalmia with linear skin defects syndrome. *Am J Hum Genet* 96:640–650, 2015.

Van Roode T, Dickson NP, Righarts AA, Gillett WR. Cumulative incidence of infertility in a New Zealand birth cohort to age 38 by sex and the relationship with family formation. *Fertil Steril* 103:1053–1058.e2, 2015.

Van Saen D, Tournaye H, Goossens E. Presence of spermatogonia in 47,XXY men with no spermatozoa recovered after testicular sperm extraction. *Fertil Steril* 97:319–323, 2012.

Van Santen HM, van de Wetering MD, Bos AME, Vd Heuvel-Eibrink MM, van der Pal HJ, Wallace WH. Reproductive complications in childhood cancer survivors. *Pediatr Clin North Am* 67:1187–1202, 2020.

Van Schie JJM, Faramarz A, Balk JA, et al. Warsaw Breakage Syndrome associated DDX11 helicase resolves G-quadruplex structures to support sister chromatid cohesion. *Nat Commun* 11:4287, 2020.

Van Sluis M, van Vuuren C, Mangan H, McStay B. NORs on human acrocentric chromosome p-arms are active by default and can associate with nucleoli independently of rDNA. *PNAS* 117:10368–10377, 2020.

Vandepoele K, Andries V, Van Roy N, et al. A constitutional translocation t(1;17)(p36.2;q11.2) in a neuroblastoma patient disrupts the human NBPF1 and ACCN1 genes. *PLoS One* 3:e2207, 2008.

Vanlerberghe C, Petit F, Malan V, et al. 15q11.2 microdeletion (BP1-BP2) and developmental delay, behaviour issues, epilepsy and congenital heart disease: A series of 52 patients. *Eur J Med Genet* 58:140–147, 2015.

Varela M, Shapira E, Hyman DB. Ullrich-Turner syndrome in mother and daughter: Prenatal diagnosis of a 46,X,del(X)(p21) offspring from a 45,X mother with low-level mosaicism for the del(X)(p21) in one ovary. *Am J Med Genet* 39:411–412, 1991.

Varvagiannis K, Stefanidou A, Gyftodimou Y, et al. Pure de novo partial trisomy 6p in a girl with craniosynostosis. *Am J Med Genet* 161A:343–351, 2013.

Vasani A, Kumar MS. Advances in the proteomics of amniotic fluid to detect biomarkers for chromosomal abnormalities and fetomaternal complications during pregnancy. *Expert Rev Proteomics* 16:277–286, 2019.

Vasilyeva TA, Marakhonov AV, Sukhanova NV, Kutsev SI, Zinchenko RA. Preferentially paternal origin of de novo 11p13 chromosome deletions revealed in patients with congenital aniridia and WAGR syndrome. *Genes (Basel)* 11:812, 2020.

Vassos E, Collier DA, Holden S, et al. Penetrance for copy number variants associated with schizophrenia. *Hum Mol Genet* 19:3477–3481, 2010.

Vaz I, Larkins SA, Norman A, Green SH. Mild developmental delay due to ring chromosome 19 mosaicism. *Dev Med Child Neurol* 41:48–50, 1999.

Vázquez-Cárdenas A, Vásquez-Velásquez AI, Barros-Núñez P, Mantilla-Capacho J, Rocchi M, Rivera H. Familial whole-arm translocations (1;19), (9;13), and (12;21): A review of 101 constitutional exchanges. *J Appl Genet* 48:261–268, 2007.

Vears DF, Delany C, Massie J, Gillam L. Parents' experiences with requesting carrier testing for their unaffected children. *Genet Med* 18:1199–1205, 2016.

Vears DF, Delany C, Massie J, Gillam L. "They Just Want to Know"—Genetic health professionals' beliefs about why parents want to know their child's carrier status. *J Genet Couns* 26:1314–1323, 2017.

Vega H, Trainer AH, Gordillo M, et al. Phenotypic variability in 49 cases of *ESCO2* mutations, including novel missense and codon deletion in the acetyltransferase domain, correlates with *ESCO2* expression and establishes the clinical criteria for Roberts syndrome. *J Med Genet* 47:30–37, 2010.

Velagaleti GVN, Lockhart LH, Schmalstieg FC, Goldman AS. Trisomy 4 pter-q12 and monosomy of chromosome 13 pter-q12 in a male with deficiency of all blood lymphocyte populations. *Am J Med Genet* 102:139–145, 2001.

Veld PA, Weber RF, Los FJ, et al. Two cases of Robertsonian translocations in oligozoospermic males and their consequences for pregnancies induced by intracytoplasmic sperm injection. *Hum Reprod* 12:1642–1644, 1997.

Velinov M, Ahmad A, Brown-Kipphut B, et al. A 0.7 Mb de novo duplication at 7q21.3 including the genes DLX5 and DLX6 in a patient with split-hand/split-foot malformation. *Am J Med Genet* 158A:3201–3206, 2012.

Vendola C, Canfield M, Daiger SP, et al. Survival of Texas infants born with trisomies 21, 18, and 13. *Am J Med Genet* 152A:360–366, 2010.

Venter PA, Dawson B, Du Toit JL, et al. A familial paracentric inversion: A short review of the current status. *Hum Genet* 67:121–125, 1984.

Vera-Carbonell A, López-González V, Bafalliu JA, et al. Pre- and postnatal findings in a patient with a novel rec(8)dup(8q)inv(8)(p23.2q22.3) associated with San Luis Valley syndrome. *Am J Med Genet* 161A:2369–2375, 2013.

Verbesselt J, Solot CB, Van Den Heuvel E, et al. Language profiles of school-aged children with 22q11.2 copy number variants. *Genes (Basel)* 14:679, 2023.

Verbesselt J, Zink I, Breckpot J, Swillen A. Cross-sectional and longitudinal findings in patients with proximal 22q11.2 duplication: A retrospective chart study. *Am J Med Genet* 188A:46–57, 2022.

Verdoni A, Hu J, Surti U, Babcock M, et al. Reproductive outcomes in individuals with chromosomal reciprocal translocations. *Genet Med* 23:1753–1760, 2021.

Verdyck P, Altarescu G, Santos-Ribeiro S, et al. Aneuploidy in oocytes from women of advanced maternal age: Analysis of the causal meiotic errors and impact on embryo development. *Hum Reprod* 38:2526–2535, 2023.

Verebi C, Caumes R, Chantot-Bastaraud S, et al. How a paternal uniparental isodisomy of chromosome 17 leads to autosomal recessive limb-girdle muscular dystrophy R3. *Neuromuscul Disord* 33:367–370, 2023.

Vergés L, Molina O, Geán E, Vidal F, Blanco J. Deletions and duplications of the 22q11.2 region in spermatozoa from DiGeorge/velocardiofacial fathers. *Mol Cytogenet* 7:86, 2014.

Vergult S, Leroy B, Claerhout I, Menten B. Familial cases of a submicroscopic Xp22.2 deletion: Genotype-phenotype correlation in microphthalmia with linear skin defects syndrome. *Mol Vis* 19:311–318, 2013.

Verhoeven WMA, Egger JIM, van den Bergh JPW, van Beek R, Kleefstra T, de Leeuw N. A 12q24.31 interstitial deletion in an adult male with *MODY3*: Neuropsychiatric and neuropsychological characteristics. *Am J Med Genet* 167A:169–173, 2015.

Verlinsky Y, Rechitsky S, Schoolcraft W, Strom C, Kuliev A. Preimplantation diagnosis for Fanconi anemia combined with HLA matching. *J Am Med Assoc* 285:3130–3133, 2001.

Verloes A, Gillerot Y, Van Maldergem L, et al. Major decrease in the incidence of trisomy 21 at birth in south Belgium: Mass impact of triple test? *Eur J Hum Genet* 9:1–4, 2001.

Verma RS, Rodriguez J, Dosik H. The clinical significance of pericentric inversion of the human Y chromosome: A rare "third" type of heteromorphism. *J Hered* 73:236–238, 1982.

Vermeesch JR, Petit P, Speleman F, Devriendt K, Fryns JP, Marynen P. Interstitial telomeric sequences at the junction site of a jumping translocation. *Hum Genet* 99:735–737, 1997.

Vermeulen MC, Pearse R, Young-Pearse T, Mostafavi S. Mosaic loss of chromosome Y in aged human microglia. *Genome Res* 32:1795–1807, 2022.

Vernon HJ, Bytyci Telegrafi A, Batista D, Owegi M, Leigh R. 6p25 microdeletion: White matter abnormalities in an adult patient. *Am J Med Genet* 161A:1686–1689, 2013.

Verp MS, Bombard AT, Simpson JL, Elias S. Parental decision following prenatal diagnosis of fetal chromosome abnormality. *Am J Med Genet* 29:613–622, 1988.

Verpoest W, Okutman Ö, Van Der Kelen A, Sermon K, Viville S. Genetics of infertility: A paradigm shift for medically assisted reproduction. *Hum Reprod* 38:2289–2295, 2023.

Verpoest W, Staessen C, Bossuyt PM, et al. Preimplantation genetic testing for aneuploicy by microarray analysis of polar bodies in advanced maternal age: A randomized clinical trial. *Hum Reprod* 33:1767–1776, 2018.

Vervoort L, Dierckxsens N, Sousa Santos M, et al. Multiple paralogues and recombination mechanisms contribute to the high incidence of 22q11.2 deletion syndrome. *Genome Res* 13:gr.279331.124, 2025.

Vetro A, Dehghani MR, Kraoua L, et al. Testis development in the absence of *SRY*: Chromosomal rearrangements at *SOX9* and *SOX3*. *Eur J Hum Genet* 23:1025–1032, 2015.

Veyt N, Van Buggenhout G, Devriendt K, Van Den Bogaert K, Brison N. Expanding the phenotype of copy number variations involving NR0B1 (DAX1). *Eur J Hum Genet* 32:421–425, 2024.

Vialard F, Nouchy M, Malan V, Taillemite JL, Selva J, Portnoï MF. Whole-arm translocations between chromosome 1 and acrocentric G chromosomes are associated with a poor prognosis for spermatogenesis: Two new cases and review of the literature. *Fertil Steril* 86:1001, e1–5, 2006a.

Vialard F, Petit C, Bergere M, Gomes DM, et al. Evidence of a high proportion of premature unbalanced separation of sister chromatids in the first polar bodies of women of advanced age. *Hum Reprod* 21:1172–1178, 2006b.

Viana MM, Vianna GS, Carvalho ERF, da Costa HBBLM, de Aguiar MJB. High-level mosaic monosomy 21 in a 13-year-old girl: Case report and review of the literature. *Am J Med Genet* 188A:953–958, 2022.

Vichinsartvichai P. Primary ovarian insufficiency associated with autosomal abnormalities: From chromosome to genome-wide and beyond. *Menopause* 23:806–815, 2016.

Vicidomini C, Ponzoni L, Lim D, et al. Pharmacological enhancement of mGlu5 receptors rescues behavioral deficits in *SHANK3* knock-out mice. *Mol Psychiatr* 22:689–702, 2017.

Vickers S, Dahlitz M, Hardy C, Kilpatrick M, Webb T. A male with a de novo translocation involving loss of 15q11q13 material and Prader-Willi syndrome. *J Med Genet* 31:478–481, 1994.

Victor AR, Griffin DK, Brake AJ, et al. Assessment of aneuploidy concordance between clinical trophectoderm biopsy and blastocyst. *Hum Reprod* 34:181–192. 2019.

Vieira GH, Rodriguez JD, Carmona-Mora P, et al. Detection of classical 17p11.2 deletions, an atypical deletion and *RAI1* alterations in patients with features suggestive of Smith-Magenis syndrome. *Eur J Hum Genet* 20:148–154, 2012.

Vieira JP, Lopes F, Silva-Fernandes A, et al. Variant Rett syndrome in a girl with a pericentric X-chromosome inversion leading to epigenetic changes and overexpression of the *MECP2* gene. *Int J Dev Neurosci* 46:82–87, 2015.

Villa N, Bentivegna A, Ertel A, et al. A de novo supernumerary genomic discontinuous ring chromosome 21 in a child with mild intellectual disability. *Am J Med Genet* 155A:1425–1431, 2011.

Villavicencio-Lorini P, Klopocki E, Trimborn M, Koll R, Mundlos S, Horn D. Phenotypic variant of brachydactyly-mental retardation syndrome in a family with an inherited interstitial 2q37.3 microdeletion including *HDAC4*. *Eur J Hum Genet* 21:743–748, 2013.

Vincent KM, Stavropoulos DJ, Beaulieu-Bergeron M, et al. A 79-kb paternally inherited 7q32.2 microdeletion involving MEST in a patient with a Silver-Russell syndrome-like phenotype. *Am J Med Genet* 188A:2421–2428, 2022.

Viotti M, Greco E, Grifo JA, et al. Chromosomal, gestational, and neonatal outcomes of embryos classified as a mosaic by preimplantation genetic testing for aneuploidy. *Fertil Steril* 120:957–966. 2023.

Viotti M, Victor AR, Barnes FL, et al. Using outcome data from one thousand mosaic embryo transfers to formulate an embryo ranking system for clinical use. *Fertil Steril* 115:1212–1224, 2021.

Visootsak J, Graham JM. Klinefelter syndrome and other sex chromosomal aneuploidies. *Orphanet J Rare Dis* 1:42, 2006.

Vissers LELM, van Ravenswaaij CMA, Admiraal R, et al. Mutations in a new member of the chromodomain gene family cause CHARGE syndrome. *Nat Genet* 36:955–957, 2004.

Vloeberghs V, Verheyen G, Santos-Ribeiro S, et al. Is genetic fatherhood within reach for all azoospermic Klinefelter men? *PLoS One* 13:e0200300, 2018.

Vockley J, Inserra JA, Breg WR, Yang-Feng TL. "Pseudomosaicism" for 4p- in amniotic fluid cell culture proven to be true mosaicism after birth. *Am J Med Genet* 39:81–83, 1991.

Voiculescu I, Barbi G, Wolff G, Steinbach P, Back E, Schempp W. Familial pericentric inversion of chromosome 12. *Hum Genet* 72:320–322, 1986.

Vona B, Nanda I, Neuner C, et al. Terminal chromosome 4q deletion syndrome in an infant with hearing impairment and moderate syndromic features: Review of literature. *BMC Med Genet* 15:72, 2014.

Vorstman JA, Breetvelt EJ, Duijff SN, et al. Cognitive decline preceding the onset of psychosis in patients with 22q11.2 deletion syndrome. *JAMA Psychiatry* 72:377–385, 2015.

Vos N, Kleinendorst L, van der Laan L, van Uhm J, et al. Evaluation of 100 Dutch cases with 16p11.2 deletion and duplication syndromes; from clinical manifestations towards personalized treatment options. *Eur J Hum Genet* 32:1387–1401, 2024.

Voullaire L, Collins V, Callaghan T, McBain J, Williamson R, Wilton L. High incidence of complex chromosome abnormality in cleavage embryos from patients with repeated implantation failure. *Fertil Steril* 87:1053–1058, 2007.

Voullaire L, Gardner RJM, Vaux C, Robertson A, Oertel R, Slater H. Chromosomal duplication of band 10p14 segregating through four generations. *J Med Genet* 37:233–237, 2000a.

Voullaire LE, Slater HR, Petrovic V, Choo KHA. A functional marker centromere with no detectable alpha-satellite, satellite III, or CENP-B protein: Activation of a latent centromere? *Am J Hum Genet* 52:1153–1163, 1993.

Voullaire L, Slater H, Williamson R, Wilton L. Chromosome analysis of blastomeres from human embryos by using comparative genomic hybridization. *Hum Genet* 106:210–217, 2000b.

Vozdova M, Horinova V, Wernerova V, et al. der(4)t(Y;4): Three-generation transmission and sperm meiotic segregation analysis. *Am J Med Genet* 155A:1157–1161, 2011.

Vranekovic J, Božovic IB, Grubic Z, et al. Down syndrome: Parental origin, recombination, and maternal age. *Genet Test Mol Biomarkers* 16:70–73, 2012.

Vreeburg M, van Steensel MA. Genodermatoses caused by genetic mosaicism. *Eur J Pediatr* 171:1725–1735, 2012.

Vujisic S, Korac P, Pavlica M, Vujnovic N, Dmitrovic R. Chromosomal segregation in sperm of the Robertsonian translocation (21;22) carrier and its impact on IVF outcome. *J Assist Reprod Genet* 37:231–238, 2020.

W

Wagner T, Wirth J, Meyer J, et al. Autosomal sex reversal and campomelic dysplasia are caused by mutations in and around the *SRY*-related gene *SOX9*. *Cell* 79:1111–1120, 1994.

Wahab MA, Nickless EM, Najar-M'Kacher R, Parmentier C, Podd JV, Rowland RE. Elevated chromosome translocation frequencies in New Zealand nuclear test veterans. *Cytogenet Genome Res* 121:79–87, 2008.

Wakeling EL, Abu-Amero S, Alders M, et al. Epigenotype-phenotype correlations in Silver-Russell syndrome. *J Med Genet* 47:760–768, 2010.

Wakeling EL, Brioude F, Lokulo-Sodipe O, et al. Diagnosis and management of Silver-Russell syndrome: First international consensus statement. *Nat Rev Endocrinol* 13:105–124, 2017.

Wakui K, Gregato G, Ballif BC, et al. Construction of a natural panel of 11p11.2 deletions and further delineation of the critical region involved in Potocki-Shaffer syndrome. *Eur J Hum Genet* 13:528–540, 2005.

Walczak C, Enders H, Grissinger K, Dufke A. Retrospective diagnosis of trisomy 15 in formalin-fixed, paraffin-embedded placental tissue in a newborn girl with Prader-Willi syndrome. *Prenat Diagn* 20:914–916, 2000.

Walczak-Sztulpa J, Wisniewska M, Latos-Bielenska A, et al. Chromosome deletions in 13q33-34: Report of four patients and review of the literature. *Am J Med Genet* 146A:337–342, 2008.

Wald N, Bestwick J, Morris J. Risk or chance. *J Med Screen* 29:68, 2022.

Walker LC, Krause L; kConFab Investigators; Spurdle AB, Waddell N. Germline copy number variants are not associated with globally acquired copy number changes in familial breast tumours. *Breast Cancer Res Treat* 134:1005–1011, 2012.

Walkinshaw SA. Fetal choroid plexus cysts: Are we there yet? *Prenat Diagn* 20:657–662, 2000.

Walknowska J, Conte FA, Grumbach MM. Practical and theoretical implications of fetal-maternal lymphocyte transfer. *Lancet* 1:1119–1122, 1969.

Wallace BMN, Hultén MA. Triple chromosome synapsis in oocytes from a human foetus with trisomy 21. *Ann Hum Genet* 47:271–276, 1983.

Wallace WHB, Kelsey TW. Human ovarian reserve from conception to the menopause. *PLoS One* 5:e8772, 2010.

Wallerstein R, Oh T, Durcan J, Abdelhak Y, Clachko M, Aviv H. Outcome of prenatally diagnosed trisomy 6 mosaicism. *Prenat Diagn* 22:722–724, 2002.

Wallerstein R, Twersky S, Layman P, et al. Long term follow-up of developmental delay in a child with prenatally-diagnosed trisomy 20 mosaicism. *Am J Med Genet* 137:94–97, 2005.

Wallerstein R, Yu MT, Neu RL, et al. Common trisomy mosaicism diagnosed in amniocytes involving chromosomes 13, 18, 20 and 21: Karyotype-phenotype correlations. *Prenat Diagn* 20:103–122, 2000.

Wallis M, Pope-Couston R, Mansour J, Amor DJ, Tang P, Stock-Myer S. Lymphedema distichiasis syndrome may be caused by FOXC2 promoter-enhancer dissociation and disruption of a topological associated domain. *Am J Med Genet* 185A:150–156, 2021.

Wallon D, Boluda S, Rovelet-Lecrux A, et al. Clinical and neuropathological diversity of tauopathy in MAPT duplication carriers. *Acta Neuropathol* 142:259–278, 2021.

Walters, S. (1995). Down's tests are a right. *Sunday Age* (Melbourne), July 23, 1995.

Walters-Sen LC, Windemuth K, Angione K, Nandhlal J, Milunsky JM. Familial transmission of 5p13.2 duplication due to maternal der(X)ins(X;5). *Eur J Med Genet* 58:305–309, 2015.

Walzer S, Bashir AS, Silbert AR. Cognitive and behavioral factors in the learning disabilities of 47,XXY and 47,XYY boys. *Birth Defects Orig Artic Ser* 26:45–58, 1990.

Wakeling EL, Brioude F, Lokulo-Sodipe O, et al. Diagnosis and management of Silver-Russell syndrome: First international consensus statement. *Nat Rev Endocrinol* 13:105–124, 2017.

Wang BT, Chong TP, Boyar FZ, et al. Abnormalities in spontaneous abortions detected by G-banding and chromosomal microarray analysis (CMA) at a national reference laboratory. *Mol Cytogenet* 7:33, 2014a.

Wang H, Dong Z, Zhang R, et al. Low-pass genome sequencing versus chromosomal microarray analysis: Implementation in prenatal diagnosis. *Genet Med* 22:500–510, 2020a.

Wang J, Li D, Xu Z, et al. Analysis of meiotic segregation modes in biopsied blastocysts from preimplantation genetic testing cycles of reciprocal translocations. *Mol Cytogenet* 12:11, 2019.

Wang J, Xiao L, Wang J, Ding Z, Ni J, Long X. Mosaic ring chromosome 18 in a Chinese child with epilepsy: A case report and review of the literature. *Neurol Sci* 42:5231–5239, 2021.

Wang JC, Fisker T, Dang L, Teshima I, Nowaczyk MJ. 4.3-Mb triplication of 4q32.1-q32.2: Report of a family through two generations. *Am J Med Genet* 149A:2274–2279, 2009.

Wang JCC, Mamunes P, Kou SY, Schmidt J, Mao R, Hsu WT. Centromeric DNA break in a 10;16 reciprocal translocation associated with trisomy 16 confined placental mosaicism and maternal uniparental disomy for chromosome 16. *Am J Med Genet* 80:418–422, 1998.

Wang L, Iqbal F, Li G, et al. Abnormal meiotic recombination with complex chromosomal rearrangement in an azoospermic man. *Reprod Biomed Online* 30:651–658, 2015.

Wang NJ, Liu D, Parokonny AS, Schanen NC. High-resolution molecular characterization of 15q11-q13 rearrangements by array comparative genomic hybridization (array CGH) with detection of gene dosage. *Am J Hum Genet* 75:267–281, 2004.

Wang T, Lian J, Ren C, et al. Prenatal diagnosis of mosaic trisomy 2 and literature review. *Mol Cytogenet* 25;13:36, 2020b.

Wang X, Zhang Z, Zuo W, et al. Case report: Identification of microduplication in the chromosomal 2p16.1p15 region in an infant suffering from pulmonary arterial hypertension. *Front Cardiovasc Med* 10:1219480, 2023a.

Wang Y, Chen Y, Tian F, et al. Maternal mosaicism is a significant contributor to discordant sex chromosomal aneuploidies associated with noninvasive prenatal testing. *Clin Chem* 60:251–259, 2014b.

Wang Y, Lazier J, Myles-Reid D, Noor A, Chitayat D, Greenfeld E. Role of comprehensive cytogenomic investigation in successful reproductive outcome of parental small neocentromeric supernumerary ring chromosome: A case report. *Clin Case Rep* 11:e6632, 2023b.

Wang Y, Zhang B, Zhang L, et al. The 3D Genome Browser: A web-based browser for visualizing 3D genome organization and long-range chromatin interactions. *Genome Biol* 19:151, 2018.

Wang Z, Cody JD, Leach RJ, O'Connell P. Gene expression patterns in cell lines from patients with 18q-syndrome. *Hum Genet* 104:467–475, 1999.

Wapner RJ, Martin CL, Levy B, et al. Chromosomal microarray versus karyotyping for prenatal diagnosis. *N Engl J Med* 367:2175–2184, 2012.

Warburton D. Genetic factors influencing aneuploidy frequency. In Dellarco VL, Voytek PE, Hollaender A (eds.), *Aneuploidy: Etiology and Mechanisms.* New York, NY: Plenum, 1985.

Warburton D. De novo balanced chromosome rearrangements and extra marker chromosomes identified at prenatal diagnosis: Clinical significance and distribution of breakpoints. *Am J Hum Genet* 49:995–1013, 1991.

Warburton D. Trisomy 7 mosaicism: Prognosis after prenatal diagnosis. *Prenat Diagn* 22:1239–1240, 2002.

Warburton D, Dallaire L, Thangavelu M, Ross L, Levin B, Kline J. Trisomy recurrence: A reconsideration based on North American data. *Am J Hum Genet* 75:376–385, 2004.

Warburton D, Twersky S. Risk of phenotypic abnormalities in paracentric inversion carriers. *Am J Med Genet* 69:219, 1997.

Wartosch L, Schindler K, Schuh M, et al. Origins and mechanisms leading to aneuploidy in human eggs. *Prenat Diagn* 41:620–630, 2021.

Wasielak-Politowska M, Kordowitzki P. Chromosome segregation in the oocyte: What goes wrong during aging. *Int J Mol Sci* 23:2880, 2022.

Waters JJ, Campbell PL, Crocker AJM, Campbell CM. Phenotypic effects of balanced X-autosome translocations in females: A retrospective survey of 104 cases reported from UK laboratories. *Hum Genet* 108:318–327, 2001.

Watkins C, Lazzarini A, McCormack M, Reid CS. Genetic counseling for the mildly mentally retarded client: Three case reports. In Zellers N (ed.), *Strategies for Genetic Counseling: Tools for Professional Advancement*. New York, NY: Human Services Press, 1989:219–234.

Watson CM, Crinnion LA, Harrison SM, et al. A chromosome 7 pericentric inversion defined at single-nucleotide resolution using diagnostic whole genome sequencing in a patient with hand-foot-genital syndrome. *PLoS One* 11:e0157075, 2016.

Watson P. Legal and ethical issues in wrongful life actions. *Melbourne Univ Law Rev* 26:14, 2002.

Watt AJ, Devereux FJ, Monk NA, Myers CJ, Gardner RJM. The phenotype in placental trisomy 7. *Aust NZ J Obstet Gynaecol* 31:246–248, 1991.

Wattanasirichaigoon D, Promsonthi P, Chuansumrit A, et al. Maternal uniparental disomy of chromosome 16 resulting in hemoglobin Bart's hydrops fetalis. *Clin Genet* 74:284–287, 2008.

Wawrocka A, Sikora A, Kuszel L, Krawczynski MR. 11p13 deletions can be more frequent than the *PAX6* gene point mutations in Polish patients with aniridia. *J Appl Genet* 54:345–351, 2013.

Weaver MS, Anderson V, Beck J, et al. Interdisciplinary care of children with trisomy 13 and 18. *Am J Med Genet* 185A:966–977, 2021.

Webb GC, Voullaire LE, Rogers JG. Duplication of a small segment of 5p due to maternal recombination within a paracentric shift. *Am J Med Genet* 30:875–881, 1988.

Weber W. France's highest court recognises "the right not to be born." *Lancet* 358:1972, 2001.

Webster A, Schuh M. Mechanisms of aneuploidy in human eggs. *Trends Cell Biol* 27:55–68, 2017.

Wegiel J, Kaczmarski W, Barua M, et al. Link between DYRK1A overexpression and several-fold enhancement of neurofibrillary degeneration with 3-repeat tau protein in Down syndrome. *J Neuropathol Exp Neurol* 70:36–50, 2011.

Wegner RD, Entezami M, Knoll U, Horn D, Sohl S, Becker R. Prenatal diagnosis of fetal trisomy 6 mosaicism and phenotype of the affected newborn. *Am J Med Genet* 124A:85–88, 2004.

Wegner RD, Kistner G, Becker R, et al. Fetal 46,XX/69,XXY mixoploidy: Origin and confirmation by analysis of fetal urine cells. *Prenat Diagn* 29:287–289, 2009.

Wei HJ, Chiang HS, Lin WM, Wen JY. Pregnancy after preimplantation genetic diagnosis by fluorescence in situ hybridization using 18-, X-, and Y-chromosome probes in an infertile male with mosaic trisomy 18. *J Assist Reprod Genet* 17:229–231, 2000.

Wei S, Djandji A, Lattin MT, et al. Rapid nanopore sequencing-based screen for aneuploidy in reproductive care. *N Engl J Med* 387:658–660, 2022.

Wei S, Weiss ZR, Gaur P, Forman E, Williams Z. Rapid preimplantation genetic screening using a handheld, nanopore-based DNA sequencer. *Fertil Steril* 110:910–916.e2, 2018.

Weil D, Wang I, Dietrich A, Poustka A, Weissenbach J, Petit C. Highly homologous loci on the X and Y chromosomes are hot-spots for ectopic recombinations leading to XX maleness. *Nat Genet* 7:414–419, 1994.

Weisz B, Rodeck CH. An update on antenatal screening for Down's syndrome and specific implications for assisted reproduction pregnancies. *Hum Reprod Update* 12:513–518, 2006.

Weksberg R, Shuman C, Beckwith JB. Beckwith-Wiedemann syndrome. *Eur J Hum Genet* 18:8–14, 2010.

Wells D, Alfarawati S, Fragouli E. Use of comprehensive chromosomal screening for embryo assessment: Microarrays and CGH. *Mol Hum Reprod* 14:703–710, 2008.

Wenger SL, Boone LY, Cummins JH, et al. Newborn infant with inherited ring and de novo interstitial deletion on homologous chromosome 22s. *Am J Med Genet* 91:351–354, 2000.

Wenger SL, Sell SL, Painter MJ, Steele MW. Inherited unbalanced subtelomeric translocation in a child with 8p- and Angelman syndromes. *Am J Med Genet* 70:150–154, 1997.

Wenger SL, Steele MW, Boone LY, Lenkey SG, Cummins JH, Chen XQ. "Balanced" karyotypes in six abnormal offspring of balanced reciprocal translocation normal carrier parents. *Am J Med Genet* 55:47–52, 1995.

Weremowicz S, Sandstrom DJ, Morton CC, Niedzwiecki CA, Sandstrom MM, Bieber FR. Fluorescence in situ hybridization (FISH) for rapid detection of aneuploidy: Experience in 911 prenatal cases. *Prenat Diagn* 21:262–269, 2001.

Werner-Lin A, Barg FK, Kellom KS, et al. Couple's narratives of communion and isolation following abnormal prenatal microarray testing results. *Qual Health Res* 26:1975–1987, 2016a.

Werner-Lin A, McCoyd JL, Bernhardt BA. Balancing genetics (science) and counseling (art) in prenatal chromosomal microarray testing. *J Genet Couns* 25:855–867, 2016b.

Werner-Lin A, Walser S, Barg FK, Bernhardt BA. "They can't find anything wrong with him, yet": Mothers' experiences of parenting an infant with a prenatally diagnosed copy number variant (CNV). *Am J Med Genet* 173A:444–451, 2017.

Wessels MW, Los FJ, Frohn-Mulder IME, Niermeijer MF, Willems PJ, Wladimiroff JW. Poor outcome in Down syndrome fetuses with cardiac anomalies or growth retardation. *Am J Med Genet* 116A:147–151, 2003.

White LM, Treat K, Leff A, Styers D, Mitchell M, Knoll JHM. Exclusion of uniparental inheritance of chromosome 15 in a fetus with a familial dicentric (Y;15) translocation. *Prenat Diagn* 18:111–116, 1998.

White M, Zacharin MR, Fawcett S, McGillivray G. Klinefelter Syndrome: What should we tell prospective parents? *Prenat Diagn* 43:240–249, 2023.

Whiteford ML, Baird C, Kinmond S, Donaldson B, Davidson HR. A child with bisatellited, dicentric chromosome 15 arising from a maternal paracentric inversion of chromosome 15q. *J Med Genet* 37:E11, 2000.

Wieczorek D, Prott EC, Robinson WP, Passarge E, Gillessen-Kaesbach G. Prenatally detected trisomy 4 and 6 mosaicism—Cytogenetic results and clinical phenotype. *Prenat Diagn* 23:128–133, 2003.

Wieland I, Schanze D, Schanze I, Volleth M, Muschke P, Zenker M. A cryptic unbalanced translocation der(4)t(4;17)(p16.1;q25.3) identifies Wittwer syndrome as a variant of Wolf-Hirschhorn syndrome. *Am J Med Genet* 164A:3213–3214, 2014.

Wiersma R. True hermaphroditism in southern Africa: The clinical picture. *Pediatr Surg Int* 20:363–368, 2004.

Wigby K, D'Epagnier C, Howell S, et al. Expanding the phenotype of triple X syndrome: A comparison of prenatal versus postnatal diagnosis. *Am J Med Genet* 170A:2870–2881, 2016.

Wiktor AE, Van Dyke DL. Detection of low level sex chromosome mosaicism in Ullrich-Turner syndrome patients. *Am J Med Genet* 138A:259–261, 2005.

Wiland E, Midro AT, Panasiuk B, Kurpisz M. The analysis of meiotic segregation patterns and aneuploidy in the spermatozoa of father and son with translocation t(4;5)(p15.1;p12) and the prediction of the individual probability rate for unbalanced progeny at birth. *J Androl* 28:262–272, 2007.

Wiland E, Olszewska M, Woźniak T, Kurpisz M. How much, if anything, do we know about sperm chromosomes of Robertsonian translocation carriers? *Cell Mol Life Sci* 77:4765–4785, 2020.

Wilbur AK. Possible case of Rubinstein-Taybi syndrome in a prehistoric skeleton from west-central Illinois. *Am J Med Genet* 91:56–61, 2000.

Wilkins EJ, Archibald AD, Sahhar MA, White SM. "It wasn't a disaster or anything": Parents' experiences of their child's uncertain chromosomal microarray result. *Am J Med Genet* 170A:2895–2904, 2016.

Willemsen MH, Beunders G, Callaghan M, et al. Familial Kleefstra syndrome due to maternal somatic mosaicism for interstitial 9q34.3 microdeletions. *Clin Genet* 80:31–38, 2011a.

Willemsen MH, Vallès A, Kirkels LAMH, et al. Chromosome 1p21.3 microdeletions comprising *DPYD* and *MIR137* are associated with intellectual disability. *J Med Genet* 48:810–818, 2011b.

Williams J, Dear PRF. An unbalanced t(X;10) mat translocation in a child with congenital abnormalities. *J Med Genet* 24:633, 1987.

Williamson EM, Miller JF, Seabright M. Pericentric inversion (13) with two different recombinants in the same family. *J Med Genet* 17:309–312, 1980.

Willis MJH, Bird LM, Dell'Aquilla M, Jones MC. Natural history of prenatally diagnosed 46,X,isodicentric Y. *Prenat Diagn* 26:134–137, 2006.

Willis MJH, Bird LM, Dell'Aquilla M, Jones MC. Expanding the phenotype of mosaic trisomy 20. *Am J Med Genet* 146:330–336, 2008.

Wilson GR, Sim JC, McLean C, et al. Mutations in RAB39B cause X-linked intellectual disability and early-onset Parkinson disease with α-synuclein pathology. *Am J Hum Genet* 95:729–735, 2014.

Wilson MG, Lin MS, Fujimoto A, Herbert W, Kaplan FM. Chromosome mosaicism in 6,000 amniocenteses. *Am J Med Genet* 32:506–513, 1989.

Wilton L, Williamson R, McBain J, Edgar D, Voullaire L. Birth of a healthy infant after preimplantation confirmation of euploidy by comparative genomic hybridization. *N Engl J Med* 345:1537–1541, 2001.

Wimalasundera RC, Gardiner HM. Congenital heart disease and aneuploidy. *Prenat Diagn* 24:1116–1122, 2004.

Wimmer R, Neumann U, Weber A, et al. Intersexual twins due to tetragametic chimerism. *Cytogenet Genome Res* 162:378–385, 2022.

Wimplinger I, Rauch A, Orth U, Schwarzer U, Trautmann U, Kutsche K. Mother and daughter with a terminal Xp deletion: Implication of chromosomal mosaicism and X-inactivation in the high clinical variability of the microphthalmia with linear skin defects (MLS) syndrome. *Eur J Med Genet* 50:421–431, 2007.

Wincent J, Helgadóttir HT, Sergouniotis F, et al. Genome sequencing differentiates a paracentric inversion from a balanced insertion enabling more accurate preimplantation genetic testing. *Acta Obstet Gynecol Scand* 103:1564–1569, 2024.

Winter JSD. Androgen therapy in Klinefelter syndrome during adolescence. *Birth Defects Orig Artic Ser* 26:235–245, 1990.

Wischmeijer A, Magini P, Giorda R, et al. Olfactory receptor-related duplicons mediate a microdeletion at 11q13.2q13.4 associated with a syndromic phenotype. *Mol Syndromol* 1:176–184, 2011.

Witters I, Devriendt K, Legius E, et al. Rapid prenatal diagnosis of trisomy 21 in 5049 consecutive uncultured amniotic fluid samples by fluorescence in situ hybridisation (FISH). *Prenat Diagn* 22:29–33, 2002.

Witters I, Fryns JP. Follow-up of a child with trisomy 17 mosaicism. *Prenat Diagn* 28:1080, 2008.

Witteveen JS, Willemsen MH, Dombroski TC, et al. Haploinsufficiency of *MeCP2*-interacting transcriptional co-repressor *SIN3A* causes mild intellectual disability by affecting the development of cortical integrity. *Nat Genet* 48:877–887, 2016.

Wójcik C, Volz K, Ranola M, et al. Rubinstein-Taybi syndrome associated with Chiari type I malformation caused by a large 16p13.3 microdeletion: A contiguous gene syndrome? *Am J Med Genet* 152A:479–483, 2010.

Wójtowicz A, Madetko-Talowska A, Wójtowicz W, Szewczyk K, Huras H, Bik-Multanowski M. Cardiovascular anomalies among 1005 fetuses referred to Invasive prenatal testing—A comprehensive cohort study of associated chromosomal aberrations. *Int J Environ Res Public Health* 19:10019, 2022.

Wolff DJ, Miller AP, Van Dyke DL, Schwartz S, Willard HF. Molecular definition of breakpoints associated with human Xq isochromosomes: Implications for mechanisms of formation. *Am J Hum Genet* 58:154–160, 1996.

Wolstenholme J. Confined placental mosaicism for trisomies 2, 3, 7, 8, 9, 16, and 22: Their incidence, likely origins, and mechanisms for cell lineage compartmentalization. *Prenat Diagn* 16:511–524, 1996.

Wolstenholme J, Webb AL, English CJ, Evans J. Prenatal diagnosis of chromosome 22 mosaicism with extensive investigation of placental and fetal tissues. *Ann Génét* 44 (Suppl 1):14s, 2001a.

Wolstenholme J, White I, Sturgiss S, Carter J, Plant N, Goodship JA. Maternal uniparental heterodisomy for chromosome 2: Detection through "atypical" maternal AFP/hCG levels, with an update on a previous case. *Prenat Diagn* 21:813–817, 2001b.

Won RH, Currier RJ, Lorey F, Towner DR. The timing of demise in fetuses with trisomy 21 and trisomy 18. *Prenat Diagn* 25:608–611, 2005.

Woodage T, Prasad M, Dixon JW, et al. Bloom syndrome and maternal uniparental disomy for chromosome 15. *Am J Hum Genet* 55:74–80, 1994.

Woods CG, Bankier A, Curry J, et al. Asymmetry and skin pigmentary anomalies in chromosome mosaicism. *J Med Genet* 31:694–701, 1994.

Woods CG, Noble J, Falconer AR. A study of brothers with Klinefelter syndrome. *J Med Genet* 34:702, 1997.

Woodward ER, Skytte AB, Cruger DG, Maher ER. Population-based survey of cancer risks in chromosome 3 translocation carriers. *Genes Chromosomes Cancer* 49:52–58, 2010.

Woodward KJ, Stampalia J, Vanyai H, et al. Atypical nested 22q11.2 duplications between LCR22B and LCR22D are associated with neurodevelopmental phenotypes including autism spectrum disorder with incomplete penetrance. *Mol Genet Genomic Med* 7:e00507, 2019.

Worsham MJ, Miller DA, Devries JM, et al. A dicentric recombinant 9 derived from a paracentric inversion: Phenotype, cytogenetics, and molecular analysis of centromeres. *Am J Hum Genet* 44:115–123, 1989.

Warton C, Johnston M, Mills C. Reproductive deliberation: Supporting autonomous decision making in prenatal genetic counseling. *J Genet Couns* 32:576–583, 2023.

Worton RG, Stern R. A Canadian collaborative study of mosaicism in amniotic fluid cell cultures. *Prenat Diagn* 4:Spec No. 131–144, 1984.

Wright DJ, Day FR, Kerrison ND, et al. Genetic variants associated with mosaic Y chromosome loss highlight cell cycle genes and overlap with cancer susceptibility. *Nat Genet* 49:674–679, 2017.

Wright JR, Astrovskaya I, Barns SD, et al. Return of genetic research results in 21,532 individuals with autism. *Genet Med* 26:101202, 2024.

Wu C, Wang L, Iqbal F, et al. Preferential Y-Y pairing and synapsis and abnormal meiotic recombination in a 47,XYY man with non obstructive azoospermia. *Mol Cytogenet* 9:9, 2016.

Wu L, Jin L, Chen W, et al. The true incidence of chromosomal mosaicism after preimplantation genetic testing is much lower than that indicated by trophectoderm biopsy. *Hum Reprod* 36:1691–1701, 2021.

Wu T, Yin B, Zhu Y, et al. First report on an X-linked hypohidrotic ectodermal dysplasia family with X chromosome inversion: Breakpoint mapping reveals the pathogenic mechanism and preimplantation genetics diagnosis achieves an unaffected birth. *Clin Chim Acta* 475:78–84, 2017.

Wu YC, Yu MT, Chen LC, Chen CL, Yang ML. Prenatal diagnosis of mosaic tetrasomy 10p associated with megacisterna magna, echogenic focus of left ventricle, umbilical cord cysts and distal arthrogryposis. *Am J Med Genet* 117A:278–281, 2003.

Wyrobek AJ, Adler ID. Detection of aneuploidy in human and rodent sperm using FISH and applications of sperm assays of genetic damage in heritable risk evaluation. *Mutat Res* 352:173–179, 1996.

X

Xanthopoulou L, Mantzouratou A, Mania A, et al. Male and female meiotic behaviour of an intrachromosomal insertion determined by preimplantation genetic diagnosis. *Mol Cytogenet* 8:2, 2010.

Xi H, Qiu L, Yao Y, et al. Noninvasive chromosome screening for evaluating the clinical outcomes of patients with recurrent pregnancy loss or repeated implantation failure. *Front Endocrinol (Lausanne)* 13:896357, 2022.

Xiao P, Liu P, Weber JL, Papasian CJ, Recker RR, Deng HW. Paternal uniparental isodisomy of the entire chromosome 3 revealed in a person with no apparent phenotypic disorders. *Hum Mutat* 27:133–137, 2006.

Xiao B, Luo X, Liu Y, et al. Combining optical genome mapping and RNA-seq for structural variants detection and interpretation in unsolved neurodevelopmental disorders. *Genome Med* 16:113, 2024.

Xie P, Hu L, Peng Y, Tan YQ, et al. Risk factors affecting alternate segregation in blastocysts from preimplantation genetic testing cycles of autosomal reciprocal translocations. *Front Genet* 13:880208, 2022.

Xie P, Hu L, Tan Y, et al. Retrospective analysis of meiotic segregation pattern and interchromosomal effects in blastocysts from inversion preimplantation genetic testing cycles. *Fertil Steril* 112:336–342.e3, 2019.

Xie P, Li Y, Cheng D, et al. Preimplantation genetic testing results of blastocysts from 12 non-Robertsonian translocation carriers with chromosome fusion and comparison with Robertsonian translocation carriers. *Fertil Steril* 116:174–180, 2021.

Xin S, Zhang X. Case report: Diabetes mellitus type MODY5 as a feature of 17q12 deletion syndrome with diabetic gastroparesis. *Front Endocrinol (Lausanne)* 14:1205431, 2023.

Xing XH, Takam R, Bao XY, Ba-Alwi NA, Ji H. Methyl-CpG-Binding protein 2 duplication syndrome in a Chinese patient: A case report and review of the literature. *World J Clin Cases* 11:6505–6514, 2023.

Xu F, Zhang YN, Cheng DH, et al. The first patient with a pure 1p36 microtriplication associated with severe clinical phenotypes. *Mol Cytogenet* 7:64, 2014.

Xu HH, Zhang Y, He ZH, Di XH, Pan FY, Shi WW. Familial 5.29 Mb deletion in chromosome Xq22.1-q22.3 with a normal phenotype: A rare pedigree and literature review. *BMC Med Genomics* 16:111, 2023.

Xu J, Chernos J, Roland B. Trisomy 16pter to 16q12.1 and monosomy 22pter to 22q11.2 resulting from adjacent-2 segregation of a maternal complex chromosome rearrangement. *Am J Med Genet* 73:327–329, 1997.

Xu J, Fang R, Chen L, et al. Noninvasive chromosome screening of human embryos by genome sequencing of embryo culture medium for in vitro fertilization. *Proc Natl Acad Sci USA* 113:11907–11912, 2016.

Xu J, Zhang Z, Niu W, et al. Mapping allele with resolved carrier status of Robertsonian and reciprocal translocation in human preimplantation embryos. *Proc Natl Acad Sci USA* 114:E8695–E8702, 2017.

Xu W, Robert C, Thornton PS, Spinner NB. Complete androgen insensitivity syndrome due to X chromosome inversion: A clinical report. *Am J Med Genet* 120A:434–436, 2003.

Xu Z, Liu N, Gao L, Yu D. Application of chromosomal microarray analysis in genetic reasons of miscarriage tissues. *Appl Clin Genet* 17:85–93, 2024a.

Xu Z, Luo H, Li M, OuYang L, Xia Z. Prenatal diagnosis and molecular cytogenetic analyses of a homozygous Robertsonian translocation family with novel mosaic Robertsonian fission karyotype. *Psychiatr Genet* 34:106–110, 2024b.

Y

Yaegashi N, Senoo M, Uehara S, et al. Age-specific incidences of chromosome abnormalities at the second trimester amniocentesis for Japanese mothers aged 35 and older: Collaborative study of 5484 cases. *J Hum Genet* 43:85–90, 1998.

Yakut S, Clarck OA, Sanhal C, et al. A familial interstitial 4q35 deletion with no discernible clinical effects. *Am J Med Genet* 167A:1836–1841, 2015.

Yamamoto T, Dowa Y, Ueda H, et al. Tetralogy of Fallot associated with pulmonary atresia and major aortopulmonary collateral arteries in a patient with interstitial deletion of 16q21-q22.1. *Am J Med Genet* 146A:1575–1580, 2008.

Yamamoto T, Wilsdon A, Joss S, et al. An emerging phenotype of Xq22 microdeletions in females with severe intellectual disability, hypotonia and behavioral abnormalities. *J Hum Genet* 59:300–306, 2014.

Yamanaka M, Setoyama T, Igarashi Y, et al. Pregnancy outcome of fetuses with trisomy 18 identified by prenatal sonography and chromosomal analysis in a perinatal center. *Am J Med Genet* 140:1177–1182, 2006.

Yamashita D, Muramatsu H, Narita A, et al. Hematological abnormalities in Jacobsen syndrome: Cytopenia of varying severities and morphological abnormalities in peripheral blood and bone marrow. *Haematologica* 108:3438–3443, 2023.

Yamazawa K, Inoue T, Sakemi Y, et al. Loss of imprinting of the human-specific imprinted gene *ZNF597* causes prenatal growth retardation and dysmorphic features: Implications for phenotypic overlap with Silver-Russell syndrome. *J Med Genet* 58:427–432, 2021.

Yamazawa K, Ogata T, Ferguson-Smith AC. Uniparental disomy and human disease: An overview. *Am J Med Genet Semin Med Genet* 154C:329–334, 2010.

Yan D, Ouyang XM, Angeli SI, Du LL, Liu XZ. Paternal uniparental disomy of chromosome 13 causing homozygous 35delG mutation of the *GJB2* gene and hearing loss. *Am J Med Genet* 143A:385–386, 2007.

Yanagishita T, Yamamoto-Shimojima K, Nakano S, et al. Phenotypic features of 1q41q42 microdeletion including WDR26 and FBXO28 are clinically recognizable: The first case from Japan. *Brain Dev* 41:452–455, 2019.

Yang L, Zhan GD, Ding JJ, et al. Psychiatric illness and intellectual disability in the Prader-Willi syndrome with different molecular defects—A meta analysis. *PLoS One* 8:e72640, 2013.

Yang M, Rito T, Metzger J, et al. Depletion of aneuploid cells in human embryos and gastruloids. *Nat Cell Biol* 23:314–321, 2021.

Yang Q, Sherman SL, Hassold TJ, et al. Risk factors for trisomy 21: Maternal cigarette smoking and oral contraceptive use in a population-based case-control study. *Genet Med* 1:80–88, 1999.

Yang SP, Bidichandani SI, Figuera LE, et al. Molecular analysis of deletion (17)(p11.2p11.2) in a family segregating a 17p paracentric inversion: Implications for carriers of paracentric inversions. *Am J Hum Genet* 60:1184–1193, 1997.

Yang X, Li M, Qi Q, et al. Prenatal diagnosis of recurrent Kagami-Ogata syndrome inherited from a mother affected by Temple syndrome: A case report and literature review. *BMC Med Genomics* 17:222, 2024.

Yang Y, Yang C, Zhu Y, et al. Intragenic and extragenic disruptions of *FOXL2* mapped by whole genome low-coverage sequencing in two BPES families with chromosome reciprocal translocation. *Genomics* 104:170–176, 2014.

Yang YF, Ai Q, Huang C, et al. A 1.1Mb deletion in distal 13q deletion syndrome region with congenital heart defect and postaxial polydactyly: Additional support for a CHD locus at distal 13q34 region. *Gene* 528:51–54, 2013.

Yao Q, Wang L, Yao B, et al. Meiotic prophase I defects in an oligospermic man with Wolf-Hirschhorn syndrome with ring chromosome 4. *Mol Cytogenet* 7:45, 2014.

Yao Z, Zeng J, Zhu H, et al. Mutation analysis of the TUBB8 gene in primary infertile women with oocyte maturation arrest. *J Ovarian Res* 15:38, 2022.

Yapan C, Beyazyurek C, Ekmekci C, Kahraman S. The largest paracentric inversion, the highest rate of recombinant spermatozoa—Case report: 46,XY, inv(2)(q21.2q37.3) and literature review. *Balkan J Med Genet* 17:55–62, 2014.

Yardin C, Esclaire F, Gilbert B, Brosset P, Hugon J, Barthe D. Identical chromosome imbalance in two siblings born to a mother with a double reciprocal translocation. *Ann Genet* 40:232–234, 1997.

Yardin C, Esclaire F, Terro F, Baclet MC, Barthe D, Laroche C. First familial case of ring chromosome 18 and monosomy 18 mosaicism. *Am J Med Genet* 104:257–259, 2001.

Yaron Y, Feldman B, Kramer RL, et al. Prenatal diagnosis of 46,XY/46,XX mosaicism: A case report. *Am J Med Genet* 84:12–14, 1999.

Yaron Y, Hyett J, Langlois S. Current controversies in prenatal diagnosis 2: For those women screened by NIPT using cell free DNA, maternal serum markers are obsolete. *Prenat Diagn* 36:1167–1171, 2016.

Yauk CL, Aardema MJ, Benthem JV, et al. Approaches for identifying germ cell mutagens: Report of the 2013 IWGT workshop on germ cell assays. *Mutat Res Genet Toxicol Environ Mutagen* 783:36–54, 2015.

Yauy K, de Leeuw N, Yntema HG, Pfundt R, Gilissen C. Accurate detection of clinically relevant uniparental disomy from exome sequencing data. *Genet Med* 22:803–808, 2020.

Ye M, Yeh J, Kosteria I, Li L. Progress in fertility preservation strategies in Turner syndrome. *Front Med (Lausanne)* 7:3. 2020.

Ye Y, Qian Y, Xu C, Jin F. Meiotic segregation analysis of embryos from reciprocal translocation carriers in PGD cycles. *Reprod Biomed Online* 24:83–90, 2012.

Yenamandra A, Deangelo P, Aviv H, Suslak L, Desposito F. Interstitial insertion of Y-specific DNA sequences including *SRY* into chromosome 4 in a 45,X male child. *Am J Med Genet* 72:125–128, 1997.

Yeung A, Francis D, Giouzeppos O, Amor DJ. Pallister-Killian syndrome caused by mosaicism for a supernumerary ring chromosome 12p. *Am J Med Genet* 149A:505–509, 2009.

Yeung KS, Ho MSP, Lee SL, et al. Paternal uniparental disomy of chromosome 19 in a pair of monochorionic diamniotic twins with dysmorphic features and developmental delay. *J Med Genet* 55:847–852, 2018.

Yin X, Tan K, Vajta G, et al. Massively parallel sequencing for chromosomal abnormality testing in trophectoderm cells of human blastocysts. *Biol Reprod* 88:69, 2013.

Yokoyama Y, Narahara K, Teraoka M, et al. Cryptic pericentric inversion of chromosome 17 detected by fluorescence in situ hybridization study in familial Miller-Dieker syndrome. *Am J Med Genet* 71:236–237, 1997.

Yong PJ, Barrett IJ, Kalousek DK, Robinson WP. Clinical aspects, prenatal diagnosis, and pathogenesis of trisomy 16 mosaicism. *J Med Genet* 40:175–182, 2003.

Yong PJ, Marion SA, Barrett IJ, Kalousek DK, Robinson WP. Evidence for imprinting on chromosome 16: The effect of uniparental disomy on the outcome of mosaic trisomy 16 pregnancies. *Am J Med Genet* 112:123–132, 2002.

Youings S, Ellis K, Ennis S, Barber J, Jacobs P. A study of reciprocal translocations and inversions detected by light microscopy with special reference to origin, segregation, and recurrent abnormalities. *Am J Med Genet* 126A:46–60, 2004.

Young D, Klepacka D, McGarvey M, Schoolcraft WB, Katz-Jaffe MG. Infertility patients with chromosome inversions are not susceptible to an inter-chromosomal effect. *J Assist Reprod Genet* 36:509–516. 2019.

Yu C, Tian Y, Qi L, Wang B. Prenatal diagnosis and genetic counseling of a uniparental isodisomy of chromosome 8 with no phenotypic abnormalities. *Mol Cytogenet* 15:18, 2022

Yu MHC, Chau JFT, Au SLK, et al. Evaluating the clinical utility of genome sequencing for cytogenetically balanced chromosomal abnormalities in prenatal diagnosis. *Front Genet* 11:620162, 2021.

Yu N, Kruskall MS, Yunis JJ, et al. Disputed maternity leading to identification of tetragametic chimerism. *N Engl J Med* 346:1545–1552, 2002.

Yu S, Cox K, Friend K, et al. Familial 22q11.2 duplication: A three-generation family with a 3-Mb duplication and a familial 1.5-Mb duplication. *Clin Genet* 73:160–164, 2008.

Yu YR, You LR, Yan YT, Chen CM. Role of *OVCA1/DPH1* in craniofacial abnormalities of Miller-Dieker syndrome. *Hum Mol Genet* 23:5579–5596, 2014.

Yuan B, Harel T, Gu S, et al. Nonrecurrent 17p11.2p12 rearrangement events that result in two concomitant genomic disorders: The *PMP22-RAI1* contiguous gene duplication syndrome. *Am J Hum Genet* 97:691–707, 2015.

Yuan B, Neira J, Gu S, et al. Nonrecurrent *PMP22-RAI1* contiguous gene deletions arise from replication-based mechanisms and result in Smith-Magenis syndrome with evident peripheral neuropathy. *Hum Genet* 135:1161–1174, 2016.

Yuan J, Jin L, Wang M, Wei S, Zhu G, Xu B. Detection of chromosome aberrations in 17 054 individuals with fertility problems and their subsequent assisted reproductive technology treatments in Central China. *Hum Reprod* 38(Suppl ii):34–46, 2023.

Yuan S, Cheng D, Luo K, et al. Reproductive risks and preimplantation genetic testing intervention for X-autosome translocation carriers. *Reprod Biomed Online* 43:73–80, 2021.

Zhou J, Zheng Y, Liang G, et al. Atypical deletion of Williams-Beuren syndrome reveals the mechanism of neurodevelopmental disorders. *BMC Med Genomics* 15:79, 2022.

Zhou R, Cheng J, Ma D, et al. Identifying novel copy number variants in azoospermia factor regions and evaluating their effects on spermatogenic impairment. *Front Genet* 10:427, 2019.

Zhou W, Machiela MJ, Freedman ND, et al. Mosaic loss of chromosome Y is associated with common variation near *TCL1A*. *Nat Genet* 48:563–568, 2016.

Zhu S, Zhu Y, Zhang F, et al. FISH analysis of numerical chromosomal abnormalities in the sperm of robertsonian translocation der(13;14)(q10;q10) carriers. *Front Genet* 13:1010568, 2022a.

Zhu S, Zhu Y, Zhang F, Wu J, Lei C, Jiang F. Comprehensive chromosome FISH assessment of sperm aneuploidy in normozoospermic males. *J Assist Reprod Genet* 39:1887–1900, 2022b.

Zhuang B, Shang J, Yao Y. HLA-G: An important mediator of maternal-fetal immune-tolerance. *Front Immunol* 12:744324, 2021.

Ziats CA, Jain L, McLarney B, et al. Neurofibromatosis type 2 in Phelan-McDermid syndrome: Institutional experience and review of the literature. *Eur J Med Genet* 63:104042, 2020.

Ziats MN, Goin-Kochel RP, Berry LN, et al. The complex behavioral phenotype of 15q13.3 microdeletion syndrome. *Genet Med* 18:1111–1118, 2016.

Ziegler BM, Abelleyro MM, Marchione VD, et al. Comprehensive genomic filtering algorithm to expose the cause of skewed X chromosome inactivation. The proof of concept in female haemophilia expression. *J Med Genet* 61:769–776, 2024.

Zielinska AP, Bellou E, Sharma N, et al. Meiotic kinetochores fragment into multiple lobes upon cohesin loss in aging eggs. *Curr Biol* 29:3749–3765.e7, 2019.

Zietkiewicz E, Wojda A, Witt M. Cytogenetic perspective of ageing and longevity in men and women. *J Appl Genet* 50:261–273, 2009.

Žilina O, Reimand T, Tammur P, Tillmann V, Kurg A, Õunap K. Patient with dup(5)(q35.2-q35.3) reciprocal to the common Sotos syndrome deletion and review of the literature. *Eur J Med Genet* 56:202–206, 2013.

Zinn AR, Ouyang B, Ross JL, Varma S, Bourgeois M, Tonk V. Del (X)(p21.2) in a mother and two daughters with variable ovarian function. *Clin Genet* 52:235–239, 1997.

Zirn B, Arning L, Bartels I, et al. Ring chromosome 22 and neurofibromatosis type II: Proof of two-hit model for the loss of the NF2 gene in the development of meningioma. *Clin Genet* 81:82–87, 2012.

Zollino M, Ponzi E, Gobbi G, Neri G. The ring 14 syndrome. *Eur J Med Genet* 55:374–380, 2012.

Zollino M, Tiziano F, Di Stefano C, Neri G. Partial duplication of the long arm of chromosome 15: Confirmation of a causative role in craniosynostosis and definition of a 15q25-qter trisomy syndrome. *Am J Med Genet* 87:391–394, 1999.

Zou W, Li M, Wang X, et al. Preimplantation genetic testing for monogenic disorders (PGT-M) offers an alternative strategy to prevent children from being born with hereditary neurological diseases or metabolic diseases dominated by nervous system phenotypes: A retrospective study. *J Assist Reprod Genet* 41:1245–1259, 2024.

Zou YS, McGrann PS, Uphoff TS, Van Dyke DL. A case of mosaic supernumerary ring chromosome 15 with two copies of the segment 15p11.1-q14. *Am J Med Genet* 40A:1663–1668, 2006.

Zuccarello D, Dallapiccola B, Novelli A, Foresta C. Azoospermia in a man with a constitutional ring 22 chromosome. *Eur J Med Genet* 53:389–391, 2010.

Zuffardi O, Bonaglia M, Ciccone R, Giorda R. Inverted duplications deletions: Underdiagnosed rearrangements? *Clin Genet* 75:505–513, 2009.

Zühlke C, Thies U, Braulke I, Reis A, Schirren C. Down syndrome and male fertility: PCR-derived fingerprinting, serological and andrological investigations. *Clin Genet* 46:324–326, 1994.

INDEX

For the benefit of digital users, indexed terms that span two pages (e.g., 52–53) may, on occasion, appear on only one of those pages.